IMAGING *in* ONCOLOGY
Second Edition

IMAGING *in* ONCOLOGY

Second Edition

Edited by

Janet E Husband OBE, FMedSci, FRCP, FRCR

Academic Department of Diagnostic Radiology
The Royal Marsden NHS Trust, London, UK

and

Rodney H Reznek FRCP, FRCR

Academic Department of Radiology
Barts and The London NHS Trust, London, UK

Medical Illustrations by
Dee McLean

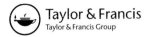
Taylor & Francis
Taylor & Francis Group

© 2004 Taylor and Francis

First published in the United Kingdom in 1998
by Isis Medical Media Ltd.

Second edition published in 2004 by Taylor and Francis,
an imprint of the Taylor & Francis Group
11 New Fetter Lane, London EC4P 4EE
Tel.: +44 (0) 20 7583 9855
Fax.: +44 (0) 20 7842 2298
E-mail: info@dunitz.co.uk
Website: http://www.dunitz.co.uk

Although every effort has been made to ensure that all owners of copyright material have been acknowledged in this publication, we would be glad to acknowledge in subsequent reprints or editions any omissions brought to our attention.

Although every effort has been made to ensure that drug doses and other information are presented accurately in this publication, the ultimate responsibility rests with the prescribing physician. Neither the publishers nor the authors can be held responsible for errors or for any consequences arising from the use of information contained herein. For detailed prescribing information or instructions on the use of any product or procedure discussed herein, please consult the prescribing information or instructional material issued by the manufacturer.

A CIP record for this book is available from the British Library.

ISBN 1-84184-421-7

Distributed in North and South America by
Taylor & Francis
2000 NW Corporate Blvd
Boca Raton, FL 33431, USA

Within Continental USA
Tel.: 800 272 7737; Fax.: 800 374 3401

Outside Continental USA
Tel.: 561 994 0555; Fax.: 561 361 6018

E-mail: orders@crcpress.com

Distributed in the rest of the world by
Thomson Publishing Services
Cheriton House
North Way
Andover, Hampshire SP10 5BE, UK
Tel.: +44 (0)1264 332424
E-mail: salesorder.tandf@thomsonpublishingservices.co.uk

Composition by Phoenix Photosetting, Chatham, UK

Printed and bound in Spain by Grafos S.A. Arte Sobre Papel

Contents

Contents

Suzanne L Aquino, MD
Assistant Professor of Radiology, Department of Radiology, FND 202, Massachusetts General Hospital, Boston, Massachusetts, USA

Peter Armstrong, MB BS, FMedSci, FRCP, FRCR
Professor of Radiology, Academic Department of Radiology, Barts and the London NHS Trust, London, UK

Syed Babar, MB BS, FCPS, DMRD, FRCR
Radiology Department, Queen Elizabeth II Hospital, London, UK

Jelle Barentsz, PhD, MD
Professor of Radiology, Department of Diagnostic Radiology, University Hospital Nijmegen, Nijmegen, The Netherlands

Richard L Baron, MD
Professor & Chairman, Department of Radiology, University of Chicago, Chicago, Illinois, USA

Ann Barrett, MD, FRCR, FRCP, FMed
Professor of Oncology, School of Medicine, Health Policy & Practice, University of East Anglia, Norwich, UK

Jonathan W Berlin, MD, MBA
Professor of Oncology, School of Medicine, Health Policy & Practice, University of East Anglia, Norwich, UK

Juliet Britton, MB BS, FRCR, FRCP
Consultant Neuroradiologist, Atkinson Morley Wing, St George's Hospital, London, UK

Keith E Britton, MD, MSc, FRCR, FRCP
Professor in Nuclear Medicine, Queen Mary Hospital, Honorary Director Cancer Research, UK Medicine Group, Physician in Charge, Department of Nuclear Medicine, Barts and the London NHS Trust, London, UK

Gina Brown, MB, MD, MRCP, FRCR
Consultant Radiologist and Honorary Senior Lecturer, Academic Department of Radiology, Royal Marsden Hospital, Sutton, Surrey, UK

Guy J C Burkill, BSc, MBBS, MRCP, FRCR
Consultant Radiologist, Department of Radiology, The Royal Sussex County Hospital, Brighton Hospital, Sussex, UK

Bernadette M Carrington, MB ChB, MRCP, FRCR
Consultant Radiologist, Dept of Diagnostic Radiology, Christie Hospital NHS Trust, Withington, Manchester, UK

Helen Carty, MB, BCh, DMRD, FFR, FRCR, FRCPI, FRCP (Lond), FRCPCH
Professor of Paediatric Radiology, Royal Liverpool Children's NHS Trust, Alder Hey, Liverpool, UK

Paul Caruso, MD
Instructor, Staff Radiologist, Harvard Medical School, Radiology Department, Boston, Massachusetts, USA

Richard H Cohan, MD
Professor of Radiology, Department of Radiology, University of Michigan Hospital, Ann Arbor, Michigan, USA

Michel P Coleman, BA, BM, BCh, MSc, FPHM
Professor of Epidemiology and Vital Statistics, London School of Hygiene & Tropical Medicine, Deputy Chief Medical Statistician, Office for National Statistics, London School of Hygiene & Tropical Medicine, London, UK

Conor D Collins, BSc, FRCPI, FRCR, FFRRCSI
Consultant Radiologist, Department of Radiology, St Vincent's University Hospital, Dublin, Ireland

Gary J R Cook, MBBS, MSc, MD, FRCP, FRCR
Consultant Radiologist, Royal Marsden Hospital, Sutton, Surrey, UK

Hugh D Curtin, MD
Chief of Radiology, Department of Radiology, Massachusetts Eye and Ear Infirmary, Boston, Massachusetts, USA

Sujal R Desai, MD, MRCP, FRCR
Consultant Radiologist, Department of Radiology, King's College Hospital, London, UK

Willem Deserno, MD, MSc
Consultant Radiologist, Department of Diagnostic Radiology, University Hospital Nijmegan, Nijmegan, The Netherlands

H Jane Dobbs, MB, BChir, MA, FRCP, FRCR
Consultant in Clinical Oncology, Guy's & St Thomas' Cancer Centre, Guy's & St Thomas' Hospital, London, UK

Andrzej Dzik-Jurasz, PhD, MB BS, FRCS (Lond), FRCR
Cancer Research UK, Clinical MR Research Group, Royal Marsden NHS Trust, Sutton, Surrey, UK

Jacques Estève, PhD
Professor, Claud Bernard University, Lyon, France

Jane Evanson, MRCP, FRCR
Consultant Neuroradiologist, Department of Neuroradiology, The Royal London Hospital, London, UK

James V Ferris, MD
Assistant Professor of Radiology, University of Pittsburgh Medical Center, Pittsburgh, Pennsylvania, USA

Isaac R Francis, MD
Professor of Radiology, Department of Radiology, University of Michigan Health System, Ann Arbor, Michigan, USA

Christopher J Gallagher, MBChB, PhD, FRCP
Honorary Senior Lecturer Medical Oncology, St Bartholomew's Hospital, London, UK

Alice R Gillams, MBChB, MRCP, FRCR
Senior Lecturer, The Royal Free and University College, London Medical School, Honorary Consultant, Medical Imaging, The Middlesex Hospital, London, UK

Richard M Gore, MD
Professor of Radiology, Northwestern University Medical School, Chief Gastrointestinal Radiology Evanstown Northwestern Healthcare, Evanstown, Illinois, USA

Ashley B Grossman, BA, BSc, MD, FRCP, FMedSci
Professor of Neuroendocrinology, Department of Neuroendocrinology, St Bartholomew's Hospital, London, UK

Nishi Gupta, MBBS, MRCP, FRCR
Clinical Research Fellow, PET Oncology Group, Imperial College London, London, UK

David Hansell, MD, FRCP, FRCR
Professor of Thoracic Imaging, Imperial College, London. Consultant Radiologist, Royal Brompton Hospital, London, UK

Mukesh G Harisinghani, MD
Assistant Professor, Department of Radiology, Massachusetts General Hospital, Boston, Massachusetts, USA

Jane Hawnaur, MB ChB, MRCP, FRCR, DMRD
Consultant Radiologist, Department of Clinical Radiology, Manchester Royal Infirmary, Manchester, UK

Jeremiah C Healy, MA, MB BChir, MRCP, FRCR
Honorary Senior Lecturer, Imperial College School of Medicine, London. Consultant Radiologist, Chelsea & Westminster Hospital, London, UK

Robert Hermans, MD, PhD
Professor at the Faculty of Medicine, Department of Radiology, University Hospitals Leuven, Leuven, Belgium

Alan Horwich, PhD, MB BS, FRCP, FRCR
Academic Unit of Radiotherapy & Oncology, Royal Marsden NHS Trust, Sutton, Surrey, UK

Paul A Hulse, MRCP, FRCR
Consultant Radiologist, Christie Hospital NHS Trust, Withington, Manchester, UK

Janet E Husband, OBE, FMedSci, FRCP, FRCR
Academic Department of Diagnostic Radiology, The Royal Marsden NHS Trust, London, UK

Hero K Hussain, MD, FRCR
Assistant Professor, Department of Radiology, University of Michigan Health System, Ann Arbor, Michigan, USA

Revathy B Iyer, MD
Associate Professor of Radiology, Diagnostic Imaging, MD Anderson Cancer Center, Houston, Texas, USA

R Brooke Jeffrey, Jr MD
Professor of Radiology, Chief of Abdominal Imaging Section, Department of Radiology, Stanford University School of Medicine, Stanford, California, USA

Peter Johnson, MA, MD, FRCP
Professor of Medical Oncology, Cancer Research UK Oncology Unit, Southampton General Hospital, Southampton, UK

D Michael King, MB BS, DMRD, FRCR
Consultant Radiologist, Royal Marsden Hospital, London, UK

Dow-Mu Koh, MRCP, FRCR
Consultant Radiologist, Royal Marsden Hospital, Sutton, Surrey, UK

Janet E Kuhlman, MD, MS
Professor of Radiology, Department of Radiology, University of Wisconsin Medical School, Wisconsin, USA

Jérôme Leclère, MD
Department of Diagnostic Imaging, nstitut Gustave Roussy, Villejuif, France

Michael H Lev, MD
Director, Neurovascular Lab and Emergency Neuroradiology, Massachusetts General Hospital, Assistant Professor of Radiology, Harvard Medical School, Boston, Massachusetts, USA

Herman I Libshitz, MD, FACR
2637 University Boulevard, Houston, Texas, USA

Anthony J Lopez, BSc, MRCP, FRCR
Honorary Senior Lecturer, University of Surrey, Consultant Radiologist, Department of Diagnostic Imaging, The Royal Surrey County Hospital & St Luke's Cancer Centre, Guildford, UK

Sarah Lowndes, BM BCh, MA, MRCP
Department of Medical Oncology, Southampton General Hospital, Southampton, UK

Evelyne M Loyer, MD
Associate Professor and Radiologist, University of Texas MD Anderson Cancer Center, Houston, Texas, USA

Alison McLean, FRCP, FRCR
Consultant Radiologist, Department of Radiology, Barts and the London NHS Trust, London, UK

Theresa McLoud, MD
Department of Radiology, Massachusetts General Hospital, Boston, Massachusetts, USA

David MacVicar, MA, MRCP, FRCR
Honarary Senior Lecturer, Consultant Radiologist, Royal Marsden Hospital, Surrey, UK

James S Malpas, Dphil, FRCP, FRCR, FRCPCH
Emritus Professor of Medical Oncology, 253 Lauderdale Tower, Barbican, London, UK

Alec J Megibow, MD, MPH, FACR
Professor and Vice Chairman, Department of Radiology, New York University Medical Center, New York, USA

Stephen Morris, FRCR
Specialist Registrar, Academic Unit of Radiotherapy and Oncology, Royal Marsden NHS Trust, Sutton, Surrey, UK

Eleanor Moskovic, FRCP, FRCR
Consultant Radiologist, Royal Marsden Hospital, London, UK

Lia Moulopoulos, MD
Assistant Professor, Department of Radiology, University of Athens, Athens, Greece

Reginald F Munden, MD, DMD
Associate Professor, Section Chief, Thoracic Imaging, UT MD Anderson Cancer Center, Houston, Texas, USA

Anthony J Neal, MD, MRCP,FRCR
Consultant Clinical Oncologist, St Luke's Cancer Centre, Royal Surrey County Hospital, Guildford, UK

Geraldine M Newmark, MD
Section Head, Body Imaging, Director of Education, Evanstown Northwestern Healthcare, Department of Radiology

Liliane Ollivier, MD
Department of Radiology, Institut Curie, Paris, France

Anwar R Padhani, MBBS, MRCP, FRCR
Honorary Senior Lecturer, University College London, Consultant Radiologist, West Hertfordshire NHS Trust, Mount Vernon Hospital, Middlesex, UK

Jacqueline M Parkin, MBBS, PhD, FRCP
Honorary Consultant in Clinical Immunology, Barts and the London NHS Trust, London, UK

Patricia Price, MA, MD, FRCR, FRCP
Ralston Paterson Professor of Radiation Oncology. Director of The Wolfson Molecular Imaging Centre. Honorary Consultant, Christie Hospital, Manchester, UK

Sheila C Rankin, DCH, FRCR
Consultant Radiologist, ,Radiology Department, Guy's Hospital, London, UK

Rodney H Reznek, FRCP, FRCR
Academic Department of Radiology, Barts and the London NHS Trust, London, UK

Philip J A Robinson, FRCP, FRCR
Professor of Clinical Radiology, Dept of Clinical Radiology, St James' University Hospital, Leeds, UK

Andrea G Rockall, BSc, MBBS, MCRP, FRCR
Senior Lecturer, Academic Department of Radiology, Barts and the London NHS Trust, London, UK

Timothy A Rockall, MD, FRCS
Visiting Senior Fellow, University of Surrey, Guildford, London, UK. Honorary Senior Lecturer, Imperial College, London, UK

Eric M Rohren, MD, PhD
Assistant Professor of Radiology and Nuclear Medicine, Mayo Clinic, Rochester, Minnesota, USA

Laura V Romo, MD
Instructor, Harvard Medical School, Staff Radiologist, Massachusetts Eye and Ear Infirmary, Boston, Massachusetts, USA

Anju Sahdev, MBBS, MRCP, FRCR
Consultant Radiologist, Homerton University and St Bartholomew's Hospitals, Homerton Hospital, London, UK

Amita Sharma, MBBS, MRCP, FRCR
Instructor of Radiology, Harvard Medical School, Assistant Radiologist, Department of Radiology, Massachusetts General Hospital, Boston, Massachusetts, USA

Marilyn J Siegel, MD
Washington University School of Medicine, Mallinckrodt Institute of Radiology, St Louis, Missouri, USA

Paul Silverman, MD
Professor of Radiology, Gerald D Dodd, Jr Distinguished Chair, Diagnostic Imaging, Director, Academic Development, Chief, Section, Body Imaging, Dept of Radiology, MD Anderson Cancer Center, Houston, Texas, USA

S Aslam A Sohaib, BSc, MRCP, FRCP
Consultant Radiologist, Department of Radiology, Royal Marsden Hospital, London, UK

Vernon K Sondak, MD
Professor of Surgery, University of Michigan Medical Center, Ann Arbor, Missouri, USA

John A Spencer, MA, MD, MRCP, FRCR
Consultant Radiologist, Department of Clinical Radiology, St James' University Hospital, Leeds, UK

Murali Sundaram, MBBS, FRCR
Professor of Radiology, Senior Associate Consultant, Department of Radiology, Mayo Clinic, Minnesota, USA

M Ben Taylor, MRCP, FRCR
Consultant Radiologist, Christie Hospital, Manchester, UK

Daniel Vanel, MD
Professor of Radiology, Department of Radiology, Institut Gustave-Roussy, Villejuif Cedex, France

Datla G K Varma, MD
Professor of Radiology, University of Texas, Houston, Texas, USA

Sarah J Vinnicombe, BSc(Hons), MRCP, FRCR
Consultant Radiologist, Department of Radiology, Barts and the London NHS Trust, London, UK

Judith A W Webb, BSc, MD, FRCP, FRCR
Consultant Radiologist, Radiology Department, Queen Elizabeth II Wing, Barts and the London NHS Trust, London, UK

Louise Wilkinson, BA, BM, BCh, FRCR
Consultant Radiologist, St George's Hospital, London, UK

Helen Williams, MB ChB, MRCP, FRCR
Research Fellow Paediatric Radiology, Royal Liverpool Children's NHS Trust, Alder Hey, Liverpool, UK

Vahid Yaghmai, MD, MS
Assistant Professor and Medical Director of CT, Feinberg School of Medicine, Northwestern University, Chicago, Illinois, USA

As with the first edition of '*Imaging in Oncology*', the aim of this edition is to provide radiologists and other clinicians with a state-of-the-art text which addresses in depth all aspects of cancer imaging from diagnosis through to long-term follow-up. Since the first edition of '*Imaging in Oncology*' was published in 1998 there have been major advances in the development of highly sophisticated imaging technology such as the introduction of multi-detector CT, enhanced MR techniques and the advent of positron emission tomography (PET). PET and PET/CT are evolving as robust diagnostic tools, providing added value in the management of cancer.

Together with these developments, the last five years has seen an increased awareness of the central role of imaging in cancer management. It is now well established that the radiologist plays a key role providing critical information for management decisions within the multidisciplinary team made up of oncologists, surgeons and others.

In order to achieve the highest possible standards of patient care, the cancer radiologist requires not only a detailed knowledge of the imaging findings in different tumours but also understanding of current concepts of cancer development and growth, and must be familiar with different staging classifications and treatment options. Increasingly too, the pivotal role of imaging in monitoring response to therapy must be appreciated and the appearances of recurrent disease recognised. This text will endeavour to meet all these needs and to evaluate the role of different imaging techniques in all the common cancers. We hope that the new edition of '*Imaging in Oncology*' will provide a valuable framework for setting standards of imaging practice and guidelines for protocols.

'*Imaging in Oncology*' comprises two volumes and is divided into nine sections. As in the previous edition the first section provides a general overview of cancer and discusses imaging strategies in oncology, cancer incidence, staging methods, principles of treatment, assessment of response and second malignancies. Complications of therapy are more frequently seen today because patients are undergoing more aggressive treatment and are surviving longer. Therefore imaging is increasingly required both to investigate complex clinical problems and to guide therapeutic intervention. With improved patient survival in many cancers, imaging has become important in early recognition of recurrent disease, appearances which are often confusing. These issues are addressed in expanded chapters in all the common tumours. Similarly new data is included on the late development of second malignancies following successful therapy. Several of these chapters have been expanded to deal broadly with changes in therapy that have evolved since publication of the first edition. While the diagnosis of cancer is of critical importance this task usually falls within the context of general radiology and for this reason investigations leading to the diagnosis of cancer and its differential diagnosis are not considered in detail in this text. In '*Imaging in Oncology*' emphasis has been placed on image interpretation for tumour staging and follow-up.

New chapters in the text reflect the ever widening application of imaging to different cancers. We have therefore included additional chapters on imaging adrenal tumours, neuroendocrine tumours, splenic malignancy and malignant melanoma metastases. We have expanded the section on imaging the immunocompromised host with new chapters on general clinical considerations and on imaging the central nervous system.

The elucidation of the complete sequence of the human genome now presents an unparalleled opportunity to determine the genetic basis of cancer in many different tumour types. This breakthrough for cancer research is already driving new initiatives in cancer therapy. Thus novel drugs directed at molecular targets now are being tested in Phase I clinical trials. As functional imaging becomes established in clinical practice there will be increasing use of these techniques in the assessment of Phase I trials. Thus today radiologists working in the field of cancer should become familiar with basic molecular biology and keep abreast of developing knowledge regarding the genetic basis of cancer as well as new approaches to treatment directed at molecular targets. For this reason this second edition of '*Imaging in Oncology*' contains a new section entitled '*New Horizons in Imaging*' in which molecular imaging in cancer treatment is discussed in relation to PET and MRI, and a separate chapter on imaging angiogenesis is also included. MR lymphography remains within the research arena but its potential impact on clinical practice in the assessment of lymph node disease is enormous and we have therefore included a chapter on this new development.

All chapters in the second edition of '*Imaging in Oncology*' have been revised and edited during 2003 and many of the images have been replaced with state-of-the-art imaging on multi-channel CT and MR. Positron emission tomography has been introduced into the text where relevant. '*Imaging in Oncology*' therefore contains the most up-to-date information and reflects authors' current views of the role of imaging in this ever expanding field.

Where relevant, each chapter is accompanied by colour diagrams of tumour staging, anatomy or other aspects of tumour imaging. These illustrations have been produced by Dee McLean to whom we are indebted for her beautiful work. In this text MR images have been annotated according to the sequence used but the precise detailed sequence information including repetition time and echo time has not been included as a general rule. This is a decision based on the fact that 'Imaging in Oncology' represents a multi-modality approach to cancer imaging and therefore we did not wish to enter into a detailed discussion of magnetic resonance techniques, a topic considered in detail in the numerous textbooks dedicated to magnetic resonance imaging which are available today. In each chapter we have highlighted the text with a system of key points as well as a summary of the salient issues covered. The 2002 UICC TNM Staging Classification of Malignant Tumours has been used throughout the book.

We would like to warmly acknowledge all those who have worked so hard to bring the second edition of 'Imaging in Oncology' to fruition. Mrs. Maureen Watts and Mrs. Julie Jessop have spent many hours typing and updating the manuscript as well as deciphering the editors' often illegible handwriting and even more doubtful expertise on the keyboard of their laptops! Mrs. Maureen Watts has co-ordinated the whole project for Janet Husband and Mrs. Julie Jessop for Rodney Reznek. Mrs. Janet Macdonald has taken a major role in production of the images and has worked with individual authors to produce the best possible results. We would also like to thank the Medical Illustration Department of Barts and the London NHS Trust for their meticulous high quality work.

We are most grateful to all our contributors who have found the time within their busy working lives to provide us with such excellent contributions and for generously giving their own special expertise to this project.

Finally, we would like to express our gratitude to Mr. John Harrison of ISIS Medical Media for his generosity, vision and enthusiasm which underpinned the success of the first edition. We hope that 'Imaging in Oncology' will continue to make a valuable contribution to the radiological literature and will allow those caring for patients with cancer to have a greater understanding of imaging within this complex and rapidly changing specialty.

Janet E Husband
Rodney H Reznek

More than 100 years after the discovery of x-rays, we are witnessing the rebirth of medical imaging. As the scope of imaging has broadened from anatomy to metabolism and function, its actual and potential applications have expanded immeasurably. The progress in medical imaging has been driven largely by increases in computer power, advances in micro-processing, the rapid expansion of communication technology, and the resurgence of biomedical science.

Cancer imaging, in particular, is benefiting enormously from all of these advances. The spatial and temporal resolution of anatomic images has reached new levels of excellence, making it possible to identify and characterize fine details of even small tumours. As a result, patients benefit from earlier tumour detection and more accurate staging and treatment follow-up.

Imaging paradigms are changing. The 3-D displays of computed tomography (CT) and magnetic resonance imaging (MRI) are replacing a number of conventional diagnostic studies, such as conventional angiography, intravenous urography, and, in the near future, barium enema. The fusion of images from different modalities, such as MR imaging and MR spectroscopic imaging, or CT and positron emission tomography (PET), now permits the single-platform display of anatomy, metabolism and function.

Physicians in all specialties have embraced minimally invasive, image-guided diagnostic and therapeutic techniques that have transformed cancer care. Novel methods for image-guided tracking and interventions, including robotics, navigation and intra-procedural visualization are being developed. The use of virtual reality to guide laparoscopic surgery is generating new oncological applications for thermal, laser or other types of ablation. A new subspecialty called Image-Guided Intervention—a hybrid of radiology and surgery—is being born.

Perhaps most exciting of all are the increasingly powerful imaging paradigms that permit non-invasive, in vivo assessment of metabolic processes at the cellular and molecular levels. The surging biomedical research discipline of molecular imaging combines basic cell and molecular biology, chemistry, medicine, pharmacology, medical physics, biomathematics and bioinformatics. With the ability to monitor multiple molecular events nearly simultaneously and follow the trafficking and targeting of cells, molecular imaging provides the tools to rapidly expand our understanding of disease processes, closely monitor and fine-tune treatment, and develop more effective drug and gene therapies. Indeed, it should be possible within the next decade to visualize and determine which genes are being expressed in a specific cancer and translate this information directly into better clinical management of the individual patient.

Any physician who wishes to provide cancer patients with the best possible quality of life and the greatest chances of survival needs to keep abreast of these rapid changes in imaging. But how does one stay informed and still have enough time to sleep, eat, and practice medicine? This updated edition of *Imaging in Oncology* is part of the answer.

Editors Husband and Reznek have once again recruited superb authors from all over the world and shaped their contributions into a wonderfully readable textbook. They themselves have contributed numerous outstanding chapters concerning the specialties in which they are internationally recognized leaders. *Imaging in Oncology* is thorough, well organized, and superbly illustrated. The introductory chapters provide basic tools essential to the practice of oncology. The middle chapters on specific cancer sites combine the latest advances in imaging and therapy, describing the most clinically relevant uses of imaging and their practical integration into overall patient management. Moreover, to help readers prepare for the next wave of changes, imaginative concluding chapters peer into the future of molecular and genetic imaging.

Imaging in Oncology is the culmination of the dedication and hard work of two remarkable clinician-scientists. Those who seek solutions and ideas in its pages will be amply rewarded.

Hedvig Hricak

HAEMATOLOGICAL MALIGNANCY

Chapter 32

Lymphoma

Rodney H Reznek, Sarah J Vinnicombe and Janet E Husband

Introduction

The lymphomas, Hodgkin's disease (HD) and non-Hodgkin's lymphoma (NHL) are a diverse group of neoplasms that vary widely in age of presentation, patterns of tumour growth and survival rates. Hodgkin's disease was first described by Thomas Hodgkin in 1832, but it is only during the last 2 decades that the prognosis has improved so that currently Hodgkin's disease is curable in the majority of patients. Non-Hodgkin's lymphoma has a variable course, ranging from slow and indolent to aggressive and rapidly fatal. As in Hodgkin's disease, improvements in survival are attributed to advancements in therapy but the use of modern imaging methods to delineate the extent of disease with a high degree of accuracy is also an important factor.

In the lymphomas, imaging plays a vital role in the correct deployment of combined modality treatment at the time of diagnosis and staging, in monitoring response to therapy and in the detection of relapse.

The objectives of initial staging are to define as accurately as possible the local extent of clinically overt disease and to search for occult disease elsewhere with a full knowledge of the likely pattern of tumoural spread.[1] The choice of the appropriate imaging method requires an appreciation of:

- the likelihood of particular sites being affected
- the sensitivity and specificity of particular tests chosen to investigate those sites
- the likely impact of a positive result on treatment choice

Incidence

Lymphoma accounts for 5–6% of malignancy in adults in the UK and about 10% of all childhood cancers.[2,3] In the USA in 2003 it is estimated that 53,400 new cases of NHL were diagnosed and that the total number of deaths was 23,400.[4] Each year in the USA NHL accounts for 5% of new cancers in men and 4% of new cancers in women. According to the National Cancer Institute, the USA age-adjusted incidence rate for NHL was 15.5 per 100,000 peo-

ple in 1996.[5] Hodgkin's disease is less common than NHL and it is estimated that in the USA there were 7,600 new cases of HD in 2003 and 1,300 deaths.[4] In the UK there were 10,100 new cases of non-Hodgkin's lymphoma in 1999 and 2,215 new cases of Hodgkin's disease; there were 4,630 deaths from NHL and 264 deaths from HD in 2001. The lifetime risk of developing NHL is approximately one in 83, and males are affected slightly more often than females in both types of lymphoma:[2]

- Hodgkin's disease M:F 1.4:1
- Non-Hodgkin's lymphoma M:F 1.1:1

While the incidence of Hodgkin's disease remains approximately stable, that of NHL has risen by approximately 60% in the USA since 1960. The increased incidence is evident for all age groups, but is much more marked with increasing age.[6] This marked increase has been noted in international cancer registries of seven European countries[7] and also in all geographical areas of the USA.[5] The mortality rate for NHL has also increased steadily over the last few decades. Several hypotheses have been used to explain the striking increase. Some may be artifactual, where new NHL classification techniques and systems have led to a diagnosis of NHL in some patients who would previously have had other diagnoses;[8] improved imaging techniques have undoubtedly led to more NHL diagnoses, particularly lymphoma of the central nervous system (CNS);[8] it has also been estimated that in 10–15% of cases a reclassification of cases previously called HD contributes to the apparent increase in NHL incidence.[9] Part of the increase is a consequence of the increased incidence of lymphomas associated with immune deficiency, particularly secondary to human immunodeficiency virus (HIV) infection. Nevertheless, even when factors such as accuracy and completeness of diagnosis, the effect of HIV and occupational exposures are considered, the reason for most of the increase in NHL remains unexplained.[10]

Hodgkin's disease shows a bimodal peak distribution, the first in the third decade of life, and the second between 65 and 75 years of age; but in recent years this has become less obvious, with a decrease in the incidence in patients over 55 years. However, NHL is a disease mainly of the elderly with an increasing incidence over the age of 50 years[11] and a median age at diagnosis of 65 years.[12]

Key points: incidence

- The incidence of NHL has increased by 60% over the last 2 decades in the USA and UK, while the incidence of HD is stable

- Hodgkin's disease has a peak incidence between the ages of 30 and 40 years, and also in those aged over 65 years. Non-Hodgkin's lymphoma is seen in children and in those over 50 years of age

- There is a link between the Epstein–Barr virus (EBV) and HD as well as NHL. Genetic dysfunction is an important aetiological factor

Aetiology

There is an association between EBV and HD but debate continues regarding the exact aetiological role of EBV in this disease. It is interesting that the suggestion of infection having a causal relationship with HD was originally made by Hodgkin himself at the time of his first description of the morbid anatomy of the condition. Patients with HD have a higher antibody titre to the EBV viral capsular antigen than normal adults and there is also an increased risk of HD amongst patients who have had infectious mononucleosis.[13]

Genetic studies have revealed the importance of mutation, altered expression and loss of function of genes in the development and progression of NHL, largely accounting for the diversity of clinical presentations and clinical course of this disease.[14] In NHL, immunosuppression is an important aetiological factor, the disease having a high incidence in patients with acquired immune deficiency syndrome (AIDS) and those on long-term immunosuppressant therapy, for example, following renal transplantation.[15,16] Epstein–Barr virus may be an important aetiological factor in Burkitt's lymphoma (BL), whereas the rare primary effusion lymphomas (Table 32.1) are associated with human herpes virus (HHV). *Helicobacter pylori* infection is necessary for the development of gastric lymphoma of mucosa-associated lymphoid tissue (MALT) type, whereas organ-specific autoimmune diseases predispose to the development of extranodal marginal zone lymphomas of MALT type within the affected organs (for example, the thyroid and salivary glands). The HTLV-1 retrovirus is known to have a causal relationship with adult T-cell leukaemia/lymphoma.[14,17]

Pathology

Classification

Non-Hodgkin's lymphoma

The importance of any classification is first its clinical relevance and second its translatability to allow communication of new knowledge and comparison of clinical results.[18] In this context, the reproducibility and widespread use of the Rye modification of the Luke–Butler classification introduced in 1966 has proved to be reliable for HD (Table 32.1).[19,20] This contrasts greatly with the profusion of classifications for NHL, although since its introduction in 1982 the working formulation has resulted in some degree of consensus.[21] The functional anatomy of the lymph node and its relationship to lymphoma is shown in Figure 32.1. The recognition that most NHLs arise from the cells of the germinal follicle of the lymph node led to the development of a Working Formulation of NHL for clinical usage (Table 32.2).[21] This classification was widely employed, until the introduction of the REAL (Revised European American Classification of Lymphoid Neoplasms) classification, and completely superseded the plethora of previous classifications, which were largely unsatisfactory.[22,23] The Working Formulation was based upon the idea that lymphoma is a result of clonal expansion of T or B lymphocytes at a particular point in their normal maturation.[24] B lymphocytes (bone marrow derived) are concerned with antibody production and develop into plasma cells that produce immunoglobulin. If normal maturation is prevented, the arrested cell multiplies, resulting in lymphoma; the type and grade of lymphoma which results depends on the stage of maturation at the time of insult. T lymphocytes (thymic derived) do not contain immunoglobulin but are also concerned with

Table 32.1. *Rye classification of Hodgkin's disease with approximate distribution of frequency*[19,20]

Histology	Frequency (%)
Lymphocyte predominance	5
Nodular sclerosis	65
Mixed cellularity	25
Lymphocyte depletion	5

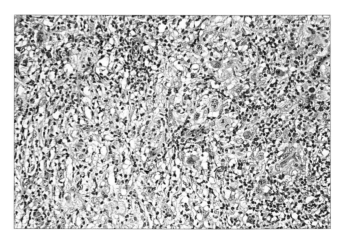

Figure 32.1. *Relationship of functional lymph node anatomy to normal cell type and lineage of the NHLs.*

Table 32.2. *A Working Formulation of NHL for clinical usage*[21,22]

Low grade	
A	Small lymphocytic: consistent with chronic lymphocytic leukaemia or with plasmacytoid features
B	Follicular, small cleaved cell
C	Follicular, mixed small cleaved and large cell
Intermediate grade	
D	Follicular, large cell
E	Diffuse, small cleaved cell
F	Diffuse, mixed small and large cell
G	Diffuse, large cell
High grade	
H	Large cell immunoblastic
I	Lymphoblastic (convoluted or non-convoluted)
J	Small non-cleaved cell (Burkitt or non-Burkitt type)
Miscellaneous	
Composite	
Histiocytic	
Mycosis fungoides	
Extramedullary plasmacytoma	
Hairy cell	
Unclassifiable	

immune response. T-cell lymphomas are either central T-cell lymphomas that are immature (e.g. diffuse lymphoblastic lymphoma), or those derived from more mature T lymphocytes, which are termed peripheral T-cell lymphomas. Histiocytic lymphomas do not fall into either of these categories.

The majority of NHLs (over 90%) are B-cell lymphomas. Non-Hodgkin's lymphomas, which arise at stages of development occurring within the germinal centre of the node, have a follicular pattern, whereas lymphomas that arise outside the germinal centre have a diffuse architectural pattern. The Working Formulation designated each lymphoma according to characteristics of the cell type at the time of arrested maturation and overall divided NHL into low-grade, intermediate and high-grade tumours. The 'miscellaneous' group did not fulfil all the requirements of the main three categories.[25]

The Working Formulation had important practical implications:

- Therapy was based on the grade of lymphoma
- The grade of lymphoma carried important prognostic significance
- The classification of lymphoma predicted possible transformation into a higher grade

- The detailed subclassification of lymphomas allowed standardization of therapies and comparison of results from different centres

More recently, in 1994, improvement in the understanding of NHL and the recognition of new clinico-pathological entities resulted in the introduction of the REAL classification by the International Lymphoma Study Group, which is now being adopted internationally.[26]

The REAL classification is a consensus list of all lymphoid neoplasms that appear to be distinct clinical entities. Unlike the Working Formulation, it utilizes all available features (morphology, immunophenotype, genetics and clinical features) to define each entity. This practical consensus approach differentiates it from previous morphological classifications and should enable widespread usage by pathologists and clinicians.

In 1995, under the auspices of the WHO, the European Association for Haematopathology and the Society for Haematopathology collaborated on a project to classify all tumours of haematopoietic and lymphoid lineages. The proposals were reviewed by a Clinical Advisory Committee (CAC) and the result is the WHO Classification of Tumours of Haematopoietic and Lymphoid Tissues,[27] which is an updated version of the REAL classification (Table 32.3).

The WHO classification stratifies neoplasms by lineage: myeloid, lymphoid, histiocytic/dendritic and mast cell. The classification is a list of distinct disease entities that are defined by a combination of morphology, immunophenotype, and genetic features, and which have distinct clinical features. It recognizes three major groups of lymphoid neoplasms: B cell, T cell and NK cell; and Hodgkin's lymphoma (HL). It includes the leukaemias, as they represent circulating phases of particular neoplasms. Thus B-cell chronic lymphocytic leukaemia and B-cell small lymphocytic lymphoma are the same entity, as are lymphoblastic lymphoma and lymphoblastic leukaemia. The definition of distinct clinical diseases means that classification by histological grade of aggressiveness is neither helpful nor possible. However, within the B and T/NK categories two major groups are recognized – precursor neoplasms (corresponding to the early stages of differentiation) and mature or peripheral neoplasms, corresponding to more differentiated stages. The main lymphoid groups are shown in Table 32.1.

The approach is thought to represent a significant advance in the ability to identify and treat disease entities, with international consistency. A study to address this issue of consistency showed that expert haematopathologists, given adequate material, could correctly classify the entity in over 95% of cases.[28,29]

Hodgkin's disease

Biological and clinical studies have shown that HD is a true lymphoma and the term HL is now preferred by many pathologists. Central to the diagnosis of HD is the demon-

Table 32.3. *Summary of the WHO classification of tumours of lymphoid tissues*

B-cell neoplasms	T-cell and NK-cell neoplasms
Precursor B-cell neoplasm	*Precursor T-cell neoplasms*
Precursor B lymphoblastic leukaemia/lymphoma	Precursor T lymphoblastic leukaemia/lymphoma
	Blastic NK cell lymphoma
Mature B-cell	*Mature T-cell & NK neoplasms*
CLL/small lymphocytic lymphoma	T-cell prolymphocytic leukaemia
B-cell prolymphocytic leukaemia	T-cell large granular lymphocytic leukaemia
Lymphoplasmacytic lymphoma	Aggressive NK cell leukaemia
Splenic marginal zone lymphoma	Adult T-cell leukaemia/lymphoma
Hairy cell leukaemia	Extranodal NK/T-cell lymphoma, nasal type
Plasma cell myeloma	Enteropathy-type T-cell lymphoma
Solitary plasmacytoma of bone	Hepatosplenic T-cell lymphoma
Extraosseous plasmacytoma	Subcutaneous panniculitis-like T-cell lymphoma
Extranodal marginal zone B-cell lymphoma of mucosa associated lymphoid tissue (MALT)	Mycosis fungoides
Nodal maginal zone B-cell lymphoma	Sezary syndrome
Follicular lymphoma	Primary cutaneous anaplastic large cell lymphoma
Mantle cell lymphoma	Peripheral T-cell lymphoma, unspecified
Diffuse large B-cell lymphoma	Angioimmunoblastic T-cell lymphoma
Mediastinal (thymic) large B-cell lymphoma	Anaplastic large cell lymphoma
Intravascular large B-cell lymphoma	
Primary effusion lymphoma	
Burkitt's lymphoma/leukaemia	
B-cell proliferations of uncertain malignant potential	*T-cell proliferation of uncertain malignant potential*
Lymphomatoid granulomatosis	Lymphoid papulosis
Post-transplant lymphoproliferative disorder, polymorphic	
	Hodgkin's lymphoma
	Nodular lymphocyte predominant HL
	Classical HL
	Nodular sclerosis classical HL
	Lymphocyte rich classical HL
	Mixed cellularity classical HL
	Lymphocyte depleted classical HL

stration of neoplastic Reed–Sternberg (Fig. 32.2) and Hodgkin cells, in a background of non-neoplastic inflammatory cells. The Rye modification of the Luke–Butler classification divides HD into four subgroups, based on the proportion of lymphocytes in relation to the number of Hodgkin and Reed–Sternberg cells, and the type of connective tissue background. However, as recognized in the REAL and WHO classifications, HD comprises two distinct entities:

- Nodular lymphocyte predominant Hodgkin's lymphoma (NLPHL)
- Classical Hodgkin's lymphoma (CHL)

These two differ in clinical features, behaviour, morphology and immunophenotype, whereas the four CHL subtypes all share the same immunophenotype.

Most cases of NLPHL were probably misclassified as lymphocyte predominance Hodgkin's disease in the past. It represents 5% of all HD. Patients are mostly male in the 30–50-year age group. Most patients present with Stage I or II peripheral adenopathy; mediastinal, splenic, and marrow involvement are rare. Latent EBV infection is not seen in the malignant cells.

Classical HL accounts for 95% of all cases. Patients with infectious mononucleosis have a higher incidence and familial and geographic clustering is seen.

In nodular sclerosing HD, nodules of lymphoid tissue are separated by dense bands of collagen. It is the most frequent subgroup, accounting for 70% of classical HD. The median age is around 25 years and it is the only form of HD without a male preponderance. Mediastinal disease occurs in 80% of cases, bulky disease in around 50%, splenic and/or lung involvement in 10%. Most patients are Stage II at presentation and B symptoms are seen in 40%.

Mixed cellularity HD comprises 20–25% of classical HD and is commoner in patients with HIV infection and in developing countries. Of those affected, 70% are male. Stage III or IV disease is common, as are B symptoms. Peripheral nodal disease is frequent, splenic involvement occurs in up to 30%, and marrow involvement in 10% of affected individuals. Mediastinal disease is uncommon.

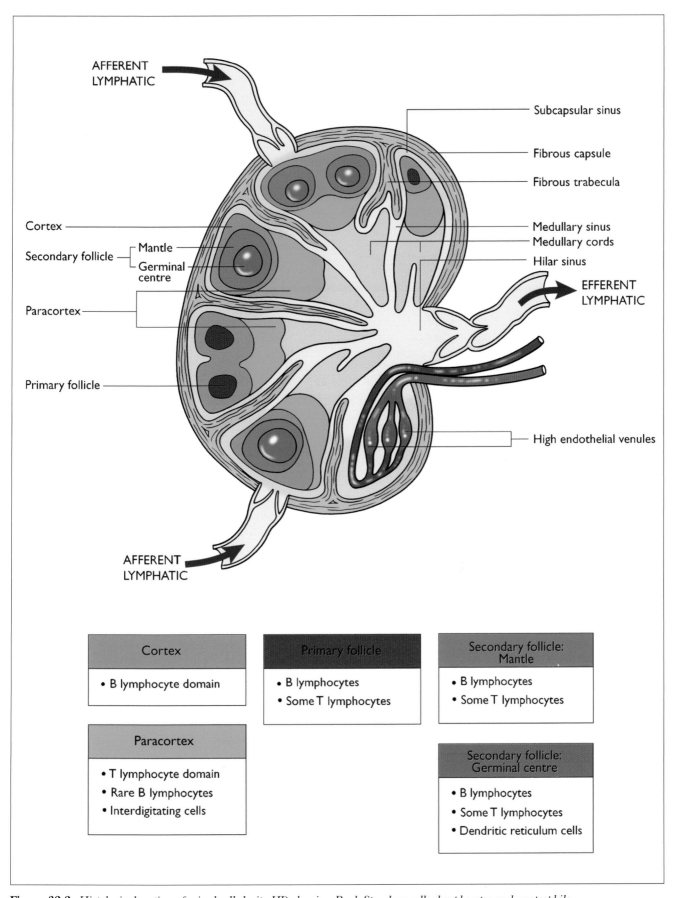

AFFERENT LYMPHATIC

Subcapsular sinus

Fibrous capsule

Fibrous trabecula

Cortex

Secondary follicle — Mantle
— Germinal centre

Medullary sinus
Medullary cords
Hilar sinus

EFFERENT LYMPHATIC

Paracortex

Primary follicle

High endothelial venules

AFFERENT LYMPHATIC

Cortex
• B lymphocyte domain

Primary follicle
• B lymphocytes
• Some T lymphocytes

Secondary follicle: Mantle
• B lymphocytes
• Some T lymphocytes

Paracortex
• T lymphocyte domain
• Rare B lymphocytes
• Interdigitating cells

Secondary follicle: Germinal centre
• B lymphocytes
• Some T lymphocytes
• Dendritic reticulum cells

Figure 32.2. *Histological section of mixed cellularity HD showing Reed–Sternberg cells, lymphocytes and neutrophils.*

Lymphocyte-rich classical HD comprises 5% of all HD; 70% are male, with a higher median age. Stage I or II peripheral nodal disease is typical, without mediastinal involvement or B symptoms.

Lymphocyte-depleted classical HD is the rarest subtype, accounting for less than 5% of cases; 75% of the affected individuals are male, with a median age of 35–40 years. It is often associated with HIV infection and is seen more often in developing countries. Peripheral lymph nodes are relatively spared, with involvement instead of abdominal organs, retroperitoneal nodes and bone marrow. Stage III or IV disease is common (70%) as are B symptoms (80%). Most HIV-positive cases are EBV infected and have relatively aggressive courses.

Key points: classification of lymphomas

- Hodgkin's disease comprises two distinct entities: NLPHL and CHL

- Classical Hodgkin's disease is made up of four subtypes: nodular sclerosing (70%), mixed cellularity (20–25%), lymphocyte rich (5%), and lymphocyte depleted (<5%)

- The WHO update of the Revised European American Lymphoma (REAL) classification stratifies lymphoma by myeloid, lymphoid, histiocytic/dendritic and mast cell lineage, and provides a list of distinct disease entities

Staging classifications

The Ann Arbor staging system was introduced for HD in 1970 and takes into account the extent of nodal disease and the presence of extranodal extension. However, an increasing recognition of the influence of tumour bulk as an independent prognostic indicator within each stage, and the routine application of new diagnostic techniques, such as computed tomography (CT) or magnetic resonance imaging (MRI) led to a modification of the Ann Arbor classification in 1989, known as the Cotswolds classification (Table 32.4).[30] This system is similar to the Ann Arbor classification, but Stage III is subdivided and an additional qualifier 'X' denotes bulky disease. Both the Ann Arbor and Cotswolds systems are applied to NHL, but are of less value, as the prognosis in NHL is more dependent on histological grade and other parameters such as tumour bulk and specific organ involvement, than on stage.[31,32] In NHL, the critical question is whether or not disease is limited and, therefore, potentially treatable with radiotherapy, or whether it is disseminated.

Childhood NHL exhibits a clinical spectrum somewhat different to adult lymphoma with more frequent extranodal involvement, there being a very high incidence of lymphoma in the gastrointestinal tract, solid abdominal viscera including the kidneys and pancreas, and extranodal sites in the head and neck.[33,34] The staging system of Murphy is most widely used (Table 32.5).

Table 32.4. *Staging of lymphoma (Cotswolds Classification)*[31]

Stage	Area of involvement
I	One lymph node region or extralymphatic site
II	Two or more lymph node regions on the same side of the diaphragm
III	Involvement of lymph node region or structures on both sides of diaphragm, subdivided thus:
III(1[1])	With involvement of spleen and/or splenic hilar, coeliac and portal nodes
III(2[1])	With para-aortic, iliac or mesenteric nodes
IV	Extranodal sites beyond those designated E

Additional qualifiers	
A	No symptoms
B	Fever, sweats, weight loss (to 10% of body weight)
E	Involvement of single extranodal site, contiguous in proximity to a known nodal site
X[1]	Bulky disease Mass >1/3 thoracic diameter at T5 Mass >10 cm maximum dimension
CE[1]	Clinical stage
PS[1]	Pathological stage: PS at a given site denoted by a subscript (i.e. M = marrow, H = liver, L = lung, O = bone, P = pleural, D = skin

[1]Modifications from Ann Arbor system.

Clinical features

Hodgkin's disease and NHL are diseases of the lymph nodes, both of which may present as truly localized processes involving a single nodal group or organ, or as widely disseminated disease. However, recognizable differences distinguish the clinical presentation in the two diseases (Table 32.6).

Hodgkin's disease

Most patients with HD present with painless asymmetrical lymph node enlargement, which may be accompanied with sweats, fever, weight loss, and pruritus in about 40% of patients. Alcohol-induced pain is a rare complaint.

On clinical examination the commonest site of nodal involvement is the cervical region, which is seen in 60–80% of patients. Axillary nodal involvement is also common, occurring in 6–20% of patients, and inguinal/femoral nodal disease is seen in 6–15%. Exclusive infradiaphragmatic lymphadenopathy only occurs in less than 10% of

Table 32.5. *Murphy's staging system for childhood NHL*

Stage	Criteria for extent of disease
I	A single tumour (extranodal) or single anatomical area (nodal) with the exclusion of the mediastinum or abdomen
II	A single tumour (extranodal) with regional nodal involvement
	Two or more nodal areas on the same side of the diaphragm
	Two single (extranodal) tumours with or without regional node involvement of the same side of the diaphragm
	A primary GI tract tumour, usually in the ileocaecal area, with or without involvement of associated mesenteric nodes only, grossly completely resected
III	Two single tumours (extranodal) on opposite sides of the diaphragm
	Two or more nodal areas above and below the diaphragm
	ALL primary intrathoracic tumours (mediastinal, pleural, thymic)
	ALL extensive primary intra-abdominal disease, unresected
	ALL paraspinal or epidural tumours, regardless of other tumour site(s)
IV	Any of the above with initial CNS and/or bone marrow involvement

Table 32.6. *Key differences between the clinical features of HD and NHL*

	HD	NHL
Clinical features		
Fever, night sweats, loss of weight	40%	20%
Spread	Tends to be by contiguous spread	Multiple remote nodal groups are often involved
Age	Uncommon in childhood	More frequent 40–70 years
Nodal groups		
Thoracic	65–85%	25–40%
Para-aortic	25–35%	45–55%
Mesenteric	5%	50–60%
Extranodal disease		
CNS	<1%	2%
GI tract	<1%	5–15%
Genitourinary tract	<1%	1–5%
Bone marrow	3%	20–40%
Lung parenchyma	8–12%	3–6%
Bone	<1%	1–2%
Stage at diagnosis	>80% Stages I–II	>85% Stages III–IV

patients at diagnosis. Splenomegaly is found on clinical examination in about one third of patients.

Hodgkin's disease tends to spread in a contiguous fashion from one lymph node group to the next adjacent group. Primary extranodal HD is very rare and can only be diagnosed after a thorough search for disease in other sites.

Non-Hodgkin's lymphoma

As in HD, the majority of patients with NHL present with nodal enlargement, but extranodal disease is far commoner.

In low-grade lymphoma, lymphadenopathy may be intermittent and the median age at diagnosis is between 55 and 60 years. They are rarely diagnosed under the age of 30 years and account for 30–45% of all lymphomas.

Intermediate-grade lymphoma usually includes both follicular and diffuse forms. The diffuse large-cell lymphoma is the most common NHL subtype and usually presents with rapidly enlarging lymph nodes. Together with follicular large cell lymphoma, these tumours comprise 50% of all lymphomas. They usually present between the ages of 50 and 55 years and may be associated with extranodal disease at presentation.

High-grade lymphomas are the most aggressive tumour subtype but most patients have apparently localized disease at the time of presentation. Overall, approximately 20% of patients with NHL have systemic symptoms such as fever, sweats and weight loss, compared with 40% of patients with HD. Non-Hodgkin's lymphoma is a disseminated disease involving lymph node groups haphazardly, and multiple organs may be involved as well as the bone marrow.[35]

Key points: clinical aspects

■ The majority of patients with HD and NHL present with painless enlargement of a group of lymph nodes

■ In HD, most patients present with Stage I or II disease, and in NHL the majority of patients have Stage III or IV disease at diagnosis

■ Systemic symptoms are seen more frequently in HD than NHL

Prognosis and treatment options

Hodgkin's disease

The prognosis of HD depends upon a number of factors,[13] including:

- Age. Older patients have a worse prognosis
- Tumour subtype. Those with mixed cellularity and lymphocyte depletion have a worse prognosis than with nodular sclerosis and lymphocyte-predominant HD
- Raised erythrocyte sedimentation rate (ESR)
- Multiple sites of involvement
- Bulky mediastinal disease
- Systemic symptoms

Patients with HD have traditionally been divided into two or three prognostic groups, chiefly according to stage and B symptoms, but also taking various other factors into consideration. Each group is associated with a typical standard treatment strategy:

- Early stages, favourable: radiation alone (extended field)
- Early stages, unfavourable: moderate amount of chemotherapy plus radiation
- Advanced stages: extensive chemotherapy with or without consolidatory (usually local) radiation

The standard treatment for early-stage HD is radiotherapy to the involved nodes as well as the adjacent lymph node

chains. These tumours are highly radiosensitive and can be cured by radiotherapy alone.[30] Administration of mantle radiotherapy for cervical lymphadenopathy has stood the test of time and includes irradiation to the bilateral cervical nodes, the supraclavicular and axillary nodes, together with mediastinal nodes, extending down to the lower border of the vertebral body of T10.

Until relatively recently, staging laparotomy was routinely undertaken in patients with HD to identify splenic involvement and intra-abdominal lymph node spread. Although it is known that the spleen is involved in about 30% of patients with Stage I and Stage II HD, the technique has been abandoned for the following reasons:

- Even if the laparotomy is negative, relapse in the abdomen is common following mantle radiotherapy
- Combination chemotherapy is more frequently used in the treatment of HD, thereby obviating the need for splenectomy
- Patients with undiagnosed infradiaphragmatic disease who are treated with mantle radiotherapy can be salvaged with subsequent chemotherapy
- Staging laparotomy is a major procedure, and splenectomy increases the risk of infection and may have a causal relationship with the subsequent development of leukaemia[36]

Hodgkin's disease is chemosensitive and chemotherapy combined with radiotherapy is widely used in patients with adverse prognostic indicators in early-stage disease, for example, those presenting with bulky mediastinal masses or multiple sites of involvement. Chemotherapy with or without irradiation is also the standard approach for the treatment of Stages III and IV disease. The aim in patients with bulky disease is to use chemotherapy to reduce bulk, followed by radiotherapy to that site, in order to avoid excessive irradiation of lung parenchyma and subsequent radiation fibrosis. There is long-term toxicity from radiotherapy including an excess of breast cancer in women who have received mantle radiotherapy.[37]

Major developments in treatment have been aimed at reducing toxicity while at the same time maintaining efficacy. The different regimes have different side effects ranging from nausea, vomiting, and hair loss to bone marrow suppression, sterility and leukaemogenesis.[38–40] The overall 10-year survival rate in patients with Stages I and II HD treated with radiotherapy is greater than 90%.[41,42]

In patients with more advanced disease (bulky Stage II, Stage III and IV), overall between 50% and 80% will achieve complete remission following multi-agent chemotherapy, but of these between 30% and 50% will subsequently relapse within 5 years.[30] Combination chemotherapy for recurrence after primary treatment with radiotherapy alone is successful in achieving a prolonged second remission.[43] Patients failing initial chemotherapy for advanced HD have a poor prognosis but high-dose chemotherapy with haemopoietic stem cell rescue is being increasingly employed, although its long-term benefits are not yet established.[44]

Non-Hodgkin's lymphoma

The prognosis of NHL varies tremendously. Unlike HD, histological subtype is the major determinant of treatment, and prognosis and treatment is dependent on a combination of histological subtype and stage. Low-grade lymphomas, although incurable, often have a prolonged indolent course. Low-grade lymphoma, for example follicular lymphoma, is slowly progressive and has a tendency to become more diffuse with a greater number of large cells. Such transformation has important implications for prognosis and therefore an impact on treatment strategy. Intermediate and high-grade lymphomas carry a worse prognosis, especially those with larger cells and blast forms. In these patients, however, cure is possible with advanced chemotherapeutic regimens. The International Prognostic Index (IPI) was developed by an international collaborative group in recognition of the fact that appropriate choice of therapy for a patient and comparison of therapies can only be achieved with a uniform prognostic system in place.[45] For diffuse large B-cell lymphoma, five factors were found to have prognostic significance:

- Age > 60 years
- Elevated serum lactate dehydrogenase (LDH)
- Eastern Cooperative Oncology Group (ECOG) performance status >1 (i.e. non-ambulatory)[46]
- Advanced Stage (III or IV)
- Presence of >1 extranodal site of disease

Prognostic stratification enables choice of more aggressive therapies for those at higher risk. However, the applicability of the IPI to other more rare forms of NHL and to follicular NHL is uncertain.

Although the REAL classification has changed our understanding of the clinical pattern and prognosis of the disease, the treatment in the individual NHL subtypes is still largely dictated by the previous broad categorization into low- and high-grade lymphomas, as well as the sites of involvement. At one end of the scale, patients presenting with low-grade lymphomas who are asymptomatic may simply be followed without treatment until symptoms develop or transformation occurs. At the other end of the scale, patients presenting with high-grade disease may be successfully treated with multi-agent chemotherapy with most attaining a remission and up to 50% of patients achieving long-term disease-free survival.[47] The development of antibody therapies has added a new dimension to NHL and the immunological subtype is now an additional important consideration in defining treatment, particularly for B-cell lymphomas. However, once relapse occurs, particularly if

remission is short, further response to salvage chemotherapy is difficult to sustain. Current investigation is directed towards high-dose therapy with autologous bone marrow transplant.[48]

Radiotherapy has a role in low and intermediate-grade NHL but is usually inappropriate for treatment of high-grade lymphomas, which are frequently widely disseminated tumours.

Overall, 10-year survival in patients treated with radiotherapy for low-grade Stages I and II disease are in the order of 90%.[41,42]

The major differences between the clinical features of HD and NHL are shown in Table 32.6.

Broadly, NHL is disseminated at presentation more frequently than HD and, although the majority of adult patients with NHL present with superficial lymphadenopathy, involvement of the viscera is more common in all types of NHL than it is in HD.

Nodal disease

Lymph node enlargement tends to be greater in NHL than HD, but both types may produce huge conglomerate tumour masses or may not produce any significant nodal enlargement. In nodular sclerosing HD and lymphocyte-depleted HD, involved nodes tend to be normal in size or only moderately enlarged. Typically, high-grade NHL produces large-volume nodal disease. A characteristic feature of lymphoma is that involved nodes tend to displace structures rather than invade them and in this respect they differ from carcinomas, an exception being the large cell high-grade lymphomas that are often locally invasive.

Imaging techniques

Cross-sectional imaging

The ability of CT to demonstrate enlarged lymph nodes throughout the body and detect associated pathology in soft tissue structures, together with its reproducibility, have all contributed to CT becoming the modality of choice for the staging and follow-up of lymphoma. Not only does it accurately demonstrate the full extent of disease, it also enables localization of the most appropriate lesion for consideration of percutaneous image-guided biopsy. Ultrasound will readily show lymph node enlargement in the coeliac region, splenic hilum and porta hepatis.[49–53] Frequently, however, the entire retroperitoneum cannot be shown, limiting its value in staging. Typically, lymphomatous nodal involvement produces uniformly hypoechoic, lobulated masses, appearances that are non-specific. The pattern of nodal vascular perfusion as assessed by power Doppler sonography may suggest a diagnosis of lymphoma, lymphomatous nodes being highly perfused in both the nodal centre and periphery (Fig. 32.3).[54] The main value of ultrasound in lymphoma lies not in routine staging,[55] for

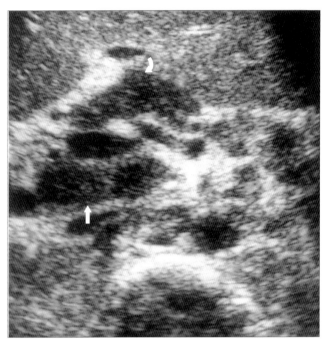

Figure 32.3. *Nodal enlargement on ultrasound. A transverse scan through the upper abdomen showing multiple hypoechoic lobulated masses consistent with lymph node enlargement located between the inferior vena cava and portal vein (arrow) and within the porta hepatis (curved arrow).*

which it is not sufficiently reliable, but in confirming that a palpable mass is in fact nodal or in solving specific problems in the liver, spleen or kidneys.[56] Although the accuracy of MRI in detecting lymph node involvement is equal to that of CT,[57–59] it has no particular advantage over CT, and its role is essentially adjunctive, used to solve problems in the identification of lymph node pathology or in monitoring response to treatment.[60] Involved lymph nodes cannot

be diagnosed other than by size criteria.[61] They are easily identified as relatively low/intermediate signal intensity masses on T1-weighted images and are of intermediate/high signal intensity in T2-weighted images (Fig. 32.4). At present, MRI-specific lymphographic agents in the form of ultrasmall superparamagnetic iron oxide particles do not have a role in the detection of lymphomatous involvement of normal-sized nodes.[62,63] On short tau inversion recovery (STIR) sequences, enlarged nodes may have very high signal intensity. Treated nodes, particularly in nodular sclerosing HD, may become necrotic and the nodes then have a signal intensity similar to that of fluid (Fig. 32.5). Calcification may occasionally develop following treatment for HD, which is clearly seen on CT. On MRI the signal intensity of calcified nodes is reduced.

Radioisotopes

For all three of the cross-sectional imaging modalities, recognition of nodal disease depends almost entirely on size criteria, and detection of disease in normal-sized nodes is not possible (though clustering of multiple small prominent nodes is suggestive). Conversely, it is not possible to differentiate between nodes that are enlarged by lymphoma or reactive hyperplasia. Both distinctions are theoretically possible with functional radioisotope studies. Gallium-67 (Ga-67) and the positron emitter 2-[F-18]fluoro-2-deoxy-D-glucose ([18]FDG) can demonstrate viable tumour cells within nodes with high sensitivity.[64,65] The accuracy of Ga-67 is dependent on several factors including cell type, and the location and size of the lesions. Its accuracy is greater for HD and high-grade lymphoma than for other forms; its accuracy decreases when the lesion is <2 cm or >5 cm. It is poor below the diaphragm, because of confounding bowel and splenic uptake, and some lymphomas, especially low-grade NHL, are non-gallium avid,

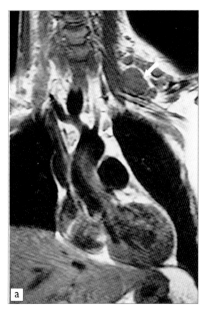

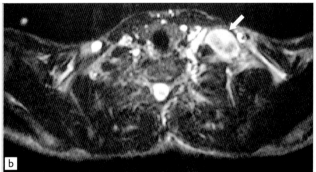

Figure 32.4. *MR image in a patient with HD showing enlarged lymph nodes in the left supraclavicular fossa. (a) T1-weighted paracoronal image showing the involved nodes (arrowed) as low signal intensity masses. (b) An axial T2-weighted image shows that the enlarged nodes have a high signal intensity (arrowed). Note a high signal intensity node measuring 1 cm is also visible on the right.*

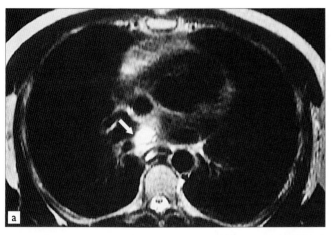 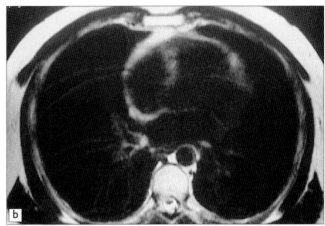

Figure 32.5. *MR images of a patient with HD. (a) Pretreatment turbo spin-echo T2-weighted image shows a high signal intensity residual lymph node in the subcarinal space (arrowed). No further treatment was given. (b) A follow-up examination 4 months later shows complete resolution of the node, presumed to be necrotic.*

resulting in too many false-negative studies to render it effective as an isolated staging tool in NHL or HD.[66–68]

Positron emission tomography

In the last decade there have been numerous studies of the efficacy of 2-[F-18]fluoro-2-deoxy-D-glucose positron emission tomography (FDG PET) in the staging and re-staging of HD and NHL. Recent studies give results at least comparable to or better than CT for the detection of nodal and extranodal disease,[69,70] with a trend to greater positivity for FDG PET on a lesion-by-lesion or site-based analysis. FDG PET tends to demonstrate a higher site positivity rate than Ga-67,[71,72] resulting in clinically significant upstaging in 10–20% of patients. It is more sensitive than Ga-67 for small masses (1–2 cm), below the diaphragm, and in the assessment of low-grade lymphomas.[73–75]

In HD, upstaging as a result of FDG PET can lead to changes in therapy, for example, from radiotherapy to chemotherapy, or alteration of radiotherapy portals,[76,77] but few authorities would recommend the use of FDG PET in isolation as a staging tool.[76]

In NHL, staging FDG PET gives important information for all grades of tumours by indicating tumour burden as well as the presence of extranodal disease. Most low-grade tumours do show uptake, the occasional exceptions being mucosa-associated lymphoid tissue (MALT) type and small lymphocytic types.[78,79]

The recent introduction of PET/CT heralds a new era in staging HD and NHL, allowing accurate localization of morphological abnormalities together with their associated functional changes.

Lymphangiography

During the 1980s, several studies showed that lymphangiography was equal to or slightly superior to CT for detecting nodal lymphoma.[80–87] However, lymphangiography does have several disadvantages; most significant is its inability to demonstrate lymph nodes above the level of the second lumbar vertebra and outside the retroperitoneum as well as the true extent of a nodal mass once it is has broken through the lymph node capsule (Fig. 32.6). Its advantages have become limited due to the development of newer generation CT scanners, which permit the detection of smaller degrees of lymphadenopathy. Another important factor is the increasing efficacy of chemotherapy, which is now able to salvage patients with apparent early-stage supradiaphragmatic disease, but who actually harbour microscopic foci of tumour in the spleen and/or infra-diaphragmatic nodes. Thus, although lymphangiography remains the only imaging method that visualizes nodal architecture, the complementary yield of lymphangiography over CT in HD is negligible and it is estimated that in only 5% of cases of HD will lymphangiography show true-positive abnormalities in lymph nodes <1 cm. Another problem with lymphangiography is the general lack of expertise currently available both in carrying out the procedure and in interpretation of the results. Even with lymphangiography, false-negative examinations are inevitable due to microscopic deposits in normal-sized nodes, but in addition false-positive examinations result from nodal enlargement due to benign hyperplasia.[88] Although some specialized centres continue to undertake lymphangiography in HD, it is generally only recommended when immediate detection of tumour in a normal-sized retroperitoneal node is considered essential for patient management and local expertise is available.[88]

Nodal disease in HD and NHL may involve any site where lymph nodes are found anatomically but for convenience this description is divided into the following sections: neck, thorax, abdomen and pelvis.

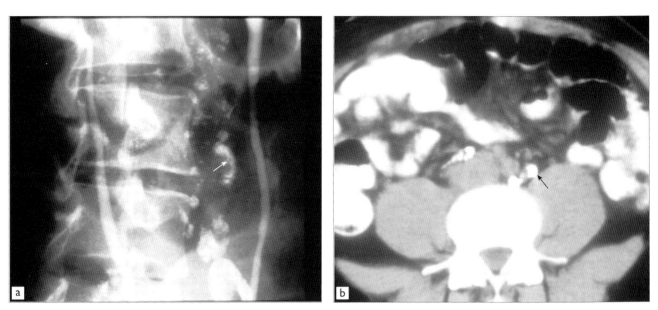

Figure 32.6. *Lymphangiogram in Hodgkin's disease. (a) Oblique view of the lumbar spine showing filling defects in involved left para-aortic lymph nodes (arrow). (b) Computed tomographic scan in the same patient as (a) performed on the same day, showing opacified unenlarged lymph nodes shown to be involved on LAG (arrow).*

Neck

A group of enlarged lymph nodes in the neck is the commonest presentation in HD seen in 60–80% of cases and this may also be the presenting feature in NHL. Hodgkin's disease typically involves the internal jugular chain of nodes first, but further spread is to the spinal accessory chain and the transverse cervical chain, these nodes forming the deep lymphatic chains of the neck.[89] The internal jugular chain follows the course of the internal jugular vein, the spinal accessory nodes are found between the sternocleidomastoid and trapezius muscles in the posterior triangle, and the transverse cervical nodes join the internal jugular and spinal accessory nodes in the lower neck (Fig. 32.7). Nodes in the submandibular, submental, parotid and retropharyngeal regions are occasionally involved. Patients with bulky supraclavicular or bilateral neck adenopathy are at increased risk of infradiaphragmatic disease. The pattern of NHL is more haphazard than HD because of haematogenous spread and is more likely to be associated with extranodal and bulky disease.

Lymph nodes >1 cm in diameter are generally considered enlarged on CT. Minimally enlarged discrete lymph nodes seen in the neck in patients with lymphoma usually have a well-defined contour, but once the tumour has broken beyond the confines of the node, the fat planes between the nodal mass and adjacent structures are lost.

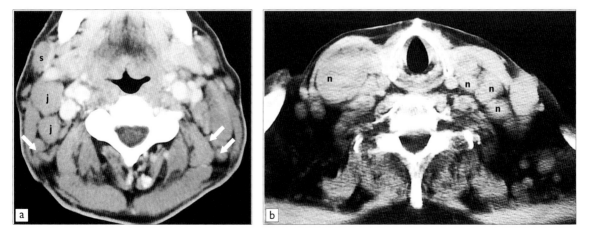

Figure 32.7. *NHL involving lymph nodes in the neck. (a) Contrast-enhanced CT shows discrete enlargement of lymph nodes bilaterally at presentation. The involved nodes are larger on the right. Submandibular nodes (s), jugular node (j), spinal accessory node (arrows); (b) unenhanced CT in a patient with intermediate-grade NHL showing bilateral involvement of midjugular nodes bilaterally (n). The sternocleidomastoid muscle on the right is displaced by a node measuring 3 × 2 cm in diameter.*

Fibrosis following radiotherapy may also eliminate the fat planes, making post-treatment assessment difficult on clinical examination and CT. Central necrosis within a lymph node is rarely seen in the lymphomas, a striking contrast to the typical features seen in squamous carcinoma nodal metastasis on contrast-enhanced CT. Enhancement following IV injection of contrast medium is usually mild to moderate though occasionally marked.[90]

Imaging, particularly CT, has a useful role in evaluating the neck in patients with lymphoma as it may:

- Identify involved nodes that are clinically impalpable
- Assess treatment response, particularly in patients treated with radiotherapy
- Identify recurrence in patients with thickened tissues due to previous radiotherapy (Fig. 32.8)

Magnetic resonance imaging may be particularly useful for defining the extent of lymphomatous masses in the lower neck and supraclavicular fossa (Fig. 32.9).

Thorax

The frequency and distribution of intrathoracic lymph node involvement in HD and NHL differ, although the appearances on imaging are similar. As in the neck, lymph nodes >1 cm in diameter are considered enlarged both on CT and MRI. However, account should also be given to the number of nodes present; multiple nodes, although <1 cm in diameter within the anterior mediastinum, should certainly be regarded as suspicious (Fig. 32.10). Nodes within the thorax are involved at the time of presentation in 60–85% of patients with HD and 25–40% of patients with NHL.[32,91–93] Any intrathoracic group of nodes may be

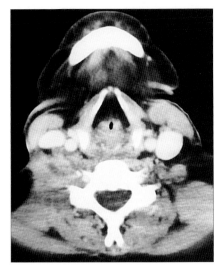

Figure 32.8. *Recurrent low-grade NHL. A nodal mass on the right side of the neck is seen on contrast-enhanced CT, which has an ill-defined contour and is closely applied to the sternocleidomastoid muscle. The patient had previously been treated with radiotherapy.*

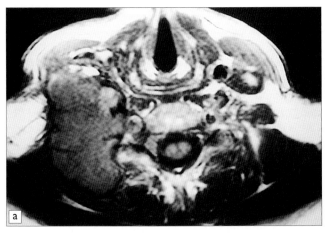
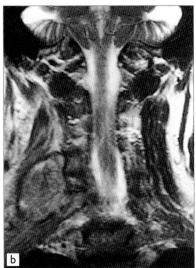

Figure 32.9. *MR images in a patient with NHL showing a large mass in the right lower neck extending into the supraclavicular fossa. (a) An axial turbo spin-echo T1-weighted image clearly shows the lobulated low-signal intensity mass on the right side of the neck; (b) a coronal turbo spin-echo T2-weighted image shows that the mass has a heterogeneous intermediate/high signal intensity. The mass is surrounded by a well-defined low signal intensity rim.*

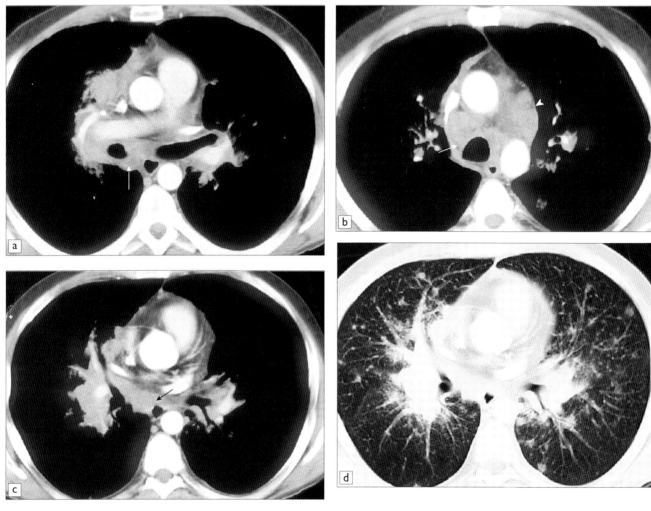

Figure 32.10. *Extensive mediastinal lymph node and lung parenchymal involvement in NHL. (a) Subcarinal lymph node enlarged (arrowed). (b) Scan above the level at (a) showing lymph node enlargement in the paratracheal region (arrow) and in the aortopulmonary region (arrowhead). (c) Lymph node enlargement in the azygo-oesophageal region in the same patient as (a). (d) In the same patient as shown in (a–c) when viewed on lung settings, there is peribronchial and juxtamediastinal lung parencymal involvement with linear shadowing and more discrete peripheral nodularity also shown in Figure 28.10(e).*

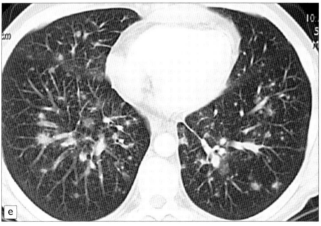

involved in patients with lymphoma, but all the mediastinal sites are more frequently involved by HD than NHL, except the paracardiac and posterior mediastinal nodes. The frequency of nodal involvement in HD is as follows:[92]

- Prevascular and paratracheal (84%)
- Hilar (28%)
- Subcarinal (22%) (Fig. 32.10)

- Other sites (approx. 5%)
  - Aortopulmonary window
  - Anterior diaphragmatic
  - Internal mammary
  - Posterior mediastinal

The frequency of intrathoracic nodal involvement in NHL has recently been analysed by Castellino et al.[94]

- Superior mediastinal (34%)
- Hilar (9%)
- Subcarinal (13%)
- Other sites (up to 10%) (Fig. 32.10)

In most cases lymphadenopathy is bilateral but asymmetric. Almost all patients with nodular sclerosing HD have disease in the anterior mediastinum.[93] The great majority of cases of HD show enlargement of two or more nodal groups, whereas only one nodal group is involved in up to half of the cases of NHL. Hilar nodal enlargement is rare without associated mediastinal involvement, particularly in HD. The posterior mediastinum is infrequently involved but if disease is present in the lower part of the mediastinum, contiguous retrocrural disease is likely.[95] Although nodes in the internal mammary chains and paracardiac regions are rarely involved at presentation, they become important as sites of recurrence as they may not be included in the conventional radiation field (Fig. 32.11).[96]

On CT, enlarged nodes may be discrete or matted together, and usually show only minor enhancement after injection of IV contrast medium (Fig. 32.12). Calcification prior to therapy is extremely rare, and does not appear to have any prognostic implications, though it is commoner in more aggressive subtypes.[93,97,98] It is seen occasionally following therapy. Cystic degeneration may be seen rarely in both HD and NHL, which may persist following therapy when the rest of the nodal masses shrink away (Fig. 32.5).[99] Cystic change is more likely with large anterior mediastinal masses, but again this does not have any prognostic significance, nor does it indicate a particular pathological sub-

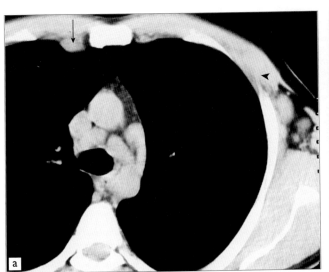
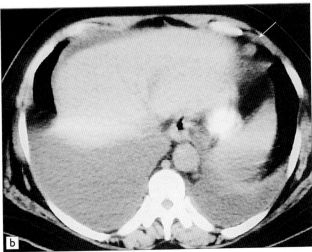

Figure 32.11. *CT scan showing right internal mammary lymph node enlargement (arrowed) together with left axillary (arrowhead) and middle mediastinal lymph node enlargement. (b) CT scan of a patient with NHL with bilateral pleural effusions. There is a 1 cm diaphragmatic lymph node adjacent to the left cardiac border (arrowed).*

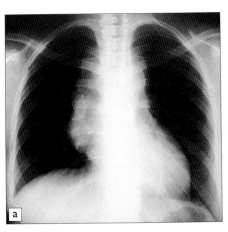
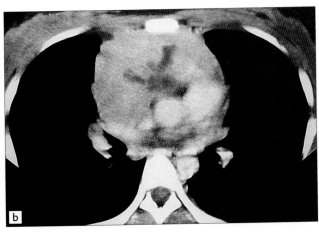

Figure 32.12. *Massive lymph node enlargement in a patient presenting with HD. (a) Plain chest radiograph. (b) Contrast-enhanced CT scan showing anterior mediastinal lymph node mass. Note low-density area centrally, probably representing necrosis.*

type, occurring in both nodular sclerosing HD and mediastinal large B-cell lymphoma (Fig. 32.13).[99]

In about 10% of patients with HD, CT demonstrates enlarged mediastinal nodes despite a normal chest radiograph (Fig. 32.14).[92] Patients with HD who have even a moderate volume of unsuspected intrathoracic disease at CT have a poorer prognosis.[100] CT will change clinical stage in up to 16% of patients with lymphoma and management may be altered in up to 25%, particularly where radiotherapy is planned. Thus, the effect of CT is more pronounced in patients with HD than NHL.[92,94,101–103]

Even in patients with bulky disease, CT frequently provides additional information such as:

- The inferior extent of the mass and its relationship to the heart
- The presence of pericardial thickening and effusion, which can be distinguished from lymphadenopathy

Large anterior mediastinal masses usually represent thymic infiltration as well as a nodal mass[104] (Fig. 32.15a). Enlarged nodes can usually be distinguished from a thymic mass but on occasion thymic involvement can only be definitely recorded on evaluation of follow-up studies after treatment, when the thymus has resumed its normal shape in up to 30% of patients[105] (Fig. 32.15b). Thymic infiltration may be

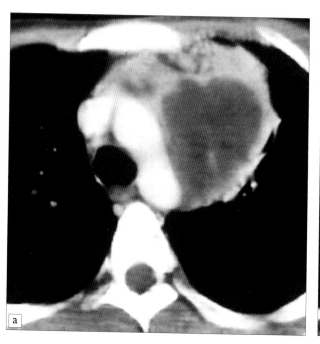

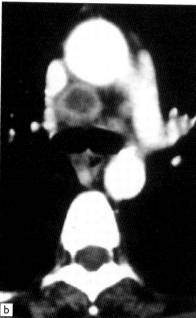

Figure 32.13. *Cystic change within lymph nodes. (a) Cystic change within a mediastinal mass of nodes. (b) Ring enhancement following IV injection of contrast medium due to cystic change within a paratracheal lymph node.*

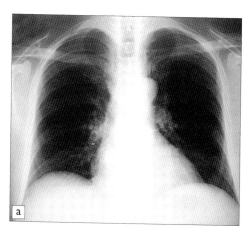

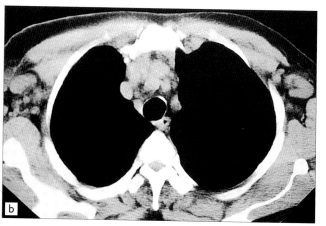

Figure 32.14. *(a) Plain chest radiograph and (b) CT scan in a patient with NHL. The plain chest radiograph appears normal but CT shows multiple enlarged lymph nodes in the mediastinum, indicating intrathoracic disease. Note left internal mammary and bilateral axillary lymph node enlargement.*

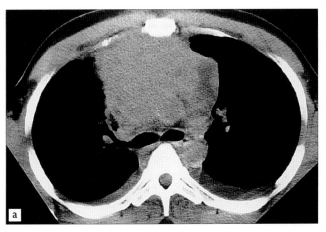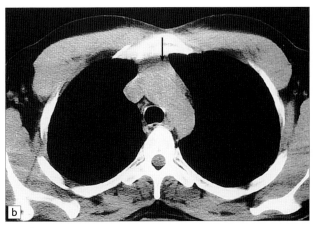

Figure 32.15. *CT scan in a patient with HD. (a) Before treatment there is a large anterior mediastinal mass, probably involving the thymus. Note an area of low density within the mass on the left which either represents necrosis or cystic change. (b) Following treatment the mass has shown an excellent response to treatment and the thymus has resumed its normal shape (arrowed), indicating that the mass almost certainly represented thymic infiltration.*

seen in both HD and NHL. Although the thymus is usually seen on CT as a homogeneous soft tissue mass, cystic areas within the mass may be identified both on CT and MRI, especially with mediastinal large B-cell lymphoma (previously called sclerosing diffuse large B-cell lymphoma (Fig. 32.15).[106] These cysts are more frequently detected on MRI.[107] Some research indicates that in NHL high-grade tumours tend to be more heterogeneous on pre- and post-contrast CT scans than low-grade tumours of comparable size, but the clinical relevance of this is uncertain.[108] Similarly, there is some evidence that heterogeneous high T2 signal intensity within mediastinal masses is associated with high-grade tumours and poorer survival.[109,110] A large anterior mediastinal mass, especially over one third of the transthoracic diameter at the level of T6, is an adverse prognostic factor in Hodgkin's disease, as recognized in the Ann Arbor classification.

Impalpable axillary nodal enlargement is also frequently detected on CT in HD and NHL, and may be unilateral or bilateral (Figs. 32.10a and 32.14b). Occasionally nodes contain fat centrally, which is helpful in distinguishing those involved by lymphoma from those with enlargement due to benign hyperplasia.

Magnetic resonance imaging of the chest may provide additional information to CT in a problem-solving role, for example in the demonstration of nodal enlargement in areas where evaluation with CT is difficult, such as the subcarinal space and aortopulmonary window (Fig. 32.16). Magnetic resonance imaging is also helpful for defining the full extent of disease, for example infiltration of the chest wall.

When reporting thoracic CT for staging HD or NHL, it is always important to check all possible sites of involvement because minimally enlarged nodes in such sites as the internal mammary group or diaphragmatic nodes are easily overlooked (Fig. 32.11a,b).

Key points: supradiaphragmatic nodal disease

- 60–80% of patients with HD present with enlarged neck nodes. It is also a common presentation in NHL

- 60–80% of those with HD and 25–40% of patients with NHL have prevascular and paratracheal lymphadenopathy at diagnosis

- 10% of patients with HD have enlarged nodes detected on CT but a normal chest radiograph

- Hilar lymphadenopathy is rarely seen in isolation

- A large anterior mediastinal mass may represent lymphomatous infiltration of the thymus

- Enlarged axillary nodes are found in 6–20% of HD at diagnosis

Abdomen and pelvis

At presentation, the retroperitoneal nodes are involved in 25–35% of patients with HD, and 45–55% of patients with NHL.[111–113] Mesenteric lymph nodes are involved in more than half of patients with NHL and <5% of patients with HD.[111–114] Other sites, as in the porta hepatis and around the splenic hilum, are also less frequently involved in HD than NHL. In HD, nodal spread is predictably from one lymph node group to contiguous groups.[115,116] In this context, the term 'contiguous' does not mean physical contiguity but through directly connected lymphatic pathways. Nodes are frequently of normal size or only minimally enlarged.[87] In NHL, nodal involvement is frequently non-contiguous, bulky and is more frequently associated with extranodal disease. Enhancement following IV injection of contrast medium is mild and calcification is rare before treatment.

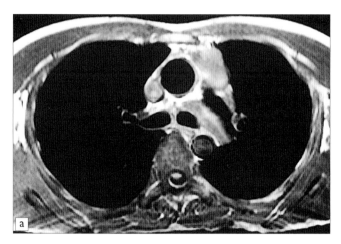

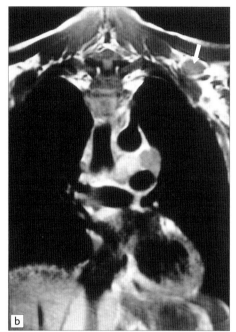

Figure 32.16. *MR images in a patient with HD showing nodal enlargement in the anterior mediastinum and aortopulmonary window. Turbo spin-echo T1-weighted images: (a) axial; (b) coronal. The enlarged nodes have an intermediate signal intensity lower than that of fat but higher than that of muscle. Note an enlarged lymph node in the left supraclavicular fossa (arrowed).*

In HD the coeliac axis, splenic hilar and porta hepatis nodes are involved in about one third of patients, and splenic hilar nodal involvement is almost always associated with diffuse splenic infiltration (Figs. 32.17 and 32.18). In the porta hepatis, an important node is the node of the foramen of Winslow (portocaval node), which lies between the portal vein and inferior vena cava (Fig. 32.19). This node has a triangular or lozenge shape; its normal trans-

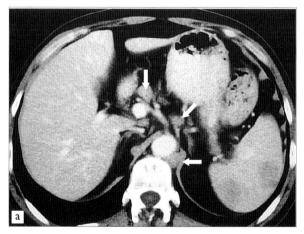

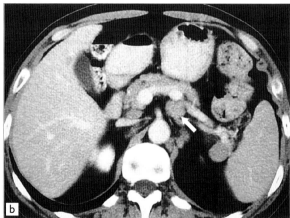

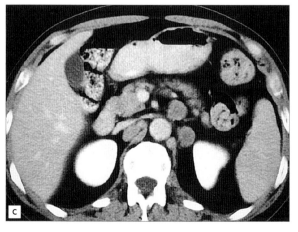

Figure 32.17. *HD. CT scans showing involvement of (a) coeliac axis lymph nodes and a retrocrural lymph node on the left (arrowed). Note focal deposits in the spleen. (b) At a lower level there is an enlarged lymph node at the splenic hilum and a further enlarged node is seen in the superior mesenteric group (arrowed). The portal node is prominent but not enlarged on CT criteria. (c) At the level of the upper poles of the kidneys, enlarged retroperitoneal lymph nodes are seen.*

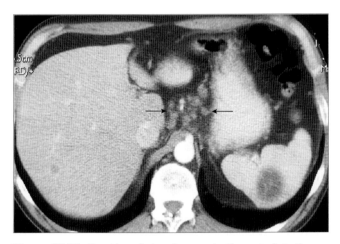

Figure 32.18. *Lymph node involvement in the gastrohepatic ligament (arrowed). Note the focal lesion in the spleen.*

verse diameter is up to 3 cm and in the anterio-posterior plane is approximately 1 cm.[117] Enlargement of this portocaval node is easily overlooked, which is particularly important if it is the only site of relapse. Spread from the mediastinum occurs through lymphatic vessels to the retrocrural nodes, coeliac axis, and so on. In the coeliac axis, multiple normal-sized nodes may be seen, which can be difficult to evaluate because involved normal-sized nodes are frequent in HD.[116]

In NHL, nodal involvement is frequently non-contiguous and bulky. Discrete mesenteric nodal enlargement or masses may be seen with or without retroperitoneal nodal enlargement (Fig. 32.20). Large-volume nodal disease in both the mesentery and retroperitoneum, may give rise to the so-called 'hamburger' sign, in which a loop of bowel is compressed between the two large nodal masses (Fig. 32.20c). In NHL, regional nodal involvement is frequently seen in patients with primary extranodal lymphoma involving an abdominal viscus. Analysis of post-contrast enhance-

ment characteristics of nodes may help differentiate lymphoma from infectious causes such as TB or atypical infections. Central necrosis, peripheral or multilocular enhancement favour infection.[118] Multiple normal-sized

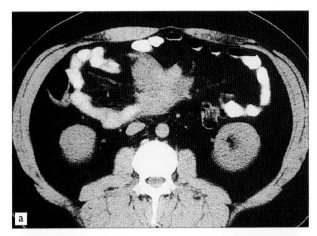

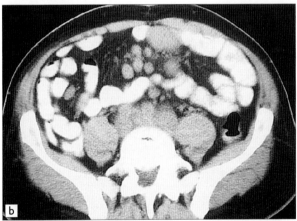

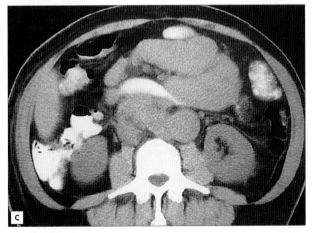

Figure 32.20. *CT scans in three different patients with NHL. (a) A large mesenteric mass without evidence of retroperitoneal lymph node involvement. (b) Discrete nodal enlargement of mesenteric lymph nodes associated with retroperitoneal lymphadenopathy. (c) A large mass in the mesentery associated with a mass of retroperitoneal lymph nodes. These masses compress an opacified loop of bowel, giving rise to the 'hamburger' sign.*

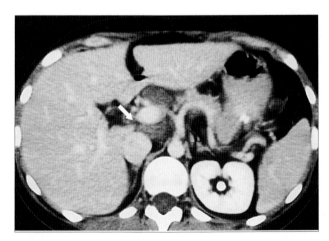

Figure 32.19. *A patient with NHL showing an enlarged portocaval lymph node (arrowed). There is also an enlarged node anterior to the portal vein in the porta hepatis.*

mesenteric nodes should be regarded with suspicion for the diagnosis of lymphoma, as should nodularity and streakiness within the mesentery, the latter presumably reflecting dilatation and obstruction of lymphatic vessels.

In the pelvis all nodal groups may be involved in both HD and NHL (Fig. 32.21). Presentation with enlarged inguinal/femoral lymphadenopathy is seen in less than 20% of cases of HD, but when it does occur careful attention must be paid to the evaluation of pelvic nodes on imaging as these will be the next contiguous sites of tumour spread. In patients with massive pelvic disease, MRI is helpful for delineating the full extent of tumour in the coronal and axial planes. It can also help differentiate between engorged venous tributaries and lymph nodes, and in problem solving.[57,59]

Key points: abdominal nodal disease

- ■ Retroperitoneal lymphadenopathy is more commonly seen in NHL than HD

- ■ In NHL, mesenteric lymphadenopathy is seen in over 50% of cases

- ■ In HD, the coeliac, splenic hilar, and porta hepatis nodes are involved in about 30% of patients

- ■ Splenic hilar lymphadenopathy is almost invariably accompanied by splenic infiltration

Extranodal disease

In about 40% of cases, the vast majority of which are NHL, lymphoma arises in extranodal sites.[119] There is a propensity for lymphomas associated with immunodeficiency and also those that develop in childhood to arise extranodally. Secondary extranodal lymphoma occurs due to spread of lymph node disease into adjacent structures and organs, and may be seen in both HD and NHL. The presence of extranodal disease is an adverse prognostic factor as recognized in the IP Index.[45] The increase in incidence of NHL has been much more marked for extranodal sites, especially in the gastro-intestinal (GI) tract, central nervous system (CNS) and eye.[6] Furthermore, visceral lymphoma can mimic many other disease entities, making recognition of the radiological appearances of extranodal lymphoma increasingly important. As with nodal disease, CT is generally excellent in the depiction of extranodal lymphoma. There are specific areas where MRI and ultrasound perform better, as indicated in the relevant sections. In addition, FDG PET is generally more sensitive and accurate in the staging of extranodal disease and splenic infiltration, largely because of its ability to demonstrate bone marrow involvement.[70] However, it has yet to replace CT as a primary staging modality.

Thorax

Lung

Secondary involvement of the lung parenchyma at presentation in HD is most commonly by direct invasion from involved hilar and mediastinal nodes, hence the frequent perihilar or juxtamediastinal location. In this situation, there is no effect on staging: the 'E' lesion. However, peripheral subpleural masses or consolidation without visible connection to enlarged nodes in the mediastinum or hila also occur in both HD and NHL. On chest radiography, lung parenchymal involvement is seen three times more frequently in HD (12%) than in NHL[88,93,119] (Fig. 32.22). Parenchymal involvement in HD is almost invariably accompanied by intrathoracic adenopathy, whereas in NHL pulmonary or pleural lesions may be seen without

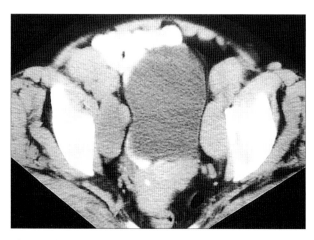

Figure 32.21. *Pelvic lymph node involvement in NHL. Gross bilateral enlargement of external iliac and obturator lymph nodes.*

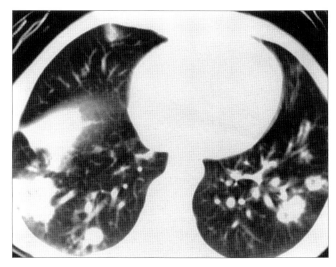

Figure 32.22. *CT scan showing pulmonary involvement in a patient with HD. There are multiple ill-defined nodules, several of which show cavitation, particularly those at the left lung base.*

mediastinal or hilar lymphadenopathy in as many as 50% of cases.[120] However, if the mediastinal and hilar nodes have been previously irradiated, recurrence confined to the lungs is seen in both HD and NHL.[121] Thus, in a patient with HD who has not received radiotherapy, in whom there is no evidence of hilar or mediastinal disease, a pulmonary abnormality probably represents pathology other than HD.[93,120] In the presence of widespread extrathoracic disease, parenchymal involvement is commoner, especially in AIDS-related lymphoma (ARL).[122]

The radiographic changes in both HD and NHL are varied and difficult to characterize. Pulmonary involvement is frequently perihilar or juxtamediastinal (Fig. 32.10).[123] The most common pattern is one or more discrete nodules resembling primary or metastatic carcinoma, but usually less well-defined, which may also cavitate (Figs. 32.10, 32.23 and 32.24).[91,124–126] Rounded or segmental consolidation with visible air bronchograms, often subpleural, is another common pattern (Figs. 32.24 and 32.25). Peribronchial pulmonary nodules (Fig. 32.26) extending from the hila, or focal streaky shadowing, also peribronchial, may be seen in association with the consolidation, reflecting spread along the peribronchial lymphatics (Fig. 32.26). The least common pattern is widespread reticulonodular (lymphangitic) shadowing. This is sufficiently rare in HD to necessitate other conditions causing interstitial lung disease to be excluded. Endobronchial disease causing atelectasis is extremely rare, but is still more likely than extrinsic occlusion by neighbouring lymph node enlargement.[127]

Primary (or isolated) pulmonary lymphoma is uncommon, and is usually due to NHL. Low-grade B-cell lymphomas comprise the majority of primary NHL of the lung. These are neoplasms of small lymphoid cells. Currently, most of the low-grade lymphomas of the lung are believed

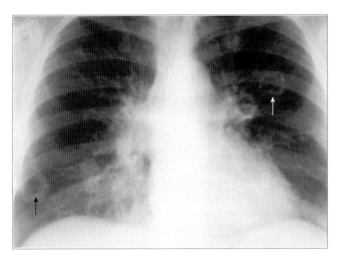

Figure 32.23. *Chest radiograph on a patient with HD, bilateral hilar lymph node enlargement and cavitating lung nodules in both lungs (arrowed).*

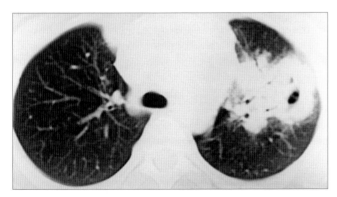

Figure 32.24. *Pulmonary involvement in a patient with high-grade NHL. The CT scan shows consolidation with air bronchograms and cavitation.*

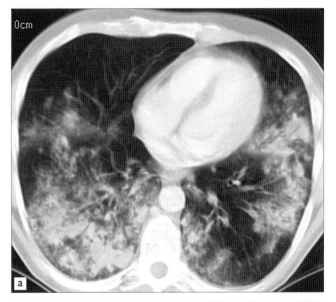

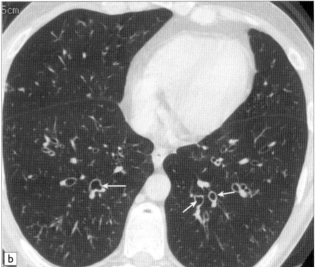

Figure 32.25. *(a) Segmental consolidation bilaterally in a patient with NHL. (b) The same patient as in (a) following treatment showing almost complete resolution of the parenchymal disease, but with residual mild bilateral bronchiectasis (arrowed).*

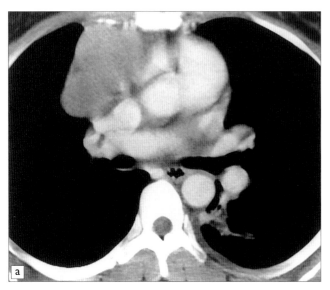
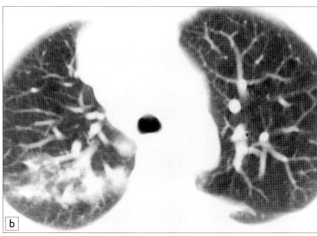

Figure 32.26. *Pulmonary involvement in a patient with HD. (a) A predominantly right-sided anterior mediastinal mass. (b) A CT scan showing peribronchial pulmonary nodules extending from the hila.*

to represent lymphomas of mucosa- (or bronchus-) associated lymphoid tissue (MALT or BALT).[128,129] These low-grade lymphomas occur most frequently in patients in their fifth to sixth decades of life, the clinical course is indolent, and there is an 80–90% survival rate at 5 years. The radiographic findings are non-specific as described previously. Solitary nodules are identified on chest radiographs in >50% of cases, ranging from 2–20 cm. Multiple nodules may occur, or there may be localized or multiple areas of consolidation.[130] Ill-defined alveolar multifocal opacities are also seen.[131] Hilar or mediastinal lymph nodes are rarely involved.

Although MALT lymphoma constitutes the majority of primary pulmonary lymphomas, high-grade NHL accounts for the remaining 15–20% of primary lung lymphomas.[130] These patients are usually symptomatic with dyspnoea, cough and B symptoms. Solitary or multiple nodules are the most common radiographic pattern, and rapid growth is a feature that can cause diagnostic confusion.[132] Primary pulmonary HD is an extremely rare entity.[130] The commonest findings are single or multiple nodules with an upper zone predominance and a relatively high incidence of cavitation.[133,134]

The diverse appearances of pulmonary lymphoma provide a particular challenge to diagnosis because many of these patients have other reasons for developing lung disease, such as:

- Opportunistic infection either following or during chemotherapy
- Pneumonitis following radiotherapy
- Drug-related pulmonary fibrosis

However, the differential diagnosis is difficult and the diagnosis of pulmonary lymphoma, particularly in previously treated patients, must be made in the light of full clinical information. In one study of 60 patients with HIV, cavitation size <1 cm and centrilobular distribution favoured infection rather than lymphoma.[135] Percutaneous or transbronchial biopsy will often be necessary to establish the diagnosis.

Pleural disease

Pleural effusions due to lymphoma occur in up to 10% of patients at presentation and are nearly always accompanied by mediastinal lymph node enlargement, and sometimes by pulmonary involvement, visible on a chest radiograph.[91] Most effusions are unilateral, are usually exudates and may disappear with irradiation of mediastinal nodes. Such effusions probably result from venous or lymphatic obstruction by enlarged mediastinal nodes, rather than direct neoplastic involvement, and may be detected on CT in over 50% of patients with mediastinal nodal involvement (Fig. 32.27).[125] Chylothorax is only occasionally encountered. Solid soft tissue pleural masses are rare at presentation and are seen more often in recurrent disease, usually accompanied by an effusion. In one review, 40% of patients with an effusion had adjacent extrapleural or pleural soft tissue disease, with nodules or thickening of the parietal pleura being a common finding.[136]

Chest wall

Involvement of the chest wall occurs most commonly in HD as a result of direct extension from an anterior mediastinal mass. Less commonly, large masses of NHL may arise primarily in the soft tissues of the thoracic wall. Both direct invasion and primary chest wall lymphoma are better demonstrated on MRI than CT. T2-weighted images are preferable to T1-weighted images because tumour is seen as a high signal intensity mass, well contrasted against the low

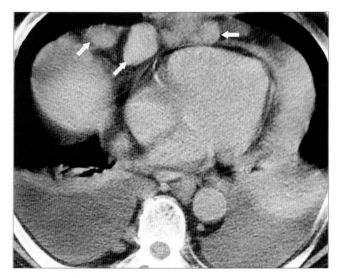

Figure 32.27. *Pericardial involvement in a high-grade NHL. The CT scan shows massive pericardial disease with a large soft tissue mass encasing the pericardium. There is also discrete paracardiac lymph node enlargement (arrows). Note too, the bilateral pleural effusions.*

signal intensity of the normal muscles of the chest wall. In this way MRI may allow more accurate planning of radiotherapy portals.[137,138] Bony destruction is uncommon and suggests infection or carcinoma.

Pericardium and heart

Pericardial effusions are seen on CT in 6% of patients with HD at presentation.[139] Effusions are presumptive evidence of pericardial involvement and in all such patients there is coexistent large mediastinal adenopathy extending over the cardiac margins.[91] Pericardial effusions are frequently seen in patients undergoing therapy for HD and NHL.

They are usually distinguishable from pericardial lymphomatous involvement (Fig. 32.27) because they develop when the patient is on chemotherapy, are usually small and resolve spontaneously.

Direct invasion of the heart may be seen in patients with aggressive, bulky mediastinal masses and in this rare situation MRI is probably the best technique for defining the presence and extent of cardiac involvement (Fig. 32.28).[140] Intracardiac masses can occur with high-grade T-cell lymphomas and large B-cell lymphoma, especially in the setting of ARL or post transplant lymphoproliferative disorder (PTLD).

Thymus

Thymic involvement occurs in 30–50% of patients with newly diagnosed HD.[104] It may be impossible to distinguish the enlarged thymus on CT or MRI from adjacent lymphadenopathy, which is usually but not invariably present (Fig. 32.15). Mediastinal LBCL also involves the thymus, and in contradistinction to most other types of lymphoma can cause vascular occlusion and airway obstruction; SVCO is present in up to 40% of affected individuals. On CT, the gland may be of homogeneous soft tissue density, similar to adjacent lymph nodes. On MRI too the signal intensity on both T1- and T2-weighted images is similar to that of enlarged nodes. Cysts and calcification may be seen within the enlarged gland, either at presentation or during follow-up on both CT and MRI.[105,107] Cysts are better appreciated on MRI but calcification is more easily recognized on CT.[107] As with other malignancies, benign thymic rebound hyperplasia can develop after completion of chemotherapy, which can be difficult to differentiate from recurrent disease. Unfortunately, functional imaging with Ga-67 or FDG PET may not always differentiate between the two and clinical correlation combined with follow-up studies may be necessary.

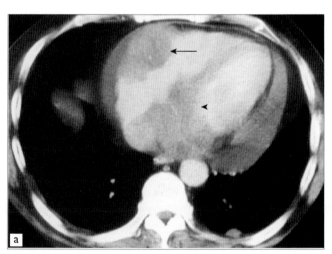 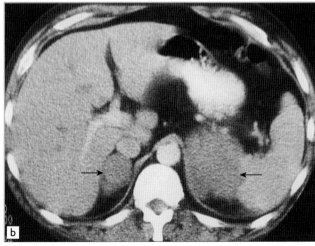

Figure 32.28. *Pericardial, cardiac and adrenal involvement in NHL. (a) CT scan through the heart following IV injection of contrast medium showing a moderate-sized pericardial effusion and mass lesions involving the right ventricle (arrow) and left ventricle (arrowhead). (b) CT scan of the abdomen in the same patient showing lymphomatous masses in both adrenal glands (arrowed).*

Key points: extranodal thoracic disease

- Secondary involvement of the lung parenchyma is seen three times more frequently in HD than NHL. Lung involvement in HD is almost invariably associated with mediastinal lymphadenopathy

- Most primary low-grade lymphomas of the lung are believed to represent MALT or BALT tumours

- Pleural effusions are associated with mediastinal lymphadenopathy in over 50% of cases

- Chest wall invasion occurs most commonly in HD by direct extension of a mediastinal mass

- Thymic infiltration occurs in 30–50% of patients newly diagnosed with HD

Breast

Primary breast lymphoma is rare, accounting for less than 1% of all breast tumours and approximately 2% of all lymphomas. In the majority of cases of primary breast lymphoma, masses are solitary, but synchronous bilateral disease and metachronous contralateral disease are well recognized. Ultrasound demonstrates fairly well-defined hypoechoic lesions with posterior acoustic enhancement.[141] A more diffuse pattern is occasionally seen resembling inflammatory carcinoma.[142] This is well recognized in pregnancy and lactation, especially in cases of Burkitt's and other high-grade lymphomas. In secondary lymphoma, multiple masses (not infrequently impalpable) with associated large volume axillary adenopathy are seen. Masses tend to be better defined than in primary disease.[143] Calcification and distortion are rare in primary and secondary forms.

Abdomen

Spleen

The spleen is involved in 30–40% of patients with HD.[113,144] In the majority of cases this occurs in the presence of nodal disease above and below the diaphragm,[145] but it is the sole abdominal focus of disease in 10% of adults presenting with HD clinically confined to sites above the diaphragm. To date, all imaging techniques have been unreliable in the detection of splenic involvement, partly because in the vast majority of cases of splenic HD, nodules are <1 cm in size. An enlarged spleen is not a reliable indicator of disease; one third of patients with HD and splenomegaly do not have enlargement of the spleen; however, one third of normal-sized spleens in patients with either HD or NHL are found to contain tumour at laparotomy.[112]

Occasionally, focal splenic nodules >1 cm are seen on cross-sectional imaging (Figs. 32.18 and 32.29). These lesions have a non-specific appearance, are usually hypoechoic on ultrasound, isodense on unenhanced CT, and enhance to a lesser extent than normal parenchyma following IV injection of contrast medium (Fig. 32.17). Splenic lymphoma can take the form of a solitary lesion, miliary nodules or multiple low-attenuation masses. Detection of such lesions has improved with the advent of multislice CT, since the entire spleen can be imaged in the portal venous phase of enhancement, and lesions of a few millimetres in

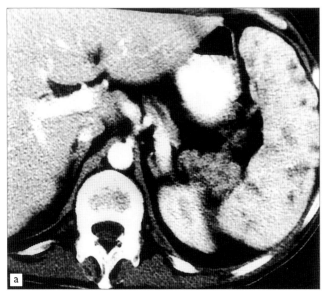
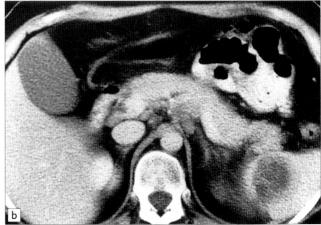

Figure 32.29. *Splenic involvement in lymphoma. (a) Postcontrast CT scan showing multiple small focal abnormalities of similar size within the spleen. The patient had HD. (b) CT scan showing a solitary large focal abnormality within the spleen in a patient with NHL. Note too the presence of paracoeliac lymph node enlargement.*

size can be identified. The differential diagnosis of focal lesions includes opportunistic infection, and occasionally sarcoid or metastases, which can appear identical. Infectious nodules tend to be smaller and more uniform in size.[146]

In early studies, the sensitivity of ultrasound in demonstrating splenic involvement was extremely low (not exceeding 35%),[49,82,84] although in a more recent study ultrasound was more sensitive than CT (63 vs. 37%), detecting nodules down to 3 mm in size and identifying diffuse infiltration more often than CT.[51] Although this low accuracy for the detection of splenic involvement on imaging is disappointing, failure to detect splenic infiltration in HD is now of less clinical disadvantage than before. This is because patients with early-stage disease who relapse due to untreated splenic infiltration can be salvaged by multi-agent chemotherapy, following primary treatment with radiotherapy. This has also resulted in the cessation of staging laparotomy for Stages I and II HD in most European centres.

Up to 40% of patients with NHL have splenic involvement at some stage. Primary splenic NHL is rare, accounting for 1–2% of all NHL. It is a particular feature of mantle cell and splenic marginal zone lymphomas, where massive splenomegaly can occur. In contradistinction to HD, the presence of splenomegaly generally indicates involvement, and infarction is a frequent complication (Fig. 32.30). Primary disease usually presents as a mass or masses rather than splenomegaly alone.[147] Where there is diffuse infiltration, serial measurements of splenic volume during treatment may be helpful in the assessment of response to treatment.[148] However, despite excellent results in some series, splenic volumes and indices have not gained widespread acceptance, being somewhat cumbersome.[149–151] Unfortunately, the intrinsic tissue contrast of MRI is insufficient for consistent recognition of diffuse infiltration,[61] though IV superpara-

magnetic iron oxide (SPIO) may improve detection of diffuse and focal infiltration, as may ultrasmall SPIO.[152–154] Finally, FDG PET may detect splenic infiltration more accurately than CT or Ga-67 scintigraphy.[70,155]

Liver

In HD, nearly 5% of patients have liver involvement, nearly always associated with splenic involvement.[145,156] In NHL, at presentation, about 15% of patients have hepatic infiltration though the incidence is higher in the paediatric population and in recurrent disease. True primary lymphoma of the liver is extremely rare, though the incidence is increasing, especially in immunocompromised patients. It is indistinguishable radiologically from other forms of hepatic malignancy such as hepatocellular carcinoma or metastatic disease. Up to 25% of patients are hepatitis B or C positive.

As with splenic disease, in untreated patients,[157] liver lymphoma usually occurs as microscopic or small macroscopic foci of tumour confined to the portal triad.

Detection of liver involvement by cross-sectional imaging is usually difficult. Large focal areas of involvement, detectable on ultrasound, CT or MRI, are seen in only 5–10% of patients with liver disease and resemble metastatic disease from other sources (Fig. 32.31). In both HD and NHL, the lesions are well-defined, frequently large, hypoechoic on ultrasound and hypodense relative to the normal parenchyma on both enhanced and unenhanced CT scans. As in metastatic disease, on T1-weighted MR images, the lesions are hypointense and on T2-weighted images they are hyperintense relative to the liver. It has been suggested that MRI may be more sensitive than CT in the detection of focal hepatic pathology.[158] Occasionally, especially in children, a form of liver infiltration is demonstrated as low density soft tissue infiltrating the porta hepatis and the margins of the portal veins (Fig. 32.32).[34,159]

Cross-sectional imaging is relatively insensitive to the detection of the more common diffuse microscopic liver infiltration. However, in contradistinction to the unreliability of splenomegaly, liver enlargement is strongly suggestive of infiltration in NHL particularly. To date, despite initial enthusiasm,[160] attempts to detect the diffuse form on MRI have not been successful,[61,161] though some work suggests that SPIO may increase the sensitivity of MRI for focal lesions.[162]

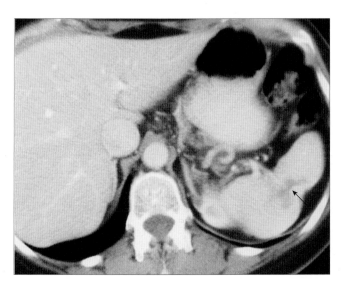

Figure 32.30. *Post contrast CT scan showing splenic infarction (arrow) in a patient with mantle-cell NHL.*

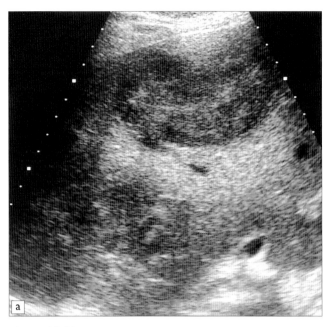

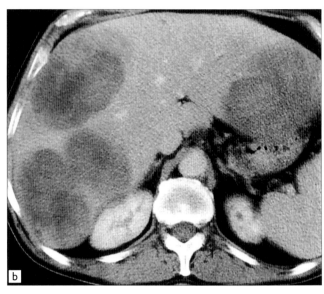

Figure 32.31. *Liver involvement in a patient with NHL. (a) Transverse ultrasound scan showing multiple large inhomogeneous focal abnormalities of varying echogenicity. (b) Post contrast CT scan in the same patient also showing multiple focal partially enhancing lesions of decreased echogenicity within the liver.*

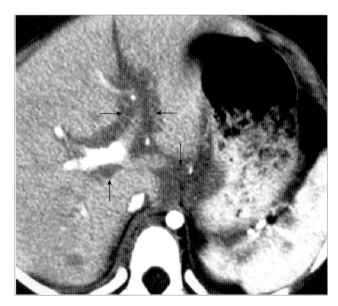

Figure 32.32. *CT in a child with NHL, showing periportal infiltration by low-density lymphomatous tissue (arrowed).*

Involvement of the bile ducts and gall bladder is rare, but has been described in AIDS-related lymphoma (see section on AIDS).

Key points: liver involvement

- Liver involvement is almost invariably associated with splenic infiltration

- Only 5–10% of patients with liver disease have focal lesions detectable on cross-sectional imaging

- Enlargement of the liver is a strong indicator of lymphomatous infiltration

- Periportal low attenuation may be a feature of NHL

Gastro-intestinal tract

The GI tract (GIT) is the most common site of primary extranodal lymphoma, being the initial site of involvement in 5–10% of adult patients.[163] Hodgkin's disease of the GIT is extremely rare.

Primary GI lymphomas develop from the lymphoid elements in the lamina propria and constitute about 1% of GI tumours; these occur most frequently in two age-related peaks, the first below the age of 10 years Burkitt's lymphoma (BL) and a second between the ages of 50 and 60 years (most of which are the GALT type and also high-grade intestinal T cell type associated with enteropathy). Primary lymphomas of the GIT usually involve only one site. The criteria for the diagnosis of primary GI lymphoma include:

- Absence of superficial or intrathoracic lymph nodes
- Normal white cell count
- No involvement of liver or spleen
- Lymph node involvement, if present, must be confined to the drainage area of the involved segment of gut.[164]

A modified Ann Arbor staging system takes account of these criteria. Stage I is where disease is confined to the visceral wall, and Stage II where there is local extension to adjacent organs (IIE) or draining lymph nodes.[165]

Secondary gastrointestinal involvement is common because of the frequent origin of lymphoma in the mesenteric or retroperitoneal nodes. Typically, multiple sites are involved.

In both the primary and secondary forms, the stomach is the most commonly involved organ (51%), followed by the small bowel (33%), large bowel (16%), and oesophagus (<1%). In 10–50% of cases the involvement is multicentric.[163] In children, the disease appears almost exclusively in the ileum and ileocaecal region.

Stomach (see also Chapter 11, Gastric cancer

Primary lymphoma of the stomach accounts for about 2–5% of gastric tumours.[163,166] Radiologically, the appearances reflect the gross pathological findings: common appearances are multiple nodules, some with central ulceration, seen readily at endoscopy or barium meal, or a large fungating lesion with or without ulceration. About one third of cases present with diffuse infiltration with marked thickening of the wall and narrowing of the lumen, sometimes with extension into the duodenum, indistinguishable from scirrhous carcinoma. Localized polypoid forms have also been described.[167] Only about one tenth are characterized by diffuse enlargement of the gastric folds (Fig. 32.33), similar to the pattern seen in hypertrophic gastritis and Ménétrier's disease.

Because the disease originates in the submucosa, these signs are best demonstrated endoscopically or on barium studies, but do not reflect the extent of the disease (Fig.

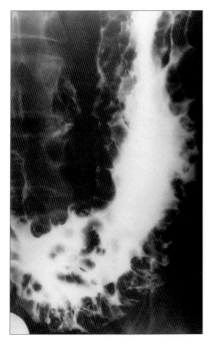

Figure 32.33.
Stomach involvement in NHL. The barium meal shows diffuse enlargement of the gastric folds due to submucosal infiltration.

32.33). Computed tomography has proved particularly valuable, often showing extensive gastric wall thickening with a smoothly lobulated border. Unlike gastric carcinoma, the walls of the stomach are usually clearly separable from the surrounding organs (Fig. 32.34).[168] The presence of associated bulky retroperitoneal adenopathy extending below the renal hilum should suggest the correct diagnosis.

Gastric MALT lymphomas, especially low grade ones, usually result in minimal gastric mural thickening, which may not even be recognizable even with dedicated CT studies utilizing an oral water load and IV smooth muscle relaxants.[169] Endoscopic ultrasound is of more value in local staging and assessment of response to treatment, but multiorgan involvement occurs in up to 25% of patients, so extensive staging may be necessary.[170,171]

Small bowel

Lymphoma accounts for up to 50% of all primary tumours of the small bowel,[164] occurring most frequently in the terminal ileum and becoming less frequent proximally. Of the tumours in this region, 60% are of B-cell lineage. Patients with AIDS are prone to lymphoma and the pattern resembles that found in immunocompetent patients.[172] Multifocal disease is present in up to 50% of cases. As it usually originates in the lymphoid follicles, mural thickening is typical and results in constriction of segments of bowel with obstructive symptoms, which are common at presentation. Thickening of the bowel is well demonstrated on CT (Figs. 32.35 and 32.36) with displacement of adjacent loops. As the tumour spreads through the submucosa and muscularis propria, it creates a tube-like segment that ultimately becomes aneurysmal, presumably because of destruction of the muscularis and autonomic plexus in the affected segment. Alternating areas of dilatation and constriction are the most common manifestation.[164] Occasionally, the lymphomatous infiltration is predominantly submucosal, resulting in multiple nodules or polyps of varying size, scattered throughout the small bowel but predominantly in the terminal ileum. This form is particularly prone to intussusception, which is a classical mode of presentation (Fig. 32.37), usually ileocaecal or ileoileal. This is the commonest cause of intussusception in children older than 6. Barium studies may show multiple polypoid filling defects, with or without irregular thickening and ulceration of the valvulae.

Enteropathy-associated T-cell lymphoma (associated with gluten-sensitive enteropathy) and immunoproliferative small intestinal disease (alpha-chain disease) affect the jejunum and ileum; malabsorption and acute abdominal presentations secondary to perforation are common.

Secondary invasion of the small bowel by large mesenteric lymph node masses causing displacement, encasement or compression may also be seen. Omental thickening, peritoneal enhancement and ascites cannot be differentiated from peritoneal carcinomatosis and usually occur in advanced abdominal disease, though it may be seen at presentation in BL.[173]

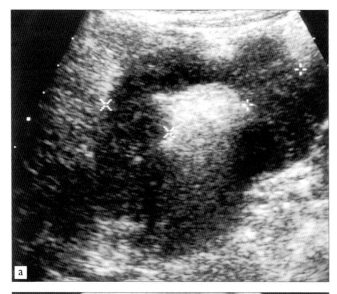

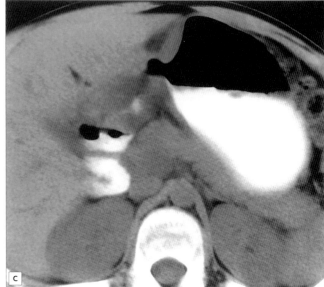

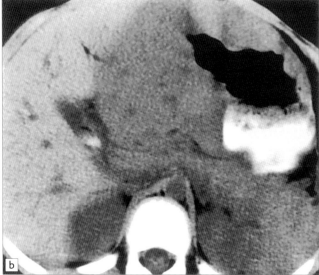

Figure 32.34. *Burkitt's lymphoma of the stomach in a child. (a) Transverse ultrasound scan showing massive thickening of the wall of the body of the stomach. (b) CT scan correlating with the ultrasound appearances in (a), again showing massive thickening of the wall, which is clearly separable from the surrounding organs. (c) Follow-up CT scan following chemotherapy 2 months after (b) showing an excellent response to chemotherapy. Only a minor amount of thickening of the wall of the gastric antrum persists.*

Colon and rectum

Primary lymphoma accounts for only 0.05% of all colonic neoplasms and usually involves the caecum and rectum rather than other parts of the colon. Conversely, secondary involvement is usually widely distributed and multicentric. The most common form of the disease is a diffuse or segmental distribution of nodules 0.2–2 cm in diameter, typically with the mucosa intact (Fig. 32.35). A focal form appears as a large polypoid mass, often in the caecum, and is indistinguishable from colonic cancer, unless there is concomitant involvement of the terminal ileum, which is more suggestive of lymphoma. The mass may have a large intraluminal component. In very advanced disease, there may be marked thickening of the colonic or rectal folds, resulting in focal strictures or ulcerative masses with fistula formation (Fig. 32.38). Colonic involvement is a particular feature of ARL and BL, but MALT types also occur, usually causing nodularity (see section on MALT lymphomas) (Fig. 32.38).

Oesophagus

Intrinsic oesophageal involvement is extremely uncommon, usually involves the distal third of the oesophagus and can result in a smooth tapered narrowing. Occasionally, both the fundus and distal oesophagus are involved by a bulky fungating tumour.

Pancreas

Primary pancreatic lymphoma is extremely rare and accounts for only 1.3% of all cases of pancreatic malig-

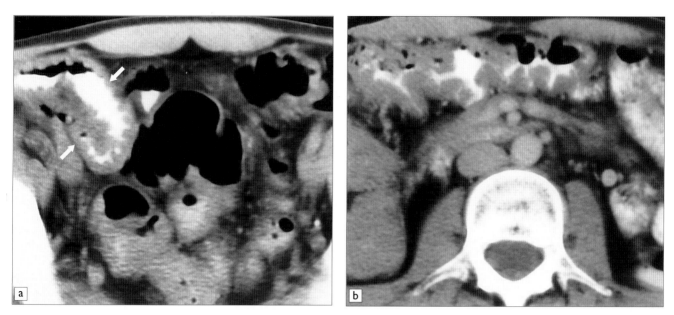

Figure 32.35. *Involvement of the bowel by NHL. (a) This shows marked uniform thickening of the wall of a loop of ileum in the right iliac fossa (arrows). (b) CT scan of the same patient showing diffuse uniform thickening of the transverse colon due to infiltration by NHL.*

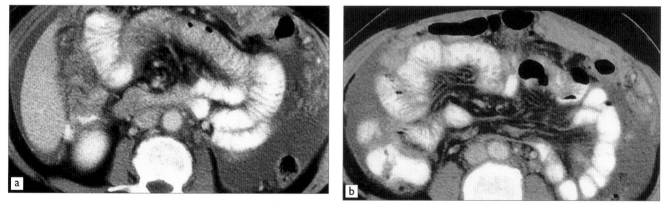

Figure 32.36. *Small bowel infiltration in NHL. (a) Marked thickening of the valvulae conniventes in a loop of jejunum. (b) CT scan performed slightly inferior to (a) also shows thickening of the valvulae in the ileum. Note in (a) and (b) the extensive infiltration of the omentum, perivascular thickening and thickening of the peritoneum.*

nancy[174] and 2% of patients with NHL.[175] Secondary pancreatic involvement usually occurs in association with disease elsewhere, most commonly due to direct infiltration from adjacent nodal masses, which may be focal or massive.[176] Intrinsic involvement of the pancreas most commonly results in a solitary mass lesion, indistinguishable from a primary adenocarcinoma on ultrasound, CT or MRI (Fig. 32.39).[176] Biliary and pancreatic ductal obstruction as well as invasion or narrowing of the portal vein are commonly seen at CT.[177] Calcification and necrosis are rare. The presence of a large mass in the head of the pancreas, with only mild biliary or pancreatic ductal dilatation, should raise the possibility of lymphoma, especially if there is retroperitoneal nodal enlargement below the level of the renal veins.[178] Less commonly, diffuse palpable masses or diffuse uniform enlargement of the pancreas is seen. Involvement is far more common in NHL than HD, particularly in ARL.

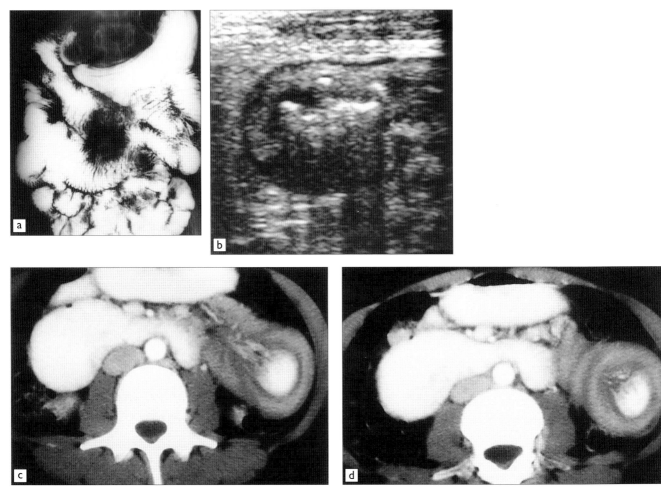

Figure 32.37. *Duodeno-jejunal intussusception due to lymphoma. (a) A barium follow-through examination showing an apparent mass lesion in the region of the jejunum with dilatation of the jejunum proximal to this 'mass'. Note too the thickening of the valvulae conniventes. (b) Ultrasound examination in the mid-abdomen in the region of the 'mass' showing marked thickening of the wall of the loop of small bowel. (c and d) CT scans showing thickening of the wall of the loop of jejunum with a classic 'coiled spring' appearance due to intussusception.*

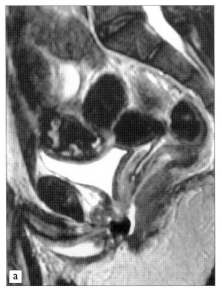

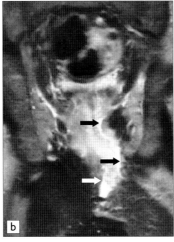

Figure 32.38. *Rectal involvement in a patient with lymphoma and AIDS. (a) A sagittal fast spin-echo T2-weighted MR image showing thickening of the rectal wall and a high-signal intensity fistula extending into the perineum. (b) A coronal STIR image in the same patient showing the marked thickening and a marked increase in signal intensity of the rectal wall. This scan also shows the high signal intensity of the complex fistula extending from the left side of the rectal wall into the perineum (arrowed).*

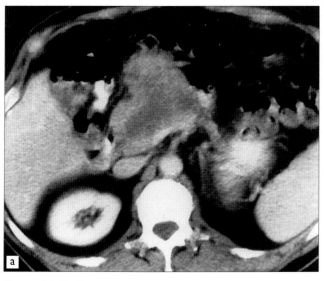
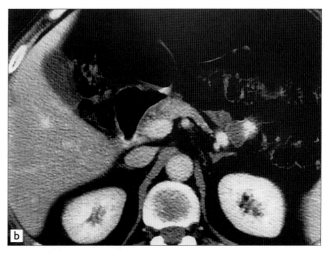

Figure 32.39. *Primary pancreatic lymphoma. (a) Note a large mass of decreased attenuation following contrast medium replacing the normal body and head of the pancreas due to primary pancreatic NHL. (b) A CT scan performed 3 months following chemotherapy shows complete resolution of the lymphomatous mass with marked atrophy of the remaining pancreas.*

Key points: gastro-intestinal tract

- The stomach is the most frequent site of GI lymphoma, and it may be primary or secondary

- Lymphoma accounts for up to 50% of all primary tumours of the small bowel and is multifocal in 50% of cases

- Intussusception is a characteristic feature at presentation with predominantly submucosal nodular/polypoid lymphoma

- Involvement of the colon and rectum accounts for only 0.5% of colonic neoplasms

- Pancreatic lymphoma is usually secondary due to invasion by adjacent lymph node masses

---

Genitourinary tract

The genitourinary tract is very rarely involved at the time of presentation, although in end-stage disease more than 50% of cases will have involvement of some part of the genitourinary tract. The testicle is the most commonly involved organ, followed by the kidney and perirenal space. Involvement of the bladder, prostate, uterus, vagina and ovaries is extremely rare.[179]

Kidney

Renal involvement is detected in about 3% of all patients undergoing abdominal scans for the staging of lymphoma.[180–182] Primary or isolated renal lymphoma is extremely rare. Although CT is more sensitive in identifying lymphomatous renal masses than ultrasound or urography, a large discrepancy exists between the radiological detection and incidence at autopsy (up to 50% having involvement in autopsy series), presumably because renal involvement is a late phenomenon. It is extremely unusual for the detection of renal involvement to alter the disease stage close to 90% of cases are due to high-grade NHL, renal function is usually normal and in more than 40% of patients the disease occurs at the time of recurrence only. Diffuse large B-cell lymphoma and BL are the histological subtypes that most commonly involve the kidneys.

Multiple masses is the most frequent pattern of disease seen in up to 60% of cases, which on CT may show a typical 'density reversal pattern' before and after contrast administration, with the lesions being more dense than the surrounding parenchyma before contrast medium administration and less dense after (Fig. 32.40).[180]

Solitary masses occur less frequently (10–20%) and may be indistinguishable from renal cell carcinoma.[180] An important feature of renal masses occurring in NHL is that in over 50% of cases there is no evidence of retroperitoneal lymph node enlargement on CT, suggesting that the kidneys are involved by haematogenous spread.

Direct infiltration of the kidney is the second most common type of renal involvement, occurring in 25% of cases. Invasion occurs from the retroperitoneum into the renal hilum and sinus, encasing the renal vessels and simulating a transitional cell carcinoma, an important differential diagnosis (Fig. 32.41). Frequently, a soft tissue mass is seen in the perirenal space, occasionally encasing the kidney without evidence on CT of invasion of the parenchyma (Fig. 32.42).

Diffuse infiltration of the kidneys (Fig. 32.43) with global renal enlargement without focal nodules is a less

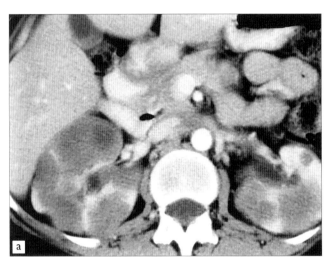 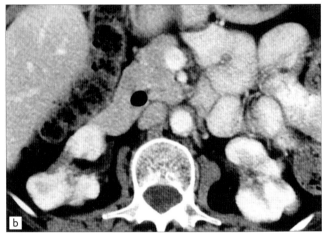

Figure 32.40. *Renal lymphoma. (a) CT scan showing multiple masses enhancing less than the adjacent renal parenchyma following IV injection of contrast medium. Note the absence of retroperitoneal lymph node enlargement. (b) CT scan performed 4 months after (a) following chemotherapy shows complete resolution of the multiple renal masses with marked scarring of the kidneys following treatment.*

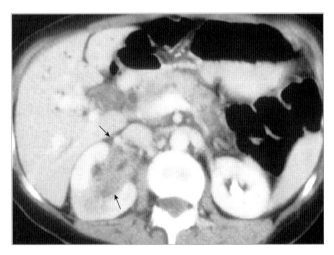 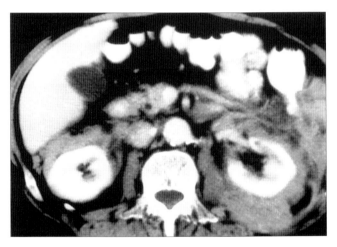

Figure 32.41. *Renal lymphoma simulating transitional cell tumour. CT scan on a patient with NHL showing a mass within the right renal pelvis (arrowed), extending into the renal parenchyma.*

Figure 32.42. *Perirenal lymphomatous infiltration. CT scan following IV injection of contrast medium shows low-density masses infiltrating the perirenal and pararenal space bilaterally, with thickening of Gerota's fascia. The renal parenchyma appears normal bilaterally. Note the absence of retroperitoneal (para-aortic) lymph node enlargement.*

common manifestation, usually without lymph node enlargement. The appearance after IV contrast medium injection is variable, but usually the normal parenchymal enhancement is replaced by homogeneous non-enhancing tissue. This pattern can be seen with BL. After successful treatment, the appearance can revert entirely to normal. A particularly rare form of disease is isolated periureteric lymphoma, which has been described in NHL and HD.

Bladder and prostate

Although primary lymphoma of the bladder is extremely rare, secondary lymphoma of the bladder is more common and is found in 10–15% of patients with lymphoma at autopsy.[179,183] Such secondary involvement can affect the wall of the bladder intrinsically or in contiguity from the adjacent involved nodes. Microscopic involvement is far more common than gross involvement, but this too can be associated with haematuria. The appearances on CT and MRI are non-specific (Fig. 32.44) with either diffuse widespread thickening of the bladder wall or a large nodular mass, both patterns indistinguishable from transitional cell carcinoma.[184]

Primary bladder lymphoma accounts for less than 1% of all bladder tumours. There is a female preponderance in

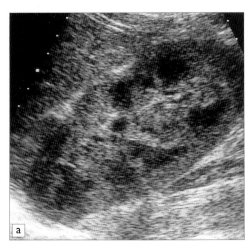
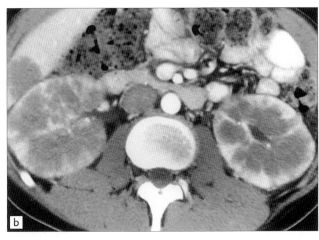

Figure 32.43. *Diffuse lymphomatous infiltration of the kidney in a patient with high-grade NHL. (a) Longitudinal ultrasound scan through the right kidney showing marked enlargement of the kidney (the right kidney measures 16 cm, the left 16.5 cm). There is diffuse increased reflectivity of the renal parenchyma with resultant prominent lucency of the renal papillae. The normal outline of the kidney is preserved. (b) CT scan following IV injection of contrast medium in the same patient as (a), showing diffuse infiltration of both kidneys by lymphomatous tissue. There is preservation of a rim of normal renal parenchyma. Note the absence of retroperitoneal lymph node enlargement and the presence of a focal lesion in the inferior aspect of the right lobe of the liver.*

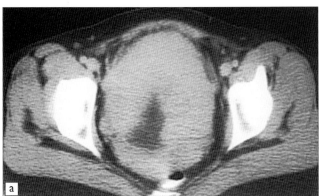

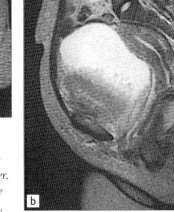

Figure 32.44. *NHL of the bladder. (a) CT scan showing large soft tissue mass occupying a major part of the base of the bladder. (b) Sagittal spin-echo T2-weighted MR image showing extensive involvement of the anterior abdominal wall in the same patient.*

the sixth and seventh decades, and a history of cystitis is common, explaining the high incidence of MALT-type lymphomas. Solitary or occasionally multiple sessile masses are most often seen.[185]

Unlike primary lymphoma of the bladder, where the response to chemotherapy/radiotherapy is good, lymphomatous involvement of the prostate carries a poor prognosis. It is usually intermediate or high grade and produces irritative obstructive symptoms. Solitary nodules are uncommon and in the majority of cases involvement is diffuse, with infiltration throughout the prostate and periprostatic tissue. Secondary involvement of the prostate is far

more common than primary prostatic involvement and direct extension into the prostate from pelvic lymph nodes is often seen in very advanced disease.

Testis

Testicular lymphoma is the most common testicular tumour occurring in individuals over the age of 60, but accounts for only 5% of all testicular neoplasms.[186] At presentation it is seen in about 1% of men with NHL (more commonly in BL) but is practically non-existent in HD. As in other sites of lymphomatous involvement of the genitourinary tract, the frequency of involvement discovered at autopsy is much higher: 18% of men with NHL. There is an association with lymphoma of Waldeyer's ring, the CNS, and skin.

On ultrasound, the lesions usually have a non-specific appearance, with focal areas of decreased echogenicity. However, a well-recognized pattern is a diffuse decrease in reflectivity of the testicle without any focal abnormality. As involvement is bilateral in 10–25% of cases, it is extremely important to examine the contralateral side. MRI offers little advantage over ultrasound in evaluation of the testis.[187]

Female genitalia

In advanced, widespread lymphomatous disease, the female genital organs are frequently involved secondarily.[22] However, isolated lymphomatous involvement is rare, accounting for approximately 1% of extranodal NHL. Most are diffuse large B cell in type. Around 70% of women affected are postmenopausal and present with vaginal bleeding. The tumours originate predominantly in the uterine cervix, where on CT and MRI a large mass can be seen (Fig. 32.45). Involvement of the uterine body usually produces diffuse enlargement, often with a lobular contour similar to a fibroid, with a relatively homogeneous signal intensity in spite of large tumour size.[188] Similarly, primary lymphoma of the cervix and/or vagina is characterized by a large, exophytic, soft tissue mass. Involvement of these gynaecological organs is best demonstrated by MRI, since masses are seen as high signal intensity lesions on T2 weighting and are therefore clearly distinguished from the surrounding normal tissues, including the uterus, cervix, and vaginal wall. Characteristically, the mucosa is spared and the low signal intensity junctional zone is intact. MRI is excellent in follow-up and assessment of response to treatment.[189] Ovarian lymphoma is less common and carries a

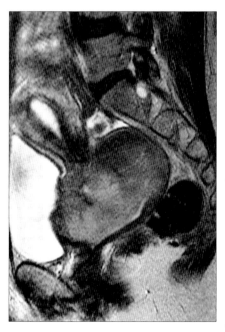

Figure 32.45.
Primary NHL of the cervix. Sagittal fast spin-echo T2-weighted MR image showing a very large mass in the uterine cervix due to high-grade NHL. There was no evidence of disease elsewhere in this patient.

worse prognosis than uterine lymphoma because the tumours are more advanced at the time of discovery. The appearance on cross-sectional imaging is indistinguishable from primary ovarian carcinoma.[190] Disease is often bilateral, and DLBCL or BL are the usual subtypes. The presence of large bilateral homogeneous masses with moderate enhancement on MRI, without haemorrhage, necrosis or calcification, may suggest this diagnosis.[191]

Key points: genitourinary tract

■ Renal involvement is seen in about 3% of cases undergoing abdominal CT

■ Lymphomatous involvement of the kidneys is not usually associated with renal impairment

■ Primary lymphoma of the prostate carries a poor prognosis whereas primary lymphoma of the bladder has a good prognosis

■ The testes is the most frequent site of involvement of the genitourinary tract with lymphoma

■ Lymphoma of the testis accounts for only 5% of all testicular tumours

■ Primary lymphoma of the female genital tract is rare and is best demonstrated on MRI

Adrenal glands

Primary adrenal lymphoma is rare, occurring in men over the age of 60. Secondary involvement of the adrenal glands in lymphoma is usually demonstrated on routine abdominal CT for staging (where it is seen in up to 6% of cases of NHL) as presentation with adrenal insufficiency is extremely rare.[179,190] Involvement is usually bilateral and the appearances are indistinguishable from bilateral metastases, but readily distinguishable from adenomas (Fig. 32.28b). Non-lymphomatous bilateral hyperplasia of the adrenal glands has been described.[192] The reason for this is unclear.

Central nervous system

Primary

Primary CNS lymphoma is initially localized to the CNS at presentation. It occurs almost exclusively within the brain, as the spinal cord is only very rarely the site of origin (<1%).[193,194] Although in the mid-1980s primary lymphoma accounted for only 1.5% of all brain tumours, its frequency is increasing, which is in part due to an association with immunosuppression therapy following cardiac or renal transplants and immunodeficiency. Up to 6% of AIDS patients can be expected to develop primary CNS lymphoma during the course of the disease.[195] Cases of primary CNS lymphoma have been reported from the age of 2 months to 90 years, but presentation between the fourth and sixth decades appears to be the most frequent. There is a separate peak in the first decade of life. It now accounts for over 3% of brain tumours and up to 30% of cases of NHL in some series.

On CT or MRI, more than 50% of lesions occur within the cerebral white matter, close to or within the corpus callosum.[194] Most touch the ependyma of the ventricles or the ependymal surface. A butterfly distribution with spread across the corpus callosum is seen.[196] In about 15% of cases, the deep cortical grey matter of the basal ganglia, thalamus and hypothalamus are involved. In 11% of cases, lymphoma develops in the posterior fossa and is multifocal in about 15% of cases. On CT, the tumour mass is typically of increased density on unenhanced CT and the majority of lesions enhance homogeneously after IV injection of contrast medium. Only about 10% of lesions do not enhance.[193]

Calcification is very rare and surrounding vasogenic oedema relatively mild.[196] On MRI, the typical appearance is of a tumour mass hypo- or isointense, relative to the surrounding normal tissue on T1-weighted sequences. As after injection of X-ray contrast medium, IV injection of gadolinium–DTPA also results in enhancement on T1-weighted sequences (Fig. 32.46). Ring enhancement can be a feature of AIDS-related primary CNS lymphoma. The appearance of primary and secondary lymphoma within the brain is essentially similar on CT and MRI.

Secondary
Cerebral involvement occurs in 10–15% of patients with NHL at some time during the course of their disease.[59,197] Certain

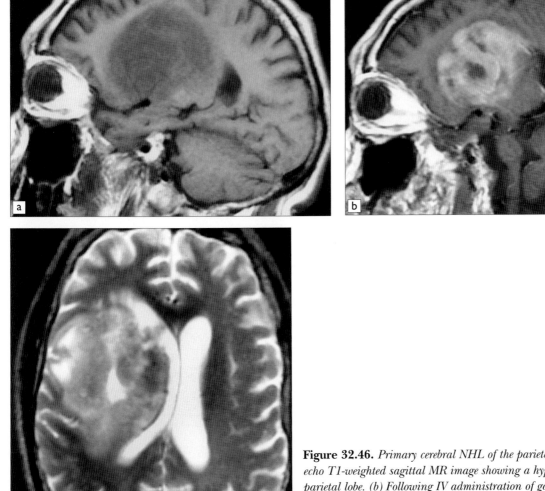

Figure 32.46. *Primary cerebral NHL of the parietal lobe. (a) A fast spin-echo T1-weighted sagittal MR image showing a hypointense mass in the parietal lobe. (b) Following IV administration of gadolinium-DTPA, the mass enhances intensely. (c) An axial fast spin-echo T2-weighted MR image showing a typical parietal lobe mass resulting in marked mass effect with compression of the right lateral ventricle.*

groups are at risk: those with stage IV disease, testicular or ovarian presentations, high-grade T-cell lymphomas, immunoblastic, and BL.[198] Secondary cerebral involvement is so rare in HD that a space-occupying lesion in the brain of a patient with known HD should prompt a second diagnosis.[199] Secondary lymphoma is distinguishable from the primary form to some extent by its propensity to involve the extracerebral spaces (epidural, subdural and subarachnoid) (Fig. 32.47) and the spinal epidural and subarachnoid spaces.[193] Magnetic resonance imaging with direct multiplanar imaging is ideal for detecting extracerebral plaque-like tumour deposits in the subdural or epidural spaces. Typically, these plaques are hypo- to isodense on all pulse sequences, but they are made more obvious on gadolinium–DTPA-enhanced T1-weighted images (Fig. 32.47). Computed tomography is less sensitive, not only in the detection of these extracerebral lesions, but also in demonstrating leptomeningeal deposits of lymphoma coating the cranial nerves,[200] particularly when resulting in cranial nerve palsies.

Gadolinium-enhanced MRI is also a relatively sensitive, non-invasive method for demonstrating spinal leptomeningeal involvement by lymphoma and involvement of the spinal cord and nerve roots. Nonetheless, there is a significant false-negative rate that is higher than that for leptomeningeal carcinomatosis.[201] Epidural extension of tumour into the spinal canal from a paravertebral nodal mass may also be elegantly demonstrated on MRI. Although extension through the intervertebral foramina

may also be clearly depicted on CT, subtle disease is easily missed (Fig. 32.48).[202]

Compression of the spinal cord or cauda equina due to lymphomatous disease is a late manifestation of HD, but is often an earlier manifestation of NHL. In both types of lymphoma, extension of nodal spread through the intervertebral neural foramina is the most common cause. Tumour compresses the dura, but the dura itself usually acts as an effective barrier to the intrathecal spread of tumour. Vertebral collapse with cord compression may be seen in some of the aggressive forms of NHL, but it is less common than compression due to an epidural mass (Fig. 32.48). On occasion, patients can present with epidural disease causing back pain and paresis, for example in endemic BL.

The orbit

Non-Hodgkin's lymphoma is the most common primary orbital malignancy in adults and accounts for 10–15% of orbital masses.[193] Primary orbital lymphomas occur most commonly in patients between 40 and 70 years of age, and most typically present as a slow-growing, diffusely infiltrative tumour for which the main differential diagnosis is from the non-malignant condition known as 'orbital pseudotumour'. Retrobulbar lymphoma infiltrates around and through the extraocular muscles causing proptosis and ophthalmoplegia, but, visual acuity is rarely disturbed. In patients with an orbital lymphomatous mass, about half will be found to have an extracentral nervous system primary site of origin. Secondary orbital involvement occurs in approximately 3.5–5% of both HD and NHL. In both the primary and secondary forms, the clinical manifestations will depend on the site of involvement. Involvement of the lacrimal glands is frequently bilateral; the presenting features are those of bilateral masses with downward displacement of the globe (Fig. 32.49). The prognosis is generally good (even with bilateral disease). Relapse in the contralateral orbit is not uncommon. Involvement of the eyelids and subconjunctival spaces is readily assessed on clinical examination, whereas MRI best depicts the presence and extent of any intracranial extension.

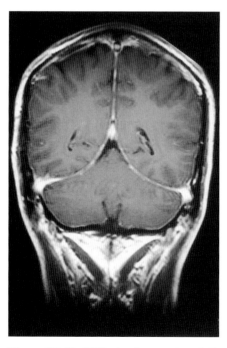

Figure 32.47. *NHL showing meningeal disease on a coronal MR image using a T1-weighted sequence following injection of IV contrast medium (gadolinium–DTPA). Note intense enhancement of the thickened meninges over the cerebral hemispheres, cerebellum and tentorium.*

Key points: central nervous system

- Primary CNS lymphoma almost exclusively involves the cerebral white matter

- Primary cerebral lymphoma is increasing in incidence

- Secondary lymphoma preferentially involves the extracerebral spaces and the spinal epidural and subarachnoid spaces

- Spinal cord compression results from nodal spread through the intervertebral neural foramina in both HD and NHL

- NHL is the most common primary orbital malignancy in adults

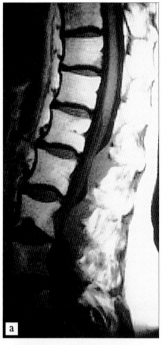
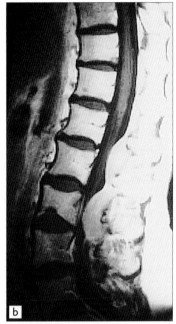

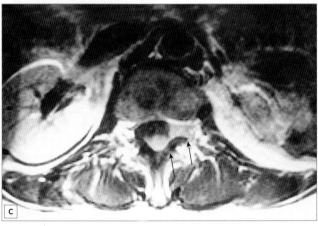

Figure 32.48. *T1-weighted MR images showing extradural disease in a patient with NHL: (a) precontrast, (b and c) postcontrast. In the sagittal plane, the extradural mass is clearly shown on both the pre- and postcontrast images extending from the level of the first lumbar vertebra to the level of the fourth lumbar vertebra. In the axial plane, extension of enhancing tissue into the spinal canal is clearly seen.*

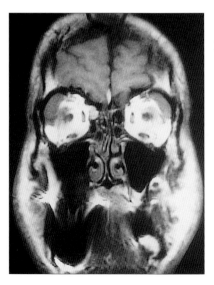

Figure 32.49. *Orbital lymphoma. T1-weighted coronal MR image. There are bilateral orbital masses of homogeneous low signal intensity. The masses are symmetrical and occupy the superolateral orbital compartments. There is no evidence of bone erosion.*

Head and neck lymphoma

Although HD typically involves the cervical lymph nodes as the presenting feature, true extranodal involvement of sites in the head and neck region is rare. Extension from nodal masses in the neck to Waldeyer's ring may occur, but this is seen in less than 1% of patients.

In NHL, extranodal head and neck tumour involvement is relatively common and indeed 10% of patients present with extranodal disease in the head and neck; on investigation about half will have disseminated lymphoma. Extranodal NHL accounts for approximately 5% of head and neck cancers.[203]

Waldeyer's ring is the commonest site of head and neck lymphoma and there is a close link with involvement of the

GIT, which may be synchronous, or metachronous (Fig. 38.50); this probably a reflection of the fact that many are of the MALT type. Hence some centres include abdominal CT and/or endoscopy as part of staging, since up to 30% will have advanced disease at presentation. Waldeyer's ring comprises lymphoid tissue in the nasopharynx, oropharynx, the faucal and palatine tonsil, and the lingual tonsil on the posterior third of the tongue. A diagnosis of NHL is suggested by circumferential involvement or multifocality. Middle-aged women are most often affected. Many tumours are of the low-grade MALT type, and a history of Sjögren's syndrome should be sought (see earlier). Secondary invasion from adjacent nodal masses is also a common occurrence.

NHL comprises 8% of tumours of the paranasal sinuses.[204] In the West, the disease affects middle-aged men and the maxillary sinus is most commonly involved, whereas the aggressive diffuse T-cell type (that formed part of the 'lethal midline granuloma' syndrome) affects younger Asians. Whilst paranasal sinus involvement often presents with acute facial swelling and pain, and disease often spreads from one sinus to the other in a contiguous fashion, bony destruction is considerably less marked than in squamous cell carcinomas.[204]

Magnetic resonance imaging is the preferred imaging technique for evaluating head and neck lymphoma due to high tissue contrast between tumour adjacent to normal structures; its multiplanar capability allows clear demonstration of the full extent of disease within the intricate anatomy of the facial region. It also permits detection of tumour spread into the cranial cavity from the infratemporal fossa, orbit and soft tissue of the face.

Salivary glands

All the salivary glands may be involved in lymphoma but the parotid gland is the most frequently involved.[205] The patient presents with single or multiple well-defined masses that are of higher density than the surrounding gland on CT, hypoechoic on ultrasound, and of intermediate signal intensity on T1- and T2-weighted MRI sequences.

Thyroid

Non-Hodgkin's lymphoma accounts for 2% of malignant tumours of the thyroid.[206] There is an association with Hashimoto's disease, so the disease tends to occur in women in their 60s with MALT types. However, DLBCL also occurs, and these patients present with a rapidly growing mass and obstructive symptoms. Direct spread of tumour beyond the gland and involvement of adjacent lymph nodes is common. On CT these masses usually have a lower attenuation than the normal gland and they may show peripheral enhancement following injection of IV contrast medium (Fig. 32.51).

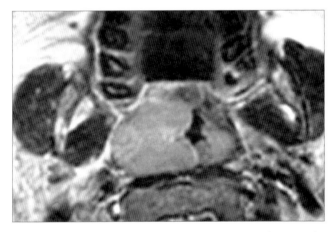

Figure 32.50. *Axial T1-weighted MRI showing involvement of Waldeyer's ring with massive soft tissue thickening of the parapharyngeal tissues.*

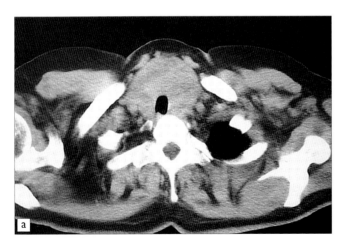
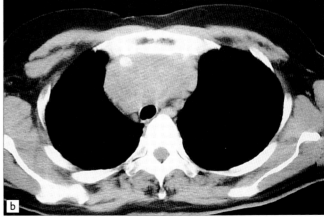

Figure 32.51. *CT scans showing primary lymphoma of the thyroid. On staging, no other evidence of disease was found in this patient with biopsy-proven disease.*

Key points: head and neck

- Extranodal NHL accounts for approximately 5% of all head and neck cancers

- Waldeyer's ring is the most common site of head and neck lymphoma

- The parotid is the most frequent salivary gland involved by lymphoma

- Non-Hodgkin's lymphoma accounts for 2% of all malignant thyroid tumours

Musculoskeletal system

Skeletal involvement may occur in both HD and NHL. Since the bone marrow is an integral part of the reticuloendothelial system, lymphomas may arise within the marrow as a true primary disease. It is then categorized as Stage IE disease. More often, however, the marrow is involved as part of a disseminated process. In this instance bone marrow involvement is categorized as Stage IV disease. The majority of those with 'apparent' primary lymphomas usually have widespread disease and therefore in reality have secondary lymphomas. This is particularly true in children. Hence this diagnosis is made less often nowadays, probably because better imaging enables detection of synchronous disease elsewhere.

Bone and bone marrow are important sites of disease relapse and any skeletal symptoms following previous treatment for lymphoma should raise the suspicion of bone disease. Involvement of osseous bone is less widespread, does not necessarily imply bone marrow involvement,[207] and skeletal radiography has no predictive value in determining marrow involvement. Infiltration of bone may also occur by direct invasion of adjacent soft tissue masses. This is designated with the suffix 'E' after the appropriate stage of disease elsewhere, e.g. Stage IIE. For the purposes of clarity, involvement of the bone is distinguished in this description from diffuse involvement of the bone marrow.

Bone

Primary lymphoma of bone is almost exclusively due to NHL as primary HD of bone is extremely rare. The criteria for the diagnosis of primary lymphoma require that:

- Only a single bone is involved
- There is unequivocal histological evidence of lymphoma
- Other disease is limited to regional areas at the time of presentation
- The primary tumour precedes metastasis by at least 6 months

The average age at presentation is 24 years; 50% of cases occur in patients between 10 and 30 years of age. Males are affected more often than females. Primary lymphoma affects the appendicular skeleton involving the femur, tibia and humerus, in descending order of frequency. Primary lymphoma of bone accounts for about 1% of all NHL.[208]

Secondary involvement of bones is present in 5–6% of patients with NHL,[207,208] although less present with symptoms due to a skeletal lesion. Bone involvement is more frequent in children with NHL.[34] Radiographic evidence of bone involvement is present in 20% of patients, with HD appearing in 4% as the initial presentation.[207] Systemic (secondary) NHL involves the axial skeleton more frequently than the appendicular skeleton.

Appearances

Primary NHL of bone is radiologically indistinguishable from systemic NHL, HD and other bone tumours. However, whereas the bone lesions in NHL (primary or secondary) are usually permeative osteolytic (77%) (Fig. 32.52), sclerotic in only 4% and mixed in 16%, bony involvement in HD typically gives a sclerotic or mixed sclerotic and lytic (86%) and infrequently lytic (14%) picture.[209] Isotope scintigraphy is more sensitive than plain radiography, but MRI is the imaging modality of choice for staging and follow-up, depicting the extent of marrow involvement and muscle infiltration much more accurately.[210] It has been suggested that FDG PET is more sensitive and specific than bone scintigraphy, with a high positive predictive value (PPV) for the detection of osseous involvement.[211]

In HD, soft tissue disease typically may involve adjacent bones; anterior mediastinal and paravertebral masses frequently invade the sternum and vertebrae, respectively, resulting either in destruction or scalloping. A classic finding is the sclerotic 'ivory vertebra'. Direct invasion of bone by local lymph node disease is denoted by the suffix 'E' added to the appropriate stage.

Because of the relatively low incidence of bone lesions at presentation, screening for bone involvement is not routine but is reserved for patients with specific complaints. Bone scintigraphy has a sensitivity of close to 95% in the detection of bone involvement,[212] but is relatively non-specific so that plain films are used to investigate areas that are positive on the bone scans.

Bone marrow

Involvement of the bone marrow indicates Stage IV disease. It is rare at presentation in HD but is found in 20–40% of patients with NHL at presentation[115,213–215] and is associated with a worse prognosis than involvement of the liver, lung or osseous bone.[216] During the course of HD, marrow involvement occurs in 5–15% of patients.[217]

Because of these figures, bone marrow biopsies are not indicated as part of the initial staging of HD, but the high incidence in NHL justifies its use as a staging procedure,[218] increasing the stage in up to 30% of cases, mainly from Stage III to Stage IV.[218] Bone marrow involvement in low-grade NHL is typically diffuse but in intermediate- and

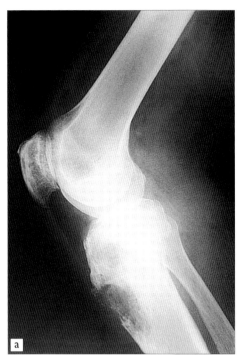

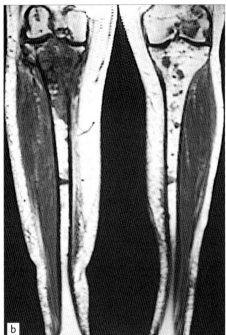

Figure 32.52. *NHL of upper tibia. (a) Lateral plain radiograph showing a destructive lesion in the upper aspect of the tibia. (b) Coronal T1-weighted MR image showing a large area of abnormal low signal intensity in the upper tibia that corresponds to the abnormal bone on the plain radiograph. However, in addition, multiple lesions of low signal intensity are seen throughout both femoral condyles and tibiae, indicating much more extensive disease than had been appreciated clinically and on skeletal radiographs.*

high-grade lymphoma it is more likely to be focal. Therefore, not surprisingly, the performance of bilateral rather than single-site biopsies increases the pick-up rate substantially.[219] Magnetic resonance imaging is undoubtedly an extremely sensitive technique in the demonstration of bone marrow involvement (Fig. 32.53). On T1-weighted images, tumour infiltration is of low signal (Figs. 32.52 and 32.53)[219] and of high signal intensity on STIR. In one recent study, T1-weighted spin-echo was the most sensitive sequence, whereas fast STIR and ecto-planar imaging (EPI) sequences were most specific for infiltration.[220,221] Magnetic resonance imaging can upstage as many as 33% of patients with negative iliac crest biopsies. Focal desposits as small as 5 mm can be identified though false-negative studies do occur with microscopic infiltration (under 5%) and low-grade lymphoma. Compared to CT, whole-body MRI can upstage nearly 20% of patients through demonstration of bone marrow disease.[217,219,220,222]

Patients with a positive MRI study appear to have a poorer prognosis, regardless of bone marrow biopsy findings.[223] Immunoscintigraphy with technetium-99m (^{99m}Tc)-labelled monoclonal antibodies compares favourably with MRI in the depiction of bone marrow disease,[224] but there is far more interest in the use of FDG PET, which to date has shown high sensitivity and specificity for bone marrow disease. A small number of false-negative scans occur with low-grade lymphoma, often PET negative elsewhere,[225] or with microscopic infiltration. In one study, FDG PET alone resulted in change of stage twice as often as bone marrow biopsy.

Preliminary data suggest that superparamagnetic iron oxides may have a role in the differentiation of normo- and hypercellular marrow after treatment from persistent or residual infiltration, a distinction which is difficult with conventional MR imaging and FDG PET scanning (particularly if granulocyte colony-stimulating factor has been administered).[226]

Despite the sensitivity (and in some cases specificity) of these imaging techniques to detect bone marrow infiltration their precise role in the staging of patients with lymphoma has not yet been defined, given the obvious need to examine the cytology of bone marrow in these patients.

Soft tissues

Soft tissue masses may develop in both HD and NHL, either as tumour extension from bone involvement, or as an isolated mass within the muscles. Primary muscle lymphoma is extremely rare and is based on the absence of clinical or imaging features of lymphoma elsewhere. Patients with soft tissue lymphoma usually present with pain or neurological deficit, but occasionally a palpable mass may be present.[227] The commonest radiological manifestation is muscle enlargement secondary to diffuse infiltration, with or without regional adenopathy.[228] Without question, MRI is the technique of choice for investigating patients with persistent pain, and even though a mass may be detected in retrospect on CT, the lack of contrast between the mass and adjacent muscle groups may lead to difficulties in diagnosis (Fig. 32.54).

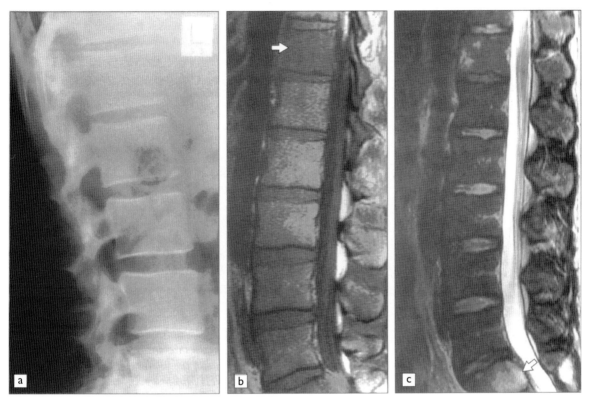

Figure 32.53. *Bone involvement in a patient with NHL. (a) Normal skeletal radiograph in a patient with NHL and back pain. The radio-isotope scan was also normal. (b) T1-weighted sagittal MR image showing loss of the normal high-signal intensity of fat in the body of L1 (arrowed). (c) Fast spin-echo T2-weighted sagittal MR image showing areas of high-signal intensity within the body of L1 vertebra and also the body of S1 (arrowed). A bone biopsy of S1 showed involvement of the cortical bone as well as of the bone marrow.*

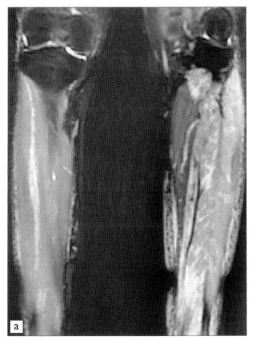

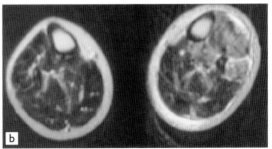

Figure 32.54. *Soft tissue involvement by lymphoma. (a) Coronal STIR MR image showing marked thickening and increased signal intensity of the muscles of the lateral aspect of the leg due to diffuse infiltration by NHL. (b) Fast spin-echo T2-weighted axial MR image of the same patient as (a), showing increased signal intensity of the involved muscles on the left and providing the exact distribution of muscle involvement.*

■ Primary lymphoma of bone accounts for only 1% of all cases of NHL, whereas secondary involvement is seen in 5–6% of cases

■ Secondary bone involvement is seen in 20% of patients with HD. Primary HD of bone is extremely rare

■ In HD, soft tissue disease may invade adjacent bone but this is rare in NHL

■ Bone scintigraphy has a sensitivity approaching 95% but is relatively non-specific

■ Bone marrow involvement indicates Stage IV disease and is present in 20–40% of patients with NHL at presentation

■ Bone marrow biopsy in NHL increases the stage of disease in up to 30% of cases (Stage III to IV)

■ In HD, bone marrow involvement occurs in 5–15% of patients during the course of disease

■ MRI is the method of choice for detecting soft tissue lymphomatous masses, which are usually due to secondary NHL

Mucosa-associated lymphoid tissue lymphoma

Whilst extranodal involvement can be seen in any subtype of NHL, some forms of B-cell NHL occur exclusively in extranodal locations – the extranodal marginal zone lymphomas. They represent around 8% of all types of lymphoma and, for convenience, are divided into MALT types and generic types.[28,29]

Pathology and clinical features

The MALT lymphomas arise from mucosal sites that normally have no organized lymphoid tissue, but within which acquired lymphoid tissue has arisen as a result of chronic inflammation or autoimmunity. Examples include Hashimoto's thyroiditis, Sjögren's syndrome and *Helicobacter*-induced chronic follicular gastritis. The association between gastric MALT lymphoma and *H. pylori* infection was established in 1991 by Wotherspoon et al.,[229] who found the organism in over 90% of cases. The detectability of *H. pylori* has been shown to diminish as lymphoma evolves from chronic gastritis.[230]

Patients with Sjögren's syndrome or lymphoepithelial sialadenitis have 44 times the risk of developing lymphoma, of which over 80% are MALT type. Patients with Hashimoto's thyroiditis have a 70 fold increased risk of thyroid lymphoma.

The histological hallmark of MALT lymphoma is the presence of lymphomatous cells in a marginal zone around reactive follicles, which can spread into the epithelium of glandular tissues to produce the characteristic lymphoepithelial lesion. In up to 30%, transformation to large cell lymphoma occurs.

The commonest site of involvement is the GIT (50% of cases) and within the GIT, the stomach is most often affected (around 85% of cases). The small bowel and colon are involved in immunoproliferative small intestinal disease (IPSID), previously known as alpha-chain disease. Other sites commonly affected include the lung, head, neck, ocular adnexae, skin, thyroid, and breast.

Most cases occur in adults with a median age of 60 and a slight female preponderance. Most patients present with stage IE or IIE disease, which tends to be indolent. Bone marrow involvement is seen in 20%, but the frequency varies depending on the primary site, being higher with MALT lymphoma of the lung and ocular adnexae. Multiple extranodal sites are involved in up to 10%, but this does not appear to have the same poor prognostic import as in other forms of NHL, as it may not reflect truly disseminated disease.[231] Nonetheless, extensive staging investigations may be necessary.[171]

Imaging features

GI tract

Often gastric MALT lymphoma, especially low grade, causes minimal mucosal thickening, and CT may be normal,[169] even if dedicated gastric CT is carried out with an oral water load and IV smooth muscle relaxants.[232] A recent study suggested that low-grade MALT lymphoma was more likely to cause shallow ulceration and nodulation, whereas higher grade ones were more likely to produce more massive gastric infiltration and polypoid masses.[233] Endoscopic ultrasound is more accurate than CT pre and post treatment, defining wall depth and lymph node involvement (Fig. 32.55).[170,171,234] In addition, staging with EUS can help predict response to treatment of *H. pylori*.[235]

In the colon and small bowel, MALT lymphoma is manifest as mucosal nodularity, which can be appreciated in barium studies.[236]

Respiratory tract

Mucosa-associated lymphoid tissue or BALT lymphoma represents 60% of all primary pulmonary lymphomas. The radiological pattern is similar to that of other lymphomas, being quite variable. The commonest patterns are masses, areas of consolidation and nodules with or without air bronchograms, and the CT angiogram sign.[237–239] Multiple lesions are present in up to 80% and lesions are often bilateral. Peribronchovascular nodularity and thickening is less common. Lesions tend to be indolent, whether nodular or

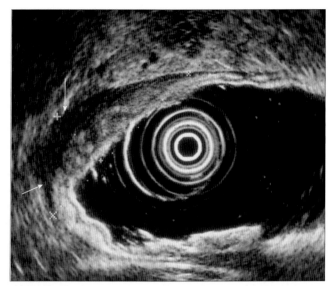

Figure 32.55. *MALT lymphoma of the stomach. Endoscopic ultrasound examination showing a submucosal mass of low reflectivity (arrowed).*

consolidative. Associated pleural effusions occur in up to 20%.

Other sites

In the thyroid, MALT lymphomas can present as diffuse enlargement or as large nodules that are hypoechoic at ultrasound and relatively hypodense at CT.

Mucosa-associated lymphoid tissue lymphomas of the lacrimal glands present as a mass or periorbital swelling. Computed tomography and MRI depict uni- or bilateral enhancing masses with a non-specific appearance.

Up to 20% of lymphomas involving Waldeyer's ring are of MALT type. The tonsils are most commonly affected, the commonest pattern being asymmetric thickening of the pharyngeal mucosa. This is well shown by CT and MRI.

Key points: MALT lymphoma

- These arise from mucosal sites that normally have no organized lymphoid tissue, but arise as a result of chronic inflammation or autoimmunity

- The commonest site of involvement is the GI tract; the stomach is involved in 85% of cases

- Other sites include the thyroid (Hashimoto's), respiratory tract, and lacrimal gland (Sjögren's)

Burkitt's lymphoma (BL)

Burkitt's lymphoma is a highly aggressive B-cell variant of NHL, associated with EBV in a variable proportion of cases.

Three clinical variants are recognized:

- Endemic (African) type[240]
- Sporadic (non-endemic)[241]
- Immunodeficiency associated

Though these tumours are extremely aggressive and rapidly growing, they are potentially curable. Though they account for only 2–3% of NHL in immunocompetent adults, 30–50% of all childhood lymphoma is BL. Immunodeficiency associated BL is seen chiefly in association with HIV infection and may be the initial manifestation of AIDS. EBV is identified in up to 40% of cases. Extranodal disease is common and all three variants are at risk for CNS disease.[242]

In the endemic form, the jaws, maxilla and orbit are involved in 50% of cases, producing the 'floating tooth sign' on plain radiography. The ovaries, kidneys and breast may be involved. The sporadic forms have a predilection for the ileocaecal region and patients can present with acute abdominal emergencies such as intussusception. Again, ovaries, kidneys and breasts are commonly involved. Retroperitoneal and paraspinal disease can cause paraplegia, the presenting feature in up to 15% of affected individuals. Thoracic disease is rare; in a recent series, 50% had disease confined to the abdomen.[243] Leptomeningeal disease can be seen at presentation and is a site of relapse.

Lymphoma in the immunocompromised
(see also chapters 56, and 57)

The WHO classification recognizes four broad groupings associated with an increased incidence of lymphoma and lymphoproliferative disorders:[244]

- Primary immunodeficiency syndromes
- Infection with HIV
- Iatrogenic immunosuppression after solid organ or bone marrow allografts
- Iatrogenic immunosuppression from methotrexate (usually for autoimmune disorders)

The development of lymphoma in these settings is multifactorial, but mostly related to defective immune surveillance, with or without chronic antigenic stimulation.

Lymphomas associated with HIV (human immunodeficiency virus)

Lymphoma is the first AIDS-defining illness in up to 5% of HIV patients. The incidence of all subtypes of NHL is increased 60–200fold. Various types are seen, including those seen in immunocompetent patients, such as BL, DLBCL (especially in the CNS), but some occur much more frequently in the HIV population (e.g. primary effusion lymphoma and plasmablastic lymphoma of the oral cavity). The incidence of HD is also increased up to eightfold.

Most have a marked propensity to involve extranodal sites, especially the GI tract, CNS (less frequent with the advent of highly active antiretroviral therapy), liver, and bone marrow. Multiple sites of extranodal involvement are seen in over 75% of cases.[245] Peripheral lymph node enlargement is seen in only 30% at presentation.

Most tumours are aggressive, with advanced stage, bulky disease and a high serum LDH at presentation. DLBCL tends to occur later on, when CD4 counts are under 100×10^6/l, whereas BL occurs in less immunodeficient patients. EBV positivity occurs in up to 70% depending on the precise morphological variant, whereas primary CNS DLBCL is associated with EBV in over 90% of cases; interestingly, EBV positivity is seen in nearly all cases of HD associated with HIV.

In the chest, NHL is usually extranodal; pleural effusion and lung disease are common, with nodules, acinar and interstitial opacity being described. Hilar and mediastinal nodal enlargement is generally mild. There is a wide differential diagnosis and in one study the presence of cavitation and nodal necrosis predicted for mycobacterial infection rather than lymphoma.[246]

Within the abdomen, the GI tract, liver, kidneys, adrenal glands and lower genitourinary tract are commonly involved. Mesenteric and retroperitoneal nodal enlargement is less common than in immunocompetent patients, but there are no apparent differences in the CT features of patients with or without AIDS, at least in relation to the small bowel.[172]

Regarding primary CNS lymphoma (PCNSL), certain features such as rim enhancement and multifocality are seen more often than in the immunocompetent population. This can cause confusion with cerebral toxoplasmosis, though the location of PCNSL in the deep white matter is suggestive.[247] Quantitative FDG PET uptake can help in the differentiation of PCNSL, toxoplasmosis and progressive multifocal leucoencephalopathy (PML).[248]

Post-transplant lymphoproliferative disorders
(Fig. 32.56)

These occur in 2–4% of solid organ transplant recipients, depending on the type of transplant, the lowest frequency being seen in renal transplant recipients (1%) and the highest in heart–lung or liver–bowel allografts (5%). Marrow allograft recipients in general have a low risk (1%). Most are associated with EBV infection and appear to represent EBV-induced monoclonal or, more rarely, polyclonal B-cell or T-cell proliferation in a setting of reduced immune surveillance as a consequence of immune suppression. The clinical features are variable, correlating with the type of allograft and type of immunosuppression. Post-transplant lymphoproliferative disorders develop earlier in patients receiving cyclosporin A (mean 15 months) rather than azathioprine (mean interval 48 months). Epstein–Barr-positive cases occur earlier than EBV-negative cases, the latter occurring 4–5 years after transplantation. In all cases, extranodal disease is disproportionately commoner. In patients receiving azathioprine, the allograft itself and the CNS are often involved, whereas in patients who have received cyclosporin A, the GI tract is affected more often than the CNS. The bone marrow, liver and lung are often affected, as are the tonsils.

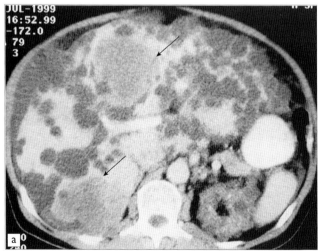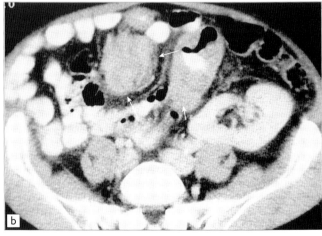

Figure 32.56. *Post-transplant lymphoproliferative disorder of the liver. (a) CT scan in patient with known autosomal dominant cystic disease of the kidneys who underwent a renal transplant (see b). Multiple lymphomatous foci are demonstrated within the liver (arrowed) together with the associated benign liver cysts. Note the associated ascites and the cystic disease of the native left kidney. (b) Renal transplant in the left iliac fossa. A large mesenteric mass is also demonstrated (arrowed) together with infiltration of the small bowel.*

In the lung, multiple or solitary pulmonary nodules occur, with or without mediastinal adenopathy. Reticulonodular opacity is rare, whereas pleural effusions are common and a confluent, patchy airspace opacity is another pattern.[249–251]

Abdominal PTLD is characterized by a relatively high frequency of extranodal disease, especially of the GI tract and liver. Multiple segments of bowel may be affected and there is a propensity for PTLD to develop in the allograft.[252,253]

Key points: lymphoma in the immunocompromised

- Lymphomas associated with HIV have a propensity to involve extranodal sites (especially the GI tract, CNS, liver, and bone marrow) and multiple sites. Most tumours are aggressive with advanced stage, bulky disease

- Post-transplant lympoproliferative disorder occurs in 2–4% of solid organ and 1% of marrow allograft recipients and typically causes solitary or multiple lung nodules. In the abdomen this disorder is characterized by involvement of the GI tract and liver

Post-treatment evaluation

Imaging plays an extremely important role in monitoring response to therapy. Also, once treatment is completed, periodic surveillance studies help in detection of potential relapse. In clinical evidence of relapse, imaging studies are performed to evaluate the extent of the disease.

Monitoring response to therapy

Achievement of a complete remission following treatment is the most important factor for prolonged survival in both HD and NHL. Thus, final evaluation of response at or within 1 month of completion of therapy is critical.

'Complete remission' is diagnosed only when no abnormality is seen at the site of previously demonstrated disease. The chest radiograph is useful in assessing response when there is intrathoracic disease and is repeated at each monthly visit. Although the chest radiograph will show response early in the treatment, changes due to radiotherapy often make the mediastinum difficult to assess. Other mediastinal changes associated with treatment such as rebound hyperplasia or thymic cyst formation cannot be reliably identified on the chest radiograph and therefore response cannot be monitored reliably. A CT scan therefore remains essential in the monitoring of response to treatment for mediastinal disease, especially when the chest radiograph is indeterminate.[254] In patients with intra-abdominal disease, serial CT is essential in monitoring

response. For the purpose of assessment of response to treatment, it is often necessary to measure a number of marker lesions before and after therapy. Modern CT scanners permit accurate reproducible measurements of well defined nodal masses provided scan parameters (narrow collimation slices, with overlapping reconstructions) and techniques are optimized. However, there is significant interobserver variation, which is even more pronounced with irregular masses or when there is poor lesion–background contrast, which may occur even with adequate bowel and vascular opacification.[255]

The optimal and exact timing of such scans for reassessment has not been widely investigated.[256,257] In many centres, the practice is to assess patients fully 1 month after completion of therapy. Others favour an interim CT study during initial chemotherapy for lymphoma after two cycles of chemotherapy; the timing will often depend on local clinical practice and on the availability of resources. The speed of modern CT scanners has largely removed the need for limited scans advocated by some. Though in the past it has been argued that routine administration of IV contrast medium is unnecessary for follow-up scans, in practice, multislice technology allows the acquisition of scans with optimal vascular and parenchymal enhancement throughout the neck, chest, abdomen, and pelvis, facilitating follow-up of nodal and extranodal disease.

Criteria of response

International standardized response criteria are essential for clinical research, facilitating data interpretation and comparison of therapies. A report published in 1999 set out new criteria for assessment of response in NHL, bringing it into line with those already in use for HD.[258] The radiological criteria are defined as follows:

- Complete remission (CR): complete disappearance of all radiographic evidence of disease. Nodes and nodal masses of disease regressed to <1.5 cm in greatest transverse diameter for nodes >1.5 cm before therapy. Previously involved nodes 1.1–1.5 cm in greatest transverse diameter regressed to ≤1 cm in greatest transverse diameter after therapy. The spleen, if enlarged by CT criteria, must have regressed
- Complete remission, unconfirmed (CRu): where there is a residual nodal mass >1.5 cm maximum transverse diameter that has regressed by >75% of sum of products of greatest diameters
- Partial remission (PR): ≥50% decrease in SPD of largest nodes/masses. No increase in size of spleen, lymph nodes, liver. Splenic and hepatic nodules decreased by 50%
- Stable disease (SD): less than a PR and no evidence of progressive disease
- Progressive disease (PD): 50% or greater increase from nadir in the SPD of any previously identified

abnormal node for PRs or non-responders – appearance of any new lesion during or at the end of therapy

- Relapse from CR or CRu requires: appearance of any new lesion or increase by 50% or more in the size of previously involved sites. 50% increase in greatest diameter of any previously identified node >1 cm in its short axis or in the SPD of more than one node

FDG PET in assessing response

Recently, there has been considerable interest in the use of functional imaging (Ga-67 SPECT and, notably, FDG PET) after a few cycles of chemotherapy for the purposes of prognostication. The value of gallium scanning is limited by its lower sensitivity and by the significant proportion of non-gallium-avid tumours.[67,259–261] FDG PET scans performed after one to three cycles of chemotherapy appear to predict eventual outcome in NHL more accurately than scans at the end of treatment and conventional imaging, especially with diffuse histologies.[262–264] In one study, all patients with a positive PET scan relapsed, and under 50% would have been predicted by conventional imaging.[265] This allows a change in therapy and may avoid potential toxicity from ineffective therapy.[266] FDG PET prior to high-dose treatment may also predict outcome.[267]

Assessment of residual masses

Although successfully treated enlarged nodes often return to normal, in HD and NHL a residual mass of 'sterilized' fibrous tissue can persist. On a chest radiograph such a residual mass may remain following treatment in 12–88% of patients.[55,268] Such residual masses occur more frequently in patients with bulky rather than non-bulky disease, in HD and NHL. Residual masses are seen at CT in up to 20–50% of patients in clinical CR after treatment for NHL.[269,270] It is uncertain whether relapse is more common in patients with residual masses; the literature on this subject is conflicting.[257,271] There is no obvious correlation between the size of the residual mass and the relapse rate. Determining the nature of such residual masses and excluding the possibility of active disease by imaging is one of the major challenges in oncological radiology today.

Computed tomography

Using the new criteria, residual masses at CT are those that have reduced by up to 75% but which are nonetheless more than 1.5 cm in maximum transverse diameter. Computed tomography cannot distinguish between fibrotic tissue, necrosis, and residual active disease on the basis of density alone, hence the very low specificity and PPV of CT after treatment in every series published to date. Nevertheless, serial CT performed every 2–3 months is the most widely used method of determining the true nature of a residual mass. Masses that remain static after 1 year are considered

to be inactive, whereas any increase in size is highly suggestive of relapse. Relapse following satisfactory response to initial treatment occurs in 10–40% of patients with HD and in around 50% of patients with NHL.[115] In HD, relapse usually occurs within the first 2 years following treatment and patients are followed up closely during this period, although CT examinations are not usually required unless clinical features suggest the possibility of recurrence.

Magnetic resonance imaging

There is now substantial data investigating the value of MRI in identifying residual active neoplasm within residual masses.[59,60,272,273] In general, a reduction in signal intensity on T2-weighted images is seen during or following successful treatment (Fig. 32.57). Persistent heterogeneous or recurrent high signal intensity on T2-weighted sequences following treatment appears to have a high specificity and PPV for residual active disease.[273] False positives do arise due to inflammatory oedema or cyst formation.[107,272,274] However, not surprisingly, the sensitivity for the detection of active disease is low, as small foci of persistent tumour within a low signal intensity mass cannot be identified reliably on T2-weighted images.[59–60,274]

Gallium-67

Gallium-67 scanning can be helpful. If no uptake is shown in a mass that initially showed substantial activity, it can be inferred that it represents residual fibrosis with over 80% specificity.[275–277] Conversely, persistent positive uptake usually indicates persistent active neoplasm reflected in a PPV for relapse double that of CT.[259,278] However, the sensitivity of Ga-67 in the initial detection of lymphoma will depend on cell type, location, and size of the lesion; sensitivity is lower in lymphocytic lymphoma, in masses <2.5 cm, and in those masses below the diaphragm. Its value in monitoring response is therefore diminished by these factors. Absence of activity on a Ga-67 scan, without a pretreatment scan to identify non-gallium-avid tumours, is thus of limited value. Conversely, non-specific inflammation, rebound thymic hyperplasia, and benign hilar uptake can all cause false-positive scans.[275] For all these reasons, Ga-67 today is not widely used to evaluate the residual mass.

Positron emission tomography

Positron emission tomography FDG has also been investigated (Figs. 32.58 and 32.59).[65] FDG PET has been shown to have a high PPV for relapse, with or without a residual mass at CT, allowing directed biopsies, or consolidative therapy as appropriate.[262,279–284] As with Ga-67, there are pitfalls in that small volumes of disease can produce false-negative examinations (in around 5%), whereas reactive and inflammatory changes (for example in the lungs, thymus and bone marrow) are causes of false-positive examinations. Thus it is essential that clinical correlation be made when interpreting scan results.[285] In one study directly comparing Ga-67 and FDG PET, the latter showed more extensive disease, but

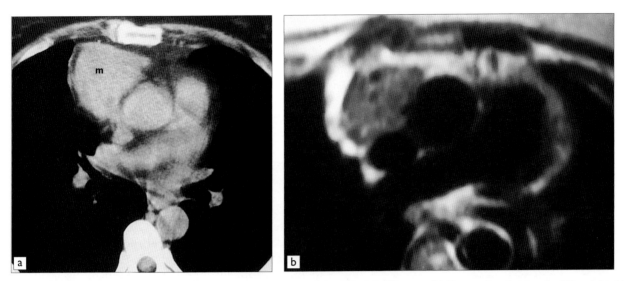

Figure 32.57. *A residual mediastinal mass in a patient treated for HD. (a) CT scan. (b) Conventional spin-echo T2-weighted MR image. The residual mass (m) measures approximately 5 × 5 cm in diameter and has a homogeneous intensity, suggesting that the mass is inactive. A CT-guided core biopsy was obtained. On histological examination there was no evidence of active HD.*

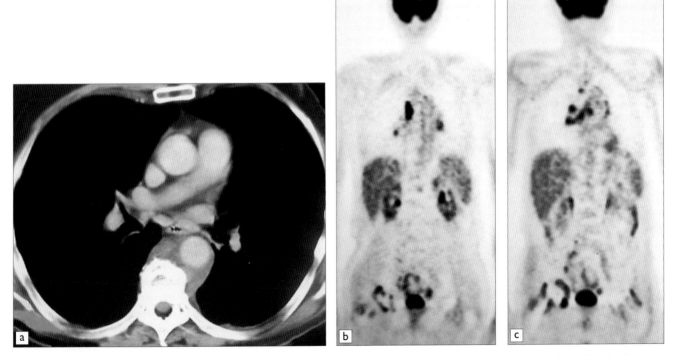

Figure 32.58. *Hodgkin's disease in a 66-year-old male patient. Following chemotherapy there is a residual posterior mediastinal mass on CT that had remained stable for over 6 months. A PET scan performed at the same time as the CT scan shows increased uptake of ^{18}FDG in multiple nodal sites within the mediastinum, which is presumed to represent activity of disease.*

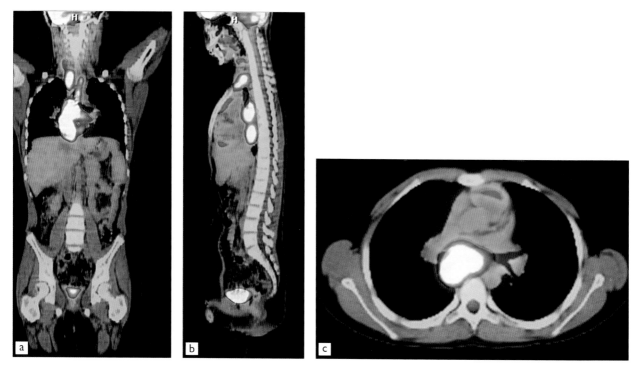

Figure 32.59. *(a–c) Hodgkin's disease. A staging PET/CT scan showing high [18]FDG uptake in nodal masses within the mediastinum.*

there were false-positive examinations (correctly interpreted as such when reference was made to the clinical history and other findings).[286]

As discussed earlier, a positive FDG PET scan at the end of therapy strongly predicts for early relapse[282] for HD and NHL. In one follow-up study, all PET-positive/CT-negative patients relapsed, as did 60% of PET-positive/CT-positive patients, whereas only 5% of PET-negative/CT-positive patients relapsed.[287] The same is true of Ga-67,[259,278,288] but the greater sensitivity of FDG PET means that the negative predictive value of FDG PET is greater than that of gallium scintigraphy.

Follow-up and surveillance

Strategies for follow-up with imaging vary between institutions and, in addition, in patients with residual masses in HD and NHL, follow-up depends on the size of the mass, the sites of involvement, and the extent of disease; it is therefore impossible to define strict guidelines for each clinical situation.

For patients who attain CR or CRu (i.e. where there is a Ga-67 or a FDG PET-negative residual mass), it has been argued that routine imaging is desirable to detect asymptomatic early relapse, so that salvage therapy can be offered. In this situation, CT may be of limited value, since it may take some time before there is an appreciable increase in the size of the residual mass.

In one series of patients with NHL who attained CR, only two of 36 relapses were diagnosed before patients were symptomatic, and only one was identified by imaging alone. This study did not include functional imaging. Of the relapses, 25% were in new sites alone, whereas the previous site was involved in the remainder.[289] The findings of Front et al.[64] were similar, but they found that Ga-67 scintigraphy indicated relapse on average 7 months before the development of clinical signs or an abnormality on CT. In this setting, the sensitivity of Ga-67 was 95%.

In another study, the quoted sensitivities and specificities for recurrence were 59% and 72% for CT, and 88% and 100% for Ga-67, respectively.[290]

There are other studies that also suggest that conventional imaging follow-up with CT is rarely rewarding. Radford et al. found that 86% of relapses in a cohort of patients with HD were detected as a result of investigation of new symptoms rather than by routine follow-up studies.[290,291]

In another series of patients with treated intermediate and high-grade NHL, only 17% of relapses were detected by routine CT (13%) or laboratory tests (4%) alone.[292]

Given the wealth of comparative data consistently showing a higher sensitivity for [18]FDG in the detection of disease compared to CT, especially at extranodal sites, and the lower radiation dose (9 mSv vs. 30 mSv), there are theoretical reasons for choosing PET as a routine surveillance procedure – but there is as yet no evidence to support the role of PET in this situation. However, in cases of suspected relapse, the development of a positive PET scan is highly suggestive.

Role of percutaneous biopsy

Percutaneous core biopsy using imaging guidance is now established as a valuable method of determining the nature of soft tissue masses in lymphoma. The indications for its use include:

- Defining the nature of a residual mass following treatment
- Detection of transformation of NHL to a higher grade[293,294]
- Primary diagnosis in patients who present with unusual manifestations of disease

Two large studies have demonstrated that core biopsy is sufficient for management in just under 90%, enabling around 80% to avoid open surgical biopsy.[294,295]

Key points: post-treatment evaluation

- Achievement of CR following treatment is the most important prognostic indicator in both HD and NHL

- Relapse following initial treatment occurs in 40% of patients with HD and over 50% of patients with NHL

- Relapse usually occurs within the first 2 years following treatment of HD

- Residual masses in HD and NHL may contain active malignancy that cannot yet reliably be detected on imaging

Summary

- NHL and HD are a heterogeneous diverse group of malignancies that predominantly involve the lymph nodes.

- In HD, most patients present with early-stage malignancy, whereas in NHL most patients present with advanced disease.

- The incidence of NHL is increasing but the incidence of HD is stable.

- In NHL, the prognosis varies widely according to tumour grade and stage at diagnosis.

- HD tends to spread from one lymph node to the next in a contiguous manner, whereas NHL spreads in a more haphazard manner.

- Involvement of intrathoracic lymph nodes is more common in HD than NHL.

- Involvement of retroperitoneal and mesenteric nodes is more common in NHL than HD.

- Extranodal sites of involvement are more common in NHL than HD.

- The spleen is involved in 10% of patients with HD as isolated infradiaphragmatic disease.

- Splenomegaly is an unreliable indicator of splenic lymphoma.

- Primary extranodal lymphoma is almost exclusively seen in NHL.

References

1. Reznek R H, Richards M A. The radiology of lymphoma. Baillière's Clin Haematol 1987; 1: 77–107
2. CancerStats – Incidence UK, April 2003. Cancer Research UK
3. Callender S T, Vaneghan R I. The lymphomas. In: Weatherall D J, Ledingham J G, Warrell D A (eds) Oxford Textbook of Medicine. Oxford: Oxford University Press, 1983: 160–174
4. American Cancer Society. Cancer Facts and Figures, 2003. Atlanta: American Cancer Society Inc, 2003
5. Ries L A, Kosary C L, Hankey B F et al. SEER Cancer Statistics Review, 1999. Bethesda, MD
6. Devesa S S, Fears T. Non-Hodgkin's lymphoma time trends: United States and international data. Cancer Res 1992; 52: 5432s–5440s
7. Cartwright R, Brincker H, Carli P M et al. The rise in incidence of lymphomas in Europe 1985–1992. Eur J Cancer 1999; 35: 627–633
8. Rabkin C S, Devesa S S, Zahm S H, Gail M H. Increasing incidence of non-Hodgkin's lymphoma. Semin Hematol 1993; 30: 286–296
9. Banks P M. Changes in diagnosis of non-Hodgkin's lymphomas over time. Cancer Res 1992; 52: 5453s–5455s
10. Hartge P, Devesa S S. Quantification of the impact of known risk factors on time trends in non-Hodgkin's lymphoma incidence. Cancer Res 1992; 52: 5566s–5569s
11. Barnes N, Cartwright R A, O'Brien C et al. Rising incidence of lymphoid malignancies – true or false? Br J Cancer 1986; 53: 393–398
12. Glass A G, Karnell L H, Menck H R. The National Cancer Data Base report on non-Hodgkin's lymphoma. Cancer 1997; 80: 2311–2320

13. Horwich A. Hodgkin's disease. In: Horwich A (ed) Oncology: A Multidisciplinary Textbook. London: Chapman and Hall, 1995: 235–250

14. Graser S, Lin R, Stewart S et al. Epstein–Barr virus associated Hodgkin's disease: epidemiologic characteristics in international data. Int J Cancer 1997; 70: 375

15. Ballerini P, Gaidano G, Gong J Z et al. Multiple genetic lesions in acquired immunodeficiency syndrome-related non-Hodgkin's lymphoma. Blood 1993; 81: 166–176

16. Cleary M L, Sklar J. Lymphoproliferative disorders in cardiac transplant recipients are multiclonal lymphomas. Lancet 1984; 2: 489–493

17. Kuefler P R, Bunn P A Jr. Adult T cell leukaemia/lymphoma. Clin Haematol 1986; 15: 695–726

18. Osborne B M. Contextual diagnosis of Hodgkin's disease and non-Hodgkin's lymphoma. Radiol Clin North Am 1990; 28: 669–682

19. Lukes R J, Butler J J. The pathology and nomenclature of Hodgkin's disease. Cancer Res 1966; 26: 1063–1083

20. Lukes R J, Craver L F, Hall T C et al. Report of the Nomenclature Committee. Cancer Res 1966; 26: 1311

21. National Cancer Institute sponsored study of classifications of non-Hodgkin's lymphomas: summary and description of a working formulation for clinical usage. The Non-Hodgkin's Lymphoma Pathologic Classification Project. Cancer 1982; 49: 2112–2135

22. Rosenberg S A, Diamond H D, Jaslowitz B, Craver L F. Lymphosarcoma: a review of 1269 cases. Medicine 1961; 40: 31–84

23. Rappaport H. Tumors of the hematopoietic system. Atlas of Tumor Pathology. Washington DC: Armed Forces Institute of Pathology, 1966; Section 2, Fasicle 8

24. Cossman J, Uppenkamp M, Sundeen J et al. Molecular genetics and the diagnosis of lymphoma. Arch Pathol Lab Med 1988; 112: 117–127

25. American Cancer Society. Cancer Facts and Figures, 1997. Atlanta: American Cancer Society Inc, 1997

26. Harris N L, Jaffe E S, Stein H et al. A revised European-American classification of lymphoid neoplasms: a proposal from the International Lymphoma Study Group. Blood 1994; 84: 1361–1392

27. Harris N L, Jaffe E S, Diebold J et al. World Health Organization classification of neoplastic diseases of the hematopoietic and lymphoid tissues: report of the Clinical Advisory Committee meeting – Airlie House, Virginia, November 1997. J Clin Oncol 1999; 17: 3835–3849

28. A clinical evaluation of the International Lymphoma Study Group classification of non-Hodgkin's lymphoma. The Non-Hodgkin's Lymphoma Classification Project. Blood 1997; 89: 3909–3918

29. Armitage J O, Weisenburger D D. New approach to classifying non-Hodgkin's lymphomas: clinical features of the major histologic subtypes. Non-Hodgkin's Lymphoma Classification Project. J Clin Oncol 1998; 16: 2780–2795

30. Lister T A, Crowther D, Sutcliffe S B et al. Report of a committee convened to discuss the evaluation and staging of patients with Hodgkin's disease: Cotswolds meeting. J Clin Oncol 1989; 7: 1630–1636

31. Cabanillas F, Fuller L M. The radiologic assessment of the lymphoma patient from the standpoint of the clinician. Radiol Clin North Am 1990; 28: 683–695

32. Marglin S I, Castellino R A. Selection of imaging studies for the initial staging of patients with Hodgkin's disease. Semin Ultrasound CT MR 1985; 6: 393

33. Murphy S B. Childhood non-Hodgkin's lymphoma. N Engl J Med 1978; 299: 1446–1448

34. Ng Y Y, Healy J C, Vincent J M et al. The radiology of non-Hodgkin's lymphoma in childhood: a review of 80 cases. Clin Radiol 1994; 49: 594–600

35. Price C G. Non-Hodgkin's lymphoma. In: Price C G, Sikora K (eds) Treatment of Cancer. London: Chapman and Hall, 1995: 881–897

36. Gupta R K, Lister T A. Hodgkin's disease. In: Price C G, Sikora K (eds) Treatment of Cancer. London: Chapman and Hall Medical, 1995: 851–880

37. Henry-Amar M. Second cancer after the treatment for Hodgkin's disease: a report from the International Database on Hodgkin's Disease. Ann Oncol 1992; 3(Suppl. 4): 117–128

38. Chabner B A, Fisher R I, Young R C, DeVita V T. Staging of non-Hodgkin's lymphoma. Semin Oncol 1980; 7: 285–291

39. Bonadonna G, Santoro A, Bonfante V, Valagussa P. Cyclic delivery of MOPP and ABVD combinations in Stage IV Hodgkin's disease: rationale, background studies, and recent results. Cancer Treat Rep 1982; 66: 881–887

40. Canellos G P, Anderson J R, Propert K J et al. Chemotherapy of advanced Hodgkin's disease with MOPP, ABVD, or MOPP alternating with ABVD. N Engl J Med 1992; 327: 1478–1484

41. Hellman S, Mauch P. Role of radiation therapy in the treatment of Hodgkin's disease. Cancer Treat Rep 1982; 66: 915–923

42. Tubiana M, Henry-Amar M, Carde P et al. Toward comprehensive management tailored to prognostic factors of patients with clinical stages I and II in Hodgkin's disease. The EORTC Lymphoma Group controlled clinical trials: 1964–1987. Blood 1989; 73: 47–56

43. Healey E A, Tarbell N J, Kalish L A et al. Prognostic factors for patients with Hodgkin disease in first relapse. Cancer 1993; 71: 2613–2620

44. Desch C E, Lasala M R, Smith T J, Hillner B E. The optimal timing of autologous bone marrow transplantation in Hodgkin's disease patients after a chemotherapy relapse. J Clin Oncol 1992; 10: 200–209

45. Shipp M A, Harrington D P, Anderson J R et al. A predictive model for aggressive non-Hodgkin's lymphoma. The International Non-Hodgkin's Lymphoma Prognostic Factors Project. N Engl J Med 1993; 329: 987–994

46. Oken M M, Creech R H, Tormey D C et al. Toxicity and response criteria of the Eastern Cooperative Oncology Group. Am J Clin Oncol 1982; 5: 649–655

47. Dyer M J. Non-Hodgkin's lymphoma. In: Horwich A (ed) Oncology: A Multidisciplinary Textbook. London: Chapman and Hall, 1995: 251–259

48. Goldstone A H, McMillan A K, Chopra R. High-dose therapy for the treatment of non-Hodgkin's lymphoma. In: Armitage J O, Antman K H (eds) High-dose Cancer Therapy. Pharmacology, Hematopoietins, Stem Cells. Baltimore: Williams and Wilkins, 1992

49. Carroll B A. Ultrasound of lymphoma. Semin Ultrasound 1982; III: 114–122

50. Beyer D, Peters P E. Real-time ultrasonography – an efficient screening method for abdominal and pelvic lymphadenopathy. Lymphology 1980; 13: 142–149

51. Munker R, Stengel A, Stabler A et al. Diagnostic accuracy of ultrasound and computed tomography in the staging of Hodgkin's disease. Verification by laparotomy in 100 cases. Cancer 1995; 76: 1460–1466

52. Clouse M E, Harrison D A, Grassi C J et al. Lymphangiography, ultrasonography, and computed tomography in Hodgkin's disease and non-Hodgkin's lymphoma. J Comput Tomogr 1985; 9: 1–8

53. Magnusson A, Erikson B, Hemmingsson A. Investigation of retroperitoneal lymph nodes in Hodgkin's disease. Ups J Med Sci 1984; 89: 205–212

54. Steinkamp H J, Wissgott C, Rademaker J, Felix R. Current status of power Doppler and color Doppler sonography in the differential diagnosis of lymph node lesions. Eur Radiol 2002; 12: 1785–1793

55. Neumann C H, Robert N J, Rosenthal D, Canellos G. Clinical value of ultrasonography for the management of non-Hodgkin lymphoma patients as compared with abdominal computed tomography. J Comput Assist Tomogr 1983; 7: 666–669

56. Reznek R H, Husband J E. The radiology of lymphoma. Curr Imaging 1990; 2: 9–17

57. Lee J K, Heiken J P, Ling D et al. Magnetic resonance imaging of abdominal and pelvic lymphadenopathy. Radiology 1984; 153: 181–188

58. Dooms G C, Hricak H, Crooks L E, Higgins C B. Magnetic resonance imaging of the lymph nodes: comparison with CT. Radiology 1984; 153: 719–728

59. Greco A, Jelliffe A M, Maher E J, Leung A W. MR imaging of lymphomas: impact on therapy. J Comput Assist Tomogr 1988; 12: 785–791

60. Hill M, Cunningham D, MacVicar D et al. Role of magnetic resonance imaging in predicting relapse in residual masses after treatment of lymphoma. J Clin Oncol 1993; 11: 2273–2278

61. Nyman R, Rhen S, Ericsson A et al. An attempt to characterize malignant lymphoma in spleen, liver and lymph nodes with magnetic resonance imaging. Acta Radiol 1987; 28: 527–533

62. Weissleder R, Elizondo G, Wittenberg J et al. Ultrasmall superparamagnetic iron oxide: an intravenous contrast agent for assessing lymph nodes with MR imaging. Radiology 1990; 175: 494–498

63. Bellin M F, Roy C, Kinkel K et al. Lymph node metastases: safety and effectiveness of MR imaging with ultrasmall superparamagnetic iron oxide particles – initial clinical experience. Radiology 1998; 207: 799–808

64. Front D, Bar-Shalom R, Epelbaum R et al. Early detection of lymphoma recurrence with gallium-67 scintigraphy. J Nucl Med 1993; 34: 2101–2104

65. Newman J S, Francis I R, Kaminski M S, Wahl R L. Imaging of lymphoma with PET with 2-[F-18]-fluoro-2-deoxy-D-glucose: correlation with CT. Radiology 1994; 190: 111–116

66. Front D, Israel O, Epelbaum R et al. Ga-67 SPECT before and after treatment of lymphoma. Radiology 1990; 175: 515–519

67. Gallamini A, Biggi A, Fruttero A et al. Revisiting the prognostic role of gallium scintigraphy in low-grade non-Hodgkin's lymphoma. Eur J Nucl Med 1997; 24: 1499–1506

68. Hussain R, Christie D R, Gebski V, Barton M B, Gruenewald S M. The role of the gallium scan in primary extranodal lymphoma. J Nucl Med 1998; 39: 95–98

69. Moog F, Bangerter M, Diederichs C G et al. Lymphoma: role of whole-body 2-deoxy-2-[F-18]fluoro-D-glucose (FDG) PET in nodal staging. Radiology 1997; 203: 795–800

70. Moog F, Bangerter M, Diederichs C G et al. Extranodal malignant lymphoma: detection with FDG PET versus CT. Radiology 1998; 206: 475–481

71. Wirth A, Seymour J F, Hicks R J et al. Fluorine-18 fluorodeoxyglucose positron emission tomography, gallium-67 scintigraphy, and conventional staging for Hodgkin's disease and non-Hodgkin's lymphoma. Am J Med 2002; 112: 262–268

72. Kostakoglu L, Leonard J P, Kuji I et al. Comparison of fluorine-18 fluorodeoxyglucose positron emission tomography and Ga-67 scintigraphy in evaluation of lymphoma. Cancer 2002; 94: 879–888

73. Bangerter M, Moog F, Buchmann I et al. Whole-body 2-[18F]-fluoro-2-deoxy-D-glucose positron emission tomography (FDG-PET) for accurate staging of Hodgkin's disease. Ann Oncol 1998; 9: 1117–1122

74. Hoh C K, Glaspy J, Rosen P et al. Whole-body FDG-PET imaging for staging of Hodgkin's disease and lymphoma. J Nucl Med 1997; 38: 343–348

75. Jerusalem G, Warland V, Najjar F et al. Whole-body ^{18}F-FDG PET for the evaluation of patients with Hodgkin's disease and non-Hodgkin's lymphoma. Nucl Med Commun 1999; 20: 13–20

76. Weihrauch M R, Re D, Bischoff S et al. Whole-body positron emission tomography using ^{18}F-fluorodeoxyglucose for initial staging of patients with Hodgkin's disease. Ann Hematol 2002; 81: 20–25

77. Menzel C, Dobert N, Mitrou P et al. Positron emission tomography for the staging of Hodgkin's lymphoma – increasing the body of evidence in favor of the method. Acta Oncol 2002; 41: 430–436

78. Hoffmann M, Kletter K, Diemling M et al. Positron emission tomography with fluorine-18-2-fluoro-2-deoxy-D-glucose (F18-FDG) does not visualize extranodal B-cell lymphoma of the mucosa-associated lymphoid tissue (MALT)-type. Ann Oncol 1999; 10: 1185–1189

79. Jerusalem G, Beguin Y, Najjar F et al. Positron emission tomography (PET) with ^{18}F-fluorodeoxyglucose (^{18}F-FDG) for the staging of low-grade non-Hodgkin's lymphoma (NHL). Ann Oncol 2001; 12: 825–830

80. Lee J K, Stanley R J, Sagel S S, Levitt R G. Accuracy of computed tomography in detecting intraabdominal and pelvic adenopathy in lymphoma. Am J Roentgenol 1978; 131: 311–315

81. Best J J, Blackledge G, Forbes W S et al. Computed tomography of abdomen in staging and clinical management of lymphoma. Br Med J 1978; 2: 1675–1677

82. Earl H M, Sutcliffe S B, Fry I K et al. Computerised tomographic (CT) abdominal scanning in Hodgkin's disease. Clin Radiol 1980; 31: 149–153

83. Marglin S, Castellino R. Lymphographic accuracy in 632 consecutive, previously untreated cases of Hodgkin disease and non-Hodgkin lymphoma. Radiology 1981; 140: 351–353

84. Castellino R A, Hoppe R T, Blank N et al. Computed tomography, lymphography, and staging laparotomy: correlations in initial staging of Hodgkin disease. Am J Roentgenol 1984; 143: 37–41

85. Enig B, Bjerregaard J B, Hjollund M E et al. Detection of neoplastic lymph nodes in Hodgkin's disease and non-Hodgkin lymphoma. Comparison between tomography and lymphography. Acta Radiol Oncol 1985; 24: 491–495

86. Strijk P. Lymphography and abdominal computed tomography in the staging of non-Hodgkin lymphoma. With an analysis of discrepancies. Acta Radiol 1987; 28: 263–269

87. Stomper P C, Cholewinski S P, Park J et al. Abdominal staging of thoracic Hodgkin disease: CT-lymphangiography-Ga-67 scanning correlation. Radiology 1993; 187: 381–386

88. Libson E, Polliack A, Bloom R A. Value of lymphangiography in the staging of Hodgkin lymphoma. Radiology 1994; 193: 757–759

89. DePena C A, Van Tassel P, Lee Y Y. Lymphoma of the head and neck. Radiol Clin North Am 1990; 28: 723–743

90. Pombo F, Rodriguez E, Caruncho M V et al. CT attenuation values and enhancing characteristics of thoracoabdominal lymphomatous adenopathies. J Comput Assist Tomogr 1994; 18: 59–62

91. Filly R, Bland N, Castellino R A. Radiographic distribution of intrathoracic disease in previously untreated patients with Hodgkin's disease and non-Hodgkin's lymphoma. Radiology 1976; 120: 277–281

92. Castellino R A, Blank N, Hoppe R T, Cho C. Hodgkin disease: contributions of chest CT in the initial staging evaluation. Radiology 1986; 160: 603–605

93. Bragg D G. Radiology of the lymphomas. Curr Probl Diagn Radiol 1987; 16: 177–206

94. Castellino R A, Hilton S, O'Brien J P, Portlock C S. Non-Hodgkin lymphoma: contribution of chest CT in the initial staging evaluation. Radiology 1996; 199: 129–132

95. Grossman H, Winchester P H, Bragg D G et al. Roentgenographic changes in childhood Hodgkin's disease. Am J Roentgenol Radium Ther Nucl Med 1970; 108: 354–364

96. Jochelson M S, Balikian J P, Mauch P, Liebman H. Peri- and paracardial involvement in lymphoma: a radiographic study of 11 cases. Am J Roentgenol 1983; 140: 483–488

97. Strijk S P. Lymph node calcification in malignant lymphoma. Presentation of nine cases and a review of the literature. Acta Radiol Diagn (Stockh) 1985; 26: 427–431

98. Apter S, Avigdor A, Gayer G et al. Calcification in lymphoma occurring before therapy: CT features and clinical correlation. Am J Roentgenol 2002; 178: 935–938

99. Hopper K D, Diehl L F, Cole B A et al. The significance of necrotic mediastinal lymph nodes on CT in patients with newly diagnosed Hodgkin disease. Am J Roentgenol 1990; 155: 267–270

100. North L B, Fuller L M, Hagemeister F B et al. Importance of initial mediastinal adenopathy in Hodgkin disease. Am J Roentgenol 1982; 138: 229–235

101. Gallagher C J, White F E, Tucker A K et al. The role of computed tomography in the detection of intrathoracic lymphoma. Br J Cancer 1984; 49: 621–629

102. Khoury M B, Godwin J D, Halvorsen R et al. Role of chest CT in non-Hodgkin lymphoma. Radiology 1986; 158: 659–662

103. Hopper K D, Diehl L F, Lesar M et al. Hodgkin disease: clinical utility of CT in initial staging and treatment. Radiology 1988; 169: 17–22

104. Heron C W, Husband J E, Williams M P. Hodgkin disease: CT of the thymus. Radiology 1988; 167: 647–651

105. Wernecke K, Vassallo P, Rutsch F et al. Thymic involvement in Hodgkin disease: CT and sonographic findings. Radiology 1991; 181: 375–383

106. Shaffer K, Smith D, Kirn D et al. Primary mediastinal large-B-cell lymphoma: radiologic findings at presentation. Am J Roentgenol 1996; 167: 425–430

107. Spiers A S, Husband J E, MacVicar A D. Treated thymic lymphoma: comparison of MR imaging with CT. Radiology 1997; 203: 369–376

108. Rodriguez M, Rehn S M, Nyman R S et al. CT in malignancy grading and prognostic prediction of non-Hodgkin's lymphoma. Acta Radiol 1999; 40: 191–197

109. Rehn S, Sperber G O, Nyman R et al. Quantification of inhomogeneities in malignancy grading of non-Hodgkin lymphoma with MR imaging. Acta Radiol 1993; 34: 3–9

110. Rehn S M, Nyman R S, Glimelius B L et al. Non-Hodgkin lymphoma: predicting prognostic grade with MR imaging. Radiology 1990; 176: 249–253

111. Harell G S, Breiman R S, Glatstein E J et al. Computed tomography of the abdomen in the malignant lymphomas. Radiol Clin North Am 1977; 15: 391–400

112. Castellino R A, Marglin S, Blank N. Hodgkin disease, the non-Hodgkin lymphomas, and the leukemias in the retroperitoneum. Semin Roentgenol 1980; 15: 288–301

113. Kadin M D, Glatstein E J, Dorfman R F. Clinicopathologic studies in 117 untreated patients subject to laparotomy for the staging of Hodgkin's disease. Cancer 1980; 27: 1277–1294

114. Goffinet D R, Warnke R, Dunnick N R et al. Clinical and surgical (laparotomy) evaluation of patients with non-Hodgkin's lymphomas. Cancer Treat Rep 1977; 61: 981–992

115. Rosenberg S A, Kaplan H S. Evidence for an orderly progression in the spread of Hodgkin's disease. Cancer Res 1966; 26: 1225–1231

116. Urba W J, Longo D L. Hodgkin's disease. N Engl J Med 1992; 326: 678–687

117. Weinstein J B, Heiken J P, Lee J K et al. High resolution CT of the porta hepatis and hepatoduodenal ligament. Radiographics 1986; 6: 55–74

118. Yang Z G, Min P Q. Sone S et al. Tuberculosis versus lymphomas in the abdominal lymph nodes: evaluation with contrast-enhanced CT. Am J Roentgenol 1999; 172: 619–623

119. Kilgore T L, Chasen M H. Endobronchial non-Hodgkin's lymphoma. Chest 1983; 84: 58–61

120. Kaplan H S. Contiguity and progression in Hodgkin's disease. Cancer Res 1971; 31: 1811–1813

121. Cobby M, Whipp E, Bullimore J et al. CT appearances of relapse of lymphoma in the lung. Clin Radiol 1990; 41: 232–238

122. Eisner M D, Kaplan L D, Herndier B, Stulbarg M S. The pulmonary manifestations of AIDS-related non-Hodgkin's lymphoma. Chest 1996; 110: 729–736

123. MacDonald J B. Lung involvement in Hodgkin's disease. Thorax 1977; 32: 664–667

124. Burgener F A, Hamlin D J. Intrathoracic histiocytic lymphoma. Am J Roentgenol 1981; 136: 499–504

125. Lewis E R, Caskey C I, Fishman E K. Lymphoma of the lung: CT findings in 31 patients. Am J Roentgenol 1991; 156: 711–714

126. Jackson S A, Tung K T, Mead G M. Multiple cavitating pulmonary lesions in non-Hodgkin's lymphoma. Clin Radiol 1994; 49: 883–885

127. Isaacson P G, Norton A J. General features of extranodal lymphoma. Extranodal Lymphomas. London: Churchill-Livingstone, 1994: 1–14

128. Cordier J F, Chailleux E, Lauque D et al. Primary pulmonary lymphomas. A clinical study of 70 cases in nonimmunocompromised patients. Chest 1993; 103: 201–208

129. Peterson H, Snider H L, Yam L T et al. Primary pulmonary lymphoma. A clinical and immunohistochemical study of six cases. Cancer 1985; 56: 805–813

130. Murray K A, Chor P J, Turner J F Jr. Intrathoracic lymphoproliferative disorders and lymphoma. Curr Probl Diagn Radiol 1996; 25: 78–106

131. Ooi G C, Ho J C, Khong P L et al. Computed tomography characteristics of advanced primary pulmonary lymphoepithelioma-like carcinoma. Eur Radiol 2003; 13: 522–526

132. Dunnick N R, Parker B R, Castellino R A. Rapid onset of pulmonary infiltration due to histiocytic lymphoma. Radiology 1976; 118: 281–285

133. Radin A I. Primary pulmonary Hodgkin's disease. Cancer 1990; 65: 550–563

134. Cartier Y, Johkoh T, Honda O, Muller N L. Primary pulmonary Hodgkin's disease: CT findings in three patients. Clin Radiol 1999; 54: 182–184

135. Edinburgh K J, Jasmer R M, Huang L et al. Multiple pulmonary nodules in AIDS: usefulness of CT in distinguishing among potential causes. Radiology 2000; 214: 427–432

136. Celikoglu F, Teirstein A S, Krellenstein D J, Strauchen J A. Pleural effusion in non-Hodgkin's lymphoma. Chest 1992; 101: 1357–1360

137. Bergin C J, Healy M V, Zincone G E, Castellino R A. MR evaluation of chest wall involvement in malignant lymphoma. J Comput Assist Tomogr 1990; 14: 928–932

138. Carlsen S E, Bergin C J, Hoppe R T. MR imaging to detect chest wall and pleural involvement in patients with lymphoma: effect on radiation therapy planning. Am J Roentgenol 1993; 160: 1191–1195

139. North L B, Libshitz H I, Lorigan J G. Thoracic lymphoma. Radiol Clin North Am 1990; 28: 745–762

140. Tesoro-Tess J D, Biasi S, Balzarini L et al. Heart involvement in lymphomas. The value of magnetic resonance imaging and two-dimensional echocardiography at disease presentation. Cancer 1993; 72: 2484–2490

141. Tohno E, Cosgrove D O, Sloan J P. Malignant disease – local recurrence and metastases. In: Tohno E, Cosgrove D O, Sloan J P (eds) Ultrasound Diagnosis of Breast Diseases. Edinburgh: Churchill Livingstone, 1994: 186

142. Paulus D D. Lymphoma of the breast. Radiol Clin North Am 1990; 28: 833–840

143. Sabate J M, Gomez A, Torrubia S et al. Lymphoma of the breast: clinical and radiologic features with pathologic correlation in 28 patients. Breast J 2002; 8: 294–304

144. Thomas J L, Bernardino M E, Vermess M et al. EOE-13 in the detection of hepatosplenic lymphoma. Radiology 1982; 145: 629–634

145. Bonadonna G, Santoro A. Clinical evolution and treatment of Hodgkin's disease. In: Wiernik P H, Canellos G, Kyle R A, Schiffer C A (eds) Neoplastic Disease of the Blood. Edinburgh: Churchill Livingstone, 1985: 789

146. Warshauer D M, Molina P L, Worawattanakul S. The spotted spleen: CT and clinical correlation in a tertiary care center. J Comput Assist Tomogr 1998; 22: 694–702

147. Dachman A H, Buck J L, Krishnan J et al. Primary non-Hodgkin's splenic lymphoma. Clin Radiol 1998; 53: 137–142

148. Daskalogiannaki M, Prassopoulos P, Katrinakis G et al. Splenic involvement in lymphomas. Evaluation on serial CT examinations. Acta Radiol 2001; 42: 326–332

149. Strijk S P, Wagener D J, Bogman M J et al. The spleen in Hodgkin disease: diagnostic value of CT. Radiology 1985; 154: 753–757

150. Strijk S P, Boetes C, Bogman M J et al. The spleen in non-Hodgkin lymphoma. Diagnostic value of computed tomography. Acta Radiol 1987; 28: 139–144

151. Hess C F, Kurtz B, Hoffmann W, Bamberg M. Ultrasound diagnosis of splenic lymphoma: ROC analysis of multidimensional splenic indices. Br J Radiol 1993; 66: 859–864

152. Harisinghani M G, Saini S, Weissleder R et al. Splenic imaging with ultrasmall superparamagnetic iron oxide ferumoxtran-10 (AMI-7227): preliminary observations. J Comput Assist Tomogr 2001; 25: 770–776

153. Weissleder R, Elizondo G, Stark D D et al. The diagnosis of splenic lymphoma by MR imaging: value of superparamagnetic iron oxide. Am J Roentgenol 1989; 152: 175–180

154. Weissleder R, Hahn P F, Stark D D et al. Superparamagnetic iron oxide: enhanced detection of focal splenic tumors with MR imaging. Radiology 1988; 169: 399–403

155. Rini J N, Manalili E Y, Hoffman M A et al. F-18 FDG versus Ga-67 for detecting splenic involvement in Hodgkin's disease. Clin Nucl Med 2002; 27: 572–577

156. Kaplan H S, Dorfman R F, Nelsen T S, Rosenberg S A. Staging laparotomy and splenectomy in Hodgkin's disease: analysis of indications and patterns of involvement in 285 consecutive, unselected patients. Natl Cancer Inst Monogr 1973; 36: 291–301

157. Maher M M, McDermott S R, Fenlon H M et al. Imaging of primary non-Hodgkin's lymphoma of the liver. Clin Radiol 2001; 56: 295–301

158. Weissleder R, Stark D D, Elizondo G et al. MRI of hepatic lymphoma. Magn Reson Imaging 1988; 6: 675–681

159. Coakley F V, O'Reilly E M, Schwartz L H et al. Non-Hodgkin lymphoma as a cause of intrahepatic periportal low attenuation on CT. J Comput Assist Tomogr 1997; 21: 726–728

160. Richards M A, Webb J A, Reznek R H et al. Detection of spread of malignant lymphoma to the liver by low field strength magnetic resonance imaging. Br Med J (Clin Res Ed) 1986; 293: 1126–1128

161. Weinreb J C, Brateman L, Maravilla K R. Magnetic resonance imaging of hepatic lymphoma. Am J Roentgenol 1984; 143: 1211–1214

162. Stark D D, Weissleder R, Elizondo G et al. Superparamagnetic iron oxide: clinical application as a contrast agent for MR imaging of the liver. Radiology 1988; 168: 297–301

163. Brady L W, Asbell S O. Malignant lymphoma of the gastrointestinal tract. Erskine Memorial Lecture, 1979. Radiology 1980; 137: 291–298

164. Dodd G D. Lymphoma of the hollow abdominal viscera. Radiol Clin North Am 1990; 28: 771–783

165. Rohatiner A, d'Amore F, Coiffier B et al. Report on a workshop convened to discuss the pathological and staging classifications of gastrointestinal tract lymphoma. Ann Oncol 1994; 5: 397–400

166. Dragosics B, Bauer P, Radaszkiewicz T. Primary gastrointestinal non-Hodgkin's lymphomas. A retrospective clinicopathologic study of 150 cases. Cancer 1985; 55: 1060–1073

167. Fishman E K, Urban B A, Hruban R H. CT of the stomach: spectrum of disease. Radiographics 1996; 16: 1035–1054

168. Megibow A J, Balthazar E J, Naidich D P, Bosniak M A. Computed tomography of gastrointestinal lymphoma. Am J Roentgenol 1983; 141: 541–547

169. Kessar P, Norton A, Rohatiner A Z et al. CT appearances of mucosa-associated lymphoid tissue (MALT) lymphoma. Eur Radiol 1999; 9: 693–696

170. Fujishima H, Chijiiwa Y. Endoscopic ultrasonographic staging of primary gastric lymphoma. Abdom Imaging 1996; 21: 192–194

171. Raderer M, Vorbeck F, Formanek M et al. Importance of extensive staging in patients with mucosa-associated lymphoid tissue (MALT)-type lymphoma. Br J Cancer 2000; 83: 454–457

172. Balthazar E J, Noordhoorn M, Megibow A J, Gordon R B. CT of small-bowel lymphoma in immunocompetent patients and patients with AIDS: comparison of findings. Am J Roentgenol 1997; 168: 675–680

173. Kim Y, Cho O, Song S et al. Peritoneal lymphomatosis: CT findings. Abdom Imaging 1998; 23: 87–90

174. Reed K, Vose P C, Jarstfer B S. Pancreatic cancer: 30 year review (1947 to 1977). Am J Surg 1979; 138: 929–933

175. Webb T H, Lillemoe K D, Pitt H A et al. Pancreatic lymphoma. Is surgery mandatory for diagnosis or treatment? Ann Surg 1989; 209: 25–30

176. Shirkhoda A, Ros P R, Farah J, Staab E V. Lymphoma of the solid abdominal viscera. Radiol Clin North Am 1990; 28: 785–799

177. Van Beers B, Lalonde L, Soyer P et al. Dynamic CT in pancreatic lymphoma. J Comput Assist Tomogr 1993; 17: 94–97

178. Prayer L, Schurawitzki H, Mallek R, Mostbeck G. CT in pancreatic involvement of non-Hodgkin lymphoma. Acta Radiol 1992; 33: 123–127

179. Charnsangavej C. Lymphoma of the genitourinary tract. Radiol Clin North Am 1990; 28: 865–877

180. Reznek R H, Mootoosamy I, Webb J A, Richards M A. CT in renal and perirenal lymphoma: a further look. Clin Radiol 1990; 42: 233–238

181. Hartman D S, David C J Jr, Goldman S M et al. Renal lymphoma: radiologic-pathologic correlation of 21 cases. Radiology 1982; 144: 759–766

182. Heiken J P, Gold R P, Schnur M J et al. Computed tomography of renal lymphoma with ultrasound correlation. J Comput Assist Tomogr 1983; 7: 245–250

183. Aigen A B, Phillips M. Primary malignant lymphoma of urinary bladder. Urology 1986; 28: 235–237

184. Yeoman L J, Mason M D, Olliff J F. Non-Hodgkin's lymphoma of the bladder – and MRI appearances. Clin Radiol 1991; 44: 389–392

185. Tasu J P, Geffroy D, Rocher L et al. Primary malignant lymphoma of the urinary bladder: report of three cases and review of the literature. Eur Radiol 2000; 10: 1261–1264

186. Mostofi F K. Proceedings: Testicular tumors. Epidemiologic, etiologic, and pathologic features. Cancer 1973; 32: 1186–1201

187. Thurnher S, Hricak H, Carroll P R et al. Imaging the testis: comparison between MR imaging and US. Radiology 1988; 167: 631–636

188. Kim Y S, Koh B H, Cho O K, Rhim H C. MR imaging of primary uterine lymphoma. Abdom Imaging 1997; 22: 441–444

189. Jenkins N, Husband J, Sellars N, Gore M. MRI in primary non-Hodgkin's lymphoma of the vagina associated with a uterine congenital anomaly. Br J Radiol 1997; 70: 219–222

190. Glazer H S, Lee J K, Balfe D M et al. Non-Hodgkin lymphoma: computed tomographic demonstration of unusual extranodal involvement. Radiology 1983; 149: 211–217

191. Ferrozzi F, Tognini G, Bova D, Zuccoli G. Non-Hodgkin lymphomas of the ovaries: MR findings. J Comput Assist Tomogr 2000; 24: 416–420

192. Vincent J M, Morrison I D, Armstrong P, Reznek R H. Computed tomography of diffuse, non-metastatic enlargement of the adrenal glands in patients with malignant disease. Clin Radiol 1994; 49: 456–460

193. Zimmerman R A. Central nervous system lymphoma. Radiol Clin North Am 1990; 28: 697–721

194. Hobson D E, Anderson B A, Carr I, West M. Primary lymphoma of the central nervous system: Manitoba experience and literature review. Can J Neurol Sci 1986; 13: 55–61

195. Snider W D, Simpson D M, Nielsen S et al. Neurological complications of acquired immune deficiency syndrome: analysis of 50 patients. Ann Neurol 1983; 14: 403–418

196. Jenkins C N, Colquhoun I R. Characterization of primary intracranial lymphoma by computed tomography: an analysis of 36 cases and a review of the literature with particular reference to calcification haemorrhage and cyst formation. Clin Radiol 1998; 53: 428–434

197. Herman T S, Hammond N, Jones S E et al. Involvement of the central nervous system by non-Hodgkin's lymphoma: the Southwest Oncology Group experience. Cancer 1979; 43: 390–397

198. Kotasek D, Albertyn L E, Sage R E. A five-year experience with central nervous system lymphoma. Med J Aust 1986; 144: 299–303

199. Bragg D G, Colby T V, Ward J H. New concepts in the non-Hodgkin lymphomas: radiologic implications. Radiology 1986; 159: 291–304

200. Chamberlain M C, Sandy A D, Press G A. Leptomeningeal metastasis: a comparison of gadolinium-enhanced MR and contrast-enhanced CT of the brain. Neurology 1990; 40: 435–438

201. Yousem D M, Patrone P M, Grossman R I. Leptomeningeal metastases: MR evaluation. J Comput Assist Tomogr 1990; 14: 255–261

202. MacVicar D, Williams M P. CT scanning in epidural lymphoma. Clin Radiol 1991; 43: 95–102

203. Evans C. A review of non-Hodgkin's lymphomata of the head and neck. Clin Oncol 1981; 7: 23–31

204. Robbins K T, Fuller L M, Vlasak M et al. Primary lymphomas of the nasal cavity and paranasal sinuses. Cancer 1985; 56: 814–819

205. Shikhani A, Samara M, Allam C et al. Primary lymphoma in the salivary glands: report of five cases and review of the literature. Laryngoscope 1987; 97: 1438–1442

206. Takashima S, Ikezoe J, Morimoto S et al. Primary thyroid lymphoma: evaluation with CT. Radiology 1988; 168: 765–768

207. Braunstein E M. Hodgkin disease of bone: radiographic correlation with the histological classification. Radiology 1980; 137: 643–646

208. Cooley B L, Higinbotham N L, Groesbeck H P. Primary reticulum cell sarcoma of bone: classification. Radiology 1950; 50: 641–658

209. Ngan H, Preston B J. Non-Hodgkin's lymphoma presenting with osseous lesions. Clin Radiol 1975; 26: 351–356

210. Stroszczynski C, Oellinger J, Hosten N et al. Staging and monitoring of malignant lymphoma of the bone: comparison of ^{67}Ga scintigraphy and MRI. J Nucl Med 1999; 40: 387–393

211. Moog F, Kotzerke J, Reske S N. FDG PET can replace bone scintigraphy in primary staging of malignant lymphoma. J Nucl Med 1999; 40: 1407–1413

212. Anderson K C, Kaplan W D, Leonard R C et al. Role of ^{99m}Tc methylene diphosphonate bone imaging in the management of lymphoma. Cancer Treat Rep 1985; 69: 1347–1351

213. Castellino R A, Goffinet D R, Blank N et al. The role of radiography in the staging of non-Hodgkin's lymphoma with laparotomy correlation. Radiology 1974; 110: 329–338

214. Chabner B A, Johnson R E, Young R C et al. Sequential nonsurgical and surgical staging of non-Hodgkin's lymphoma. Ann Intern Med 1976; 85: 149–154

215. Glatstein E, Guernsey J M, Rosenberg S A, Kaplan H S. The value of laparotomy and splenectomy in the staging of Hodgkin's disease. Cancer 1969; 24: 709–718

216. Kaplan H S. Essentials of staging and management of the malignant lymphomas. Semin Roentgenol 1980; 15: 219–226

217. Linden A, Zankovich R, Theissen P et al. Malignant lymphoma: bone marrow imaging versus biopsy. Radiology 1989; 173: 335–339

218. Pond G D, Castellino R A, Horning S, Hoppe R T. Non-Hodgkin lymphoma: influence of lymphography, CT, and bone marrow biopsy on staging and management. Radiology 1989; 170: 159–164

219. Döhner H, Gückel F, Knauf W et al. Magnetic resonance imaging of bone marrow in lymphoproliferative disorders: correlation with bone marrow biopsy. Br J Haematol 1989; 73: 12–17

220. Hoane B R, Shields A F, Porter B A, Shulman H M. Detection of lymphomatous bone marrow involvement with magnetic resonance imaging. Blood 1991; 78: 728–738

221. Yasumoto M, Nonomura Y, Yoshimura R et al. MR detection of iliac bone marrow involvement by malignant lymphoma with various MR sequences including diffusion-weighted echo-planar imaging. Skeletal Radiol 2002; 31: 263–269

222. Shields A F, Porter B A, Churchley S et al. The detection of bone marrow involvement by lymphoma using magnetic resonance imaging. J Clin Oncol 1987; 5: 225–230

223. Tsunoda S, Takagi S, Tanaka O, Miura Y. Clinical and prognostic significance of femoral marrow magnetic resonance imaging in patients with malignant lymphoma. Blood 1997; 89: 286–290

224. Altehoefer C, Blum U, Bathmann J et al. Comparative diagnostic accuracy of magnetic resonance imaging and immunoscintigraphy for detection of bone marrow involvement in patients with malignant lymphoma. J Clin Oncol 1997; 15: 1754–1760

225. Moog F, Bangerter M, Kotzerke J et al. 18-F-fluorodeoxyglucose-positron emission tomography as a new approach to detect lymphomatous bone marrow. J Clin Oncol 1998; 16: 603–609

226. Daldrup-Link H E, Rummeny E J, Ihssen B et al. Iron-oxide-enhanced MR imaging of bone marrow in patients with non-Hodgkin's lymphoma: differentiation between tumor infiltration and hypercellular bone marrow. Eur Radiol 2002; 12: 1557–1566

227. Williams M P, Olliff J F. Magnetic resonance imaging in extranodal pelvic lymphoma. Clin Radiol 1990; 42: 264–268

228. Malloy P C, Fishman E K, Magid D. Lymphoma of bone, muscle, and skin: CT findings. Am J Roentgenol 1992; 159: 805–809

229. Wotherspoon A C, Ortiz-Hidalgo C, Falzon M R, Isaacson P G. *Helicobacter pylori*-associated gastritis and primary B-cell gastric lymphoma. Lancet 1991; 338: 1175–1176

230. Nakamura S, Aoyagi K, Furuse M et al. B-cell monoclonality precedes the development of gastric MALT lymphoma in *Helicobacter pylori*-associated chronic gastritis. Am J Pathol 1998; 152: 1271–1279

231. Thieblemont C, Bastion Y, Berger F et al. Mucosa-associated lymphoid tissue gastrointestinal and nongastrointestinal lymphoma behavior: analysis of 108 patients. J Clin Oncol 1997; 15: 1624–1630

232. Vorbeck F, Osterreicher C, Puspok A et al. Comparison of spiral-computed tomography with water-filling of the stomach and endosonography for gastric lymphoma of mucosa-associated lymphoid tissue-type. Digestion 2002; 65: 196–199

233. Park M S, Kim K W, Yu J S et al. Radiographic findings of primary B-cell lymphoma of the stomach: low-grade versus high-grade malignancy in relation to the mucosa-associated lymphoid tissue concept. Am J Roentgenol 2002; 179: 1297–1304

234. Palazzo L, Roseau G, Ruskone-Fourmestraux A et al. Endoscopic ultrasonography in the local staging of primary gastric lymphoma. Endoscopy 1993; 25: 502–508

235. Sackmann M, Morgner A, Rudolph B et al. Regression of gastric MALT lymphoma after eradication of *Helicobacter pylori* is predicted by endosonographic staging. MALT Lymphoma Study Group. Gastroenterology 1997; 113: 1087–1090

236. Lee H J, Han J K, Kim T K et al. Primary colorectal lymphoma: spectrum of imaging findings with pathologic correlation. Eur Radiol 2002; 12: 2242–2249

237. King L J, Padley S P, Wotherspoon A C, Nicholson A G. Pulmonary MALT lymphoma: imaging findings in 24 cases. Eur Radiol 2000; 10: 1932–1938

238. Lee D K, Im J G, Lee K S et al. B-cell lymphoma of bronchus-associated lymphoid tissue (BALT): CT features in 10 patients. J Comput Assist Tomogr 2000; 24: 30–34

239. Vincent J M, Ng Y Y, Norton A J, Armstrong P. CT 'angiogram sign' in primary pulmonary lymphoma. J Comput Assist Tomogr 1992; 16: 829–831

240. Burkitt D P. Classics in oncology. A sarcoma involving the jaws in African children. CA Cancer J Clin 1972; 22: 345–355

241. O'Connor G T, Rappaport H, Smith E B. Childhood lymphoma resembling 'Burkitt tumour' in the United States. Cancer 1965; 18: 411–417

242. Ziegler J L, Bluming A Z, Morrow R H et al. Central nervous system involvement in Burkitt's lymphoma. Blood 1970; 36: 718–728

243. Johnson K A, Tung K, Mead G, Sweetenham J. The imaging of Burkitt's and Burkitt-like lymphoma. Clin Radiol 1998; 53: 835–841

244. World Health Organization Classification of Tumours. Pathology & Genetics. Tumours of Haematopoietic and Lymphoid Tissues. Lyon: IARC Press, 2001

245. Radin D R, Esplin J A, Levine A M, Ralls P W. AIDS-related non-Hodgkin's lymphoma: abdominal CT findings in 112 patients. Am J Roentgenol 1993; 160: 1133–1139

246. Jasmer R M, Gotway M B, Creasman J M et al. Clinical and radiographic predictors of the etiology of computed tomography-diagnosed intrathoracic lymphadenopathy in HIV-infected patients. J Acquir Immune Defic Syndr 2002; 31: 291–298

247. Cordoliani Y S, Derosier C, Pharaboz C et al. Primary cerebral lymphoma in patients with AIDS: MR findings in 17 cases. Am J Roentgenol 1992; 159: 841–847

248. O'Doherty M J, Barrington S F, Campbell M et al. PET scanning and the human immunodeficiency virus-positive patient. J Nucl Med 1997; 38:1575–1583

249. Dodd G D III, Ledesma-Medina J, Baron R L, Fuhrman C R. Posttransplant lymphoproliferative disorder: intrathoracic manifestations. Radiology 1992; 184: 65–69

250. Carignan S, Staples C A, Muller N L. Intrathoracic lymphoproliferative disorders in the immunocompromised patient: CT findings. Radiology 1995; 197: 53–58

251. Lim G Y, Newman B, Kurland G, Webber S A. Posttransplantation lymphoproliferative disorder: manifestations in pediatric thoracic organ recipients. Radiology 2002; 222: 699–708

252. Lee D A, Hartman R P, Trenkner S W et al. Lymphomas in solid organ transplantation. Abdom Imaging 1998; 23: 553–557

253. Pickhardt P J, Siegel M J. Abdominal manifestations of posttransplantation lymphoproliferative disorder. Am J Roentgenol 1998; 171: 1007–1013

254. Heron C W, Husband J E, Williams M P, Cherryman G R. The value of thoracic computed tomography in the detection of recurrent Hodgkin's disease. Br J Radiol 1988; 61: 567–572

255. Hopper K D, Kasales C J, Van Slyke M A et al. Analysis of interobserver and intraobserver variability in CT tumor measurements. Am J Roentgenol 1996; 167: 851–854

256. DeVita V T Jr, Hellman S, Rosenberg S A (eds) Non-Hodgkin's lymphomas (Ch 45.3) and Lymphoma (Ch 45.6) In: Cancer – Principles and Practice of Oncology. Toronto: J B Lippincott Co, 2001, pp 2339, 2256

257. North L B, Fuller L M, Sullivan-Halley J A, Hagemeister F B. Regression of mediastinal Hodgkin disease after therapy: evaluation of time interval. Radiology 1987; 164: 599–602

258. Cheson B D, Horning S J, Coiffier B et al. Report of an international workshop to standardize response criteria for non-Hodgkin's lymphomas. NCI Sponsored International Working Group. J Clin Oncol 1999; 17: 1244

259. Kaplan W D, Jochelson M S, Herman T S et al. Gallium-67 imaging: a predictor of residual tumor viability and clinical outcome in patients with diffuse large-cell lymphoma. J Clin Oncol 1990; 8: 1966–1970

260. Janicek M, Kaplan W, Neuberg D et al. Early restaging gallium scans predict outcome in poor-prognosis patients with aggressive non-Hodgkin's lymphoma treated with high-dose CHOP chemotherapy. J Clin Oncol 1997; 15: 1631–1637

261. Vose J M, Bierman P J, Anderson J R et al. Single-photon emission computed tomography gallium imaging versus computed tomography: predictive value in patients undergoing high-dose chemotherapy and autologous stem-cell transplantation for non-Hodgkin's lymphoma. J Clin Oncol 1996; 14: 2473–2479

262. Mikhaeel N G, Timothy A R, O'Doherty M J et al. 18-FDG-PET as a prognostic indicator in the treatment of aggressive non-Hodgkin's lymphoma – comparison with CT. Leuk Lymphoma 2000; 39: 543–553

263. Romer W, Hanauske A R, Ziegler S et al. Positron emission tomography in non-Hodgkin's lymphoma: assessment of chemotherapy with fluorodeoxyglucose. Blood 1998; 91: 4464–4471

264. Spaepen K, Stroobants S, Dupont P et al. Early restaging positron emission tomography with (18)F-fluorodeoxyglucose predicts outcome in patients with aggressive non-Hodgkin's lymphoma. Ann Oncol 2002; 13: 1356–1363

265. Spaepen K, Stroobants S, Dupont P et al. Prognostic value of positron emission tomography (PET) with fluorine-18 fluorodeoxyglucose ([18F]FDG) after first-line chemotherapy in non-Hodgkin's lymphoma: is [18F]FDG-PET a valid alternative to conventional diagnostic methods? J Clin Oncol 2001; 19: 414–419

266. Kostakoglu L, Coleman M, Leonard J P et al. PET predicts prognosis after 1 cycle of chemotherapy in aggressive lymphoma and Hodgkin's disease. J Nucl Med 2002; 43: 1018–1027

267. Becherer A, Mitterbauer M, Jaeger U et al. Positron emission tomography with [18F]2-fluoro-D-2-deoxyglucose (FDG-PET) predicts relapse of malignant lymphoma after high-dose therapy with stem cell transplantation. Leukemia 2002; 16: 260–267

268. Radford J A, Cowan R A, Flanagan M et al. The significance of residual mediastinal abnormality on the chest radiograph following treatment for Hodgkin's disease. J Clin Oncol 1988; 6: 940–946

269. Surbone A, Longo D L, Devita V T Jr et al. Residual abdominal masses in aggressive non-Hodgkin's lymphoma after combination chemotherapy: significance and management. J Clin Oncol 1988; 6: 1832–1837

270. Lewis E, Bernardino M E, Salvador P G et al. Post-therapy CT-detected mass in lymphoma patients: is it viable tissue? J Comput Assist Tomogr 1982; 6: 792–795

271. Coiffier B, Gisselbrecht C, Herbrecht R et al. LNH-84 regimen: a multicenter study of intensive chemotherapy in 737 patients with aggressive malignant lymphoma. J Clin Oncol 1989; 7: 1018–1026

272. Nyman R S, Rehn S M, Glimelius B L et al. Residual mediastinal masses in Hodgkin disease: prediction of size with MR imaging. Radiology 1989; 170: 435–440

273. Rahmouni A, Tempany C, Jones R et al. Lymphoma: monitoring tumor size and signal intensity with MR imaging. Radiology 1993; 188: 445–451

274. Rodriguez M. Computed tomography, magnetic resonance imaging and positron emission tomography in non-Hodgkin's lymphoma. Acta Radiol Suppl 1998; 417: 1–36

275. Drossman S R, Schiff R G, Kronfeld G D et al. Lymphoma of the mediastinum and neck: evaluation with Ga-67 imaging and CT correlation. Radiology 1990; 174: 171–175

276. Israel O, Front D, Epelbaum R et al. Residual mass and negative gallium scintigraphy in treated lymphoma. J Nucl Med 1990; 31: 365–368

277. Weiner M, Leventhal B, Cantor A et al. Gallium-67 scans as an adjunct to computed tomography scans for the assessment of a residual mediastinal mass in pediatric patients with Hodgkin's disease. A Pediatric Oncology Group study. Cancer 1991; 68: 2478–2480

278. Front D, Ben Haim S, Israel O et al. Lymphoma: predictive value of Ga-67 scintigraphy after treatment. Radiology 1992; 182: 359–363

279. Cremerius U, Fabry U, Neuerburg J et al. Positron emission tomography with ^{18}F-FDG to detect residual disease after therapy for malignant lymphoma. Nucl Med Commun 1998; 19: 1055–1063

280. de Wit M, Bumann D, Beyer W et al. Whole-body positron emission tomography (PET) for diagnosis of residual mass in patients with lymphoma. Ann Oncol 1997; 8(Suppl. 1): 57–60

281. Jerusalem G, Beguin Y, Fassotte M F et al. Whole-body positron emission tomography using ^{18}F-fluorodeoxyglucose for posttreatment evaluation in Hodgkin's disease and non-Hodgkin's lymphoma has higher diagnostic and prognostic value than classical computed tomography scan imaging. Blood 1999; 94: 429–433

282. Naumann R, Vaic A, Beuthien-Baumann B et al. Prognostic value of positron emission tomography in the evaluation of post-treatment residual mass in patients with Hodgkin's disease and non-Hodgkin's lymphoma. Br J Haematol 2001; 115: 793–800

283. Schoder H, Meta J, Yap C et al. Effect of whole-body (18)F-FDG PET imaging on clinical staging and management of patients with malignant lymphoma. J Nucl Med 2001; 42: 1139–1143

284. Weihrauch M R, Re D, Scheidhauer K et al. Thoracic positron emission tomography using ^{18}F-fluorodeoxyglucose for the evaluation of residual mediastinal Hodgkin disease. Blood 2001; 98: 2930–2934

285. Bakheet S M, Powe J. Benign causes of 18-FDG uptake on whole body imaging. Semin Nucl Med 1998; 28: 352–358

286. Van Den B B, Lambert B, De Winter F et al. [18]FDG PET versus high-dose ^{67}Ga scintigraphy for restaging and treatment follow-up of lymphoma patients. Nucl Med Commun 2002; 23: 1079–1083

287. Zinzani P L, Chierichetti F, Zompatori M et al. Advantages of positron emission tomography (PET) with respect to computed tomography in the follow-up of lymphoma patients with abdominal presentation. Leuk Lymphoma 2002; 43: 1239–1243

288. Gasparini M, Bombardieri E, Castellani M et al. Gallium-67 scintigraphy evaluation of therapy in non-Hodgkin's lymphoma. J Nucl Med 1998; 39: 1586–1590

289. Weeks J C, Yeap B Y, Canellos G P, Shipp M A. Value of follow-up procedures in patients with large-cell lymphoma who achieve a complete remission. J Clin Oncol 1991; 9: 1196–1203

290. Setoain F J, Pons F, Herranz R et al. [67]Ga scintigraphy for the evaluation of recurrences and residual masses in patients with lymphoma. Nucl Med Commun 1997; 18: 405–411

291. Radford J A, Eardley A, Woodman C, Crowther D. Follow up policy after treatment for Hodgkin's disease: too many clinic visits and routine tests? A review of hospital records. Br Med J 1997; 314: 343–346

292. Elis A, Blickstein D, Klein O et al. Detection of relapse in non-Hodgkin's lymphoma: role of routine follow-up studies. Am J Hematol 2002; 69: 41–44

293. Whelan J S, Reznek R H, Daniell S J et al. Computed tomography (CT) and ultrasound (US) guided core biopsy in the management of non-Hodgkin's lymphoma. Br J Cancer 1991; 63: 460–462

294. Pappa V I, Hussain H K, Reznek R H et al. Role of image-guided core-needle biopsy in the management of patients with lymphoma. J Clin Oncol 1996; 14: 2427–2430

295. Ben Yehuda D, Polliack A, Okon E et al. Image-guided core-needle biopsy in malignant lymphoma: experience with 100 patients that suggests the technique is reliable. J Clin Oncol 1996; 14: 2431–2434

Chapter 33

Multiple myeloma

Conor D Collins

Introduction

Multiple myeloma is the third most common form of haematological malignancy after non-Hodgkin's lymphoma and leukaemia, accounting for approximately 14,600 new cases per annum in the USA and almost 3,500 in the UK (58 per million people).[1,2] The condition is rare in Asians but roughly twice as common in Afro-Caribbean ethnic groups compared with Caucasians. The prognosis is poor; the most recent statistics from the USA between 1992–1997 show a relative 5-year survival of only 29% and there has been little improvement in outcome over the last few decades.[2] At any one time in the UK there are about 10,000–15,000 patients with the disease.[3] Multiple myeloma is a disease of later life, with 98% of patients aged 40 or older. The only unequivocal cause of myeloma is exposure to high levels of ionizing radiation. Certain chemical exposures are reported to increase the risk and an increased incidence is seen in agricultural workers.[4]

Multiple myeloma is characterized by uncontrolled proliferation of a single clone of plasma cells within the bone marrow, the cells of the bone marrow that make immunoglobulins (mature antibody-producing B cells). As a result, a monoclonal protein in the form of an intact immunoglobulin (Ig) is produced and secreted (M protein). Immunoglobulin (Ig)G paraprotein is present in 60% of patients, IgA in 20–25% and free immunoglobulin light chains alone in 15–20% of patients. The latter are detectable in the urine as Bence Jones protein; the former are demonstrable by serum protein electrophoresis. The malignant transformation of a single clone of plasma cells is manifest as a monoclonal gammopathy and demonstrable by serum protein electrophoresis. A wide range of chromosomal abnormalities are associated with myeloma, which suggests that when the affected cell becomes malignant, it is already committed to becoming a plasma cell.[5] A striking feature of myeloma is the interaction between myeloma cells, osteoblasts and osteoclasts.[6] Myeloma cells are capable of recruiting osteoclasts to tumour sites and increasing their bone-destroying activity. They also recruit osteoblasts, which help to create a microenvironment that is hospitable to the myeloma cells but inhibits the formation of new bone.[7,8]

Myeloma should not be confused with the condition known as monoclonal gammopathy of undetermined significance (MGUS). In this disease the serum paraprotein level is <3 g/dl with no evidence of myeloma or a related disorder. Although a small percentage of patients with MGUS go on to develop myeloma, most do not. MGUS is not rare and is often detected on a routine screen. It occurs in 1% of people aged over 50 years and in 3% of people aged over 70 years.[9] The risk of MGUS progressing to myeloma or a related condition is low: 16% at 10 years, 33% at 20 years and 40% at 25 years.[9]

The presence of large numbers of plasma cells in the peripheral bloodstream is rare and usually indicates late-stage disease. Where plasma cells are primarily present in the blood and marrow without localized bone lesions the condition is classified as plasma cell leukaemia.[10] Where there is a single tumour (in bone or soft tissue) containing plasma cells and the other features of myeloma are present, this is called a solitary plasmacytoma.[11]

Clinical features

Myeloma may present in a number of different ways. Some patients are asymptomatic, with abnormalities being identified as a result of routine screening or following investigations relating to another illness. Where clinical features are present these may include (singly or together):

- Bone pain – often manifest as persistent unexplained backache associated with loss of height and osteoporosis (especially in men)
- Recurrent or persistent infection – due to impaired production of normal immunoglobulin
- Anaemia – due to accumulation of plasma cells in marrow
- Symptoms of renal impairment – due to tubular protein deposition of M protein
- Symptoms associated with hyperviscosity (impaired vision, purpura, neuropathy), spinal cord compression, hypercalcaemia or amyloidosis. These are less common.

The incidence of various presenting features is shown in Table 33.1.[12]

Diagnosis is based on laboratory and radiographical findings and depends on three abnormal results:

Table 33.1. *Incidence of presenting features of myeloma*

Presenting feature	%
≥40 years old	98
Proteinuria	88
Monoclonal heavy chain on serum immunoelectrophoresis	83
Skeletal radiographic abnormalities	79
Spike on serum protein electrophoresis	76
Spike on urinary electrophoresis	75
Bone pain	68
Anaemia	62
Men	61
Renal insufficiency	55
Bence Jones proteinuria	49
Hypercalcaemia	30
Hepatomegaly	21

- Bone marrow containing >15% plasma cells (normally no more than 4% of the cells in the bone marrow are plasma cells)
- Generalized osteopenia and/or lytic bone deposits on plain film radiography
- Blood serum and/or urine containing an abnormal protein

Normal blood contains a mixture of immunoglobulin of different types (IgM, IgG, IgA, IgD, IgE) and specificities. After protein separation (electrophoresis) these show up as various bands or spikes. When most or all of the immunoglobulin present is of one type, this will produce a single band on separation. The presence of such a band is called paraproteinaemia or a monoclonal spike or M band. In about 75% of all cases of multiple myeloma the paraprotein present will correspond with one type of immunoglobulin. The disease may therefore be referred to as IgG, IgA, IgD or IgE myeloma. IgD myeloma is rarely seen. In about 60% of cases an abnormal protein, known as Bence Jones protein, may also be found in the urine. Measuring the amount of paraprotein in the blood or urine is of value in the diagnosis of myeloma and in monitoring the response to treatment.

Treatment

Treatment strategy is directed towards adequate analgesia, rehydration, management of hypercalcaemia and renal impairment, and treatment of infection. Chemotherapy is indicated for management of symptomatic myeloma. Oral melphalan and prednisolone produce a greater than 50% reduction in paraprotein concentration in 50% of patients. Combination regimens are more effective in younger

patients and may produce a higher response rate (up to 70% of patients). In recent years thalidomide has been recognized as a valuable drug for the treatment of myeloma.[13] The most serious morbidity invariably results from destructive bone deposits, which cause severe intractable pain, pathological fractures and often deformity and disability. The introduction of the bisphosphonate group of drugs has transformed this aspect of the condition. They bind to bone at sites of active bone remodelling and can therefore inhibit myelomatous bone damage.[14] Autologous transplantation has an established place in the treatment of myeloma. It is the treatment of choice for patients under the age of 60 and should be considered for those aged between 60 and 70 who have a good performance status. The mortality from donor stem cell transplantation has decreased with improved conditioning regimens and this option is now frequently considered for patients under the age of 50, particularly women (who have a lower transplant-related mortality rate than men). In the UK a set of guidelines on all aspects of the diagnosis and treatment of myeloma has been published by the UK Myeloma Forum,[3] with the support of the British Committee for Standards in Haematology.

Myeloma is generally considered to be incurable. It is a slowly progressing disease with long periods of relative inactivity. Relapse occurs in virtually all cases. The median survival with conventional therapy is about 3 years, whilst stem cell transplantation can achieve a median survival rate of more than 5 years.[15]

Key points: general features

- Multiple myeloma is an uncontrolled proliferation of a clone of plasma cells

- Myeloma is characterized by (1) plasma cell proliferation of the bone marrow, (2) lytic bone deposits and (3) myeloma protein in the serum or urine

- Myeloma should not be confused with MGUS

Staging

The staging system devised by Durie and Salmon is the most widely used (Table 33.2).[16] This system is based on the serum concentration of haemoglobin, calcium and paraprotein, urinary Bence Jones protein excretion and the number of skeletal lesions seen on plain radiographs.

Radiology and cross-sectional imaging

Radiology plays an important role in staging, monitoring treatment response, detection of relapse, and assessing

Table 33.2. *Durie and Salmon staging system for multiple myeloma*

Stage[1]	Criteria	Cell mass
I	All of the following:	Low
	Haemoglobin >10 g/100 ml	<0.6 × 10^{12} cells per mm^2
	Normal serum calcium <12 mg/100 ml	
	Normal bone structure or solitary bone lesion only on radiography	
	Low M component production rates IgG <5 g/100 ml IgA <3 g/100 ml Urine light chain M component on electrophoresis <4 g/24 hr	
II	Fitting neither Stage I nor Stage III	Intermediate
III	One or more of the following:	High
	Haemoglobin <8.5 g/100 ml	>1.2 × 10^{12} cells per mm^2
	Serum calcium >12 mg/100 ml	
	Advanced lytic bone lesion	
	High M component production rates IgG >7 g/100 ml IgA >5 g/100 ml Urine light chain M component on electrophoresis >12 g/24 hr	

[1] Subclassifications: A = relatively normal renal function (serum creatinine value <20 mg/100 ml [175 mmol/l]); B = abnormal renal function (serum creatinine value >20 mg/100 ml [175 mmol/l]).

complications. The various imaging techniques employed and their associated findings are described more fully later. The radiological features of multiple myeloma versus bone metastases are shown in Table 33.3.

Plain film radiography

Almost 80% of patients with multiple myeloma will have radiological evidence of skeletal involvement and the plain film radiograph (skeletal survey) is the best method of identifying lytic deposits within bone.[9] The most common sites include the vertebrae, ribs, skull, and pelvis, whereas involvement of the distal bones is unusual (Figs. 33.1–33.3). Sites involved include:

- Vertebrae (66% of patients)
- Ribs (45%)
- Skull (40%)
- Shoulder (40%)
- Pelvis (30%)
- Long bones (25%)

Myeloma lesions are sharply defined, small lytic areas (average size 20 mm) of bone destruction with no reactive bone formation. At postmortem these lesions are due to nodular replacement of marrow and bone by plasma cells. Although myeloma arises within the medulla, disease progression may produce infiltration of the cortex, invasion of the periosteum and large extra-osseous soft tissue masses. The pattern of destruction may be geographic, moth eaten or permeated. Pathological fractures are common (Fig. 33.2).[17]

Generalized osteopenia may be the only bone manifestation of myeloma in up to 15% of patients. At postmortem these patients show diffuse replacement of marrow with plasma cells but have less severe bone resorption when compared with lytic deposits.[17] Vertebral body collapse is the usual manifestation of this subtype, which should not

Table 33.3. *Multiple myeloma vs. bone metastases*

Radiological features	Multiple myeloma	Bone metastases
Involvement of intervertebral discs	Yes	No
Involvement of mandible	Yes	No
Involvement of vertebral pedicles	No	Yes
Associated paraspinal soft tissue mass	Yes	No
Isotope bone scan	Frequently negative	Frequently positive

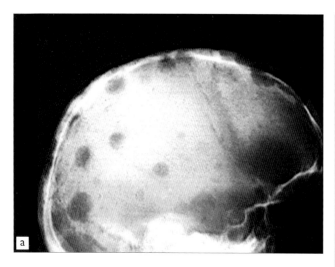

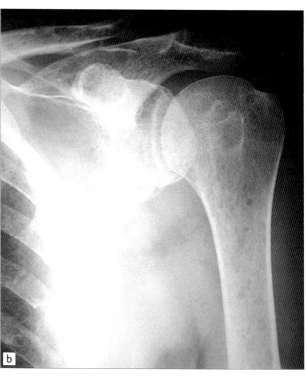

Figure 33.1. *(a) Plain radiograph of skull (lateral view) demonstrating multiple lytic deposits. (b) Plain radiograph of left shoulder demonstrating multiple lytic deposits in left humerus, clavicle and scapula.*

be confused with non-myelomatous osteoporosis, which occurs in many older patients. Normal bone surveys are noted in 10% of myeloma patients, though this has not always been associated with an improved rate of survival.[18]

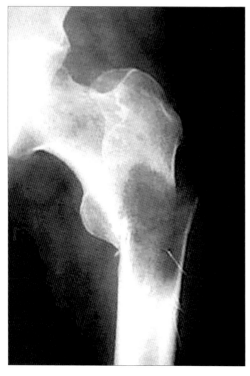

Figure 33.2. *Plain radiograph of proximal left femur (AP view) demonstrating a large lytic deposit associated with a pathological fracture.*

Radionuclide imaging

Plain film radiography can significantly underestimate the extent and magnitude of bone and bone marrow involvement. Technetium-99m (^{99m}Tc)-labelled diphosphonate is adsorbed onto the hydroxyapatite crystals of bone, depending on the degree of osteoblastic activity. However, in multiple myeloma the osteoblastic response to bone destruction is negligible. The bone scan is often therefore normal or may show areas of decreased uptake (photopenia) (Fig. 33.3). Most studies have shown that the sensitivity of skeletal scintigraphy for detecting individual deposits ranges from 40–60%.[19,20] However, skeletal scintigraphy may be helpful in evaluating areas not well visualized on plain film radiographs such as the ribs and the sternum.

^{99m}-Technetium-2-methoxy-2-isobutyl-isonitrile (^{99m}Tc-MIBI) has been shown to be superior to plain film radiography and skeletal scintigraphy in detecting bone and bone marrow involvement.[21,22] Alterations in cell metabolism that occur in malignant cells (including plasma cells) can affect the membrane potential of the cell wall and mitochondrion, leading to accumulation of ^{99m}Tc-MIBI within the cell.[23] Different patterns of ^{99m}Tc-MIBI uptake have been described with multiple myeloma (negative, diffuse, focal, combined focal, and diffuse) and semi-quantitative evaluation of these patterns showed a significant correlation with clinical status and stage of the disease.[24] A negative scan in a patient with multiple myeloma indicates early-stage disease or post-treatment remission, while the presence of focal uptake and/or intense diffuse bone marrow uptake suggests an advanced stage of active disease (91% of patients with a positive scan had active myeloma). The semi-quantitative score of diffuse ^{99m}Tc-MIBI bone

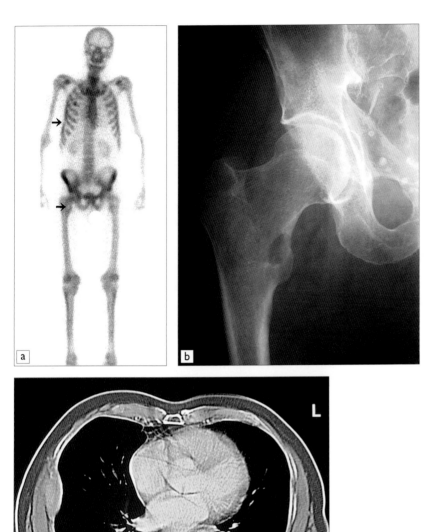

Figure 33.3. *(a) Technetium-99m diphosphonate isotope bone scan showing photopenic regions affecting mid-right rib (arrow) and lesser trochanter of right femur (arrow). There is also a recent fracture affecting third right anterior rib. (b) Plain radiograph confirms presence of lytic deposit in lesser trochanter of right femur. (c) CT scan demonstrates an expansile myelomatous deposit arising from mid-right rib.*

marrow uptake (based on intensity and extension of uptake) correlates with the amount of monoclonal component and percentage of bone marrow plasma cells. These results suggested a potential role for ^{99m}Tc-MIBI in the prognosis and follow-up of patients with multiple myeloma (currently based on measurement of the monoclonal component, skeletal survey and bone marrow biopsy). A subsequent follow-up study involving 22 patients showed a significant correlation between the scintigraphic findings and clinical status post chemotherapy.[25]

Thallium-201 has also been described in multiple myeloma but due to limitations of the isotope, its use has not been widespread nor has it been shown to be superior to ^{99m}Tc-MIBI.[26,27]

Positron emission tomography (PET) using the glucose analogue fluorine-18 fluorodeoxyglucose (^{18}FDG PET) has both the functional and morphological capacity to identify the extent and activity of multiple myeloma for staging and monitoring purposes. The ability of PET to perform whole-body examinations is a major advantage over conventional imaging techniques. In one series comprising 28 patients, PET was true positive in almost 93% of the radiographically documented osteolytic deposits and demonstrated a greater extent of disease than plain film radiography in 61% of patients.[28] Another recent study confirmed the reliability of PET in detecting active myeloma both within bone and in extramedullary sites, and its ability to differentiate between new active disease and inactive (treated) sites.[29] PET is extremely useful in the evaluation of non-secretory myeloma and in identifying patients with a poor prognosis (residual myeloma post stem cell transplantation and extramedullary myeloma). A negative ^{18}F-FDG PET strongly supports the diagnosis of MGUS.[29] Positron emission tomography scanning is complementary to plain film radiography, CT and MRI because anatomical assessment of myeloma deposits will still be necessary. However, PET/CT provides combined morphological and functional information and thus this dual-modality scanner is likely to have an important role in staging and follow-up of patients with multiple myeloma.

Key points: radiological and radionuclide features

- Almost 80% of patients have radiographic evidence of skeletal disease

- Vertebral deposits are present in 66% of patients

- Bone deposits are typically small (20 mm) and sharply defined with no reactive bone formation

- Conventional bone scintigraphy may be helpful in evaluating the ribs and sternum

- Different patterns of ^{99m}Tc-MIBI uptake have been described, which correlates with the clinical status and stage of disease

- [18]FDG PET reliably detects active myeloma within bone and at extramedullary sites

- A negative ^{18}F-FDG indicates MGUS

Cross-sectional imaging

Computed tomography

CT is a well-established but rarely used technique for imaging multiple myeloma.[30] Unlike plain radiographs, where approximately 50% of bone must be resorbed or destroyed in order to visualize bone destruction, CT can detect small lytic deposits. CT is not suitable as a screening imaging technique in myeloma due to limited power of the X-ray tube and the necessity to have collimation >5 mm to cover the large volume required. Most reports concern the use of axial CT images for analysing small, well-defined regions of the spine. It enables more precise analysis of bone destruction and assessment of the presence and extent of soft tissue involvement than plain radiographs. CT can be used to direct needle biopsy for histological diagnosis. A wide range of CT findings in bone have been described in multiple myeloma. These include sharp, lytic foci of small and relatively homogeneous size with no sclerotic rim, diffuse faint osteolysis, an angioma-like appearance due to the presence of thickened vertical trabeculae and expansile deposits (Fig. 33.3).[31,32] Myelomatous bone marrow often shows an abnormally high attenuation value compared with normal marrow. Discrete interruption of the cortical contour may be seen.

For detection of small lytic bone deposits of <1 cm, narrow collimation protocols at a high tube current and tube voltage are mandatory, because these parameters determine the resolution and image noise. This has been a limiting factor in the widespread use of helical CT. Recent advances in X-ray tube technology with high heat storage capacities enable examination of the whole spine to be undertaken. Simultaneous acquisition of multiple slices per rotation allows scanning time to be shortened significantly to less than 1 minute for a complete body scan. Patient cooperation is also markedly improved, particularly in those with advanced disease and severe back pain.

A recent study using multidetector CT (MDCT) in patients with Stage III myeloma provided more detailed information on the risk of vertebral fractures compared with plain film radiography and MRI (Fig. 33.4). Upward stage migration occurred in 17% of patients.[33] MDCT also allows for improved imaging of patients with scoliosis due to its ability to adapt the data set to the individual patient's features. As the degree of osseous infiltration in myeloma has a significant influence on therapy it is likely there will be an increasing role for this technique in patients who are severely disabled or who are unable to undergo an MRI examination. As most patients are elderly, dose considerations are not a major drawback and its ability to image well the ribs, sternum, shoulders, and sacrum in addition to the fact that IV contrast is not necessary makes it a realistic alternative in the clinical scenarios outlined earlier.

Key points: computed tomography features

- CT allows more precise assessment of bone destruction than plain radiographs or MRI

- CT can accurately depict the presence and extent of an associated soft tissue mass

- CT is helpful for performing percutaneous biopsy

- Multidetector CT allows high-quality sagittal imaging of the spine to be performed

Magnetic resonance imaging

Magnetic resonance imaging is used routinely in many centres as a diagnostic technique due to its high sensitivity and ability to directly visualize bone marrow. In patients with suspected epidural involvement it is the examination of first choice. Bone deposits have been shown by MRI in about 50% of asymptomatic myeloma patients with normal plain radiographs. Nonetheless, despite the increased availability of MRI, plain film radiography retains an important role in myeloma.[34]

Sagittal MRI studies of the spine enable screening of a

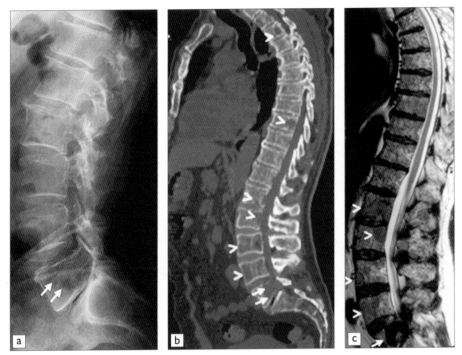

Figure 33.4. *68-year-old man with newly diagnosed multiple myeloma, Stage III (Durie and Salmon criteria). (a) Lateral radiograph of lumbar spine corresponding to multidetector CT (MDCT) and MR image shows large osteolytic deposit affecting L5 (arrows). Further deposits >1 cm in diameter in lumbar spine and in T3 and T9 are not recognizable on conventional radiographs. (b) Multidetector CT scan reconstruction in the sagittal plane depicts deposits with diameter <10 mm in L5 (arrows) as well as L1–L4, T3 and T9 (arrowheads). Diffuse osteopenia or deposits with diameters between 5 mm and 1 cm are visible in all vertebrae depicted. Depression of the vertebral end-plate is visible in L1. (c) Sagittal T2-weighted MR image shows tumour infiltration of all depicted vertebrae. Lesions >1 cm in lumbar spine (arrowheads), especially in L5 (arrow), are clearly depicted. (From Ref 33, with permission).*

high proportion of haematopoietic marrow in a limited time and detection of any potential threat to the spinal cord. Additional coronal images of the pelvis and proximal femora enable evaluation of about an extra one third of red marrow in an adult. These images may enable detection of deposits potentially at risk of fracture. Total body MRI can be performed but its clinical benefit has not yet been fully evaluated in myeloma.

The imaging patterns in multiple myeloma can be classified as follows:[35,36]

- Normal
- Focal
- Diffuse
- Variegated

Normal marrow is present on MRI at diagnosis in 50–75% of patients with early untreated (Stage I) myeloma and in about 20% of patients with advanced and treated (Stage III) disease. Monoclonal plasma cells arrange themselves so as not to displace the fat cells and the ratio of haematopoietic (and myeloma) to fat cells in bone marrow does not exceed that of healthy individuals.[37] In adults between 40 and 70 years old, haematopoietic marrow is composed of

approximately 20–25% bone substance, 40–45% fat and 30–35% cellular marrow.[38]

The focal pattern consists of localized areas of decreased signal intensity on T1-weighted images and increased signal intensity on T2-weighted images or on short tau inversion recovery (STIR) sequences (Fig. 33.5). Myelomatous deposits are generally sharply demarcated on a background of an otherwise normal-appearing bone marrow. Homogeneous enhancement occurs on T1-weighted images following IV contrast medium injection.

The diffuse pattern is characterized by diffuse and homogeneous decrease in marrow signal intensity, which becomes identical to or lower than that of adjacent intervertebral discs on T1-weighted images. On T2-weighted or on STIR images there is diffuse or patchy increase in signal intensity (Fig. 33.6a). Marked enhancement is usually seen on T1-weighted images following IV contrast. The increased contrast between enhancing marrow and the lower signal intervertebral discs allows more subtle forms of infiltration to be identified.[39]

The variegated pattern is characterized by the presence of multiple foci of low signal intensity on T1-weighted images, intermediate to high signal intensity on T2-weighted images and enhancement following IV contrast

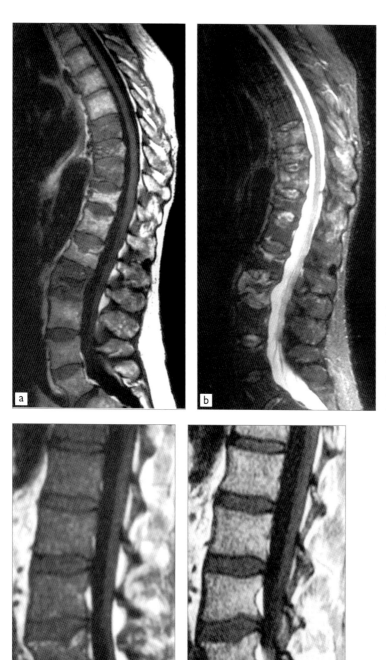

Figure 33.5. *MR images of thoracic and lumbar spine prior to treatment (sagittal view using a phase array coil). (a) T1-weighted spin-echo sequence. (b) Fat suppression STIR sequence. There is partial collapse of several thoracic and lumbar vertebrae, many of which have low signal intensity on T1 and high signal intensity on STIR, representing active disease.*

Figure 33.6. *(a) Sagittal T1-weighted MR image of lumbar spine pre-transplantation, demonstrating diffuse abnormal low signal intensity in vertebral bodies. (b) Sagittal T1-weighted MR image of lumbar spine post-transplantation shows conversion to normal high signal marrow. (From ref 52, with permission).*

T1-weighted images. This pattern is seen almost exclusively in an early stage of the disease.[40]

These patterns of marrow involvement do not seem to correlate with the interstitial, nodular and diffuse patterns of marrow infiltration seen at microscopy. However, they show a positive correlation with some laboratory parameters. Patients with the normal and variegated patterns tend to have a lower tumour burden than those with the focal and diffuse marrow involvement patterns. Higher cellularity, higher plasmacytosis and more severe signs of bone failure are usually found in patients with the diffuse pattern.[41]

The lack of specificity of the MRI patterns of myelomatous disease should be noted. The focal and diffuse patterns may be observed in both metastatic disease from primary solid tumours and in other haematological malignancies, especially lymphoma and leukaemia. Differentiation between red marrow hyperplasia secondary to anaemia, infection, malignant or treated marrow infiltration can be extremely difficult. Normal marrow heterogeneities may mimic the variegated pattern. However in most cases, high signal intensity on T2-weighted images and contrast enhancement on T1-weighted images help distinguish bone marrow abnormalities from normal haematopoietic foci. The latter usually show an intermediate signal intensity on T2-weighted images and no contrast enhancement on T1-weighted images.

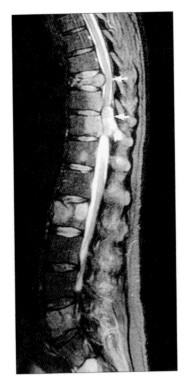

Figure 33.7. *Sagittal MRI STIR image of the spine, showing malignant vertebral body compression at T9 and T11 in addition to cord compression at these sites (arrows).*

Key points: magnetic resonance imaging findings

- MR imaging shows bone abnormalities in 50% of asymptomatic patients with normal plain radiographs

- MR imaging patterns can be classified as normal, focal, diffuse, and variegated

- Myeloma deposits are of low signal intensity on T1 weighting and high signal intensity on T2 weighting

- Myeloma deposits enhance with IV contrast medium

- There is no correlation between MRI and microscopic patterns of infiltration

- The MRI patterns are not specific and may be observed in both metastatic disease from primary solid tumours and other haematological malignancies

Compression fractures in multiple myeloma

Compression fractures arise from extensive osteoclastic bone resorption or replacement of bone by a growing plasma cell tumour mass. Several criteria exist for differentiating benign from malignant vertebral body compression fractures[4] (Table 33.4, Fig. 33.7). However, these criteria should be applied with caution to patients with multiple myeloma as normal signal intensity within a compressed vertebral body on spinal MR images does not preclude the

diagnosis of multiple myeloma. In a study of 224 vertebral fractures in patients with known multiple myeloma, Lecouvet et al found that 67% appeared benign on MRI and 38% of their 37 patients had benign fractures only at diagnosis.[42]

In patients with osteoporotic or post-traumatic vertebral compression of recent onset, MRI will usually show signal alteration that parallels one of the end-plates, involves less than half of the vertebral body, does not extend to the pedicles and enhances homogeneously following IV contrast. Diffusion-weighted MRI may also prove to be a useful method to apply to the differential diagnosis of compression fractures.[43]

Patients being treated for multiple myeloma may suffer acute back pain secondary to vertebral body collapse, even after effective chemotherapy. This is due to resolution of the tumour mass that was supporting the bony cortex. On the post-treatment images of 29 patients with multiple

Table 33.4. *MRI criteria for the differential diagnosis of benign versus malignant vertebral fractures*[45]

Variable	Osteoporotic fractures	Malignant fractures
Marrow signal	Normal on all sequences (old fracture) Band-like low single intensity (SI) adjacent to fracture (acute) Normal SI preserved opposite the fractured end-plate	Diffusely low on T1-weighted images High or heterogeneous on T2-weighted images Round or irregular foci of marrow replacement Posterior elements involved Soft tissues/epidural involvement
Contrast enhancement	Homogeneous 'return to normal' SI after injection	High or heterogeneous
Vertebral contours	Retropulsion of a posterior bone fragment (often posterosuperior)	Convex posterior cortex

myeloma in remission, 35 new vertebral compression fractures were discovered.[44] In another study, 131 vertebral compression fractures appeared in 37 patients with multiple myeloma after the onset of therapy.[43] Conversely, progression of disease may also be responsible for a new compression fracture and MRI may be useful in differentiating between these two clinical settings. It has been shown that patients with either normal marrow appearance or <10 focal lesions on pre-treatment MR images had significantly longer fracture-free survival times than patients with >10 focal lesions or with diffuse patterns on pre-treatment MR images.[41]

Key points: compression fractures

■ Criteria for differentiating benign and malignant vertebral compression fractures should be applied with caution in patients with multiple myeloma

■ New compression fractures may arise following treatment as a result of resolving soft tissue masses that formerly supported bone

■ Compression fractures occur significantly less frequently in patients with a normal MRI pattern or less than ten focal deposits

Assessment of response to treatment and post-treatment evaluation

For many years, treatment of multiple myeloma relied on a combination of melphalan and prednisone and then, during the last decade, various other multiagent combination chemotherapy regimens have undergone clinical trials. However none of these regimens has made a significant impact on outcome, with reported 5-year survival rates of only about 25%.[46]

Recently development of high-dose myeloablative chemotherapy in combination with haematopoietic growth factors and with marrow or blood stem cell transplantation led to a substantial improvement in response rate and relapse-free and overall survival rates.[47] The addition of bisphosphonate compounds as antiosteoclast agents leads to bone strengthening, which may become evident on plain film radiographs.

The role of radiology in the assessment of treatment response is limited and sequential quantification of biological markers of disease (monoclonal protein levels and bone marrow plasmacytosis) are sufficient to assess response to chemotherapy. On plain film radiography, shrinking or sclerosing deposits indicate a response to therapy. Persistence of radiological abnormalities should not be considered evidence of active disease, since they may represent residual osteolysis in the absence of plasma cell proliferation. Although conventional skeletal scintigraphy is not routinely performed, the presence of abnormal uptake has been shown to indicate residual activity.[20] A more recent study, reported by Pace et al. in 2001, demonstrated conversion from a positive to negative isotope scan using ^{99m}Tc-MIBI in successfully treated patients.[25] [18]FDG PET can also differentiate between active and treated sites of disease.[29]

Computed tomography

Disappearance of soft tissue masses and reappearance of a continuous cortical contour and of a fatty marrow content may be observed in treated lytic lesions.

Magnetic resonance imaging

Interpretation of post-treatment MRI changes can be difficult as there is a wide spectrum of possible treatment-induced changes on MRI depending on the pattern of bone marrow infiltration (Fig. 33.8). There has also been little long-term follow-up of these patients. Changes in contrast enhancement between the pre- and post-treatment MRI examinations have been studied. The lack of lesion enhancement or only a peripheral rim enhancement seen after treatment can be indicative of responsive deposits. Focal marrow lesions may remain identical or decrease in size.[44,48,49] Local radiation therapy of focal complex deposits induces a rapid decrease in the soft tissue extension and appearance of presumably necrotic, avascular central areas within the deposit on T1-weighted images, with a later decrease in lesion size.[50]

In diffuse marrow abnormalities, increased marrow signal is usually observed on post-treatment T1-weighted images due to reappearance of fat cells within more hydrated cellular components. Conversion of a diffuse to a focal or variegated pattern is also frequent.[44] Post-treatment MRI of the bone marrow may provide important information in patients with equivocal clinical and laboratory results as well as in patients with non-secretory myeloma.

After bone marrow transplantation, bone marrow generally has a high signal intensity on T1-weighted images but focal residual deposits are frequent (Fig. 33.6).[51] The prognostic significance of these abnormalities is uncertain. In one series, patients with residual bone marrow abnormalities did not have a poorer outcome than those with normal post-transplantation MRI scans.[52] Increased marrow cellularity due to marrow-stimulating factors and decreased signal intensity due to marrow haemosiderosis resulting from repeated transfusions may also be present on post-transplantation MR images. Distinction between all these pathophysiological processes may be impossible on MRI.

Key points: assessment of response and post-treatment evaluation

■ The role of radiology in assessment of treatment is limited

■ Sequential analysis of biological markers is more frequently employed

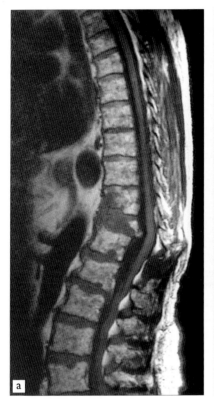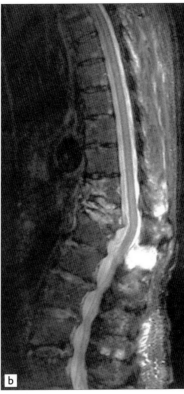

Figure 33.8. *MR images of the thoracic and lumbar spine following chemotherapy (sagittal view using phased array coil). (a) T1-weighted spin-echo sequence. (b) Fat suppression STIR sequence. There is a complete collapse of T11 vertebral body associated with posterior displacement of the spinal cord. The increased signal intensity on the STIR sequence within T10, T11 and T12 indicates active disease in this region. The lack of increased signal within the remaining vertebrae indicates inactive disease.*

- Both plain film radiographs and CT demonstrate shrinkage of lytic deposits and sclerosis in patients responding to treatment

- A wide spectrum of findings is present on post-treatment MRI scans

- Conversion of diffuse to a focal or variegated pattern on MRI scans is frequent

- Lack of contrast enhancement on MRI scans can be indicative of responsive deposits

- Focal residual deposits are frequent on MRI scans following bone marrow transplantation

- Marrow deposits post transplantation are not necessarily associated with a poorer outcome

Relationship of radiology to laboratory values and prognosis

Plain film radiographs retain a key role for staging patients with newly diagnosed myeloma. The clinical staging system devised by Durie and Salmon distinguishes different patient subgroups in terms of tumour mass and disease aggression and is still used to determine management.[16] Patients with at least two lytic foci are classified in advanced disease subgroups and aggressive systemic treatment is usually indicated. Although absence of lytic deposits on skeletal radiography is associated with a lower stage and improved survival, Smith et al. found only 11% of such patients were alive at 3 years. In that study patients with osteopenia alone and those with extensive lytic deposits had an intermediate survival rate of 32% and 33% at 3 years, respectively, whereas the 3-year survival rate was 44% in patients with minimum lytic changes.[18]

In early asymptomatic stages of the disease with no (or only one) lytic deposit(s) on plain film radiographs, patients with relevant abnormalities at MRI have a significantly shorter time lag before the onset of more aggressive disease than those with normal-appearing marrow at MRI.[34,40,53] As stated previously, patients with the normal and variegated patterns tend to have a lower tumour burden than those with the focal and diffuse marrow involvement patterns. Higher cellularity, higher plasmacytosis and more severe signs of bone failure are usually found in patients with the diffuse pattern.[41] In patients with advanced-stage disease, those with normal MRI findings at diagnosis have better response to conventional chemotherapy with a longer survival rate than those with focal or diffuse marrow abnormalities at MRI treated with conventional chemotherapy.[39] This feature has not yet been assessed in patients treated with marrow transplantation.

In the spine and pelvis, MRI consistently demonstrated more numerous marrow lesions and more patients with marrow involvement than the corresponding conventional radiographs.[54] Despite the superiority of MRI over plain radiographs for spinal and pelvic lesion detection, an MRI survey limited to these areas may be less sensitive than the conventional skeletal survey, which may detect deposits in the skull and ribs.[54]

In patients with a solitary bone plasmacytoma, MR screening of the spine and pelvis will usually reveal radiographically unsuspected deposits in up to 80% of patients, thus suggesting true myeloma from the outset. This finding is associated with a poor response to localized radiotherapy and earlier development of systemic disease than in patients with a negative MRI survey.[55]

High levels of serum beta-2 microglobulin correlate with a poor prognosis and remain the single most powerful determinant of outcome.[56] No correlation between this finding and appearances on MRI has yet been demonstrated.

Long-term prospective studies are required to establish the significance and prognostic value of the different MRI patterns of marrow involvement and their correlation with various laboratory values, particularly in patients undergoing transplantation.

Key points: radiology and laboratory tests

- Patients with at least two lytic deposits on skeletal survey are classified as having advanced disease

- Asymptomatic patients with abnormal MRI are at significant risk of early disease progression

- Patients with normal and variegated patterns on MRI tend to have a lower tumour burden than those with focal and diffuse patterns

- Serum beta-2 microglobulin level is the single most powerful determinant of outcome

- There is no correlation between serum beta microglobulin levels and MRI patterns of marrow infiltration

Complications

The complications of multiple myeloma can be summarized as:

- Spinal cord compression
- Pathological fractures
- Secondary amyloidosis
- Renal impairment
- Predilection for recurrent pneumonia due to leucopenia
- Thromboembolism

A pathological fracture affects about 50% of patients during the course of their disease, with many of the fractures affecting the vertebral bodies. Spinal cord compression resulting from vertebral body collapse may occur in up to 25% of patients and has been described as the presenting feature in 12% of patients (Fig. 33.7).[57–59] Early recognition of back pain and neurological symptoms is essential. Magnetic resonance is the imaging investigation of choice. Fractures of the tubular bones heal readily with normal amounts of callus but extensive fractures may require insertion of intramedullary nails.

Renal impairment is common in myeloma and affects up to half of all patients at some stage in their illness. Up to 20% present with renal failure while 3–12% experience advanced renal failure that requires dialysis or another intervention.[3] This may be a consequence of paraproteinaemia, leading to proximal tubular damage or to protein cast nephropathy. Other possible causes include hypercalcaemia, dehydration, hyperuricaemia, infection or the action of nephrotoxic drugs. Unfortunately several of the drugs that are used to treat myeloma have an adverse effect on kidney function. Secondary amyloid occurs in approximately 10% of cases and in the early stages ultrasound demonstrates enlarged kidneys with increased cortical reflectivity. Amyloid protein is deposited mainly in the cortex so that corticomedullary differentiation is preserved and the pyramids are normal in size.[60] Radiolabelled serum amyloid P component scintigraphy is a non-invasive and quantitative method for imaging amyloid deposits, though it is less effective in myeloma-associated amyloid than other forms of amyloid.[61]

Patients with myeloma have a predilection for recurrent pneumonia due to associated leucopenia. These patients can be assessed using plain chest radiography and thin-section high-resolution CT (HRCT) as required.

The major causes of death in myeloma are recurrent infection, renal impairment and thromboembolism.

Uncommon variants of myeloma

Extra-osseous myeloma
Clinical manifestations of extra-osseous myeloma are rare, occurring in less than 5% of patients with multiple myeloma. Extra-osseous myeloma deposits have been reported at multiple sites, with the breast, lymph nodes and spleen most frequently involved. Extra-osseous myeloma is more aggressive, occurs in a younger age group (average age 50 years) and is associated with a worse rate of survival than conventional myeloma.[62]

Sclerotic myeloma
Primary sclerotic manifestations are rare and occur only in 3% of patients. It may take the form of diffuse osteosclerosis, patchy sclerotic areas throughout the skeleton or very small numbers of focal sclerotic lesions.[63]

Summary

- Multiple myeloma is characterized by the classic triad of bone marrow infiltration by plasma cells, lytic bone deposits on plain film radiographs (skeletal survey) and the presence of M protein in serum or urine.

- The staging system devised by Durie and Salmon is based on serum haematological, urinary Bence Jones protein and skeletal survey findings.

- Myeloma should not be confused with MGUS – the risk of MGUS progressing to myeloma is low (16% at 10 years)

- Several differential points help to (1) distinguish lytic deposits of multiple myeloma from bone metastases, and (2) benign from malignant vertebral compression fractures.

- Multidetector CT is a realistic alternative for spinal imaging in severely disabled patients or those unable to have an MRI scan.

- ^{18}FDG PET reliably detects active myeloma within bone and at extramedullary sites.

- Several different patterns of marrow infiltration appear on MRI – these are not specific and do not correlate with microscopic patterns of infiltration.

- Role of radiology in the assessment of treatment response is limited – sequential analysis of biological markers is preferred.

- Marrow deposits on post-transplantation MRI are not necessarily associated with a poorer outcome.

- Serum beta microglobulin levels are the single most powerful prognostic determinant.

References

1. CancerStats Incidence – UK, April 2003. Cancer Research UK, 2003

2. Cancer Facts & Figures 2003. American Cancer Society Inc., 2003

3. UK Myeloma Forum. The diagnosis and management of multiple myeloma. Br J Haematol 2001; 115: 522–540

4. Nanni O, Falcini F, Buiatti E et al. Multiple myeloma and work in agriculture: results of a case–control study in Forli, Italy. Cancer Causes Control 1998; 9: 277–283

5. Bersgagel P L, Kuehl W M. Chromosome translocations in multiple myeloma. Oncogene 2001; 20: 5611–5622

6. Callander N S, Roodman E D. Myeloma bone in disease. Semin Haematol 2001; 38: 276–285

7. Kanis J A, McCloskey E V. Bisphosphonates in multiple myeloma. Cancer 2000; 88: 3022–3032

8. Roodnam G D. Biology of osteoclastic activation in cancer. J Clin Oncol 2001; 19: 3562–3571

9. Kyle R A. Multiple myeloma, macroglobulinaemia and the monocloncal gammopathies. Curr Pract Med 1999; 2: 1131–1137

10. Costello R, Sainty D, Fermand J P et al. Primary plasma cell leukaemia: a report of 18 cases. Leuk Res 2001; 25: 103–107

11. Dimopoulos M A, Moulopoulos L A, Maniatis A, Alexanian R. Solitary plasmacytoma of bone and asymptomatic multiple myeloma. Blood 2000; 96: 2037–2044

12. Kyle R A. Multiple myeloma: review of 869 cases. Mayo Clin Proc 1975; 50: 29–40

13. Barlogie B, Zangari M, Spencer T et al. Thalidomide in the management of multiple myeloma. Sem Haematol 2001; 38: 250–259

14. Theriault R L, Hortobagyi G N. The evolving role of bisphosphonates. Oncology 2001; 28: 284–290

15. Zaidi A A, Vesole D H. Multiple myeloma: an old disease with new hope for the future. CA: A cancer journal for clinicians 2001; 51: 273–285

16. Durie B G M, Salmon S E. A clinical staging system for multiple myeloma: correlation of measured myeloma cell mass with presenting clinical features, response to treatment and survival. Cancer 1975; 36: 842–854

17. Kapadia S B. Multiple myeloma: a clinicopathologic study of 62 consecutively autopsied cases. Medicine 1980; 59: 380–392

18. Smith D B, Scarffe J H, Eddleston B. The prognostic significance of X-ray changes at presentation and reassessment in patients with multiple myeloma. Haematol Oncol 1988; 6: 1–6

19. Ludwig H, Kupman W, Sinzinger H. Radiography and bone scintigraphy in multiple myeloma: a comparative analysis. Br J Radiol 1982; 55: 173–181

20. Bataille R, Chevalier J, Rossi M, Sany J. Bone scintigraphy in plasma cell myeloma. A prospective study of 70 patients. Radiology 1982; 145: 801–804

21. Catalano L, Pace L, Califano C et al. Detection of focal myeloma lesions by Tc-99m sestaMIBI scintigraphy. Haematologica 1999; 84: 119–124

22. Alexandrakis M G, Kyriakou D S, Passam F et al. Value of Tc-99m sestamibi scintigraphy in the detection of bone lesions in multiple myeloma: comparison with Tc99m methylene diphosphonate. Ann Haematol 2001; 80: 349–363

23. Fonti R, Del Vecchio S, Zannetti A et al. Bone marrow uptake of Tc-99m MIBI in patients with multiple myeloma. Eur J Nucl Med 2001; 28: 214–220

24. Pace L, Catalano L, Pinto A M et al. Different patterns of

technetium 99m-sestamibi uptake in multiple myeloma. Eur J Nucl Med 1998; 25: 714–720

25. Pace L, Catalano L, Del Vecchio S et al. Predictive value of technetium-99m sestamibi in patients with multiple myeloma and potential role in follow-up. Eur J Nucl Med 2001; 28: 304–312

26. Ishibashi M, Nonoshita M, Uchida M. Bone marrow uptake of thallium-201 before and after therapy in multiple myeloma. J Nucl Med 1998; 39: 473–476

27. Chun K A, Cho I H, Won K C et al. Comparison of Tc99m MIBI and Tl-201 uptake in multiple myeloma. Clin Nucl Med 2001; 26: 212–215

28. Schirrmeister H, Bommer L, Buck A K et al. Initial results in the assessment of multiple myeloma using ^{18}F-FDG PET. Eur J Nucl Med Molec Imag 2002; 29: 361–366

29. Durie B G M, Waxman A D, D'Agnolo A, Williams C M. Whole body ^{18}F-FDG PET identifies high risk myeloma. J Nucl Med 2002; 43: 1457–1463

30. Schreiman J S, McLeod R A, Kyle R A, Beabout J W. Multiple myeloma: evaluation by CT. Radiology 1985; 154: 483–486

31. Helms C A, Genant H K. Computed tomography in the early detection of skeletal involvement with multiple myeloma. J Am Med Assoc 1982; 248: 2886–2887

32. Laroche M, Assoun J, Sixou L, Attal M. Comparison of MRI and computed tomography in the various stages of plasma cell disorders: correlations with biological and histological findings. Clin Exp Rheumatol 1996; 14: 171–176

33. Mahnken A H, Wildberger J E, Gehbauer G et al. Multidetector CT of the spine in multiple myeloma: comparison with MR imaging and radiography. Am J Roentgenol 2002; 178: 1429–1436

34. Moulopoulos L A, Dimopoulos M A, Smith T L. Prognostic significance of magnetic resonance imaging in patients with asymptomatic multiple myeloma. J Clin Oncol 1995; 13: 251–256

35. Dimopoulos M A, Moulopoulos L A, Datseris I et al. Imaging of myeloma bone disease. Acta Oncol 2000; 39: 823–827

36. Lecouvet F E, van de Berg B C, Malghem J, Maldague B E. Magnetic resonance and computed tomography imaging in multiple myeloma. Semin Musculoskel Radiol 2001; 5: 43–55

37. Stabler A, Baur A, Bard R et al. Contrast enhancement and quantitative signal analysis in magnetic resonance imaging of multiple myeloma: assessment of focal and diffuse growth patterns in marrow correlated with biopsies and survival rates. Am J Roentgenol 1996; 167: 1029–1036

38. Bartl R, Frisch B, Fateh-Moghadam A. Histological classification and staging of multiple myeloma. Am J Clin Pathol 1987; 87: 342–355

39. Lecouvet F E, van de Berg B C, Michaux L et al. Stage III multiple myeloma: clinical and prognostic value of spinal bone marrow MR imaging. Radiology 1998; 209: 653–660

40. van de Berg B C, Lecouvet F E, Michaux L et al. Stage I multiple myeloma: value of MR imaging of the bone marrow in the determination of prognosis. Radiology 1996; 201: 243–246

41. Lecouvet F E, Malghem J, Michaux L et al. Vertebral compression fractures in multiple myeloma. Part II. Assessment of fracture risk with MR imaging of spinal bone marrow. Radiology 1997; 204: 201–205

42. Lecouvet F E, van de Berg B C, Maldage B E et al. Vertebral compression fractures in multiple myeloma. Part I. Distribution and appearance at MR imaging. Radiology 1997; 204: 195–199

43. Baur A, Stabler A, Bruning R et al. Diffusion weighted MR imaging of bone marrow: differentiation of benign versus pathologic compression fractures. Radiology 1998; 207: 349–356

44. Moulopoulos L A, Dimopoulos M A, Alexanian R et al. MR patterns of response to treatment. Radiology 1994; 193: 441–446

45. Cuenod C A, Laredo J D, Chevret S et al. Acute vertebral collapse due to osteoporosis or malignancy: appearances on unenhanced and gadolinium-enhanced MR images. Radiology 1996; 199: 541–549

46. Boccadero M, Palumbo A, Argentino C et al. Conventional induction treatments do not influence overall survival in multiple myeloma. Br J Haematol 1997; 96: 336–337

47. Barlogie B, Jagannath S, Vesole D H et al. Superiority of tandem autologous transplantation over standard therapy for previously untreated multiple myeloma. Blood 1997; 89: 789–793

48. Rahmouni A, Divine M, Mathieu D et al. MR appearance of multiple myeloma of the spine before and after treatment. Am J Roentgenol 1993; 160: 1053–1057

49. Lecouvet F E, De Nayer P, Garber C et al. Treated plasma cell lesions of bone with MRI signs of response to treatment: unexpected pathological findings. Skeletal Radiol 1998; 27: 692–695

50. Lecouvet F E, Richard F, van de Berg B C et al. Long term effects of localised spinal radiation therapy on vertebral fractures and focal lesions: appearance in patients with multiple myeloma. Br J Haematol 1997; 96: 743–745

51. Agren B, Reidberg U, Isberg B et al. MR imaging of multiple myeloma patients with bone marrow transplants. Acta Radiol 1998; 39: 36–42

52. Lecouvet F E, Dechambre S, Malghem J et al. Bone marrow transplantation in patients with multiple myeloma: prognostic significance of MR imaging. Am J Roentgenol 2001; 176: 91–96

53. Weber D M, Dimopoulos M A, Moulopoulos L A et al. Prognostic features of asymptomatic multiple myeloma. Br J Haematol 1997; 97: 810–814

54. LeCouvet F E, Malghem J, Michaux L et al. Skeletal survey in multiple myeloma: radiographic versus MR imaging survey. Br J Haematol 1999; 106: 35–39

55. Moulopoulos L A, Dimopoulos M A, Weber D et al. Magnetic resonance imaging in the staging of solitary plasmacytoma of bone. J Clin Oncol 1993; 11: 1311–1315

56. Sezer O, Niemoller K, Jakob C et al. Relationship between bone marrow angiogenesis and plasma cell infiltration and serum beta 2 microglobulin levels in patients with multiple myeloma. Ann Haematol 2001; 80: 598–601

57. Woo E, Yu Y L, Ng M. Spinal cord compression in multiple myeloma. Who gets it? Aus NZ J Med 1986; 16: 671–675

58. Speiss J L, Adelstein D J, Hines F D. Multiple myeloma presenting with spinal cord compression. Oncology 1988; 45: 88–92

59. Loughrey G J, Collins C D, Todd S M et al. MRI in the management of suspected spinal canal disease in patients with known malignancy. Clin Radiol 2000; 55: 849–855

60. Subramanyam B R. Renal amyloidosis–sonographic features. Am J Roentgenol 1981; 136: 411–412

61. Hawkins P. Serum amyloid P component scintigraphy for diagnosis and monitoring amyloidosis. Curr Opin Nephrol Hypertens 2002; 11: 649–655

62. Patlas M, Hadas-Halpern I, Libson E. Imaging findings of extraosseous multiple myeloma. Cancer Imaging 2002; 2: 120–122

63. Grover S B, Dhar A. Imaging spectrum in sclerotic myelomas. Eur Radiol 2000; 10: 1828–1831

Chapter 34

Leukaemia

Janet E Husband and Dow-Mu Koh

Introduction

The leukaemias are a group of diverse neoplasms which are derived from the arrested or aberrant development of a clone of normal haemopoietic cells. These immature cells proliferate progressively within the bone marrow replacing normal haemopoietic tissue and circulate within the peripheral blood becoming deposited in various organs and tissues. Leukaemic cells are incapable of normal function and many of the clinical features and complications of leukaemia are a direct result of the failure of normal haemopoietic activity.

There are four major groups of leukaemia, categorized according to the predominant type of proliferating cell:

- Acute myelogenous leukaemia (AML)
- Acute lymphoblastic leukaemia (ALL)
- Chronic myelocytic leukaemia (CML)
- Chronic lymphocytic leukaemia (CLL)

Full classification of the leukaemias has become increasingly complex as methods of discriminating different subtypes, such as immunophenotyping and cytogenetic studies, have been developed. Thus the subclassification and characterization of the leukaemias continues to evolve.[1,2] The classification shown in Table 34.1 illustrates the wide ranging heterogeneity of these diseases.

While the radiologist working in oncological practice does not need to have a full knowledge of the different subtypes of leukaemia, some subtypes manifest different radiological appearances.

There is some overlap between the leukaemias and the lymphomas but, in general, ALL is distinguished from lymphomas on the basis of cellular maturity and by the fact that lymphomas mainly involve extramedullary sites, at least initially. The lymphoblastic lymphomas and Burkitt's lymphoma have features of both leukaemia and lymphoma. Adult T cell leukaemia/lymphoma (ATLL) is a distinct variety of leukaemia/lymphoma that is characterized by lymphadenopathy and hepatosplenomegaly and is endemic in certain parts of the world including Japan and the Caribbean basin.

Myelodysplasia is a syndrome characterized by pancytopenia or chronic anaemia which results from dysfunction of

Table 34.1. *Classification of leukaemia*

Acute

Acute myelogenous leukaemia (AML)
Acute myeloblastic leukaemia
Acute promyelocytic leukaemia
Acute myelomonocytic leukaemia
Acute monoblastic leukaemia
Acute erythroleukaemia
Acute megakaryoblastic leukaemia

Acute lymphoblastic leukaemia (ALL)
Pre-B-cell acute lymphoblastic leukaemia
Common acute lymphoblastic leukaemia
Cytoplasmic immunoglobulin (+) ALL
Philadelphia chromosome (+) ALL
T-cell
B-cell

Acute unclassifiable leukaemia (AUL)

Chronic

Chronic myelocytic leukaemia (CML)
Chronic phase of CML
Metamorphosis of CML
Accelerated ± myelofibrosis
Lymphoblastic transformation
Myeloblastic transformation
Megakaryoblastic transformation

Juvenile chronic granulocytic leukaemia

Chronic eosinophilic leukaemia

Chronic lymphocytic leukaemia (CLL)
B-cell
T-cell

Hairy cell leukaemia

Polymorphocytic leukaemia

Plasma cell leukaemia

Sézary syndrome*

Adult T-cell leukaemia/lymphoma

*Leukaemic phase of mycosis fungoides.

the bone marrow. Transformation into acute leukaemia may develop during the course of disease.

Cross-sectional imaging, as well as conventional radiology, has an important place in the management of this disease. However, it is impossible to define strict algorithms for the use of imaging because the disease is manifested in many different organs and organ systems and the complications of leukaemia are common and diverse. As in other malignant tumours, close liaison between clinician and radiologist is essential to determine the most appropriate use of imaging for individual patient care.

Incidence and aetiology

The acute leukaemias account for less than 3% of all cancers in the USA but are a leading cause of cancer death in patients under the age of 35 years. It is estimated that there were approximately 30,500 new cases of leukaemia diagnosed in the USA in 2003, of which about half were acute leukaemias and half were chronic subtypes. The total number of deaths is estimated at approximately 21,900:[3]

Subtype	New cases	Deaths
Acute myeloid leukaemia	10,500	7,800
Chronic lymphatic leukaemia	7,300	4,400
Chronic myeloid	4,300	1,700
Acute lymphocytic leukaemia	3,600	1,400
Other leukaemias	4,900	6,600

Acute myelogenous leukaemia is more common than ALL in adults, but ALL is the most common subtype seen in childhood. In adults, the most common subtypes of leukaemia are AML and CLL.

In the UK, the incidence of leukaemia in relation to other cancers and the distribution of subtypes is similar to the USA; there are about 3,000 new cases diagnosed annually and over 1,500 deaths.[4] The current overall lifetime risk of developing leukaemia is 1.0% in males and 0.8% in females.

Over recent years enormous strides have been made in understanding the molecular biology and cytogenetics of leukaemia. Various chromosomal abnormalities have been identified which have helped to define the subsets of AML and ALL listed in the classification (e.g. Philadelphia chromosome-positive). These subsets of leukaemia have various clinical features and different patterns of response to therapy. Such information is used to direct patients to particular therapeutic regimens and, in the longer-term, may allow appropriate targeting of new therapies.

While the importance of genetic changes in the development of the leukaemias is well-recognized, the underlying causes initiating these changes are largely unknown. Down's syndrome and certain other genetic syndromes are linked with leukaemia, and excessive exposure to ionizing radiation is now established as an important cause,[5] as are chronic exposure to low-dose radiation in the environment, chemicals and smoking.[6]

Secondary AML may develop after treatment of childhood acute leukaemia and following therapy for other cancers such as tumours of the breast and ovary, and Hodgkin's disease.[7–10]

A human retrovirus (HTLV-1) has been identified as a cause of human T cell leukaemia/lymphoma (ATLL).[11,12] The cumulative risk of an infected individual developing ATLL is estimated to be between 0.5 and 5%.[13,14]

Key points: general features

- The leukaemias are derived from the arrested or aberrant development of a clone of normal haemopoietic cells

- Various subtypes are recognized which have different clinical features, radiological features, prognosis and therapeutic implications

- ALL is the most common subtype in childhood

- AML and CLL are the most common subtypes in adults

- Various chromosomal abnormalities have been identified in the leukaemias

- Down's syndrome is strongly linked with acute leukaemia

- Ionizing radiation, chemicals and smoking have a causal relationship with leukaemia

- The human retrovirus (HTLV-1) infection is a known cause of human T cell leukaemia/lymphoma

Clinical features

The replacement of normal haemopoietic cells within the bone marrow by an excessive number of abnormal functionless cells is responsible for the major clinical features of the leukaemias:

- Anaemia
- Infection
- Haemorrhage

In acute leukaemia, patients usually present with a 1- to 3-month history of weight loss, fatigue, bruising or signs of infection such as fever. In the chronic leukaemias, the onset of disease is more insidious but fever may be observed without an obvious infective cause. Occasionally, the diagnosis of chronic leukaemia is made on routine examination of the peripheral blood in an otherwise asymptomatic patient.

In all patients, the diagnosis is confirmed by examination of the peripheral blood and bone marrow biopsy.

Immunophenotyping and cytogenetic studies are performed to discriminate between the different subsets of the disease. In the majority of patients, anaemia and thrombocytopenia are present. The peripheral white cell blood count may be normal, raised or reduced but blast cells are seen in the peripheral blood in practically all patients.

There are certain clinical features of leukaemia which are more prevalent in one subtype than another, and the frequency of involvement of different organs and sites also varies (Table 34.2).[15]

In the acute leukaemias, central nervous system (CNS) involvement is more common in ALL than AML but is also seen in the chronic leukaemias. The CNS is resistant to chemotherapy and is therefore termed a sanctuary site of disease.

Hepatosplenomegaly due to leukaemia infiltration is seen in practically all cases of leukaemia but in the chronic forms of the disease the degree of enlargement is greater than in the acute leukaemias (Fig. 34.1).

Lymphadenopathy is most frequently seen in CLL and in juvenile CML (Figs. 34.2 and 34.3). It is rare in adult Philadelphia chromosome-positive CML. The incidence of enlarged lymph nodes at presentation in the acute leukaemias is as follows:

- Acute lymphoblastic leukaemias (50%) (usually T cell or B cell)
- Acute monoblastic leukaemias (15–20%)
- Other subtypes of acute myelogenous leukaemia (8%)[16]

Fever is a common feature of all the leukaemias whether due to infection or not. In those without documented infection, fever may arise as a result of increased metabolism due to the leukaemic process.

Anaemia is present in the majority of patients and is caused by inadequate erythrocyte production, bleeding, hypersplenism or haemolysis.

Bleeding is more common in the acute leukaemias than in the chronic subtypes and usually takes the form of small petechial haemorrhages. Occasionally, a patient may present with a catastrophic intracranial haemorrhage.

In the acute leukaemias, haemorrhage is a major cause of death and morbidity. Haemorrhage results from coagulation defects associated with the disease, thrombocytopenia and the effects of chemotherapy. The acute promyelocytic form of leukaemia is particularly prone to haemorrhage and, in one study, intracranial haemorrhage

Table 34.2. *Organ involvement by leukaemia cell type (1958–1982) (Adapted from ref. 15)*

Organ/Sites	AML (%)	CML (%)	ALL (%)	CLL[§] (%)
CNS (sanctuary sites)				
Brain	9	11	14	7
Dura mater	14	14	26	21
Leptomeninges	12	10	34	8
Lymphoreticular sites				
Liver	41	55	63	83
Lymph nodes	45	59	55	76
Spleen	58	68	70	76
Cardiopulmonary				
Pericardium	8	6	11	14
Heart	15	11	21	22
Pleura	8	5	11	16
Lungs	28	29	41	41
Gastro-intestinal				
Oesophagus	17	9	16	19
Stomach	11	11	17	11
Large bowel	15	9	20	15
Pancreas	8	6	18	12
Endocrine				
Pituitary	9	10	15	20
Thyroid	6	3	5	7
Adrenals	15	22	21	33
Genito-urinary				
Kidneys	33	38	53	63
Bladder	7	6	9	8
Prostate	9	5	12	22
Uterus	11	4	25	14
Gonads (sanctuary sites)				
Testes	20	16	40	15
Ovaries	11	9	21	22
Total number of cases	585	204	308	109

[§]Percentage of all cases examined.

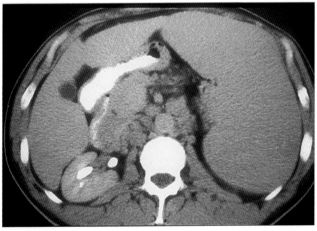

Figure 34.1. *A post-contrast CT scan in a 62-year-old male patient with CLL, showing a huge spleen and multiple enlarged retroperitoneal lymph nodes.*

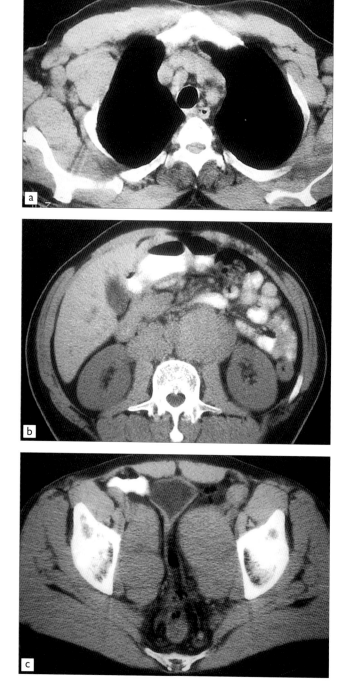

Figure 34.2. *A male patient with CLL showing multiple enlarged lymph nodes on CT: (a) in the mediastinum and axillae; (b) in the retroperitoneum; (c) in the pelvis.*

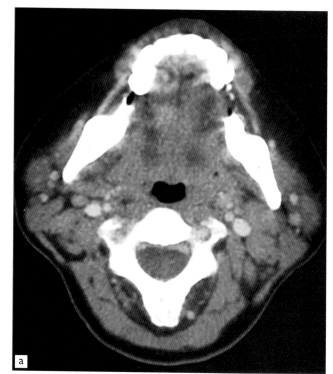

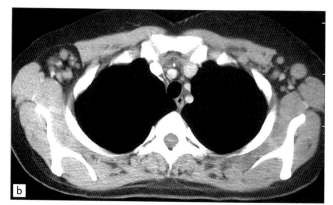

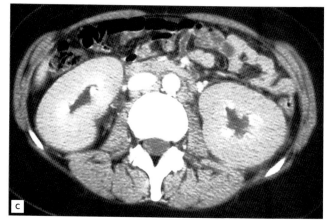

Figure 34.3. *In this 24-year-old man with ALL, there is nodal enlargement seen (a) along the deep cervical chain of lymph nodes in the neck, (b) both axillae and (c) within the retroperitoneum. Note also the diffusely enlarged kidneys due to leukaemic infiltration.*

was the cause of death in 60% of patients.[17] Another group of patients at particularly high risk of intracranial haemorrhage are those with acute leukaemia in 'blast' crisis. In such patients the excessive numbers of leucocytes form tiny foci which plug small arterioles and destroy the vascular walls, leading to haemorrhage.[18]

Patients with intracranial haemorrhage present acutely with headaches, seizures and deterioration of neurological function. Rarely, intracranial haemorrhage may herald the diagnosis of acute leukaemia.

Bone pain is a common presenting feature in children with ALL, occurring in 25–30% of cases, whereas in adults it is only seen in approximately 5% of patients.[19,20] Bone pain is characteristically migratory and periarticular.[21] It is probably due to lifting of the periosteum by infiltration of leukaemic cells or to the development of bone infarction.[22] Monoarthralgia or polyarthralgia is not an uncommon presenting feature.

Abdominal pain and chest pain are also relatively common and are related to a variety of problems. For example, abdominal pain may result from stretching of the splenic capsule due to rapid enlargement or from intestinal obstruction due to leukaemic infiltration of the bowel wall. Chest pain may be caused by a large mediastinal mass compressing adjacent structures.

Granulocytic sarcoma (chloroma) is a mass composed of leukaemic cells. These tumours are usually seen in patients with AML but may also occur in CML and other myeloprolific disorders such as polycythaemia rubra vera.[23] They consist of myeloblasts, promyelocytes and myelocytes and are most frequently found in the orbits, subcutaneous tissues, paranasal sinuses, lymph nodes and bones but many other sites have also been described.[24] In a series of 728 patients with childhood myelogenous leukaemia, Pui et al. found an incidence of 4.7% of granulocytic sarcoma developing at some point during the course of disease. Others have reported an incidence ranging from 2.5 to 8%.[25,26] Rarely, these tumours may be the presenting feature of leukaemia occurring before the onset of clinically overt disease.[27] They were first described by Burns in 1811[28] but it was not until 1853 that the term chloroma was coined by King to describe their typical greenish colour.[29] However, in 1966, the term chloroma was replaced by granulocytic sarcoma because fewer than half of them actually display the characteristic greenish colour.

Key points: clinical features

- The major clinical features of leukaemia are anaemia, infection and haemorrhage

- CNS involvement is more common in ALL than AML

- Lymphadenopathy is most frequently seen in CLL

- Bone pain is a common presenting feature in childhood leukaemia, occurring in about 25% of cases. Bone pain occurs in only 5% of adults

- Granulocytic sarcoma is a mass composed of leukaemic cells which occurs most frequently in AML. The incidence ranges from 2.5 to 8%

- The most common sites of granulocytic sarcoma are the orbits, subcutaneous tissues, paranasal sinuses and bones

Treatment

Treatment of acute leukaemia aims to induce a remission as quickly as possible and then to maintain remission. The success of therapy depends as much on the treatment of non-leukaemic-related problems as on the eradication of leukaemia itself.

In the acute leukaemias, certain features are important prognostic factors and determine the detailed approach to management. These include patient age (older patients are less likely to achieve complete remission) or previous myelodysplasia. Certain cytogenetic subtypes have a poorer prognosis (B-cell and unclassified leukaemias are rarely controlled in the long term).

Acute lymphoblastic leukaemia (common ALL) is the most successfully treated of all the leukaemias.[30–33] Complete remission can be achieved in over 90% of children and in up to 80% of adults.[30] The cure rates in childhood ALL have continued to improve, and the expected current cure rates approach 75–80% of all children with ALL, including T-ALL and mature B-cell ALL, the two variants that, not too long ago, had a considerably poorer prognosis compared with the common form of BpALL.[34] However, adult ALL has a higher likelihood of relapsing following initial cure.[35] Treatment of common ALL includes induction chemotherapy, which is followed by consolidation therapy and maintenance therapy for a period of up to two years. Prophylactic intrathecal chemotherapy with or without cranial irradiation is used for CNS prophylaxis.[31]

The prognosis of AML depends on the age of the patient at presentation. Elderly patients have a worse prognosis, which is related to the high incidence of death from infection or other problems related to the disease. Patients with AML are treated with induction chemotherapy using a combination of drugs followed by intensive post-remission therapy.[34,36,37] This is either in the form of high-dose chemotherapy supported by bone marrow transplantation or intensive short-term consolidation therapy to prevent relapse.[38–40]

Chronic myelogenous leukaemia is caused by expression of the Bcr-Abl tyrosine kinase oncogene, the product of the t(9;22) Philadelphia translocation. The aim of treatment in CML is to reduce the number of Bcr-Abl-expressing cells to as low a level as possible. The therapy should strive to achieve complete haematological, cytogenetical and molecular remission, with evidence of inhibiting Bcr-Abl expression by polymerase chain reaction.

In the past year, a novel drug, Imatinib, an orally administered inhibitor of the Bcr-Abl kinase, has been widely evaluated in the treatment of CML. Imatinib has been found to be superior to the combination of alpha interferon (IFN-α) and low-dose cytarabine as first-line therapy in newly diagnosed chronic-phase CML, in terms of haematological and cytogenetical responses, tolerability and the likelihood of progression to accelerated-phase or blast-crisis.[41] There is also evidence that Imatinib can induce haematological and cytogenetical improvement in patients with accelerated-phase CML, although such response may not be sustained.[42] At present, allogenic stem cell transplantation is the only known curative treatment for CML, as well as the only treatment that induces molecular remission in a large number of patients.

The survival of leukaemia varies according to the category of leukaemia as well as its subtype. In ALL, the relative 5-year survival rates are between 50 and 80% for children and 20 and 40% for adults.[30] In AML, patients under 60 years of age have a better outlook than older patients but the 5-year actuarial survival for all age groups is between 40 and 50%.[34,43] In a follow-up of 716 patients with AML diagnosed between 1980 and 1982 with a median follow-up of 14.7 years, complete remission and survival varied significantly depending on the cytogenetic classification and induction chemotherapy. Only 8.9% of patients were alive 5 years following diagnosis, but 5 years of continuous remission was synonymous with cure.[44]

In the chronic leukaemias, cure is usually impossible but prolonged survival can be achieved in certain subtypes using conventional chemotherapy, bone marrow transplantation (BMT), allogenic stem cell transplantation and novel therapies such as IFN-α and Imatinib.[41,45,46]

Key points: treatment

■ The success of therapy in leukaemia depends as much on the treatment of non-leukaemic-related problems as on the eradication of leukaemia itself

■ Acute lymphoblastic leukaemia (common ALL) is the most successfully treated of all the leukaemias. Complete remission is achieved in over 90% of children and in up to 80% of adults

■ The 5-year survival of common ALL is 50–80% for children and 20–40% for adults

■ In AML, the 5-year survival for all age groups is 40–50%

■ The acute leukaemias are treated with induction chemotherapy followed by consolidation therapy. Prophylactic CNS treatment is required in ALL

■ The chronic leukaemias are traditionally treated with chemotherapy but recently IFN-α has shown encouraging results

■ Allogeneic BMT has an important role in the treatment of leukaemias. Graft rejection is a major complication

Imaging in leukaemia

Leukaemia is diagnosed and monitored by haematological studies of the peripheral blood and bone marrow and imag-ing therefore plays a lesser role in the diagnosis and staging of this disease than in the lymphomas. However, the importance of radiology in the management of leukaemia has increased over the last two decades, mainly due to the advent of cross-sectional imaging and also to improvements in therapy. Imaging is used to evaluate the leukaemic process itself or to investigate its complications. Thus the imaging findings in leukaemia can be broadly categorized into two groups, those related to:

- Direct involvement of organs and tissues by leukaemic cells
- Indirect involvement of organs and tissues due to complications

In this text, direct and indirect imaging findings will be discussed in relation to different anatomical sites and organ systems.

Central nervous system

Direct involvement by leukaemia

Central nervous system involvement is usually seen in acute leukaemia. It may be a manifestation of disease at diagnosis or may herald relapse in patients believed to be in remission. At diagnosis, approximately 3% of children with ALL have CNS disease[47] but the number of patients who relapse with CNS involvement has been dramatically reduced by the introduction of CNS prophylactic therapy.[48]

Leukaemic spread to the CNS is presumed to be by direct infiltration from involved bone marrow of the cranium (or vertebrae) or by the haematogenous route whereby circulating leukaemia cells enter the CNS by migration through spaces in the venous endothelium.[49,50]

The leukaemic process may involve the leptomeninges, dura or both, and may be diffuse or focal. Meningeal involvement occurs in up to 10% of patients with acute leukaemia and begins in the superficial arachnoid membrane; leukaemic cells then invade the cerebrospinal fluid (CSF) space and pia mater.[51,52] Extradural (para-meningeal) masses (granulocytic sarcoma) may also be observed in intracranial or intraspinal sites. Involvement of the brain parenchyma is rare but when it does occur, it probably results from perivascular extension of disease across the Virchow–Robin spaces through the pia–glial membrane.[53] Intracerebral and meningeal granulocytic sarcomas are a rare occurrence in the myelogenous leukaemias.

Meningeal and dural disease

Symptoms of meningeal involvement of the brain include headache, nausea, vomiting and lethargy. Signs of intracranial pressure and cranial nerve palsies may be apparent on clinical examination.[48] The diagnosis of meningeal involvement is made on the finding of leukaemic cells within CSF. However, analysis of the CSF is often negative and several repeat lumbar punctures may be required to establish the diagnosis of meningeal disease.

Imaging is complementary to lumbar puncture but the detection of diffuse meningeal involvement with computed tomography (CT) has been disappointing due to insufficient contrast enhancement of the abnormal meninges.[54] Computed tomography is more accurate in carcinomatous meningitis and inflammatory conditions because the contrast enhancement is usually more intense.[53]

Magnetic resonance (MR) imaging is the method of choice for the detection of intracranial and spinal leptomeningeal disease and on occasion may demonstrate leukaemic infiltration in the presence of multiple negative cytological analyses.[48] The technique is considerably more sensitive than CT, myelography or CT myelography, and MR has replaced these techniques in the investigation of CNS leukaemia.[55,56] Although T2-weighted spin-echo sequences may reveal abnormal signal intensity within the CSF space, meningeal disease is best demonstrated on gadolinium-enhanced T1-weighted images. Axial and coronal images of the head, and sagittal images of the spine, provide the best imaging planes to survey all the meningeal surfaces. Leukaemic infiltration is seen as abnormal nodular thickening of the meninges which enhances after injection of intravenous (IV) contrast medium (Fig. 34.4). Thickening and enhancement of nerve roots, particularly in the region of the cauda equina, is shown on MR but may also be demonstrated on CT myelography. Diffuse dural infiltration is less common than leptomeningeal disease but is also seen as thickening and enhancement of the dural surfaces. In patients with leukaemia, the observation of thickened enhancing meninges is not pathognomonic of leukaemic infiltration as it may also be seen in other conditions associated with leukaemia such as infectious meningitis, drug reactions and meningeal fibrosis following haemorrhage.[48]

Parameningeal disease

Intracranial and spinal parameningeal disease usually take the form of a mass of leukaemic cells known as granulocytic sarcoma (chloroma).

The majority of intracranial granulocytic sarcomas are dural-based lesions and are believed to develop by direct spread from the bone marrow. The CT and MR appearances of granulocytic sarcomas are variable and they may mimic meningiomas, other tumours or abscesses.[57,58] Recently, Ahn et al. described a case of granulocytic sarcoma in ALL mimicking a falx meningioma.[59]

On unenhanced CT, intracranial granulocytic sarcomas are isodense or slightly hyperdense compared with normal brain but frequently show intense enhancement following injection of IV contrast medium (Fig. 34.5).[60] On MR, these lesions may be of high signal intensity on T1-weighted images, they are bright on T2 weighting and, as with CT, show intense contrast enhancement.[57]

Spinal granulocytic sarcomas may be paraspinal or intraspinal (Fig. 34.6). Soft tissue masses in the paravertebral region extend into the spinal canal via the intervertebral foraminae (Fig. 34.7).[61] These masses invade the dura and may cause spinal cord compression, nerve root compression and bone destruction.

Although CT may show paravertebral masses and extension into the spinal canal or discrete intraspinal masses

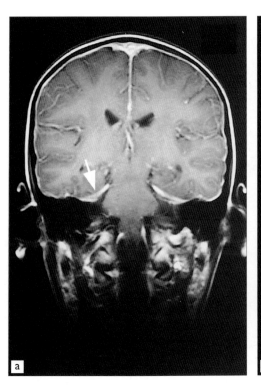
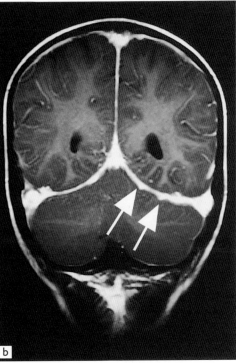

Figure 34.4. *(a and b) Contrast-enhanced T1-weighted coronal MR images in a 9-year-old boy with AML. There is extensive contrast-enhanced nodular thickening of the leptomeninges (arrows), representing leukaemic infiltration.*

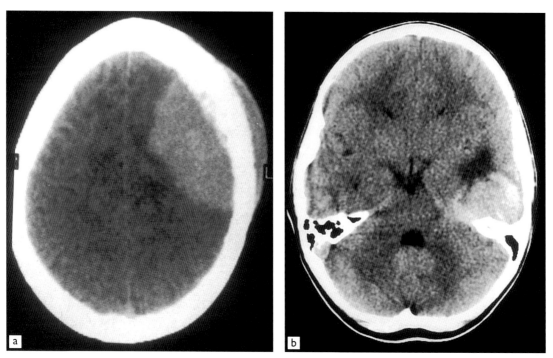

Figure 34.5. *Intracranial granulocytic sarcoma. (a) CT scan of the brain in a 14-year-old boy with relapsed ALL. The mass which probably arises from the left parietal bone extends both intracranially and into the subcutaneous soft tissues. There is homogeneous intense contrast enhancement (from ref. 61, with permission); (b) CT scan of an 8-year-old girl who relapsed following initial therapy for ALL with a large durally based lesion in the temporal lobe. Note homogeneous enhancement and surrounding oedema.*

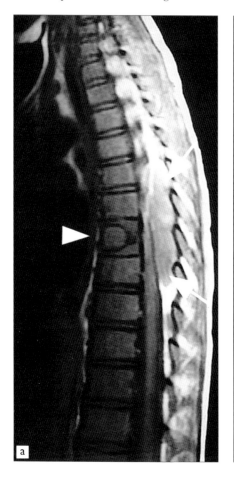

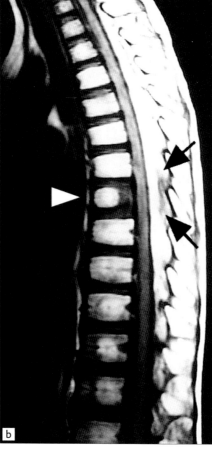

Figure 34.6. *A 9-year-old boy who presented with acute back pain and signs of spinal cord compression. (a) T1-weighted sagittal MR showing an intraspinal extradural soft tissue mass in the mid-thoracic region (arrows). Note partial collapse of the vertebral body of T5. A diagnosis of AML with a granulocytic sarcoma was made on investigation. There is diffuse abnormally low signal intensity throughout the vertebral bodies indicating diffuse leukaemic infiltration. (b) Repeat T weighted MR scan 6 weeks later shows an excellent response to treatment. The granulocytic sarcomatous mass has almost completely resolved (arrows) and the signal intensity of the bone marrow has increased markedly indicating reduction in bone marrow infiltration. The vertebral body of T5 still shows abnormal signal intensity posteriorly.*

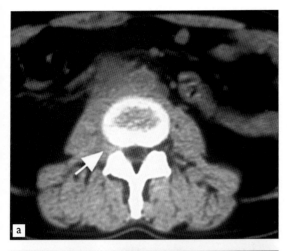

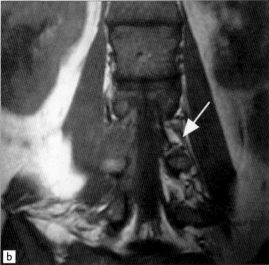

Figure 34.7. *An adult male patient who presented with back pain due to a granulocytic sarcoma before clinical manifestation of AML. (a) CT scan; (b) T1-weighted coronal MR. In (a) a soft tissue mass is seen surrounding the inferior vena cava and obscuring the contour of the aorta. The mass extends posteriorly deep to the right psoas muscle and enters the spinal canal through the intervertebral foramen (arrow). In (b) the coronal MR image shows the cranio-caudal extent of the mass and clearly delineates the intraspinal component at the level of L3/L4 and L4/L5 intervertebral foraminae. Tumour surrounds the exit nerve roots. Note normal nerve roots on the left side (arrow).*

(Fig. 34.7a), MR is the preferred imaging technique for demonstrating these lesions because the whole spine can be examined at a single investigation (Fig. 34.7b). The multiplanar capability of MR is also an advantage as it allows clear delineation of tumour extent. Granulocytic sarcomas have a low signal intensity on T1-weighted images and a relatively high or intermediate signal intensity on T2-weighted images.[61] They often show intense contrast enhancement.

Key points: central nervous system

- CNS involvement is usually a manifestation of acute leukaemia

- Approximately 3% of all children with ALL have CNS disease

- The leukaemic process may involve the leptomeninges, dura or extradural space

- Disease may be diffuse or focal

- Granulocytic sarcomas are usually dural based lesions

- MR is the best imaging method for detecting intracranial meningeal and dural infiltration as well as granulocytic sarcoma

Indirect effects of leukaemia

The indirect effects of leukaemia on the CNS include vascular events, infection and toxic effects related to therapy.

Vascular complications

Haemorrhage CT or MR is essential in patients suspected of intracranial haemorrhage. In most cases, CT will be undertaken, as this is more readily available and generally quicker than MR examinations. Unenhanced CT will show the classic features of subarachnoid and/or intracerebral haemorrhage, which includes the presence of high-density material in the subarachnoid space, in the brain parenchyma and ventricular system. There may be mass effect with some surrounding oedema. On MR, fresh blood has a high signal intensity on T1 weighting and, on T2 weighting, the appearances are also those of high signal intensity. Breakdown products of haemoglobin (haemosiderin) may also be present giving a low signal intensity on T2 weighting.

CT and MR are not only valuable for demonstrating the presence of intracranial haemorrhage but also for excluding haemorrhage in patients in whom the diagnosis is questionable on clinical grounds. Furthermore, imaging may show other associated abnormalities such as sinovenous thrombosis.

Sinovenous thrombosis Sinovenous thrombosis, another vascular complication of acute leukaemia, may be related to treatment with L-asparaginase as well as to leukaemic infiltration.[54,61] Both CT and MR are useful non-invasive methods of detecting sinovenous thrombosis. On CT, postcontrast-enhanced images may show a low density filling defect within the sinus and, on precontrast images, the sinus may be abnormally hyperdense. On MR, loss of the normal signal void is apparent on T2-weighted sequences and, on postcontrast images, a filling defect may be observed, as on CT. Gradient-echo or other flow sensitive techniques such as fast fluid-attenuated inversion recovery (FLAIR) may also demonstrate sinovenous thrombosis on MR.[54,62] Leukaemic infiltration of meninges and sinus thrombosis may coexist.

Cerebral infarction Patients with leukaemia are at an increased risk of cerebral infarction for several reasons, which include: [54]

- General risks – patient age, atherosclerosis
- Intravascular coagulation
- Sinovenous occlusion
- Tumour emboli
- Septic emboli
- Effects of therapy[17]

As in the diagnosis of intracranial haemorrhage, CT and MR are valuable for demonstrating the presence of cerebral infarction and for distinguishing infarcts from other intracranial lesions such as haemorrhage, infection and drug-related toxicity. Perfusion studies of the brain using MR or single-photon emission computed tomography (SPECT) are of particular value in the early phase of development of the lesion.

Infection

In leukaemic patients, intracranial infection results from direct spread of infection from the paranasal sinuses or by the haematogenous route. Sinusitis is usually aggressive in immunocompromised patients and infection with organisms such as Aspergillus results in invasion of local structures and destruction of bone (Fig. 34.8), thereby giving access to the dura, meninges and underlying brain parenchyma. Other organisms including bacteria (e.g. *Klebsiella pneumonii*) and viruses are also associated with intracranial infection in leukaemia.[63] Abscesses may develop and, whether solitary or multiple, may simulate parenchymal leukaemic deposits.[63] On CT, abscesses usually show rim enhancement with a relatively low-density centre; on MR, these masses have a high signal intensity on T2 weighting and a relatively low signal intensity on T1 weighting. As on CT, rim enhancement is noted following injection of IV contrast medium.

Treatment-related complications

There are many neurological complications associated with the treatment of leukaemia but such complications are especially related to the treatment or prophylaxis of the CNS. Different syndromes and clinical features are associated with particular drugs or radiotherapy. In general, CNS toxicity can be divided into acute, subacute and chronic forms.

Acute or subacute neurological complications are more likely to be reversible than the complications which develop in the longer term. Patients present with symptoms and signs of raised intracranial pressure, and on examination

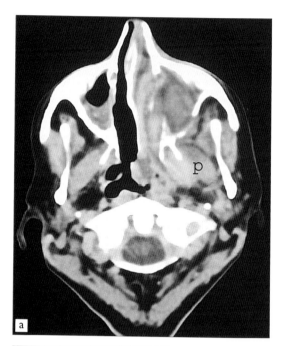

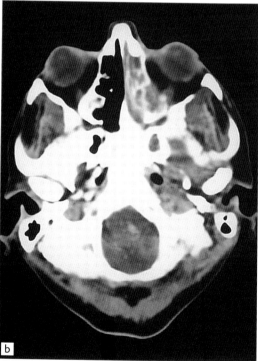

Figure 34.8. *CT scan in a 53-year-old male patient with relapsed AML showing extensive paranasal sinus infection with Aspergillus. (a) The soft tissue mass occupies the left maxillary sinus. There is almost complete destruction of the medial wall of the maxillary sinus with extension of the soft tissue mass into the nasal cavity and nasopharynx. There is also destruction of the lateral wall of the maxillary sinus with extension of disease into the pterygoid region. Note enlargement and poor definition of the lateral pterygoid muscle (p). (b) The soft tissue mass is also seen extending into the posterior aspect of the left orbit. The left ethmoid sinuses are replaced by soft tissue and there is destruction of the medial wall of the orbit.*

neurological deficit is common.[64] After BMT for CML, MR may show acute ventricular enlargement and cortical atrophy which progress over time.[65] On clinical evaluation, it may be impossible to distinguish CNS leukaemic relapse from the effects of therapy and, in this situation, imaging plays a key role. Delayed or chronic toxic effects are more likely to be irreversible and may develop several years after initial treatment.

Radiotherapy neurotoxicity is usually subacute, developing several weeks after treatment. It is characterized by drowsiness, nausea and malaise, as well as somnolence.[48] Imaging is not usually required to reach a definitive diagnosis.

The delayed effects of radiotherapy include cerebral atrophy and even necrosis. This results in growth disturbance, intellectual impairment and neuroendocrine problems. Magnetic resonance shows abnormally high signal intensity in the white matter following cranial irradiation and may demonstrate abnormalities even in patients without clinical evidence of toxicity. Computed tomography may reveal areas of low attenuation within the white matter and calcifications. Long-term survivors of childhood ALL treated with cranial irradiation and intrathecal methotrexate frequently show abnormalities on MR; this is more common in patients treated with both modalities than with intrathecal methotrexate alone.[66,67] The incidence of long-term effects of cranial irradiation has not been widely studied. A recent study reported by Laitt and colleagues[68] revealed an inci-

dence of significant abnormalities in the brain on MR in 26% of 35 long-term survivors. These abnormalities included three tumours (meningioma, rhabdomyosarcoma, anaplastic astrocytoma) as well as large vessel vasculopathy, small cystic infarcts and diffuse white matter change. Recently, long-term cerebral metabolic changes have been demonstrated with proton MR spectroscopy (MRS) in patients treated with intrathecal methotrexate and cranial irradiation prophylaxis for ALL. These abnormalities were found in brains with haemosiderin and were reflected by decreasing *N*-acetylaspartate (NAA)/creatine(Cr) and choline(Cho)/creatine(Cr) since diagnosis.[69]

Intrathecal methotrexate may cause acute arachnoiditis and imaging is not required in the diagnostic work-up. Subacute neurotoxicity and delayed reactions are characterized by seizures and other manifestations of motor dysfunction such as paraplegia. Imaging may be required to exclude direct involvement of the CNS by leukaemia, for example the presence of a granulocytic sarcoma. Delayed effects of methotrexate include white matter ischaemia and imaging shows intracerebral calcifications and cerebral atrophy. Both CT and MR are useful for demonstrating the extent of these abnormalities.

Disseminated necrotizing leucoencephalopathy is more likely to develop when CNS irradiation is combined with intrathecal methotrexate and high-dose methotrexate (Fig. 34.9).[48,64,70] This condition may be fulminating and rapidly fatal, or less severe leading to chronic neurological

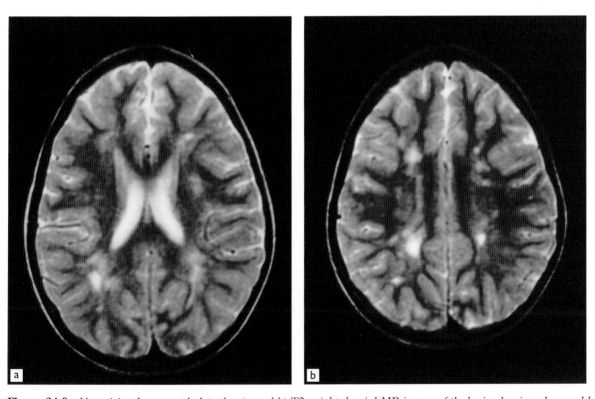

Figure 34.9. *Necrotizing leucoencephalopathy. (a and b) T2-weighted axial MR images of the brain showing abnormal high signal intensity in the white matter following cranial irradiation and methotrexate therapy.*

deficit. Leucoencephalopathy affects the white matter of the brain and is seen on CT as multifocal areas of low attenuation and, on MR, as areas of high signal intensity on spin-echo T2-weighted images. Enhancement of these lesions can sometimes be seen on MR.[71-73] Calcification may also be observed in the basal ganglia and in the subcortical white matter.

Other drugs such as cytarabine and cyclosporin A are also associated with severe neurotoxicity.[48] Vera et al.[74] investigated SPECT in the diagnosis of CNS toxicity following therapy with a cytarabine-containing regimen and found that diffuse heterogeneous low perfusion levels may be the only abnormal feature on imaging.

Neuropsychological disorders developing as a result of treatment of childhood leukaemia are well-recognized but imaging appears to have little role in the routine follow-up of these children. Harila-Saari et al.[75] showed no significant correlation between neuropsychological outcome and MR findings of white matter change, atrophy, old haemorrhage and calcifications. However, investigation of the long-term cognitive effects of intrathecal methotrexate and cranial irradiation in a group of 21 children cured of ALL showed that poor performance was associated with white matter changes in 50% of cases.[76] Furthermore, there was good correlation between the presence of calcifications and the number of methotrexate injections.

Key points: CNS complications

- Haemorrhage is a major cause of death in acute leukaemia, particularly in acute promyelocytic leukaemia and patients in 'blast' crisis

- Sinovenous thrombosis may be demonstrated by MR and CT but may co-exist with leukaemic meningeal infiltration

- Cerebral infarction has an increased incidence in patients with leukaemia

- Intracranial infection usually results from spread of infection from paranasal sinuses directly by organisms such as Aspergillus

- CNS toxicity is related to irradiation, intrathecal methotrexate and high-dose methotrexate

- Disseminating necrotizing leucoencephalopathy affects the white matter of the brain and is demonstrated on MR as areas of high signal intensity with foci on T2-weighted images. Enhancement of the lesions may be seen

- Long-term cognitive changes are associated with abnormalities due to methotrexate and cranial irradiation. These can be demonstrated on CT and MR

Head and neck

Direct involvement by leukaemia

The most important extracranial site of leukaemia of the head and neck region is the orbit. Leukaemic deposits may infiltrate around the optic nerve, often in association with meningeal disease and the choroid and retina may also be involved by diffuse infiltration. The orbit is a well-recognized site of granulocytic sarcoma (chloroma).[58] On both CT and MR, intra-orbital granulocytic sarcomas enhance with IV contrast medium and are usually seen as soft tissue masses related to the intraocular muscles (Fig. 34.10).[24] Granulocytic sarcoma in the paranasal sinuses may spread by direct extension into the orbit.

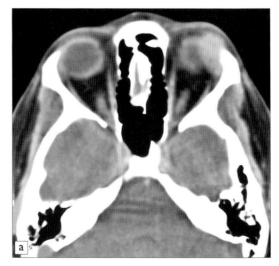

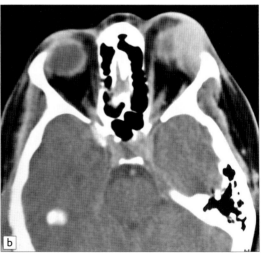

Figure 34.10. *Orbital chloroma in a young man with ALL. (a) Contrast media-enhanced CT image showing an enhancing mass arising from the superolateral corner of the left orbit, with displacment of the underlying globe. The appearance is typical for orbital granulocytic sarcoma. (b) Computed tomography of the orbits obtained 3 months later showed progression of disease.*

Indirect effects of leukaemia

Major indirect effects of leukaemia in the head and neck are haemorrhage and infection. Infection of the paranasal sinuses may be extremely aggressive, resulting in intracranial disease as described above. Imaging with CT or MR may be required to define the extent of infection extracranially as well as the presence of meningeal or brain involvement.

Intrathoracic disease

The vast majority of pulmonary abnormalities detected in leukaemic patients are due to indirect causes related to complications of therapy, whereas mediastinal abnormalities, although much less common, are usually the result of nodal involvement. Chest radiographs play an important role in the assessment of leukaemic patients, especially during therapy at the time of immunosuppression. High resolution CT (HRCT) of the lungs can also provide additional useful information in selected cases but should be used as an adjunct to plain chest radiographs and not as a substitute investigation.[77]

Direct involvement by leukaemia

Mediastinal lymphadenopathy is a common feature of ALL as well as CLL (Fig. 34.11). A large anterior mediastinal mass on plain chest films is a characteristic feature of childhood T-cell leukaemia, and indeed over 50% of patients with adult T-cell leukaemia have mediastinal disease (Fig 34.12).[16,78]

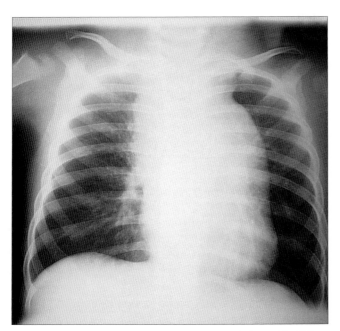

Figure 34.11. *Chest radiograph in a 4-year-old boy with ALL showing a large mediastinal mass at presentation.*

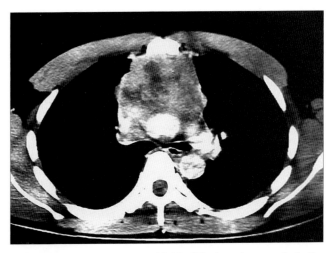

Figure 34.12. *In this man with T-cell leukaemia, note the bulky heterogeneous anterior mediastinal lymphadenopathy, resulting in widening of the mediastinum.*

These large masses may cause superior vena caval obstruction or tracheal compression. Hilar lymphadenopathy may also be seen.

Pulmonary leukaemic infiltration is only rarely diagnosed on plain chest radiographs but is found more commonly at autopsy.[79] On a plain chest film, leukaemic infiltration appears as diffuse peribronchial infiltration accompanied by septal lines. The findings are usually indistinguishable from infection or pulmonary edema and therefore the diagnosis is rarely made radiologically. In those cases detected during life, the diagnosis is readily made at transbronchial biopsy and bronchial lavage.[80] In a series of 109 patients reported by Green and Nichols, 30 had autopsy evidence of pulmonary infiltration but only two of these patients showed evidence of infiltration on chest radiographs.[81]

Indirect effects of leukaemia

Mediastinal widening may be due to haemorrhage within the mediastinum, thrombus within the superior vena cava (usually as a result of central line insertion) or to mediastinitis (this may be associated with central line insertion due to an extraluminal placement of a catheter tip or infection). The cause can be detected on contrast-enhanced CT and is readily distinguished from lymphadenopathy (Fig. 34.13).

Pulmonary infection is a major cause of abnormal shadowing detected on plain chest radiographs in leukaemic patients. These infections result from immunosuppression and may be bacterial, viral or fungal (Fig. 34.14). The most common organisms which have a predilection for immunosuppressed hosts include cytomegalovirus (CMV), *Pneumocystis carinii* and fungal infection by organisms such as Aspergillus and Cryptococcus.[82–84] On occasion, CT may be useful in the differential diagnosis of pulmonary infiltration, for example CT may demonstrate the rounded lesions

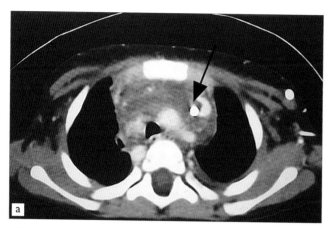

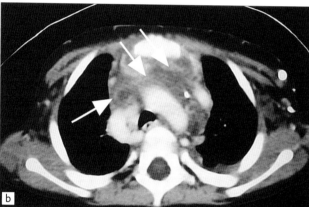

Figure 34.13. *(a and b) Contrast-enhanced CT scans in a 3-year-old child with massive mediastinal widening due to extrusion of the central line from the left innominate vein into the mediastinal soft tissues. Note thrombus in the left innominate vein shown as tubular low attenuation (arrows). Thrombus is also present in the superior vena cava (arrow). The mediastinum is widened and contains generalized increased soft tissue density due to mediastinitis. Note the central line (black arrow).*

of *Aspergillus fumigatus* not visualized on plain chest films. Oropharyngeal and oesophageal infection with *Candida albicans* is common and results from antibiotic therapy as well as the impaired immune response.[82] These complications of treatment are discussed further in Chapter 52.

Pulmonary haemorrhage should be considered in the differential diagnosis of abnormal air space pulmonary shadowing on plain chest films, particularly if accompanied by haemoptysis. Pulmonary oedema may mimic infection and indeed may coexist with an inflammatory process.

Treatment-related pulmonary damage is important in the differential diagnosis of abnormal pulmonary shadowing and chest symptoms in the leukaemic patient.

Drugs cause pulmonary oedema and vasculitis. In the early stages of lung toxicity, plain chest radiographs are usually normal. Alveolar damage is usually a generalized process at the lung bases and, in moderate to severe cases, is seen as bilateral abnormal non-specific shadowing both

on plain films and on CT. Such injury may be caused by busulphan, carmustine (BCNU) and methotrexate. Pulmonary vasculitis leads to infarction and, in some cases, cavitation may result. Pulmonary vascular damage may occur with busulphan therapy.[85]

Chronic graft versus host disease (GVHD) is characterized by lymphocytic infiltration of the interstitial tissues and bronchial walls. Bronchiolitis obliterans is also seen.[86] Plain chest radiographs may be normal but on CT abnormal shadowing around peripheral bronchi may be observed.[87]

Key points: thoracic manifestations

- Mediastinal lymphadenopathy is a common feature of ALL and CLL

- Mediastinal lymphadenopathy is also seen in T-cell childhood leukaemia and in adult T-cell leukaemia/lymphoma

- Leukaemic infiltration of the lungs is rarely diagnosed during life. The appearances are often indistinguishable from infection or pulmonary oedema

- Mediastinal widening may be due to mediastinitis, haemorrhage or superior vena caval thrombosis as well as lymphadenopathy

- Pulmonary infection is a major cause of morbidity in leukaemic patients. Organisms include CMV, *Pneumocystis carinii* and fungal infections such as invasive pulmonary aspergillosis

Abdomen and pelvis

Direct involvement by leukaemia

Hepatosplenomegaly due to diffuse involvement of the liver and spleen is a frequent manifestation of leukaemia (Fig. 34.1). Imaging is not usually undertaken to evaluate these organs but both CT and ultrasound will demonstrate hepatosplenomegaly. Focal lesions within the liver and spleen due to leukaemia are rarely seen. Splenic infarction may be associated with gross splenomegaly and, on CT, these lesions appear as an irregular, relatively low-density area within a massively enlarged spleen and as hypoechoic lesions on ultrasound.

Renal involvement in leukaemia is common, occurring in approximately 50% of cases at autopsy.[16] As in patients with lymphoma, leukaemia may involve the kidneys by:

- Diffuse parenchymal infiltration (bilateral or unilateral) (Fig. 34.15)
- Discrete renal mass or masses
- Obstruction due to lymphadenopathy at the hilum

In a recent review of 700 cases of the renal manifestations of non-Hodgkin's lymphoma and lymphocytic leukaemia,

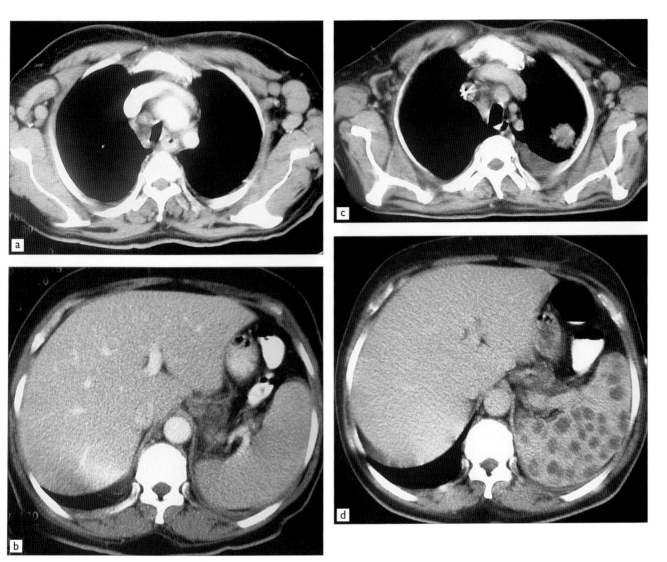

Figure 34.14. *(a and b) CT images in a 41-year-old man with ALL obtained prior to treatment showing bilateral axillary lymphadenopathy. The spleen was normal in appearance. (c and d) CT imaging was performed 2 months after commencing chemotherapy. Imaging revealed improvement in the axillary lymphadenopathy, but a new mass was visible within the left upper lobe associated with a small pleural effusion (c). In addition, multiple low attenuation lesions were also noted within the spleen (d). Biopsy of the lung mass confirmed infection with mycobacterium tuberculosis.*

Da'as et al.[88] found that no cases of primary renal involvement were found. Acute renal failure was seen in 83 patients but leukaemic infiltration was found to be the cause in only five.[88]

Ultrasound is a useful technique for detecting leukaemic infiltration. The kidneys are diffusely enlarged and show patchy areas of low echogenicity. On contrast-enhanced CT, the parenchyma shows an inhomogeneous pattern with areas of diminished density interspersed with areas of enhancement, findings which are similar to those seen in lymphoma.[89] Solid renal masses may also be observed on CT.

The gastro-intestinal tract is involved in leukaemia in about 25% of cases.[90] Leukaemia infiltrates spread through the lamina propria or submucosa of the bowel wall producing localized areas of bowel wall thickening. Imaging is seldom required as it is unusual for such lesions to become clinically manifest. Occasionally, a granulocytic sarcoma may develop within the bowel wall and may present as abdominal pain or intestinal obstruction.

As in other anatomical sites, abdominal lymph node involvement is more commonly seen in the acute lymphoblastic and chronic lymphocytic leukaemias than in the myelogenous leukaemias. Multiple enlarged nodes may be seen within the retroperitoneum, mesentery, splenic hilum, porta hepatis and other intra-abdominal and pelvic sites (Figs. 34.2 and 34.15). Nodes are usually discretely enlarged and, on imaging, the appearances are indistinguishable from those of non-Hodgkin's lymphoma.

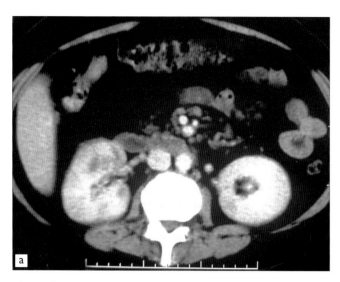
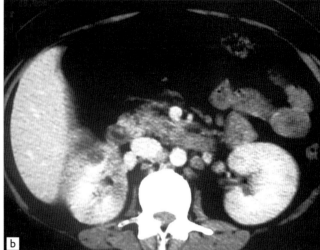

Figure 34.15. *CT scan images in a 40-year-old female patient with AML showing bilateral renal infiltration. Both kidneys are enlarged and demonstrate multiple ill-defined low attenuation areas in keeping with leukaemic infiltration. Note the presence of small volume retroperitoneal lymph nodes.*

Other sites of involvement in the abdomen and pelvis include the prostate gland, uterus and adrenal glands. The testis and ovary are sanctuary sites and are therefore relatively resistant to chemotherapy (Table 34.2).[15]

Key points: abdominal/pelvic manifestations

- Hepatosplenomegaly is a common feature of all the leukaemias

- Splenic infarcts may be demonstrated on imaging

- Renal involvement is seen in 50% of cases at autopsy

- Renal involvement may be diffuse or focal

- Enlarged lymph nodes in the abdomen and pelvis occur in multiple sites in ALL and CLL

- The gastro-intestinal tract is involved in approximately 25% of cases. In the majority of patients the disease is silent

Indirect effects of leukaemia

The most important indirect effects of leukaemia within the abdomen and pelvis are GVHD, neutropenic enterocolitis, haemorrhage and infection.

Graft versus host disease

Graft versus host disease most commonly affects the skin, gastro-intestinal tract and liver. This disease is a major complication of allogeneic BMT, occurring in about 50% of patients. The phenomenon is a manifestation of graft rejec-tion in which the immunocompetent donor lymphoid cells react against host antigens. The principal bowel abnormal-ities are those of lymphocytic infiltration of the lamina pro-pria, crypt dilatation and necrosis and focal micro-abscess formation.[91,92] Involvement of the bowel can be demon-strated on conventional plain abdominal radiographs, bar-ium studies and on CT.

On plain radiography, air–fluid levels, bowel wall and mucosal fold-thickening and ascites may be seen.[93] On bar-ium studies, the small bowel shows thickening and flatten-ing of the mucosal folds, a rapid transit time and air–fluid levels.[94] Pneumatosis intestinalis may be observed in severe cases.[95] Graft versus host disease may resolve completely, in which case the abnormal plain film and barium findings return to normal. Computed tomography findings of GVHD include bowel wall thickening, stenosis of small bowel loops and oedema of the bowel wall. Oedema is typi-cally seen as a 'target sign' with decreased attenuation cen-trally bounded by high attenuation on both the serosal and mucosal surfaces of the bowel (Fig 34.16). In addition, there is usually generalized increased density within the mesenteric fat.[96] These findings are non-specific and may be seen in other benign and malignant conditions.

Neutropenic enterocolitis

Neutropenic enterocolitis is a severe complication of inten-sive chemotherapy for acute leukaemia and is difficult to diagnose with confidence clinically. Patients present with abdominal pain, fever and diarrhoea, and imaging with ultrasound and CT can play a useful role in the diagnosis by demonstrating bowel wall thickening. Cartoni et al.[97] found that ultrasound was able to determine bowel wall thickening and that the degree of thickness correlated well with the clin-ical course and disease outcome. Patients with bowel wall

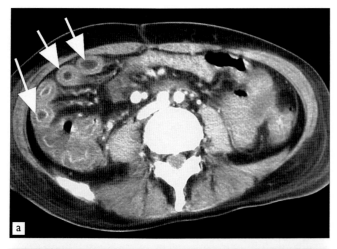

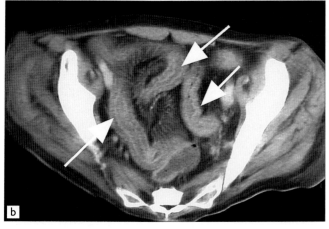

Figure 34.16. *In this 38-year-old man with previous history of an allogenic bone marrow transplant for CML, CT (a and b) shows multiple thickened small bowel loops exhibiting 'target sign' (arrows), due to low attenuation oedema within the bowel wall adjacent to the enhancing mucosal and serosal surfaces. The CT appearance is suggestive of graft versus host disease.*

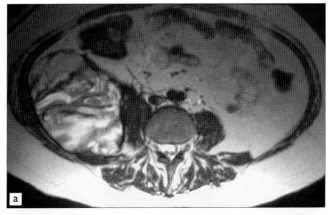

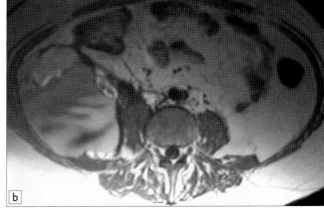

Figure 34.17. *(a) T1-weighted and (b) T2-weighted axial MR images in a 35-year-old man with ALL, presenting with acute right flank pain. The images show a large right retroperitoneal haematoma, which appears of high signal intensity on both T1- and T2-weighted imaging, indicating the presence of blood within the lesion.*

thickening greater than 10 mm had a significantly poorer prognosis than those with lesser degrees of thickening.

Haemorrhage

Occasionally, imaging is required to investigate clinical features suggestive of intra-abdominal haemorrhage in leukaemic patients. This is usually manifested by acute abdominal pain together with clinical features of blood loss. Retroperitoneal haemorrhage may present as acute back pain and, in such patients, CT is the ideal imaging modality to demonstrate the presence of fresh blood and the extent of haemorrhage (Fig. 34.17).

Infection

Intra-abdominal infection is an important cause of abdominal pain in leukaemic patients. Infectious cecitis (typhli-tis), perirectal abscesses and appendicitis may all complicate the clinical picture of leukaemia. Computed tomography may be helpful in the management of these patients because haemorrhage may be distinguished from infection and the site of infection localized.

Liver infection is a serious complication of treatment. Candidiasis may involve the liver and spleen and is recognized on imaging as multiple small focal lesions throughout the organ parenchyma. Diagnosis must be made by biopsy or blood culture in the presence of abnormal imaging findings. Magnetic resonance is a sensitive method of identifying these focal liver abnormalities and may also be used to monitor therapy. In one study, the median time to disappearance of all lesions on MR was 9 weeks in the patients who responded to therapy (86%).

Key points: abdominal/pelvic complications

- ■ GVHD is a major complication of allogeneic BMT
- ■ Acute GVHD most commonly affects the skin, liver and gastro-intestinal tract
- ■ Plain radiographs, barium studies and CT may all show dilatation, stenosis and thickening of small bowel loops with air–fluid levels
- ■ Ascites and pneumatosis intestinalis are seen in severe cases
- ■ Neutropenic enterocolitis is a serious complication of intensive treatment as is manifested by bowel wall thickening
- ■ Intra-abdominal/retroperitoneal haemorrhage may account for the onset of abdominal pain in leukaemic patients
- ■ Intra-abdominal infection such as cecitis (typhlitis) may complicate acute leukaemia
- ■ Liver infection with candidiasis can be detected and monitored with imaging; MR is a sensitive technique to monitor response

Skeletal system

Direct involvement of leukaemia

The incidence and radiographic manifestations of skeletal involvement in leukaemia vary with patient age and subtype of the disease.

Radiographic findings

In children, leukaemic infiltration of the long bones produces characteristic appearances on plain radiographs (Fig. 34.18), which include:

- • Diffuse osteoporosis
- • Transverse metaphyseal bands of diminished density
- • Dense transverse metaphyseal lines of arrested growth
- • Subperiosteal new bone formation
- • Osteolytic lesions
- • Osteosclerotic lesions in less than 2% of patients[20]

Diffuse osteoporosis is the most common skeletal abnormality in childhood ALL, occurring in up to 60% of cases, and is most obvious in the spine.

In adults, osteoporosis and cortical thinning of long bones due to expansion of the marrow space are common. Other features such as metaphyseal bands, so characteristic of childhood leukaemia, are not seen in adults. In adult T-cell leukaemia/lymphoma, lytic bone lesions are common.[78] Subperiosteal bone resorption may be seen in this subtype of leukaemia and probably results from hypercalcaemia.[78]

In children with acute leukaemia presenting with back ache, plain radiographs may show collapse of one or several vertebral bodies (Fig. 34.19a). This is either due to vertebral compression fractures as a result of osteoporosis or from destruction of bone trabeculae by leukaemic infiltration. With treatment, remodelling of the vertebral body with reconstitution of the vertebral height may be observed

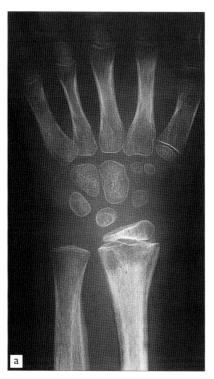
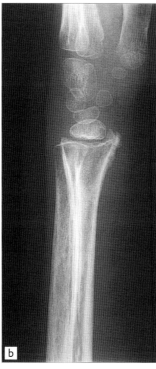

Figure 34.18. *Plain radiographs of the wrist in a 4-year-old boy with ALL. (a) Anterior/posterior view; (b) lateral view, showing diffuse osteoporosis throughout the radius and ulna as well as the bones of the wrist. Transverse metaphyseal bands of diminished density are noted. There is an extensive periosteal reaction on the distal surfaces of the radius and ulna.*

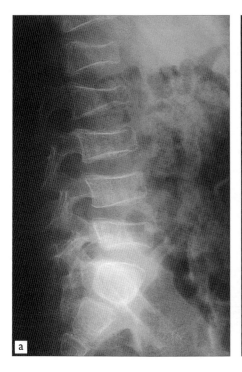
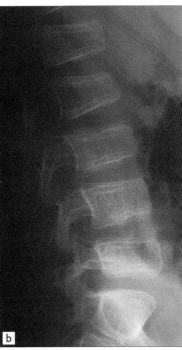

Figure 34.19. *Lateral plain radiographs in a 4-year-old boy who presented with back pain due to ALL. (a) At presentation, partial collapse of the lumbar vertebral bodies is noted. The most severely affected vertebra is L2. (b) Two years later following treatment, there has been remodelling of the bone. Note the thin dense lines adjacent to the vertebral end-plates giving the appearance of a bone within a bone. There is still extensive osteoporosis.*

(Fig. 34.19b). A characteristic but unusual feature is that of a 'bone' within a bone.[98]

Submetaphyseal bands are seen in approximately 40% of children and probably represent osteoporosis in the rapidly growing region of the long bone. They are seen most frequently in the distal femur, proximal tibia, proximal humerus and vertebral bodies.

Focal lytic lesions are less common in AML than in ALL (Fig. 34.20) but may develop in CML during the accelerated growth phase and, in this group of patients, hypercalcaemia may also be evident.[99] Focal lesions are usually permeative and may show cortical destruction with pathological fracture. In the skull, lucent areas with a 'moth-eaten' appearance may be identified due to leukaemic infiltration and in

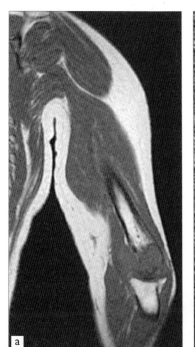
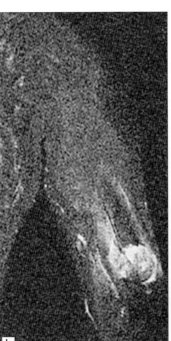
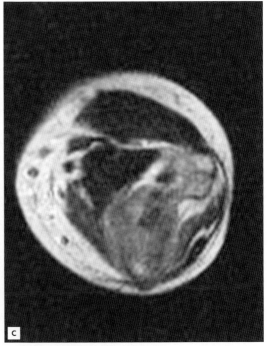

Figure 34.20. *A 42-year-old man with ALL. (a) T1-weighted coronal, (b) STIR coronal and (c) T1-weighted axial images, showing a focal leukaemic deposit replacing the normal marrow signal within the condyles of the distal left humerus. The mass infiltrates into the adjacent soft tissues.*

children, widening of the sutures is associated with underlying meningeal disease. This has been less commonly observed since the introduction of CNS prophylaxis.

Bone is one of the most frequent sites for development of granulocytic sarcoma. An area of bone destruction is seen on plain radiographs which may be accompanied by a soft tissue mass. The lesions are most commonly found in the skull, spine, ribs and sternum.[100]

Computed tomography is indicated for the evaluation of leukaemic masses (granulocytic sarcoma) in various sites, as the technique can define the soft tissue disease as well as the extent of bone destruction.

Radionuclide bone scanning either with technetium-99m-diphosphonate, or bone marrow imaging with colloid, is not required in the routine management of leukaemia[101,102] but bone scans may be helpful in patients suspected of harbouring occult bone infection.

When MR was first introduced into clinical practice over a decade ago there was considerable enthusiasm regarding its potential to evaluate diffuse bone marrow disease. Certainly, diffuse infiltration of the bone marrow can be elegantly demonstrated on spin-echo imaging as diffuse abnormally low signal intensity on T1-weighted images accompanied by an intermediate signal intensity on T2-weighted images. In leukaemia, the axial skeleton is mainly involved (Fig. 34.21). However, MR is non-specific, and benign and malignant disorders give similar appearances (Fig. 34.22).[103,104] Clear advantages of MR are the ability to

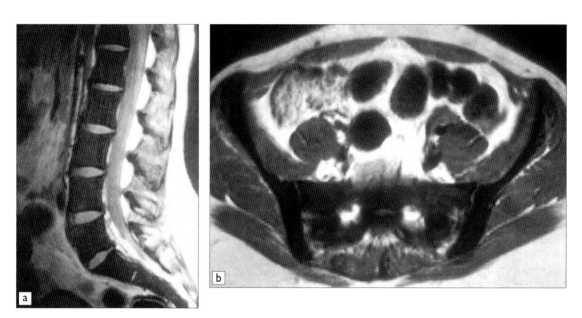

Figure 34.21. *T1-weighted spin-echo MR images in a 21-year-old female with ALL. (a) Sagittal image of the spine; (b) axial image through the pelvis. The MR examination shows widespread diffuse abnormal low signal intensity throughout the vertebral bodies and pelvis, indicating extensive bone marrow infiltration.*

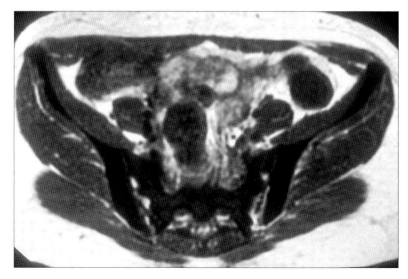

Figure 34.22. *A 50-year-old female patient with myelofibrosis. The spin-echo T1-weighted axial MR image of the pelvis shows diffuse abnormal low signal intensity throughout the iliac bones and sacrum. The appearances are identical to those of leukaemic infiltration.*

survey large volumes of the bone marrow at a single investigation and the high sensitivity of the technique in detecting bone marrow pathology.

Magnetic resonance may demonstrate changes within the bone marrow in leukaemic patients in response to treatment (Fig. 34.23) and some authors have used quantitative measurements of T1 relaxation times to evaluate therapeutic response.[105,106] In a recent study, van de Berg et al.[107] showed that sequential quantitative MR during therapy for ALL and AML revealed significant differences in the initial bulk values of T1 relaxation between these subtypes of leukaemia and also in the changes observed in T1 between the two groups during therapy. As a result, these authors suggest that bone marrow imaging with MR may be a useful method of predicting response in ALL.[107] However, Lecouvet et al.[108]

have shown that quantitative MR failed to identify bone marrow abnormalities in 41% of patients with CLL. Recently, diffusion-weighted imaging has been applied to examination of the bone marrow in leukaemic patients.[109] Measured signal-to-noise ratios agreed with an estimate of percentage cellularity and, in addition, the signal-to-noise ratios were also dependent on time after commencement of treatment.[109]

Despite these interesting results, the current role of MR in the evaluation of leukaemia is limited as clinical and haematological investigations usually direct patient management. Although MR seems to have little role in the routine evaluation of the bone marrow in leukaemia, it is useful in patients suspected of relapse, for example, in patients believed to be in remission who represent with bone pain (Fig. 34.24), or in patients at high risk of

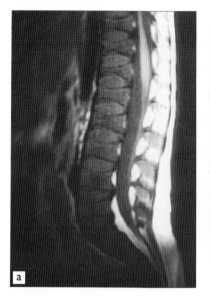 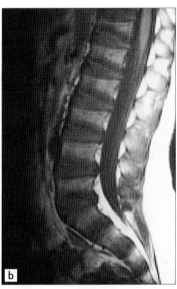

Figure 34.23. *MR images in a 4-year-old boy with ALL. This is the same patient as shown in Figure 34.17. T1-weighted sagittal images through the thoracic and lumbar spine: (a) before treatment; (b) 2 years after treatment. The MR image at presentation shows diffuse abnormal low signal intensity throughout the vertebral bodies indicating leukaemic infiltration. Note that the signal intensity of the bone marrow is lower than that of the adjacent intervertebral discs. There is partial collapse of multiple vertebrae. Two years later the signal intensity of the vertebral bodies is higher than the adjacent intervertebral discs. This represents response to treatment.*

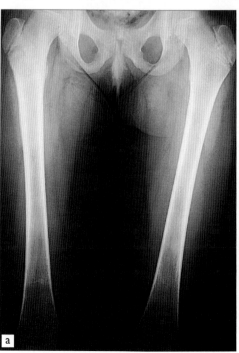 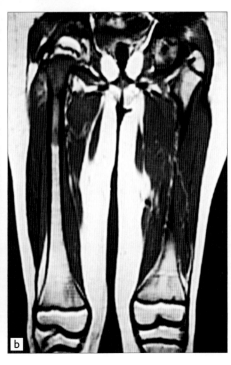

Figure 34.24. *A 10-year-old boy treated three years previously for ALL with CNS relapse. He represented with right leg pain: (a) plain radiograph of the femora did not reveal any abnormality; (b) coronal T1-weighted MR image of the femora showing extensive abnormal low signal intensity throughout the metaphyseal region and upper diaphysis of the right femur. This represented leukaemic relapse.*

relapse in whom serial bone marrow biopsies are negative.

Key points: skeletal involvement

- In childhood ALL, osteoporosis occurs in up to 60% of cases

- Metaphyseal translucencies are seen in the long bones in approximately 40% of children with ALL

- Focal bone lesions are more common in ALL than AML

- Granulocytic sarcoma in AML occurs most frequently in the skull, ribs and sternum

- MR shows diffuse bone marrow abnormality in acute leukaemia but the appearances are non-specific

- MR has a valuable role in the detection of leukaemic relapse in patients with bone pain

Indirect effects of leukaemia

Following therapy with BMT, repopulation of the bone marrow gives rise to striking appearances with bands of low signal intensity adjacent to the vertebral end-plates with higher signal intensity centrally on MR (Fig. 34.25).

These appearances are related to repopulation of the marrow in the region of the capillary network which lies adjacent to the vertebral end-plates.[110,111] Treatment with steroids may lead to avascular necrosis of the femoral head (Fig. 34.26). Magnetic resonance is well-established as the best imaging technique for detecting avascular necrosis and is indicated in all symptomatic patients with normal plain films. As in other areas of the body, infection is a major hazard in the acute leukaemias and bone pain may represent osteomyelitis as well as leukaemic relapse (Fig. 34.27).

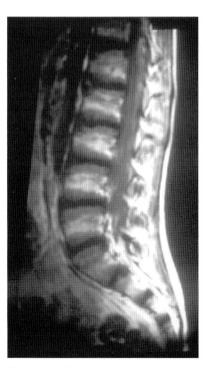

Figure 34.25. *MR image in a 21-year-old male patient following bone marrow transplant. T1-weighted sagittal image showing typical 'bandlike' pattern of repopulation of bone marrow with areas of low signal intensity adjacent to the vertebral end-plates. Higher signal intensity centrally represents fat.*

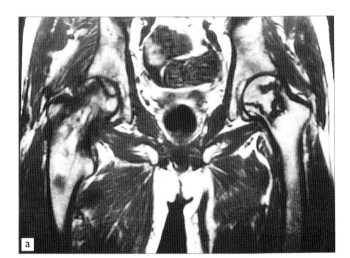

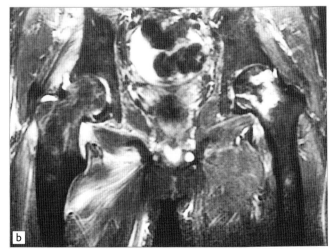

Figure 34.26. *An adult male patient with ALL with bilateral avascular necrosis of the femoral heads. (a) Coronal T1-weighted MR image, (b) turbo STIR image. The T1-weighted image shows classic signs of avascular necrosis with irregular areas of low signal intensity within the femoral heads bilaterally. The STIR image shows abnormal high signal intensity areas within the femoral heads and also in the femoral neck on the right, indicating associated oedema.*

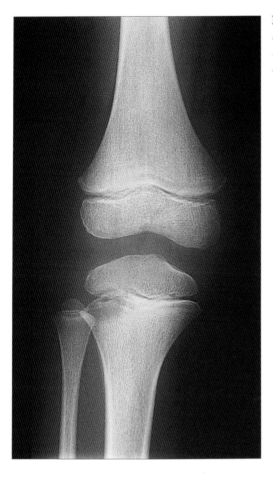

Figure 34.27. *Plain film of the right knee in a 5-year-old boy with ALL complaining of severe bone pain around the knee joint. There is a destructive lytic lesion in the lateral aspect of the tibial metaphysis. This was due to osteomyelitis and was surgically drained.*

Conclusion

Leukaemia comprises a heterogeneous group of neoplasms for which the investigation and treatment has changed markedly over recent years. Cross-sectional imaging, as well as conventional radiology, has an important place in the management of this disease. However, it is impossible to define strict algorithms for the use of imaging because the disease is manifested in many different organs and organ systems and the complications of leukaemia are common and diverse. As in other malignant tumours, close liaison between clinician and radiologist is essential to determine the most appropriate use of imaging for individual patient care.

Summary

- There are four major groups of leukaemia which are categorized according to the predominant type of proliferating cell – ALL, AML, CML, CLL

- Acute lymphoblastic leukaemia (ALL) is the most common subtype in childhood

- Acute myelogenous leukaemia (AML) and chronic lymphocytic leukaemia (CLL) are the most common subtypes in adults

- Chromosomal abnormalities have been identified in many of the subtypes of leukaemia

- The major clinical features of leukaemia relate to anaemia, infection and haemorrhage

- Bone pain is a common presenting feature in children with ALL but is uncommon in adults

- Granulocytic sarcoma (chloroma) is a mass composed of precursors of myelocytes. It occurs in AML disorders but also occurs in other myeloprolific disorders

- Granulocytic sarcoma most commonly involves the orbits, subcutaneous tissues, paranasal sinuses and bones

- Leukaemia is primarily treated with combination chemotherapy. Bone marrow transplantation, craniospinal irradiation and Interferon-α (IFN-α) all have a place in patient management

- The 5-year survival rate of ALL in children is 50–80% and in adults it is 20–40%

- The 5-year survival in AML is 40–50%

- Imaging findings in leukaemia are related to direct involvement of organs and tissues by the disease and to indirect involvement of organs due to complications

- In the CNS, leukaemia involves the leptomeninges, dura and, rarely, the brain parenchyma. It may be diffuse or focal

- Haemorrhage, sinovenous thrombosis and cerebral infarction, as well as infection, are all indirect effects of leukaemia on the CNS

- Intrathoracic leukaemia usually involves mediastinal and hilar lymph nodes. Pulmonary complications include infection, haemorrhage, oedema and graft versus host disease (GVHD)

- Diffuse involvement of intra-abdominal organs is common (liver, spleen, kidneys, gastro-intestinal tract, intra-abdominal lymph nodes)

- GVHD and neutropenic enterocolitis are important intra-abdominal complications which can be assessed with CT and ultrasound

- Skeletal manifestations of childhood leukaemia are seen in up to 60% of patients and include osteoporosis, transmetaphyseal bands and subperiosteal new bone formation

- Focal lytic lesions in the bone are more common in AML than ALL

- MR may demonstrate diffuse bone marrow abnormalities, both in acute and chronic leukaemia, but is not widely used for routine evaluation

- MR is useful in the investigation of pain in patients suspected of relapse with bone pain

References

1. Caligiuri M A, Ritz J. Immunology. In: Henderson E S, Lister T A (eds). Leukaemia, 5th edn. Philadelphia: W B Saunders, 1990; 103–130

2. Garson C M. Cytogenetics of leukemic cells. In: Henderson E S, Lister T A (eds). Leukaemia, 5th edn. Philadelphia: W B Saunders, 1990; 131–152

3. Cancer Facts and Figures 2003. American Cancer Society, Inc, 2003

4. CancerStats Incidence UK – April 2003. Cancer Research UK, 2003

5. Preston D L, Kusumi S, Tomonaga M et al. Cancer incidence in atomic bomb survivors. Part III. Leukemia, lymphoma and multiple myeloma, 1950–1987. Radiat Res 1994; 137: S68–97

6. Sandler D P. Recent studies in leukemia epidemiology. Curr Opin Oncol 1995; 7: 12–18

7. Arseneau J C, Sponzo R W, Levin D L et al. Nonlymphomatous malignant tumors complicating Hodgkin's disease. Possible association with intensive therapy. N Engl J Med 1972; 287: 1119–1122

8. Aisenberg A C. Acute nonlymphocytic leukemia after treatment for Hodgkin's disease. Am J Med 1983; 75: 449–454

9. Curtis R E, Boice J D Jr, Stovall M et al. Risk of leukemia after chemotherapy and radiation treatment for breast cancer. N Engl J Med 1992; 326: 1745–1751

10. Kaldor J M, Day N E, Pettersson F et al. Leukemia following chemotherapy for ovarian cancer. N Engl J Med 1990; 322: 1–6

11. Robert-Guroff M, Reitz M S Jr, Robey W G et al. In vitro generation of an HTLV-III variant by neutralizing antibody. J Immunol 1986; 137: 3306–3309

12. Kalyanaraman V S, Sarngadharan M G, Nakao Y et al. Natural antibodies to the structural core protein (p24) of the human T-cell leukemia (lymphoma) retrovirus found in sera of leukemia patients in Japan. Proc Natl Acad Sci USA 1982; 79: 1653–1657

13. Weber J. HTLV-I infection in Britain. Br Med J 1990; 301: 71–72

14. Anonymous. HTLV-1 comes of age. Lancet 1988; 1: 217–219

15. Barcos M, Lane W, Gomez G A et al. An autopsy study of 1206 acute and chronic leukemias (1958–1982). Cancer 1987; 60: 827–837

16. Henderson E S, Afshani E. Clinical manifestation and diagnosis. In: Henderson E S, Lister T A (eds). Leukaemia, 5th edn. Philadelphia: W B Saunders, 1990; 291–359

17. Graus F, Rogers L R, Posner J B. Cerebrovascular complications in patients with cancer. Medicine (Baltimore) 1985; 64: 16–35

18. Freireich E J, Thomas L B, Frei E et al. A distinctive type of intracerebral haemorrhage associated with "blastic crisis" in patients with leukaemia. Cancer 1960; 13: 146–154

19. Fernbach D J. Natural history of acute leukemia. In: Sutow W, Vietti TJ, Fernbach DJ (eds). Pediatric Oncology, 2nd edn. St Louis: Mosby, 1977; 291–333

20. Thomas L G, Forkner C E J, Frei E. The skeletal lesions of acute leukemia. Cancer 1961; 14: 608

21. Hann I M, Gupta S, Palmer M K et al. The prognostic significance of radiological and symptomatic bone involvement in childhood acute lymphoblastic leukaemia. Med Pediatr Oncol 1979; 6: 51–55

22. Nies B A, Kundel D W, Thomas L B et al. Leucopenia, bone pain, and bone necrosis in patients with acute leukemia. A clinicopathological complex. Ann Intern Med 1965; 62: 698

23. Neiman R S, Barcos M, Berard C et al. Granulocytic sarcoma: a clinicopathologic study of 61 biopsied cases. Cancer 1981; 48: 1426–1437

24. Pui M H, Fletcher B D, Langston J W. Granulocytic sarcoma in childhood leukemia: imaging features. Radiology 1994; 190: 698–702

25. Muss H B, Moloney W C. Chloroma and other myeloblastic tumors. Blood 1973; 42: 721–728

26. Liu P I, Ishimaru T, McGregor D H et al. Autopsy study of granulocytic sarcoma (chloroma) in patients with myelogenous leukemia, Hiroshima-Nagasaki 1949–1969. Cancer 1973; 31: 948–955

27. Krause J R. Granulocytic sarcoma preceding acute

leukemia: a report of six cases. Cancer 1979; 44: 1017–1021

28. Burns A. Observation of the Surgical Anatomy of the Head and Neck. Edinburgh, Scotland: Thomas Bryce, 1811

29. King A. A case of chloroma. Monthly J Med Soc 1853; 17: 97

30. Henderson E S, Hoelzer D, Freeman A I. The treatment of acute lymphoblastic leukaemia. In: Henderson E S, Lister T A (eds). Leukaemia, 5th edn. Philadelphia: W B Saunders, 1990; 443–482

31. Ortega J A, Nesbit M E, Sather H N et al. Long-term evaluation of a CNS prophylaxis trial–treatment comparisons and outcome after CNS relapse in childhood ALL: a report from the Children's Cancer Study Group. J Clin Oncol 1987; 5: 1646–1654

32. de Vries E G, Mulder N H, Houwen B et al. Combination chemotherapy for acute lymphocytic leukaemia in 25 adults. Blut 1982; 44: 151–158

33. Veerman A J, Hahlen K, Kamps W A et al. High cure rate with a moderately intensive treatment regimen in non-high-risk childhood acute lymphoblastic leukemia. Results of protocol ALL VI from the Dutch Childhood Leukemia Study Group. J Clin Oncol 1996; 14: 911–918

34. Ravindranath Y. Recent advances in pediatric acute lymphoblastic and myeloid leukemia. Curr Opin Oncol 2003; 15: 23–35

35. Zhang M J, Hoelzer D, Horowitz M M et al. Long-term follow-up of adults with acute lymphoblastic leukemia in first remission treated with chemotherapy or bone marrow transplantation. The Acute Lymphoblastic Leukemia Working Committee. Ann Intern Med 1995; 123: 428–431

36. Lister T A, Whitehouse J M, Oliver R T et al. Chemotherapy and immunotherapy for acute myelogenous leukemia. Cancer 1980; 46: 2142–2148

37. Weinstein H J, Mayer R J, Rosenthal D S et al. The treatment of acute myelogenous leukemia in children and adults: VAPA update. Hamatol Bluttransfus 1983; 28: 41–45

38. Gale R P, Champlin R E. Bone marrow transplantation in acute leukaemia. Clin Haematol 1986; 15: 851–872

39. Gale R P, Foon K A, Cline M J et al. Intensive chemotherapy for acute myelogenous leukemia. Ann Intern Med 1981; 94: 753–757

40. Tricot G, Boogaerts M A, Vlietinck R et al. The role of intensive remission induction and consolidation therapy in patients with acute myeloid leukaemia. Br J Haematol 1987; 66: 37–44

41. O'Brien S G, Guilhot F, Larson R A et al. Imatinib compared with interferon and low-dose cytarabine for newly diagnosed chronic-phase chronic myeloid leukemia. N Engl J Med 2003; 348: 994–1004

42. Sawyers C L, Hochhaus A, Feldman E et al. Imatinib induces hematologic and cytogenetic responses in patients with chronic myelogenous leukemia in myeloid blast crisis: results of a phase II study. Blood 2002; 99: 3530–3539

43. Goldman J M. Leukaemia. In: Price P, Sikora K (eds). Treatment of Cancer, 3rd edn. London: Chapman and Hall, 1995; 835–839

44. Bloomfield C D, Shuma C, Regal L et al. Long-term survival of patients with acute myeloid leukemia: a third follow-up of the Fourth International Workshop on Chromosomes in Leukemia. Cancer 1997; 80: 2191–2198

45. Kantarjian H M, Talpaz M, Keating M J et al. Intensive chemotherapy induction followed by interferon-alpha maintenance in patients with Philadelphia chromosome-positive chronic myelogenous leukemia. Cancer 1991; 68: 1201–1207

46. Deininger M, Lehmann T, Krahl R et al. No evidence for persistence of BCR-ABL-positive cells in patients in molecular remission after conventional allogenic transplantation for chronic myeloid leukemia. Blood 2000; 96: 779–780

47. Coccia P F, Bleyer W A, Siegel S E et al. Development and preliminary findings of Children's Cancer Study Group Protocols (#161,162,163) for low-, average- and high-risk acute lymphoblastic leukemia in children. In: Murphy S, Gilbert J R (eds). Leukemia Research – Advances in Cell Biology and Treatment. Amsterdam: Elsevier/North Holland, 1983; 241

48. Bleyer W A. Central nervous system leukemia. In: Henderson E S, Lister T A (eds). Leukaemia, 5th edn. Philadelphia: W B Saunders, 1990; 733–768

49. Price R A, Johnson W W. The central nervous system in childhood leukemia. I. The arachnoid. Cancer 1973; 31: 520–533

50. Azzarelli V, Roessmann U. Pathogenesis of central nervous system infiltration in acute leukemia. Arch Pathol Lab Med 1977; 101: 203–205

51. Brant-Zawadzki M, Enzmann D R. Computed tomographic brain scanning in patients with lymphoma. Radiology 1978; 129: 67–71

52. Enzmann D R, Krikorian J, Yorke C et al. Computed tomography in leptomeningeal spread of tumor. J Comput Assist Tomogr 1978; 2: 448–455

53. Pagani J J, Libshitz H I, Wallace S et al. Central nervous system leukemia and lymphoma: computed tomographic manifestations. Am J Roentgenol 1981; 137: 1195–1201

54. Ginsberg L E, Leeds N E. Neuroradiology of leukemia. Am J Roentgenol 1995; 165: 525–534

55. Paakko E, Patronas N J, Schellinger D. Meningeal Gd-DTPA enhancement in patients with malignancies. J Comput Assist Tomogr 1990; 14: 542–546

56. Sze G, Abramson A, Krol G et al. Gadolinium-DTPA in the evaluation of intradural extramedullary spinal disease. Am J Roentgenol 1988; 150: 911–921

57. Kao S C, Yuh W T, Sato Y et al. Intracranial granulocytic sarcoma (chloroma): MR findings. J Comput Assist Tomogr 1987; 11: 938–941

58. Pomeranz S J, Hawkins H H, Towbin R et al. Granulocytic sarcoma (chloroma): CT manifestations. Radiology 1985; 155: 167–170

59. Ahn J Y, Kwon S O, Shin M S et al. Meningeal chloroma (granulocytic sarcoma) in acute lymphoblastic leukemia mimicking a falx meningioma. J Neurooncol 2002; 60: 31–35

60. Barnett M J, Zussman W V. Granulocytic sarcoma of the brain: a case report and review of the literature. Radiology 1986; 160: 223–225

61. Williams M P, Olliff J F, Rowley M R. CT and MR findings in parameningeal leukaemic masses. J Comput Assist Tomogr 1990; 14: 736–742

62. Ho C L, Chen C Y, Chen Y C et al. Cerebral dural sinus thrombosis in acute lymphoblastic leukemia with early diagnosis by fast fluid-attenuated inversion recovery (FLAIR) MR image: a case report and review of the literature. Ann Hematol 2000; 79: 90–94

63. Henderson E S. Complications of leukaemia: a selective overview. In: Henderson E S, Lister T A (eds). Leukaemia, 5th edn. Philadelphia: W B Saunders, 1990; 671–685

64. Bleyer W A. Neurologic sequelae of methotrexate and ionizing radiation: a new classification. Cancer Treat Rep 1981; 65 Suppl 1: 89–98

65. Jager H R, Williams E J, Savage D G et al. Assessment of brain changes with registered MR before and after bone marrow transplantation for chronic myeloid leukemia. Am J Neuroradiol 1996; 17: 1275–1282

66. Packer R J, Zimmerman R A, Bilaniuk L T. Magnetic resonance imaging in the evaluation of treatment-related central nervous system damage. Cancer 1986; 58: 635–640

67. Duffner P K, Cohen M E, Brecher M L et al. CT abnormalities and altered methotrexate clearance in children with CNS leukemia. Neurology 1984; 34: 229–233

68. Laitt R D, Chambers E J, Goddard P R et al. Magnetic resonance imaging and magnetic resonance angiography in long term survivors of acute lymphoblastic leukemia treated with cranial irradiation. Cancer 1995; 76: 1846–1852

69. Chan Y L, Roebuck D J, Yuen M P et al. Long-term cerebral metabolite changes on proton magnetic resonance spectroscopy in patients cured of acute lymphoblastic leukemia with previous intrathecal methotrexate and cranial irradiation prophylaxis. Int J Radiat Oncol Biol Phys 2001; 50: 759–763

70. Rubinstein L J, Herman M M, Long T F et al. Disseminated necrotizing leukoencephalopathy: a complication of treated central nervous system leukemia and lymphoma. Cancer 1975; 35: 291–305

71. Price R A, Birdwell D A. The central nervous system in childhood leukemia. III. Mineralizing microangiopathy and dystrophic calcification. Cancer 1978; 42: 717–728

72. Ito M, Akiyama Y, Asato R et al. Early diagnosis of leukoencephalopathy of acute lymphocytic leukemia by MRI. Pediatr Neurol 1991; 7: 436–439

73. Bjorgen J E, Gold L H. Computed tomographic appearance of methotrexate-induced necrotizing leukoencephalopathy. Radiology 1977; 122: 377–378

74. Vera P, Rohrlich P, Stievenart J L et al. Contribution of single-photon emission computed tomography in the diagnosis and follow-up of CNS toxicity of a cytarabine-containing regimen in pediatric leukemia. J Clin Oncol 1999; 17: 2804–2810

75. Harila-Saari A H, Paakko E L, Vainionpaa L K et al. A longitudinal magnetic resonance imaging study of the brain in survivors in childhood acute lymphoblastic leukemia. Cancer 1998; 83: 2608–2617

76. Iuvone L, Mariotti P, Colosimo C et al. Long-term cognitive outcome, brain computed tomography scan, and magnetic resonance imaging in children cured for acute lymphoblastic leukemia. Cancer 2002; 95: 2562–2570

77. Lee W A, Hruban R H, Kuhlman J E et al. High resolution computed tomography of inflation-fixed lungs: pathologic–radiologic correlation of pulmonary lesions in patients with leukemia, lymphoma, or other hematopoietic proliferative disorders. Clin Imaging 1992; 16: 15–24

78. George C D, Wilson A G, Philpott N J et al. The radiological features of adult T-cell leukaemia/lymphoma. Clin Radiol 1994; 49: 83–88

79. Armstrong P, Dyer R, Alford B A et al. Leukemic pulmonary infiltrates: rapid development mimicking pulmonary edema. Am J Roentgenol 1980; 135: 373–374

80. Berkman N, Polliack A, Breuer R et al. Pulmonary involvement as the major manifestation of chronic lymphocytic leukemia. Leuk Lymphoma 1992; 8: 495–499

81. Green R A, Nichols N J. Pulmonary involvment in leukemia. Am Rev Resp Dis 1959; 80: 833–844

82. Schimpff S C. Infection in the leukaemia patient: diagnosis, therapy and prevention. In: Henderson E S, Lister T A (eds). Leukaemia, 5th edn. Philadelphia: W B Saunders, 1990; 687–709

83. DeGregorio M W, Lee W M, Linker C A et al. Fungal infections in patients with acute leukemia. Am J Med 1982; 73: 543–548

84. Olliff J F, Williams M P. Radiological appearances of cytomegalovirus infections. Clin Radiol 1989; 40: 463–467

85. Dee P. Drug- and radiation-induced lung disease. In: Armstrong P, Wilson A G, Hansell D M (eds). Imaging Diseases of the Chest, 2nd edn. St Louis: Mosby, 1995; 461–484

86. Chan C K, Hyland R H, Hutcheon M A et al. Small-airways disease in recipients of allogeneic bone marrow transplants. An analysis of 11 cases and a review of the literature. Medicine 1987; 66: 327–340

87. Graham N J, Muller N L, Miller R R et al. Intrathoracic complications following allogeneic bone marrow transplantation: CT findings. Radiology 1991; 181: 153–156

88. Da'as N, Polliack A, Cohen Y et al. Kidney involvement and renal manifestations in non-Hodgkin's lymphoma and lymphocytic leukemia: a retrospective study in 700 patients. Eur J Haematol 2001; 67: 158–164

89. Gore R M, Shkolnik A. Abdominal manifestations of pediatric leukemias: sonographic assessment. Radiology 1982; 143: 207–210

90. Boggs D A, Wintrobe M M, Cartwright G E. The acute leukaemias. Analysis of 322 cases and review of the literature. Medicine 1962; 41: 163

91. Epstein R J, McDonald G B, Sale G E et al. The diagnostic accuracy of the rectal biopsy in acute graft-versus-host disease: a prospective study of thirteen patients. Gastroenterology 1980; 78: 764–771

92. Slavin R E, Woodruff J M. The pathology of bone marrow transplantation. In: Somers S C (ed). Pathology Annual. New York: Appleton-Century Crofts, 1974; 291

93. Belli A M, Williams M P. Graft-versus-host disease: findings on plain abdominal radiography. Clin Radiol 1988; 39: 262–264

94. Fisk J D, Shulman H M, Greening R R et al. Gastrointestinal radiographic features of human graft-versus-host disease. Am J Roentgenol 1981; 136: 329–336

95. Maile C W, Frick M P, Crass J R et al. The plain abdominal radiograph in acute gastrointestinal graft-versus-host disease. Am J Roentgenol 1985; 145: 289–292

96. Jones B, Fishman E K, Kramer S S et al. Computed tomography of gastrointestinal inflammation after bone marrow transplantation. Am J Roentgenol 1986; 146: 691–695

97. Cartoni C, Dragoni F, Micozzi A et al. Neutropenic enterocolitis in patients with acute leukemia: prognostic significance of bowel wall thickening detected by ultrasonography. J Clin Oncol 2001; 19: 756–761

98. deCastro L A, Kuhn J P, Freeman A I et al. Complete remodeling of the vertebrae in a child successfully treated for acute lymphocytic leukemia (ALL). Cancer 1977; 40: 398–401

99. Tricot G, Boogaerts M A, Broeckaert-Van Orshoven A et al. Hypercalcemia and diffuse osteolytic lesions in the acute phase of chronic myelogenous leukemia. A possible relation between lymphoid transformation and hypercalcemia. Cancer 1983; 52: 841–845

100. Van Slyck E J. The bony changes in malignant hematologic disease. Orthop Clin North Am 1972; 3: 733–734

101. Goergen T G, Alazraki N P, Halpern S E et al. 'Cold' bone lesions: a newly recognized phenomenon of bone imaging. J Nucl Med 1974; 15: 1120–1124

102. Parker B R, Marglin S, Castellino R A. Skeletal manifestations of leukemia, Hodgkin disease, and non-Hodgkin's lymphoma. Semin Roentgenol 1980; 15: 302–315

103. Porter B A, Shields A F, Olson D O. Magnetic resonance imaging of bone marrow disorders. Radiol Clin North Am 1986; 24: 269–289

104. Jones R J. The role of bone marrow imaging. Radiology 1992; 183: 321–322

105. Moore S G, Gooding C A, Brasch R C et al. Bone marrow in children with acute lymphocytic leukemia: MR relaxation times. Radiology 1986; 160: 237–240

106. McKinstry C S, Steiner R E, Young A T et al. Bone marrow in leukemia and aplastic anemia: MR imaging before, during, and after treatment. Radiology 1987; 162: 701–707

107. van de Berg B C, Michaux L, Scheiff J M et al. Sequential quantitative MR analysis of bone marrow: differences during treatment of lymphoid versus myeloid leukemia. Radiology 1996; 201: 519–523

108. Lecouvet F E, van de Berg B C, Michaux L et al. Chronic lymphocytic leukemia: changes in bone marrow composition and distribution assessed with quantitative MRI. J Magn Reson Imaging 1998; 8: 733–739

109. Ballon D, Dyke J, Schwartz L H et al. Bone marrow segmentation in leukemia using diffusion and T(2)-weighted echo planar magnetic resonance imaging. NMR Biomed 2000; 13: 321–328

110. Stevens S K, Moore S G, Amylon M D. Repopulation of marrow after transplantation: MR imaging with pathologic correlation. Radiology 1990; 175: 213–218

111. Tanner S F, Clarke J, Leach M O et al. MRI in the evaluation of late bone marrow changes following bone marrow transplantation. Br J Radiol 1996; 69: 1145–1151

Part IV

PAEDIATRICS

Chapter 35

General principles in paediatric oncology

Helen Williams and Helen Carty

Introduction

Children with cancer place significant demands on a department of paediatric radiology. The children are often ill and there is considerable parental and family anxiety while awaiting the outcome of the radiological investigations. There is an urgency of response required by the oncologist, anxious to reach a diagnosis and plan the patient's treatment. In providing this service, the radiologist should be objective, decisive, sensitive and diagnostically accurate.

For the complete assessment of children with cancer, the radiology department must have on site access to or easy availability of all five main imaging modalities:

- Plain radiography
- Ultrasound
- Nuclear medicine
- Computed tomography (CT)
- MR imaging

The Department

In this section, points are highlighted which are often overlooked in non-specialized paediatric departments. Children are best managed in departments of paediatric radiology where the ambient environment is designed for children, where staff are familiar with handling children and communicating with them. Successful examinations are more readily achieved if the child's full cooperation is obtained. There should be explanatory books and leaflets available, written with the child in mind. The procedures should be explained in a language that the child can understand, and explained to the child and not just the parent. Knowledge allays anxiety and fear.

Heat loss

Most modern computer-controlled equipment requires an air-conditioned, stable environmental temperature for its operation. Heat loss in children in relation to body surface area is greater than in adults. Children who are cold become restless. In small infants, hypothermia can be dangerous. Heat loss can be combated by covering the child with blankets and other heat-retaining devices.

Injections

Most children fear pain and are aware that they need intravenous (IV) injections for many of their examinations. The discomfort of an injection can be minimized by a combination of prior application of a local anaesthetic cream to a suitable vein and ensuring that children's injections are done by a radiographer or doctor skilled in obtaining IV access in children. In most departments, even within paediatric departments, needle skills are variable and it is only fair that the most skilled should undertake the difficult patient. Intravenous injection of any contrast medium can be satisfactorily achieved with 23 and 25 French gauge needles, though with difficult veins, 27 G needles may be required. A butterfly system should be used because needle stability is better controlled.

Once a cancer is diagnosed and the child is on treatment, IV access via a long line such as a Hickman or Broviac catheter is almost invariably established. When these are used for IV access there must be clear protocols in place, agreed with the oncology ward, to avoid cross infection. In general, the parents are fully versed with the management of central lines and can be consulted if in doubt.

Before embarking on an IV puncture, the radiologist should always check that there is no requirement for blood samples or subsequent chemotherapy that day. The insertion of an IV cannula instead of a simple butterfly system may avert a second venepuncture.

There are a group of children who require regular scanning with the use of IV contrast but do not have long lines, who are absolutely terrified at the prospect of the venepuncture in spite of all the best care. Consideration should be given to referring these children for psychological support and play therapy in an effort to help them overcome their fears. This type of service is increasingly available in children's hospitals.

Sedation and general anaesthesia for imaging

Some children are uncooperative either due to their age, level of development or medical condition and require sedation or general anaesthesia in order to remain stationary for an investigation. This is often required for MR examinations, and sometimes for CT in order to obtain an adequate examination. A requirement for general anaesthesia further increases the demand on resources and requires close cooperation with anaesthetic and theatre staff and availability of day case beds. Children who are sedated need close monitoring of their pulse rate and oxygen saturation in order to detect any respiratory compromise. This requires a dedicated nurse or doctor and cannot be the responsibility of the radiographer performing the scan. It is essential that adequate provision of nursing staff, monitoring equipment and day case beds are available when considering sedation in children. Sedation regimens should be prescribed according to defined hospital or departmental protocols developed with input from anaesthetic, paediatric medical, radiology and nursing staff.

Equipment

The equipment used in imaging children with oncological problems has by definition to be that which is commercially available and is designed mainly for the adult population. When choosing equipment for mixed adult and childhood use, the requirements of the child should be considered.

Ultrasound

It is essential that a full range of probes is available, including a high-frequency linear array probe. Colour Doppler is essential. There should be high-quality mobile ultrasound facilities available as well as the departmental machines. It is important that machines and probes are carefully cleaned between patients in order to avoid cross infection.

Nuclear medicine

Nuclear medicine facilities are required as an integral part of imaging children with cancer. The camera head should not be placed over the child – it frightens them. Anterior views can be obtained by placing the child prone. High-resolution collimation must be available for bone imaging. A liberal supply of videos and CDs played during the examination help to allay boredom. This type of distraction therapy also works with CT and MR.

There is currently very little clinical experience in the use of 2-[F-18]fluoro-2-deoxy-D-glucose positron emission tomography ([18]FDG PET) scanning in paediatric oncology. Presently it is used in selected cases, for example in lymphoma where there is a residual mass following treatment. Current constraints include the need for sedation/general anaesthesia for young children and limited availability of scanners. It is likely that as further experience of [18]FDG PET in children develops its role will expand.

Computed tomography scanner

The choice of a CT scanner should be influenced by the availability of fast scan times which reduce sedation and general anaesthetic requirements, and detector systems, which minimize radiation dose.. Multidetector CT (MDCT) scanners with dose modulation technology are well suited to paediatric practice. CT scan planes should be chosen to minimize radiation dose to critical structures consistent with obtaining accurate information. For example, angling the gantry away from the orbitomeatal line during head scanning reduces the lens dose and reduces the number of slices for a head scan when compared with scanning in the orbitomeatal plane. Scan protocols should be designed in order to answer specific clinical questions.

Dose considerations in paediatric computed tomography

Children are more sensitive to radiation than adults and there has recently been increased awareness of the risks of low level radiation from CT in children.[1,2] Each CT examination confers an excess risk of inducing cancer and of cancer mortality in later life. For a single examination, this risk is small and the benefits far outweigh the risks, but in patients undergoing multiple examinations for reassessment of disease the risk increases. As new treatments have resulted in better survival of children with cancer, this assumes increased importance. Radiologists have a responsibility to reduce the dose from paediatric CT to a minimum. This can be accomplished by reducing the total number of CT examinations performed, substituting ultrasound or MR for staging or reassessment where possible. Dose reduction can also be achieved by changing scan parameters, reducing mAs and kVp according to patient weight and increasing slice thickness or scan pitch whilst maintaining the overall diagnostic accuracy of the examination.[3,4] Modern scanners are equipped with algorithms for paediatric protocols so that dose is effectively controlled for a given examination.

Magnetic resonance equipment

The main MR equipment requirements are that the system should be as non-intimidating as possible, with maximum tunnel width and openness, good air flow within the tube, and the ability to leave several coils in situ at the same time, so that moving a child to change a coil is avoided. For example, routine scanning of the head and spine may be required in the follow-up of a child with medulloblastoma. Moving a sedated child to change from a head to spinal coil may awaken them. Prior play therapy with mock-ups of the scanner and familiarization with the noise by playing audio tapes will improve the success rate of non-sedated scanning. Ease and reliability in achieving cardiac and respiratory gating must also be ensured.

Radiographers

Radiographers at ease with children and with good communication skills will achieve a higher success rate in scanning children without sedation than those who only occasionally examine children. In mixed adult and children's units, children should be scanned by a small number of specially trained radiographers.

Principles of imaging

Certain principles underpin diagnostic imaging of children with cancer:

- Diagnosis
- Staging
- Tissue diagnosis
- Communication
- Research

Diagnosis

The ultimate diagnosis of a tumour depends on tissue histology, but while awaiting this, patterns of imaging are sufficiently diagnostic in most childhood cancers that a working diagnosis can be established by imaging, and initial patient management planned on this basis. In arranging imaging for a child with a suspected cancer, tests should be arranged using the most appropriate, least invasive, first. In general, the initial imaging of such a child needs plain films of the suspect area, ultrasound of any palpable mass lesion and a chest radiograph. When planning cross-sectional imaging if a general anaesthetic is required, arrangements should be made following discussion between the radiologist and oncologist. Thus, where appropriate, bone marrow aspiration, lumbar puncture, insertion of a long line and biopsy may all be done at the same time, thereby maximizing the scope of investigation under general anaesthesia and avoiding the need to repeat it.

Imaging protocols must be designed to yield maximum information with minimum invasiveness and discomfort for the patient.

Once a decision to image is made, it should be done once, properly. In general, this is best done in the centre in which the child is to be treated. Tempting though it may be for a peripheral unit to want to image an 'interesting' case, knowing that the child will require transfer to a specialist unit, it could be argued that it is a waste of resources to use a slot on a hard-pressed CT or MR schedule when the examination done outside the specialist centre is often inadequate, does not answer the specific diagnostic questions and may have to be repeated.

Staging

Imaging is required to stage a tumour. The pattern of this imaging should be designed knowing the pattern of spread of the disease. For example, children with neuroblastoma do not require routine chest CT as the tumour rarely metastasizes to the lungs. The choice of CT or MR for cross-sectional imaging and staging depends on ease of local availability, tumour type and the requirement to obtain lung parenchymal images for identification of metastases. In a child with a Wilms' tumour, staging by CT alone is satisfactory, as both abdominal and chest imaging is required. Staging of a child with osteosarcoma will require both CT

and MR; CT is needed for identification of any lung metastases, MR for staging of the primary bone lesion.

Tumours in which MR is considered to be mandatory include tumours of the:

- Brain
- Spine
- Liver
- Bone
- Soft tissue

Magnetic resonance is the preferred technique for staging:

- All pelvic tumours
- Neuroblastomas
- Lymphoma follow-up [preferred technique of authors; short tau inversion recovery (STIR) sequence is particularly helpful in the abdomen]

Computed tomography is still considered satisfactory for Wilms' tumour, ovarian tumours and lymphoma if MR is not easily available.

Tissue diagnosis

Where technically feasible and medically appropriate, tissue diagnosis by excision of the primary tumour or an accessible lymph node is the primary choice. In many tumours, the appropriate management of the primary tumour is by neo-adjuvant chemotherapy with excision of residual tumour later. A biopsy is required for tissue diagnosis. The basic principles underlying tumour biopsy are:

- The choice of biopsy route, open or closed, is dictated by safety with avoidance of complications
- In general, open surgical biopsy by laparotomy should be avoided. Adequate tissue can be obtained by image-guided biopsies or by laparoscopy or thoracoscopy
- Prior to biopsy the child should have a clotting screen, and any identified deficiency corrected by the haematologist
- Imaging is required to establish the safest biopsy route. For example, if a child has chest lymphoma, no palpable nodal disease but splenic or renal involvement, it may be preferable to biopsy the spleen or kidney instead of the mediastinum to obtain tissue
- Biopsy tissue must be obtained from viable and not necrotic tumour
- Tissue samples must be sufficiently large to enable the pathologist to undertake all the required stains, immunohistochemistry and cytogenetic studies required for diagnosis. Also, ideally, there should also be enough tumour tissue to store in a tissue bank for further research. Primary diagnosis takes precedence if tissue is sparse

- The handling of the tissue must be agreed in advance by radiologist and pathologist. Placing tissue in formalin will destroy it for cytogenetic studies
- When carrying out the biopsy, the radiologist must be familiar with the subsequent surgical requirements, such as excision of the biopsy track if this is appropriate

Communication

Reference has already been made to the importance of good communication between the radiographer and the child when carrying out the technical aspects of scanning. Just as important are clear lines of communication between radiologist and oncologist as to the information the parent is given at the end of an examination.

Research

Much of the improvement in survival and cure of children with cancer is attributable to collaborative research and multicentre therapy trials. Imaging to monitor progress of disease is important in this research, and will on occasion entail imaging for research purposes alone. This is acceptable but, in designing these trials, the tolerance of the child and their family in coping with these tests, in addition to the cost-effectiveness, must be borne in mind. Families, though grateful for the success of the treatment and cure, have a finite tolerance for being part of research programmes and require great sensitivity in their handling.

Key points: general considerations

- Precautions should be taken to prevent heat loss, particularly in small infants and babies

- Clear protocols should be in place for the use of IV central lines for the administration of contrast medium

- Imaging and other tests such as bone marrow biopsy should all be performed as a single procedure under the same sedation or general anaesthesia

- Percutaneous biopsy under imaging control should obviate the need for surgical open biopsy or laparotomy in a high proportion of patients

- Even in mixed adult and paediatric scanning units, radiographers should be specially trained for paediatric scanning

Acute complications

There are certain acute complications of cancer treatment in children common to many types of cancer. Many of these are either directly related to the toxic effects of the drugs used in treatment or the neutropenia and immunosuppression associated with the drug treatment. These include:

- Intravenous access complications
- Abdominal complications
- Chest infection
- Haemorrhagic complications

Intravenous access complications

Most children will have some form of long line inserted for chemotherapy and, on occasion, parenteral nutrition. Fracture of the line will lead to extravasation of infused substances and may cause pain during infusion with or without visible soft tissue swelling. Fluoroscopy during infusion of radio-opaque contrast is the best method of identifying the site of the fracture or line blockage. All such studies must be performed with a rigorous aseptic technique and non-ionic contrast media.

Venous thrombosis distal to the catheter tip is clinically manifest by pain on infusion, difficulty in aspirating blood and frequent stoppage of the infusion pump. More rarely, there are signs of obstruction with limb oedema or symptoms of superior vena cava obstruction. Initial assessment of such a problem should be by Doppler ultrasound but venous angiography either by digital subtraction angiography or MR angiography (MRA) may be needed for complete assessment. Doppler ultrasound and MRA are both very helpful in identifying venous anatomy and patency in order to aid placement of a new central venous line (Figs. 35.1 and 35.2).[5,6]

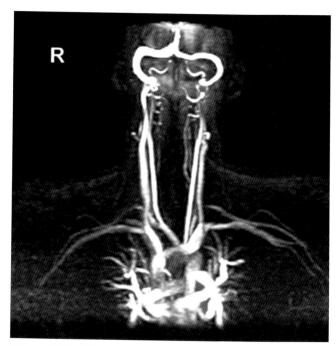

Figure 35.1. *Phase-contrast MR of the neck and mediastinum showing normal central venous anatomy.*

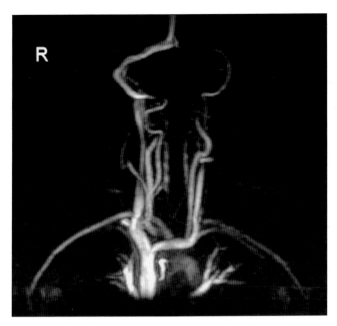

Figure 35.2. *Phase-contrast MR in a patient with an occluded right subclavian vein.*

Line infection

This is a frequent cause of pyrexia in neutropenic children. Bacterial thrombi can form on the line and lead to bacterial endocarditis and septic emboli. Echocardiography is the method of choice for the identification of bacterial thrombi on the line tip or the heart valves. Septic emboli to the brain are best imaged by MR or CT depending on what is easily locally available. Suspect septic emboli to the lung leading to perfusion defects are best imaged by a perfusion lung scan. Computed tomography may be needed to assess any abscess formation. A potential pitfall of CT is that such lesions may in theory be multiple and can, of course, resemble metastases.

If the tumour undergoing treatment is not one that metastasizes to the lungs, caution in interpretation should be exercised. Review of the current scan with previous imaging and correlating the scan and clinical details should avoid confusion. This complication is more a theoretical than a practical reality.

Abdominal complications

A full review of these conditions is outside the scope of this chapter. The imaging approach to the common lesions is described which include:

- Neutropenic colitis
- Pseudomembranous colitis
- Graft versus host disease (GVHD)

Neutropenic colitis

Any child who is immunosuppressed on chemotherapy is potentially at risk for the development of neutropenic coli-

tis (or typhlitis) but it is most commonly seen in children with leukaemia.[7] Clinical presentation is with abdominal pain and fever. There may be associated diarrhoea which may be bloody. The pain, though often generalized, may be localized to the right lower quadrant and simulate appendicitis. The abdomen is tender on palpation and there is often ileus and peritonism. Bowel sounds are diminished. Initial imaging is by plain abdominal radiography. On plain abdominal radiograph, the appearances are variable. Thickened bowel may be visible but this is unusual. More commonly there is distended bowel with a pattern of ileus. A distended abdomen, with displacement of bowel gas centrally and distension of the flank stripes will be present if there is sufficient ascites. Perforation, though unusual, is manifest by free intra-abdominal air. The best further method of investigation is by bowel and abdominal ultrasound.[8] Ultrasonic findings mirror the combination of the clinical features and plain radiographs. The bowel wall is thickened, the right colon and caecum being most affected (Fig. 35.3). These features are also seen on CT but this is usually not necessary.[9] Free fluid, which is usually clear and not turbulent, is present in variable quantity. Ileus of the bowel is noted. This thickened bowel may act as the lead point of an intussusception. The ultrasonic findings will then be those of intussusception, with the intussuscipiens lying in the thickened bowel (Fig. 35.4). Unless there is perforation, hydrostatic or air reduction of the intussusception should be undertaken. As the bowel is already compromised, if using contrast this should be water-soluble to avoid barium contamination of the peritoneum should a perforation occur (Fig. 35.5). The child will, in general, require analgesia for the reduction. It is one occasion in which reduction under general anaesthesia may be indicated with a view to proceeding to surgery if the reduction fails.

Monitoring of the progress of neutropenic colitis is by ultrasound and plain films, as clinically indicated. Abscess

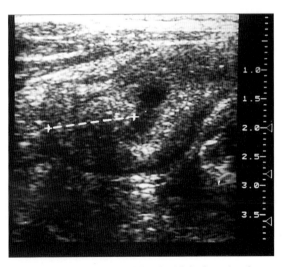

Figure 35.3. *Nine-year-old girl with leukaemic relapse. Ultrasound of the caecum. Note the thickened wall between crosses. The bowel wall measured 2.0 cm.*

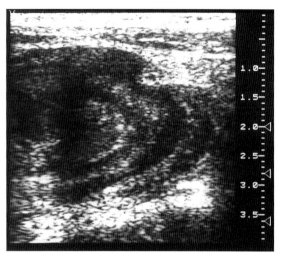

Figure 35.4. *Same child as Fig. 35.3; 2 days later. Typical appearances of ileo–ileo-colic intussusception. Note the multiple layers of bowel wall.*

formation is most easily detected by ultrasound or CT; perforation by plain radiographs. Children who are immunocompromised are, in theory, at risk from many other abdominal inflammatory conditions, though in practice these are quite rare. Neutropenic colitis is the most frequent.

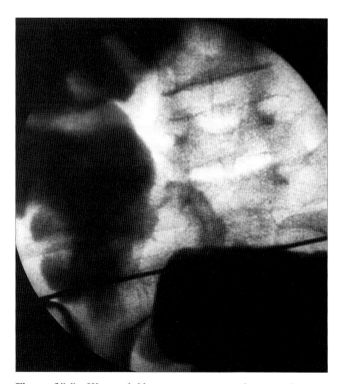

Figure 35.5. *Water-soluble contrast enema under general anaesthetic. Same child as Figs. 35.3 and 35.4. The intussusception was reduced. There is a little caecal oedema but marked oedema of the terminal ileum.*

Pseudomembranous colitis

Pseudomembranous colitis due to overgrowth with *Clostridium difficile* and its toxin is caused by antibiotic therapy. There is diffuse thickening of the colonic wall seen on ultrasound or CT, which may be seen on plain radiographs as thumbprinting. Contrast enema demonstrates marked coarse mucosal irregularity,[10,11] although this is contraindicated in severe forms of the disease because of the risk of perforation. Pneumatosis intestinalis may be seen in association with pseudomembranous colitis.[12]

Graft versus host disease

Graft versus host disease is unique to children who have had a bone marrow transplant. Target organs of acute GVHD are the skin, liver and the gastro-intestinal tract. On the plain abdominal radiograph, bowel wall thickening and non-specific dilatation may be seen. On sonographic examination, there is marked bowel wall thickening, mainly due to increased thickness of the submucosa.[13] Pneumatosis intestinalis is a recognized feature.[14,15] This may be evident on the plain radiograph but may also be detected using ultrasound. Gas bubbles within the bowel wall are seen as an intramural echogenic circle on ultrasound.[16] On CT examination, there is abnormal bowel wall enhancement in a central mucosal location, a fluid-filled bowel due to ileus and increased attenuation of the mesenteric fat due to infiltration and oedema.[9,17] Magnetic resonance features of intestinal GVHD have been described.[18] In addition to wall-thickening, abnormal mucosal enhancement, on T1-weighted fat-saturated images, three layers of the bowel wall are identified, with hyperintense outer and inner zones surrounding a hypointense middle zone.

Infectious enteritis may occur due to a whole host of organisms. The imaging features are non-specific and include mild bowel wall thickening, ileus and variable amounts of free intra-abdominal fluid. As for neutropenic colitis, primary imaging should be by plain radiograph and abdominal and bowel ultrasound, supplemented by CT if the information is inadequate or conflicts with clinical assessment.

In all these children, management is conservative, surgery being reserved for perforation, obstruction or abscess drainage if the latter cannot be drained percutaneously.

Chest infection

Children undergoing chemotherapy are neutropenic and therefore prone to developing infection. The infection may be a simple common viral or bacterial infection. The radiological appearance of these does not differ from patterns seen in the non-compromised child. The dilemma for the clinician is to diagnose opportunistic infections such as *Pneumocystis carinii* pneumonia, (Fig. 35.6), fungal and viral infection, tuberculosis or aspergillosis, and to institute appropriate antimicrobial treatment as early as possible. Many of these infections have characteristic radiographic patterns, well-described in standard texts, which will not be

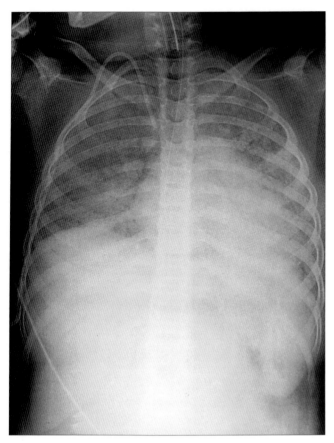

Figure 35.6. *Typical appearance of* Pneumocystis carinii *pneumonia.*

repeated here.[19–21] The patterns in immunocompromised children on chemotherapy are similar to those in children with autoimmunodeficiency syndrome (AIDS) or other immune deficiency syndromes. Most of these radiographic patterns are only seen when infection is well established. Early diagnosis is best achieved by bronchial lavage and, once a diagnosis of opportunistic infection is suspected, this is indicated.

If there is doubt about pulmonary infiltration on a chest radiograph, high-resolution CT (HRCT) is invaluable in assessing pulmonary parenchymal infiltration.[22] Computed tomography is also excellent in showing the extent of mycetoma in cavities and assessment of mediastinal nodal disease (Fig. 35.7).

Lung GVHD is a recognized complication of bone marrow transplantation and may be acute or chronic. Symptoms include cough and bronchospasm. There is an obstructive pattern to pulmonary function. Radiographic findings are variable and range from a normal appearance to mild hyperinflation (Fig. 35.8). There may be patchy perihilar infiltrations, which in severe cases progress to a diffuse interstitial pattern.[23] The underlying pathology is that of lymphocytic infiltrates, with the development of broncholitis obliterans in severe cases. Once suspected, the child requires HRCT, but the diagnosis is confirmed by biopsy.

Haemorrhagic complications

These are relatively infrequent in spite of the low platelet counts that accompany the chemotherapy. Imaging will depend on the location. In the brain, non-contrast-enhanced CT is the method of choice. Elsewhere in the body, initial investigation is with plain radiographs, ultrasound and CT, with MR being the imaging technique of choice for suspected intramuscular haemorrhage.

Long-term effects of treatment of children with cancer

As children survive their primary oncological disease, there are a number of important effects of treatment that may affect almost any body organ.[24,25] These complications may be due to radiation therapy or potent anticancer drugs. Imaging of these effects will depend on the nature and location of the clinical problem and, as for imaging of the primary disease, full diagnostic facilities are required. A multidisciplinary approach to the management of the child's problem is also essential. Routine surveillance for most of these long-term complications is not indicated. Each is imaged as it clinically presents. Radiologists must be familiar with these known complications so that they can advise the most appropriate investigations. When a child with a previous history of cancer treatment is referred for imaging, a proper history of the drugs and the radiation field used must be available to the radiologist so that a correct interpretation of imaging findings is made. Great confusion can be caused by the incorrect interpretation of imaging findings, which if interpreted out of context, may be misconstrued and mistakenly diagnosed as other diseases. Conversely, the radiologist must always be careful not to miss a new disease if imaging findings are not compatible with the late effects of cancer therapy. An increasingly important late effect is the development of second primary cancers.

The main regions affected by therapy that will be considered are:

- Central nervous system (CNS)
- Musculoskeletal system
- Cardiopulmonary system
- Gonads
- Thyroid
- Kidneys

Central nervous system effects

Central nervous system effects of treatment can be divided into general effects on brain function and specific injury to the special senses and neuroendocrine function. The main

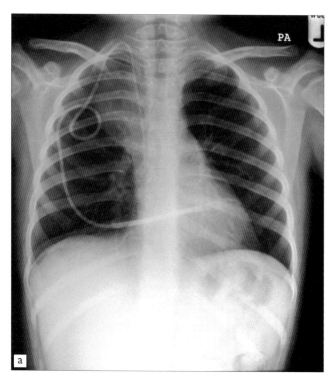

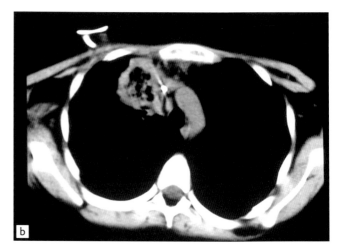

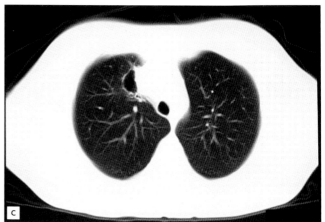

Figure 35.7. *(a) Chest radiograph of a child with leukaemia showing a well-defined right paratracheal mass. (b) Computed tomography (soft tissue window) demonstrates this to be a thick-walled cavity in the right upper lobe, containing some debris. There was no demonstrable abnormality in the surrounding lung parenchyma. The patient was treated for presumed pulmonary fungal infection. (c) Computed tomography (lung window) following prolonged antifungal treatment. There is a thin-walled residual cavity.*

effect of radiation and chemotherapy on general brain function is a resultant deterioration in intellectual ability. Imaging studies may show varying degrees of generalized cerebral atrophy with ventricular dilatation, with further focal damage at the site of the primary brain tumour. Cerebral atrophy may also occur in children with leukaemia who have CNS irradiation even though there is no focal primary tumour. Cerebral calcification may develop in either group. The best imaging technique for the demonstration of the late effects of treatment is MR. These late effects of treatment are discussed fully in Chapter 30.

Damage to the hypothalamus or pituitary gland may occur from irradiation, not just to primary central brain tumours but also in those children with tumours of the orbit or nasopharynx. The damage is usually functional rather than physical, but if imaging of the hypothalamus or pituitary gland is indicated, MR is the technique of choice. Suspected damage to the auditory or optic nerves is also best imaged by MR. Radiation-induced cataracts are best imaged by ultrasound.

Radiation-induced musculoskeletal disease

Radiation to the growing skeleton may damage growth of both bones and soft tissues. This can lead to complications such as scoliosis, limb shortening and asymmetry of development of the structures in the irradiated field. Imaging of these complications is similar to imaging of the lesions if they were a primary disease. Scoliosis monitoring is by plain posterior–anterior (PA) full spinal radiographs with special lateral bending and traction views preoperatively if surgery is being planned. Leg asymmetry is monitored by leg length monitoring. Facial asymmetry may result from irradiation. If surgical correction of this is contemplated, three-dimensional craniofacial CT will be required.

Late cardiopulmonary effects

Mediastinal irradiation may rarely result in radiation-induced constrictive pericarditis.[24] This is increasingly rare as mediastinal irradiation is used less frequently since the advent of chemotherapeutic drugs for the treatment of mediastinal tumours, notably Hodgkin's disease.

The main long-term cardiac effect of cancer treatment

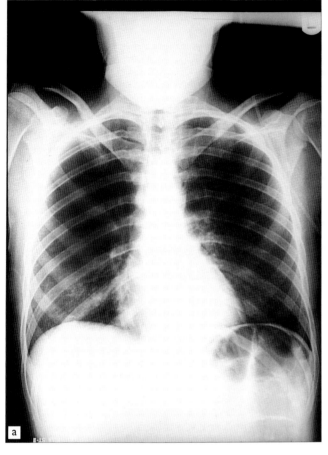

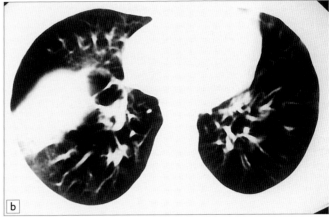

Figure 35.8. *Graft versus host disease, biopsy proven. (a) Plain radiograph. There is non-specific right middle lobe infiltrate; (b) CT scan. There is paucity of vessel markings on the left due to bronchiolitis obliterans but without hyperinflation. On the right side there is segmental consolidation of the right middle lobe and patchy infiltration in the right lower lobe. The appearances of both the radiograph and CT scan are non-specific.*

is related to drug treatment, especially the anthracyclines.[26] Left ventricular function is impaired. Monitoring of cardiac function is predominantly by echocardiography but nuclear medicine studies have a part to play, especially if there is difficulty in obtaining good echo studies due to the patient's habitus or the results are equivocal. Radiation pneumonitis and fibrosis has long been recognized and is best imaged by HRCT. Pulmonary toxicity with infiltration and basal fibrosis may also result from chemotherapeutic drugs such as methotrexate, bischloroethyl nitrosurea (BCNU), busulphan and bleomycin. If suspected, HRCT is indicated, but should only be repeated, once a diagnosis is made, for clinical deterioration. Ventilation/perfusion (V/Q) nuclear medicine studies will also show the functional distribution of the disease.

Gonadal dysfunction

This is a well-recognized complication of both irradiation and chemotherapy. In general, no radiological imaging of the affected gonad is required. Gonadal dysfunction may be associated with growth failure and delayed bone matu-ration. Bone maturation is assessed by hand and wrist radiography. The most sensitive and widely accepted method of assessment for height prediction is the TW2 method (Tanner Whitehouse System 2).[27] This, where necessary, can be repeated at yearly intervals until skeletal maturity.

Thyroid dysfunction

Thyroid dysfunction may result from radiation to the neck. Monitoring is by biochemical studies but, if required, these can be correlated with imaging of the thyroid by nuclear medicine studies. These latter are indicated if there is any palpable nodularity of the gland to show whether the nod-ules are functional or not. Ultrasound of the thyroid gland will identify cystic nodules. Both are only indicated in symp-tomatic patients.

Nephrotoxicity

Radiation nephritis has long been recognized to cause hypertension. Monitoring of general renal function is mainly by biochemistry. If there is any reason to suspect unilateral disease then nuclear medicine studies are indicated for divided renal function. Radiation-induced renal artery stenosis has been described. Duplex Doppler ultrasound should be the initial investigation, followed by captopril renography and MRA. The gold standard for the detection of renal artery stenosis is by catheter angiography. Angioplasty of the stenosed segment may result in the relief of hypertension.

Chemotherapy with *cis*-platinum, BCNU, ifosfamide and methotrexate may cause acute nephrotoxicity. Long-term effects may persist but as both kidneys are affected, monitoring of renal function is, in general, non-radiological.

Cyclophosphenol and ifosfamide may both cause damage to the bladder wall with telangiectatic lesions. These may cause haematuria. The lesions are seen at cystoscopy. Radiation cystitis will cause thickening of the bladder wall and a small volume bladder. The thickening is well-demonstrated by ultrasound. Bladder volume pre- and post-micturition may be measured by ultrasound.

Summary

- Children are most appropriately imaged in paediatric centres where treatment will be given

- Techniques and protocols of examination should be defined according to pattern of tumour spread

- A multidisciplinary approach to obtain all the information at a single investigation is essential if general anaesthesia or sedation is used – e.g. imaging, bone marrow biopsy, etc

- Acute complications of therapy include IV access blockage, abdominal infections, GVHD, chest infections and haemorrhage

- Long-term complications include cerebral atrophy, musculoskeletal growth problems, cardiopulmonary effects, thyroid and gonadal dysfunction and nephrotoxicity. The development of second primary tumours is becoming increasingly important

References

1. Brenner D J, Elliston C D, Hall E J, Berdon W E. Estimated risks of radiation induced fatal cancer from pediatric CT. Am J Roentgenol 2002; 176: 289–296

2. Paterson A, Frush D P, Donnelly L F. Helical CT of the body: are settings adjusted for paediatric patients? Am J Roentgenol 2002; 176: 297– 301

3. Donnelly L F, Emery K H, Body A S et al. Minimising radiation dose for pediatric body applications of single-detector helical CT: strategies at a large children's hospital. Am J Roentgenol 2002; 176: 303–306

4. Frush D P. Pediatric CT: practical approach to diminish the radiation dose. Paediatr Radiol 2002; 32: 714–717

5. Shinde T S, Lee V S, Rofsky N M et al. Three-dimensional gadolinium-enhanced MR venographic evaluation of patency of central veins in the thorax: initial experience. Radiology 1999; 213: 555–560.

6. Rose S C, Gomes A S, Yoon H C. MR angiography for mapping potential central venous access sites in patients with advanced venous occlusive disease. Am J Roentgenol 1996; 166: 1181–1187

7. Baerg J, Murphy J J, Anderson R, Magee J F. Neutropenic enteropathy: a 10-year review. J Pediatr Surg 1999; 34: 1068–1071

8. Cartoni C, Dragoni F, Micozzi A et al. Neutropenic enterocolitis in patients with acute leukaemia: prognostic significance of bowel wall-thickening detected by ultrasonography. J Clin Oncol 2001; 19: 756–761

9. Donnelly L F. CT Imaging of immunocompromised children with acute abdominal symptoms. Am J Roentgenol 1996; 167: 909–913

10. Ros P R, Buetow P C, Pantograg-Brown L et al. Pseudomembranous colitis. Radiology 1996; 198: 1–9.

11. Zamora S, Coppes M J, Scott R B, Mueller D L. *Clostridium difficile*, pseudomembranous enterocolitis: striking CT and sonographic features in a pediatric patient. Eur J Radiol 1996; 23: 104–106

12. Gillett P M, Russell R K, Wilson D C, Thomas A E. *C. difficile*-induced Pneumatosis intestinalis in a neutropenic child. Arch Dis Child 2002; 87: 85

13. Haber H P, Schlegel P G, Dette S et al. Intestinal acute graft-versus-host disease: findings on sonography. Am J Roentgenol 2000; 174: 118–120

14. Jones B, Wall S D. Gastrointestinal disease in the immunocompromised host. Radiol Clin North Am 1992; 30: 555–577

15. Yeager A M, Kanof M E, Kramer S S et al. Pneumatosis intestinalis in children after allogenic bone marrow transplantation. Pediatr Radiol 1987; 17: 18–22

16. Goske M J, Goldblum J R, Applegate K E et al. The 'circle sign': a new sonographic sign of Pneumatosis intestinalis: clinical, pathologic and experimental findings. Pediatr Radiol 1999; 29: 530–535

17. Donnelly L F, Morris C L. Acute graft-versus-host disease in children: abdominal CT findings. Radiology 1996; 199: 265–268

18. Mentzel H-J, Kentouche K, Kosmehl H et al. US and MRI of gastrointestinal graft-versus-host disease. Pediatr Radiol 2002; 32: 195–198

19. Markowitz R I, Kramer S S. The spectrum of pulmonary infection in the immunocompromised child. Semin Roentgenol 2000; 2: 171–180.

20. Jeanes A C, Owens C M. Chest imaging in the immuno-compromised child. Pediatr Respir Rev 2002; 3: 59–69

21. Donnelly L F. CT of acute pulmonary infection/trauma. In: Lucaya J, Strife JL (eds). Pediatric Chest Imaging. Chest Imaging in Infants and Children. Berlin: Springer-Verlag, 2002: 113–127

22. Hiorns M P, Screaton N J, M?ller N L. Acute lung disease in the immunocompromised host. Radiol Clin North Am 2001; 39: 1137–1151

23. Armstrong P, Dee P. AIDS and other forms of immunocompromise. In: Armstrong P, Wilson AG, Dee P, Hansell DM (eds). Imaging of Diseases of the Chest. London: Mosby, 2000: 255–304

24. Malpas J S. Clinical review: Long-term effects of treatment of childhood malignancy. Clin Radiol 1996; 51: 466–474

25. Schwartz C L. Long-term survivors of childhood cancer: the late effects of therapy. Oncologist 1999; 4: 45–54

26. Lipscultz S E, Colan S D, Gelber R D et al. Late cardiac effects of doxorubicin therapy. New Engl J Med 1991; 324: 808–815

27. Tanner J M, Whitehouse R H, Marshall W A et al. Assessment of Skeletal Maturity and Prediction of Adult Height (TW2 Method). London: Academic Press, 1975

Chapter 36

Wilms' tumour and associated neoplasms of the kidney

Helen Williams and Helen Carty

Wilms' tumour

Incidence and epidemiology

Wilms' tumour or nephroblastoma is the most common primary malignant renal tumour of childhood, with an incidence of 1 per 10,000 live births per year[1] and 6% of all childhood malignancies. Its peak incidence is at 3–4 years of age[2] and 80% of patients present before 5 years of age.[3] The sex incidence is reported to be equal in most series but, in the USA, the incidence of unilateral Wilms' tumour in girls is 22% higher than that in boys.[4] The tumour is most frequently unilateral but in approximately 5% of cases is bilateral.[5,6] Children with bilateral tumours tend to present at a slightly earlier age than those with unilateral disease. Population studies have shown a relatively increased incidence of Wilms' tumour in black children relative to Asian or Caucasian children.[1,7]

Biology and genetics of Wilms' tumour

It is generally accepted that cancers occur as a result of changes in the DNA composition in the cells of origin. This may result in direct mutation of the cell or a change in protein synthesis that leads to dysregulation of growth and increased mitotic activity. The change in DNA composition may alternatively produce a decrease in tumour suppressor activity, resulting in the development of malignancy. Some tumours are the result of mutations in germ cells, which can either be inherited from a parent or arise *de novo*. Like other cancers, Wilms' tumour is characterized by alterations in genes that regulate cell growth, proliferation and differentiation. Much of the understanding of the genetics of Wilms' tumour has come from its association with several congenital anomalies and syndromes. *WT1* was the first Wilms' tumour gene to be identified and has been extensively investigated. The discovery of this gene stemmed from the observation that patients with aniridia, genito-urinary malformations and mental retardation are at high risk for Wilms' tumour (>30%). Individuals with this syndrome were found to have a large deletion at chromosome 11p13. Gene *WT1* is also associated with Denys–Drash and Frasier syndromes. The second but less well understood Wilms' tumour gene, *WT2*, located on chromosome 11p15, is implicated in patients with Beckwith–Wiedemann syndrome. Other sites known to be associated with genetic alterations in children with Wilms' tumour include chromosomes 16, 1p, 7p and 17p.[8] Loss of heterozygosity for chromosome 16q has been linked with a higher mortality rate in Wilms' tumour patients.[9]

Studies have shown that there is a definite relationship between the response to treatment, recurrence rate and tumour grade.[8] Tumours are classified on the basis of histology into favourable or unfavourable types. In the last 50 years, many advances have been made in the detection, diagnosis and treatment of Wilms' tumour, improving the 5-year survival for unilateral tumours, with favourable histology to approximately 90%.[10] This is compared with a 5-year survival of 30% in the 1950s. In the USA, most children with Wilms' tumour are managed according to clinical trials developed by the National Wilms' Tumour Study Group (NWTSG), whilst in Europe most children are managed according to studies designed by the International Society of Paediatric Oncology (SIOP). Incorporation of patients into large, multicentre therapeutic trials increases the statistical significance of the results. Over the last 30 years the results of prospective clinical trials by these two groups has led to the development of evidence-based treatment protocols which have ultimately resulted in improved survival from this tumour. Goals of current research include the identification of molecular or genetic markers that predict outcome so that more intensive treatment can be reserved for children who are identified as having more aggressive disease and at the same time morbidity of treatment for low-risk patients can be reduced. Controversies remain concerning the management of bilateral tumours and the role of partial nephrectomy.

Key points: general features

- Wilms' tumour is the most common renal tumour of childhood
- Wilms' tumours are bilateral in 5% of cases
- Genetic mutations have been identified in Wilms', e.g. *WT1* and *WT2*
- 5-year survival rates are about 95% in children with favourable histology

Associations of Wilms' tumour

There are a number of syndromes associated with Wilms' tumour:

- WAGR syndrome
- Denys–Drash syndrome
- Beckwith–Wiedemann syndrome
- Perlman syndrome
- Hemihypertrophy/hemihyperplasia

Aniridia and WAGR syndrome

Patients with aniridia characterized by iris hypoplasia and other ocular defects have an increased incidence of Wilms' tumour compared with the general population. Two thirds of patients with aniridia have a familial form and one third are sporadic. The majority show an autosomal dominant pattern of inheritance with almost complete penetrance but variable expression. In some rare syndromes, aniridia is transmitted as autosomal recessive, and two thirds of new sporadic cases represent a new autosomal dominant condition.[11] There is an increased incidence of Wilms' tumour in patients with sporadic aniridia and the tumour usually presents before 3 years of age. Patients with familial forms of aniridia do not have an increased risk of developing Wilms' tumour.[11]

WAGR syndrome consists of Wilms' tumour, aniridia, genito-urinary anomalies and mental retardation. Some authors propose renaming the syndrome 'AGR triad with an increased incidence of Wilms' tumour'. The WAGR syndrome usually occurs sporadically and may be only partially manifest in different combinations. In this syndrome, there is a deletion at chromosome 11p13 which encompasses a contiguous set of genes including *PAX6*, the gene responsible for aniridia, and *WT1*.[11,12]

Denys–Drash syndrome

The association of male pseudohermaphroditism, glomerulopathy and Wilms' tumour was first reported by Denys et al. in 1967.[13] Drash et al. suggested this triad as a syndrome in 1970.[14] Since then there have been several more reports of both the complete and incomplete syndrome.[15–17] When two components are present, the syndrome is regarded as being incomplete. One variant of the incomplete syndrome including renal disease, XY gonadal dysgenesis, with streak gonads and frequent gonadoblastoma but without Wilms' tumour is known as Frasier syndrome.[18] Although the two syndromes can be distinguished by differences in nephropathy, it is now considered that these two syndromes can be regarded as part of a spectrum of related conditions caused by mutations in the *WT1* gene.[19] The most frequent genito-urinary tumour occurring in patients with Denys–Drash syndrome is Wilms' tumour, but clear cell sarcoma has also been described.[16]

Beckwith–Wiedemann syndrome

The main characteristics of this syndrome are macroglossia, omphalocele, umbilical hernia, visceromegaly, gigantism, ear pits and creases and asymmetry of the limbs (hemihypertrophy). Hypoglycaemia may occur in the neonatal period. All features are not present in every patient. The incidence of Wilms' tumour is said to be less than 5%[1] but patients with hemihypertrophy as part of the syndrome have a threefold increase in neoplasms. Other neoplasms associated with Beckwith–Wiedemann syndrome include rhabdosarcoma, hepatoblastoma and adrenal carcinoma; renal cell carcinoma has also been reported.[20]

Perlman syndrome

This rare, autosomal recessive syndrome has many features in common with Beckwith–Wiedemann syndrome. Children with Perlman syndrome have characteristic facial and somatic features, a high neonatal mortality rate, mental retardation and renal abnormalities including a high risk of developing Wilms' tumour. The distinctive facial features include a small, short nose with depressed nasal bridge, an inverted 'v'-shaped upper lip and a serrated alveolar margin. Macrocephaly and low-set ears are also found. There is often macrosomia and organomegaly but macroglossia, ear creases and pits, omphalocele and umbilical hernia are found only in association with Beckwith–Wiedemann syndrome.[21] The risk of developing Wilms' tumour is high – 45% in the reported cases, but there is no apparent increased risk of other neoplasms.[21]

Hemihypertrophy/hemihyperplasia

Hemihypertrophy (hemihyperplasia) is characterized by asymmetric growth of cranium, face, trunk, limbs and/or digits with or without visceral involvement. It may be an isolated finding or occur with certain syndromes. An association between isolated hemihyperplasia and neoplasms in childhood has been long recognized, Wilms' tumour being the most frequent of these. The incidence of Wilms' tumour associated with hemihyperplasia is 3–4%.[22] There is also an increased incidence of hepatoblastoma and adrenocortical neoplasms. A recent study has found an overall incidence of embryonal tumours to be 5.9% in children with isolated hemihypertrophy.[23] Children with solid tumours usually have the mass on the same side as the hemihypertrophy.[22]

Clinical presentation

The most common initial clinical presentation of Wilms' tumour is the incidental finding of an abdominal mass, usually by a parent or carer whilst bathing or dressing the child. Usually the child is asymptomatic although the tumours are frequently large at presentation. Other presenting features include an increasing abdominal girth, abdominal pain, anorexia, vomiting, fever of unknown origin and frank haematuria. Macroscopic haematuria is a rare primary presentation but can occur following trauma to the affected kidney, with resultant tumour rupture or haemorrhage into the tumour. Haemorrhage into the tumour may also occur spontaneously and is accompanied by rapid abdominal enlargement, anaemia, hypotension and fever. A non-reducible varicocele secondary to obstruction of the testicular vein can occur with tumour thrombus in the renal vein or inferior vena cava (IVC)[24,25] and has been reported in association with Budd–Chiari syndrome.[26] Tumour thrombus in the IVC can extend into the right atrium. Primary presentation with metastatic disease is rare.

Staging

The prognosis for and treatment of children with Wilms' tumour depends on staging and histological type. Preoperative staging is clinical and radiological with further assessment being visually carried out during surgery. The surgeon plays a central role in the proper staging of children with Wilms' tumour. The standard surgical approach is transabdominal–transperitoneal to allow thorough inspection of the intra-abdominal contents, including the contralateral kidney. The presence of bilateral disease affects both surgical and oncological management. Despite improved imaging techniques, preoperative imaging may miss bilateral disease that is subsequently detected at surgery.[27] The internationally accepted staging system for Wilms' tumour is the NWTSG system (Table 36.1).

Bilateral Wilms' tumour

Synchronous bilateral disease occurs in approximately 5% of patients with Wilms' tumour.[28] There is a higher incidence of associated abnormalities such as aniridia, Beckwith–Wiedemann syndrome, genito-urinary malformation and hemihypertrophy than in the children presenting with unilateral disease. Children with synchronous bilateral lesions also tend to present at a younger age than patients with unilateral disease.[29] Metachronous bilateral disease, which is either a new tumour or relapse presenting in the contralateral kidney, is less common than synchronous bilateral tumours, with an incidence of about 1%.[28]

Treatment for children with bilateral Wilms' tumour must be individualized. These patients are at high risk of renal failure but multidisciplinary treatment has resulted in a markedly improved outcome. The goal of treatment is to remove tumour whilst preserving as much functioning renal tissue as possible thus avoiding bilateral nephrectomy with the subsequent requirement for dialysis and possible transplant. Bilateral renal biopsies to confirm the diagnosis and establish the histological type of each tumour are recommended.[28,30] The imaging of bilateral tumours is similar to that for unilateral disease, but each kidney is staged separately (Fig. 36.1). Pre-resection chemotherapy has become acceptable treatment, particularly in the case of bilateral tumours. Reduction in tumour volume of up to or in excess of 50% has been reported.[31] Re-evaluation following chemotherapy is then performed to determine if tumour resection with significant renal preservation is possible,

Table 36.1. *National Wilms' Tumour Study Group clinico-pathological staging system*

I.	Tumour limited to kidney and completely excised. The surface of the renal capsule is intact. Tumour was not ruptured before or during removal. There is no residual tumour apparent beyond the margins of resection
II.	Tumour extends beyond the kidney but is completely removed. There is regional extension of the tumour (i.e. penetration through the outer surface of the renal capsule into perirenal soft tissues). Vessels outside the kidney substance are infiltrated or contain tumour thrombus. A biopsy from the tumour may have been taken, or there has been local spillage of tumour confined to the flank. There is no residual tumour apparent at or beyond the margins of excision
III.	Residual non-haematogenous tumour confined to abdomen. Any one or more of the following occur:

   1. Lymph nodes on biopsy are found to be involved in the hilum, the periaortic chains, or beyond

   2. There has been diffuse peritoneal contamination by tumour such as by spillage of tumour beyond the flank before or during surgery, or by tumour growth that has penetrated through the peritoneal surface

   3. Implants are found on the peritoneal surfaces

   4. The tumour extends beyond the surgical margins either microscopically or grossly

   5. The tumour is not completely resectable because of local infiltration into vital structures

IV.	Haematogenous metastases
	Deposits beyond Stage III (i.e. lung, liver, bone, and brain)
V.	Bilateral renal involvement at diagnosis
	An attempt should be made to stage each side according to the above criteria on the basis of extent of disease before biopsy

although ultimately this is determined at surgical exploration.

Partial nephrectomy may be considered for patients with unilateral tumours but in whom there are known risk factors for bilateral disease.[29] Some patients with Wilms' tumour in a solitary kidney but without associated risk factors for bilateral disease may also be suitable for partial nephrectomy but this is controversial.[28,30] The overall survival of children with bilateral tumours is high, at about 70% at 10 years[32] and 82% at 2 years.[33] As with unilateral tumours, survival is dependent on stage at presentation and histological type.

Wilms' tumour occurring in a horseshoe kidney

An increased incidence of neoplasia developing in horseshoe kidneys is known (Fig. 36.2).[34] These include renal cell carcinoma, renal pelvic tumours and Wilms' tumour. A recent retrospective study of all Wilms' tumours arising from a horseshoe kidney over a 29-year period has demonstrated an increased risk of Wilms' tumour in horseshoe

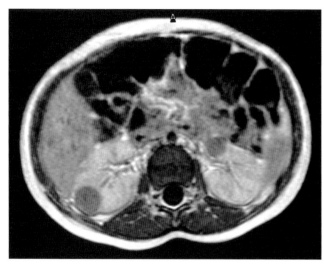

Figure 36.1. *An 18-month-old child with hemihypertrophy and synchronous bilateral Wilms' tumour subsequently treated by partial nephrectomies. Contrast-enhanced T1-weighted MR. (Courtesy of Dr K. Johnson, Birmingham Children's Hospital. UK.)*

kidneys.[35] Although horseshoe kidneys are common, the risk of development of Wilms' tumour is very low. It is estimated that Wilms' tumour is 1.96 times more frequent in horseshoe kidneys compared with normal kidneys. Wilms' tumour occurring in a horseshoe kidney presents a unique surgical challenge. There is the challenge of tumour removal whilst preserving renal function, similar to bilateral Wilms' tumour or tumour occurring in a single kidney. But horseshoe kidneys often have anomalous renal arteries and this, combined with the frequently large size of the tumour at presentation, makes surgery more difficult. Preoperative MR angiography (MRA) or catheter angiography may aid surgical planning. A horseshoe kidney may not be detected on preoperative imaging because a large

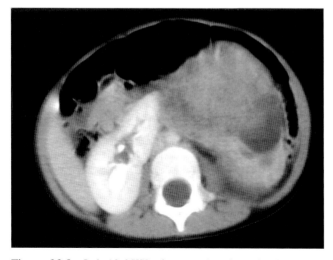

Figure 36.2. *Left-sided Wilms' tumour in a horseshoe kidney. Contrast-enhanced CT.*

tumour extending across the midline may obscure the isthmus. It is helpful to divide the horseshoe kidney into two halves and treat each as a separate kidney for the purpose of staging and treatment planning.

Key points: considerations for surgery

- Surgical resection through a thoraco-abdominal approach is the treatment of choice for unilateral Wilms' tumours

- Bilateral tumours occur in 5% of cases; most are synchronous

- Neo-adjuvant chemotherapy and partial nephrectomy have a place in management of bilateral tumours

- There is an increased risk of Wilms' tumour in horseshoe kidneys. The goal is to excise the primary tumour completely while maintaining as much normal renal parenchyma as possible

Diagnostic imaging techniques

The principles of imaging the child presenting with an abdominal mass are:

- Identification of the organ of origin of the lesion
- Characterization of the mass
- Assessment of its extent for staging
- Assessment of suitability for primary excisional surgery
- Detection of metastatic disease

The accepted initial investigation of the child presenting with an abdominal mass is a plain radiograph of the chest and ultrasound examination of the abdomen.

Plain abdominal radiograph

On abdominal radiography, the tumour will be seen to lie predominantly in a flank, displacing the bowel gas laterally or medially and inferiorly (Fig. 36.3). Very large tumours may displace the diaphragm upwards and occasionally cause respiratory embarrassment. Calcification is rarely seen on the radiograph. If the tumour has ruptured into the peritoneum, there may be evidence of ascites. Other than showing the mass, the radiographic appearance is non-specific.

Intravenous urography

The intravenous urogram (IVU) was once the gold standard for evaluation of patients suspected of having Wilms' tumour. It now remains primarily of historical interest as children with Wilms' tumour now undergo more sophisticated imaging studies, better able to define the extent of the mass as well as determine internal characteristics, its relationship to adjacent abdominal structures and vascular

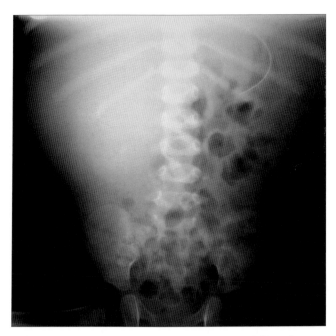

Figure 36.3. *Plain abdominal radiograph in a child with a right-sided Wilms' tumour. Note the displacement of the hepatic flexure. The clinical presentation was with an abdominal mass.*

invasion. The appearance of a Wilms' tumour at urography is that of an intrarenal mass lesion with displacement of the collecting system by the mass (Fig. 36.4). In between 3 and 18% of patients, the affected kidney is non-functioning at urography due to renal vein invasion, obstructive uropathy

or, rarely, complete replacement of the kidney by tumour.[36] Bleeding from the tumour may appear as filling defects in the calyces and renal pelvis due to clot. The child may present with renal colic due to clot as well as haematuria. In the context of the appropriate clinical presentation, the IVU appearances are characteristic. The main differential diagnosis is a renal abscess or benign cyst.

Ultrasound

Ultrasound is often the first study obtained in patients with Wilms' tumour. It has the advantage of being able to differentiate between cystic and solid lesions. Another important role of ultrasound is the evaluation of the renal vein and IVC both with real-time ultrasound and duplex to exclude or define tumour extension. At ultrasound, the tumour is typically a heterogeneous intrarenal mass with distortion of the renal parenchyma and collecting system (Fig. 36.5). The mass, if large, may be exophytic. There may be a predominantly solid mass with hypoechoic or cystic areas due to tumour necrosis or haemorrhage (Fig. 36.6). Cystic areas, primarily due to tumour necrosis, are common in Wilms' tumour, but there are rare cases of predominantly cystic Wilms' tumour that are ultrasonically indistinguishable from multilocular cystic nephroma – a benign tumour. The identification of cysts within the septa of neoplastic lesions is a useful discriminating feature.[37] Areas of increased echogenicity within the tumour may be due to calcium or fat.[6] The tumour–kidney interface is often sharply defined by an echogenic rim representing the tumour pseudocapsule or a rim of compressed renal tissue. Examination of the IVC to detect tumour thrombus and define its extent is essential because it may alter staging or modify the surgical approach. The renal vein and even the IVC may be difficult to visualize adequately, with large tumours causing vascular compression; however, the portion of the IVC entering the right atrium is usually

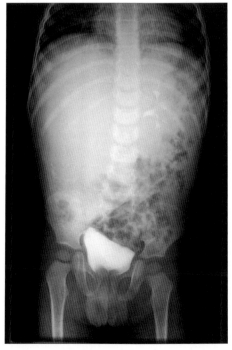

Figure 36.4. *Fifteen-minute film from IVU in a child with a right-sided Wilms' tumour. There is distortion and displacement of the right collecting system by the large upper pole mass.*

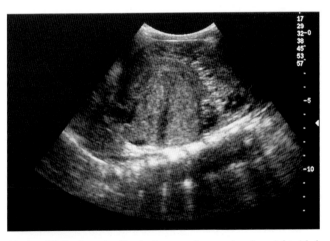

Figure 36.5. *Longitudinal ultrasound scan showing right-sided Wilms' tumour which appears encapsulated on this image. The tumour is mainly solid. The bright echoes may represent haemorrhage or microcalcification.*

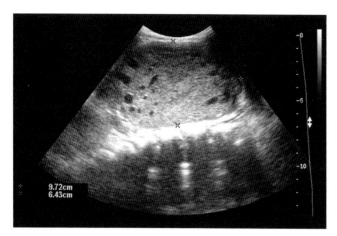

Figure 36.6. *Longitudinal ultrasound scan of right kidney in a patient with Wilms' tumour. There is a large central mass replacing most of the right kidney. The hypoechoic areas represent areas of necrosis.*

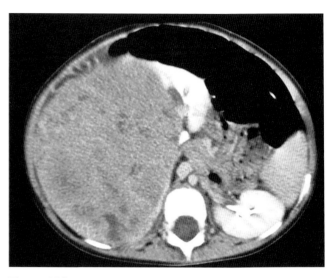

Figure 36.7. *Large right-sided predominantly solid Wilms' tumour. Contrast-enhanced CT. Note the marked anterior and medial displacement of normal renal tissue.*

visible so that tumour extension to this level can usually be identified at ultrasound. Patency of a compressed IVC can often be confirmed using Doppler and leg vein compression but small amounts of tumour thrombus may be missed. Another important role of the initial ultrasound is to examine the contralateral kidney. This should be inspected carefully for evidence of synchronous tumour, congenital abnormalities or other pathology. Liver metastases are rarely found with Wilms' tumour and are mainly associated with rhabdoid and anaplastic lesions. Wilms' tumours occasionally rupture into the peritoneum and cause ascites.

Computed tomography

Computed tomography (CT) is the primary cross-sectional imaging technique to establish tumour extent and is more sensitive than ultrasound. At contrast-enhanced CT, the tumour is of lower density than the normal kidney tissue (Fig. 36.7). Tumour necrosis, which may be hyperechoic due to haemorrhage and therefore mistaken as solid tumour at ultrasound, does not enhance and is easier to appreciate than on ultrasound (Figs. 36.8 and 36.9). Calcification is appreciated on unenhanced scans. The staging scan should extend from diaphragm to the bottom of the tumour and include both kidneys. Opacification of aorta and IVC makes it easier to appreciate nodal disease (Fig. 36.10) and tumour invasion of the IVC, although the latter is easier to appreciate with ultrasound. Computed tomography (and MR) may give a false impression of tumour invasion of the liver due to a partial volume effect (Fig. 36.11). The dynamic movement of a right Wilms' tumour relative to the liver, and therefore lack of invasion, is easier to appreciate with ultrasound.

Chest CT has been shown to be superior to chest radiographs in the detection of lung metastases from Wilms' tumour. Computed tomography scan can identify small lesions not visible on the chest radiograph and also is more

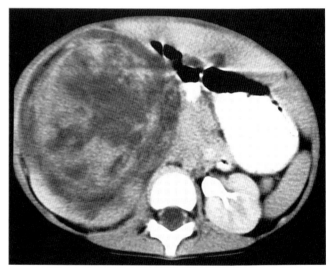

Figure 36.8. *Enhanced CT scan of right-sided Wilms' tumour. The tumour enhances heterogeneously and the low attenuation areas are necrotic. Note the thin rim of residual renal tissue posteriorly.*

sensitive in the identification of small amounts of calcification within lung nodules that may not be appreciated radiographically. These nodules may represent metastatic disease or benign lung pathology. About 10% of patients with Wilms' tumours have lung metastases at diagnosis and several studies have shown that between 7 and 33% of nodules seen on CT are not visible on chest radiography.[36] The role of chest CT scanning in the initial staging of Wilms' tumour has been widely debated. The staging system for Wilms' tumour was based on data collected before CT scanning was available and relies primarily on operative findings plus radiographic examination of the chest. Staging and

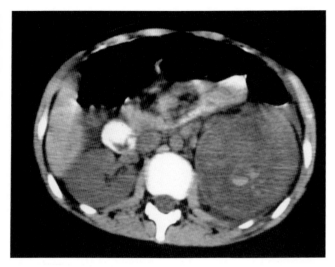

Figure 36.9. *Unenhanced CT scan showing a left Wilms' tumour. The tumour is haemorrhagic as indicated by the areas of high attenuation within the mass and fluid–fluid levels.*

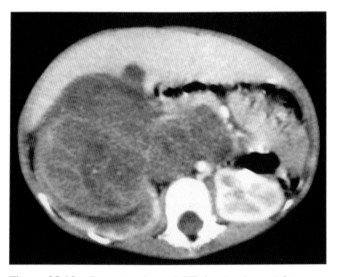

Figure 36.10. *Contrast-enhanced CT showing large right Wilms' tumour. The tumour has breached the renal capsule anteriorly, there is bulky para-aortic nodal disease and the IVC is non-opacified. At surgery there was tumour thrombus in the IVC extending to the level of the hepatic veins.*

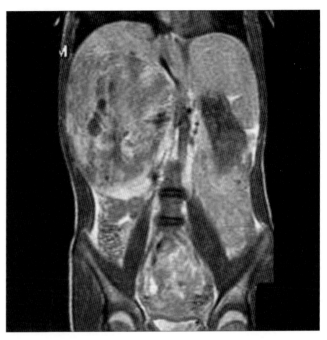

Figure 36.11. *Coronal T1-weighted postcontrast MR scan with right Wilms' tumour that indents the undersurface of the liver. Hepatic invasion could not be excluded from this examination. On ultrasound the liver and spleen appeared to move separately with respiration and at surgery there was no evidence of hepatic involvement.*

treatment protocols now include chest CT in the initial imaging of Wilms' tumour but discordant lesions (i.e. those visible on CT but not on chest radiograph) are ignored and not considered in management decisions.[6] A previous report found there was no difference in the survival of children who were 'up-staged' by virtue of CT scan results, and those in whom discordant lung lesions were ignored.[38] However, a recent study has suggested that the subgroup of patients with nodules detected on CT but a negative chest radiograph may be at increased risk of pulmonary relapse.[39] It is also suggested that pulmonary nodules identified only on CT are biopsied. Only children with confirmed metastatic disease would then undergo more intensive treatment with its inherent risks.

Magnetic resonance

There are no large series reporting on the relative merits of CT versus MR in the staging of Wilms' tumour, as both techniques are satisfactory. The known advantages of MR with direct multiplanar imaging, non-ionizing radiation and excellent soft tissue contrast have little practical advantage over CT. Computed tomography is quicker, readily accessible and can frequently be carried out without sedation. Disadvantages of MR include a longer examination time, greater cost, less availability, increased sedation requirements and more susceptibility to degradation of images by bowel or body movement. Vascular patency can be adequately assessed using MR and is not hampered by the presence of overlying bowel gas, as is often the case with ultrasound.

If MR is undertaken, T1- and T2-weighted spin-echo sequences are carried out in axial and coronal planes, together with short tau inversion recovery (STIR) sequences. Contrast-enhanced images are also required. The tumour has low to intermediate signal intensity on T1-weighted sequences, with high signal intensity on T2 (Fig. 36.12).[5] There is frequently heterogeneity within the tumour due to areas of haemorrhage and necrosis. Fresh haemorrhage will appear as high signal intensity on T1-

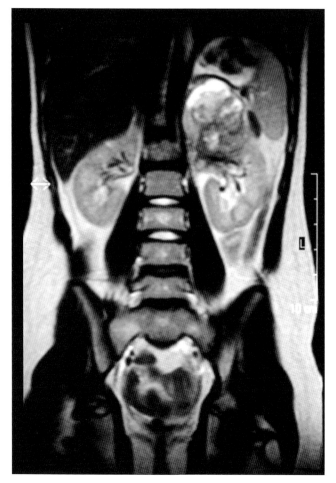

Figure 36.12. *Coronal T2-weighted MR scan showing left Wilms' tumour. The tumour is heterogeneous with areas of high signal intensity representing necrosis.*

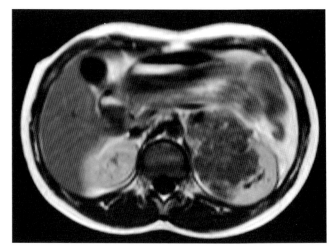

Figure 36.13. *Contrast-enhanced T1-weighted MR scan showing left Wilms' tumour. There is non-enhancement of the majority of the tumour due to necrosis.*

Radionuclide studies

There is no indication for either renal or bone studies in the routine preoperative assessment of children with Wilms' tumour. Bone scanning should only be performed if the child presents with bone pain. Radionuclide studies are useful in establishing preoperative differential renal function in children in whom the Wilms' tumour arises in an otherwise normal kidney but there is an abnormal contralateral kidney. This gives a guide to prognosis for long-term renal function and potential need for renal dialysis or transplant.

Key points: radiological investigation

- Plain abdominal radiography shows a mass predominantly in the flank with displacement of bowel gas

- Ultrasound is frequently the first investigation performed

- Ultrasound can demonstrate the heterogeneous nature of the mass and invasion of the IVC, and examine the contralateral kidney

- Chest CT is superior to chest radiography for identifying pulmonary nodules but discordant results are ignored for staging purposes

- MR may be used for staging but as yet no large series have been published comparing MR with CT

- Vascular mapping with conventional angiography or MR is indicated if partial nephrectomy is planned or removal of a tumour within a horseshoe kidney is required

- Radionuclide studies may be useful to assess renal function in children with congenital abnormalities in the contralateral kidney

weighted sequences. Tumour enhancement with gadolinium is heterogeneous and reflects the heterogeneity of the mass composition. The tumour has a diminished enhancement pattern compared with the brightly enhancing normal renal tissue (Fig. 36.13).[6]

Angiography

There is no role for preoperative angiography in the routine assessment of children with Wilms' tumour. If partial nephrectomy is being considered, especially in children with bilateral tumours, or in the case of a tumour arising in a horseshoe kidney, then vascular mapping may be indicated. A decision is made for each individual patient. Magnetic resonance angiography is an alternative to catheter arteriography and the quality of MRA is now such that it is probably appropriate to do this initially and proceed to catheter arteriography if the information is deemed inadequate. Magnetic resonance venography is an alternative to ultrasound in detecting thrombus in the IVC and should be attempted if ultrasound is equivocal or inconclusive. It has been claimed that MR is the best non-invasive method of demonstrating IVC tumour thrombus.[5]

Reassessment of disease following preoperative chemotherapy

There are some fundamental differences in the management of Wilms' tumour between NWTSG and SIOP.

NWTSG recommends primary nephrectomy prior to adjuvant chemotherapy or irradiation,[40] whereas the SIOP trials are based on the use of preoperative chemotherapy.[31] Both groups use preoperative chemotherapy for patients with bilateral tumours, tumours in a solitary kidney, tumours with extension into the IVC above the hepatic veins and tumours found to be unresectable at operation. The management of massive tumours also differs, with NWTSG recommending initial surgical exploration to determine resectability and SIOP recommending routine preoperative chemotherapy without initial biopsy followed by nephrectomy. The advantage of preoperative chemotherapy in these cases is reduction in tumour bulk, which in turn reduces the risk of tumour rupture at operation.[41] The primary concern over these differences in management is the effect that preoperative chemotherapy has on staging. Because staging of the disease remains primarily surgical, the use of preoperative treatment may result in a different stage being assigned to the tumour than would otherwise have been designated. These issues remain controversial.

Imaging has an important role in the assessment of tumour response to chemotherapy. The imaging modalities used prior to and following chemotherapy should be comparable. Some patients may not have a measurable response; however, failure of the mass to shrink does not necessarily mean that there is persistence of viable tumour. Change in the tumour imaging characteristics may indicate response such as necrosis.

The role of imaging in preoperative biopsy

Because the majority of patients enrolled in the NWTSG study protocols undergo primary tumour resection, the need for a preoperative biopsy only arises in the minority of patients who will receive pre-resection chemotherapy. Patients enrolled in SIOP protocols usually undergo pre-resection chemotherapy without prior biopsy. Therefore, classification of tumour histology is not obtained before initiation of therapy. In this situation there is always the risk that chemotherapy with its potentially toxic side-effects may be given to patients with benign disease such as congenital mesoblastic nephroma. Furthermore, lack of histological information of the tumour may result in less potent chemotherapy being given to patients with more malignant tumours that would respond better to more aggressive chemotherapeutic agents. Again, these are controversial issues and policies for obtaining a pretreatment biopsy vary. As treatment regimens become more tailored to tumour histology, the value of pretreatment biopsy may increase.

Open surgical biopsy under general anaesthesia has been the traditional method of obtaining tissue for histology but other less invasive methods are now available. Radiologists frequently perform percutaneous biopsy of suspected Wilms' tumour under ultrasound or CT guidance. The disadvantages of obtaining a percutaneous biopsy are insufficient tissue retrieval and the risk of tumour seeding in the biopsy tract. The biopsy should be taken from viable tumour tissue, which is usually present peripherally; necrotic areas of the tumour lie more centrally. There should be agreement about the handling of specimens between the departments of oncology, surgery, radiology and pathology.

Imaging during treatment and follow-up

During neo-adjuvant chemotherapy for localized disease, 3-monthly abdominal ultrasound and chest radiography is recommended. For patients with Stage IV disease due to lung metastases, chest radiography is recommended at 6 weeks to assess response and at 12 weeks to confirm that response is maintained. Following this, a 3-monthly chest radiograph and abdominal ultrasound throughout treatment is acceptable.[42]

Most Wilms' tumour relapses occur within the first 2 years after nephrectomy. In addition to regular clinical examination of children following treatment for Wilms' tumour, imaging studies are required in order to detect recurrence. The optimum imaging examination during follow-up will depend on the original stage of disease at presentation. Children with Stage I and Stage II disease have a very low incidence of local or intra-abdominal tumour recurrence. In these patients, the most frequent site of recurrence is the lung (Fig. 36.14).[43] Chest radiographs at 3-monthly intervals are indicated for 3 years from the end of treatment and abdominal ultrasound at 3-monthly intervals for 2 years from the end of treatment.[42] This also

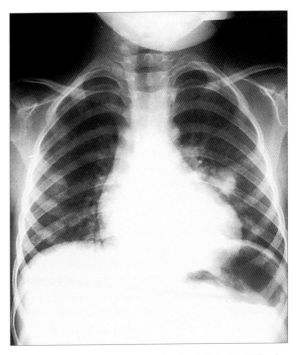

Figure 36.14. *Chest radiograph of a child with Wilms' tumour. Note the bilateral pulmonary metastases.*

applies to higher stage tumours, but patients with haematogenous metastases at presentation require regular evaluation of the affected sites. Metastatic disease to the brain is best evaluated with MR, and to the lungs with CT, although not all lesions seen on CT represent metastatic disease. Ultrasound or MR have the advantage over CT of being non-ionizing and are therefore preferable in the follow-up of patients with liver metastases. Plain radiographs and bone scintigraphy are used to detect bone metastases, although these are rare in Wilms' tumour. The frequency will depend on the length of time off treatment and clinical signs and symptoms. Irradiated bony structures are monitored for life for the possible development of radiation-associated neoplasms, chondromas and chondrosarcomas being the two main lesions.

Monitoring of children at increased risk for Wilms' tumour

It is generally accepted that children with syndromes that put them at high risk for developing Wilms' tumour should be monitored at intervals frequent enough to detect the occurrence of Wilms' tumour in its early stages. In patients with Beckwith–Wiedemann and other predisposing syndromes, both kidneys are assumed to be at equal risk for the development of Wilms' tumour and therefore it is particularly important to detect tumour when it is small and localized. This increases the likelihood that kidney-sparing approaches can be used, which in turn increases the options for managing any subsequently developing Wilms' tumour. Renal sonography is the method usually advised for routine monitoring of children for Wilms' tumour, but unfortunately there are no reliable long-term prospective trials that predict the frequency and duration of monitoring and most advice is based on anecdotal statements. It is well-recognized that as the mass of a Wilms' tumour appears rapidly, an interval of even 6 months between sonograms will not detect lesions at a time when they are clinically silent.[44–46]

Up to 95% of children with Wilms' tumour associated with hemihypertrophy syndromes will develop the tumour before their 8th birthday and 92% of children with aniridia develop their tumour under the age of 5 years.[44] There is some evidence that a subset of patients with Beckwith–Wiedemann syndrome and nephromegaly at risk of developing Wilms' tumour may be identified on scans in early infancy.[47]

Currently, most would accept that sonography at 3-monthly intervals up to the age of 5 years in children with aniridia and 8 years in children with hemihypertrophy is generally safe.[48] Because Beckwith–Wiedemann syndrome is also associated with increased risk of other abdominal neoplasms, sonography provides the significant advantage of screening the other upper abdominal organs. The disadvantages of this policy are the cost of screening and the anxiety and inconvenience of such regular attendance at hospital for the patient and their family, as well as false positive findings that may result in further imaging and possibly surgical intervention. As yet there is no reliable serological or urine test to screen for the development of Wilms' tumour but new developments in the field of genetics and molecular biology may provide new methods for identifying patients at risk for developing Wilms' tumour and other malignancies in the future.[49]

Key points: imaging and assessment of treatment

- Chemotherapy may be given in the neoadjuvant or adjuvant setting according to different study protocols (NWTSG or SIOP)

- Preoperative percutaneous biopsy under ultrasound or CT control is required for certain protocols

- Disadvantages of biopsy include inadequate tissue sampling and the risk of tumour seeding in the needle track

- Most Wilms' tumour relapses occur in the first 2 years after nephrectomy and optimum follow-up depends on the stage of disease

- During chemotherapy for localized disease, 3-monthly follow-up with abdominal ultrasound and chest radiography is indicated

- Ultrasound is the method of choice for routine monitoring of children at risk, e.g. those with syndromes associated with an increased incidence of Wilms' tumours

Other renal tumours of childhood

- Nephroblastomatosis
- Clear cell sarcoma of the kidney (CCSK)
- Rhabdoid tumour of the kidney (RTK)
- Renal cell carcinoma (RCC)
- Renal lymphoma
- Multilocular cystic renal tumour
- Congenital mesoblastic nephroma (CMN)
- Angiomyolipoma

Nephroblastomatosis

Nephroblastomatosis is defined as the presence within the kidneys of nephrogenic rests which may be multifocal or diffuse. These are islands of primitive blastemal elements that persist in the kidneys after birth and have the potential for malignant transformation into Wilms' tumour. Nephroblastomatosis has been detected in 41% of patients with unilateral Wilms' tumour and in 94% and 99% of metachronous and synchronous bilateral tumours, respectively.[50] The presence of nephroblastomatosis in association with Wilms' tumour does not affect tumour staging. Nephroblastomatosis is especially prevalent in patients with hemihypertrophy. It has been found in less than 1% of normal infants.[3] It is currently believed that nephrogenic rests give rise to approximately 30–40% of Wilms' tumours.[3]

Microscopic foci of nephroblastomatosis cannot be detected by imaging, but macroscopic foci act as space-occupying lesions within the kidney and can be detected. The affected kidney may be enlarged and have an indistinct cortico-medullary junction. It may contain focal areas of reduced echogenicity but the lesions may be iso- or even hyperechoic compared with normal renal parenchyma.[51] Diffuse nephroblastomatosis may mimic renal lymphoma, leukaemia or polycystic kidneys.[6] Sonography lacks the sensitivity of CT and MR for the detection of nephroblastomatosis. Palpation of the contralateral kidney at surgery in the child with a unilateral Wilms' tumour has been the traditional way to detect nephroblastomatosis rests prior to CT, but clinical palpation will miss deep-seated intralobar rests and CT is now recognized as the most sensitive method to detect them.

At CT, macroscopic nephrogenic rests appear as low-attenuation peripheral nodules with poor enhancement relative to adjacent normal renal tissue (Fig. 36.15). With MR, the nodules are low signal intensity on both T1- and T2-weighted sequences. Diffuse nephroblastomatosis is usually seen as diffuse reniform enlargement with a thick peripheral rind of tissue that may show striated enhancement.[5]

There are no imaging criteria to determine whether the rests are benign or malignant. This distinction is made only by histology but it may be impossible or impractical to biopsy all the lesions. Nephroblastomatosis is usually diagnosed when the child is under investigation for a clinically apparent Wilms' tumour and is seldom discovered by serendipity. The usual management of a patient is to treat the clinically presenting Wilms' tumour as per protocol, to biopsy accessible contralateral lesions and then to monitor the kidney by imaging surveillance. Once detected, nephroblastomatosis rests must be monitored regularly for growth, as increase in size is recognized as demonstrating malignant transformation. A suggested monitoring scheme is as follows:

- 3-monthly sonography for 1 year after diagnosis, increasing to 4-monthly intervals for a second year and then 6-monthly until the child reaches the 10th birthday
- Computed tomography at 6-monthly intervals for 2 years, increasing to yearly until the age of 10

Any change in appearance at ultrasound or change in symptoms during that period will require more intensive investigation to exclude the development of a Wilms' tumour.

Clear cell sarcoma of the kidney

Once thought to be a highly aggressive form of Wilms' tumour, this is now recognized as a distinct tumour in its own right. It accounts for approximately 4% of primary renal tumours in childhood. The peak incidence is between 1 and 4 years of age and there is a male predominance.[2] There are no syndromic associations and no reports of bilateral tumours. Presentation is non-specific, the tumour often manifesting as an abdominal mass. Imaging studies do not allow differentiation from Wilms' tumour, but the tumour is characterized by its aggressive behaviour. It may metastasize to the bone, lymph nodes, brain, liver and lungs. In some cases, metastases develop long after resection of the primary tumour (Fig. 36.16). Skeletal metastases may have osteolytic or osteoblastic appearances and reduced or increased uptake of isotope may be seen on

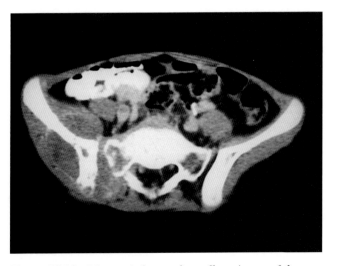

Figure 36.16. *Metastasis from a clear cell carcinoma of the kidney. There is destruction of the right hemi-sacrum and iliac blade with a large soft tissue mass.*

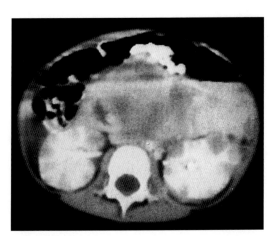

Figure 36.15. *Nephroblastoma rests appearing as focal areas of low attenuation in both kidneys on contrast-enhanced CT scan.*

bone scintigraphy.[6] Because of the high incidence of bone metastases, current recommendations from the NWTSG-V are for periodic screening with skeletal surveys and bone scintigraphy.[6] There is a higher mortality rate and a higher relapse rate than with Wilms' tumour, and the current long-term survival is in the order of 60–70%.[2]

Rhabdoid tumour of the kidney

Rhabdoid tumour (RTK) is a rare highly aggressive malignancy of early childhood accounting for approximately 2% of all primary renal tumours. It occurs exclusively in children. Approximately 80% of tumours present under the age of 2 years, but the majority occur in the first year of life[2] and there is a male predominance. There is no relationship with Wilms' tumour or rhabdomyosarcoma as was once previously thought. Rhabdoid tumour has the worst prognosis of all the primary renal tumours of childhood. It is highly aggressive and metastasizes early. Most patients present with advanced disease and 80% develop metastases most commonly to the lungs, liver, brain, lymph nodes and bone. Rhabdoid tumour is distinctive in its association with synchronous or metachronous primary intracranial neoplasms and brain metastases. The brain lesion is usually found near the midline, often in the posterior fossa. Primitive neuroectodermal tumour (PNET), ependymoma and cerebellar and brain stem astrocytoma have all been described in association with RTK.[52] This tumour is also associated with hypercalcaemia secondary to hyperparathyroidism, which usually returns to normal following removal of the tumour.[53] Imaging demonstrates a large, centrally located, heterogeneous soft tissue mass involving the renal hilum with indistinct margins. Several imaging features may suggest the diagnosis of RTK rather than Wilms' tumour:

- Subcapsular fluid collections
- Tumour lobules separated by dark areas of necrosis or haemorrhage
- Linear calcifications outlining tumour lobules
- Vascular and local invasion is common at presentation[5]

Renal cell carcinoma

Renal cell carcinoma is rare in children, accounting for less than 7% of all primary renal tumours manifesting in the first two decades of life. Less than 2% of all renal cell carcinomas occur in children, this being primarily a tumour of adults.[6] Renal cell carcinoma is associated with the von Hippel–Lindau syndrome, in which the tumours tend to be multiple and occur at a younger age. Clinical manifestations are similar to those in adult patients and include gross painless haematuria, flank pain and a palpable mass. On imaging, this lesion cannot be distinguished from Wilms' tumour; however, there is a higher incidence of calcification in renal cell carcinoma than in Wilms' tumour.[3] The tumour invades locally with spread to adjacent retroperitoneal lymph nodes. Metastases to the lungs, brain or bone are found in 20% of patients at diagnosis. The prognosis is influenced more by the stage of presentation than by the histology. The best outcomes are achieved by radical nephrectomy and clearance of regional nodes as the tumour is extremely resistant to chemotherapy, making metastatic disease difficult to treat.[5] Rests of RCC are occasionally found within Wilms' tumours at histological examination. There are rare reports of RCC arising as a recurrence of Wilms' tumour,[54] which then carry a poor prognosis.

Renal lymphoma

The kidney is a common extranodal site for lymphoma. When kidney involvement is present together with typical nodal disease, the diagnosis is obvious. In children, non-Hodgkin's lymphoma (NHL), especially Burkitt's lymphoma, is more likely to involve the kidney than in adults. Because the renal parenchyma does not contain lymphatic tissue, the existence of primary lymphoma of the kidney is debated; nevertheless there have been reports of isolated renal involvement.[55] With lymphomatous involvement, typically the kidneys are enlarged and there are multiple bilateral tumour deposits. Diffuse infiltration may also be seen (Fig. 36.17). A solitary renal mass or nodule may occur and this often leads to the presumptive diagnosis of Wilms' tumour. However, the correct diagnosis is made on histological examination. Renal lymphoma presenting as a solitary lesion with bony metastases may be misdiagnosed as a clear cell sarcoma of the kidney.[56] At sonography, the lesions are solid but of low echogenicity compared with the normal renal parenchyma and may demonstrate enhanced through-transmission. The CT appearance is non-specific with altered attenuation characteristics.[5] Lymphoma deposits are of low

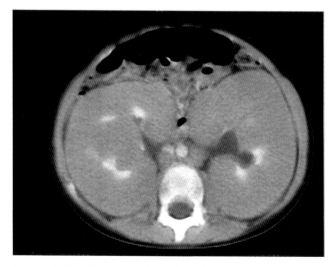

Figure 36.17. *Contrast enhanced CT in a patient with lymphoma and bilateral renal involvement. The kidneys are enlarged due to infiltration and there is abnormal enhancement. Note the para-aortic lymphadenopathy. (Courtesy of Dr K. Johnson, Birmingham Children's Hospital. UK.)*

signal intensity on T1-weighted MR sequences and of relatively high signal intensity on T2-weighted MR sequences.

Multilocular cystic renal tumour

This is a collective term for two types of uncommon renal tumour: cystic nephroma (CN) and cystic poorly differentiated nephroblastoma (CPDN). Two age peaks of multiloculated cystic renal tumours occur. The first is in children between 3 and 24 months. There is a 2 : 1 male sex predominance. A further group of patients with these tumours presents over the age of 30, with an 8 : 1 female predominance, and in this group CN is more common.[57] Most children with these conditions present in the first 2 years of life with a painless abdominal mass. The tumours are both well-circumscribed, discrete lesions consisting entirely of multiple cysts and septa, without solid tumour components except for the septa. This differentiates them from cystic forms of other renal neoplasms (Fig. 36.18). The size of the cysts varies from microscopic to several centimetres, and the cysts do not communicate with each other or with the renal collecting system. Cystic nephroma and CPDN are indistinguishable on gross examination and on imaging studies, and the distinction between these two tumour types is histological. Cystic nephromas contain fibrous tissue in their septa, and there may be well-differentiated tubular

structures present in addition. Cystic poorly differentiated nephroblastomas are similar but also contain blastemal cells and other embryonal stromal cells.[57] On imaging studies, both CN and CPDN appear as well-circumscribed, encapsulated multicystic masses. The cystic structure is best demonstrated by ultrasound although, if the cysts are very small, the lesion may appear solid (Fig. 36.19). The septa

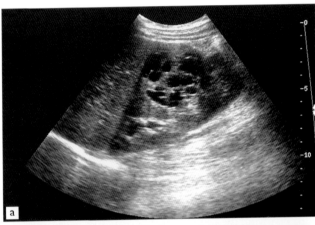

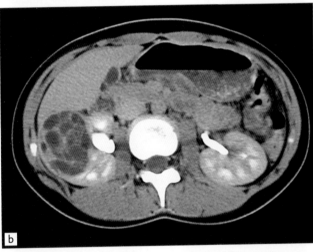

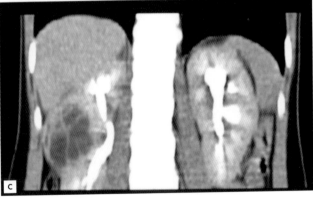

Figure 36.19. *(a) Ultrasound of a smaller cystic nephroma in a 14-year-old girl who presented with painless haematuria. The tumour is well encapsulated. (b) Enhanced CT scan, with coronal reconstruction (c) in the same patient. The septa enhance to the same degree as the surrounding renal tissue.*

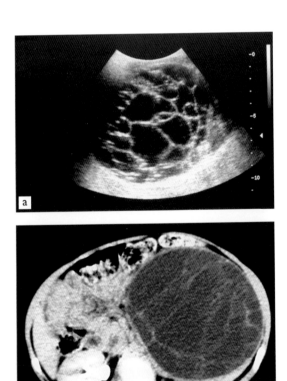

Figure 36.18. *Large left cystic nephroma; the child presented with an abdominal mass at 21 months of age. (a) Ultrasound scan shows the multiloculated cystic nature of the mass; (b) enhanced CT scan of the same patient.*

may enhance on CT.[5] Both CN and CPDN typically have a benign course and nephrectomy alone is usually curative. Local recurrence is rare but has been successfully treated with local radiotherapy or with chemotherapy. Metastases do not occur.

Congenital mesoblastic nephroma

Mesoblastic nephroma is the most common cause of a solid renal mass in the neonatal period. It was once thought to be a form of congenital Wilms' tumour but is now recognized as a distinct clinical entity with predominantly benign behaviour, although it is considered to have some malignant potential. The tumour usually presents in the first few months of life as an abdominal mass, but haematuria, hypercalcaemia or hypertension can be presenting features.[6] Some cases are detected antenatally, but the mean age of presentation is 3 months and it is more common in males. Congenital mesoblastic nephroma is believed to consist of proliferation of early nephrogenic mesenchyme and lacks a tumour capsule. Imaging studies demonstrate a large solid intrarenal mass, replacing renal tissue and typically involving the renal sinus. There may be cystic, necrotic or haemorrhagic areas. Local infiltration of the perinephric tissues is common.[5] Treatment is nephrectomy with a wide excision margin due to the infiltrative nature of the tumour. Follow-up at least in the first year of life is generally advocated as local recurrence, although rare, can occur if the tumour has been incompletely resected. Metastases to lungs, bone and brain can also occur following incomplete excision.[58]

Angiomyolipoma

Angiomyolipoma is an uncommon benign tumour consisting of a disordered arrangement of vascular, smooth muscle and fatty elements. It often occurs sporadically but is also found in association with tuberous sclerosis (TS), neurofibromatosis and von Hippel–Lindau syndrome. Angiomyolipoma is rare in children except in association with TS and 80% of children with TS will be expected to develop lesions by 10 years of age.[59] They are more often bilateral, multifocal and larger in patients with TS. Although these lesions are benign they can be symptomatic due to intratumoural haemorrhage, and the risk of haemorrhage is related to the size of the lesions. Typically, those over 4 cm in diameter have an increased risk of bleeding, whereas those under 4 cm are unlikely to bleed spontaneously.

Imaging appearance of angiomyolipoma varies depending on the amount and type of tissue elements present. Computed tomography and MR are diagnostic when fat is found within the mass. Ultrasound demonstrates highly echogenic, non-shadowing foci which correlate with the fatty elements. Although fat is occasionally found in Wilms' tumour and RCC, the diagnosis of angiomyolipoma is usually straightforward in the appropriate clinical setting.

Rarely, angiomyolipoma may become locally aggressive, invading neighbouring structures, but the main risk is of spontaneous haemorrhage which can be life-threatening. Patients with TS may undergo monitoring in order to identify growing lesions that may require prophylactic embolization or partial nephrectomy.[59–61]

Key points: other renal tumours

- Nephroblastomatosis is defined as nephrogenic rests of cells with the potential to develop into Wilms' tumours
- Macroscopic foci of nephroblastomatosis can be detected on imaging
- CCSK accounts for 4% of all primary renal tumours of childhood
- CCSK is a highly aggressive tumour which metastasizes early
- RTK is rare and highly aggressive
- RTKs are associated with primary intracranial tumours
- RCC is rare. It is associated with the von Hippel–Lindau syndrome
- Renal lymphoma is usually secondary to nodal disease
- Renal lymphoma may appear on imaging as diffuse renal enlargement or as focal renal masses
- Multilocular cystic renal tumours (CN and CPDN) are multicystic masses
- CMN is the most common cause of a solid renal mass in the neonatal period. Metastases occasionally develop
- Angiomyolipomas are benign renal neoplasms which contain fatty elements and are subject to haemorrhage
- Angiomyolipomas are benign but may become locally aggressive

Complications of treatment of Wilms' tumour

Although the survival rate of children with Wilms' tumour has increased dramatically over recent years, this has been at the expense of side-effects and long-term toxicity associated with successful therapy. The complications of treatment of Wilms' tumour are similar in principle to those of treatment of other cancers and can be divided into early and late complications. Complications occurring acutely during chemotherapy are usually related to the effects of immunosuppression. Organ damage due to chemotherapy or radiation that is noted at the end of therapy may remain stable or progress over time. Any side-effect that does not resolve completely after completion of therapy is a long-term effect and one that the patient may have to compensate for during life. However, tissue damage may not be clinically evident at the end of treatment because cytotoxic effects of chemotherapy and radiation on maturing tissues only becomes apparent with further development. This is particularly important in the treatment of paediatric malignancy.

Late effects of cancer treatment refer specifically to those unrecognized toxicities that are absent or subclinical at the end of therapy but manifest later as a result of growth, development, increased organ or tissue demand or ageing. These may impact upon physical or intellectual development and reproductive capability.[62]

The toxic effects of treatment for Wilms' tumour will be briefly discussed, with reference to specific organs.

Cardiac toxicity

The heart may be damaged by several chemotherapeutic agents, particularly the anthracyclines, which includes the drug doxorubicin used to treat high-risk patients with Wilms' tumour. Doxorubicin causes dose-related cardiomyopathy that may be increased in children.[63] Cardiac damage manifests as congestive cardiac failure, but may not become apparent until there is increased cardiac demand such as during exercise or pregnancy. The cumulative frequency of congestive cardiac failure in patients treated according to NWTSG protocols I–IV was 4.4% at 20 years after diagnosis among patients treated initially with doxorubicin and 17.4% at 20 years among those treated with doxorubicin for first and subsequent relapses of Wilms' tumour.[64]

Cyclophosphamide and radiation therapy have additive effects when combined with doxorubicin in treatment.[62] Radiation-induced cardiac damage may be a risk in patients treated with radiotherapy for lung metastases from Wilms' tumour. Cardiac damage may be pericardial, myocardial, or vascular depending on the dose and target volume and technique used.[65]

Pulmonary

Radiation and certain chemotherapeutic agents can affect pulmonary function. There may be acute effects, some of which may subside with time or long-term damage to the lungs. Long-term damage is associated with reduction in pulmonary function as a result of pneumonitis and pulmonary fibrosis induced by these agents. Thoracotomy for excision of lung metastases can further compromise lung function.[65]

Renal

Surgical treatment for Wilms' tumour with nephrectomy or partial nephrectomy can impair renal function but the use of nephrotoxic chemotherapeutic agents and antibiotics further increases the risk of renal failure. In patients treated with nephrectomy and radiation therapy, renal dysfunction is more common.[65] Radiotherapy can cause tubular damage or impaired renal function due to renal artery stenosis as a result of radiation effects on the extrarenal segment of the renal artery. Renal artery stenosis may cause hypertension requiring angioplasty. The frequency of functional impairment is dose-related.[66]

Hepatotoxicity and radiation hepatitis

The liver may be damaged by several cytotoxic agents, including actinomycin-D and irradiation. Using the currently accepted radiotherapy techniques, radiation-related hepatitis is rare in survivors of Wilms' tumour. Most early reports suggested that the main cause of hepatic damage in patients treated with multimodality treatment was radiation but it is now known to occur in patients treated with vincristine and actinomycin-D without irradiation.[67] Damage due to actinomycin-D may be dose-related as there is an increased incidence of hepatic damage in patients who receive less of this drug.[65] Hepatic veno-occlusive disease (VOD) is primarily a clinical diagnosis and manifests as hepatomegaly or right upper quadrant pain, jaundice, ascites and unexplained weight gain resulting from hepatotoxicity associated with chemotherapy or radiotherapy. It is an important complication in children with Wilms' tumour and can be fatal. Histologically, VOD is characterized by an obliteration of the small intrahepatic branches of the hepatic veins due to intimal proliferation and fibrosis associated with centrilobular hepatocellular necrosis.[68] Treatment is primarily supportive but chemotherapy is withheld until the clinical signs of VOD have subsided.

Skeletal effects

Therapeutic radiation can cause growth suppression in any bone, but this is most evident in the spine in patients with Wilms' tumour who have received trunk irradiation. This may result in the development of scoliosis severe enough to require corrective surgery.

Underdevelopment of soft tissues can also occur which may have significant cosmetic effects (Fig. 36.20). A radiation dose of 20 Gy or more is associated with increased morbidity.[69] Growth-suppression effects of radiotherapy on the paediatric spine could result in reduced adult stature, but this is dose- and age-dependent. A recent report from the NWTG has found that the average height deficit observed at maturity for children receiving the currently recommended lower doses of radiotherapy is non-significant.[70]

Osteochondromas may develop in the radiation field and may be found on the ribs or lower scapular blade in children who have received radiotherapy for Wilms' tumour.

Clinical rickets has developed in some patients treated with ifosfamide, secondary to the development of renal tubular Fanconi syndrome (Fig. 36.21). The kidneys usually recover but any persisting skeletal deformity of rickets may require corrective orthopaedic surgery.[71,72]

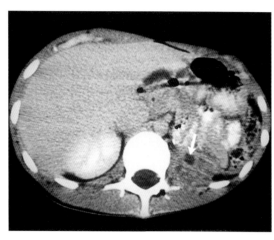

Figure 36.20. *CT scan showing postirradiation hemiatrophy of the left side of the abdomen. Left nephrectomy. There is recurrent tumour (arrow) in the left psoas muscle.*

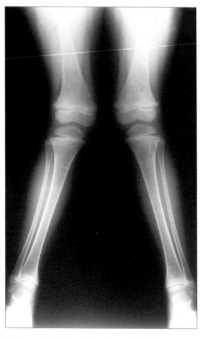

Figure 36.21. *Bowing of the legs as a result of rickets secondary to treatment with ifosfamide. Corrective osteotomies were required.*

Gonadal toxicity

Infertility is one of the main late side-effects of cytotoxic chemotherapy. Because dividing cells are more sensitive to the cytotoxic effects of alkylating agents than cells at rest, impairment of fertility is more frequent in boys than in girls.[73] Ovarian failure can result from abdominal pelvic radiotherapy but when the ovaries are outside the radiation field this is rare.[74] The outcome of pregnancies in patients who received irradiation for childhood Wilms' tumour is less successful, with increased incidence of low birth weight and an increase in perinatal deaths.[75,76] The reduced fetal size may be due to the effects of radiation on uterine vascu-

lature or on the ability of the uterus to grow with pregnancy.[77] There is no increase in congenital abnormalities and there is not an increased incidence of Wilms' tumour in the offspring of survivors.[78]

Development of a second malignancy

Both an inherited disposition towards the development of malignancy and treatment with chemotherapy and radiotherapy can put Wilms' tumour survivors at risk of developing a second malignancy. Most of the second malignancies reported such as bone tumours, breast and thyroid cancers have occurred in irradiated areas. Certain chemotherapeutic agents including doxorubicin, actinomycin-D and vincristine may contribute to an increased risk for developing second malignancies.[65] A cumulative risk of 1.6% for the development of a second neoplasm at 15 years from diagnosis has been reported among patients entered in the National Wilms' Tumour Studies.[79] Abdominal irradiation increased the risk of a second malignant neoplasm and doxorubicin potentiated the radiation effect. An increased incidence in the development of acute myelogenous leukaemia has been reported recently following treatment for Wilms' tumour with chemotherapy regimens including doxorubicin or etoposide and infradiaphragmatic radiation. The latent period between initial diagnosis of the renal tumour and development of leukaemia was 3 years.[80] This emphasizes the importance of current efforts to limit the use of intensive chemotherapy and radiotherapy in the treatment of Wilms' tumour. Now only patients with advanced stage disease or those with tumours with unfavourable histology receive intensive therapy.

> ### Key points: complications of treatment of Wilms' tumours
>
> ■ Late effects of cancer treatment impact on physical, intellectual and reproductive development
>
> ■ Cardiac toxicity manifests as cardiac failure, often at a time of increased demand, e.g. pregnancy
>
> ■ Pneumonitis and pulmonary fibrosis may result from radiation and certain chemotherapeutic agents
>
> ■ Radiotherapy may induce renal impairment. Antibiotics and chemotherapeutic agents also carry a risk of renal failure
>
> ■ Liver toxicity may occur with certain chemotherapeutic agents, e.g. vincristine and actinomycin-D
>
> ■ Spinal growth retardation may ensue after radiotherapy
>
> ■ Infertility is an important complication of chemotherapy
>
> ■ There is a cumulative risk of 1.6% of developing a second malignancy after treatment of Wilms' tumour with chemotherapy and radiotherapy

Summary

- Wilms' tumour is the most common renal tumour of childhood, with a peak incidence between 6 months and 4 years

- Bilateral tumours occur in 5–10% of cases

- Ultrasound is the method of choice for detecting Wilms' tumours

- Contrast-enhanced CT is the primary imaging method for staging the primary tumour

- Metastases are predominantly to the lungs. Routine CT of the chest is recommended

- Currently, pulmonary nodules detected on CT but not visualized on chest radiography do not impact on patient management

- Most relapses from Wilms' tumour occur within the first 2 years after nephrectomy

- Routine follow-up with chest radiographs and ultrasound at 3-monthly intervals for up to 3 years is recommended for Stage I and Stage II disease

- There is an increased risk of Wilms' tumours in patients with various syndromes, e.g. Beckwith–Wiedemann syndrome, nephromegaly and hemihypertrophy

- Nephroblastomatosis represents nephrogenic areas which are multifocal or diffuse and may transform into Wilms' tumours

- Clear cell sarcoma of the kidney is characterized by aggressive behaviour but on imaging cannot be distinguished from Wilms' tumour

- Rhabdoid tumour of the kidney can be distinguished from Wilms' tumours on imaging characteristics and is also highly aggressive

- Renal cell carcinoma is rare and is associated with von Hippel–Lindau syndrome

- Renal lymphoma in childhood is similar to adult disease and may appear as a diffuse renal enlargement or as focal renal masses

- Benign renal masses of childhood include multilocular cystic renal tumours and angiomyolipoma

- Congenital mesoblastic nephroma is the most common renal tumour of the newborn. Malignancy is uncommon but occasionally it metastasizes to distant sites

- Complications of treatment include cardiac, hepatic and pulmonary damage as well as renal impairment. Skeletal growth retardation is also a complication of therapy

- Second malignancies usually develop in the irradiated area

References

1. Julian J C, Merguerian P A, Shortliffe L M D. Pediatric genitourinary tumors. Curr Opin Oncol 1995; 7: 265–274

2. Charles A K, Vujanic G M, Berry P J. Renal tumours of childhood. Histopathology 1998; 32: 293–309

3. Lonergan G J, Martinez-Leon M I, Agrons G A et al. Nephrogenic rests, nephroblastomatosis and associated lesions of the kidney. Radiographics 1998; 18: 947–968

4. Breslow N E, Olshan A, Beckwith J B, Green D M. Epidemiology of Wilms' tumor. Med Pediatr Oncol 1993; 21: 172–181

5. Lowe L H, Isuani B H, Heller R M et al. Pediatric renal masses: Wilms' tumor and beyond. Radiographics 2000; 20: 1585–1603

6. Geller E, Smergel E M, Lowry P A. Renal neoplasms of childhood. Radiol Clin North Am 1997; 35: 1391–1413

7. Stiller C A, McKinney P A, Bunch K J et al. Childhood cancer and ethnic group in Britain: a United Kingdom Children's Cancer Study Group [UKCCSG] study. Br J Cancer 1991; 64: 543–548

8. McLowrie G. Wilms' tumor (nephroblastoma). Curr Opin Urol 2001; 11: 567–570

9. Grundy R G, Richard J, Scambler P, Cowell J K. Loss of heterozygosity on chromosome 16 in sporadic Wilms' tumor. Br J Cancer 1998; 78: 1181–1187

10. Merguerian P A, Chang B. Pediatric genitourinary tumors. Curr Opin Oncol 2002; 14: 273–279

11. Ivanov I, Shuper A, Shohat M, Snir M, Weitz R. Aniridia: recent achievements in paediatric practice. Eur J Paediatr 1995; 154: 795–800

12. Dome J S, Coppes M J. Recent advances in Wilms' tumor genetics. Curr Opin Paediatr 2002; 14: 5–11

13. Denys P, Malvaux P, van den Berghe H et al. Association d'un syndrome anatomo-pathologique de pseudohermaphroditisme masculine, d'un tumour de Wilms, d'un nephropathie parenchymateuse et d'un mosaicisme XX/XY. Arch Fr Pediatr 1967; 24: 729–739

14. Drash A, Sherman F, Hartmann W H et al. A syndrome of pseudohermaphroditism, Wilms' tumour, hypertension, and degenerative renal disease. J Pediatr 1970; 76: 585–593

15. Tank E S, Melvin T. The association of Wilms' tumour

with nephrologic disease. J Pediatr Surg 1990; 25: 724–725

16. Buyukpamukcu M, Kutluk T, Buyukpamukcu N et al. Renal tumours with pseudohermaphroditism and glomerular disease. Acta Oncol 1992; 31: 745–748

17. Schmitt K, Zabel B, Tulzer G et al. Nephropathy with Wilms' tumour or gonadal dysgenesis: incomplete Denys–Drash syndrome or separate diseases? Eur J Pediatr 1995; 154: 577–581

18. Moorthy A W, Chesney R W, Lubinsky M. Chronic renal failure and XY gonadal dysgenesis: Frasier syndrome. A commentary on reported cases. Am J Med Genet 1987; 3 (Suppl): 297–302

19. McTaggart S J, Algar E, Chow C W et al. Clinical spectrum of Denys–Drash and Frasier syndrome. Pediatr Nephrol 2001; 16: 335–339

20. Yamaguchi T, Fukuda T, Uetani M et al. Renal cell carcinoma in a patient with Beckwith–Wiedemann syndrome. Pediatr Radiol 1996; 26: 312–314

21. Grundy R G, Pritchard J, Baraitser M et al. Perlman and Wiedemann–Beckwith syndromes: two distinct conditions associated with Wilms' tumour. Eur J Pediatr 1992; 151: 895–898

22. Smith P J, Sullivan M, Algar E, Shapiro D N. Analysis of paediatric tumour types associated with hemihyperplasia in childhood. J Paediatr Child Health 1994; 30: 515–517

23. Hoyme H E, Seaver L H, Jones K L et al. Isolated hemihyperplasia (hemihypertrophy): report of a prospective multicentre study of the incidence of neoplasia and review. Am J Med Genet 1998; 79: 274–278

24. Petruzzi M J, Green D M. Wilms' tumor. Pediatr Clin North Am 1997; 44: 939–952

25. Navoy J, Royal S A, Vaid Y N et al. Wilms' tumour: unusual manifestations. Paediatr Radiol 1995; 25: 76–86

26. Jose B, Nakayan P L, Pietsch J B et al. Budd–Chiari syndrome secondary to hepatic vein thrombus from Wilms' tumour: case report and literature review. J Kentucky Med Assoc 1989; 87: 174–176

27. Ritchey M R, Green D M, Breslow N E. Accuracy of current imaging modalities in the diagnosis of synchronous bilateral Wilms' tumor. A report from the National Wilms' Tumor Study Group. Cancer 1995; 75: 600–604

28. Farhat W, McLorie G, Capolicchio G. Wilms' tumor: surgical considerations and controversies. Clin North Amer Urol Oncol 2000; 27: 455–462

29. Paya K, Horcher E, Lawrenz K et al. Bilateral Wilms' tumor: surgical aspects. Eur J Pediatr Surg 2001; 11: 99–104

30. Haase G M, Ritchey M L. Nephroblastoma. Semin Pediatr Surg 1997; 6: 11–16

31. Graf N, Tournade M-F, de Kraker J. The role of preoperative chemotherapy in the management of Wilms' tumor. The SIOP studies. International Society of Paediatric Oncology. Clin North Am Urol 2000; 27: 443–454

32. Coppes M J, de Kraker J, van Dijken P L et al. Bilateral Wilms' tumor: long-term survival and some epidemiological features. J Clin Oncol 1989; 7: 310–315

33. Ritchey M L, Coppes M J P. The management of synchronous bilateral Wilms' tumour. Hematol Oncol Clin North Am 1995; 9: 1303–1315

34. Talpallikar M C, Sawant V, Hirgad S et al. Wilms' tumor arising in a horseshoe kidney. Pediatr Surg Int 2001; 17: 465–466

35. Neville H, Ritchey M L, Shamberger R C et al. The occurrence of Wilms' tumor in horseshoe kidneys: a report from the National Wilms Tumor Study Group (NWTSG). J Pediatr Surg 2002; 37: 1134–1137

36. Babyn P, Owens C, Gyepes M et al. Imaging patients with Wilms' tumour. Haematol Oncol Clinics N Am 1995; 9: 1217–1252

37. Duncan A W, Charles A K, Berry P J. Cysts within septa: an ultrasound feature distinguishing neoplastic from non-neoplastic renal lesions in children? Pediatr Radiol 1996; 26: 315–317

38. Green D M, Fernbach D J, Norkool P et al. The treatment of Wilms' tumor patients with pulmonary metastases detected only with computed tomography: a report form the National Wilms' Tumor Study. J Clin Oncol; 1991: 1776–1781

39. Owens C M, Veys P A, Pritchard J et al. Role of chest computed tomography at diagnosis in the management of Wilms' tumor: a study by the United Kingdom Children's Cancer Study Group. J Clin Oncol 2002; 20: 2768–2773

40. Neville H L, Ritchey M L. Wilms' tumor: overview of National Wilms' Tumor Study Group results. Urol Clin North Am 2000; 27: 435–442

41. Blakely M L, Ritchey M L. Controversies in the management of Wilms' tumor. Semin Pediatr Surg 2001; 10: 127–131

42. Duncan A, on behalf of the United Kingdom Children's Cancer Study Group. UKCCSG Radiology Imaging Guidelines; June 2001

43. Egeler R M, Wolff J E A, Anderson R A, Coppes MJ. Long-term complications and post-treatment follow-up of patients with Wilms' tumor. Semin Urol Oncol 1999; 17: 55–61

44. Beckwith J B. Questions and answers. Am J Roentgenol 1995; 164: 1291–1295

45. Green D M, Breslow N E, Beckwith J B et al. Screening of children with hemihypertrophy, aniridia, and Beckwith–Wiedemann syndrome in patients with Wilms tumour: a report from the National Wilms' Tumour Study. Med Pediatr Oncol 1993; 21: 188–192

46. Garber J E, Diller L. Screening children at genetic risk of cancer. Curr Opin Pediatr 1993; 5: 712–715

47. DeBaun M R, Siegel M J, Choyke P L. Nephromegaly in infancy and early childhood: a risk factor for Wilms' tumor in Beckwith–Wiedemann syndrome. J Paediatr 1998; 132: 401–404

48. Beckwith J B. Editorial. Children at increased risk for Wilms' tumor: monitoring issues. J Paediatr 1998; 132: 377–379

49. Nichols K E, Li F P, Haber D A, Diller L J. Childhood cancer predisposition: applications of molecular testing and future implications. J Paediatr 1998; 132: 389–397

50. Beckwith J B, Kiviat N B, Bonadio J F. Nephrogenic rests, nephroblastomatosis and the pathogenesis of Wilms' tumour. Pediatr Pathol 1990; 10: 1–36

51. White K S, Kirks D R, Bove K E. Imaging of nephroblastomatosis: an overview. Radiology 1992; 182: 1–5

52. Agrons G A, Kingsman K D, Wagner B J, Sotelo-Avila C. Rhabdoid tumour of the kidney in children: a comparative study. Am J Roentgenol 1997; 168: 447–451

53. Jafri S Z H, Freeman J L, Rosenberg B F et al. Clinical and imaging features of rhabdoid tumour of the kidney. Urol Radiol 1991; 13: 94–97

54. Allsbrook W C, Boswell W C, Takahashi H et al. Recurrent renal cell carcinoma arising in Wilms' tumour. Cancer 1991; 67: 690–695

55. Dyer R B, Lowe L H, Zagoria R J, Amiss E S Jr. Mass effect in the renal sinus: an anatomic classification. Curr Prob Diagn Radiol 1994; 23: 1–28

56. Capps G W, Das Narla L. Renal lymphoma mimicking clear cell sarcoma in a pediatric patient. Pediatr Radiol 1995; 25: 87–89

57. Agrons G A, Wagner B J, Davidson A J, Suarez E S. Multilocular cystic renal tumor in children: radiologic–pathologic correlation. Radiographics 1995; 15: 653–669

58. Schlesinger A E, Rosenfield N S, Castle V P, Jasty R. Congenital mesoblastic nephroma metastatic to the brain: a report of two cases. Pediatr Radiol 1995; 25: S73–S75

59. Ewalt D H, Sheffield E, Sparagana S P et al. Renal lesion growth in children with tuberous sclerosis complex. J Urol 1998; 160: 141–145

60. Kennelly M J, Grossman H B, Cho K J. Outcome analysis of 42 cases of renal angiomyolipoma. J Urol 1994; 152: 1988–1991

61. Van Baal J G, Smits N J, Keeman J N et al. The evolution of renal angiomyolipomas in patients with tuberous sclerosis. J Urol 1994; 152: 35–38

62. Schwartz C L. Long-term survivors of childhood cancer: the late effects of therapy. Oncologist 1999; 4: 45–54

63. Green D M, Doncterwolcke R, Evans A E, D'Angio G J. Late effects of treatment for Wilms' tumor. Hematol/Oncol Clin North Am 1995; 9: 1317–1327

64. Green D M, Grigoriev Y A, Nan B et al. Congestive heart failure after treatment for Wilms' tumor: a report from the National Wilms' Tumor Study Group. J Clin Oncol 2001; 19: 1926–1934

65. Egeler R M, Wolff J E A, Anderson R A, Coppes M J. Long-term complications and post-treatment follow-up of patients with Wilms' tumor. Semin Urol Oncol 1999; 17: 55–61

66. Ludin A, Macklis R M. Radiotherapy for pediatric genitourinary tumors. Urol Clin North Am 2000; 27: 553–562

67. Green D M, Norkool P, Breslow N et al. Severe hepatic toxicity after treatment with vincristine and actinomycin-D using single dose or divided dose schedule: a report from the National Wilms' Tumor Study. J Clin Oncol 1990; 8: 1525–1530

68. Tornesello A, Piciacchia D, Mastrangelo S et al. Veno-occlusive disease of the liver in right-sided Wilms' tumors. Eur J Cancer 1998; 34: 1220–1223

69. Taylor R E. Morbidity from abdominal radiotherapy in the first United Kingdom Children's Cancer Study. United Kingdom Children's Cancer Study Group. Clin Oncol 1997; 9: 381–384

70. Hogeboom C J, Grosser S C, Guthrie K A et al. Stature loss following treatment for Wilms' tumor. Med Pediatr Oncol 2001; 36: 295–304

71. Skinner R, Pearson A D J, Price L et al. Nephrotoxicity after ifosfamide. Arch Dis Child 1990; 65: 732–738

72. Sweeney L E. Hypophosphataemic rickets after ifosfamide treatment in children. Clin Radiol 1993; 47: 345–347

73. Blumenfeld Z, Haim N. Prevention of gonadal damage during cytotoxic therapy. Ann Med 1997; 29: 199–206

74. Stillman R J, Schinfeld J S, Schiff I et al. Ovarian failure in long-term survivors of childhood malignancy. Am J Obstet Gynecol 1981; 139: 62–66

75. Hawkins M M, Smith R A. Pregnancy outcomes in childhood cancer survivors: probable effects of abdominal irradiation. Int J Cancer 1989; 43: 399–402

76. Li F P, Gimbrere K, Gelber R D et al. Outcome of pregnancy in survivors of Wilms' tumour. JAMA 1987; 257: 216–219

77. Bath L E, Chambers S E, Anderson R E et al. Ovarian and uterine function following treatment for childhood cancer. 5th International Conference on Long-Term Complications of Treatment of Children and Adolescents for Cancer. Niagara-on-the-lake, Ontario, Canada, 1998

78. Byrne J, Mulvihill J J, Connelly R R et al. Reproductive problems and birth defects in survivors of Wilms' tumour and their relatives. Med Pediatr Oncol 1988; 16: 233–240

79. Breslow N E, Takashima J R, Whitton J A et al. Second malignant neoplasms following treatment for Wilms' tumor: a report from the National Wilms' Tumor Study Group. J Clin Oncol 1995; 13: 1851–1859

80. Shearer P, Kapoor G, Beckwith J B et al. Secondary acute myelogenous leukaemia in patients previously treated for childhood renal tumours: a report from the National Wilms' Tumor Study Group. J Pediatr Hematol Oncol 2001; 23: 109–111

Chapter 37

Neuroblastoma

Marilyn Siegel

Introduction

Neuroblastoma is the most common extracranial malignant tumour of childhood. It has a spectrum of locations and degrees of histopathologic differentiation which result in a diversity of clinical and biologic features.[1-3] With the exception of infants under the age of 1 year, the prognosis of children with neuroblastoma is poor. Imaging plays a crucial role in the determination of stage and is extremely important as the stage of the tumour remains an important indicator of outcome.

Incidence

Neuroblastoma accounts for 8–10% of all childhood cancers. The prevalence is about one case per 7,000 live births and there are approximately 600 newly diagnosed cases of neuroblastoma in the USA annually.[1,3] The annual incidence rates per million for neuroblastoma in the UK (1986–1995) from 0 to 14 years is 9.3 (age-standardized to world standard population). Thus in the UK, the expected annual number of new cases of neuroblastoma is 86.[4] The median age at diagnosis of children with neuroblastoma is approximately 17 months.[1] Approximately 40% of patients are under 1 year of age, 90% are under 4 years and 98% are under 10 years of age.

Neuroblastoma can arise anywhere along the sympathetic chain, from the neck to the pelvis. Approximately two thirds of tumours occur in the abdomen, and 50–75% of these arise in the adrenal medulla. The remaining abdominal tumours arise from sympathetic ganglia. Other sites of origin are the posterior mediastinum (10–15%), neck (5%) and pelvis (5%). In approximately 1% of children, a primary tumour cannot be found. The site of origin varies with patient age. Infants have more cervical and thoracic tumours, whereas older children have more primary adrenal tumours.[5]

Clinical presentation

Most children with neuroblastoma are symptomatic. The tumour, however, can be detected incidentally on antenatal ultrasonography,[6] postnatal screening programmes,[1,7-11]

physical examination, or imaging studies obtained for other indications.

Screening programmes

Neuroblastoma *in situ* has been described in fetuses.[7-9] Clinical and radiological follow-up postnatally has demonstrated spontaneous resolution in all of these cases, confirming the benign nature of these antenatal tumours.

Postnatal screening programmes have been introduced in Canada, Europe and Japan.[10-15] The basis for introducing population screening with urinary catecholamines was that early detection of neuroblastoma could decrease the incidence of advanced stage disease in children older than 1 year of age. These screening studies increased the incidence of neuroblastoma in infants under 1 year of age without decreasing the incidence of unfavourable advanced stage disease in older children. The majority of patients identified had lower stages of disease and virtually all of the tumours were biologically favourable.

Symptoms due to local disease

The clinical presentation varies depending on the site of tumour and extent of disease.[1,2,5,16] Patients with neuroblastoma may present with clinical complaints related to the primary tumour, distant disease, or a paraneoplastic syndrome.

Tumours occurring in the abdomen are more likely to be symptomatic than those arising in the chest. Abdominal disease is likely to result in a palpable abdominal mass or abdominal pain. Sudden increase in abdominal size can result from spontaneous haemorrhage into the tumour. Pelvic tumours can result in sciatic nerve palsy, urinary and fecal incontinence, neuropathic bladder and leg weakness or nerve root injury.[17]

Primary posterior mediastinal tumours are often an incidental finding on chest radiographs obtained to evaluate respiratory symptoms or trauma. However, high thoracic and cervical neuroblastoma can be associated with dysphagia, stridor or Horner's syndrome (unilateral ptosis, pupillary constriction and anhydrosis).[18] Occasionally, thoracic tumours can result in superior vena cava syndrome.

Paraspinal tumours can result in scoliosis, back pain, urinary or fecal retention and peripheral neurologic deficits due to neural foraminal invasion and nerve root or cord compression. The neurologic manifestations are usually related to the level and extent of tumour invasion in the spinal canal and include radicular pain and subacute or acute paraplegia as well as bladder or bowel dysfunction.[1] Hypertension, due to encasement or stretching of the renal artery or to activation of the renin–angiotensin system, is an additional finding in some children with neuroblastoma. Because neuroblastoma has often disseminated at the time of diagnosis, non-specific signs and symptoms, including fever, irritability, weight loss and anaemia, are also common findings.

Symptoms due to distant disease

At least 70% of patients will have disseminated disease at the time of diagnosis, including 70% of infants and 85% of children older than 1 year of age.[1] In infants under 12 months of age, metastases are predominantly to the skin, liver, bone marrow and lymph nodes. Metastases to the skin or subcutaneous tissue cause non-tender, bluish, mobile nodules ('blueberry muffin baby'), while metastases to the liver can present as hepatomegaly. In neonates, the enlarging liver can cause severe respiratory compromise and compression of the inferior vena cava, with resultant ascites, anasarca and renal failure.[16]

In children older than 1 year of age, metastases are primarily to cortical bone, bone marrow, lymph nodes and liver. Bone metastases may cause persistent, migratory or recurrent bone pain or a palpable mass. These symptoms are often confused with leukaemia, juvenile rheumatoid arthritis or osteomyelitis.[19] Metastatic disease to the sphenoid bone or retrobulbar soft tissues can result in proptosis and ecchymosis with swelling and proptosis, creating a characteristic 'racoon eye' appearance. Metastatic lesions to the dura or brain can present with findings of increased intracranial pressure, such as widened cranial sutures, or focal neurologic signs.

Paraneoplastic syndrome

Several paraneoplastic syndromes have been associated with both localized and disseminated neuroblastoma, including opsoclonus–myoclonus syndrome, intractable diarrhoea and flushing associated with hypertension. These findings have been attributed to metabolic and immunological disturbances associated with the tumour. The opsoclonus–myoclonus syndrome, also referred to as myoclonic encephalopathy of infants, is characterized by acute cerebellar and truncal ataxia and random eye movements ('dancing eyes').[20,21] It occurs in up to 4% of patients with neuroblastoma. Conversely, up to 50% of children with this syndrome may have neuroblastoma.[1] The primary lesion is most commonly found in the posterior mediastinum (50% of cases), but it may be found anywhere along the sympathetic chain. The majority of patients with opsoclonus–myoclonus syndrome have favourable outcomes with respect to their tumour; however, most have long-term neurologic deficits that may progress even after removal of the tumour.[20,21] These deficits are presumably due to anti-neural antibodies against the primary tumour that cross-react with neural cells in the cerebellum or elsewhere in the brain.[21]

Intractable watery diarrhoea associated with hypokalaemia and dehydration is a result of tumour secretion of vasoactive intestinal peptide (VIP). Most VIP-secreting tumours are histologically mature and either ganglioneuroma or ganglioneuroblastoma.[22] Flushing with associated hypertension has been reported also in patients with neuroblastomas. This presentation is uncommon and is thought to be a manifestation of very high levels of catecholamines. Patients with tumour-related diarrhoea and hypertension usually have more mature tumours (either ganglioneuroma or ganglioneuroblastoma) and favourable outcomes.[23] Surgical resection of the tumour leads to resolution of symptoms.

Key points: incidence and clinical features

- Neuroblastoma is the most common extracranial malignant tumour of childhood accounting for 8–10% of all childhood malignancies

- 80% of tumours occur under 4 years of age

- Approximately two thirds of tumours occur in the abdomen, 50–75% in the adrenal medulla

- Most children with neuroblastoma are symptomatic at diagnosis

- Several paraneoplastic syndromes are associated with localized and disseminated neuroblastoma

- Approximately 90% of tumours result in elevated VMA, HVA and dopamine

- At least 70% of patients have disseminated disease at the time of diagnosis

- Metastases are predominantly to the skin, liver, bone marrow and lymph nodes

Pathology

Neuroblastoma arises from primitive sympathetic cells, which are derived from the embryonic neural crest. There are three histopathologic patterns of neuroblastoma, which correlate with the degree of tumour differentiation:

- Neuroblastoma
- Ganglioneuroblastoma
- Ganglioneuroma[1,2]

The neuroblastoma is composed of small round cells with scanty cytoplasm, often arranged in clusters resembling rosettes. The ganglioneuroblastoma contains rests of neuroblasts along with mature or maturing ganglion cells. The ganglioneuroma is fully differentiated and is composed of mature ganglion cells. Neuroblastoma and ganglioneuroblastoma are usually grouped together (and referred to as neuroblastoma) for purposes of staging and reporting survival statistics as well as imaging features.

Macroscopically, neuroblastomas are usually about 6–8 cm in size and are often haemorrhagic. Areas of stroma are often interposed between areas of haemorrhagic tissue, giving the tumour a lobular appearance. Distinguishing neuroblastoma from other small, round blue cell tumours of childhood, including Ewing's sarcoma, primitive neuroectodermal tumour, rhabdomyosarcoma, leukaemia and lymphoma, can be difficult on routine light microscopy and often requires the adjunctive use of electron microscopy or immunohistochemistry.

Key points: pathology

- Neuroblastomas are usually 6–8 cm in diameter and are haemorrhagic

- Neuroblastoma is composed of small round cells with scanty cytoplasm, often arranged in clusters resembling rosettes

Methods of diagnosis

An unequivocal pathologic diagnosis can be made based on tissue sampling and light microscopy, electron microscopy or immunohistology. A diagnosis also can be established by the combination of a bone marrow aspirate or biopsy that shows unequivocal tumour cells *and* increased serum or urinary catecholamines or metabolites. Percutaneous biopsy of the primary tumour or liver metastases in children with advanced disease (Stages 3, 4, or 4S disease) is a feasible alternative to open biopsy for diagnosis and determination of prognostic information.[24]

Staging

In the past, there were two major staging systems used for neuroblastoma: the Evans system and the system used by Pediatric Oncology Group. The Evans system described in 1971 was based on disease extent as determined by physical examination, imaging evaluation and bone marrow biopsy. This staging system did not consider surgical resectability of the tumour, which has been shown to be an important prognostic factor.[25] The Pediatric Oncology Group staging system described in 1983 was based on surgical findings.[26,27]

The most recent staging system for neuroblastoma is the International Neuroblastoma Staging System (INSS) (Table 37.1).[28,29] This classification takes into account radi-

Table 37.1. INSS staging system for neuroblastoma

Stage	Definition
I	Localized tumour with complete resection, with or without microscopic residual disease; representative ipsilateral lymph nodes negative for tumour microscopically
IIA	Localized tumour with incomplete gross excision; representative ipsilateral non-adherent lymph nodes negative for tumour microscopically
IIB	Localized tumour with or without complete gross excision, with representative ipsilateral non-adherent lymph nodes positive for tumour. Enlarged contralateral lymph nodes must be negative microscopically.
III	Unresectable unilateral tumour infiltrating across the midline, with or without regional lymph node involvement; or localized unilateral tumour with contralateral regional lymph node involvement; or midline tumour with bilateral extension by infiltration (unresectable) or by lymph node involvement.
IV	Any primary tumour with dissemination to distant lymph nodes, bone, bone marrow, liver, skin and/or other organs (except as defined for Stage IVS)
IVS	Localized primary tumour (as defined for stage I, IIA, or IIB), with dissemination limited to skin, liver, and/or bone marrow. Bone marrow involvement should be minimal (<10% of total nucleated cells identified as malignant on bone marrow biopsy or on marrow aspirate). Limited to infants <1 year of age

ological findings, surgical resectability, lymph node involvement and bone marrow involvement and provides more uniformity in the interpretation of clinical studies and staging patients with neuroblastoma.

Key point: staging

- The International Neuroblastoma Staging System (INSS) is now the most widely used staging classification

Treatment

The treatment of neuroblastoma is determined by the stage of the tumour at diagnosis. Patients with localized tumour (Stages I and II) are candidates for primary surgical resection. In patients with Stage I tumours with good biologic markers, surgery alone is usually curative.[30,31] Patients with Stage II disease usually also receive chemotherapy.

Patients with unresectable local disease that encases vessels (Stage III) and those with metastatic disease at diagnosis (Stage IV) are treated with chemotherapy initially to shrink the tumour and eradicate metastatic deposits. Percutaneous biopsy of the lesions may provide the necessary tissue for diagnosis and determination of prognosis, thus obviating open biopsy.[24] Debulking surgery can be necessary at time of diagnosis if the tumour is compressing a vital organ. Once the tumour decreases sufficiently in volume, delayed surgical resection is performed. Following this, any residual tumour is treated with one or a combination of the following: chemotherapy, radiation therapy and total body irradiation followed by autologous bone marrow transplantation.

Recently, targeted therapy with radiolabelled meta-iodobenzylguanidine (MIBG),[32,33] [131]I-3F8 monoclonal antibody,[34] or cis-retinoic acid[35] has been used to treat localized bulky disease residua. In some patients, ^{131}I MIBG is being used as initial therapy prior to surgery.[32,33]

Occasionally, neuroblastoma will regress spontaneously. Spontaneous regression occurs most commonly in infants and is also seen in about 1% of children with gross residual disease following surgical excision of tumour. Neuroblastoma cells also may differentiate into more benign ganglion cells, either spontaneously or after chemotherapy.[1]

When disease recurs, it may be in the primary tumour site with extension into surrounding tissues or in other areas of the body. Bone and bone marrow relapses are common sites of relapse.

Prognostic considerations

A variety of independent clinical, biologic and genetic variables have been shown to correlate directly with patient prognosis and survival.[36] The two most important clinical predictors of survival from neuroblastoma are the stage of disease and age of the patient at diagnosis.[36] Survival is longer in lower stage disease and younger patients. Patients with Stage I or II disease have greater than a 90% survival rate,[36] whereas those with Stage III and Stage IV disease have survival rates of approximately 64% and 24%, respectively. Most children diagnosed with neuroblastoma under 1 year of age have an excellent long-term survival (almost 75%).[37] Site of the primary tumour also can have prognostic importance, although it is not independent of age and stage.[38] Patients with thoracic neuroblastomas have a better prognosis than those with non-thoracic neuroblastomas.[38]

Certain biologic markers, including serum levels of lactate dehydrogenase, ferritin and neurone-specific enolase, also provide useful information in the determination of prognosis.[1,39,40] In general, low levels of any of these serum markers predicts a good outcome, whereas high serum levels are associated with a poor prognosis.

Genetic markers with prognostic value include the amount of tumour cell DNA, the karyotype and N-myc amplification.[1,41–45] Up to 30% of children with neuroblastoma present with N-myc amplification in tumour cells (greater than 10 copies of a segment of DNA termed N-myc oncogene). N-myc amplification and a diploid karyotype are more often associated with disseminated disease; they also are strongly associated with rapid tumour progression and

a poor prognosis, regardless of tumour stage. A lack of N-myc amplification and hyperploidy (more DNA), by contrast, are linked to a favourable prognosis.[41,42,44,46] Allelic loss of chromosome 1p is another poor prognostic sign.[43,45]

Important histopathologic prognostic factors include the tumour stromal content, degree of mitosis[47–49] and the level of nerve growth factor TRKA expression.[50] A stroma-rich tumour matrix, low mitotic activity and a high level of expression of nerve growth factor TRKA correlate strongly with a favourable outcome.

Key point: prognosis

- Prognosis depends on multiple variables: clinical (patient age, tumour stage), biologic (lactate dehydrogenase, ferritin, neurone-specific enolase), genetic (tumour cell DNA, loss of chromosome 1p, N-myc oncogene amplification) and histopathologic (stromal content, degree of mitosis, level of nerve growth factor expression)

Imaging features of abdominal tumours

Imaging of neuroblastoma requires diagnosis of the primary tumour along with evaluation of the extent of disease. Because nearly two thirds of neuroblastomas occur in the abdomen, the imaging features of these tumours will be addressed initially, followed by a discussion of the imaging features of extra-abdominal tumours.

Plain radiographs

Plain films may be acquired for unrelated clinical indications and demonstrate an unsuspected primary tumour in the chest or abdomen or they may be obtained to further evaluate a suspected or known abdominal mass (most often diagnosed by sonography).

Plain radiographic findings of abdominal neuroblastoma include a paraspinal mass and enlargement of the intervertebral foramina or erosion of the pedicles due to intraspinal extension of tumour. The tumour may contain calcifications.

Ultrasonography

The evaluation of patients with palpable abdominal masses, including neuroblastoma, usually begins with sonography. Sonography is an excellent study to confirm the presence of an abdominal or pelvic mass and its site of origin. Neuroblastoma appears either as a suprarenal or paraspinal mass (Figs. 37.1 and 37.2). These tumours are usually heterogeneous and contain hyperechoic areas secondary to calcification, and hypoechoic areas, secondary to haemorrhage, necrosis, cystic change, or some combination thereof.[51,52] Doppler sonography may show increased peripheral or central tumour vascularity.

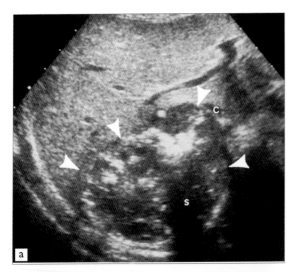

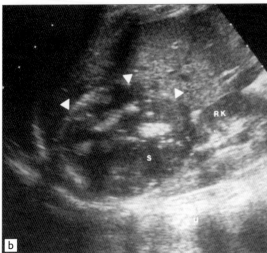

Figure 37.1. *Suprarenal neuroblastoma in a 15-month-old girl. Transverse (a) and longitudinal (b) sonograms show a hypoechoic right suprarenal mass (arrowheads) with scattered hyperechoic areas, representing calcification. Some of the calcified areas cast an acoustic shadow (S). Pathologically, most of the tumour was solid and contained clumps of calcification. C, inferior vena cava; RK, right kidney. (Reprinted with permisssion from reference 52.)*

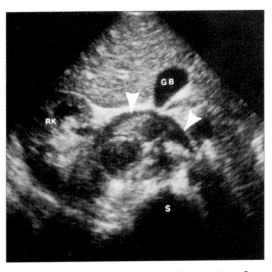

Figure 37.2. *Extra-adrenal neuroblastoma in a 3-year-old boy. Transverse sonogram shows a complex right paraspinal mass (arrowheads) medial to the right kidney (RK). S, spine; GB, gallbladder. (Reprinted with permission from reference 52.)*

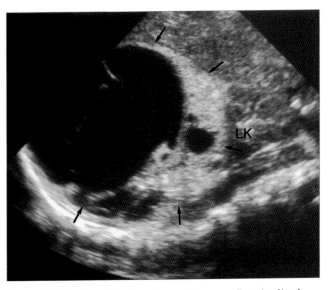

Figure 37.3. *Neonate adrenal neuroblastoma. Longitudinal views through the left upper quadrant of a 1-week-old boy show a complex suprarenal mass, containing a large cystic area. Histologic examination showed a necrotic neuroblastoma. LK, left kidney.*

In the newborn, neuroblastomas may be predominantly cystic or anechoic (Fig. 37.3).[53,54] On pathological sections, this appearance reflects either degenerative change in the tumour or, in some cases, clusters of microcysts in the tumour cells. Unfortunately, this appearance is non-specific and can mimic adrenal hematoma, another common lesion of the neonate. Differentiation requires demonstration of metastatic disease or positive laboratory studies, i.e. urinary catecholamine analysis, or serial sonographic examination. The generally excellent prognosis of neuroblastoma in this age group makes observation rather than surgery a reasonable alternative.

Computed tomography

After the presence of an abdominal mass has been confirmed by sonography, patients undergo further imaging with either computed tomography (CT) or magnetic resonance (MR) imaging to determine the extent of disease and guide staging. On CT, neuroblastoma appears as a homogeneous or heterogeneous soft tissue mass in a suprarenal or paraspinal location (Fig. 37.4).[55,56] The tumour enhances less than that of surrounding tissues after intravenous (IV) administration of contrast material.

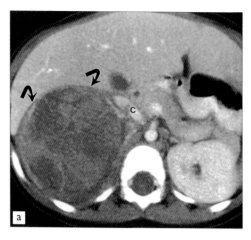
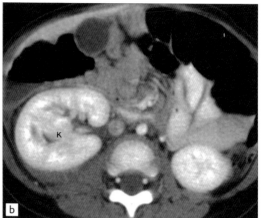

Figure 37.4. *Adrenal neuroblastoma. (a and b) CT scans in a 2-year-old girl show a large soft tissue mass (arrows) in the right suprarenal area. The tumour displaces the inferior vena cava (C) anteriorly and the right kidney (K) inferiorly. There is no midline extension. Pathologically proven Stage I tumour.*

Calcifications within the tumour, which may be coarse, mottled, solid or ring-shaped, are observed in approximately 85% of abdominal neuroblastomas (Figs. 37.4 and 37.5).

Magnetic resonance

On MR, neuroblastoma appears as an extrarenal or paraspinal mass which is predominantly iso- or hypointense to liver on T1-weighted spin-echo sequences and iso- or hyperintense to fat on T2-weighted sequences.[57–59] The margins may be smooth, irregular, or lobulated. Heterogeneity is common due to haemorrhage, necrosis, or calcification. Haemorrhage results in variable signal intensity, dependent on the age of the blood. Necrotic foci usually appear hypointense on T1-weighted sequences and hyperintense on T2-weighted sequences, while tumour calcification has low signal intensity on both pulse sequences.[57–59] Most enhance after administration of IV gadolinium chelate compounds (Fig. 37.6).

Additional findings of primary abdominal tumours

Adrenal masses commonly displace the kidney inferiorly and laterally. Occasionally, the kidney is displaced anteriorly and medially. Aggressive neuroblastoma may invade the kidney and simulate Wilms' tumour.[60,61] Renal atrophy also may be seen. Renal atrophy may be the result of infarction due to encasement or compression of the renal vessels (Fig. 37.7) by the primary tumour, surgical trauma, chemotherapy or radiation therapy.

Evaluation of local disease extent

Both local and distant extent of tumour need to be determined. With respect to local disease, the presence or absence of midline extension, vascular encasement, regional lymph node enlargement and intraspinal extension need to be determined as these factors can affect surgical planning, staging and prognosis.

Ultrasonography is seldom able to demonstrate the full extent of a very large tumour. It has limited value in demonstrating involvement of retroperitoneal and retrocrural

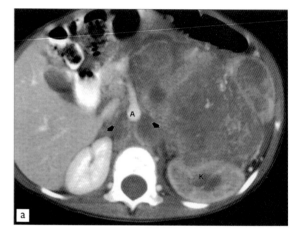

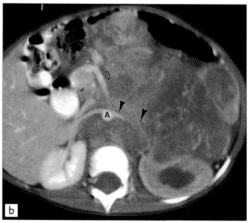

Figure 37.5. *Adrenal neuroblastoma. (a) CT scan in a 2-year-old girl shows a soft tissue mass with coarse calcifications in the left suprarenal area. The tumour displaces the left kidney (K) inferiorly, crosses the midline (arrows) anterior to the spine, and displaces and encases aorta (A). (b) At a lower level, the tumour encases the left renal artery (arrowheads), the aorta (A) and superior mesenteric artery (open arrow). Again noted is midline tumour extension and inferior displacement of the left kidney which is hydronephrotic.*

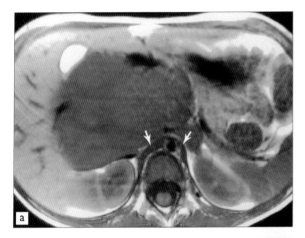

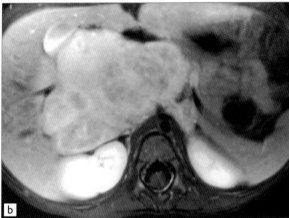

Figure 37.6. *Adrenal neuroblastoma in a 2-year-old girl. (a) Axial T1-weighted image demonstrates a large right suprarenal neuroblastoma that is hypointense to liver. The tumour crosses the midline anterior to the diaphragmatic crura (arrows). (b) On the T2-weighted image, the tumour is isodense to subcutaneous fat. Again note the midline extension.*

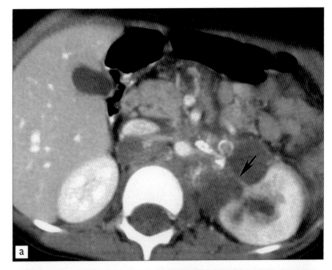

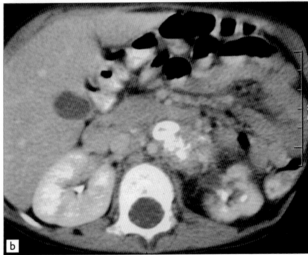

Figure 37.7. *Neuroblastoma with renal atrophy. (a) At the time of diagnosis, the left kidney is displaced laterally and the renal artery (arrow) is encased by calcified tumour. The tumour extends across the midline anterior to the spine. (b) Six-month follow-up after chemotherapy. The left kidney is small and irregular. This was thought to represent infarction from long-standing compression of the renal vessels. Also note that the primary tumour has decreased in size and is heavily calcified.*

nodes and is unable to detect extension into the spinal canal.

The choice of CT versus MR has been the subject of continuing debate. Unfortunately, there are no large prospective series that compare MR and CT in neuroblastoma for staging accuracy. Computed tomography with contrast enhancement can reliably demonstrate the primary tumour and it is superior to MR in demonstrating calcification. A multicentre study of children with newly diagnosed neuroblastoma found that, overall, CT and MR had statistically similar, but relatively poor, performance for assessing features of local disease.[62] Computed tomography was slightly more accurate than MR for determining the presence or absence of vessel encasement.

Midline extension or vascular encasement occurs in approximately 50% of cases. Midline extension is defined as tumour extending to or beyond the pedicle contralateral to the primary tumour. Vascular encasement is defined as tumour surrounding at least three fourths of the circumfer-

ence of one or more major abdominal arteries or veins, including the aorta, superior mesenteric artery and vein, IVC, or right or left renal artery and vein (Fig. 37.4). Detection of midline extension is important because it alters staging and up-grades the disease to Stage III. Vascular encasement affects management not staging. It usually is a contraindication to primary surgical resection. Vascular invasion is a rare feature of neuroblastoma.[63]

Adenopathy occurs in about 30% of patients with neuroblastoma. Lymph node involvement is defined as discrete masses separate from the main tumour mass. Detection of nodal disease is important because it alters stage. Ipsilateral nodes correspond to a Stage II disease (Fig. 37.8).

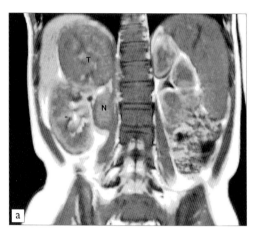
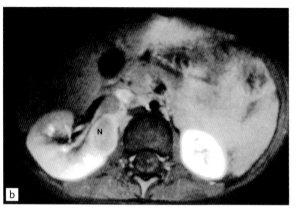

Figure 37.8. *Ipsilateral adenopathy. (a) Coronal T1-weighted MR in 3-year-old boy shows a right adrenal tumour (T) and ipsilateral lymph node (N) enlargement. (b) Fat-suppressed axial T1-weighted image after gadolinium administration also shows the enlarged ipsilateral lymph node (N). Stage II disease proven at pathological examination.*

Contralateral nodal disease indicates Stage III disease (Fig. 37.9).

Intraspinal extension of neuroblastoma occurs in about 15% of patients and is defined as a mass within the spinal canal (with or without cord displacement) that is contiguous with the main tumour mass (Fig. 37.10).[64] Intraspinal extension is important because it can cause cord compression, which requires either urgent treatment with chemotherapy and steroids to shrink the tumour or a laminectomy with tumour removal. Intraspinal extension is

particularly well-documented on MR. The presence of tumour extension into the intervertebral foramina and spinal canal and also the degree of spinal cord displacement and compression may be shown in coronal, sagittal, or axial planes.[64] The cranio-caudal extent of intraspinal tumour is best seen on sagittal images (Fig. 37.11).

Distant disease: imaging characteristics

The second part of the staging procedure is determination of the distant extent of disease. Detection of distant metas-

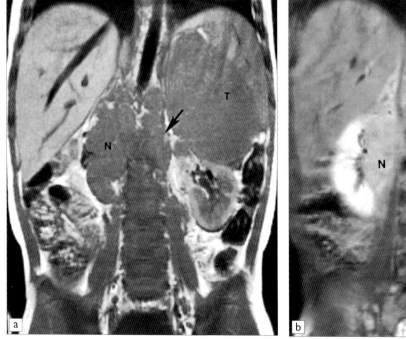
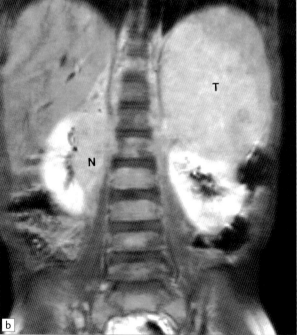

Figure 37.9. *Contralateral adenopathy. (a) Coronal T1-weighted MR in 3-year-old boy shows a left adrenal tumour (T) and both ipsilateral (arrow) and contralateral lymph node (N) enlargement. (b) Fat-suppressed coronal T1-weighted image after gadolinium administration also shows the enlarged contralateral lymph node (N). Stage III disease proven at pathological examination.*

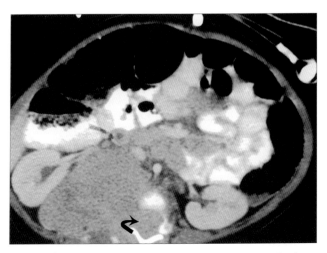

Figure 37.10. *Intraspinal extension. A large paravertebral neuroblastoma displaces the right kidney laterally and extends through the neural foramen into the spinal canal (arrow).*

tases up-stages the tumour to a Stage IV or IVS. Neuroblastoma metastasizes to liver, distant nodes, cortical bone and bone marrow.

Hepatic metastases

Hepatic metastases occur in 5–10% of children with neuroblastoma. Two common patterns of hepatic metastases have been described: focal masses, usually affecting older children, and diffuse infiltration, usually occurring in infants with stage 4S disease. Focal mass lesions tend to be well-defined and they may be single or multiple (Fig. 37.12). These lesions are equally well-recognized on CT and MR. Diffuse liver infiltration can be difficult to detect on CT unless the parenchyma is heterogeneous with a low attenuation (Fig. 37.13). The diagnosis is difficult when the parenchymal attenuation is uniformly altered. Diffuse infiltration is easier to recognize on MR, especially on T2-

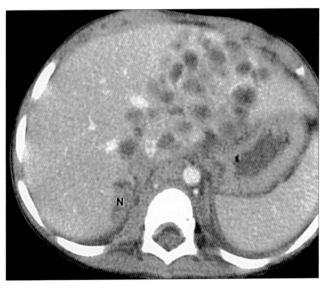

Figure 37.12. *Focal hepatic metastases. Contrast-enhanced CT shows multiple hypoattenuating hepatic metastases in the left hepatic lobe. There is a small right neuroblastoma (N).*

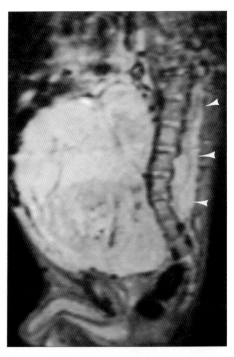

Figure 37.11. *Intraspinal invasion. Sagittal STIR image shows a large retroperitoneal neuroblastoma that arose in the pelvis and extended superiorly into the abdomen and posteriorly into the spinal canal (arrowheads).*

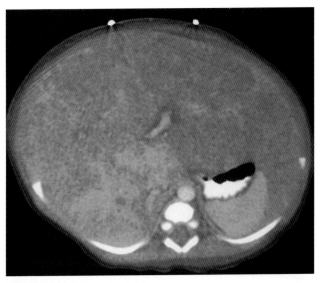

Figure 37.13. *Diffuse hepatic infiltration. Neonate with stage IVS neuroblastoma who presented with an enlarged abdomen and subcutaneous nodules. Contrast-enhanced CT shows an enlarged liver, which displaces the stomach posteriorly. The hepatic parenchyma shows heterogeneous enhancement.*

weighted sequences where hyperintense masses may be seen diffusely throughout the liver.

Distant nodal metastases

Distant nodes are those that are outside the cavity of origin of the tumour. Evaluation of the chest, abdomen and pelvis, regardless of the site of primary disease, is performed in all patients with neuroblastomas to enhance demonstration of distant nodal involvement. A common site of distant nodal spread is the supraclavicular region.[65]

Skeletal and bone marrow metastases

Skeletal metastases occur in 50–60% of patients at diagnosis, mostly in patients over 1-year-old. These can involve cortical bone or bone marrow.

Plain radiographs

While plain radiographs are not routinely used in the detection of bony metastases, the initial presentation in some patients may be with bone pain, prompting skeletal radiographs. Thus, recognition of the conventional radiographic features is important. Skull radiographs may demonstrate sutural diastasis and irregularity of the sutures secondary to infiltration of the meninges. Plain radiographs of the long bones in patients with bone metastases may show irregular submetaphyseal lucencies, focal periosteal reaction and sclerotic foci (Fig. 37.14), representing areas of tumour infarction. In other cases, a generalized reduction in bone density and a mottled trabecular pattern due to diffuse marrow infiltration can be seen.

Computed tomography

Computed tomography can be useful for confirming cortical metastases that are suspected on MR or scintigraphic studies but not confirmed by radiography. In some instances, metastases may be an unsuspected finding on CT scans obtained for evaluation of other clinical problems. Metastases are recognized because they produce destructive and less commonly sclerotic lesions, periosteal new bone, or a soft tissue mass (Fig. 37.15). In rare cases, metastatic lesions are identified only because they replace the marrow with higher attenuation tumour cells.

Skeletal scintigraphy

Until recently, skeletal scintigraphy with Tc-99m-labelled dimercaptophosphonate (MDP) had been the method of choice in the detection of bone metastases. The sensitivity of radionuclide imaging in detecting occult metastases is reported to be about 90% compared with a sensitivity of between 35 and 70% for radiographic skeletal survey.[66,67] Metastases will appear either as focal areas of increased radiopharmaceutical accumulation (Fig. 37.16) or, rarely, as photopenic or cold lesions. Asymmetrical metaphyseal uptake is typical. Common sites of metastases are the skull, facial bones, orbits, ribs and vertebral bodies. Increased tracer activity can be seen in the primary tumour and in bone, bone marrow and soft tissue metastases.

MIBG scintigraphy

More recently, MIBG has become the study of choice to image skeletal metastases.[68–72] MIBG, an analogue of catecholamine precursors, is taken up by catecholamine-producing tumours. Although other tumours, including phaechromocytoma, carcinoid tumours and medullary thyroid carcinomas, can show MIBG uptake, these lesions are extremely uncommon in the paediatric population and therefore, uptake of MIBG in a child is virtually specific for neuroblastoma. In patients with neuroblastoma, abnormal activity can be seen in the primary tumour and in bone, bone marrow and soft tissue metastases (Fig. 37.17).

MIBG is available in two forms: [131]I MIBG and ^{123}I MIBG. [123]I MIBG is preferable to ^{131}I MIBG because of lower radiation dose to the patient, better image resolution and superior sensitivity. [131]I MIBG has a sensitivity of

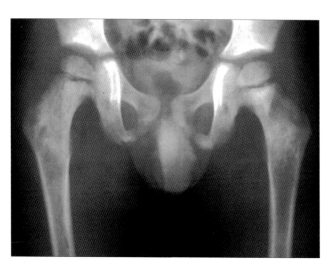

Figure 37.14. *Osseous metastases. Plain radiograph of the hips. Diffuse osteopenia and patchy sclerotic foci, representing blastic metastases, are seen in the proximal femurs.*

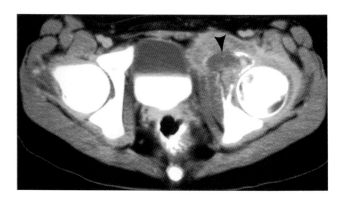

Figure 37.15. *Osseous metastasis. Computed tomography shows a destructive lesion in the left anterior acetabulum (arrowhead). There is associated soft tissue swelling anteriorly and medially.*

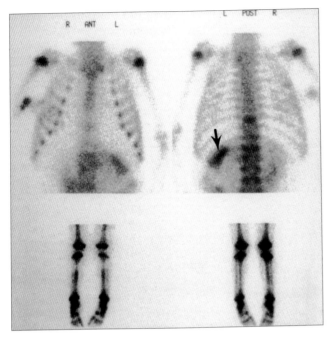

Figure 37.16. *Bone scintigraphy. Bone scintigram in a 3-year-old boy shows abnormal areas of increased osseous uptake throughout the skeleton, including the spine, flat bones, and metadiaphyseal parts of long bones, resulting from metastases from neuroblastoma. Also note tracer uptake in left adrenal gland (arrow) with displacement of left kidney inferiorly.*

approximately 70% for detection of skeletal metastases, versus an 80–95% sensitivity for ^{123}I MIBG.[70,71] The disadvantage of ^{123}I MIBG compared with ^{131}I MIBG is a shorter half-life and, therefore, it must be used on the same day it is produced, making it unavailable in many institutions and also more costly.

Occasionally, primary neuroblastomas will not take up MIBG. This can occur in more mature tumours and also in some very undifferentiated tumours. In a small number of other patients, the primary tumour and metastases may initially show MIBG uptake and then subsequently fail to take up the agent in the presence of demonstrable disease.[73] In these cases, MIBG cannot be used to document tumour response to treatment. Nevertheless, MIBG scanning remains important in diagnosis and follow-up of neuroblastoma because new areas of uptake generally indicate new active disease.

Magnetic resonance

The use of rapid MR sequence permits imaging of areas of the medullary cavity that contain large amounts of red marrow (the thoracolumbar spine, pelvis and proximal ends of the long bones) in less than 1 hour.[62,74–78] Typically, metastatic disease produces a low signal intensity on T1-weighted sequences and a high signal intensity on T2-weighted and fat-suppressed images (Fig. 37.18). The sensitivity of MR for detecting marrow involvement is between 80 and 90%.[62,78,79]

Magnetic resonance can show abnormalities not detected by bone marrow biopsy.[62]

Two morphologic patterns of bone marrow involvement have been described: focal and diffuse.[79] On MR, the diffuse form of marrow infiltration is invariably associated with cortical destruction (84% of cases) and commonly (>75% of cases) leaves residual signal abnormalities after chemotherapy. In contrast, the focal form of disease rarely has associated cortical involvement (16% of cases) and virtually always disappears after chemotherapy.

Pentetreotide scanning

Indium-111 pentetreotide (octreotide), a somatostatin receptor, also has been used to image neuroblastoma (Fig. 37.19).[80,81] These scans are more frequently positive in undifferentiated tumours and in tumours associated with elevated urinary catecholamines. Pentetreotide may be picked up in MIBG-negative tumours[82,83] and vice versa. The sensitivity of pentetreotide for detection of the primary tumour is 80–100%.[84,85] In addition to being useful for diagnosis, octreotide has the potential to provide information about prognosis. In small series, patients with receptor-positive tumours had 100% 1-year survival, while those with receptor-negative tumours had less than 60% 1-year survival.[84,85] The usefulness of octreotide for staging distant disease is still to be determined.

Positron emission tomography

In contrast to the dependence primarily on anatomic imaging features, positron emission tomography (PET) depends on the metabolic characteristics of a tissue for the detection of disease. The metabolic activity of neuroblastoma may be evaluated by utilizing 2-[fluorine-2418]-fluoro-2-deoxy-D-glucose ([18]FDG) or 11Chydioxyephedrine (HED).[86,87] Most neuroblastomas and their metastases avidly concentrate [18]FDG prior to chemotherapy or radiation therapy. The uptake after therapy is variable. These agents also may be useful in imaging tumours that do not concentrate MIBG.[86,87]

Key points: imaging of abdominal tumours

- Ultrasonography is used predominantly to confirm the presence of a mass lesion; CT and MR are used to stage the disease

- In the newborn, neuroblastomas are often cystic

- The essential staging features that need to be assessed on CT/MR for local staging are the presence of midline extension, vascular encasement, regional lymph node enlargement and intraspinal extension

- There are no large series that compare CT with MR for staging accuracy in neuroblastomas

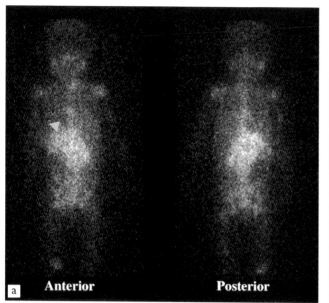

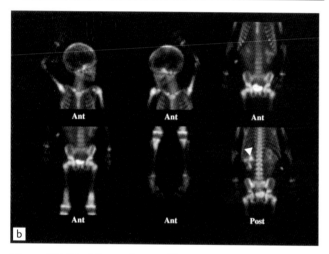

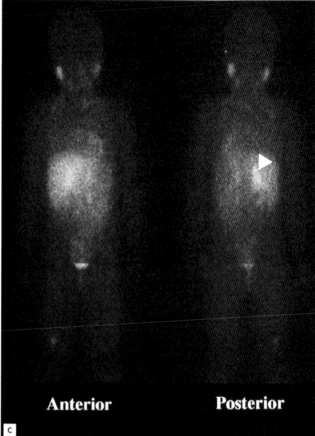

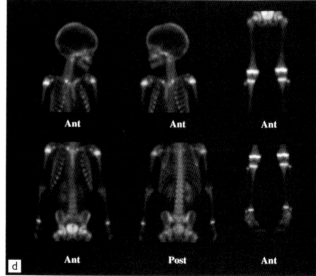

Figure 37.17. *Metastatic neuroblastoma. (a) MIBG scan – anterior and posterior scintigrams obtained 48 hours after injection of ^{131}I MIBG demonstrate large primary right adrenal neuroblastoma (arrowhead) extending into the mid abdomen and across the midline as well as heterogeneous diffuse increased activity in the skeleton consistent with bone and bone marrow metastases. (b) Bone scintigraphy at same time as MIBG scan demonstrates widespread osseous metastases most prominent in the ends of long bones and calvarium. Increased tracer uptake also noted in the right adrenal mass (arrowhead). (c) Follow-up MIBG scan 11 months later. Anterior and posterior scintigrams obtained 24 hours after injection of ^{123}I MIBG demonstrate increased activity in the right adrenal mass which is substantially smaller than on the pretreatment scan as well as a few subtle foci consistent with bone metastases in the right first rib, left medial clavicle and right distal femur. Normal tracer uptake noted in the salivary glands, myocardium and liver. Note substantially better quality with ^{123}I MIBG than with ^{131}I MIBG. (d) Follow-up bone scintigraphy demonstrates marked improvement with only subtle increased activity in the ends of the long bones.*

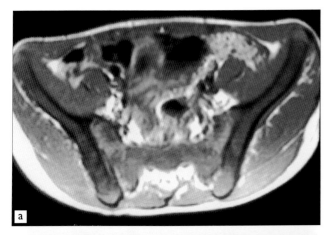

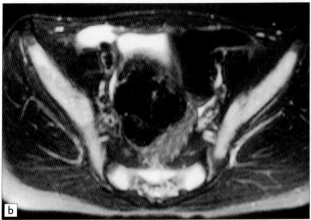

Figure 37.18. *Metastatic neuroblastoma. (a) Axial T1-weighted MR of the pelvis of a 6-year-old boy shows diffusely low signal intensity marrow. (b) Fat-suppressed T2-weighted MR abnormally bright signal shows diffuse marrow infiltration. By comparison, normal red marrow would have a signal intensity similar to that of muscle on fat-suppressed images.*

■ Midline extension occurs in 50% of cases and is defined on CT/MR as tumour extending to or across to the contralateral pedicle. This feature up stages the tumour

■ Lymphadenopathy up stages neuroblastoma and is defined as a tumour mass separate from the primary mass

■ Vascular encasement and intraspinal extension affect surgical management but do not affect stage

■ MIBG and Tc-99m-labelled MDP are the methods of choice for detecting skeletal metastases

■ Several other imaging techniques play an adjunctive role in assessing distant metastases, including MR, Indium-III pentetreotide (octreotide) and ¹⁸FDG PET imaging

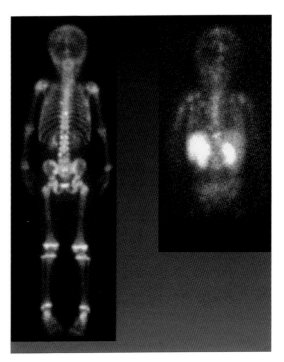

Figure 37.19. *Metastatic neuroblastoma, octreotide scan. Posterior bone scintigram (left panel) and Indium-111 pentetreotide scintigram (right panel) demonstrate multifocal osseous metastases from neuroblastoma. Normal activity seen in the spleen, kidneys and liver on the octreotide study.*

Extra-abdominal tumours

Pelvic neuroblastoma

Pelvic tumours are frequently presacral in location and are usually situated above or behind the bladder. Erosion of the sacrum and bony pelvis and extension into the lateral pelvic side walls, sacral foramina and sciatic notches is not uncommon (Fig. 37.20). The differential diagnosis includes pelvic rhabdomyosarcoma.

Thoracic neuroblastoma

A thoracic neuroblastoma is almost always paravertebral and may be associated with rib and vertebral body erosion and scoliosis. Chest radiography will demonstrate the tumour but CT or MR are required to show the extent of tumour and any extension into the spinal canal (Fig. 37.21). The tumours may be small and encapsulated, or large and demonstrate vascular encasement and neural foraminal extension. Approximately 50% of thoracic neuroblastomas demonstrate calcification on CT scans. The differential diagnosis includes other causes of posterior mediastinal masses such as neurenteric and enteric duplication cysts and thoracic meningoceles.

Pulmonary and pleural involvement are rare initial complications of neuroblastoma, occurring in fewer than 3% of children.[60] Pulmonary involvement can result from haematogenous or lymphatic spread or from direct exten-

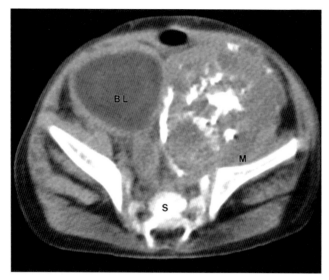

Figure 37.20. *Pelvic neuroblastoma. CT scan shows a soft tissue mass with amorphous calcifications anterior to the sacrum (S) and lateral to the bladder (BL). The tumour has invaded the left iliacus muscle (M).*

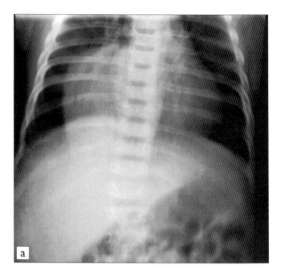

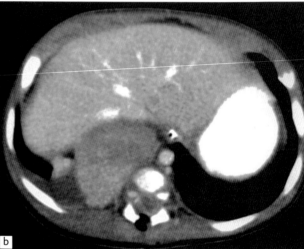

Figure 37.21. *Thoracic neuroblastoma with intraspinal extension. (a) Plain chest radiograph in a 6-month-old girl shows a right paravertebral mass. (b) CT demonstrates an elliptical, paraspinal soft tissue attenuation mass and a small pleural effusion.*

sion. On CT, parenchymal metastases appear as either focal nodules or large intraparenchymal masses. Pleural disease may manifest as either an effusion or as pleural masses.

Cervical and apical neuroblastoma

The mass seen in cervical neuroblastoma is usually well demarcated in the parapharyngeal space, displacing the carotid and jugular anteriorly (Fig. 37.22).[87–89] On ultrasonography, cervical tumour appears as an irregular solid echogenic mass. Calcification is common. Extension through the skull base into the infratemporal fossa may be seen on CT and MR.[90] The differential diagnosis of masses in the posterior parapharyngeal space includes metastases, rhabdomyosarcoma, lymphoma and other neurogenic tumours, especially neurofibromas.

Cerebral neuroblastoma

Intracranial involvement is generally confined to the dura and leptomeninges, with parenchymal disease usually attributed to direct extension from adjacent skull or dura.[91,92] Isolated parenchymal brain metastases from extracranial primary neuroblastoma without associated calvarial or dural involvement are rare, but can occur. Parenchymal brain metastases are usually solid and show heterogeneous contrast enhancement on CT and MR. Haemorrhagic and cystic metastases occur but are less common.[93] Cerebral metastatic disease is usually seen at the time of relapse, rather than at the time of diagnosis.

Metastases to the skull and orbit have been reported in up to 25% of cases of neuroblastoma, often being the first evidence of the primary tumour.[94] Four patterns of calvarial involvement have been described: sutural diastasis secondary to dural involvement, periosteal reaction ('sunburst'

appearance) (Fig. 37.23), lytic defects and thickened bone. CT or MR can show extension into the soft tissues of the scalp or through the inner table of the skull. When there is sphenoid bone involvement, the tumour can extend into the orbits and cause proptosis.

Key points: extra-abdominal tumours

- Pelvic tumours are frequently presacral

- Thoracic neuroblastomas are almost always paravertebral

- Cervical tumours usually arise in the parapharyngeal space

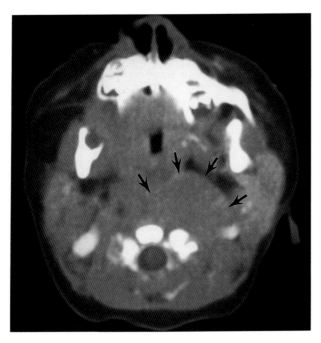

Figure 37.22. *Cervical neuroblastoma in a 7-month-old with left neck mass. Contrast-enhanced CT scan reveals a left-sided prevertebral soft tissue mass (arrows), extending just beyond the midline. The tumour was completely excised.*

- MR is advisable to show extension of tumour into the spinal canal

- Cerebral neuroblastomas rarely extend outside the cranial vault

Response to treatment

The International Neuroblastoma Response Criteria (INRC) were established in 1988 and subsequently modified in 1993.[28,29] Response to treatment consists of response of the primary tumour and also the metastatic sites. The INRC requires that the primary tumour lymph nodes and liver metastases be evaluated by CT and/or MR and that distant metastases be evaluated using MIBG scans, Tc-99m bone scans and bilateral iliac crest marrow aspirates and trephine biopsies. Because of the difficulties in making accurate measurements of a tumour with an irregular shape, the volume (three dimensions rather than the product of the two largest diameters) is used to assess response.

A complete response (CR) indicates complete disappearance of all primary and metastatic disease. A very good partial response (VGPR) indicates a 90–99% volume reduction in the primary tumour with resolution of pre-existing metastatic disease and no new bone lesions. The only exception to this is that there can be residual abnormality on technetium bone scintigraphy attributable to incomplete healing of the bone at sites of previous metastases.

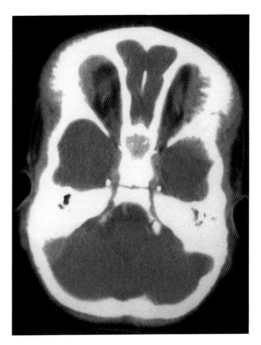

Figure 37.23. *Calvarial metastases. CT scan shows spiculated periosteal new bone formation along the orbits bilaterally ('sunburst' appearance).*

The MIBG scan should be negative at all metastatic sites. A partial response (PR) indicates a 50–90% reduction in both the primary tumour and all measurable metastatic sites. No response (NR) indicates a less than 50% reduction of some or all measurable lesions, but no increase of greater than 25% in any existing lesion and no new lesions. Progressive disease (PD) indicates the presence of any new lesion, increase of any measurable lesion by greater than 25%, or conversion of marrow from negative to positive.[28,29]

Most tumours that are going to respond to treatment do so by 3–4 months and, therefore, it is recommended that evaluations for response be performed at approximately 4 months from the initiation of chemotherapy. Further evaluation is recommended at the end of treatment, before and after surgical procedures, before stem cell transplantation and as clinically indicated.[1]

Key points: follow-up

- Measurement of response requires monitoring change in the primary tumour and in the metastases

- The primary tumour, lymph nodes and liver metastases are monitored using CT and metastases using MIBG, Tc-99m bone scans and bone marrow biopsies

- Response is assessed at approximately 4 months after initiation of chemotherapy. Further evaluation is recommended at the end of treatment, before and after surgical procedures, before stem cell transplantation and as clinically indicated

Summary

- Neuroblastoma is the most frequent extracranial malignancy of childhood; median age of diagnosis is approximately 17 months

- Although in most cases the diagnosis is based on conventional staging with haematoxylin and eosin using light microscopy, it can be made on the demonstration of bone marrow involvement combined with significantly raised urinary catecholamines or metabolites (VMA and HVA)

- Neuroblastomas can arise anywhere in the sympathetic chain; approximately two thirds arise in the abdomen. Most of these originate in the adrenal medulla

- Three major staging systems have been in use, but the recently promulgated International Neuroblastoma Staging System is now the most widely used

- Ultrasonography is an excellent screening tool for detection of abdominal tumour

- The presence of midline extension, vascular encasement, regional lymph node enlargement and intraspinal extension are important imaging features for local staging

- There are no large prospective series comparing CT with MR for local staging accuracy. However, MR is the preferred technique for showing intraspinal extension

- Most common sites of metastases are the liver, lymph nodes, cortical bone and bone marrow

- Imaging is vital in the detection of distant metastases. These are chiefly to bone and/or bone marrow, occurring in over half the children with neuroblastoma. Tc99m-laballed MDP and MIBG remain the techniques of choice in their detection. Magnetic resonance also plays a complementary role in the detection of bone lesions. Magnetic resonance, Indium-III pentetreotide (octreotide) and ^{18}FDG PET can play a role in detection of distant metastases

- The INRC (1993) require that the volume of the primary tumour, the liver and lymph nodes be evaluated by CT and/or MR and that metastases be evaluated with MIBG scans and Tc99m MDP bone scans and in bone marrow by bilateral iliac crest marrow aspirates and trephine biopsies

- Primary surgical resection is the treatment of choice for Stage I and II tumours; advanced tumours are treated with a combination of chemotherapy and surgery and radiotherapy

References

1. Brodeur G M, Maris J M. Neuroblastoma. In: Devita V T, Hellman S, Rosenberg S A (eds). Cancer Principles and Practice of Oncology. Lippincott Williams & Wilkins: Philadelphia, 2001; 895–933

2. Brodeur G M, Castleberry R P. Neuroblastoma. In: Pizzo P A, Poplack D G (eds). Principles and Practice of Pediatric Oncology. JB Lippincott Co: Philadelphia, 1997; 761–797

3. Gurney J G, Davis S, Severson R K et al. Trends in cancer incidence among children in the US. Cancer 1996; 78: 532–541

4. Stiller C A. Aetiology and epidemiology. In: Pinkerton C R, Plowman N (eds). Paediatric Oncology, 3rd edn. Hodder Arnold Health Sciences: London, 2004 (in press)

5. Lonnergan G J, Schwab C M, Suarez E S, Carlson C L. Neuroblastoma, ganglioneuroblastoma and ganglioneuroma: radiologic–pathologic correlation. Radiographic 2002; 22: 911–934

6. Lukens J N. Neuroblastoma in the neonate. Semin Perinatol 1999; 23: 263–273

7. Granata C, Fagnani A M, Gambini C et al. Features and outcome of neuroblastoma detected before birth. J Pediatr Surg 2000; 35: 88–91

8. Ho P T C, Estroff J A, Kozakewich H et al. Prenatal detection of neuroblastoma: a 10-year experience from the Dana–Farber Cancer Institute and Children's Hospital. Pediatrics 1993; 92: 358–364

9. Erttmann R, Tafese T, Berthold F et al. Ten years' neuroblastoma screening in Europe: preliminary results of a clinical and biological review from the study group for evaluation of neuroblastoma screening in Europe (SENSE). Eur J Cancer 1998; 34: 1391–1397

10. Nishi M, Miyake H, Takeda T et al. Mass screening of neuroblastoma in Sapporo City, Japan. Am J Pediatr Hematol Oncol 1992; 14: 327–331

11. Nishihira H, Toyoda Y, Tanaka Y et al. Natural course of neuroblastoma detected by mass screening: a 5-year prospective study at a single institution. J Clin Oncol 2000; 18: 3012–3017

12. Toma P, Lucigrai G, Marzoli A et al. Prenatal diagnosis of metastatic adrenal neuroblastoma with sonography and MR imaging. Am J Roentgenol 1994; 162: 1183–1184

13. Woods W G, Tuchman M, Robison L L et al. Screening for neuroblastoma is ineffective in reducing the incidence of unfavourable advanced stage disease in older children. Eur J Cancer 1997; 33: 2106–2112

14. Woods S G, Tuchman M, Robson L L et al. A population-based study of the usefulness of screening for neuroblastoma. Lancet 1996; 348: 1682–1687

15. Yamatoo K, Hayashi Y, Hanada R et al. Mass screening and age-specific incidence of neuroblastoma in Saitame Prefecture, Japan. J Clin Oncol 1995; 13: 2033–2038

16. Abramson S J. Adrenal neoplasms in children. Radiol Clin North Am 1997; 35: 1415–1453

17. Cruccetti A, Kiely E M, Spitz L et al. Pelvic neuroblastoma: low mortality and high morbidity. J Ped Surg 2000; 35: 724–728

18. Abramson S J, Berdon W E, Ruzal-Shapiro C et al. Cervical neuroblastoma in eleven infants–tumor with favorable prognosis. Clinical and radiologic (US, CT, MRI) findings. Pediatr Radiol 1993; 23: 253–257

19. Applegate K, Connolly L, Treves S. Neuroblastoma presenting clinically as hip osteomyelitis: a 'signature' diagnosis on skeletal scintigraphy. Pediatr Radiol 1995; 25: 93–96

20. Koh P S, Raffensperger J G, Berry S et al. Long-term outcome in children with opsoclonus–myoclonus and ataxia and coincident neuroblastoma. J Pediatr 1994; 125: 712–716

21. Mitchell W G, Snodgrass S R. Opsoclonus–ataxia due to childhood neural crest tumors: a chronic neurologic syndrome. J Child Neurol 1990; 5: 153

22. Tiedeman K, Pritchard J, Long R et al. Intractable diarrhoea in a patient with vasoactive intestinal peptide-secreting neuroblastoma. Eur J Pediatr 1981; 137: 217–219

23. Mendelsohn G, Eggleston J C, Olson J L et al. Vasoactive intestinal peptide and its relationship to ganglion cell differentiation in neuroblastoma. Cancer 1976; 37: 846

24. Hoffer F A, Chung T, Diller L et al. Percutaneous biopsy for prognostic testing of neuroblastoma. Radiology 1996; 200: 213–216

25. Evans A E, D'Angio G J, Randolph J. A proposed staging for children with neuroblastoma. Cancer 1971; 27: 374–378

26. Hayes F A, Green A, Husto H O et al. Surgicopathologic staging of neuroblastoma: Prognostic significance of regional lymph node metastases. J Pediatr 1983; 102: 59–62

27. Nitschke R, Smith E I, Shochat S et al. Localized neuroblastoma treated by surgery: a Pediatric Oncology Group Study. J Clin Oncol 1988; 6: 1271–1279

28. Brodeur G M, Seeger R C, Barrett A et al. International criteria for diagnosis, staging and response to treatment in patients with neuroblastoma. J Clin Oncol 1988; 6: 1874–1881

29. Brodeur G M, Pritchard J, Berthold F et al. Revision of the international criteria for neuroblastoma diagnosis, staging and response to treatment. J Clin Oncol 1993; 11: 1466–1477

30. Kiely E M. The surgical challenge of neuroblastoma. J Pediatr Surg 1994; 29: 128–133

31. Nitschke R, Smith E I, Shochat S et al. Localized neuroblastoma treated by surgery: a Pediatric Oncology Group study. J Clin Oncol 1988; 6: 1271

32. Mastrangelo R, Lasorella A, Iavarone A et al. Critical observations on neuroblastoma treatment with 131-I-metaiodobenzylguanidine at diagnosis. Med Pediatr Oncol 1993; 21: 411–415

33. Gaze M N, Wheldon T E. Radiolabeled MIBG in the treatment of neuroblastoma. Eur J Cancer 1996; 32A: 93–96

34. Cheung N K, Yeh S D J, Gulati S et al. 131 I-3F8 targeted radiotherapy of neuroblastoma (NB): a phase I clinical trial [abstract]. Proceedings of the American Association for Cancer Research 1990; 31: 284

35. Villablanca J G, Avramims V I, Khan A A et al. Phase I trial of 13-cis-retinoic acid (cis-RA) in neuroblastoma patients following bone marrow transplantation (BMT). Proceedings of the American Society of Clinical Oncology Annual Meeting 1992; 11: 366

36. Evans A E, D'Angio G J, Propert K et al. Prognostic factors in neuroblastoma. Cancer 1987; 59: 1853–1859

37. Grosfeld J L, Rescorla F J, West K W et al. Neuroblastoma in the first year of life: clinical and biologic factors influencing outcome. Semin Pediatr Surg 1993; 2: 37–46

38. Morris J A, Shochat S J, Smith E I et al. Biological variables in thoracic neuroblastoma: a Pediatric Oncology Group study. J Pediatr Surg 1995; 30: 296–302

39. Berthold F, Trechow R, Utsch S, Zieschang J. Prognostic factors in metastatic neuroblastoma. A multivariate analysis of 182 cases. Am J Pediatr Hematol Oncol 1992; 4: 207–215

40. Zeltzer P M, Marangos P J, Evans A E, Schneider S L. Serum neuron-specific enolase in children with neuroblastoma: relationship to stage and disease course. Cancer 1986; 57: 1230–1234

41. Brodeur G M, Seeger R C, Schwab M et al. Amplification of N-myc in untreated human neuroblastomas correlates with advanced disease stage. Science 1984; 224: 1121–1124

42. Brodeur G M. Molecular basics for heterogeneity in human neuroblastomas. Euro J Cancer 1995; 31A: 505–51

43. Caron H, van Sluis P, de Kraker J et al. Allelic loss of chromosome 1p as a predictor of unfavourable outcome in patients with neuroblastoma. N Engl J Med 1996; 334: 225–230

44. Look A T, Hayes A, Shuster J J et al. Clinical relevance of tumour cell ploidy and N-myc gene amplification in childhood neuroblastoma: a Pediatric Oncology Group study. J Clin Oncol 1991; 9: 581–591

45. Maris J M, White P S, Beltinger C P et al. Significance of chromosome 1p loss of heterozygosity in neuroblastoma. Cancer Res 1995; 55: 4664–4669

46. Kaneko Y, Kanda N, Maseki N et al. Different karyotypic patterns in early and advanced stage neuroblastomas. Cancer Res 1987; 47: 311

47. Joshi V, Cantor A B, Altshuler G et al. Recommendations for modification of terminology of

neuroblastic tumors and prognostic significance of Shimada classification. Cancer 1992; 69: 2183–2196

48. Shimada H, Chatten J, Newton W A et al. Histopathologic prognostic factors in neuroblastic tumours: Definition of subtypes of ganglioneuroblastoma and age-linked classification of neuroblastomas. J Natl Cancer Inst 1984; 73: 405–416

49. Shimada H, Stram D O, Chatten J et al. Identification of subsets of neuroblastomas by combined histopathologic and N-*myc* analysis. J Natl Cancer Inst 1995; 87: 1470–1476

50. Nakagawara A, Arima-Nakagawara M, Scavarda N J et al. Association between high levels of expression of the TRK gene and favorable outcome in human neuroblastoma. New Engl J Med 1993; 328: 847–854

51. Berdon W, Ruzal-Shapiro C, Abramson S. The diagnosis of abdominal neuroblastoma: Relative roles of ultrasonography, CT and MR. Urol Radiol 1992; 14: 252–262

52. Siegel M J. Adrenal glands, pancreas and retroperitoneum. In: Siegel M J (ed) Pediatric Sonography. Lippincott Williams & Wilkins: Philadelphia, 2002

53. Cassady C, Winters W D. Bilateral cystic neuroblastoma: imaging features and differential diagnosis. Pediatr Radiol 1997; 27: 758–759

54. Teoh S K, Whitman G J, Chew F S. Neonatal neuroblastoma. Am J Roentgenol 1997; 168: 54

55. Merten D F, Gold S H. Radiologic staging of thoracoabdominal tumors in childhood. Radiol Clin N Am 1994; 32: 133–149

56. Siegel M J. Retroperitoneum. In: Siegel M J (ed) Pediatric Body CT. Lippincott-Raven: Philadelphia, 1999

57. Borrello J A, Mirowitz S A, Siegel M J. Neuroblastoma. In: Siegel B A, Proto A V (eds) Pediatric Disease (fourth series): Test and Syllabus. American College of Radiology: Reston, VA, 1993; 640–665

58. Meyer J. Retroperitoneal MR imaging in children. Pediatr MRI Clin N Am 1996; 4: 657–677

59. Siegel M J. MR imaging of pediatric abdominal neoplasms. MRI Clin N Am 2000; 8: 837–851

60. Panuel M, Bourliere-Najean B, Gentet J C et al. Aggressive neuroblastoma with initial pulmonary metastases and kidney involvement simulating Wilms' tumor. Eur J Radiol 1992; 14: 201–203

61. Rosenfield N S, Leonidas J C, Barwick K W. Aggressive neuroblastoma simulating Wilms' tumor. Radiology 1988; 166: 165–167

62. Siegel M J, Ishwaran H, Fletcher B et al. Staging of neuroblastoma by imaging: Report of the Radiology Diagnostic Oncology Group. Radiology 2002; 223: 168–175

63. Day D L, Johnson R, Cohen M D. Abdominal neuroblastoma with inferior vena caval thrombosis: report of three cases (one with right atrial extension). Pediatr Radiol 1991; 21: 205–207

64. Siegel M J, Jamroz G A, Glazer H S, Abramson C L. MR imaging of intraspinal extension of neuroblastoma. J Comput Assist Tomogr 1986; 10: 593–595

65. Abramson S J, Berdon W, Stolar C et al. Stage IV N neuroblastoma: MRI diagnosis of left supraclavicular 'Virchow's' nodal spread. Pediatr Radiol 1996; 26: 717–719

66. Howman-Giles R B, Gilday D L, Ash J M. Radionuclide skeletal survey in neuroblastoma. Radiology 1979; 131: 497–502

67. Sty J R, Kun L E, Casper J T. Bone imaging as a diagnostic aid in evaluating neuroblastoma. Am J Pediatr Hematol Oncol 1980; 2: 115–118

68. Gelfand M J. Meta-iodobenzylguanidine in children. Semin Nucl Med 1993; 23: 231–242

69. Gelfand M J, Elgazzar A H, Kriss V M et al. Iodine-123-MIBG SPECT versus planar imaging in children with neural crest tumors. J Nucl Med 1994; 35: 1753–1757

70. Gordon I, Peters A M, Gutman A et al. Skeletal assessment in neuroblastoma. The pitfalls of iodine-123-MIBG scans. J Nucl Med 1990; 31: 129–134

71. Paltiel H J, Gelfand M J, Elgazzar A H et al. Neural crest tumors: I-123 MIBG imaging in children. Radiology 1994; 190: 117–121

72. Shulkin B L, Shapiro B, Hutchinson R J. Iodine-131-metaiodobenzylguanidine and bone scintigraphy for the detection of neuroblastoma. J Nucl Med 1992; 33: 1735–1740

73. Andrich M P, Shalaby-Rana E, Movassaghi N, Majd M. The role of 131 iodine-metaiodobenzylguanidine scanning in the correlative imaging of patients with neuroblastoma. Pediatrics 1996; 97: 246–250

74. Corbett R, Olliff J, Fairly N et al. A prospective comparison between magnetic resonance imaging, meta-iodobenzylguanidine scintigraphy and marrow histology/cytology in neuroblastoma. Eur J Cancer 1991; 27: 1560–1564

75. Couanet D, Geoffray A, Hartmann O et al. Bone marrow metastases in children's neuroblastoma studied by magnetic resonance imaging. Prog Clin Biol Res 1988; 271: 547–555

76. Mazumdar O, Siegel M J, Narra V, Luchtman-Jones L. Whole-body fast inversion recovery MR imaging of small cell neoplasms in pediatric patients. Am J Roentgenol 2002; 179: 1261–1266

77. Ruzal-Shapiro C, Berdon W, Cohen M, Abramson S. MR imaging of diffuse bone marrow replacement in pediatric patients with cancer. Radiology 1991; 181: 587–589

78. Sofka C M, Semelka R C, Kelekis N L et al. Magnetic resonance imaging of neuroblastoma using current techniques. Magn Reson Imag 1999; 17: 193–198

79. Tanabe T, Ohnuma N, Iwai J et al. Bone marrow metastasis of neuroblastoma analyzed by MRI and its influence on prognosis. Med Pediatr Oncol 1995; 24: 292–299

80. Dorr U, Sautter-Bihi M L, Schilling F H et al. Somatostatin receptor scintigraphy: a new diagnostic test in neuroblastoma. Prog Clin Biol Res 1994; 385: 355

81. Sautter–Bihl M L, Dorr U, Schilling F et al. Somatostatin receptor imaging: a new horizon in the diagnostic management of neuroblastoma. Semin Oncol 1994; 21: 38–41

82. Lauriero F, Rubini G, DíAddobbo F et al. I-131 MIBG scintigraphy of neuroectodermal tumors: comparison between I-131 MIBG and In-111 DTPA octreotide. Clin Nucl Med 1995; 20: 243–249

83. Manil L, Edeline V, Lumbroso J et al. Indium-111-pentetreotide scintigraphy in children with neuroblast-derived tumors. J Nucl Med 1996; 37: 893–896

84. Moertel C L, Reubi J C, Scheithauer B S et al. Expression of somatostatin receptors in childhood neuroblastoma. Am J Clin Pathol 1994; 102: 752–756

85. O'Dorisio M S, Hauger M, Cecalupo A J. Somatostatin receptors in neuroblastoma: diagnostic and therapeutic implications. Semin Oncol 1994; 21: 33–37

86. Shulkin B L, Hutchinson R J, Castle V P et al. Neuroblastoma: positron emission tomography with 2-[Fluorine-18]-Fluoro-2-deoxy-D-glucose compared with metaiodobenzylguanidine scintigraphy. Radiology 1996; 99: 743–750

87. Shulkin B L, Wieland D M, Baro M E et al. PET hydroxyephedrine imaging of neuroblastoma. J Nucl Med 1996; 37: 16–21

88. Casselman J W, Smet M H, VanDamme B, Lemahieu S F. Primary cervical neuroblastoma: CT and MR findings. J Comput Assist Tomogr 1988; 12: 684–686

89. Herman T E, Siegel M J. Cervical neuroblastoma, Stage IV-S. Perinatololgy 2001; 21: 470–472

90. Goldberg R M, Keller I A, Schonfeld S M et al. Intracranial route of a cervical neuroblastoma through skull base foramina. Pediatr Radiol 1996; 26: 715–716

91. Kenny B, Pizer B, Duncan A, Foreman N. Cystic metastatic cerebral neuroblastoma. Pediatr Radiol 1995; 25: 97–98

92. Aronson M R, Smoker W R K, Oetting G M. Hemorrhagic intracranial parenchymal metastases from primary retroperitoneal neuroblastoma. Pediatr Radiol 1995; 25: 284–285

93. Sener R N. CT of diffuse leptomeningeal metastasis from primary extracerebral neuroblastoma. Pediatr Radiol 1993; 23: 402–403

94. Egelhoff J C, Zalles C. Unusual CNS presentation of neuroblastoma. Pediatr Radiol 1996; 26: 51–54

Chapter 38

Uncommon paediatric neoplasms

Marilyn J Siegel

Introduction

Malignant neoplasms are a major cause of mortality in children between 1 and 14 years of age.[1] The most common malignancies diagnosed in children are acute leukaemia, lymphoma, primary tumours of the central nervous system, neuroblastoma and Wilms' tumours, comprising at least 70% of all neoplasms.[1] Rhabdomyosarcomas, hepatic tumours and germ cell tumours arising in extragonadal or gonadal sites account for most of the remaining tumours diagnosed in paediatric patients. Although uncommon, these tumours offer a diagnostic challenge to the radiologist who encounters only an occasional case. This chapter reviews the clinical and imaging features of the following tumours of children and adolescents:

- Hepatic neoplasms
- Rhabdomyosarcoma
- Extragonadal germ cell tumours
- Testicular germ cell tumours
- Ovarian germ cell tumours

Hepatic neoplasms

Epidemiology

Primary hepatic tumours account for approximately 1–4% of all paediatric tumours, with an annual incidence rate of 1.5–1.6 per million children.[1–3] In the USA, approximately 100–150 new cases of liver cancer in children develop each year.[3] Between 60 and 70% of all primary liver tumours in children are malignant, with hepatoblastoma and hepatocellular carcinoma constituting the vast majority (90% or more) of these malignancies.[1–4] The remaining hepatic malignancies are usually either undifferentiated embryonal sarcoma or the embryonal rhabdomyosarcoma. Hemangioendothelioma and mesenchymal hamartoma account for nearly all the non-malignant tumours in children.

Hepatoblastoma and hepatocellular carcinoma

Epidemiology

Hepatoblastoma is more common than hepatocellular carcinoma, occurring at an annual rate of 1.3 cases per 1 million children under 15 years of age.[1] Typically, it is diagnosed in young children under 4 years of age, with a median age at diagnosis of 1 year. In contrast, hepatocellular carcinoma has an annual incidence of 0.4 cases per 1 million and is typically diagnosed in older children, between 5 and 15 years of age, with a median age of 12 years.[1] Both tumours show a male predominance, with a male to female ratio of 1.4–2.0 : 1.0.[3,4]

Clinical presentation

Infants and children with hepatoblastoma usually present with an abdominal mass or distension. Abdominal pain, anorexia, weight loss, vomiting and precocious puberty (related to the secretion of chorionic gonadotrophins) may be seen in some cases. The presenting features of hepatocellular carcinoma are similar to those of hepatoblastoma. Hepatoblastoma has been associated with Beckwith–Wiedemann syndrome, hemihypertrophy, fetal alcohol syndrome, familial polyposis coli and Gardner's syndrome.[1–3] Hepatocellular carcinoma has been associated with hepatitis B virus infection, type I glycogen storage disease, cystinosis, tyrosinaemia, Wilson's disease, α-1-antitrypsin deficiency, extrahepatic biliary atresia and giant cell hepatitis.[1–6] The serum level of alpha-fetoprotein (AFP) is elevated in 80–90% of patients with hepatoblastomas and 60–90% of those with hepatocellular carcinoma.[2,3,6]

Pathology

Hepatoblastoma tends to be a solitary mass.[1–4] The right lobe is involved more often than the left lobe. Histologically, hepatoblastoma contains small, primitive epithelial cells, resembling fetal liver at 6–8 weeks of gestation. These may be admixed with mesenchymal elements (osteoid, cartilaginous and fibrous tissue), embryonal cells, or small undifferentiated cells resembling neuroblastoma cells.[1–3] In contrast to hepatoblastoma, hepatocellular carcinoma is more often multicentric at diagnosis. Histologically, it consists of large, pleomorphic multinucleated cells with variable degrees of differentiation.[2,3]

Metastases and staging

Metastatic disease occurs in 10–40% of patients with hepatoblastomas at initial presentation.[5] The most common sites of distant spread, in order of decreasing frequency, are the lungs, bone and brain.

The two widely used systems for staging paediatric hepatic tumours are the Paediatric Oncology Group and the International Society of Paediatric Oncology systems. The Paediatric Oncology Group staging system is based on surgical findings (Table 38.1).[3] Based on this classification, 29% of tumours are Stage I at diagnosis, 11% are Stage II, 21% are Stage III and 39% are Stage IV.[2,5] The International Society of Paediatric Oncology assigns tumour stage by the number of liver segments involved, which is determined by preoperative imaging studies.[3,7,8] Studies in Europe have shown that this pretreatment classification (termed PRE-TEXT) correlates well with resection and ultimate survival.[3,7]

Table 38.1. *Paediatric Oncology Group staging of malignant hepatic tumours*

Stage	Extent of disease
Stage I	Completely resected with typical fetal histologic pattern
Stage I	Complete resection with histologic pattern other than purely fetal
Stage II	Grossly resected with evidence of microscopic residual
Stage III	Not resectable or partially resectable with measurable tumour left behind. Also includes lymph node involvement
Stage IV	Distant metastases at presentation

From reference 3.

Treatment options

Surgical excision remains the cornerstone of treatment for both hepatoblastoma and hepatocellular carcinoma. Long-term survival is directly related to successful resection.[1,3] The features that may limit surgical resection are involvement of both lobes, bulky tumour or adenopathy in the porta hepatis, extension into the inferior vena cava (IVC) and involvement of the main hepatic artery or all branches of the hepatic vein. Only 30–50% of hepatoblastomas and 30% of hepatocellular carcinomas are resectable at the time of diagnosis.[1,5–9] Adjuvant chemotherapy is routinely given to patients with both hepatoblastomas and hepatocellular carcinomas to facilitate surgical excision. With preoperative chemotherapy, the resectability rate for hepatoblastoma increases to almost 90%.[7] Radiation therapy has a limited role in the treatment of hepatoblastoma and hepatocellular carcinoma, except as an adjunct in children with residual tumour following chemotherapy.

Prognosis

Event-free survival rates of 65–87% have been reported in children with hepatoblastoma treated with chemotherapy and complete surgical excision.[3,7–9] Survival rates approach 100% in Stage I disease, 75–80% in Stage II disease, 65–68% in Stage III disease and 0–27% in Stage IV disease.[3]

Despite aggressive chemotherapy and surgical management, only a 13% survival rate has been reported in children with hepatocellular carcinoma.[1]

Imaging

Diagnosis
Sonography with Doppler interrogation is the preferred examination to screen for the presence of an intrahepatic mass and to differentiate solid and cystic masses. It also is a useful study to identify the presence and extent of vascular involvement by tumour. At ultrasonography, hepatoblastoma and hepatocellular carcinoma appear as predominantly solid masses but they may have areas of necrosis or haemorrhage. The solid components may be hypo-, iso-, or hyperechoic relative to normal parenchyma. Central calcification is present in up to 50% of tumours and appears as small hyperechoic foci with acoustic shadowing (Fig. 38.1).[10,11] By Doppler imaging, prominent internal vascularity or areas of arteriovenous shunting may be identified.

Localized staging
Computed tomography (CT) or magnetic resonance (MR) imaging is needed to assess tumour extent.[11–17] CT findings of hepatoblastoma and hepatocellular carcinoma are of a soft tissue mass, which may have well-demarcated or ill-defined margins. These tumours tend to be hypo- or isodense to liver on precontrast images. They are frequently hypervascular during the arterial phase of enhancement and usually hypodense to liver during the portal venous phase of enhancement. They also may contain focal areas

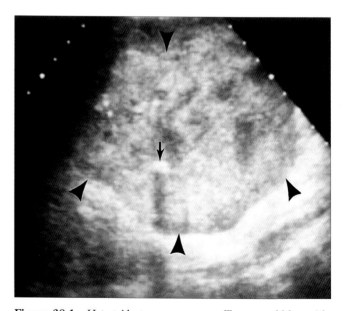

Figure 38.1. *Hepatoblastoma, sonogram. Two-year-old boy with a palpable right upper quadrant mass. Transverse view of the right lobe of the liver demonstrates a large heterogeneous mass (arrowheads) with focal calcification (arrow). The tumour is slightly hypoechoic to adjacent parenchyma.*

of decreased attenuation, due to the presence of necrosis or haemorrhage (Fig. 38.2).[18,19] On MR, hepatoblastoma and hepatocellular carcinoma are typically hypointense to normal liver on T1-weighted sequences, although they may have foci of high signal intensity, which is due to the presence of fat or haemorrhage. On T2-weighted images, these tumours are generally heterogeneous and hyperintense (Fig. 38.3). Similar to CT, early arterial enhancement with rapid wash-out is typical after administration of gadolinium chelate agents (Fig. 38.4).[15,16,19,20]

The crucial factors in assessing extent and resectability of hepatic neoplasms are the extent of the primary tumour, most importantly the presence of tumour in surgically critical areas such as the porta hepatis, portal vein and IVC, and the presence of regional extrahepatic spread or distant metastases. Tumour thrombus appears as an echogenic focus on sonography, a low attenuation filling defect on CT (Fig. 38.5), a high signal attenuation area on spin-echo MR and a signal void on gradient-echo images. Lymph node metastases have a soft tissue attenuation on CT, a low intermediate signal intensity (similar to liver) on T1-weighted images and intermediate or high signal intensity on T2-weighted images and gadolinium-enhanced images (Fig. 38.6).

With the advent of CT and MR, angiography is no longer performed in the initial staging evaluation of children with hepatic malignancy. On rare occasions, however, CT with arterial portography may be necessary for tumour mapping prior to trisegmentectomy.

Distant staging

Because the vast majority of metastases present at diagnosis are to the lungs, plain chest radiographs and chest CT are routinely obtained to detect pulmonary metastases. Skeletal involvement is assessed by scintigraphy. Because brain metastases are very rare, head CT or MR are usually reserved for patients with relevant clinical symptoms.

Follow-up evaluation

Most recurrences occur in the first two postoperative years and, therefore, CT or MR of the liver and abdomen are obtained at regular intervals up to 2 years after surgery. The exact timing of the follow-up examinations is determined by the specific treatment protocol utilized.

Key points: hepatoblastoma/ hepatocellular carcinoma

- ■ Crucial criteria for determining resectability include the presence of spread into the portal vein, IVC, porta hepatis, regional lymph nodes and distal metastases

- ■ Hepatoblastoma and hepatocellular carcinoma have similar imaging features on sonography, CT and MR

- ■ These tumours are usually solitary but occasionally are multifocal

- ■ Either CT or MR suffices for staging local tumour extent

- ■ CT is the best technique for detecting pulmonary metastases

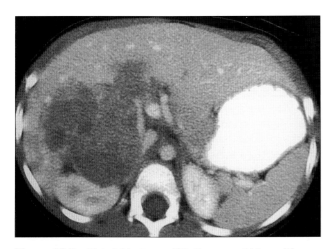

Figure 38.2. *Hepatoblastoma, CT. One-year-old boy with a palpable right upper quadrant mass; CT scan during the portal venous phase of contrast enhancement shows a low density mass in the right lobe of the liver. The tumour displaces the right kidney inferiorly.*

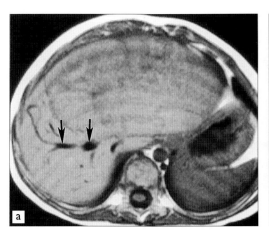 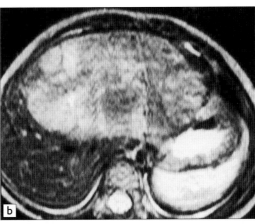

Figure 38.3. *Hepatoblastoma, MR. The mass is hypointense on a T1-weighted axial image (a) and hyperintense on a T2-weighted image (b). The right portal vein (arrows) is displaced posteriorly.*

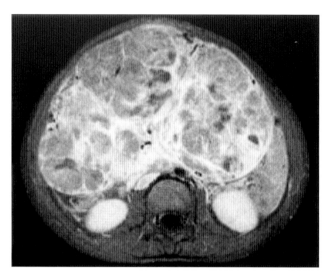

Figure 38.4. *Hepatoblastoma. Fat-suppressed T1-weighted image after gadolinium chelate administration shows heterogeneous enhancement of this large tumour. (Case courtesy of Frederic Hoffer, MD, Memphis, TN.)*

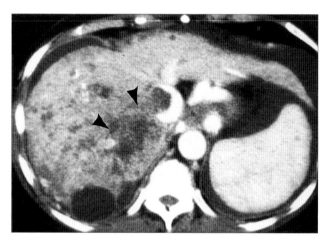

Figure 38.5. *Diffusely infiltrating hepatocellular carcinoma with portal vein invasion. Contrast-enhanced CT shows heterogeneous enhancement of the hepatic parenchyma. The enlarged portal vein (arrowheads) is filled with low density tumour thrombus. This patient had no previous history of liver disease.*

Fibrolamellar hepatocellular carcinoma

Fibrolamellar hepatocellular carcinoma is a histologic subtype of hepatocellular carcinoma that occurs predominantly in adolescent and younger adults. Histologically, it contains eosinophilic-laden hepatocytes separated by thin, fibrous bands arranged in a lamellar pattern, hence, the term 'fibrolamellar'. A central scar and calcifications are common. Fibrolamellar carcinomas arise in otherwise normal livers.[3] Hepatomegaly and abdominal pain are common presenting features. Serum AFP levels are usually normal. Fibrolamellar hepatocellular carcinoma is less aggressive than the typical variety of hepatocellular carcinoma and has a more favourable prognosis.[21–24]

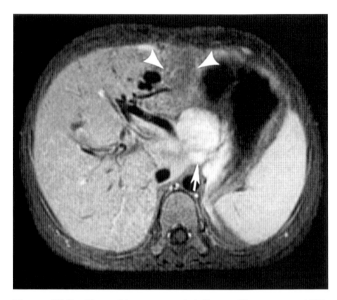

Figure 38.6. *Hepatoblastoma, nodal disease. Fat-suppressed T1-weighted MR after gadolinium chelate administration shows a low signal intensity tumour in the left hepatic lobe (arrowheads) and high signal intensity nodes (arrow) in the porta hepatis. The tumour mass was seen better on more cranial scans. (Case courtesy of Frederic Hoffer, MD, Memphis, TN.)*

Fibrolamellar carcinoma is typically a large well-demarcated tumour (mean diameter, 12 cm). On ultrasonography, it may be hyper- or isoechoic to liver. At CT, this lesion is either hypo- or isodense to liver on precontrast scans and it often shows heterogeneous enhancement during the arterial phase of enhancement. During the portal venous phase of enhancement, it is isodense to liver. The central scar is hypodense during both the arterial and portal venous phases of enhancement. On MR, fibrolamellar carcinoma is typically hypointense to liver on T1-weighted images and hyperintense on T2-weighted images. The central scar is hypointense on both sequences.[15,21–24] As is the case on CT, the tumour parenchyma, but not the central scar, enhances after administration of gadolinium chelates. Central calcifications are common (68% of cases). Associated findings include intrahepatic biliary obstruction (42%), portal or hepatic vein invasion (87%), lymphadenopathy (65%), extrahepatic tumour spread (42%) and distant metastases (29%).[22]

Key points: hepatic neoplasms

- ■ Primary hepatic tumours are the third most common paediatric cancer

- ■ The majority of hepatic tumours are hepatoblastomas and hepatocellular carcinomas

- ■ Hepatoblastoma occurs in infants and young children, whereas hepatocellular carcinoma is seen in older children

■ AFP is elevated in over 60% of patients with primary liver cancer

■ Pathological differentiation between hepatoblastoma and hepatocellular carcinoma is based on cellular maturity

■ Regional lymph node spread is common in both hepatoblastoma and hepatocellular carcinoma

■ Fibrolamellar carcinoma is rare and occurs in older children and young adults

Undifferentiated embryonal sarcoma

Undifferentiated embryonal sarcoma of the liver is the third most common hepatic malignancy in the paediatric population.[2–4,15,25,26] The tumour usually affects children between 6 and 10 years of age and it has a slight male predominance. Clinical findings include right upper quadrant pain and/or palpable mass. The serum AFP levels are normal. Association with other conditions is rare. Gross section reveals a soft lesion with solid, gelatinous or cystic areas and areas of haemorrhage and necrosis. Histologically, the tumour contains undifferentiated spindle cells in an abundant myxoid matrix.[2,25,26] Prognosis is poor, with a median survival of approximately 1 year.[2,25] Approximately 10–20%

of patients have a disease-free survival time of more than 2 years.[2,25] Metastases are to lung and bone.

At ultrasonography, embryonal sarcomas typically have a predominantly solid appearance, which is likely related to the presence of gelatinous material.[26] The solid components are iso- or hyperechoic to the surrounding hepatic parenchyma. By sonography, cystic areas compose only 20% of the tumour volume.

Computed tomography findings are those of a predominantly hypodense mass with attenuation values equal to water in almost 90% of cases.[26] Soft tissue components are usually found around the periphery of the tumour, although they may extend into the central portion of the tumour (Fig. 38.7). The solid components enhance on dynamic CT examinations. On T1-weighted images, most embryonal sarcomas are hypointense to liver. On T2-weighted sequences, they typically demonstrate high signal intensity similar to that of cerebrospinal fluid (Fig. 38.8).[15,16,26] A fluid–debris level or areas of high attenuation on CT and high signal intensity on T1-weighted images may also be seen. These areas correspond to areas of haemorrhagic tissue or fluid seen at pathologic examination. Presumably an increased water content within the myxoid stroma accounts for the lower attenuation values on CT and high signal intensity on T2-weighted MR.

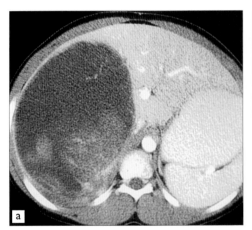
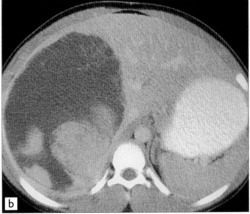

Figure 38.7. *Undifferentiated embryonal sarcoma, CT. A 10-year-old girl with abdominal pain. CT scans during (a) hepatic arterial and (b) portal venous phases of enhancement show a large, well-circumscribed, near water attenuation mass with peripheral solid nodules. The tumour is confined to the right lobe. Complete surgical resection was successful.*

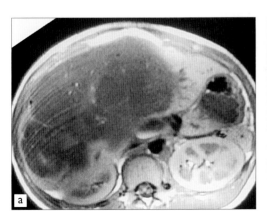
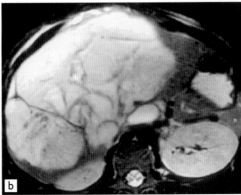

Figure 38.8. *Undifferentiated embryonal sarcoma, MR. A mass in the right hepatic lobe is hypointense on a T1-weighted image (a) and hyperintense on a T2-weighted image (b). (Case courtesy of Lane Donnelly, Cincinnati, OH.)*

Rhabdomyosarcoma of the biliary tree

Rhabdomyosarcoma of the liver accounts for about 1% of all primary liver tumours in children.[2] The tumour tends to affect children under 5 years of age (75% of cases) and is rare after the age of 15 years.[27,28] Obstructive jaundice, hepatomegaly and abdominal distension are common clinical findings. Grossly, rhabdomyosarcoma of the biliary tract presents as a botryoid, gelatinous mass occluding the right, left, or common bile ducts. Extension into the liver parenchyma is common. The histologic features are typical of the embryonal subtype of rhabdomyosarcoma.[2] Treatment is complete resection, although at presentation this is possible in only 20–40% of patients.[2] Resection rates increase with the use of pre-operative chemotherapy.

The imaging findings are those of intra- and extrahepatic ductal dilatation and a mass, which is usually in the porta hepatis. Similar to other hepatic malignancies, the tumour is iso- or hyperechoic relative to normal liver on sonography, hypodense on contrast-enhanced CT, hypointense on T1-weighted MR and hyperintense on T2-weighted images.[27] Rhabdomyosarcoma of the biliary tract spreads by direct extension to contiguous structures or by haematogenous or lymphatic dissemination. The most frequent sites of metastatic disease are the liver and lungs. Metastases can also be found on peritoneal surfaces and in lymph nodes and bone.[27]

Benign tumours of the liver

Between 30 and 40% of hepatic tumours in children are benign, with hemangio-endothelioma and multilocular cystic hamartoma accounting for over 95% of these neoplasms. Hepatic adenomas and nodular hyperplasia account for less than 5% of benign hepatic tumours in childhood.[2–4] Their imaging features are similar to those seen in adults and they will not be discussed further.

Hemangio-endothelioma is seen almost exclusively in the first 6 months of life. This tumour is rarely seen in children over 3 years of age.[29] Most infants present with symptomatic hepatomegaly or with congestive heart failure due to high-output overcirculation. Histologically, hemangio-endotheliomas contain thin-walled, endothelial-lined vascular spaces. They may be solitary or multifocal.[2]

By sonography, hemangio-endotheliomas usually are well-defined and hypoechoic. Doppler sonography usually demonstrates internal vascularity. The classic appearance on CT is a low attenuation mass or masses on precontrast scans, which demonstrate early nodular peripheral enhancement and progressive centripetal fill-in on delay images (Fig. 38.9). Small lesions may show early uniform enhancement, whereas large lesions may demonstrate persistent central low density due to the presence of fibrosis, thrombosis or degeneration. By MR, these lesions are hypointense to normal liver on T1-weighted images and hyperintense on T2-weighted images, with a signal intensity equal to that of cerebrospinal fluid.[10–14,18,20,30] The enhancement pattern after intravenous (IV) administration of gadolinium chelates is similar to that seen on CT. If the typical findings of centripetal enhancement and fill-in are present, the diagnosis of hemangio-endothelioma can be made with certainty. Biopsy is not necessary. In contrast to adults, cavernous hemangiomas are rare in children. The imaging features, however, are similar to those of hemangio-endothelioma.

Mesenchymal hamartoma, also referred to as lymphangioma, bile cell fibroadenoma, hamartoma and cystic hamartoma, is a benign lesion composed of cysts of varying size, surrounded by fibrous septations which contain a disorganized mixture of mesenchyme, abnormal bile ducts and hepatocytes.[2] Nearly 85% of lesions occur in children under 2 years of age and only 5% are seen after 5 years of age. Median patient age at diagnosis is approximately 10 months.[2] Affected patients usually present with a palpable mass or painless abdominal enlargement. The sonographic, CT and MR appearance of mesenchymal hamartoma ranges from that of a multilocular mass containing fluid-filled areas surrounded by septa (Fig. 38.10) to that of a predominantly solid mass containing multiple small cysts.[10–14,18–20,31] The solid parts of the tumour enhance following administration of contrast medium.

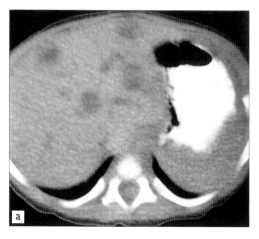
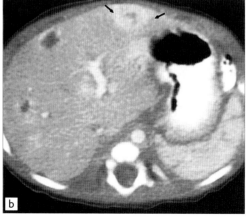

Figure 38.9. *Hemangio-endotheliomas in a neonate with hepatomegaly. (a) Precontrast CT scan shows multiple hypodense masses. (b) Postcontrast image shows multiple peripheral areas of enhancement, the density of which is similar to blood vessels. One lesion anteriorly (arrows) shows near complete enhancement. These lesions involuted completely within 6 months.*

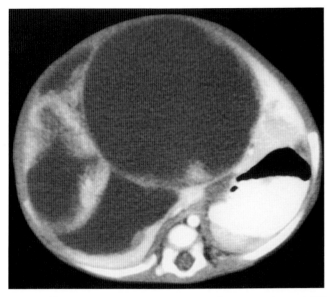

Figure 38.10. *Mesenchymal hamartoma. Contrast-enhanced CT scan shows a large mass containing near-water attenuation locules separated by soft tissue septations. (Case courtesy of James Meyer, MD.)*

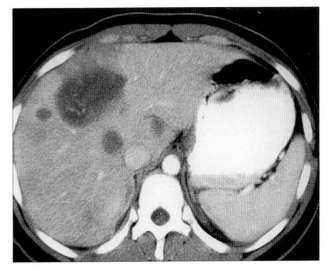

Figure 38.11. *Hepatic metastasis from rhabdomyosarcoma. Contrast-enhanced CT during the portal venous phase shows several hypoattenuating lesions in the dome of the liver. The largest lesion shows a minimal amount of internal enhancement.*

Hepatic metastases

The malignant tumours of childhood that most frequently metastasize to the liver are:

- Wilms' tumour
- Neuroblastoma
- Rhabdomyosarcoma
- Lymphoma

Neuroblastoma may affect the liver in either Stage IV or IV-S disease. Stage IV disease is characterized by the presence of a retroperitoneal mass and distant metastases to skeleton, liver, or nodes. Stage IV-S neuroblastoma occurs in patients under 1 year of age, who have small ipsilateral tumours (not crossing the midline) and metastases to liver, skin and bone marrow, but not to cortical bone. Clinically, patients with hepatic metastases present with hepatomegaly, jaundice, abdominal pain or mass, or abnormal hepatic function tests.

Hepatic metastases most often are multiple and well-circumscribed. They are hypo- or hyperechoic relative to normal liver on sonography, low attenuation on contrast-enhanced CT (Fig. 38.11), hypointense on T1-weighted MR and hyperintense on T2-weighted images (Fig. 38.12). Although the signal intensity is high on T2-weighted MR, it is not as high as that seen with hemangiomas or cysts. Other findings include mass effect with displacement of vessels and vessel invasion or amputation. Most metastases in children are hypovascular on both the arterial and portal venous phases of enhancement.

Occasionally, internal or peripheral (ring) enhancement is seen after contrast administration.

Rhabdomyosarcoma

- Prostate
- Bladder
- Vagina, uterus, cervix

Epidemiology

Rhabdomyosarcoma represents 5–10% of all malignant solid tumours of childhood and ranks fourth in frequency after central nervous system (CNS) neoplasms, Wilms' tumour and neuroblastoma.[32,33] This tumour is the most common malignant tumour of the soft tissues in infants and children. The annual incidence is 4.3–4.6 cases per 1 million children under 15 years of age, with approximately 350 new cases diagnosed in the USA per year.[1,33] Rhabdomyosarcoma has a slightly higher incidence in boys than in girls. The median age at diagnosis of children with rhabdomyosarcoma is 4 years.

Rhabdomyosarcoma can arise anywhere in the body, but the head and neck regions are most commonly involved, accounting for about 35% of all cases.[1,32,33] The genito-urinary tract is the second most common site of origin, accounting for 29% of primary rhabdomyosarcomas. The remaining tumours usually occur in the soft tissues of the thorax, trunk and extremities. Genito-urinary tumours are discussed in more detail below.

Clinical presentation

Genito-urinary tract sarcomas arise most often from paratesticular tissues and less frequently from bladder, prostate,

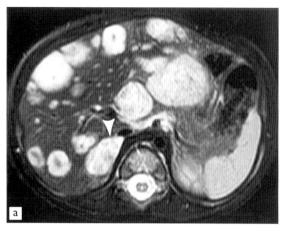

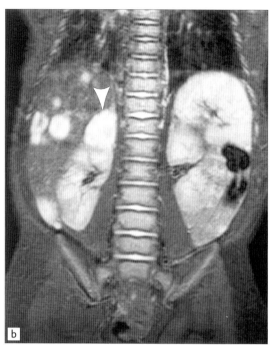

Figure 38.12. *Metastatic neuroblastoma in a neonate with hepatomegaly (Stage 4S disease). Axial (a) and coronal (b) fat-suppressed T2-weighted images show multiple high signal intensity lesions in both lobes of the liver. There is a small right adrenal neuroblastoma (arrowhead). (Case courtesy of Frederic Hoffer, MD, Memphis, TN.)*

vagina, uterus or cervix. The clinical presentation varies with the anatomic site of involvement. Children with rhabdomyosarcoma of paratesticular tissues usually present with painless scrotal enlargement. Children with bladder rhabdomyosarcoma commonly present with haematuria, dysuria, frequency or urinary tract infection, while children with prostatic rhabdomyosarcoma tend to present with urinary retention or difficulty in voiding. Flank pain can occur if there is hydronephrosis related to ureteral obstruction. Children with vaginal, cervical or uterine sarcomas come to attention because of vaginal bleeding or a vulvar, perineal or vaginal mass that may prolapse into the introitus or onto the perineum.[1,32,33]

Paratesticular rhabdomyosarcoma has a bimodal age distribution, with the first peak occurring in children 5 years or younger and the second peak occurring in adolescence. Bladder rhabdomyosarcoma typically affects patients in the first 3 years of life. Vaginal tumours are more common in infants and young children,[33] while cervical and uterine rhabdomyosarcomas are more common in adolescent girls.

Pathology

At histologic examination, rhabdomyosarcoma is classified as embryonal, alveolar or pleomorphic. The embryonal, including botryoid subtype, is more common in rhabdomyosarcoma of the genito-urinary tract, whereas the alveolar histology is most common in rhabdomyosarcoma of the trunk and extremity. The botryoid architecture arises in the bladder or vagina and is so named because it shows a polypoid growth pattern, resembling a bunch of grapes. The histologic appearance varies from primitive mesenchymal tumours with stellate cells to well-differentiated

tumours. The margins of the tumour may be infiltrative or well-defined by a compressive pseudocapsule.

Metastases and clinical staging

Approximately 25% of patients with newly diagnosed rhabdomyosarcoma have metastatic disease at diagnosis.[1] In order of decreasing frequency, the most common sites of metastatic spread are bone marrow, cortical bone and lymph nodes.[32,33] Hepatic and brain metastases are rare in newly diagnosed patients, but are common in patients who relapse. The frequency of metastatic spread varies with the anatomic location of the primary tumour. Distant spread is more frequent for tumours arising in the prostate, paratesticular and cervical sites than it is for bladder, vaginal and truncal sites.[1,32,33]

Several classifications have been used for staging rhabdomyosarcoma.[1] The two widely utilized staging systems are: (a) the TNM (i.e. tumour, nodes, metastasis) system based on the classic staging elements of the International Union Against Cancer (UICC) system and (b) the Intergroup Rhabdomyosarcoma Study Group (IRSG) system.[32–34] The TNM system is a *pretreatment* staging system. Classification of patients is based on clinical assessment of tumour (T) size (<5 cm or >5 cm), clinical status of regional lymph nodes (N), evidence of distant metastases (M) and the anatomic location of the primary tumour (at a favourable or unfavourable location) (Table 38.2).[34] The IRSG system is solely a *clinicopathologic* grouping based on surgical findings (Table 38.3).

Treatment options

Whenever possible, complete surgical excision of the tumour with negative microscopic margins is the treatment

Table 38.2. *TNM pretreatment system*

Stage	Sites	T	Tumour size	N	M
I	Orbit	TI or T2	a or b	N0 or NI or N2	M0
	Head and neck				
	Genito-urinary non-bladder/non-prostate				
II	Bladder/prostate	TI or T2	a	N0 or NX	M0
	Extremity				
	Head and neck parameningeal				
III	Bladder/prostate	TI or T2	a or b	NI	M0
	Extremity		b	N0 or NI or NX	M0
	Head and neck parameningeal				
IV	All	TI or T2	a or b	N0 or NI	MI

Definitions of T, N and M classifications

Tumour

TI	Confined to anatomic site or origin
TIa	<5 cm in size
TIb	≥5 cm in size
T2	Extension or fixation to surrounding tissues
T2a	<5 cm in size
T2b	≥5 cm in size

Regional lymph nodes

N0	Regional nodes not clinically involved
NI	Regional nodes clinically involved by tumour
NX	Clinical status of regional nodes unknown

Metastases

M0	No distant metastasis
MI	Metastases present

Pretreatment clinical staging based on tumour size (T), status of regional lymph nodes (N), evidence of metastatic disease (M) and tumour location.
From reference 34.

of choice for patients with rhabdomyosarcoma. In patients with bulky non-resectable tumour determined by imaging, biopsy of the tumour is followed by chemotherapy, radiation and future resection. The goal of treatment is to minimize radical surgery and improve long-term functional outcomes.

Prognosis

The overall 3-year survival is between 73 and 83%.[32,33] Survival in children with metastatic disease is still poor, with long-term survival between 20 and 30%.[1]

Imaging

Diagnosis

Because rhabdomyosarcoma can present as a palpable mass, it is often initially imaged by sonography. Sonographic findings include:

- An echogenic mass (Figs. 38.13 and 38.14a)
- Internal hypoechoic areas related to necrosis or haemorrhage
- Prominent internal vascularity and high diastolic flow within the tumour on Doppler interrogation

In the bladder, the tumour may be discovered incidentally on cystography or urography during the evaluation of non-specific symptoms, such as haematuria, increased frequency of urination and urinary retention. The cystographic findings are bladder wall thickening, a polypoid soft tissue mass at the bladder base, or a combination of both. With deep invasion, the bladder wall is markedly deformed and rigid and bladder capacity is diminished.

Table 38.3. *Intergroup Rhabdomyosarcoma Study Group staging: surgical–pathologic grouping system*

Stage	Extent of disease
I	Localized tumour, completely resected
A	Confined to the organ of origin
B	Infiltration outside organ; regional nodes not involved
II	Compromised or regional resection of three types:
A	Grossly resected tumour with microscopic residual
B	Regional disease, completely resected, in which lymph nodes may be involved and/or tumour extension into adjacent organ may be present
C	Regional disease or involved lymph nodes, macroscopically resected but with evidence of microscopic residual
III	Incomplete resection or biopsy with macroscopic residual tumour
A	Localized or locally extensive tumour, gross residual disease after biopsy only
B	Localized or locally extensive tumour, gross residual disease after major resection (>50% debulking)
IV	Distant metastases present at diagnosis

From reference 33.

Local staging
Preoperative evaluation of local tumour extent needs to include CT or MR.[32,37–41] Findings of rhabdomyosarcoma include:

- A soft tissue mass with a CT attenuation value approximating that of muscle (Fig. 38.14b)

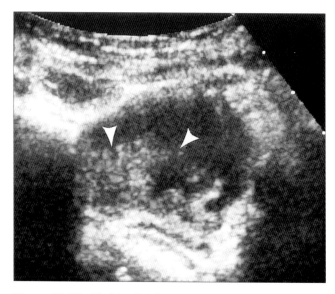

Figure 38.13. *Bladder rhabdomyosarcoma in a 10-year-old boy with haematuria. Ultrasound examination (transverse view) of the bladder shows an echogenic mass (arrowheads) projecting into the bladder lumen. The mass arose from the right trigone.*

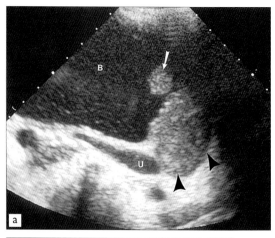

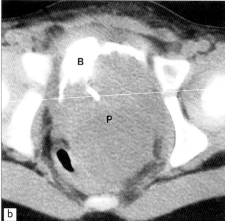

Figure 38.14. *Prostatic rhabdomyosarcoma, Stage IIIA (Intergroup classification). A 3-year-old boy with haematuria. (a) Ultrasound examination (longitudinal view) demonstrates a well-defined echogenic mass (arrowheads) at the base of the bladder (B). The mass extends into the bladder lumen (arrow) and obstructs the right ureter (U), which is dilated. (b) Contrast-enhanced CT shows a poorly marginated, enlarged prostate gland (P). The tumour invades the base of the bladder (B). Also note extension of the mass to the left internal obturator muscle. Invasion of the posterior bladder wall and pelvic sidewalls confirmed at time of open biopsy.*

- An intermediate signal intensity mass on T1-weighted images
- An intermediate or high signal intensity on T2-weighted MR
- Areas of tumour necrosis, haemorrhage and calcification

After the administration of IV iodinated contrast agent or gadolinium chelates agents, rhabdomyosarcoma usually enhances heterogeneously (Fig. 38.15).[33]

The CT and MR appearances also vary with the anatomic location of the tumour. Paratesticular rhabdomyosarcoma manifests as a scrotal mass that may surround or invade the epididymis and testis.[37] Bladder

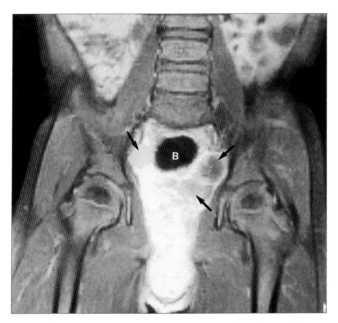

Figure 38.15. *Prostatic rhabdomyosarcoma. Fat-saturated coronal T1-weighted image following Gd-DTPA administration demonstrates a large hyperintense rhabdomyosarcoma, which surrounds the bladder (B) and extends to the pelvic sidewalls. Also noted are bilaterally enlarged internal iliac lymph nodes (arrows).*

rhabdomyosarcoma appears as a sessile or polypoid mass deforming the bladder base. It may protrude into the bladder lumen, producing the botryoid or 'bunch of grapes' appearance. Prostatic rhabdomyosarcoma appears as a mass elevating the bladder base and elongating the prostatic urethra. The precise origin of the tumour may be difficult to determine, as primary prostate lesions may invade the bladder base and, conversely, the prostate may be invaded by a tumour arising in the bladder. Vaginal rhabdomyosarcoma manifests as a soft tissue mass enlarging the vaginal lumen. Secondary findings include uterine enlargement and fluid in the endometrial cavity as a result of tumour obstruction of the cervix or vaginal canal. Both prostatic and vaginal tumours may invade the bladder base or obstruct the ureters leading to hydronephrosis.

Signs of regional spread include lymph node enlargement and invasion of adjacent pelvic organs, pelvic side walls and, in girls, the parametrium. Lymphadenopathy has a spectrum of appearances, ranging from small discrete nodules to large conglomerate masses (Fig. 38.15).

Distant staging
Imaging of the chest, abdomen and skeleton are routinely performed to search for metastases. Both CT and 2-[F-18]fluoro-2-deoxy-D-glucose positron emission tomography (^{18}FDG PET) imaging are used to determine the presence and extent of both regional and retroperitoneal lymph node enlargement (Fig. 38.16). Lymph node involvement has been documented in 10–20% of cases of rhabdomyosarcomas.[1,32,33] Computed tomography is still the study of choice to detect pulmonary metastases. Skeletal scintigraphy is the preferred study to detect bone metastases.

Follow-up evaluation
Most relapses occur within 2–3 years of diagnosis. Metastatic evaluation should include imaging examinations of the chest, abdomen, pelvis and skeleton (Fig. 38.16). CT, MR imaging and ^{18}FDG PET have been used to follow response to treatment and detect residual or recurrent disease. The timing of the follow-up imaging examinations is determined by the specific protocol to which the patient is randomized.

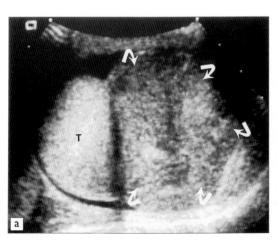
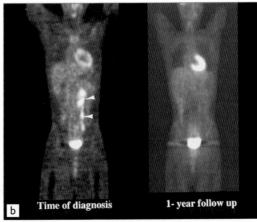

Figure 38.16. *Paratesticular rhabdomyosarcoma. A 16-year-old boy with scrotal enlargement. (a) Ultrasound examination (transverse view) of the left scrotum shows a heterogeneously hypoechoic mass (arrows) lateral to the left testis (T). (b) A coronal whole body ^{18}FDG PET image (left panel) at the time of diagnosis demonstrates multiple left para-aortic and iliac lymph node metastases (arrowheads). After completion of chemotherapy, the follow-up study at 1 year (right panel) shows no active disease.*

Comparative imaging

There have been no large studies in children comparing imaging modalities for staging and follow-up of rhabdomyosarcoma. Studies involving small number of patients have suggested that MR compared with CT improves the detection and staging of tumour.[38,39] However, results of these studies are not statistically significant. More recently, [18]FDG PET scintigraphy, whole-body MR and skeletal scintigraphy have been compared for the detection of bone metastases in children and young adults with a variety of tumours, including rhabdomyosarcoma.[42,43] In these series, sensitivity for metastasis detection was 90% for [18]FDG PET, 82–100% for whole body MR and 71% for skeletal scintigraphy.[42,43]

Key points: rhabdomyosarcoma

- Rhabdomyosarcomas of the genito-urinary tract arise in the bladder, prostate and vagina

- Rhabdomyosarcomas are the most common soft tissue tumour of childhood

- The predominant histological subtypes in the genito-urinary tract are embryonal and botryoid tumours

- Lymph node and distant metastases occur at presentation in about 25% of patients

- Ultrasonography is useful for diagnosis but CT and MR are the preferred methods for staging local spread and lymph node metastases

- CT is recommended to screen for pulmonary metastases

Other genito-urinary neoplasms

Vagina and uterus

Adenocarcinoma is a rare neoplasm of the vagina in childhood. It has been found in adolescent girls with a history of exposure to diethylstilbestrol in utero. Because this drug has not been administered for several decades, this tumour is unlikely to be seen. The imaging features are similar to those of rhabdomyosarcoma.

Gestational trophoblastic disease can be a cause of an intrauterine mass in an adolescent girl. It represents a spectrum of tumours varying from the benign hydatidiform mole to the more malignant invasive mole and choriocarcinoma.[44,45] The clinical features of trophoblastic disease are vaginal bleeding and elevated levels of serum human chorionic gonadotrophin (HCG).

Sonography is effective in the detection of trophoblastic disease, but is not as useful as CT or MR in determining tumour extent. On CT, gestational trophoblastic disease appears as a heterogeneously enhancing mass in the endometrial cavity. Myometrial tumour nodules appear as low attenuation areas on contrast enhancement scans.[44,45] On MR, the trophoblastic neoplasm appears as a heterogeneous, low signal intensity mass on T1-weighted images and as a high signal intensity mass on T2-weighted images. Other CT and MR findings include uterine enlargement, a gestational sac with or without a small fetal pole, tortuous dilated parametrial vessels, enlarged ovaries that contain thecal–lutein cysts and parametrial extension. Distant metastases to liver and lung can be seen in choriocarcinoma.

Bladder

Transitional cell carcinoma and leiomyosarcoma are rare malignant bladder neoplasms in childhood. Hemangioma, neurofibroma, paraganglioma and leiomyoma of the bladder are unusual benign neoplasms of the urinary bladder. The CT and MR features of these tumours are similar to those of rhabdomyosarcoma and include a sessile or polypoid mass arising within the bladder wall and projecting into the bladder lumen. In most cases, biopsy is required for diagnosis.

Extragonadal germ cell tumours

Germ cell tumours arising in gonadal or extragonadal sites account for approximately 3% of all paediatric malignancies. Extragonadal tumours represent nearly two thirds of all germ cell tumours in children.[1,46,47] The sacrococcygeal region is the most common site of origin for germ cell tumours in children, accounting for approximately 40% of all germ cell tumours and close to 80% of extragonadal germ cell tumours.[1,46–48] Less commonly, extragonadal tumours involve the mediastinum, retroperitoneum and head and neck area. The majority of extragonadal tumours are teratomas.

Clinical presentation

Sacrococcygeal teratomas are usually non-familial and affect females more than males (3 : 1 ratio). Most are diagnosed in neonates because the large exophytic component produces a visible mass in the sacrococcygeal or gluteal region. The diagnosis may be delayed if the tumours are small and confined to the presacral area. Presacral tumours usually present in later childhood or adolescence, producing chronic constipation, and are more likely to be malignant.

Four types of teratomas have been described based on the relative amounts of internal and external tumour (Fig. 38.17):[48]

- Type I – predominantly external; limited extension into the presacral space (47%)
- Type II – similar external and intrapelvic components (34%)
- Type III – minimal external tumour; large pelvic and abdominal components (9%)

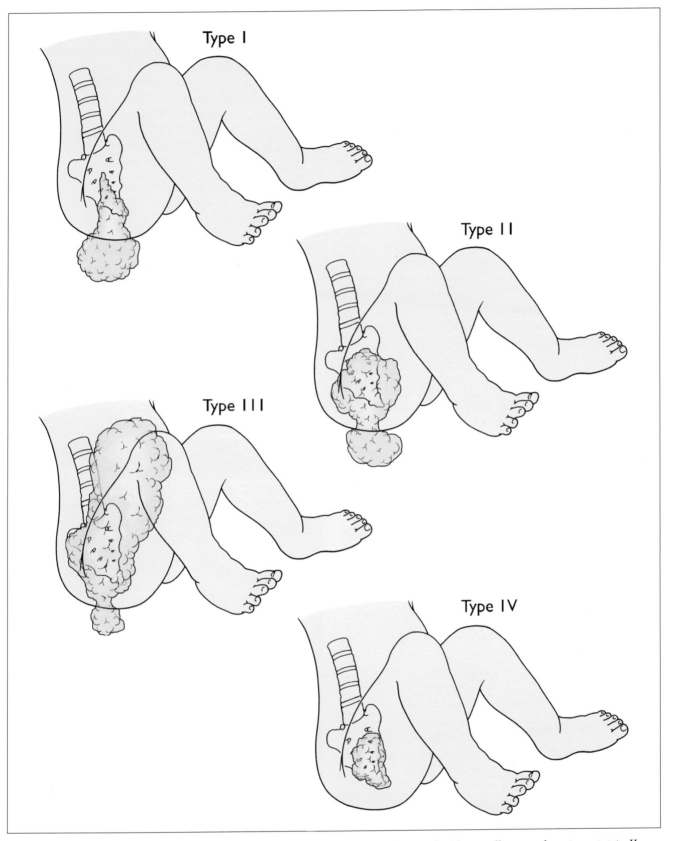

Figure 38.17. *Classification of sacrococcygeal teratomas. Type I: predominantly external with a small presacral component; type II: external with a significant intrapelvic component; type III: predominantly internal, both pelvic and intra-abdominal, with a smaller external component; and type IV, entirely presacral, without an external component or significant intraabdominal extension (Reprinted with permission from reference 49.)*

- Type IV – purely presacral tumour without an external component (10%)

The frequency of malignancy varies with the type of teratoma and age of the patient at diagnosis. Overall, about 17% of all sacrococcygeal teratomas have malignant elements.[48] The frequency of malignant elements varies from 8% for type I, 21% for type II, 34% for type III and 38% for type IV sacrococcygeal tumours.[47,48] In addition, only 2% of sacrococcygeal teratomas diagnosed in infants under 6 months of age are malignant compared with 65% of teratomas diagnosed after 6 months of age.

Pathology

The benign teratoma consists of well-differentiated tissues that are foreign to the anatomic site. The immature teratoma contains an admixture of mature and primitive neuroectodermal tissues.[46–48] Approximately 65% of sacrococcygeal tumours are mature teratomas; the remaining tumours have either immature or malignant histologies. Nearly all malignant sacrococcygeal germ cell tumours are yolk sac carcinomas.[1,47]

Metastases and staging

The most common sites of metastases are lungs and inguinal and retroperitoneal lymph nodes, followed in frequency by liver, bone and brain. Malignant sacrococcygeal teratomas are staged by the Paediatric Oncology Group/Children's Cancer Group staging system (Table 38.4).

Treatment options

Surgical excision is the mainstay of treatment. Operative management includes complete resection of the tumour and the coccyx. Complete resection suffices for benign sacrococcygeal teratomas. Malignant tumours are treated surgically and with multiagent chemotherapy.[1,47] Pelvic exenteration of malignant lesions has not been shown to increase the survival rate.

Prognosis

The long-term survival rates of children with malignant

Table 38.4. *Staging for extragonadal tumours*

Stage	Extent of disease
I	Complete resection, negative tumour margins and nodes; tumour markers positive or negative
II	Microscopic residual; lymph nodes negative; tumour markers positive or negative
III	Gross residual or biopsy only; retroperitoneal nodes negative or positive, tumour markers positive or negative
IV	Distant metastases, including liver

From reference 1.

sacrococcygeal teratomas are more than 80%.[1,47] With successful chemotherapy, malignant sacrococcygeal teratomas may regress completely, leave a small fibrotic mass, or convert to a mature teratoma.[1,50,51] An increased recurrence rate is seen if the coccyx is not resected. Immature teratomas recur more often than mature teratomas and the recurrence is more likely to be malignant.[1,47]

Imaging features

Diagnosis

Sonography is often the first study to assess pelvic and abdominal extent. Malignant tumours are likely to be either predominantly solid or complex with large areas of solid tissue. Benign sacrococcygeal tumours appear as either predominantly fluid-filled masses or as complex masses with a predominance of cystic elements and minimal amounts of solid tissue.[49]

Local staging

CT and MR imaging are superior to sonography in determining tumour extent. Malignant sacrococcygeal teratomas appear as predominantly soft tissue masses on CT (Fig. 38.18), intermediate signal intensity masses on T1-weighted images and intermediate or high signal intensity

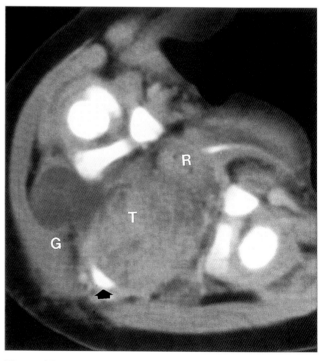

Figure 38.18. *Malignant sacrococcygeal tumour, Stage III. Computed tomography shows large soft tissue tumour (T) posterior to the rectum (R) and anterior to the sacrum (arrow). The mass invades the right internal obturator muscle, extends posteriorly behind the ischium, and invades the right gluteal muscle (G). The patient underwent biopsy for diagnosis followed by chemotherapy.*

masses on T2-weighted images and contrast-enhanced images (Fig. 38.19).[40] The tumour may contain fat, calcification, bone or teeth. Tumour margins are usually poorly defined, infiltrating adjacent soft tissue. Sacral destruction and metastatic disease are other signs of malignancy.[52] Benign teratomas, in contrast to malignant sacrococcygeal tumours, usually appear as well-defined, cystic masses con-

taining fat or a combination of fatty tissue, serous fluid, calcification, ossification, or teeth (Fig. 38.20). On T1-weighted images, fat appears as an area of high signal intensity, while serous fluid and calcifications have low signal intensity. On T2-weighted images, fat and serous fluid show high signal intensity, whereas calcifications, bone and hair demonstrate low signal intensity.

Although both CT and MR can demonstrate the extent of intrapelvic and intra-abdominal tumour, MR is better for the detection of soft tissue extension, such as the relationship of tumour to gluteal muscles and for the detection of intraspinal involvement. It is controversial whether MR is needed in neonates because most lesions are benign. Many surgeons advocate only plain radiographs and renal sonography prior to surgical resection. After 2 months of age, however, when the frequency of malignant change increases, cross-sectional imaging is recommended.

Distant staging

At the time of diagnosis, metastatic disease to abdominal viscera is evaluated by CT or MR. Potential pulmonary involvement is imaged by chest radiography and CT.

Follow-up evaluation

Follow-up evaluation includes imaging examination of the chest, abdomen and pelvis. Computed tomography is routinely performed to evaluate for pulmonary metastases and it usually suffices to image the abdomen for metastatic disease. Magnetic resonance is useful to evaluate the presence and extent of residual intraspinal, bony and soft tissue involvement. It is also used to differentiate between post-treatment fibrosis and recurrent tumour. Whereas recurrent neoplasm usually has a medium to high signal intensity on T2-weighted images, mature fibrosis (scar) has a very low signal intensity similar to that of skeletal muscle.[51]

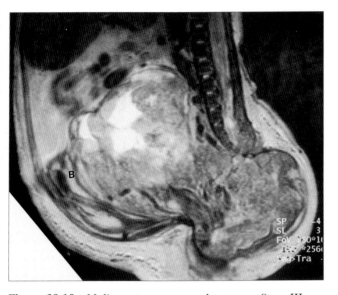

Figure 38.19. *Malignant sacrococcygeal teratoma, Stage III. Fat-suppressed T2-weighted image shows a large mass extending from the buttocks anterior to the sacrum and into the pelvis. The internal component is larger than the external component. The tumour compresses the bladder (B) and displaces it anteriorly. The predominant signal intensity of the mass is equal to that of muscle, but it contains high signal intensity areas representing necrosis. The patient underwent biopsy for diagnosis followed by chemotherapy.*

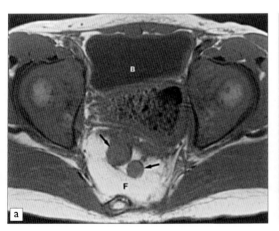 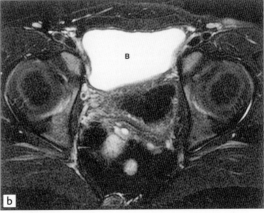

Figure 38.20. *Benign sacrococcygeal tumour. (a) Axial T1-weighted image shows a mass anterior to the sacrum and posterior to the rectum. The nodular portion of the mass (arrows) has a relatively low signal intensity equal to that of fluid, while the surrounding area has a high signal intensity equal to that of fat (F). (b) Fat-suppressed T2-weighted image. The signal intensity of the fluid components has increased, while the signal intensity of fat has decreased. B=bladder.*

Differential diagnosis

Neuroblastoma, lymphoma and anterior meningocele are other causes of a presacral mass.[40] Neuroblastoma and lymphoma appear as presacral soft tissue masses on CT and MR. Final diagnosis will require tissue sampling. Anterior meningoceles are herniations of spinal contents through a congenital defect in the vertebral body (anterior dysraphism) and are most common in the sacral region. The soft tissue contents of the herniated sac, especially the presence of a tethered cord, and the communication between the meningocele and the thecal sac can be demonstrated best with MR.

Key points: extragonadal germ cell tumours

- Sacrococcygeal tumours account for 3% of malignant neoplasms in children under the age of 17 years and 40% of all germ cell tumours

- Most sacrococcygeal tumours are benign with only 17% having malignant elements

- CT and MR are excellent for characterizing sacrococcygeal teratomas

- MR is the technique of choice for assessing local spread of malignant tumours

Testicular germ cell neoplasms

Epidemiology

With an annual incidence of 0.5–2 cases per 100,000 children, testicular tumours account for approximately 1% of all childhood malignancies and for 2–3% of solid cancers in prepubertal boys.[46,47,53] The majority of paediatric testicular tumours are of germ cell origin and most of these tumours are malignant (80%).[1] Overall, the testes account for about 20% of all germ cell tumours. Testicular tumours have a bimodal distribution, affecting very young children and adolescent boys. The median age at diagnosis of prepubertal children with malignant tumours is 2 years.[53]

Clinical presentation

Most patients with testicular tumours present with painless testicular or scrotal enlargement. If metastatic disease occurs, children may present with abdominal pain or enlargement due to nodal disease or malignant ascites or with inguinal nodes. Serum AFP and β-HCG levels are often elevated in patients with malignant testicular germ cell tumours (90% of cases).[47,53] Additional anomalies associated with testicular neoplasms include cryptorchid testes, hypospadias, contralateral testicular tumours and testicular microlithiasis.

Pathology

In prepubertal boys, testicular germ cell tumours of the testes are nearly always yolk sac tumours (endodermal sinus tumours) or benign teratomas. In adolescent boys, testicular tumours typically have histologies similar to those in adults, including embryonal carcinomas, teratocarcinomas, choriocarcinomas or seminomas.[46,47,53,54]

Metastases and clinical staging

Ninety percent or more of paediatric germ cell tumours are non-metastatic and localized to the scrotum at presentation.[1,47,53] In the remaining patients, the tumour may spread to retroperitoneal lymph nodes, lungs and liver and, rarely, to bone or brain. Right testicular tumours usually metastasize to inter-aorto-caval nodes and left testicular tumours to ipsilateral para-aortic nodes. Pulmonary metastases may occur with or without retroperitoneal nodal disease (Chapter 19).

The most widely utilized staging system for testicular germ cell tumours is one from the Children's Cancer Study Group/Paediatric Oncology Group (Table 38.5).[1,46,47,53] Approximately 80–90% of children with malignant germ cell tumours have Stage I disease; the remainder usually have Stage II or III disease. By comparison, adolescent patients with testicular tumours are more likely to have advanced stage tumour at the time of diagnosis.[47]

Treatment options

Most children and teenagers with Stage I disease are treated by radical orchidectomy alone. Chemotherapy is reserved for patients with advanced disease (e.g. metastases) and those whose tumour markers fail to decline after orchidectomy. Survival rates exceed 90%.

Imaging

Diagnosis

Sonography is the study of choice for the diagnosis of testicular tumours.[35,55–60] Sonography can define the cystic or solid

Table 38.5. *Staging of testicular germ cell tumours*

Stage	Extent of disease
I	Limited to testis (testes), completely resected with no spill; tumour markers normal
II	Trans-scrotal orchidectomy with tumour spill
	Microscopic disease in scrotum or high in spermatic cord
	Retroperitoneal lymph node involvement (≥2 cm) and/or
	Increased tumour markers after appropriate half-life decline
III	Retroperitoneal lymph node involvement (>2 cm)
	No visceral or extra-abdominal involvement
IV	Extra-abdominal lymph node metastases
	Extranodal metastases (e.g. liver, lung, peritoneum, bone, bone marrow or brain)

From references 1 and 47.

nature of a mass and its relationship to the testes. The distinction between intra- and extratesticular masses is important because the vast majority of intratesticular lesions are malignant, whereas most extratesticular lesions are benign.[37]

At sonography, CT and MR testicular tumours usually appear as discrete solid masses, but occasionally they present as diffuse testicular enlargement. On sonography, they may be hypo- or isoechoic to normal testicular tissue (Fig. 38.21). They also may be homogeneous or heterogeneous and contain calcifications or hypoechoic areas, which are due to the presence of haemorrhage or necrosis (Fig. 38.22).[35,56–58] Doppler sonography often demonstrates internal vascularity in larger tumours (> 1.5 cm); smaller tumours tend to be avascular or hypovascular.[58–60] Findings of extratesticular extension include irregularity of the tunica albuginea and reactive hydroceles. Scrotal skin thickening is rare. The combination of scrotal skin thickening and an intratesticular mass is more characteristic of an inflammatory process than a neoplasm.

Distant disease

Imaging of the chest, abdomen and pelvis are routinely performed to search for metastases. The abdomen and pelvis are evaluated by CT (Fig. 38.23) or MR. The lungs are evaluated using conventional radiographs and CT.

Follow-up evaluation

After tumour resection, sonography usually suffices for defining local scrotal recurrence, as well as assessing the status of the contralateral testis. Although the frequency is

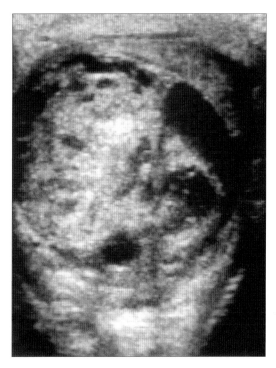

Figure 38.22. *Teratocarcinoma of the testis. A 16-year-old boy with a scrotal mass. Ultrasound scan (transverse view) of the left testis shows a heterogeneous mass composed of both solid and cystic elements. The hyperechoic foci with shadowing are calcifications.*

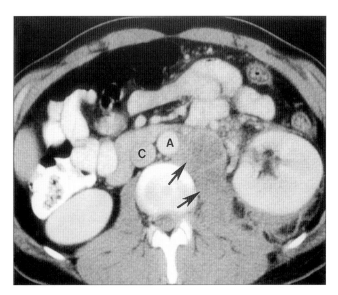

Figure 38.23. *Metastatic retroperitoneal lymphadenopathy in a patient with left testicular rhabdomyosarcoma., Stage III. Contrast-enhanced CT scan demonstrates enlarged left para-aortic lymph nodes (arrows). A=aorta; C=inferior vena cava.*

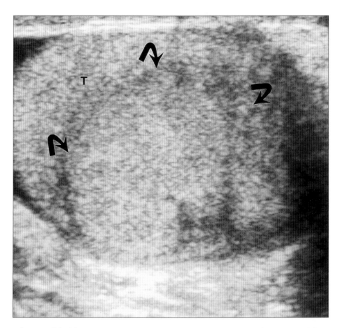

Figure 38.21. *Testicular yolk sac tumour in an 18-month-old boy with a scrotal mass, Stage I. Ultrasound scan (longitudinal view) of the right testis demonstrates a circumscribed mass (arrows) that is isoechoic to the testis (T). Tumour was localized to the testis at surgery; no extratesticular spread found.*

unknown, patients with testicular cancers are at greater risk for developing a tumour in the contralateral testis. Chest and abdominal CT are performed routinely for evaluation of lung and nodal metastases, respectively.

Differential diagnosis of primary testicular neoplasms

Approximately 10% of primary testicular neoplasms in children are stromal tumours and the vast majority of these are benign (> 90%).[53] The histologies of these tumours include Leydig cell, Sertoli cell and granulosa cell tumours. Gonadoblastoma is a rare stromal tumour (1% of all testicular tumours) that nearly always occurs in phenotypic females with streak gonads or testes and a male karyotype.[53,54,61]

Non-neoplastic intratesticular masses are rarer than primary malignant testicular tumours. These lesions include: lipoma, hemangioma, neurofibroma, cystic dysplasia, Leydig cell hyperplasia, adrenal rests, epidermoid cysts and haematomas.[35]

At sonography, the stromal and non-neoplastic testicular lesions may appear as solid, complex, or cystic masses. They cannot be differentiated on the basis of imaging, and final diagnosis requires tissue sampling.

Secondary neoplasms

Leukaemia and lymphoma are causes of secondary testicular neoplasms. Leukaemic infiltrates are found in 60–90% of children at autopsy, but they are clinically apparent only in about 8% of children.[62] Gray-scale sonography may show either a diffusely enlarged testis or focal hypoechoic lesion. Color Doppler imaging reveals intralesional flow.[35,62,63] Testicular involvement is usually bilateral, but it can be unilateral or asymmetric (Fig. 38.24).

Key points: testicular tumours

■ Testicular tumours account for 1% of all childhood malignancy, of which 80% are malignant

■ The majority of testicular neoplasms in childhood are germ cell tumours, most being yolk sac (endodermal sinus) neoplasms

■ Most children with a germ cell tumour have elevated serum alpha protein levels

■ 90% of testicular tumours are localized at diagnosis

■ Metastatic disease occurs in less than 10% of patients and is to lymph nodes and lungs

■ Ultrasonography is highly reliable in detecting testicular tumours and in distinguishing between intra- and extratesticular masses

■ CT is the technique of choice for staging testicular cancer spread to lymph nodes and distant sites

Ovarian germ cell tumours

Epidemiology

Ovarian tumours account for 1% of cancers in girls under 17 years of age and the vast majority of these are germ cell tumours.[47,64,65] Approximately two thirds are benign and one third are malignant.[1] Ovarian tumours account for about 25% of all paediatric germ cell tumours. Most ovarian germ cell tumours are diagnosed late in the first decade of life, with a peak age incidence at diagnosis of 10 years.[1]

Clinical presentation

Most patients with ovarian tumours present with a palpable abdominal or pelvic mass or pain, which may be severe if there is associated torsion of the ovarian pedicle. Other presenting findings include constipation, amenorrhoea and

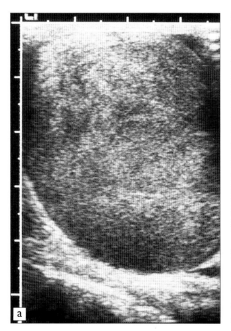
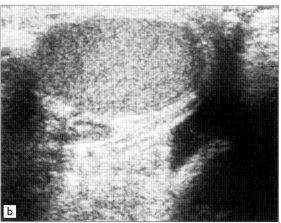

Figure 38.24. *Testicular lymphoma. Ultrasound scans of (a) longitudinal view of the scrotum shows a diffusely enlarged, mildly heterogeneous left testis. Testicular biopsy confirmed lymphoma. (b) Normal right testis for comparison.*

vaginal bleeding. In cases of metastatic disease, patients may present with abdominal swelling due to ascites. The serum levels of AFP and HCG levels usually are elevated in patients with germ cell tumours with malignant elements.

Pathology

Dysgerminoma and endodermal sinus tumour account for almost 90% of malignant ovarian neoplasms in children. Immature teratomas (containing embryonic elements, mostly prominently neural cell) account for approximately 10% of ovarian malignancies. Tumours of stromal cell origin (Sertoli–Leydig cell, granulosa–theca cell and undifferentiated neoplasms) and epithelial carcinomas are extremely rare in children.[46,47,65–68]

Clinical staging

Malignant ovarian neoplasms spread by contiguous extension, lymphogenous spread, or haematogenous dissemination. Ovarian germ cell tumours usually metastasize to liver, lungs and lymph nodes; metastases to bone and peritoneal surfaces are rare. Ovarian germ cell tumours are staged using the Children's Oncology Group system (Table 38.6). Epithelial neoplasms are staged by the International Federation of Gynecology and Obstetrics (FIGO) staging system (Table 38.7). Unlike germ cell tumours, epithelial tumours commonly metastasize to peritoneal surfaces and omentum.

Treatment

Treatment is complete resection of the primary tumour whenever possible. Otherwise, surgical debulking or biopsy is performed followed by chemotherapy and definitive resection.

Table 38.6. *Staging of ovarian germ cell tumours: Children's Oncology Group staging*

Stage	Extent of disease
I	Limited to ovary (ovaries)
	Peritoneal washings negative for malignant cells
	Tumour markers normal
II	Microscopic residual or positive lymph nodes (≤2) cm
	Negative peritoneal washings
	Tumour markers positive or negative
III	Lymph node involvement >2 cm
	Gross residual tumour or biopsy only
	Contiguous visceral involvement (omentum, intestine, bladder)
	Peritoneal washings positive for malignant cells
	Tumour markers positive or negative
IV	Distant metastases, including liver

From references 1 and 47.

Table 38.7. *Ovarian tumour staging system, after FIGO*

Stage	Extent of disease
I	Tumour limited to the ovaries
Ia	Growth limited to one ovary; no ascites. No tumour on the external surface; capsule intact
Ib	Growth limited to both ovaries; no ascites. No tumour on the external surface; capsule intact
Ic	Stage Ia or Ib but with tumour on surface of ovary; or with capsule rupture, or with ascites or with positive peritoneal washings
II	Tumour involving one or both ovaries with pelvic extension
IIa	Extension and/or metastases to the uterus and/or tubes
IIb	Extension to other pelvic tissues
IIc	Staging IIa or IIb with ascites or positive peritoneal washings
III	Tumour involving one or both ovaries with metastases outside the pelvis and/or positive nodes; extension to small bowel or omentum; superficial liver metastases
IV	Tumour involving one or both ovaries with distant metastases; parenchymal liver metastases; pleural effusion with positive cytology

From reference 47.

Prognosis

Approximately 75% of patients with malignant ovarian neoplasms have Stage I disease at diagnosis. Survival rates exceed 90% for localized disease and 80% for more advanced stage disease.[46,47,64]

Imaging

Diagnosis

The diagnosis of an ovarian mass usually is established by sonography. Sonographic findings of ovarian malignancy include a solid mass with central necrosis and thickened irregular septae or papillary projections (Fig. 38.25).[69]

Local staging

Computed tomography findings of malignant ovarian lesions include:

- A predominantly soft tissue attenuation mass (> 50% soft tissue elements)
- Thick, irregular walls
- Low-attenuation areas due to necrosis or haemorrhage (Fig. 38.26)
- Thick septa
- Papillary projections[70–73]

Irregular, coarse calcifications are common in both dysgerminomas and immature or malignant teratomas. At MR, malignant ovarian tumours commonly have a low to inter-

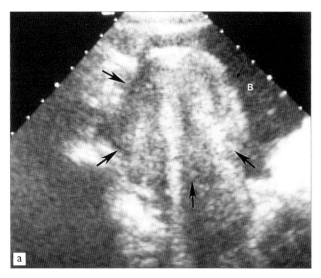

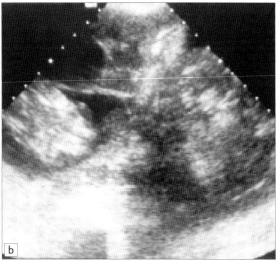

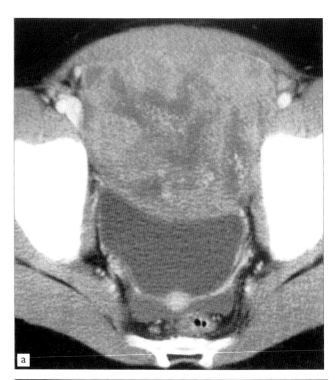

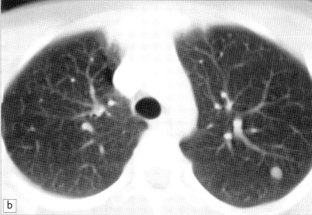

Figure 38.25. *Ovarian neoplasms, ultrasound. (a) Ovarian dysgerminoma. An 11-year-old girl with pelvic pain. Longitudinal view of the pelvis shows an echogenic mass (arrows) in the area of the right adnexa. B = bladder. (b) Teratocarcinoma. A 7-year-old girl with a pelvic mass. The transverse image of the lower abdomen shows a complex mass that is predominantly solid. The tumour contains cystic areas representing haemorrhage or necrosis. Both tumours show a predominance of soft tissue components, which is typical of malignant lesions.*

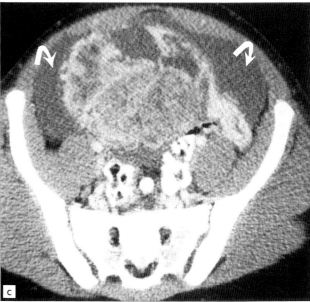

Figure 38.26. *Ovarian neoplasms, CT. (a) Ovarian dysgerminoma. Contrast-enhanced CT shows a heterogeneous mass displacing bladder posteriorly. (b) Chest CT of the same patient shows a pulmonary metastasis in the left upper lobe. (c) Ovarian yolk sac tumour. Contrast-enhanced CT shows a poorly defined tumour with solid and cystic (arrows) areas displacing bowel posteriorly.*

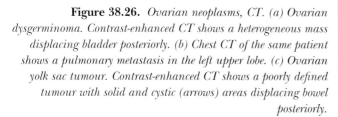

mediate signal intensity on T1-weighted images and intermediate or high signal intensity on T2-weighted and gadolinium-enhanced images (Fig. 38.27).[74–76] Multiple lobules and fibrovascular septa can be noted in ovarian dysgerminomas. These are hypo- or isointense on T1-weighted images and show marked enhancement after administration of gadolinium chelates.[76]

Distant staging

The staging evaluation should include CT of the chest and abdomen and also bone scintigraphy. CT appears to be more sensitive than MR in identifying small lymph nodes and peritoneal and mesenteric implants.[74] Peritoneal tumour implants appear as soft tissue nodules on the lateral peritoneal surfaces or in the ligaments and mesenteries of the abdomen. Omental implants appear as nodules or conglomerate masses ('omental cake') beneath the anterior abdominal wall. They may enhance after IV administration of iodinated contrast agents or gadolinium chelates. Peritoneal seeding is more common with immature teratomas than with the other germ cell neoplasms.

Follow-up evaluation

Computed tomography suffices for follow-up evaluation after surgical or medical therapy to detect residual or recurrent local disease, abdominal nodal disease and pulmonary and liver metastases.

Following chemotherapy, immature ovarian teratomas may undergo maturation. The CT findings that suggest maturation are increasing density of the tumour mass, the development of internal calcification, cystic areas or fatty areas and more sharply circumscribed tumour margins.[77]

Other ovarian neoplasms

Approximately two thirds of all ovarian tumours are benign and virtually always mature cystic teratomas. The CT diagnosis of benign teratoma is based on identification of a predominantly cystic mass containing fat or a combination of fatty tissue, calcification, ossification or teeth, and minimal soft tissue components (Fig. 38.28).[71–73] Calcific elements and fat are usually located in a Rokitansky protuberance or dermoid plug arising from the cyst wall. At MR, benign teratomas are typically hypointense relative to muscle on T1-weighted images, although they may have a higher signal intensity due to the presence of protein-filled fluid. On T2-weighted images, they generally are extremely bright with a signal intensity equal to cerebrospinal fluid.[73,75,78] Foci of fatty tissue have a high signal intensity on both T1- and T2-weighted images, while calcifications, teeth, bone, hair and fibrous tissue show low signal intensity on both pulse sequences. The presence of fat within these lesions allows a specific diagnosis of teratoma.

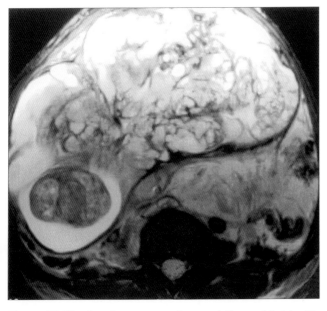

Figure 38.27. *Ovarian teratocarcinoma. A 9-year-old girl with weight loss and abdominal distension. Fat-suppressed T2-weighted MR axial image shows a large complex mass with areas of high and intermediate signal intensity, corresponding to solid tumour tissue.*

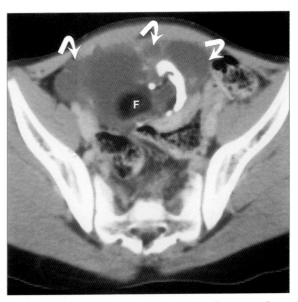

Figure 38.28. *Benign ovarian teratoma. Contrast-enhanced CT shows a complex mass (arrows) of mostly fluid attenuation in the mid pelvis. Lower attenuation density corresponding to fat (F) and thick calcifications are seen within the mass. The cystic appearance and predominantly fluid contents is characteristic of benign teratomas.*

Key points: ovarian tumours

- Ovarian tumours account for 1% of neoplasms in children under the age of 17 years, of which 30% are malignant

- Nearly all malignant neoplasms are germ cell tumours, of which dysgerminoma and yolk sac tumours are most common

- Stromal cell and epithelial tumours are extremely rare ovarian tumours in children

- AFP and HCG levels are elevated in children with malignant germ cell tumours, especially those with embryonal carcinoma

- CT is superior to sonography for characterizing ovarian masses and determining local spread

- CT of the chest is required to detect pulmonary metastases

Summary

- Malignant hepatic tumours are more common than benign; most are hepatoblastomas or hepatocellular carcinomas

- Hepatic malignancy metastasizes to portal lymph nodes, lungs and occasionally bone

- MR with contrast enhancement is the technique of choice for staging hepatic tumours in childhood

- Rhabdomyosarcoma is the most common soft tissue tumour of childhood

- Rhabdomyosarcoma metastasizes to the lungs, bone and liver

- Sacrococcygeal teratomas are the most common germ cell tumour of childhood

- Treatment of malignant sacrococcygeal tumours is complete resection with or without neoadjuvant chemotherapy depending on local extent

- MR is the best technique for assessing local extent of sacrococcygeal tumours

- Testicular tumours account for 1% of all childhood malignancies

- Metastases are predominantly to the abdominal lymph nodes and the lungs

- Ovarian tumours account for 1% of all childhood malignancies below 17 years

- 60–90% of malignant ovarian tumours are germ cell tumours

- CT is the investigation of choice for staging ovarian tumours

References

1. Ebb D H, Green D M, Shamberger R C, Tarbell N J. Solid tumors of childhood. In: DeVita V T Jr, Hellman S, Rosenberg S A (eds). Cancer: Principles and Practice of Oncology, 6th edn. Philadelphia: Lippincott Williams & Wilkins, 2001; 2169–2214

2. Stocker J T. Hepatic tumors in children. Clin Liver Dis 2001; 5: 259–281

3. Tomlinson G E, Finegold M J. Tumors of the liver. In: Pizzo P A, Poplack D C (eds). Principles and Practice of Pediatric Oncology, 4th edn. Philadelphia: Lippincott Williams & Wilkins; 2002; 847–864

4. Weinberg A G, Finegold M J. Primary hepatic tumors of childhood. Human Pathol 1983; 14: 512–537

5. Finegold M J. Tumors of the liver. Semin Liver Dis 1994; 14: 270–281

6. Chen J C, Chen C C, Chen W J et al. Hepatocellular carcinoma in children: clinical review and comparison with adult cases. J Pediatr Surg 1998; 33: 1350–1354

7. Stringer M D, Hennayake S, Howard E R et al. Improved outcome for children with hepatoblastoma. Br J Surg 1995; 82: 386–391

8. Erlich P R, Greenberg M L, Filler R M. Improved long-term survival with preoperative chemotherapy for hepatoblastoma. J Pediatr Surg 1997; 32: 999–1003

9. Reynolds M. Conversion of unresectable to resectable hepatoblastoma and long-term follow-up study. World J Surg 1995; 19: 814–816

10. Davey M S, Cohen M D. Imaging of gastrointestinal malignancy in childhood. Radiol Clin North Am 1996; 34: 717–742

11. Siegel M J. Liver. In: Siegel MJ (ed). Pediatric Sonography, 3rd edn. Philadelphia

12. Donnelly L F, Bisset G S III. Pediatric hepatic imaging. Radiol Clin North Am 1998; 36: 413–427

13. Jabra A A, Fishman E K, Taylor G A. Hepatic masses in infants and children: CT evaluation. Am J Roentgenol 1992; 158: 143–149

14. Pobiel R S, Bisset G S III. Pictorial essay: imaging of

liver tumors in the infant and child. Pediatr Radiol 1995; 25: 495–506

15. Powers C, Ross P R, Stoupis C et al. Primary liver neoplasms: MR imaging with pathologic correlation. RadioGraphics 1994: 14: 459–482

16. Rummeny E, Weissleder R, Stark D D et al. Primary liver tumors: diagnosis by MR imaging. Am J Roentgenol 1989; 152: 63–72

17. King S J, Babyn P S, Greenberg M L et al. Value of CT in determining the resectability of hepatoblastoma before and after chemotherapy. Am J Roentgenol 1993; 160: 793–798

18. Siegel M J. Liver and biliary tract. In: Siegel MJ (ed). Pediatric Body CT. Philadelphia: Lippincott Williams Wilkins, 1999; 141–174

19. Siegel M J. Pediatric liver imaging. Semin Liver Dis 2001; 21: 251–269

20. Siegel M J. Pediatric liver magnetic resonance imaging. Magn Reson Imaging Clin N Am 2002; 10: 253–273

21. Ichikawa T, Federle M P, Grazioli L et al. Fibrolamellar hepatocellular carcinoma: imaging and pathologic findings in 31 recent cases. Radiology 1999; 213: 352–361

22. Ichikawa T, Federle M P, Grazioli L, Marsh W. Fibrolamellar hepatocellular carcinoma: Pre- and post-therapy evaluation with CT and MR imaging. Radiology 2000; 217: 145–151

23. McLarney J K, Rucker P T, Bender G N et al. Fibrolamellar carcinoma of the liver: radiologic–pathologic correlation. RadioGraphics 1999; 19: 453–471

24. Stevens W R, Johnson C D, Stephens D H, Nogorney D M. Fibrolamellar hepatocellular carcinomas: stage at presentation and results of aggressive surgical management. Am J Roentgenol 1995; 164: 1153–1158

25. Lack E E, Schloo B L, Azumi N et al. Undifferentiated (embryonal) sarcoma of the liver. Clinical and pathologic study of 16 cases with emphasis on immunohistochemical features. Am J Surg Pathol 1991; 15: 1–16

26. Buetow P C, Buck J L, Pantongrag-Brown L et al. Undifferentiated (embryonal) sarcoma of the liver: pathologic basis of imaging findings in 28 cases. Radiology 1997; 203: 779–783

27. Roebuck D J, Yang W T, Lam W W M, Stanely P. Hepatobiliary rhabdomyosarcoma in children: diagnostic radiology. Pediatr Radiol 1998; 28: 101–108

28. Sanz N, de Mingo L, Florez F, Rollan V. Rhabdomyosarcoma of the biliary tree. Pediatr Surg Int 1997; 12: 200–201

29. Selby D M, Stocker J T, Waclawiw M A et al. Infantile hemangioendothelioma of the liver. Hepatology 1994; 20: 39–45

30. Kesslar P J, Buck J L, Selby D M. Infantile hemangioendothelioma of the liver revisited. RadioGraphics 1993; 13: 657–670

31. Koumanidou C, Vakaki M, Papadaki M et al. New sonographic appearance of hepatic mesenchymal hamartoma in childhood. J Clin Ultrasound 1999; 27: 164–167

32. Argons G A, Wagner B J, Lonergan G J et al. Genitourinary rhabdomyosarcoma in children: radiologic–pathologic correlation. RadioGraphics 1997; 17: 919–937

33. Wexler L H, Crist W M, Helman L J. Rhabdomyosarcoma and the undifferentiated sarcomas. In: Pizzo P A, Poplack D G (eds). Principles and Practice of Pediatric Oncology, 4th edn. Philadelphia: Lippincott Williams & Wilkins; 2002; 943–971

34. Lawrence W, Anderson J R, Gehan E A, Maurer H. Pretreatment TNM staging of childhood rhabdomyosarcoma: a report of the Intergroup Rhabdomyosarcoma Study Group. Cancer 1997; 80: 1165–1170

35. Coley B D, Siegel M J. Male genital tract. In: Siegel M J (ed). Pediatric Sonography, 3rd edn. Philadelphia. Lippincott Williams & Wilkins. 2001; 579–624

36. Frates M C, Benson C B, DiSalvo D N et al. Solid extratesticular masses evaluated with sonography: pathologic correlation. Radiology 1997; 204: 43–46

37. Woodward P J, Schwab C M, Sesterhenn I A. Extratesticular scrotal masses: radiologic–pathologic correlation. RadioGraphics 2003; 23: 215–240

38. Finelli A, Babyn P, McLorie G A et al. The use of magnetic resonance imaging in the diagnosis and follow up of pediatric pelvic rhabdomyosarcoma. J Urol 2000; 163: 1952–1953

39. Fletcher B D, Kaste S C. Magnetic resonance imaging for diagnosis and follow-up of genitourinary, pelvic, and perineal rhabdomyosarcoma. Urol Radiol 1992; 14: 262–272

40. Siegel M J, Hoffer F A. Magnetic resonance imaging of nongynecologic pelvic masses in children. Magn Reson Imaging Clin N Am 2002; 10: 325–344

41. Tannous W N, Azouz E M, Homsy Y L et al. CT and ultrasound imaging of pelvic rhabdomyosarcoma in children: a review of 56 patients. Pediatr Radiol 1989; 19: 5330–534

42. Mazumdar O, Siegel M J, Narra V, Luchtman-Jones L. Whole-body fast inversion recovery MR imaging of small cell neoplasms in pediatric patients. Am J Roentgenol 2002; 179: 1261–1266

43. Daldrup-Link H E, Franzius C, Link T M et al. Whole body MR imaging for detection of bone metastases in children and young adults: comparison with skeletal scintigraphy and FDG PET. Am J Roentgenol 2001; 177: 229–236

44. Green C L, Angtuaco T L, Shah H R, Pamley T H. Gestational trophoblastic disease: a spectrum of radiologic diagnosis. RadioGraphics 1996; 16: 1371–1384

45. Wagner B J, Woodward P H, Dickey G E. Gestational trophoblastic disease: radiologic–pathologic correlation. RadioGraphics 1996; 16: 131–148

46. Castleberry R P, Kelly D R, Joseph D B, Cain W S. Gonadal and extragonadal germ cell tumors. In: Fernbach D J,

Vietti T J (eds). Clinical Pediatric Oncology, 4th edn. St Louis: Mosby-Year Book, 1991; 577–594

47. Cushing B, Perlman E J, Marina N M, Castleberry R P. Germ cell tumors. In: Pizzo P A, Poplack D G (eds). Principles and Practice of Pediatric Oncology, 4th edn. Philadelphia: Lippincott Williams and Wilkins, 2002; 1091–1113

48. Altman R P, Randolph J G, Lilly J R. Sacrococcygeal teratoma. American Academy of Pediatrics surgical section survey – 1973. J Pediatr Surg 1974; 9: 389

49. Siegel M J. Adrenal glands, pancreas, and other retroperitoneal structures. In: Siegel M J (ed). Paediatric Sonography, 3rd edn. Philadelphia: Lippincott Williams & Wilkins, 2002

50. Cranston P E, Smith E E, Hamrick-Turner J. Emergence of mature teratoma following treatment of sacrococcygeal endodermal sinus tumor: CT and MR imaging with pathological correlation. Pediatr Radiol 1994; 24: 239–240

51. Kaste S C, Bridges J O, Marina N M. Sacrococcygeal yolk sac carcinoma: imaging findings during treatment. Pediatr Radiol 1996; 26: 212–219

52. Kesslar P J, Buck J L, Suarez E S. Germ cell tumours of the sacrococcygeal region: radiologic–pathologic correlation. RadioGraphics 1994; 14: 607–620

53. Skoog S J. Benign and malignant pediatric scrotal masses. Pediatr Clin North Am 1997;44: 1229–1250

54. Coffin C M, Dehner L P. The male reproductive system. In: Stocker J T (ed). Pediatric Pathology. Philadelphia: JB Lippincott, 1992; 905–919

55. Frush D P, Sheldon C A. Diagnostic imaging for pediatric scrotal disorders. Radiographics 1998; 18: 969–985

56. Geraghty M J, Lee F T Jr, Bernsten S A et al. Sonography of testicular tumors and tumor-like conditions: a radiologic–pathologic correlation. Crit Rev Diagn Imaging 1998; 39: 1–63

57. Hamm B. Differential diagnosis of scrotal masses by ultrasound. Eur Radiol 1997; 7: 668–679

58. Luker G D, Siegel M J. Pediatric testicular tumors: evaluation with gray-scale and color Doppler US. Radiology 1994; 191: 561–564

59. Luker G D, Siegel M J. Color Doppler sonography of the scrotum in children. Am J Roentgenol 1994; 163: 649–655

60. Luker G D, Siegel M J. Scrotal US in pediatric patients: comparison of power and standard color Doppler US. Radiology 1996; 198: 381–385.

61. Scully R E. Gonadoblastoma: review of 74 cases. Cancer 1970; 25: 1340–1356

62. Golan G, Lebensart P D, Lossos I S. Ultrasound diagnosis and follow-up of testicular monocytic leukemia. J Clin Ultrasound 1997; 25: 453–455

63. Mazzu D, Jeffrey R B, Ralls P W. Lymphoma and leukemia involving the testicles: findings on gray-scale and color Doppler sonography. Am J Roentgenol 1995; 164: 645–647

64. Miller R W, Young J L Jr, Novakovic B. Childhood cancer. Cancer 1995; 75: 395–405

65. Cronen P W, Nagaraj H S. Ovarian tumors in children. South Med J 1988; 81: 464–468

66. Brown M F, Hebra A, McGeehin K et al. Ovarian masses in children: a review of 91 cases of malignant and benign masses. J Pediatr Surg 1993; 28: 930–932

67. Gribbon M, Ein S H, Mancer K. Pediatric malignant ovarian tumors: a 43-year review. J Pediatr Surg 1992; 27: 480–484

68. Raney R B, Sinclair L, Uri A et al. Malignant ovarian tumors in children and adolescents. Cancer 1987; 59: 1214–1220

69. Siegel M J. Female pelvis. In: Siegel M J (ed). Pediatric Sonography, 3rd edn. Philadelphia: Lippincott Williams & Wilkins, 2002; 530–577

70. Brammer H M, Buck J L, Hayes W S et al. Malignant germ cell tumors of the ovary: radiologic–pathologic correlation. RadioGraphics 1990; 10: 715–724

71. Jabra A A, Fishman E K, Taylor G A. Primary ovarian tumors in the pediatric patient: CT evaluation. Clin Imaging 1993; 17: 199–203

72. Quillin S P, Siegel M J. CT features of benign and malignant teratomas in children. J Comput Assist Tomogr 1992; 16: 722–726

73. Surratt J T, Siegel M J. Imaging of pediatric ovarian masses. RadioGraphics 1991; 11: 533–548

74. Ghossain M A, Buy N J, Ligneres C et al. Epithelial tumors of the ovary: comparison of MR and CT findings. Radiology 1991; 181: 863–870

75. Siegel M J. Magnetic resonance imaging of the adolescent female pelvis. Magn Reson Imaging Clin North Am 2002; 10: 303–324

76. Tanaka Y O, Kurosaki Y, Nishida M et al. Ovarian dysgerminoma: MR and CT appearance. J Comput Assist Tomogr 1994; 18: 443–448

77. Moskovic E, Jobling T, Fisher C et al. Retroconversion of immature teratoma of the ovary: CT appearances. Clin Radiol 1991; 43: 402–408

78. Togashi K, Nishimura K, Itoh K et al. Ovarian cystic teratomas: MR imaging. Radiology 1987; 162: 669–673

Part V

METASTASES

Chapter 39

Lymph node metastases

Bernadette M Carrington

Introduction

Lymphatic dissemination is one of the three principal pathways by which tumours escape from their organ of origin, the others being direct local infiltration and haematogenous spread. Lymph node metastases are a strong adverse prognostic indicator in many tumours and identification of nodal metastases is therefore an essential part of each patient's staging procedure prior to definitive treatment. The presence of nodal involvement at the time of staging may alter patient management radically.

Lymph node metastases are frequently detected at surgery in the commoner tumours; for example, in bowel cancer, locoregional lymph node involvement is seen in 40–50% of patients at the time of surgical resection of the primary tumour.[1,2] In breast cancer, the figure is 50%[3] and, in patients thought to have surgically resectable non-small cell lung cancer, up to 20% are found to have positive nodes at surgery.[4] In the treated patient, lymph node relapse is a common finding and involved nodes occur at expected sites and sometimes in unusual locations as a result of treatment-induced modification of the disease process.

Assessment of nodal status at the same time as imaging the primary tumour for staging and follow-up is mandatory. In order to provide the best possible results it is important that the radiologist understands the physiological processes occurring in the lymphatic system, has knowledge of the preferential lymphatic drainage of each primary tumour and is familiar with the established imaging criteria for normal lymph node appearances. Furthermore, lymph nodes need to be differentiated from normal anatomical structures or variants and the more unusual sites of lymphadenopathy must also be considered and reviewed on cross-sectional imaging.

The lymphatic system

Tissue fluid accumulates in the extravascular spaces of the body due to high-pressure capillary filtration and the excess fluid is then returned to the vascular system via lymphatic pathways. En route the lymph fluid passes through a series of lymphatic channels and lymph nodes before ultimately draining into the subclavian vein through the thoracic duct. The larger lymphatics accompany the arteries and veins of a particular organ or structure and drain into the locoregional lymph nodes. Lymph nodes are situated at the confluence of several lymphatics, where they lie more or less parallel to major blood vessels and act as complex filters for antigenic material. In superficial locations, for example the neck, the number of nodes varies tremendously but in visceral sites the number of nodes is more constant.

Within each lymph node there are multiple, afferent lymphatics which pass through a collagenous capsule along the convex nodal surface. From these afferent lymphatics lymph fluid drains directly into the subcapsular sinus of the node which is located immediately deep to the capsule and extends along penetrating fibrous trabeculae to provide a route for transcortical extension of lymph into the medulla. Lymph leaves the node via a small number of efferent lymphatic ducts situated at the nodal hilum (Fig. 39.1).

Lymph nodes are in a continual state of physiological flux with varying inflow and outflow of lymph, blood and lymphocytes:

- Lymph: up to 10 ml/hr/g nodal weight
- Blood: 1 ml/min/g nodal weight
- Each node recirculates its own weight of lymphocytes every 4–12 days, depending on antigenic stimulation[5]

The anatomical site and degree of stimulation by outside factors, for example infection, influence the gross morphological appearance of lymph nodes.[5] Thus, axillary nodes may be almost entirely replaced by fat with only a thin peripheral rim of lymphatic tissue (Fig. 39.2a), inguinal nodes may have a target appearance also due to fatty infiltration (Fig. 39.2b) and focal scarring and calcification may be seen in areas of hyaline fibrosis.[5] Mesenteric nodes are extremely active, manifesting as hypercellular nodes with large numbers of follicles.[5]

Mechanism of tumour spread to lymph nodes

Most tumours do not develop new lymph vessels; lymphatic infiltration therefore occurs either by direct macroscopic tumour invasion of adjacent host lymphatics, or at the cellular level by cancer cells invaginating through the

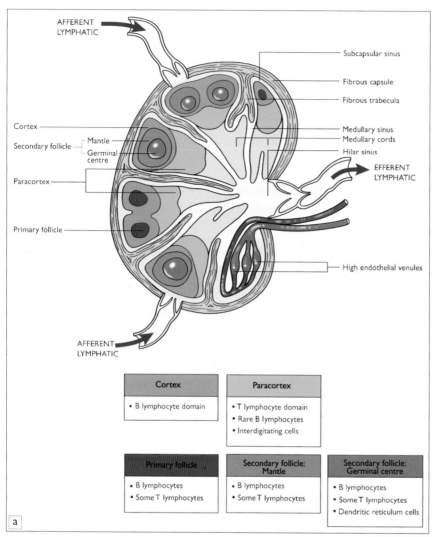

Cortex	Paracortex
• B lymphocyte domain	• T lymphocyte domain • Rare B lymphocytes • Interdigitating cells

Primary follicle	Secondary follicle: Mantle	Secondary follicle: Germinal centre
• B lymphocytes • Some T lymphocytes	• B lymphocytes • Some T lymphocytes	• B lymphocytes • Some T lymphocytes • Dendritic reticulum cells

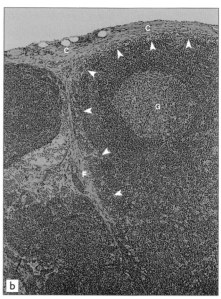

Figure 39.1. *The normal lymph node. (a) Cross-section through a normal lymph node. (b) Photomicrograph of a normal lymph node (haematoxylin and eosin). The capsule (C) is well seen as is the subcapsular sinus (arrowheads) which extends deep into the node alongside the fibrous trabecula Germinal centre.*

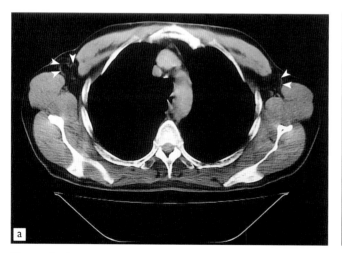

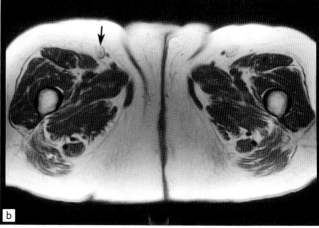

Figure 39.2. *Fatty lymph nodes. (a) Transaxial thoracic CT scan demonstrating crescents of lymphoid tissue (arrowheads) in otherwise fatty nodes. (b) Transaxial T1-weighted MR image showing a target appearance to a right inguinal node (arrow).*

lymphatic endothelium of adjacent lymphatic channels.[6] Once in the lymphatic vessel, tumour cells migrate to the nearest lymph node where they are usually arrested in the subcapsular sinus (Fig. 39.3).[5,6] Most clusters of tumour cells die rapidly[6] but a small percentage colonise the node and ultimately replace the node completely. The nodal

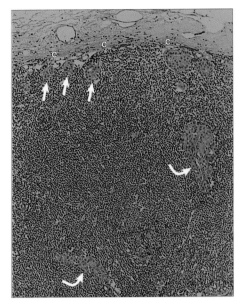

Figure 39.3. *Subcapsular sinus tumour deposits (haematoxylin and eosin). Multiple small tumour deposits (arrows) are identified within the subcapsular sinus in a patient with metastatic breast cancer. Some of these deposits measure 5 microns or less. Larger deposits are seen (curved arrows) deeper within the substance of the gland. C-capsule*

metastasis may eventually penetrate the nodal capsule and extend into the adjacent tissues. Sometimes, tumour cells pass through the lymph node without being arrested, leaving via the efferent lymphatics or venules. These cells then spread to other nodal stations or circulate within the bloodstream. The process is enhanced by the presence of preexisting deposits within the node as this reduces the involved node's filtering capability, allowing new tumour emboli effectively to bypass that node and reach other sites more easily.[7] Malignant cells within the bloodstream may then lead to the development of disseminated metastases in blood-borne sites.

Key points: general features

- Lymph node metastases are always an adverse prognostic indicator

- Most tumours cannot develop their own lymphatic system

- Tumours penetrate the lymphatic channels by direct erosion or tumour cell invagination through the lymphatic endothelium

- Tumour cells migrate to the nearest lymph node when metastatic colonies develop in the subcapsular sinus

Radiological evaluation of lymph node metastases

In clinical practice, the cross-sectional imaging modalities computed tomography (CT), ultrasound and MR imaging are widely used to assess lymph nodes and the diagnosis of nodal metastases rests on features such as nodal size and limited assessment of tissue characteristics. Unfortunately, it is well recognized that, for most primary tumours, 10–20% of normal-sized locoregional nodes will contain small tumour deposits[8–10] and, conversely, that over 30% of enlarged nodes will show only inflammatory hyperplasia.[9,11] In certain tumour types the incidence of metastatic normal-sized nodes is greater than in others; for example in colorectal cancer two thirds of nodal metastases occur in nodes <5 mm and 90% in nodes <1 cm.[1] Therefore the ideal imaging technique would allow identification of small, even microscopic, tumour deposits. Historically, lymphangiography has been used to detect tumour deposits in normal-sized nodes.[12] Advocates of lymphangiography claimed a significant advantage over CT in staging Hodgkin's disease but other studies showed poor diagnostic information from lymphangiography in Hodgkin's disease and testicular tumours.[13,14] Moreover, lymphangiography is technically demanding, not all nodal sites opacify and it requires considerable expertise in undertaking the procedure and in interpretation of the results. For all these reasons it is no longer used in most centres.

MR lymphography, using ultrasmall superparamagnetic iron oxide (SPIO) contrast agents, may be used to aid identification of intranodal metastatic deposits but is not yet available for routine use.[15,16]

The choice of imaging will depend on local expertise, the availability of each imaging modality and the primary tumour being assessed. For example, high-resolution ultrasound may be used for assessment of inguinal nodes in a patient with a peripheral melanoma, or for neck nodal status in a patient with head and neck cancer. Computed tomography or MR are the most commonly used initial imaging investigations in patients with primary malignancies of the thorax, abdomen and pelvis as, with satisfactory patient preparation and meticulous imaging technique, these modalities provide a reliable and non-invasive means of lymph node evaluation. Functional imaging techniques are assuming greater importance, particularly 2-[F-18]fluoro-2-deoxy-D-glucose positron emission tomography ([18]FDG PET), which detects metabolic changes that occur in metastatic nodes. [18]FDG PET has demonstrated advantages in lymph node assessment of several primary tumours and is likely to have an increasingly important role in the future.

Anatomical cross-sectional imaging

Computed tomography

Body coverage must include the known sites of lymph node metastases for any given tumour. For example, ovarian cancer can spread to diaphragmatic nodes,[17] so it is important that the examination extends from the xiphisternum to the pelvis. For anal canal tumours, the inferior extent of any examination must include the inguinal nodes. Meticulous radiographic technique is crucial for accurate interpretation and there must be thorough bowel preparation, contiguous or near contiguous slices and standardized window levels and window widths for all hard copy images. Intravenous (IV) contrast medium is used routinely in most centres and facilitates the distinction between lymph nodes and vessels. Efforts should be made to rule out diagnostic uncertainty; for example if, when using positive bowel contrast, the loops of bowel are poorly opacified, the patient should be rescanned through the relevant area after an interval, or scanned in the decubitus position. Water is being used increasingly as a negative oral contrast agent, because bowel wall enhancement is readily recognized, particularly when using multidetector CT. Caution should be exercised, however, when using this technique for assessing tumours which produce low density or 'cystic' nodal deposits, e.g. ovarian or testicular tumours.

Magnetic resonance

On MR, lymph nodes are best seen on T1-weighted images, where their intermediate signal intensity contrasts well with the high signal intensity of the surrounding fat.[18] Nodes become less conspicuous on T2-weighted images due to convergence of the signal intensity returned by the nodes and the surrounding fat. Short tau inversion recovery (STIR) sequences increase the signal intensity of lymph nodes relative to the adjacent suppressed pelvic fat. High-resolution images using a slice thickness of 3–4 mm also provide improved nodal delineation but usually require local surface coils to maintain a satisfactory signal-to-noise ratio.

The MR examination must cover the entire pathway of locoregional spread of the tumour being examined; for example, both the abdomen and pelvis need to be imaged in pelvic malignancies, and the entire neck for assessment of head and neck tumours. This approach may result in relatively long examination times compared with CT but advances in technology are continuing to reduce scanning times and most examinations can now be completed in an acceptable time period.

Magnetic resonance has the potential advantage that lymph nodes can be differentiated from blood vessels readily without the use of IV contrast medium because the intravascular signal void due to flowing blood is different from the signal intensity of lymph nodes (Fig. 39.4). Sometimes slow blood flow in an ectatic vein may simulate an enlarged lymph node, but this diagnostic dilemma can be solved by use of flow-sensitive techniques such as gradient recall echo imaging.

Magnetic resonance-specific bowel contrast medium is now available although it is not used routinely in most cen-

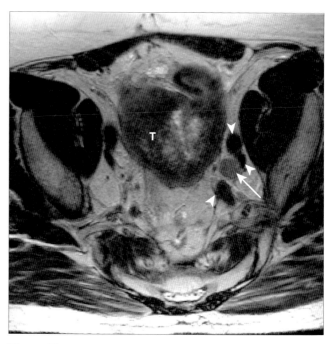

Figure 39.4. *Lymph node metastasis and signal void in adjacent vessels. Transaxial T2-weighted MR image demonstrating an enlarged left internal iliac lymph node (arrow) clearly seen separate from the signal void of the external iliac and internal iliac vessels (arrowheads). The node is of similar signal intensity to the central pelvic sigmoid colon tumour (T).*

tres. Gadolinium (Gd)-based IV contrast medium is not routinely required to identify lymph nodes but may be used to investigate nodal characteristics because nodal metastases frequently show contrast enhancement.

Identification of lymph nodes

Certain nodal sites are easily overlooked; they are listed in Table 39.1 (Fig. 39.5).[19-26] Usually, nodal metastases at these sites are not an isolated finding but their identification remains important for correct treatment and subsequent assessment of disease response.

Misdiagnosis of lymphadenopathy

Some of the normal structures and anatomical variants which may be mistaken for lymph node metastases are recorded in Table 39.2. A common cause of misinterpretation is aberrant vasculature (Fig. 39.6).[27,28] Other structures which may be confused with lymph nodes are the superior recess of the pericardium and posterior pericardial defects, dilated lymphatic trunks in the thorax or abdomen,[29,30] the diaphragmatic crura, lymphoceles, retained or transposed ovaries,[31,32] inguinal ilio-psoas bursae[33] and venous thrombi (Fig. 39.7).

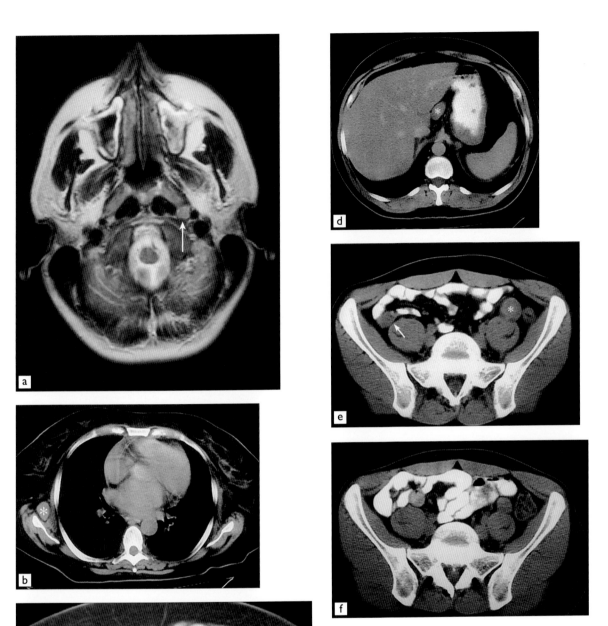

Figure 39.5. *Some overlooked lymph node sites. (a) T2-weighted MR image demonstrating a left lateral retropharyngeal node (arrow). (b) Transaxial enhanced thoracic CT scan demonstrating a right subscapular node (asterisk). (c) Transaxial contrast-enhanced abdominal CT scan demonstrating a paracardiac lymph node (arrow). (d) Transaxial contrast-enhanced abdominal CT scan showing a large hepatogastric ligament lymph node (asterisk) in a patient with Hodgkin's lymphoma. (e and f) Transaxial CT scans through the lower abdomen (e) demonstrating a left psoas node (asterisk) in a patient with teratoma. An apparent right psoas node (small arrows) is shown to represent unopacified bowel on a delayed repeat CT section (f) at the same level.*

Table 39.1. *Overlooked lymph nodes*[19–26]

Head and neck

   Lateral retropharyngeal

   Facial

   Intraparotid

Thorax

   Subpectoral/subscapular/interpectoral

   Internal mammary

   Posterior mediastinal

   Paracardiac

   Retrocrural

Abdomen

   Diaphragmatic

   Hepatogastric ligament

   Peripancreatic

   Splenic hilar

   Porta hepatis

   Porta caval

   Para caval

   Common iliac

   Psoas

Pelvis

   Obturator

   Presacral

   Paracervical

   Perirectal

   Inguinal

Table 39.2. *Mistaken for lymph nodes*

Head and neck

   Muscles – posterior belly of digastric; stylohyoid; styloglossus; stylopharyngeus

   Thrombosed internal jugular vein

   Submandibular gland – deep portion

Thorax

   Superior recess of pericardium

   Left atrial pericardial defect

   Aberrant vessels

   Coronary sinus

   Diaphragmatic crura

Abdomen

   Bowel

   Vessels, e.g. left-sided continuation of the IVC, retro-aortic left renal vein, left ascending lumbar vein

   Other structures (ureters, lymphatic trunks)

Pelvis

   Bowel

   Vessels – internal iliac branches, gonadal vessels

   Other structures (ovaries, lymphoceles, iliopsoas bursae)

- Major imaging criterion
  Size
- Minor imaging criteria
  Shape
  Site
  Number
  Nodal tissue characteristics – (attenuation/signal intensity/echogenicity)

Key points: cross-sectional imaging

- CT and MR are the preferred imaging modalities for evaluation of lymph node metastases in most anatomical sites

- MR can differentiate nodes from blood vessels without the use of IV contrast medium

- [18]FDG PET is evolving as an important diagnostic technique for nodal staging

- Common sources of error are overlooked sites of lymph node involvement and misdiagnosis of vessels as lymph nodes

- Size, site, number and tissue characteristics of nodes are all important criteria for determining whether lymph nodes are normal or abnormal

Imaging features of abnormal lymph nodes

Current criteria which are employed to differentiate between lymph nodes likely to be malignant and those considered to be benign, are as follows:

Size

Because there may be considerable interobserver variation in lymph node assessment,[34] measurement of nodes should be performed in a standard fashion to maximize reproducibility within and between examinations. Alteration of the window level and window width on CT can lead to marked variation in the apparent size of soft tissue nodules[35,36] so measurements should be made on images at a standard window level and window width. Hard copy assessment may be preferable because lesion margins have been shown to be sharper than on the computer console but the introduction of multidetector CT, together with digital archiving of all imaging data, is likely to eliminate the use of hard copy reporting in the foreseeable future. The short axis diameter should be measured (Fig. 39.8) as it has been demonstrated that the short axis diameter of a lymph node remains relatively constant irrespective of its orientation in any plane[37] and that an involved node is likely to become rounder before it elongates. Use of the short axis diameter

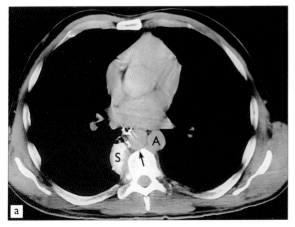

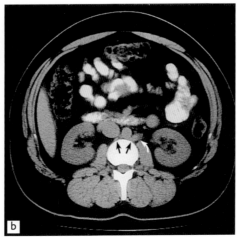

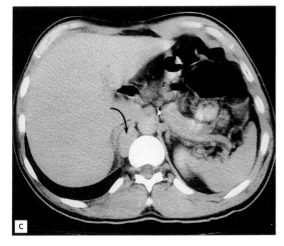

Figure 39.6. *Some vessels which may be mistaken for lymph nodes. (a and b) On a thoracic CT image, a large soft tissue nodule (black arrow in a) is shown adjacent to the descending thoracic aorta (A) and situated immediately adjacent to the surgical anastomosis in a patient who had undergone oesophagectomy with gastric pull-through for oesophageal carcinoma. Oral contrast is seen in the stomach (S). The mass could be traced inferiorly to the retrocrural region (curved arrow in b) and represented an azygous continuation of the inferior vena cava. (c) Transaxial CT scan through the upper abdomen showing a retro-aortic renal vein which may simulate a para-aortic node (white arrow). However, the vein can be traced behind the aorta (small black arrows) to its insertion with the inferior vena cava (IVC).*

as a nodal measurement may increase sensitivity, specificity, or both.[38–40] The maximum transverse diameter is preferred as the minimum short axis diameter can be misleading. Either the maximum or minimum short axis diameter has been used in different series.[38,40–42] Some authors advocate the use of the maximum to minimum short axis diameter ratio for measurement of nodal size as this provides a better assessment of overall shape related to nodal size.[43]

The upper limits of normal lymph node size have been derived from many studies, some documenting post-mortem values in normal populations,[44–46] while others deal with pathological assessment of resected specimens.[1,2,9] The majority of papers correlate cross-sectional imaging findings with pathology, other imaging modalities, biochemistry or clinical outcome[8,10,11,38–40,47–75] and one study measured nodal size on lymphangiography.[76] There have been inherent problems with some of the study populations – small patient numbers, a preponderance of North American patient groups with an increased incidence of granulomatous disease – and little allowance has been made for age and gender which also affect nodal size. Investigators have used oncological patient cohorts, sometimes in long-term remission or with tumours unlikely to affect the regions being studied, but still introducing possi-

ble bias.[73,75] Other potential errors relate to technique, particularly which nodal axis has been measured and to which anatomical subgroup the measured nodes belong. There has been difficulty in identifying which histological nodes correspond with which imaged nodes in maintaining the nodal axis between CT, surgical resection and pathological sectioning, and in quantifying the effect of histological fixation. Even in normal populations assessed at postmortem or by CT,[52,56] possible factors influencing nodal size include air pollution, pneumoconiosis, granulomatous disease and human immunodeficiency virus (HIV) status. Despite all these problems, a reasonably clear consensus is emerging as to what constitutes upper limits of normal for lymph nodes in different areas of the body (detailed in Table 39.3).

Some lymph nodes are not usually visualized on cross-sectional imaging; for example, facial, splenic hilar, central pelvic (paracervical, paravesical, perirectal) and posterior pelvic (presacral) nodes. When they are identified it is likely that they are abnormal (Fig. 39.9).

Nodal shape

Normally, lymph nodes are oval or kidney-bean-shaped and become more rounded as a consequence of metastatic infiltration. This feature is helpful in head and neck cancer,

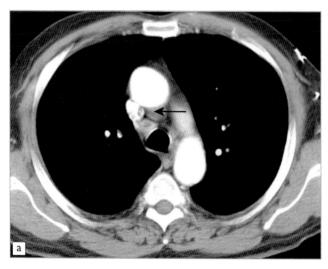

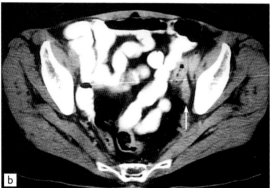

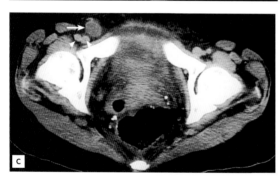

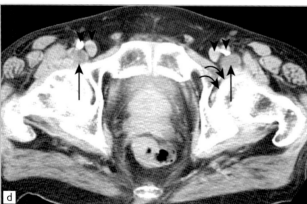

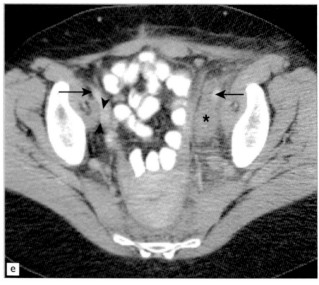

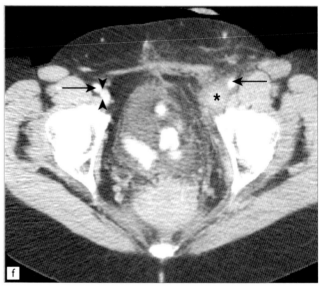

Figure 39.7. *Some structures which may be mistaken for lymphadenopathy. (a) The superior recess of the pericardium (arrow). On this transaxial contrast-enhanced CT section it is of low attenuation due to its fluid content and is always situated directly adjacent to the posterior aspect of the ascending aorta. (b) CT scan through the pelvis demonstrating a retained ovary on the left pelvic sidewall (arrow). This could easily be confused with a unilateral enlarged obturator node. The only clue that the mass may be an ovary is its pear shape, and full clinical information is required. (c) CT scan demonstrating cystic right inguinal node in a patient with a low rectal tumour. Note the position of the node (white arrows) which is anterior and medial to the femoral vein and artery (arrowheads). (d) Ilio-psoas bursae (black arrows) are situated postero-lateral to the inguinal vessels (arrowheads) on this transaxial enhanced CT scan. The bursal connection to the hip joint is just visible (curved arrows). (e and f) Venous thrombosis. Transaxial contrast-enhanced CT scans demonstrating contrast-opacified external iliac arteries (arrows), and a normal right external iliac vein (arrowheads). The thrombosed left external iliac vein (asterisk) is distended and non-opacified and mimicks a lymph node metastasis.*

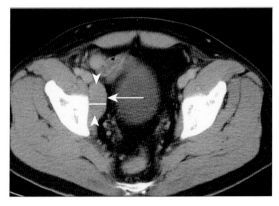

Figure 39.8. *Measurement of lymph nodes. Transaxial contrast-enhanced CT scan of the pelvis demonstrating an enlarged right obturator node (arrow). The maximum short axis is the longest measurement (line) perpendicular to the long axis (arrowheads).*

where ultrasound nodal staging sensitivity of 90% and specificity of 63% have been achieved using a criterion of nodal maximum short axis/maximum long axis diameter >0.55 to identify round nodes.[43]

Elsewhere in the body, results for nodal shape are variable with some authors reporting increased accuracy,[48,49] with helical reformations adding to the value,[77,78] and other

Table 39.3. *Size: recommendations on normal upper limit*

Site	Short axis diameter (mm)
Head and neck	10
Lateral retropharyngeal	<5
Facial	Not seen
Submental	11
Axilla	12
Mediastinum	10
Subcarinal	12
Retrocrural	6
Paracardiac	8
Abdomen	10
Gastro-hepatic ligament	8
Porta hepatis	7
Upper para-aortic	9
Lower para-aortic	11
Pelvis	10
Common iliac	9
Internal iliac	7
Obturator	8
Presacral, paracervical, perirectal	Not seen
Inguinal	15

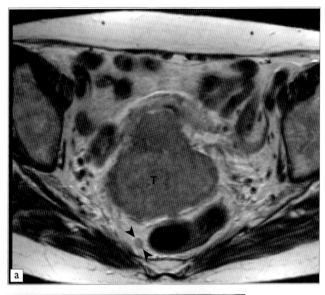

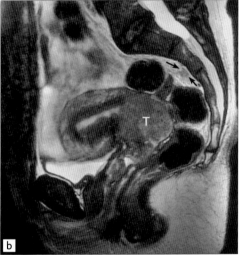

Figure 39.9. *Infrequently visualized lymph node metastases. (a) Transaxial T2-weighted MR image in a patient with a large cervical tumour (T). There is a right perirectal node (arrowheads). (b) Sagittal T2-weighted MR image in a patient with a large cervical tumour (T), in whom there is a presacral node (arrows).*

authors maintaining that a single maximum short axis diameter is the best node measurement.[38,40]

Nodal site

During radiological interpretation, more emphasis should be placed on nodes of borderline size in a recognized drainage site for a particular primary tumour. On the one hand, an asymmetrical, prominent obturator node is of great concern in bladder, prostate or cervical primary tumours, whereas on the other hand, isolated contralateral lymphadenopathy in a patient being staged for a testicular tumour is extremely rare[79] and should be interpreted with caution.

Nodal number

An asymmetrical cluster of normal-sized nodes (Fig. 39.10) is of concern but there is a paucity of data about normal nodal number in most anatomical sites. The information that does exist is recorded in Table 39.4.[51,60,73,74] In every anatomical site, fewer nodes are identified on cross-sectional imaging than at surgery or in pathological specimens, unsurprising when the smallest node may measure 1 mm, but emphasizing our current inability to provide a complete radiological evaluation of lymph nodes. In one study the number of visualized pelvic nodes on CT was increased on postlymphangiogram CT images compared with prelymphangiogram images.[73] In another study, more normal-sized pelvic nodes were demonstrated on MR than on CT.[75]

Table 39.4. *Normal number of nodes*[52,61,74,75]

Site	Range	Mean
Axilla	1–21	5
Retroperitoneum	0–4	2
Pelvis	0–28	9
Inguinal	3–8	6

Spiral and multislice CT detect increased numbers of small normal lymph nodes compared with conventional axial CT. Thus it is now possible to identify normal-sized pulmonary hilar lymph nodes on thoracic helical CT.[80] In another study, 40% of nodes measuring 5–9 mm were seen in patients undergoing surgery for gastric cancer resection using single-slice spiral CT, but only 1% of nodes <5 mm were detected.[78]

Nodal characteristics

Normal nodes may have a uniform appearance or may demonstrate an echogenic/low attenuation/high signal intensity centre due to fat (Fig. 39.2). Fatty nodes are most commonly seen in the axilla and also in the groin. Fatty nodes become partially or totally solid when involved by tumour (Fig. 39.11), often reverting back to pretreatment appearances after therapy.

Studies conducted *in vitro* on axillary nodes from patients with breast cancer suggested that MR relaxation times could be used to differentiate benign from malignant lymph nodes.[81,82] Unfortunately, *in vivo* studies have shown that there are no absolute MR criteria for lymph node involvement as there is considerable overlap in the T1 and T2 relaxation times of cancerous, lymphomatous, hyperplastic and benign nodes.[83–85] Nonetheless, when the signal intensity of a node parallels the signal intensity of the primary lesion, then this sign increases diagnostic confidence (Fig. 39.12).[86]

High-frequency ultrasound has been used to assess superficial lymph nodes, particularly in head and neck tumours, and certain factors may indicate a likely primary site. For example, uniform hypoechogenecity and posterior acoustic enhancement (pseudocystic appearance) together with a nodal distribution predominantly involving the submandibular and posterior triangle groups, are more in keeping with lymphoma than metastatic disease.[87] Metastatic papillary thyroid nodes are usually solid, hyperechoic masses, and 70% of these nodes have punctate calcification due to psammoma bodies.[88] Sonographic evidence of nodal necrosis may be identified in the head and neck and is of two types: either cystic necrosis, which appears hypoechoic, or coagulative necrosis, which appears hyperechoic though less than the echogenecity of fat (Fig. 39.13a).

The Doppler distribution of intranodal vessels differs

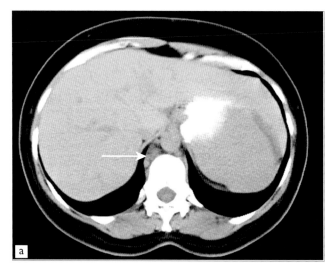

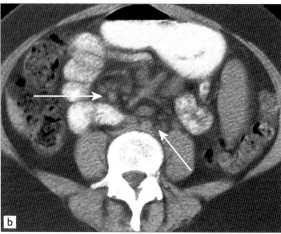

Figure 39.10. *Clusters of normal sized lymph nodes. (a and b) Contrast-enhanced CT scans demonstrating clusters of normal-sized lymph nodes in the retrocrural space, retroperitoneum and mesentery (arrows). This finding is likely to represent malignant lymph node disease, particularly as this patient has lymphoma.*

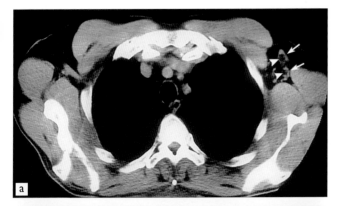

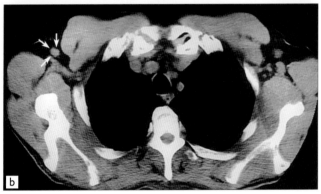

Figure 39.11. *Alteration of lymph node attenuation in disease. (a) Remission CT scan in a patient with non-Hodgkin's lymphoma demonstrating normal left axillary nodes (large arrows) which are predominantly fatty with a thin soft tissue capsule medially (arrowheads). (b) On relapse, the nodes become solid and a new node appears in the right axilla (small white arrows).*

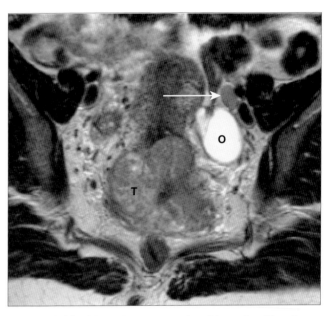

Figure 39.12. *Magnetic resonance signal intensity of lymph node metastases. Transaxial T2-weighted image in a patient with a large cervical tumour (T). The signal intensity of the left external iliac lymph node metastasis (arrow) parallels that of the primary tumour increasing diagnostic confidence that the node is metastatic. O, ovarian cyst.*

between benign and metastatic neck nodes. In benign nodes, vasculature is found at the hilum, whereas in malignant lymph nodes the vascularity is either capsular or a mix of capsular and distorted hilar vessels (Fig. 39.13b).[89] Metastatic lymph nodes generally have a higher resistive index than infective or reactive lymph nodes.[89,90]

Some characteristic features of malignant lymph nodes are discussed below.

Necrotic nodes
Central nodal necrosis may occur in metastatic nodes due to medullary invasion by tumour producing local ischaemia.[21,91] It is most frequently observed in squamous cell primary tumours of the head and neck (Fig. 39.14) and even normal sized necrotic nodes are regarded as metastatic in this patient group.[21,38] In head and neck tumours, nodal necrosis is a recognized adverse prognostic sign.[21] However, this is not true in all tumours and, in Hodgkin's lymphoma for example, nodal necrosis is not a poor prog-

nostic feature.[92] Computed tomography is superior to MR in the identification of nodal necrosis;[91,93] however, the detection rate of MR is improved by use of the contrast agent Gd-DTPA.[94]

Cystic nodes
Sometimes the consistency of the node may point to a particular primary tumour type. For example, in malignant testicular non-seminomatous germ cell tumours, involved retroperitoneal nodes are frequently of low attenuation on CT[95] (Fig. 39.15) and even non-enlarged cystic lymph nodes are likely to be involved. Furthermore, in a male patient being investigated for a retroperitoneal mass, a cystic appearance of the mass should strongly suggest the diagnosis of a primary testicular tumour.

Calcified nodes
Mediastinal or mesenteric nodes are often densely calcified due to granulomatous disease. More speckled amorphous calcification may be seen in metastatic nodes from gastrointestinal neoplasms and ovarian tumours. Calcification may persist or resolve after treatment (Fig. 39.16). In certain cancers, for example colorectal, ovarian and testicular tumours as well as in Hodgkin's disease, metastatic nodes may become densely calcified following treatment (Fig. 39.17). However, it should be noted that nodal calcification in the treated patient is not a reliable indicator of complete response.

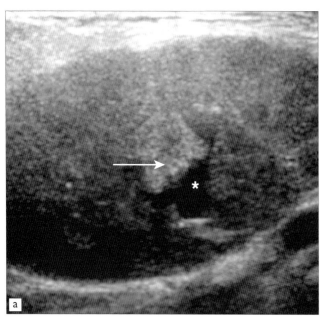

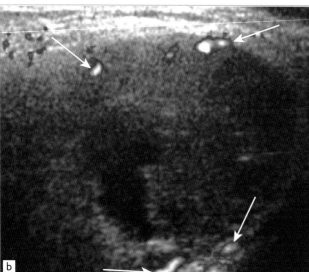

Figure 39.13. *Sonographic central nodal necrosis and Doppler characteristics of cervical lymph node metastases. (a) Ultrasound image of an enlarged level II deep cervical lymph node metastasis from a squamous cell carcinoma of the tongue. The node contains both cystic (asterisk) and coagulative (arrow) nodal necrosis. (b) Power Doppler ultrasound image of the node demonstrates enlarged capsular vessels (arrows) and absence of normal hilar vessels.*

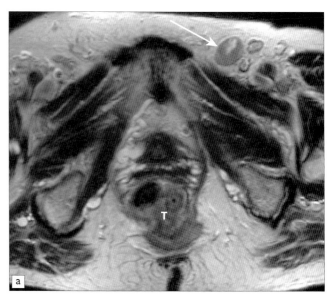

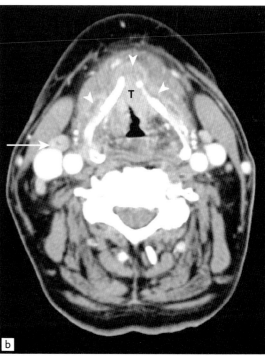

Figure 39.14. *Central cystic nodal necrosis. (a) T2-weighted MR image through the pelvis demonstrating a metastatic left inguinal node (arrow) in a patient with an anal tumour (T). The node has a high signal intensity central cystic component and the solid periphery is of similar signal to the tumour proper. (b) Transaxial contrast-enhanced CT scan showing a right level III deep cervical lymph node (arrow) with a small focus of central low attenuation due to nodal necrosis. The patient has a T4 laryngeal tumour (T) with involvement of the strap muscles of the neck (arrowheads).*

Extracapsular tumour spread

When the margins of an involved lymph node are irregular, it is likely that tumour has penetrated the capsule, providing that there is no evidence of acute inflammation in and around the nodal site (Fig. 39.18). Extracapsular spread is particularly relevant in head and neck tumours as it adversely affects prognosis.[21] It is associated with lymph node enlargement in 75% of cases.[21,91] Contrast-enhanced CT is more accurate than MR in the identification of extracapsular nodal extension of tumour.[91,92]

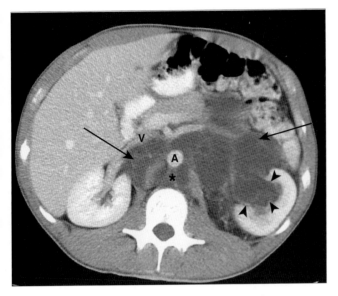

Figure 39.15. *Cystic lymph node metastases in malignant testicular teratoma. Transaxial contrast-enhanced CT section of a patient with malignant testicular teratoma demonstrating low attenuation cystic lymph node metastases in the retrocrural region (asterisk) and retroperitoneum (arrows). The inferior vena cava (V) is displaced and the left renal pelvis infiltrated (arrowheads) by the adenopathic mass. Abdominal aorta (A).*

The use of intravenous contrast media in lymph node assessment

Some lymph node masses are vascular and may enhance on CT or MR[96] (Fig. 39.19) after injection of IV contrast media but enhancement per se does not necessarily imply tumour involvement. The use of contrast medium may highlight central nodal necrosis, which can be a pointer to malignant involvement of non-enlarged nodes. Dynamic contrast-enhanced MR has been shown to facilitate the differentiation between enlarged benign and malignant nodes in a small number of patients with mediastinal lymphadenopathy from bronchogenic carcinoma.[97] In addition, the enhancement pattern of malignant nodes, as shown by signal intensity time curves, may be related to tumour aggressiveness.[86] However, the technique can only be employed over a limited body area and could not be used to assess all nodal sites.

Lymph node-specific magnetic resonance contrast medium

Ultrafine SPIO particles have been used as an MR lymph node-specific contrast medium that is injected intravenously and is taken up within the reticulo-endothelial tissue of normal lymph nodes, producing a reduction in signal intensity within the node (Fig. 39.20). Intranodal tumour replaces the reticulo-endothelial tissue, prevents SPIO uptake and results in preserved nodal signal intensity. This technique has the potential to allow differentiation between enlarged metastatic and hyperplastic nodes and

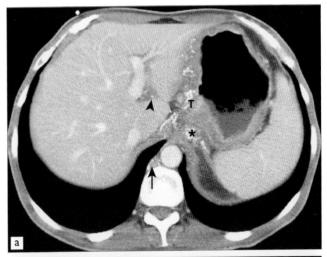

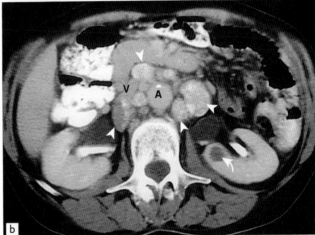

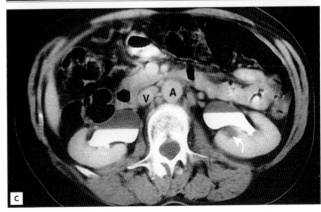

Figure 39.16. *Metastatic lymph node calcification. (a) Transaxial abdominal CT scan showing a partially calcified gastric tumour (T) and calcified lymph node metastases in the retrocrural space (arrow), porta hepatis (arrowhead) and in the coeliac axis (asterisk). (b and c) Transaxial abdominal CT scans at the same level in a patient with ovarian cancer before treatment (b) and after chemotherapy (c). Before treatment there is considerable upper retroperitoneal lymphadenopathy (arrowheads) which contains dystrophic calcification. After treatment not only do the nodes shrink but the dystrophic calcification resolves. Simple cyst in left kidney (curved arrow). A, Aorta; V, Inferior vena cava.*

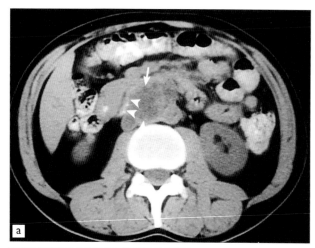

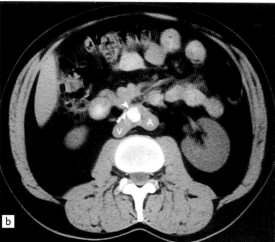

Figure 39.17. *Calcification after treatment in teratoma nodal metastases. (a and b) Transaxial CT scans demonstrating in (a) a large cystic interaortocaval nodal mass (arrows) in a patient with metastatic testicular teratoma. There is one small area of calcification (arrowheads) at the periphery of the nodal mass. (b) After treatment the residual mass is heavily calcified (arrowheads). A, Abdominal aorta; V, Inferior vena cava.*

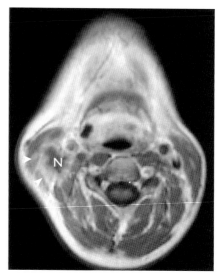

Figure 39.18. *Extracapsular nodal tumour. T1-weighted postcontrast MR image through the neck at the level of the hyoid in a patient with a metastatic deep cervical level II/III node from a head and neck primary. Central nodal necrosis (N) is seen and there is a spiculated margin to the node with enhancing soft tissue strands extending into the adjacent musculature and fat (arrowheads) due to extracapsular extension.*

allows the identification of metastases in some normal-sized nodes. Most studies to date have been performed in animals[98–103] but early reports in humans[15,104,105] show that short-term toxicity (which is proportional to the amount of injected iron) is low.[15,103,104] Superparamagnetic iron oxide-enhanced MR lymph node assessment has a high reported sensitivity of over 90% and an equally high specificity in patients with small volume nodal metastases and may be the best method of differentiating between benign and malignant lymph nodes.[15,16] This topic is further discussed in Chapter 60.

Key points: nodal characteristics

- Nodal size should be measured using the maximum short axis diameter

- Clusters of normal sized asymmetrical nodes should be regarded with suspicion for harbouring metastases

- MR demonstrates a greater number of normal sized lymph nodes than CT

- Metastatic nodes may show central necrosis, cystic change or calcification on CT

- High-frequency ultrasound may show nodal characteristics typical of a particular tumour type, e.g. lymphoma

- IV contrast medium may result in nodal enhancement on CT and MR

- Dynamic contrast-enhanced imaging has potential for differentiating enlarged benign from malignant lymph nodes

- MR lymphography is capable of identifying tumour deposits in normal sized lymph nodes

Accuracy of cro ss-sectional imaging

The literature on cross-sectional imaging accuracy for identification of lymph node metastases is confusing because patient populations, scanner sophistication, measurement methods, nodal identification and image correlation vary tremendously. For the most part, initial results have not

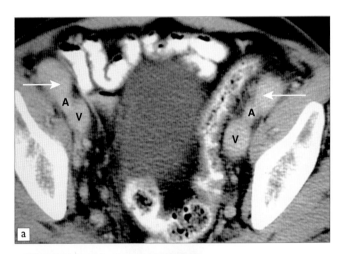

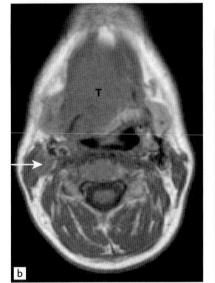

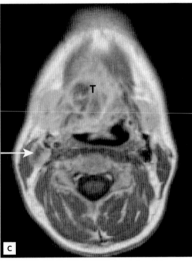

Figure 39.19. *Contrast enhancement in malignant lymph nodes. (a) Transaxial contrast-enhanced CT scan through the pelvis demonstrating enhancing external iliac lymph nodes (arrows) in a patient with metastatic malignant melanoma. A, external iliac arteries; V, external iliac veins. (b and c) Transaxial T1-weighted MR images (b) before and (c) after IV contrast injection. The right level II lymph node metastasis (arrows) demonstrates enhancement of the periphery and central non-enhancement due to nodal necrosis. The patient's extensive tongue and floor of mouth primary tumour (T) is seen. It is also shown to be partially necrotic after contrast.*

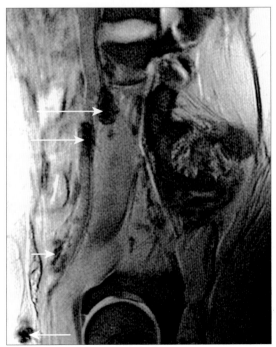

Figure 39.20. *Lymph node-specific MR contrast medium. Off-axis coronal gradient recall echo T1-weighted image 24 hr after IV injection of ultrafine superparamagnetic iron oxide (SPIO) particles. The SPIO is taken up by normal reticulo-endothelial tissue within normal lymph nodes and produces a signal drop (arrows).*

been confirmed by large prospective multicentre studies. For colorectal cancer, CT and MR have accuracies of 62% and 64%, respectively.[106] For lung cancer, respective sensitivities and specificities of 52% and 69% for CT and 48% and 64% for MR have been reported.[107] The Diagnostic Oncology Group results for head and neck tumours indicate that CT is more sensitive than MR, with false negative rates of 9% and 16% respectively.[93] Results for pelvic lymph node evaluation are more encouraging and representative figures for CT and MR accuracy are approximately 75%.[42,64,65] All studies demonstrate that reducing the size threshold for metastatic lymph nodes will increase diagnostic sensitivity but at the cost of reducing specificity.

Ultrasound is generally unreliable in the evaluation of deep metastatic nodal sites but its accuracy for detection of superficial lymph node metastases in the head and neck is high at 85%.[108] Accuracy was increased by ultrasound-guided fine-needle aspiration cytology to 100% in the same series.[108]

In the final analysis, all cross-sectional imaging assessment of nodes relies on probability rather than histological certainty and clinicians should appreciate that using the criteria outlined above will inevitably result in some false positive and false negative reports.

Key points: accuracy

- CT and MR have comparable accuracies in the detection of lymph node metastases

- MR lymphography is likely to be the most accurate imaging technique but is still undergoing clinical evaluation

Functional imaging techniques: radionuclide imaging

[67]Gallium citrate

In the 1970s and early 1980s, [67]Gallium citrate was used extensively for the clinical evaluation of oncology patients. It accumulates within lymphomatous masses and some solid tumours, particularly bronchogenic carcinoma, with reported detection rates of 70% and 90%, respectively.[109] In lung cancer, [67]Gallium was disappointing when used as a prospective preoperative staging investigation for mediastinal and hilar node involvement, with a sensitivity of only 55%.[110] Other disadvantages of [67]Gallium are high cost, the length of time of each investigation (up to 1 week), potential confusion in interpretation because inflammatory conditions are also [67]Gallium-avid and the relative lack of uptake in necrotic tumours. These factors have led to [67]Gallium falling out of favour as a diagnostic staging tool. In some centres it is still used as a predictor of disease-free status in treated lymphoma, when it may be more accurate than CT.[111]

Positron emission tomography

Clinical research has confirmed that [18]FDG PET is of value in the identification of metastatic nodal disease in breast and lung cancer (Fig. 39.21), as well as in head and neck tumours (Fig. 39.22) and lymphoma.[112–117] Involved lymph nodes are seen as focal areas of increased activity on whole-body images. Localization of involved nodes is enhanced by the recent introduction of combined [18]FDG PET–CT scanners.

In a prospective analysis of 50 patients with potentially operable non-small cell lung cancer, the sensitivity, specificity and accuracy in detecting N2 disease was 67%, 59% and 64%, respectively, for CT and 67%, 97% and 88%, respectively, for [18]FDG PET.[112] When [18]FDG PET was visually correlated with CT, sensitivity, specificity and accuracy rose

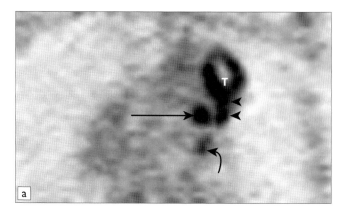

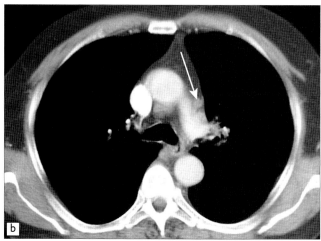

Figure 39.21. *[18]FDG PET detection of lymph node metastases in non-small cell lung cancer. (a) Coronal [18]FDG PET image (maximum intensity projection) demonstrating peripheral activity in a primary lung tumour (T) extending towards the hilum (arrowheads), with increased activity in an ipsilateral mediastinal lymph node (arrow). There is also band-like increased activity (curved arrow) beneath the node. (b) CT scan of the same patient demonstrating a small aortopulmonary lymph node metastasis (arrow). The band-like activity was subsequently shown to be due to a thoracic vertebral metastasis.*

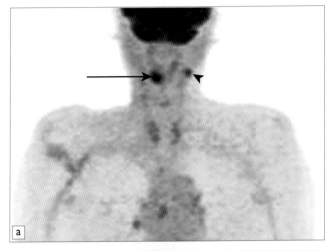

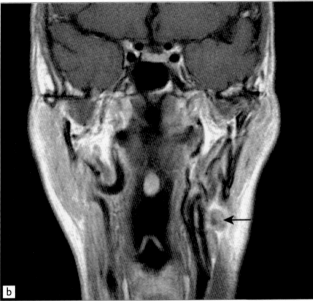

Figure 39.22. *[18]FDG PET detection of lymph node metastasis from a head and neck primary tumour. (a) Coronal [18]FDG PET image in a patient post-right-sided neck dissection for squamous cell carcinoma lymph node metastases, primary site unknown. The examination demonstrates the primary tumour in the right base of tongue (arrow) and an unrecognized left level II lymph node metastasis (arrowhead). (b) Coronal T1-weighted postcontrast MR image performed after the [18]FDG PET scan demonstrates the non-enlarged left lymph node metastasis (arrow) with a tiny focus of non-enhancing central nodal necrosis. Biopsy of this node was positive for squamous cell carcinoma.*

to 93%, 97% and 96%, respectively.[112] Two meta-analyses have shown [18]FDG PET to be superior to CT for non-small cell lung cancer staging.[116,117] In 237 patients with known non-small cell lung cancer or a suspicious lung lesion, retrospective analysis revealed that the rate of mediastinoscopy (performed to identify metastatic lymph nodes) could have been reduced by 12% when the lung lesion was not [18]FDG-avid (standardized uptake value for [18]FDG <2.5) and the mediastinum was FDG-negative.[118]

In patients with untreated lymphoma, [18]FDG PET is superior to CT in detecting disease sites, except within the abdomen, where it is equivalent.[119] After treatment, persistence of [18]FDG avidity in residual lymphomatous masses predicts for adverse progression-free survival[120,121] and overall survival.[122] [18]FDG PET has been shown to have a greater predictive value for relapse risk and survival than CT in treated lymphoma.[122]

As well as increased uptake in tumours, [18]FDG is actively taken up by inflammatory and infective lesions,[123] which could potentially result in false positive cancer staging. One way to differentiate between the two is to perform delayed imaging because [18]FDG activity characteristically continues to accumulate in tumours over time. Another source of error in [18]FDG PET is relatively poor radionuclide uptake in low-grade malignancies, particularly low-grade lymphomas. Nevertheless, [18]FDG PET is likely to have an increasing role in the routine staging of many solid tumours, not only due to its ability to detect nodal metastases in normal and minimally enlarged nodes but also because the technique can identify metastases in distant blood-borne sites as well.

Monoclonal antibody imaging

Radiolabelled-monoclonal antibodies have been raised against some tumour antigens and used to detect tumour deposits *in vivo*, for example carcinoembryonic antigen or prostate-specific antigen.[124,125] In patients with colorectal tumour, the technique has been shown to be useful in differentiating between recurrent tumour and treatment-induced fibrosis. Its accuracy in detecting involved lymph nodes is less clear, although it is theoretically capable of identifying tumour in normal sized nodes.[125] Recognized problems include non-uniform antigen expression by the tumour, the need for high-quality radionuclide imaging and false positive antibody scans due to normal radiopharmaceutical distribution and excretion.[124]

Sentinel node imaging

An alternative approach to lymph node imaging focuses on the node at greatest risk of containing metastatic tumour – known as the sentinel node. This is the first lymph node to receive lymph drainage from a given primary tumour and, once identified, can be removed and histologically examined. Those patients who are sentinel node-negative have no further surgery while those who are positive have more extensive lymph node dissection. Previously, the sentinel node has been located using peritumoural injection of blue dye;[126] more recently, lympho-scintigraphic methods have employed perilesional injection of Tc-99m-labelled human serum albumin or sulphur colloid to image the nodal drainage sites. γ-Detector-guided sentinel node resection is then performed. This technique has been used primarily in patients with breast cancer, melanoma or vulval cancer (Fig. 39.23). In a large group of breast cancer patients, ini-

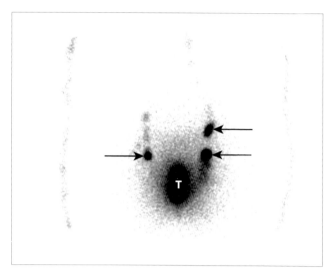

Figure 39.23. *Sentinel node imaging in vulval cancer. After injection of Tc-99m-labelled human serum albumin around a vulval tumour (T), three sentinel nodes (arrows) were demonstrated and metastatic tumour found at resection. The patient went on to have bilateral inguinal lymph node resection.*

tial results have been excellent; sentinel node status correlating with total axillary nodal status in 97% of women.[127] Early indications from current trials are that women with stage T1 or T2 early breast tumours, often screen-detected, and a negative sentinel node can be spared axillary node clearance surgery.[128] In melanoma, sentinel node identification is possible in more than 95% of patients but is in an unexpected lymph node group in 30–80% of those with head and neck or truncal lesions.[129] The technique has a low false negative rate of <4% for melanoma nodal status[130] and has been shown to be superior to [18]FDG PET for detection of melanoma metastatic regional nodes.[131]

Key points: functional imaging

■ [18]FDG PET scanning is now used for identifying nodal involvement in breast, lung and head and neck tumours as well as lymphoma

■ [18]FDG PET has a higher sensitivity and high specificity when images are correlated/fused with CT

■ After therapy, persistent [18]FDG uptake on delayed PET imaging indicates residual tumour with a high degree of accuracy

■ Radiolabelled monoclonal antibodies are currently being investigated for the detection of tumour in normal sized nodes

■ Sentinel node imaging is now routine practice in patients undergoing surgery for breast cancer. It is also useful in malignant melanoma and vulval cancer

The role of image-guided lymph node biopsy

When the radiological diagnosis of lymph node metastases is equivocal, despite careful interpretation, there are three options available to the clinician:

• Treat the suspect site
• Rescan after an interval to look for new confirmatory evidence of nodal disease
• Perform a lymph node biopsy

The choice will be governed by clinical circumstances but there is no doubt that, if an aggressive biopsy policy is adopted, then there will be increased detection of metastatic nodes over and above the detection rate from imaging alone.[132,133] Percutaneous image-guided biopsy is relatively safe, well tolerated, easy to perform and should yield a diagnostic sample in 80–90% of patients (Fig. 39.24).[134] It is usually undertaken with ultrasound for superficial nodes and with CT for deep-seated lymph nodes or nodal masses. Fine-needle aspiration biopsy is usually sufficient to allow a diagnosis of metastasis but core biopsy is required to diagnose and classify lymphomas.

Lymph node assessment following therapy

Following treatment with surgery, chemotherapy or radiotherapy for the primary tumour and locoregional lymph nodes, assessment of nodal status is required to plan further patient management. Nodal characteristics following treatment vary according to the type of treatment given, the response to treatment achieved and the presence and extent of involvement prior to treatment. For example, in a patient with nodal involvement from a testicular non-seminomatous germ cell tumour, reduction in tumour volume post-chemotherapy is the expected response but, occasionally, such nodal masses increase in size due to cystic degeneration, which results in fluid accumulation within the mass.[95] In pelvic cancers, treated nodes following radiotherapy often show a rather straight medial border, presumably due to associated radiation-induced fibrosis. The majority of treated nodes >2 cm in diameter before treatment do not return to normal size (as defined by accepted criteria) after therapy. However, it is not possible with CT or MR to determine whether active cancer persists within the treated node. [18]FDG PET scanning is developing an important role in this regard. Surgical clips following lymphadenectomy may make interpretation difficult and caution should be exercised when interpreting scans in the first few weeks after surgery as post-surgical changes may be misinterpreted as disease. In longer term follow-up, lymphocoeles may persist but are usually distinguished from tumour without difficulty as they are homogeneous cystic structures with an imperceptible wall.

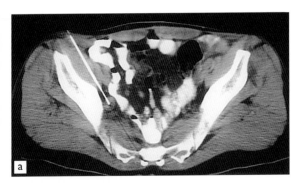

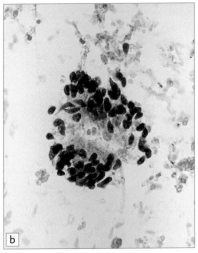

Figure 39.24. *Image-guided biopsy. (a) Percutaneous CT-guided biopsy of a right internal iliac node in a patient previously treated for rectal cancer. The needle tip is centrally positioned within the node. (b) Cytology sample of the same patient (Papanicolaou stain, magnification ×40) demonstrating pallisades of malignant glandular cells with a stromal core, compatible with a deposit of metastatic adenocarcinoma.*

Lymph node assessment in clinical trials

Defining objective tumour response to treatment has led to response criteria being developed and adopted internationally. The World Health Organization (WHO) definitions[135] have been in use for 20 years and masses are measured bidimensionally with the product of the measurements serving as a marker of tumour burden. More

recently, the Response Evaluation Criteria in Solid Tumours (RECIST)[136] requires measurement of the longest tumour diameter and, using spiral/multislice CT, lesions more than 1 cm are measured and a baseline sum longest diameter obtained. The RECIST criteria are not ideal for lymph node assessment as it is the maximum or minimum short axis diameter of the node which has been shown to best identify nodal metastases. This measurement is not allowed in the RECIST calculation and response of lymph node metastases may therefore be underestimated. Furthermore, guidelines for designating complete remission are required because a successfully treated lymph node in which tumour has been completely eradicated will remain as a soft tissue structure and is difficult or impossible to assess. Also it should be noted that none of the other cross-sectional imaging criteria for lymph node metastases can be used in clinical trial evaluation because they are qualitative rather than quantitative.

Functional imaging, using [18]FDG PET or other techniques such as dynamic contrast-enhanced MR imaging or CT, is likely to become more important in clinical trials as new anti-cancer drugs targeted to specific tumour functions, such as angiogenesis, are developed. These drugs may induce tumour response without necessarily causing reduction in tumour volume.

Conclusion

The accurate identification of lymph node metastases is an ongoing challenge in diagnostic radiology and overall lymph node assessment remains suboptimal. By understanding the physiology of the lymphatic system and by using the combination of size, site, shape, number and tissue characteristics of lymph nodes identified on cross-sectional imaging, the radiologist is better placed to indicate the likelihood of metastatic lymph node disease. Functional imaging with modalities such as [18]FDG PET adds to the sensitivity and specificity of nodal evaluation in many tumour types but also has important limitations. In some patients there is a need for percutaneous biopsy of suspicious nodal masses and this may increase diagnostic confidence. In other instances it is the responsibility of the clinician to decide whether to modify the patient's treatment so as to take account of equivocal nodal status.

Summary

- The radiologist should understand the physiology of the lymphatic system and lymphatic drainage of each primary tumour

- Using a combination of size, site, number of nodes and tissue characteristics, the radiologist can indicate the likelihood of metastatic lymph node disease

- CT and MR remain the preferred imaging modalities for lymph node staging of most solid tumours

- MR lymphography is a new and promising technique in the detection of involved lymph nodes in normal-sized nodes

- Where available, [18]FDG PET is now routinely used for staging lung, head and neck tumours

- [18]FDG PET has a valuable role in lymphoma, particularly in monitoring treatment response and in the detection of relapse

- Sentinel node imaging is an important technique for detecting nodal spread in breast cancer and is also used in malignant melanoma and vulval cancers

- Various different patterns of response to treatment of lymph nodes may be observed

- Most involved nodes greater than 2 cm in diameter do not return to normal dimensions as defined by accepted criteria

- The RECIST criteria for measurement of tumour response are not ideal for lymph node assessment as it is the maximum or minimum short axis diameter of the node which has been shown to best identify nodal metastases

Acknowledgements

I would like to acknowledge the help of the Cytology and Pathology Departments at the Christie Hospital. Yet again, I would like to thank my wonderful secretary, Mrs Kami Ramnarain, for her assistance in preparing this manuscript.

References

1. Herrera-Ornelas L, Justiniano J, Castillo N et al. Metastases in small lymph nodes from colon cancer. Arch Surg 1987; 122: 1253–1256

2. Jass J R, Morson B C. Reporting colorectal cancer. J Clin Pathol 1987; 40: 1016–1023

3. Sacks N P M, Baum M. Primary management of carcinoma of the breast. Lancet 1993; 342: 1402–1408

4. van Tinteren H, Hoekstra O S, Smit E F et al. Effectiveness of positron emission tomography in the preoperative assessment of patients with suspected non-small-cell lung cancer: The Plus Multicentre Randomised Trial. Lancet 2002; 359: 1388–1392

5. Hall J G. The functional anatomy of lymph nodes. In: Stansfield A G, d'Ardenne A J (eds). Lymph Node Biopsy Interpretation. London: Churchill Livingstone, 1992; 3–27

6. Liotta L A. Cancer cell invasion and metastasis. Sci Am 1992; 266: 54–9, 62–3

7. Fajardo L F. Lymph nodes and cancer. Front Radiat Ther Oncol 1994; 28: 1–10

8. Gross B H, Glazer G M, Orringer M B et al. Bronchogenic carcinoma metastatic to normal-sized lymph nodes: frequency and significance. Radiology 1988; 166: 71–74

9. Kayser K, Bach S, Bulzebruck H et al. Site, size and tumour involvement of resected extrapulmonary lymph nodes in lung cancer. J Surg Oncol 1990; 43: 45–49

10. Staples C A, Muller N L, Miller R R et al. Mediastinal nodes in bronchogenic carcinoma: comparison between CT and mediastinoscopy. Radiology 1988; 167; 367–372

11. McLoud T C, Bourgouin P M, Greenberg R W et al. Bronchogenic carcinoma: analysis of staging in the mediastinum with CT by correlative lymph node mapping and sampling. Radiology 1992; 182: 319–323

12. Castellino R A, Hoppe R T, Blank N et al. Computed tomography, lymphography, and staging laparotomy: initial staging of Hodgkin's disease. Am J Roentgenol 1984; 143: 37–41

13. Libson E, Polliack A P, Bloom R A. Value of lymphangiography in the staging of Hodgkin's lymphoma. Radiology 1994; 193: 757–759

14. Williams M P, Husband J E. Computed tomography scanning and post-lymphangiogram radiography in the follow-up of patients with metastatic testicular cancer. Clin Radiol 1989; 40: 47–50

15. Mack M G, Balzer J O, Straub R et al. Superparamagnetic iron oxide-enhanced MR imaging of head and neck lymph nodes. Radiology 2002; 222: 239–244

16. Harisinghani M G, Saini S, Weissleder R et al. MR lymphangiography using ultrasmall superparamagnetic iron oxide in patients with primary abdominal and pelvic malignancies: radiographic–pathologic correlation. Am J Roentgenol 1999; 172: 1347–1351

17. Johnson R J. Radiology in the management of ovarian cancer. Clin Radiol 1993; 48: 75–82

18. Dooms G C, Hricak H, Crooks L E, Higgins C B. Magnetic resonance imaging of the lymph nodes: comparison with CT. Radiology 1984; 153: 719–728

19. Mancuso A A, Harnsberger H R, Muraki A S, Stevens M H. Computed tomography of cervical and retropharyngeal lymph nodes: Normal anatomy, variants of normal, and applications in staging head and neck cancer. Radiology 1983; 148: 709–714

20. Tart R P, Mukherji S K, Avino A J et al. Facial lymph nodes: normal and abnormal CT appearance. Radiology 1993; 188: 695–700

21. Som P M. Lymph nodes of the neck. Radiology 1987; 165: 593–600

22. Callen P W, Korobkin M, Isherwood I. Computed tomographic evaluation of the retrocrural prevertebral space. Am J Radiol 1977; 129: 907–910

23. Balfe D M, Mauro M A, Koehler R E et al. Gastrohepatic ligament: normal and pathologic CT anatomy. Radiology 1984; 150: 485–490

24. Metreweli C, Ward S C. Ultrasound demonstration of lymph nodes in the hepatoduodenal ligament ('daisy chain nodes') in normal subjects. Clin Radiol 1995; 50: 99–101

25. Zirinsky K, Auh Y H, Rubenstein W A et al. The portacaval space: CT with MR correlation. Radiology 1985; 156: 453–460

26. Williams M P, Cook J V, Duchesne G M. Psoas nodes: an overlooked site of metastasis from testicular tumours. Clin Radiol 1989; 40: 607–609

27. Royal S A, Callen P W. CT evaluation of the anomalies of the inferior vena cava and left renal vein. Am J Roentgenol 1979; 132: 763–759

28. Meanock I, Ward C S, Williams M P. The left ascending lumbar vein: a potential pitfall in CT diagnosis. Clin Radiol 1988; 39: 565–566

29. Gollub M J, Castellino R A. The Cisterna Chyli: a potential mimic of retrocrural lymphadenopathy on CT scans. Radiology 1996; 199: 477–480

30. Williams M P, Olliff J F C. Case report: Computed tomography and magnetic resonance imaging of dilated lumbar lymphatic trunks. Clin Radiol 1989; 40: 321–322

31. Reed D H, Dixon A K, Williams M V. Ovarian conservation at hysterectomy: a potential diagnostic pitfall. Clin Radiol 1989; 40: 274–276

32. Bashist B, Friedman W N, Killackey M A. Surgical transposition of the ovary: radiological appearance. Radiology 1989; 173: 857–860

33. Meaney J F, Cassar-Pullicino V N, Etherington R et al. Ilio-psoas bursa enlargement. Clin Radiol 1992; 45: 161–168

34. Guyatt G H, Lefcoe M, Walter S et al. Interobserver variation in the computed tomographic evaluation of mediastinal nodal size in patients with potentially resectable lung cancer. Chest 1995; 107: 116–119

35. Koehler P R, Anderson R E, Baxter B. The effect of computed tomography viewer controls on anatomical measurements. Radiology 1979; 130: 189–194

36. Harris K M, Adams H, Lloyd D C F, Harvey D J. The effect on apparent size of simulated pulmonary nodules using three standard CT window settings. Clin Radiol 1993; 47: 241–244

37. Glazer G, Gross B H, Quint L E et al. Normal mediastinal lymph nodes: number and size according to American Thoracic Society Mapping. Am J Roentgenol 1985; 144: 261–265

38. van den Brekel M W M, Stel H V, Castelijns J A et al. Cervical lymph node metastasis: assessment of radiologic criteria. Radiology 1990; 177: 379–384

39. Platt J F, Glazer G M, Orringer M B et al. Radiologic evaluation of the subcarinal lymph nodes: a comparative study. Am J Roentgenol 1988; 151: 279–282

40. Kim S H, Kim S C, Choi B I, Han M C. Uterine cervical carcinoma: Evaluation of pelvic lymph node metastasis with MR imaging. Radiology 1994; 190: 807–811

41. Barentsz J O, Jager G J, Mugler J P III et al. Staging urinary bladder cancer: value of T1-weighted 3D MP-RAGE and 2D SE sequences. Am J Roentgenol 1995; 164: 109–115

42. Yang W T, Lam W W M, Yu M Y et al. Comparison of dynamic helical CT and dynamic MR imaging in the evaluation of pelvic lymph nodes in cervical cancer. Am J Roentgenol 2000; 175: 759–766

43. Takashima S, Sone S, Nomura N et al. Non-palpable lymph nodes of the neck: assessment with ultrasound and ultrasound guided fine needle aspiration biopsy. J Clin Ultrasound 1997; 25: 283–292

44. Genereux G P, Howie J L. Normal mediastinal lymph node size and number: CT and anatomic study. Am J Roentgenol 1984; 142: 1095–1100

45. Quint L E, Glazer G M, Orringer M B et al. Mediastinal lymph node detection and sizing at CT and autopsy. Am J Roentgenol 1986; 147: 469–472

46. Kiyono K, Sone S, Sakai F et al. The number and size of normal mediastinal lymph nodes: a postmortem study. Am J Roentgenol 1988; 150: 771–776

47. Carvalho P, Baldwin D, Carter R, Parsons C. Accuracy of CT in detecting squamous carcinoma metastases in cervical lymph nodes. Clin Radiol 1991; 44: 79–81

48. van Overhagen H, Lameris J S, Berger M Y et al. Supraclavicular lymph node metastases in carcinoma of the oesophagus and gastro-oesophageal junction: Assessment with CT, ultrasound and ultrasound-guided fine needle aspiration biopsy. Radiology 1991; 179: 155–158

49. Vassallo P, Wernecke K, Roos N, Peters P E. Differentiation of benign from malignant superficial lymphadenopathy: the role of high-resolution ultrasound. Radiology 1992; 183: 215–220

50. Ingram C E, Belli A M, Lewars M D et al. Normal lymph node size in the mediastinum: a retrospective study in two patient groups. Clin Radiol 1989; 40: 35–39

51. Parson V J, Carrington B M, Dougal M. Normal axillary lymph nodes as demonstrated by CT. (Abs) Radiology UK 1996; 702: 237

52. Murray J G, O'Driscoll M, Curtin J J. Mediastinal lymph node size in an Asian population. Br J Radiol 1995; 68: 348–350

53. Libshitz H I, McKenna R J, Haynie T P et al. Mediastinal evaluation in lung cancer. Radiology 1984; 151: 295–299

54. Buy J N, Ghossain M A, Poirson F et al. Computed tomography of mediastinal lymph nodes in non-small cell lung cancer: a new approach based on the lymphatic pathway of tumour spread. J Comp Assist Tomogr 1988; 12: 545–552

55. Seeley J M, Mayo J R, Miller R R, Muller N L. T1 lung cancer: prevalence of mediastinal nodal metastases and diagnostic accuracy of CT. Radiology 1993; 186: 129–132

56. Dorfman R E, Alpern M B, Gross B H, Sandler M A. Upper abdominal lymph nodes: criteria for normal size determined with CT. Radiology 1991; 180: 319–322

57. Thomas J L, Bernadino M E, Bracken R B. Staging of testicular carcinoma: Comparison of CT and lymphography. Am J Roentgenol 1981; 137: 991–996

58. Lien H H, Kolbenstvedt A, Talle K et al. Comparison of computed tomography, lymphography and phlebography in 200 consecutive patients with regard to retroperitoneal metastases from testicular tumour. Radiology 1983; 146: 129–132

59. Lien H H, Stenwig A E, Ous S, Fossa S D. Influence of different criteria for abnormal lymph node size on reliability of computed tomography in patients with non-seminomatous testicular tumor. Acta Radiologica Diagnosis 1986; 27: 199–203

60. Taylor A, Carrington B M, Wong-You-Cheong J J. Prospective assessment of normal abdominal lymph node size and distribution. (Abs) Roentgen Centenary Congress 1995; 396

61. Hricak H, Lacey C G, Sandles L G et al. Invasive cervical carcinoma: comparison of MR imaging and surgical findings. Radiology 1988; 166: 623–631

62. Matsukuma K, Tsukamoto N, Matsuyama T et al. Preoperative CT study of lymph nodes in cervical cancer: its correlation with histological findings. Gynecologic Oncol 1989; 33: 168–171

63. Greco A, Mason P, Leung A W L et al. Staging of carcinoma of the uterine cervix: MRI–surgical correlation. Clin Radiol 1989; 40: 401–405

64. Kim S H, Choi B I, Lee H P et al. Uterine cervical carcinoma: comparison of CT and MR findings. Radiology 1990; 175: 45–51

65. Hawnaur J M, Johnson R J, Buckley C H et al. Staging, volume estimation and assessment of nodal status in carcinoma of the cervix: comparison of magnetic resonance imaging with surgical findings. Clin Radiol 1994; 49: 443–452

66. Walsh J W, Amendola M A, Konerding K F et al. Computed tomographic detection of pelvic and inguinal lymph-node metastases from primary and recurrent pelvic malignant disease. Radiology 1980; 137: 157–166

67. Morgan C L, Calkins R F, Cavalcanti E J. Computed tomography in the evaluation, staging and therapy of carcinoma of the bladder and prostate. Radiology 1981; 140: 751–761

68. Weinerman P M, Arger P H, Coleman B G et al. Pelvic adenopathy from bladder and prostate carcinoma: detection by rapid-sequence computed tomography. Am J Roentgenol 1983; 140: 95–99

69. Amendola M A, Glazer G M, Grossman H B et al. Staging of bladder carcinoma: MRI–CT–surgical correlation. Am J Roentgenol 1986; 146: 1179–1183

70. Bryan P J, Butler H E, LiPuma J P et al. CT and MR imaging in staging bladder neoplasms. J Comp Assist Tomogr 1987; 11: 96–101

71. Buy J N, Moss A A, Guinet C et al. MR staging of bladder carcinoma: correlation with pathologic findings. Radiology 1988; 169: 695–700

72. Oyen R H, Van Poppel H P, Ameye F E et al. Lymph node staging of localized prostatic carcinoma with CT and CT-guided fine-needle aspiration biopsy: prospective study of 285 patients. Radiology 1994; 190: 315–322

73. Vinnicombe S J, Norman A R, Nicolson V, Husband J E. Normal pelvic lymph nodes: evaluation with CT after bipedal lymphangiography. Radiology 1995; 194: 349–355

74. Grey A, Carrington B M, Hulse P A, Swindell R. The inguinal region: normal anatomy and nodal distribution in an adult population. Clin Radiol 2000; 55: 124–130

75. Grubnic S, Vinnicombe S J, Norman A R, Husband J E. MR evaluation of normal retroperitoneal and pelvic lymph nodes. Clin Radiol 2002; 57: 193–200

76. Magnusson A. Size of normal retroperitoneal lymph nodes. Acta Radiol Diagn 1983; 24: 315–318

77. Steinkamp H J, Hosten N, Richter C et al. Enlarged cervical lymph nodes at helical CT. Radiology 1994; 191: 795–798

78. Fukuya T, Honda H, Hayashi T et al. Lymph-node metastases: efficacy of detection with helical CT in patients with gastric cancer. Radiology 1995; 197: 705–711

79. Dixon A K, Ellis M, Sikora K. Computed tomography of testicular tumours: distribution of abdominal lymphadenopathy. Clin Radiol 1986; 37: 519–523

80. Remy-Jardin M, Duyck P, Remy J et al. Hilar lymph nodes: identification with spiral CT and histologic correlation. Radiology 1995; 196: 387–394

81. Fossel E T, Brodsky G, Delayre J L, Wilson R E. Nuclear magnetic resonance for the differentiation of benign and malignant breast tissues and axillary lymph nodes. Ann Surg 1983; 198: 541–545

82. Wiener J I, Chako A C, Merten C W et al. Breast and axillary tissue MR imaging: correlation of signal intensities and relaxation times with pathological findings. Radiology 1986; 160: 299–305

83. Glazer G M, Orringer M B, Chenevert T L et al. Mediastinal lymph nodes: relaxation times/pathologic

correlation and implications in staging of lung cancer with MR imaging. Radiology 1988; 168: 429–431

84. Dooms G C, Hricak H, Moseley M E et al. Characterization of lymphadenopathy by magnetic resonance relaxation times: preliminary results. Radiology 1985; 155: 691–697

85. Lee J K T, Heiken J P, Ling D et al. Magnetic resonance imaging of abdominal and pelvic lymphadenopathy. Radiology 1984; 153: 181–188

86. Barentsz J O, Jager G J, van Vierzen P B J et al. Staging urinary bladder cancer after transurethral biopsy: value of fast dynamic contrast-enhanced MR imaging. Radiology 1996; 201: 185–193

87. Ahuja A, Ying M, Yang W T et al. The use of sonography in differentiating cervical lymphomatous lymph nodes from cervical metastatic lymph nodes. Clin Radiol 1996; 51: 186–190

88. Ahuja A T, Chow L, Chick W et al. Metastatic cervical nodes in papillary carcinoma of the thyroid: ultrasound and histological correlation. Clin Radiol 1995; 50: 229–231

89. Ahuja A, Ying M, Yune Y H, Metreweli C. Power Doppler sonography of cervical lymphadenopathy. Clin Radiol 2001; 56: 965–969

90. Ahuja A T, Ying M, Ho S S Y, Metreweli C. Distribution of intranodal vessels in differentiating benign from metastatic neck nodes. Clin Radiol 2001; 56: 197–201

91. Yousem D M, Som P M, Hackney D B et al. Central nodal necrosis and extracapsular neoplastic spread in cervical lymph nodes: MR imaging versus CT. Radiology 1992; 182: 753–759

92. Hopper K D, Diehl L F, Cole B A et al. The significance of necrotic mediastinal lymph nodes on CT in patients with newly diagnosed Hodgkin's disease. Am J Roentgenol 1990; 155: 267–270

93. Curtin H D, Ishwaran H, Mancuso A A et al. Comparative imaging of cancer metastasis to neck nodes: report of Radiologic Diagnostic Oncology Group III. Chicago: Radiological Society of North America Scientific Program, 1995; Abstract no. 677: 238

94. Chong V F H, Fan Y F, Khoo J B K. MR features of cervical node necrosis in metastatic disease. Clin Radiol 1996; 51: 103–109

95. Husband J E, Hawkes D J, Peckham M J. CT estimations of mean attenuation values and volume in testicular tumors: a comparison with surgical and histologic findings. Radiology 1982; 144: 553–558

96. Husband J E, Robinson L, Thomas G. Contrast enhancing lymph nodes in bladder cancer: a potential pitfall on CT. Clin Radiol 1992; 45: 395–398

97. Laissey J P, Gay-Depassier P, Soyer P et al. Enlarged mediastinal lymph nodes in bronchogenic carcinoma: assessment with dynamic contrast-enhanced MR Imaging. Radiology 1994; 191: 263–267

98. Weissleder R, Elizondo G, Josephson L et al. Experimental lymph node metastases: enhanced detection with MR lymphography. Radiology 1989; 171: 835–839

99. Weissleder R, Elizondo G, Wittenberg J et al. Ultrasmall superparamagnetic iron oxide: an intravenous contrast agent for assessing lymph nodes with MR imaging. Radiology 1990; 175: 494–498

100. Weissleder R, Elizondo G, Wittenberg C et al. Ultrasmall superparamagnetic iron oxide: characterization of a new class of contrast agents for MR imaging. Radiology 1990; 175: 489–493

101. Lee A S, Weissleder R, Brady T J, Wittenberg J. Lymph nodes: microstructural anatomy at MR imaging. Radiology 1991; 178: 519–522

102. Vassallo P, Matei C, Heston W D W et al. AMI-227-enhanced MR lymphography: usefulness for differentiating reactive from tumor-bearing lymph nodes. Radiology 1994; 193: 501–506

103. Weissleder R, Heautot J F, Schaffer B K et al. MR lymphography: study of a high-efficiency lymphotrophic agent. Radiology 1994; 191–225–230

104. Bellin M F, Roy C, Kinkel K et al. Lymph node metastases: safety and effectiveness of MR imaging with ultrasmall superparamagnetic iron oxide particles – initial clinical experience. Radiology 1998; 207: 799–808

105. Anzai Y, Blackwell K E, Hirschowitz S L et al. Initial clinical experience with dextran-coated superparamagnetic iron oxide for detection of lymph node metastases in patients with head and neck cancer. Radiology 1994; 192: 709–715

106. Zerhouni E A, Rutter C, Hamilton S R et al. CT and MR imaging in the staging of colorectal carcinoma: report of the Radiology Diagnostic Oncology Group II. Radiology 1996; 200: 443–451

107. Webb W R, Gatsonis C, Zerhouni E A et al. CT and MR imaging in staging non-small cell bronchogenic carcinoma: report of the Radiologic Diagnostic Oncology Group. Radiology 1991; 178: 705–713

108. van den Breckel M W, Castelijns J A, Stel H V et al. Modern imaging techniques and ultrasound guided aspiration cytology for the assessment of neck node metastases: a prospective comparative study. Eur Arch Otorhinolaryngol 1993; 250: 11–17

109. Bekerman C, Hoffer P B, Bitran J D. The role of gallium-67 in the clinical evaluation of cancer. Semin Nucl Med 1984; XIV: 296–323

110. Neumann R, Merino M, Hoffer P B. Gallium-67 in hilar and mediastinal staging of primary lung carcinomas. J Nucl Med 1980; 21: 32

111. Front D, Ben-Haim S, Israel O et al. Lymphoma: predictive value of Ga-67 scintigraphy after treatment. Radiology 1992; 182: 359–363

112. Vansteenkiste J F, Stroobants S G, De Leyn P R et al. The Leuven Lung Cancer Group. Mediastinal lymph node staging with FDG-PET scan in patients with potentially operable non-small cell lung cancer. Chest 1997; 112: 1480–1486

113. Albes J M, Lietzenmayer R, Schott U et al. Improvement of non-small cell lung cancer staging by means of positron emission tomography. Thorac Cardiovasc Surg 1999; 47: 42–27

114. Newman J S, Francis I R, Kaminski M S, Wahl R L. Imaging of lymphoma with PET with 2-[F-18]-fluoro-2-deoxy-D-glucose: correlation with CT. Radiology 1994; 190: 111–116

115. Jabour B A, Choi Y, Hoh C K et al. Extracranial head and neck: PET imaging with 2-[18]-fluoro-2-deoxy-D-glucose and MR imaging correlation. Radiology 1993; 186: 27–35

116. Toloza E M, Harpole L, McCrory D C. Non-invasive staging of non-small cell lung cancer. Chest 2003; 123: 137S–146S

117. Dwamena B A, Sonnad S S, Angobaldo J O, Wahl R L. Metastases from non-small cell lung cancer: mediastinal staging in the 1990s – meta-analytic comparison of PET and CT. Radiology 1999; 213: 530–536

118. Kernstine K H, McLaughlin K A, Menda Y et al. Can FDG-PET reduce the need for mediastinoscopy in potentially resectable non-small cell lung cancer? Ann Thorac Surg 2002; 73: 394–402

119. Buchmann I, Reinhardt M, Elsner K et al. 2-(Fluorine-18)fluoro-2-deoxy-D-glucose positron emission tomography in the detection and staging of malignant lymphoma. Cancer 2001; 91: 889–899

120. Naumann R, Vaic A, Beuthien-Baumann B et al. Prognostic value of positron emission tomography in the evaluation of post-treatment residual mass in patients with Hodgkin's disease and non-Hodgkin's lymphoma. Br J Haematol 2001; 115: 793–800

121. Spaepen K, Stroobants S, Dupont P et al. Can positron emission tomography with [^{18}F]-fluorodeoxyglucose after first-line treatment distinguish Hodgkin's disease patients who need additional therapy from others in whom additional therapy would mean avoidable toxicity? Br J Haematol 2001; 115: 272–278

122. Jerusalem G, Beguin Y, Fassotte M F et al. Whole-body positron emission tomography using 18F-Fluorodeoxyglucose for post-treatment evaluation in Hodgkin's disease and non-Hodgkin's lymphoma has higher diagnostic and prognostic value than classical computed tomography scan imaging. Blood 1999; 94: 429–433

123. Zhuang H, Alavi A. 18-Fluorodeoxyglucose positron emission tomographic imaging in the detection and monitoring of infection and inflammation. Semin Nucl Med 2002; 32: 47–59

124. Stomper P C, D'Souza D J, Bakshi S P et al. Detection of pelvic recurrence of colorectal carcinoma: prospective, blinded comparison of Tc-99m-IMMU-4 monoclonal antibody scanning and CT. Radiology 1995; 197: 688–692

125. Rosen S. Innovations in monoclonal antibody tumor targeting. J Am Med Assoc 1989; 261: 744–746

126. Morton D, Wen D, Wong J et al. Technical details of intraoperative lymphatic mapping for early stage melanoma. Arch Surg 1992; 127: 392–399

127. Veronesi U, Paganelli G, Galimberti V et al. Sentinel-node biopsy to avoid axillary dissection in breast cancer with clinically negative lymph nodes. Lancet 1997; 349: 1864–1867

128. Schwartz G F, Giuliano A E, Veronesi U, Consensus Conference Committee. Proceedings of the Consensus Conference on the Role of Sentinel Lymph Node Biopsy in Carcinoma of the Breast April 19–22, 2001, Philadelphia, PA, USA. Breast 2002; 8: 126–138

129. Yudd, A P, Kempf J S, Goydos J S et al. Use of sentinel node lymphoscintigraphy in malignant melanoma. RadioGraphics 1999; 19: 343–353

130. Shen J, Wallace A M, Bovet M. The role of sentinel lymph node biopsy for melanoma. Semin Oncol 2002; 29: 341–352

131. Belhocine T, Pierard G, de Labrassinne M et al. Staging of regional nodes in AJCC Stage I and II Melanoma: ^{18}FDG PET imaging versus sentinel node detection. Oncologist 2002; 7: 271–278

132. van den Brekel M W, Castelijns J A, Stel H V et al. Occult metastatic neck disease: detection with US and US-guided fine-needle aspiration cytology. Radiology 1991; 180: 457–461

133. Takes R P, Knegt P, Manni J J et al. Regional metastasis in head and neck squamous cell carcinoma: revised value of US with US-guided FNAB. Radiology 1996; 198: 819–823

134. Charboneau J W, Reading C C, Welch T J. CT and sonographically guided needle biopsy: current techniques and new innovations. Am J Roentgenol 1990; 154: 1–10

135. Miller A B, Hogestraeten B, Staquest M, Winkler A. Reporting results of cancer treatment. Cancer 1981; 47: 207–214

136. Therasse P, Arbuck S G, Eisenhauer E A et al. New guidelines to evaluate the response to treatment in solid tumours. J Natl Cancer Inst 2000; 92: 205–216

Chapter 40

Lung and pleural metastases

Suzanne L Aquino, Amita Sharma and Theresa McLoud

Introduction

Understanding the patterns of involvement of various tumours that metastasize to the lungs and pleura helps to establish a specific differential diagnosis. The purpose of this chapter is to review metastatic disease to the lungs and pleura, and to identify tumours based on their patterns of involvement that are predominantly found on computed tomography (CT). High-resolution CT (HRCT) provides better resolution of the interstitial architecture and therefore improves localization of tumour involvement. This can be particularly useful in detecting lymphangitic spread of tumour.

Historically, conventional radiologic screening for thoracic metastases relied on chest radiographs for the detection of lung nodules. Over the past decade, helical CT has replaced plain film radiography as the preferred imaging modality for surveying patients with malignancy for thoracic metastases. Helical CT provides rapid scanning of the body with minimal motion artefacts. This technology introduced interslice reconstruction in which helical data can be reconstructed into three-dimensional or volumetric datasets by overlapping image slices.[1] Small nodules lost on conventional non-helical CT due to interslice gaps were potentially retrievable.[2,3] Single detector helical CT had its limitations in slice thickness and pitch. In order to scan an entire thorax at a single breath hold, slice thickness and pitch had to be prolonged. As a trade off, resolution was compromised and small metastases could potentially still be missed. Multidetector helical CT revolutionized thoracic imaging by providing near isocubic volumetric scanning. A patient's entire thorax can be scanned in less than 10 seconds, resulting in minimal respiratory motion artefact. Slice reconstruction capabilities provided thinner slice thickness without loss of resolution. In essence, with volumetric imaging and the elimination of interscan gaps and respiratory motion, multidetector CT allowed for greater sensitivity in the detection of pulmonary metastases.[4,5]

Despite improved detection of lung metastases, there are still significant limitations. Waters et al. studied the accuracy of detection of pulmonary metastases in a radiological–pathological study of four dogs with osteosarcoma.[6] A total of 90.9% of pulmonary metastases >5 mm were detected on helical CT, but only 44% of metastases <5 mm were detected by at least one reader. The overall maximum sensitivity for CT was 56%. Surgical series, which compare preoperative CT to manual palpation at thoracotomy, have reported sensitivity rates for helical CT to be better than non-helical CT, with overall sensitivity as high as 84%.[7] Sensitivity rates of 53–62% have been reported in several surgical series for metastases <6 mm.[8,9]

2-[F-18]fluoro-2-deoxy-D-glucose positron emission tomography ([18]FDG PET) imaging for the diagnosis and staging of cancer has become well established in recent years. Many studies have reported the significance of [18]FDG PET for the detection of metastases in lung, colon, head and neck tumours, melanoma, breast and lymphoma.[10,11] Results on lung cancer patients have shown that [18]FDG PET has the additional advantage of detecting metastases that conventional diagnostic tests have missed. In Pieterman et al., 11% of their study group with lung cancer had metastases found on [18]FDG PET that were not detected on routine imaging and clinical studies.[12] In addition, indeterminate nodules found on CT of patients with lung cancer showed increased [18]FDG uptake consistent with metastases.

Diagnosis of pulmonary metastases and follow-up are vital in the monitoring of response to treatment regimens. Radiotherapy, chemotherapy and surgery are all influenced by the demonstration and confirmation of pulmonary metastatic disease. Surgical metastasectomy has been utilized in the treatment of many solid tumours of epithelial, sarcomatous and germ cell origin.[13-15] Pulmonary metastasectomy is indicated when there is complete control of the primary tumour. Provided the patient can tolerate the loss of pulmonary function, numerous nodules can be resected through median sternotomy, thoracotomy, or by video-assisted thoracoscopic surgery (VATS). The limited sensitivity of CT has led many authors to conclude that CT-guided VATS excision of pulmonary metastases is limited and that manual surgical palpation is still necessary.[7,8,16]

Key points: general

- Multidetector CT allows for greater detection of pulmonary metastases but, as most metastases are <5 mm, maximum overall sensitivity is 56–84%

- HRCT improves localization of tumour involvement within the lung parenchyma

- [18]FDG PET has become useful in differentiating benign from malignant nodules

Patterns of metastases in the lungs

Nodules

Nodular metastases are the most common pattern found in the lungs. Metastatic nodules can range from miliary in size to several centimetres (Figs. 40.1 and 40.2). Miliary nodules are more likely to be seen in tumours such as thyroid carcinoma, renal cell carcinoma and melanoma. Their distribution with respect to the interstitial compartments is random.[17,18]

Ground glass nodules

Ground glass can be seen in metastases as a result of focal interstitial infiltration, as seen with lymphoma (Fig. 40.3), or filling of the airspaces with tumour or its by-products. Ground glass nodules or nodules with surrounding ground

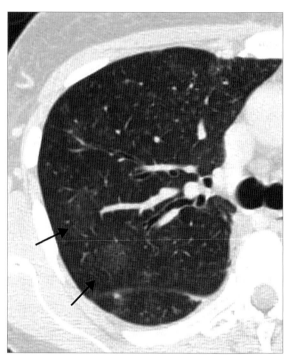

Figure 40.3. *CT scan of a 45-year-old woman with non-Hodgkin's lymphoma showing new ground glass nodules (arrows).*

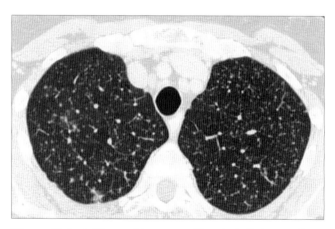

Figure 40.1. *A 60-year-old woman with metastatic pancreatic carcinoma. Multiple pulmonary nodules are present that range from miliary size, 2–3 mm to 5 mm. This patient also had lymphangitic spread to her lungs (shown in Figure 40.19).*

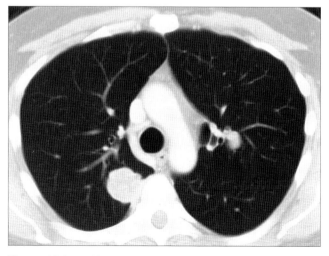

Figure 40.2. *A 49-year-old man with metastatic renal cell carcinoma. CT scan shows a 3 cm nodule in the superior segment of the right lower lobe.*

glass are seen with haemorrhagic metastases. Metastases such as choriocarcinoma, melanoma, renal cell carcinoma and angiosarcoma tend to be hypervascular, and bleed into the adjacent lungs to give this pattern (Fig. 40.4).[19,20] Mucin-producing tumours, such as adenocarcinoma from the pancreas or colon, show ground glass metastases (Fig. 40.5). In the early stages of involvement this appears as ground glass. As the disease progresses, however, areas of ground glass become consolidated and may resemble pneumonia (Fig. 40.6).

Ground glass nodules or solid nodules with surrounding ground glass are also found in diffuse bronchioloalveolar cell carcinoma. This pattern is due to both direct tumour scaffolding of the alveolar walls, termed lipidic growth, and filling of the airspaces with mucinous material.

Non-malignant lung diseases such as invasive aspergillosis or arteriovenous malformation may also develop multiple nodules with surrounding ground glass.[20] In both these disorders, the ground glass is due to surrounding haemorrhage. The distinction between invasive aspergillosis and metastases may be difficult in an immunosuppressed oncology patient who has received chemotherapy or bone marrow transplantation. In such instances, clinical information is necessary to distinguish whether the patient is febrile and more likely to have infection rather than recurrent disease.

Pulmonary epithelioid hemangio-endothelioma or intervascular bronchoalveolar tumour is a low-grade

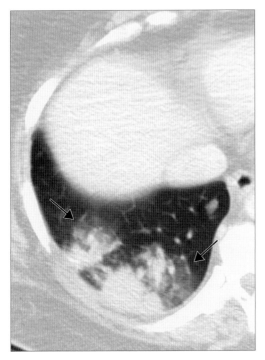

Figure 40.4. *A 53-year-old man with metastatic renal cell carcinoma. Multiple nodules show surrounding ground glass consistent with haemorrhage (arrows).*

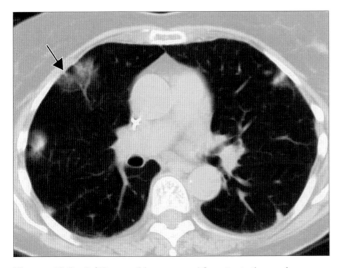

Figure 40.5. *A 73-year-old woman with metastatic mucin-producing pancreatic carcinoma. The lungs show multiple pulmonary nodules including a ground glass nodule in the right upper lobe (arrow).*

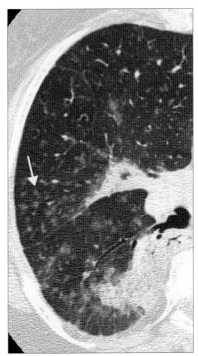

Figure 40.6. *A 70-year-old woman with mucin-producing adenocarcinoma of the caecum. Right lung shows both airspace opacities and ground glass nodules (arrow) consistent with diffuse mucinous metastases.*

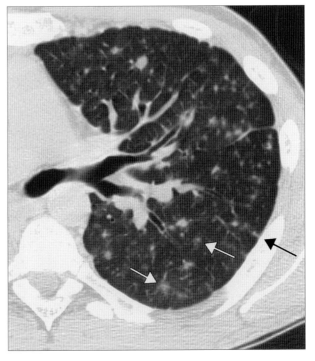

Figure 40.7. *A 23-year-old man with primary pulmonary epithelioid hemangio-endotheliosis. CT scan shows multiple ill-defined nodules (white arrows), many of which appear as ground glass. There are subpleural nodules and thickened interlobular septa (black arrow) consistent with tumour deposition along the interstitium.*

endothelial sarcoma that can arise in the lung, skeleton or soft tissues. Radiographic appearance varies and includes multiple interstitial nodules, interstitial thickening, calcified nodules, pleural thickening and effusion that tends to be a haemorrhagic or mediastinal mass. The multinodular pulmonary form is similar to metastatic angiosarcoma to the lungs. On HRCT, ill-defined ground glass nodules lie in a perivascular or centrilobular distribution (Fig. 40.7).

Thickening of the interstitium resembles lymphangitic spread of tumour.[21] These CT scan findings along with a presentation of haemoptysis may hint at the diagnosis of this unusual disease.

Nodules with calcifications

The diagnosis of a calcified metastasis is straightforward in a patient with new nodules and a history of osteosarcoma or chondrosarcoma (Fig. 40.8).[22] Without prior radiographs

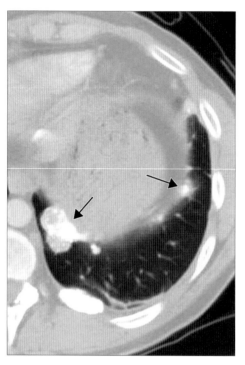

Figure 40.8. *A 26-year-old man with osteosarcoma of the femur. CT scan of the lower thorax shows multiple subpleural calcified nodules consistent with metastatic osteosarcoma (arrow).*

available to show that a nodule is new, other considerations for a calcified nodule would include a granuloma, amyloid or a hamartoma. Metastatic mucinous adenocarcinoma may also manifest as multiple pulmonary nodules containing calcification (Fig. 40.9). Dystrophic calcification can be seen in metastases from papillary thyroid carcinoma, synovial cell sarcoma and, rarely, in treated metastases (Fig. 40.10).[23]

Branching nodules

Airway metastases tend to involve the airways from the trachea to the segmental bronchi. Metastases from breast, kidney, colon, lymphoma and melanoma are the most common sources for this process.[24–27] Endobronchial metastases with complete obstruction of an airway may lead to complete collapse of the involved lung or resultant air trapping. An airway-filling defect or mass with mucus filling of a distal occluded airway is best seen on CT (Fig. 40.11). An occluded airway will appear as an arborizing opaque structure that parallels the adjacent vasculature on CT lung windows (Fig. 40.12). This has been called the 'finger-in-glove' sign on chest radiograph because the branching plugged airways resemble white-gloved fingers. If airway plugging extends to the respiratory and terminal bronchioles on CT, branching centrilobular opacities or tree-in-bud opacities will be seen (Fig. 40.13). These will be optimally seen in the subpleural regions.[28]

Tumour emboli are the result of haematogenous metastases occluding and proliferating within the small- and

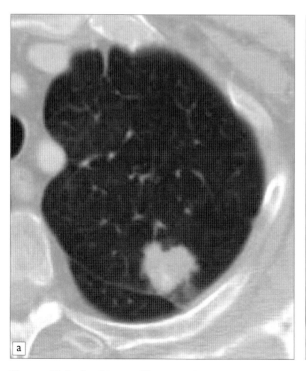
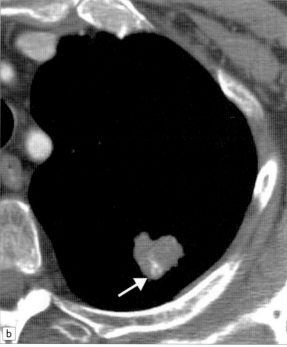

Figure 40.9. *An 80-year-old man with metastatic papillary adenocarcinoma of the colon. (a) CT scan of the thorax shows a left upper lobe nodule. (b) Soft tissue windows demonstrate calcification within the nodule (arrow).*

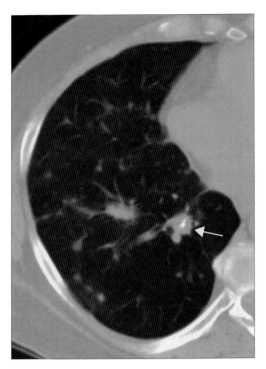

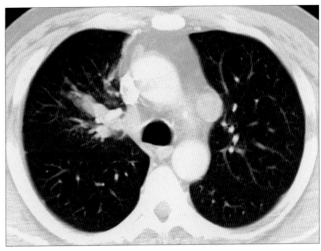

Figure 40.12. *A 47-year-old man with renal cell carcinoma and an endobronchial metastasis in the right upper lobe bronchus. Large arborizing opacity in right upper lobe correlates with an obstructed bronchus filled with tumour and mucus.*

Figure 40.10. *A 40-year-old woman with papillary thyroid carcinoma. CT scan shows multiple irregular pulmonary nodules. Intermediate windows show a focus of calcification within a nodule in the right lower lobe (arrow).*

intermediate-sized pulmonary arteries.[29] On chest radiograph, this pattern is indistinguishable from other nodular metastases. On CT, tumour emboli appear as branching lobulated enlargements or smooth symmetric beading of the small- and medium-sized pulmonary arteries (Fig. 40.14).[30] With helical CT, this pattern is now more readily detected due to thinner sequential images in which symmetric focal enlargement of a small artery is seen. Tumour emboli are associated with tumours such as soft tissue sarcomas, renal cell carcinoma, hepatoma and melanoma that spread haematogenously via the venous system. Distal infarction may occur with distal parenchymal ground glass or consolidation.

Nodular lymphangitic spread of tumour along the vascular interstitium may resemble tumour emboli. Computed tomography features, which help to identify tumour involving the interstitium rather than within the vasculature, include asymmetric and irregular nodularity along vessels, coexisting signs of lymphangitic spread in other interstitial compartments, as well as lymphadenopathy.

Branching opacities may also occur with localized dilated veins and, in the presence of metastatic disease, this can be seen with tumour venous thrombosis. This rare process is seen if tumour invades the venous system or the left atrium.[31] This has been reported with squamous cell carcinoma and sarcoma. If pulmonary infarction results, patients may present with pleuritic chest pain, cough and haemoptysis. Computed tomography findings include dilated pulmonary veins (Fig. 40.15), a filling defect in the pulmonary vein, particularly the proximal veins, and/or a filling defect in the left atrium.

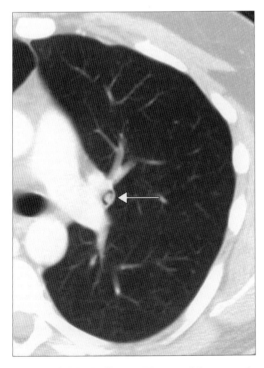

Figure 40.11. *A 49-year-old man with metastatic renal cell carcinoma. CT scan through the apical posterior segmental bronchus of the left upper lobe shows a filling defect from an endobronchial metastasis (arrow).*

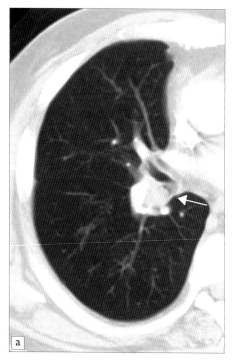 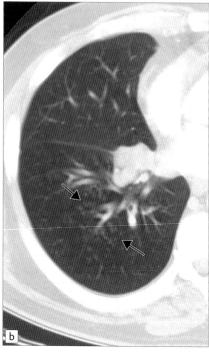

Figure 40.13. *A 47-year-old man with renal cell carcinoma (same patient as Fig. 40.15). (a) CT scan of the right lower lobe shows a filling defect in the right lower lobe bronchus consistent with an endobronchial metastasis (white arrow). (b) Computed tomography scan through the right lower lobe shows clusters of centrilobular nodules and plugged small airways consistent with a 'tree-in-bud' pattern (black arrows).*

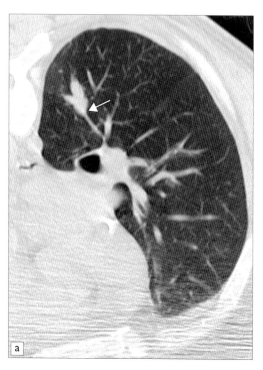 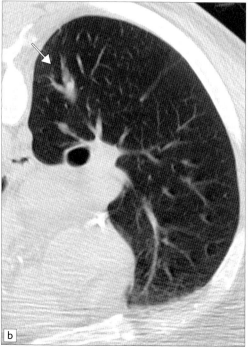

Figure 40.14. *A 48-year-old man with renal cell carcinoma and new pulmonary nodules. (a) CT scan of the thorax in the prone position shows dilatation of a small pulmonary artery in the right lower lobe consistent with a tumour embolus (arrow). (b) Sequential CT scan slice shows branching of the dilated artery (arrow).*

Key points: nodular metastases

- Nodular metastases are the most common pattern found in the lungs

- Ground glass nodules occur as a result of partial filling of the airspaces or the interstitium with tumour or haemorrhage

- Calcified nodules can be seen in metastases from osteo- or chondrosarcoma, mucin-producing adenocarcinoma and due to dystrophic calcification in metastases from thyroid carcinoma and synovial cell sarcoma

- Branching nodules may be secondary to endobronchial metastases and mucus filling of the distal airway, or due to tumour embolus in the pulmonary artery or, rarely, pulmonary vein

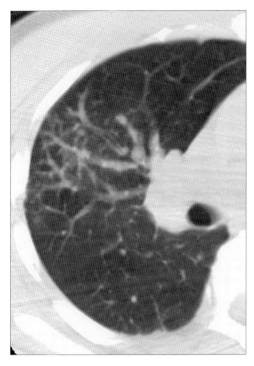

Figure 40.15. *A 45-year-old man with metastatic renal cell carcinoma. CT scan shows multiple pulmonary metastases. Scattered pulmonary veins are dilated consistent with tumour thrombosis of the pulmonary veins.*

Cystic or cavitary nodules

Cavitary metastases are most likely from metastatic squamous cell carcinoma of the cervix, head and neck (Fig. 40.16) but are also seen with colorectal carcinoma, sarcoma, transitional cell carcinoma and lymphoma.[32–34]

Non-malignant disorders such as Wegener's granulomatosis, Churg–Strauss disease, rheumatoid arthritis and amyloidosis may also present with numerous cavitary nodules.[35] Cavitary nodules associated with eosinophilic granulomatosis tend to be small at 3–4 mm with irregular thin walls. Distribution tends to be in the upper lungs and interstitial fibrosis may coexist. Fungal infection, mycobacterial infection, septic emboli and tracheobronchial papillomatosis are pulmonary infections that may give multiple pulmonary cavities and cysts. In the appropriate clinical setting, where infection is suspected, they should be included in the differential diagnosis. Pulmonary involvement of tracheo-bronchial papillomatosis manifests as multiple thin- or thick-walled cavities and may contain air–fluid levels. Transmission to the lungs is through the airways and, therefore, these cavities and cysts tend to distribute centrally in the lungs. This disease is associated with malignant degeneration to squamous cell carcinoma. Any change in cyst formation (to solid) or lymphadenopathy on CT may indicate malignant transformation.

The CT pattern of multiple nodules associated with complex cystic changes is attributed to eosinophilic granulomatosis or Langerhans' cell histiocytosis of the lungs.

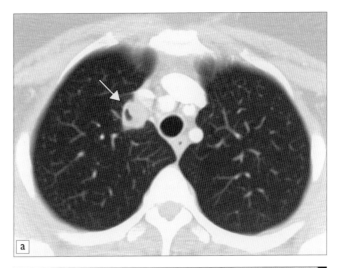

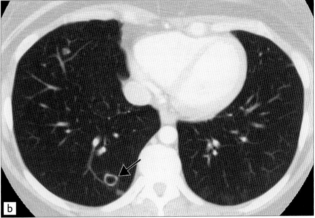

Figure 40.16. *A 48-year-old woman with metastatic squamous cell carcinoma. (a) CT scan of the upper thorax shows a cavitary nodule (white arrow) with an asymmetric thickened wall in the right upper lobe. (b) Computed tomography scan in lower thorax shows a thinner-walled nodule in the right lower lobe (black arrow). Other nodules in the lungs were solid.*

However, nodular metastases such as transitional cell carcinoma, lymphoma, renal cell carcinoma, squamous cell carcinoma can also cavitate in a similar pattern in a background of coexisting small nodules (Fig. 40.17).[36,37] Additional findings in the thorax, including lymphadenopathy, pleural effusion, bone lesions, as well as intra-abdominal metastases, may help to define the presence of metastases over a non-malignant process. Metastatic nodules may cavitate prior to chemotherapy. Cavitation and decrease in nodule size may indicate a tumour's response to therapy. Although rare, spontaneous pneumothorax may develop if a cavitary nodule is subpleural and ruptures into the pleural space.

Spontaneous pneumothorax is a well-described complication of metastatic sarcoma. The mechanism of this complication is attributed to extension of the pulmonary tumour into the pleural space, creating a communication between the airspaces and the pleura. The sarcomas associ-

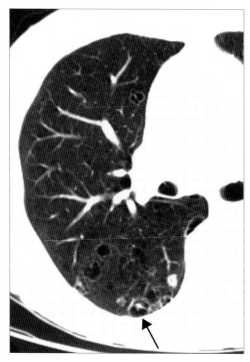

Figure 40.17. *A 63-year-old man with transitional cell carcinoma of the bladder. CT scan of the thorax shows multiple nodules and cysts. Some of the cysts are complex with central nodules and septations (arrow).*

ated with this complication include osteosarcoma, synovial cell sarcoma, angiosarcoma and leiomyosarcoma. Smevik et al. reported an increased risk for pneumothorax after the induction of chemotherapy.[38]

Key points: cystic metastases

- Cystic metastases should be differentiated from infection causing cavitary nodules

- Cystic metastases are most likely from squamous carcinoma of cervix, head and neck, but also sarcomas and transitional cell carcinoma

Reticular disease

Reticular opacities in the lungs from metastases primarily result from infiltration of tumour into the interstitial compartments. These compartments include the perihilar axial interstitium, the centrilobular interstitium, as well as the inter- and intralobular septa.[39,40] Usually, all compartments or regions of an involved lung will be infiltrated. The key feature in distinguishing lymphangitic spread from other causes of interstitial lung disease on HRCT is the preservation of lung architecture. Associated findings on CT such as lymphadenopathy, a unilateral pleural effusion, an asymmetric distribution in the lungs and lung nodules will help confirm its presence. Malignancies that

commonly involve the interstitium by lymphangitic spread include lung, breast, gastro-intestinal tract, melanoma and lymphoma.[39]

Tumour spread through the lymphatics and surrounding interstitium may initially originate either from pulmonary arterial metastases or by direct extension from hilar lymphadenopathy along the axial interstitium. The former route is most commonly seen in malignancies from the breast, gastro-intestinal tract and melanoma. Direct extension from the hilum is more likely to be seen in primary lung cancer with hilar disease, lymphoma (especially Hodgkin's disease) and, on rare occasions, leukaemia.[41]

The pattern of lymphangitic spread in the interstitium can be smooth (Fig. 40.18) or nodular (Fig. 40.19) and is best seen with thin section images. A smooth pattern may be the result of direct tumour deposit in the interstitium. Alternatively, this pattern may be the result of obstructed lymphatics from extensive lymphadenopathy with subsequent interstitial oedema. Imaging should display a proximal tumour mass or extensive hilar and mediastinal lymphadenopathy in the thorax to suggest this disease process. Nodular lymphangitic disease is easier to recognize and is indicative of tumour deposits in the interstitium or lymphatics.

Key points: reticular disease

- Malignancies which commonly involve the interstitium by lymphatic spread include lung, breast, gastro-intestinal tract, melanoma and lymphoma

- Lymphangitic spread can be nodular or smooth, and is best seen on HRCT

Reticular and nodular disease

As mentioned above, lymphangitic tumour will cause a combined nodular and reticular pattern. Tumours to be considered by this pattern, which can involve the lung, are breast, gastro-intestinal tract, melanoma and lymphoma.

Lymphocytic interstitial pneumonia, a benign disease caused by the deposit of numerous benign lymphocytes and plasma cells in the interstitium of the lung, resembles metastatic disease or diffuse lymphoma. Patients at risk for acquiring this disorder, such as those with immune deficiency disorders, are also at risk for lymphoma. Distinction between the two on a clinical and radiological basis can be difficult. A chest radiograph commonly shows reticular and/or nodular opacities in the lungs. On CT, nodules may be seen that are interstitial, including centrilobular, in distribution. These nodules may contain an air bronchogram, may be ground glass or solid and range in size from a few millimetres to 1 cm (Fig. 40.3). Although uncommon, associated parenchymal cysts may help distinguish LIP from low-grade lymphoma of the lungs (Fig. 40.20).[42] These cysts result from cellular infiltration into the walls of small

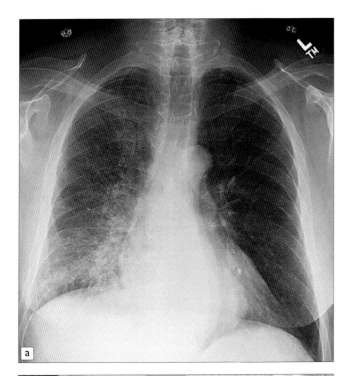

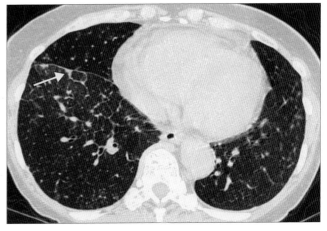

Figure 40.19. *High-resolution CT scan in a 60-year-old woman with metastatic pancreatic carcinoma. The interlobular septa show nodular thickening (arrow) consistent with tumour deposition in the interstitium.*

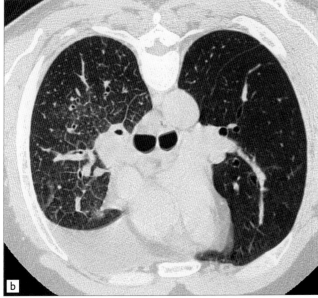

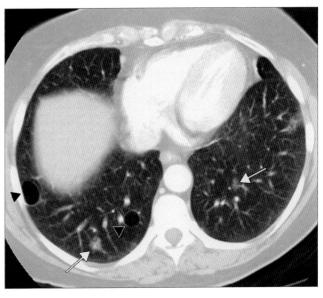

Figure 40.20. *CT scan in a 52-year-old woman with lymphocytic interstitial pneumonia. The lungs show a mixture of soft tissue nodules (arrows) and parenchymal cysts (arrowheads).*

Figure 40.18. *A 50-year-old man with non-small cell lung carcinoma. (a) Chest radiograph shows asymmetric right hilar fullness with ground glass and reticular opacities in the right lung. (b) High-resolution CT in the prone position shows smooth thickened interlobular septa with preserved lung architecture.*

Tumours with mixed nodules, airspace and interstitial disease

Lymphoma involvement of the lungs may manifest as a mixture of consolidation, nodules and interstitial disease (Fig. 40.21) (see also Chapter 32). The latter form is commonly seen as an extension of tumour along the axial bronchovascular interstitium from hilar nodal disease. The consolidative and nodular forms often have an air bronchogram that may be confused with infection. Cavitation of nodules may occur, which may be equally confusing if the clinical

airways, endoluminal obstruction and subsequent air-trapping in the distal airspaces.[43] Specific patient populations are at risk for LIP, which may help associate the CT findings with the disease. These include those with autoimmunodeficiency syndrome (AIDS), Sjögren's syndrome and primary immunodeficiency disorders.[44]

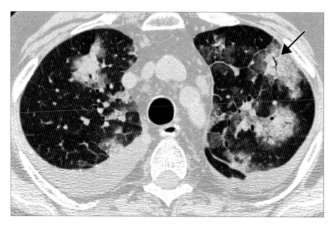

Figure 40.21. *A 54-year-old man with diffuse pulmonary non-Hodgkin's lymphoma. CT scan shows bilateral large consolidative masses (arrow) that contain air bronchograms, and have surrounding ground glass. Some of the interlobular septa are also thickened. The patient also had pleural effusions.*

(which can be ground glass and cavitary), or scattered areas of ground glass in other regions of the lung should raise suspicion for this disease (Fig. 40.23).[49,50] On rare occasions, cyst-like changes in the consolidation may develop which can be mistaken for cavitary pneumonia or bronchiectasis. Lymphadenopathy is unusual and is, therefore, not helpful in distinguishing tumour from infection. Ground glass with septal thickening, sometimes called crazy paving on HRCT, is an unusual pattern for BAC, but is well described (Fig. 40.24).[51,52] This pattern, along with other features described above, may raise the suspicion for this disease if found.

Kaposi's sarcoma involvement of the lungs commonly includes mediastinal and hilar lymphadenopathy (see Chapter 8). This tumour tends to spread from hilar nodal disease and infiltrate along the interstitial compartment of the axial bronchovasculature. Multiple flame-shaped lesions or nodules with ill-defined borders arise in the thickened interstitium (Fig. 40.25). These nodules commonly surround the bronchus and thus contain an air bron-

differential diagnosis includes infections such as invasive aspergillosis (Fig. 40.22).[45] The presence of lymphadenopathy may help, especially with Hodgkin's disease, but will not necessarily be present in primary non-Hodgkin's involvement of the lungs.[46–48]

The consolidative form of bronchoalveolar carcinoma (BAC) or adenocarcinoma with bronchoalveolar cell type is often mistakenly diagnosed as lobar pneumonia on initial chest radiographs. Many patients present with fever, cough and systemic symptoms that are consistent with infection (they can be superimposed on the tumour). Coexisting pulmonary findings on CT scan such as associated subcentimetre nodules

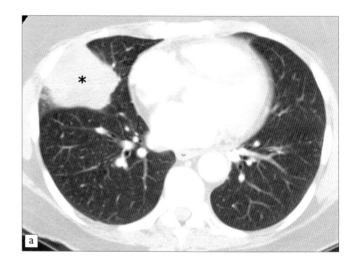

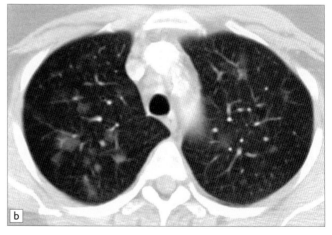

Figure 40.22. *A 21-year-old woman with progressive Hodgkin's lymphoma. CT scan of the thorax shows dense consolidative tumour in the left upper lobe (*) and cavitary nodules in the right perihilar region (arrows). There is a left pleural effusion.*

Figure 40.23. *A 55-year-old woman with bronchoalveolar cell carcinoma. (a) CT scan of the mid thorax shows a dominant mass in the middle lobe (*). (b) Computed tomography scan through the upper lobes shows multiple ground glass nodules consistent with metastases.*

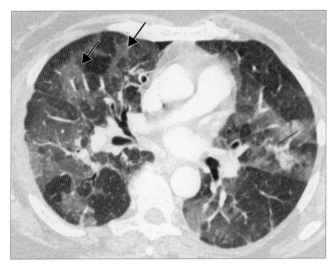

Figure 40.24. *A 50-year-old woman with mucin-producing adenocarcinoma of the lung. CT scan of the lungs shows diffuse ground glass opacities (arrows) and scattered thickened interlobular septa. Although this is not a bronchioloalveolar cell carcinoma by histopathology, its pattern is indistinguishable.*

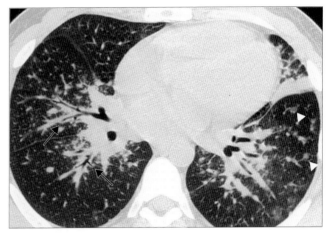

Figure 40.25. *A 40-year-old man with AIDS and Kaposi's sarcoma. Tumour extends from hilar nodal involvement along the bronchovascular bundles (arrows). Scattered nodules in the left lower lobe (arrowheads) are consistent with metastatic disease.*

chogram. High-resolution CT better displays the relationship of tumour with the bronchovasculature. Other possible patterns of Kaposi's sarcoma involvement in the thorax include a single pulmonary nodule, unilateral pleural effusion that can be bloody on thoracocentesis, or endoluminal tracheal and bronchial lesions that are best seen on bronchoscopy rather than CT scan.[53]

Pleural metastatic disease

The pleural space is involved in metastatic disease in three main ways:

- Effusions
- Thickening
- Nodules or masses

The presence of metastatic pleural disease is an ominous sign. The average time until death following the diagnosis of a malignant effusion is approximately 5–16 months.[54–56] Most malignant effusions are exudative and unilateral. In adult patients, 25% of newly diagnosed pleural effusions identified by chest radiograph are due to malignancy. The likelihood of a unilateral effusion being malignant increases with the patient's age and with the size of the effusion.[57,58] Bilateral pleural effusions with a normal heart size are reported to be secondary to malignancy in 50% of cases.[59]

Almost every tumour has been reported to metastasize to the pleura but, histologically, adenocarcinoma is responsible for over 80% of these effusions.[60] In 6–13% of patients who present with a malignant effusion, the primary site of disease is unknown.[61,62] The most common malignancy associated with pleural metastatic disease is lung cancer, which is responsible for 20–44% of all malignant pleural effusions.[62–64] Breast cancer is the second most common cause and accounts for 21–24% of all malignant effusions.[54,55,62] Lymphoma is responsible for 13–16% of all malignant effusions.[55,63] Approximately 13% of patients with both Hodgkin's and non-Hodgkin's lymphoma have an effusion at initial presentation.[64,65]

Metastatic pleural disease may also manifest with pleural thickening or nodules. Tumours most likely to demonstrate this pattern are metastatic adenocarcinoma, lymphoma and invasive thymoma (Fig. 40.26).

The role of radiology is to diagnose patients with pleural disease, identify a cause and provide aids to diagnosis and treatment, such as image-guided thoracocentesis, biopsy and pleurodesis.[66] More than 300 ml of pleural fluid is necessary for visualization on an erect chest radiograph (Fig. 40.27), but lateral decubitus films can detect as little as 5 ml of fluid.[67] Ultrasound is more sensitive in the detection and quantification of an effusion.[68] This modality also will display the presence of fluid echogenicity, which suggests exudates, pleural nodules and thickening (Fig. 40.28).[69]

In many instances, tumour deposits within the pleura and pleural space are below the resolution of CT and ultrasound.[70] The majority of malignant exudative effusions do not demonstrate pleural changes on contrast-enhanced CT.[71,72] Several studies have evaluated the use of CT in establishing criteria for detecting malignant pleural disease.[71–73] When present, the features that are most helpful are pleural nodules and nodular pleural thickening (Fig. 40.27).[72] In patients with diffuse pleural thickening, the presence of mediastinal pleural involvement, circumferential distribution or parietal thickening greater than 1 cm

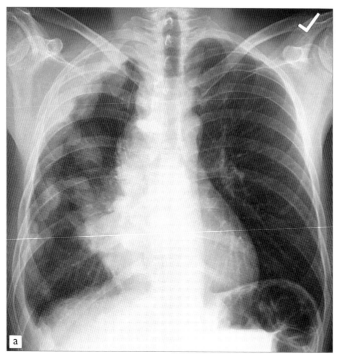

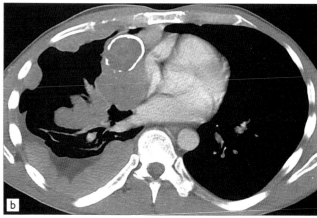

Figure 40.26. *A 23-year-old man with metastatic invasive thymoma. (a) Chest radiograph shows lobulated right pleural masses and an anterior mediastinal mass. (b) CT scan shows a heterogeneous mediastinal mass that contains curvilinear calcification. There are multiple enhancing pleural nodules and a small right pleural effusion.*

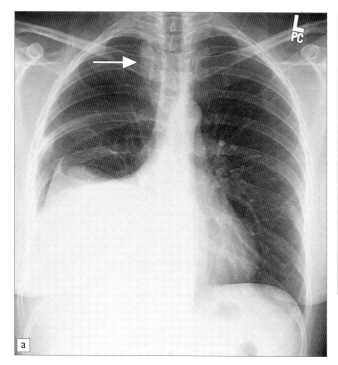

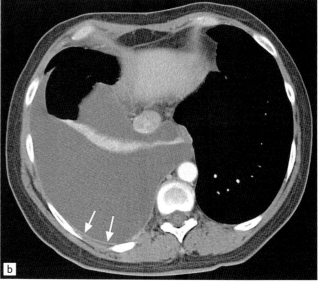

Figure 40.27a–b. *A 47-year-old woman with metastatic lung cancer. (a) Chest radiograph shows a large right pleural effusion. There is a 2 cm nodule at the right apex (arrow). (b) CT scan in the same patient confirms a large right pleural effusion with linear pleural thickening and enhancement (arrows).*

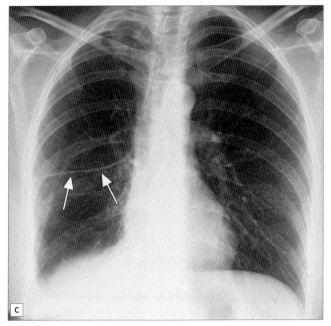

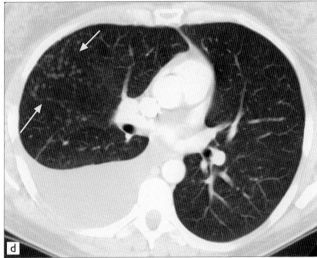

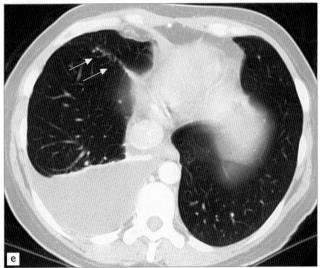

Figure 40.27c–e. *A 47-year-old woman with metastatic lung cancer. (c) Following thoracocentesis of 2 litres of fluid, the second chest radiograph shows nodular pleural thickening involving the horizontal fissure (arrows). CT scan in the same patient with selected images on lung windows confirms multiple pleural metastases involving the (d) horizontal and (e) oblique fissures (arrows).*

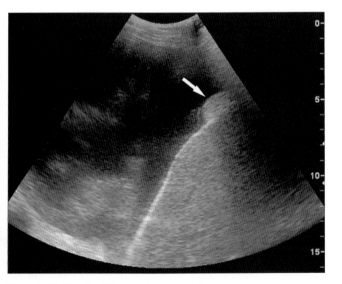

Figure 40.28. *An 82-year-old man with recurrent non-Hodgkin's lymphoma in the right pleural cavity. Ultrasound of the right hemithorax demonstrates an echogenic effusion and a diaphragmatic nodule (arrow).*

are all suggestive of malignant disease[73] (Fig. 40.29). However, metastatic pleural disease (in particular, adenocarcinoma) and malignant mesothelioma are frequently indistinguishable radiologically, and histologic confirmation is necessary.

Magnetic resonance has also been assessed in the diagnosis of metastatic pleural disease[74] and high-signal intensity in relation to intercostal muscle on T2-weighted or contrast-enhanced T1-weighted sections was found to be suggestive for malignant disease (Fig. 40.30).

There have been reports of the clinical role of [18]FDG PET in differentiating malignant from benign pleural disease. Gupta et al.[75] reported a sensitivity and specificity of 88.8% and 94.1%, respectively, of [18]FDG PET in correctly separating benign pleural disease from malignant pleural disease in patients with lung cancer. Further studies are warranted to assess the role of [18]FDG PET in the assessment of pleural disease.

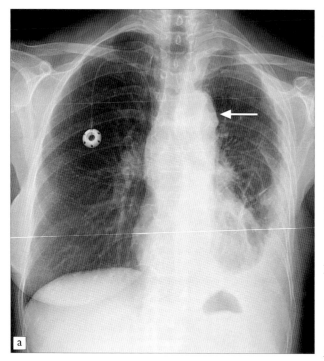

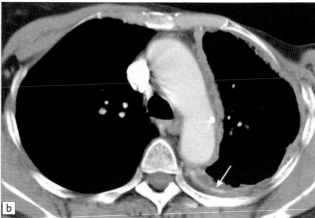

Figure 40.29. *A 46-year-old woman with metastatic breast cancer. (a) Chest radiograph shows lobulated left pleural thickening which extends along the mediastinal border and distorts the outline of the aortic arch (arrow). (b) CT scan shows mediastinal pleural thickening along the aortic arch. There is high-density material (arrow) within the left pleural cavity, which is consistent with talc from prior pleurodesis.*

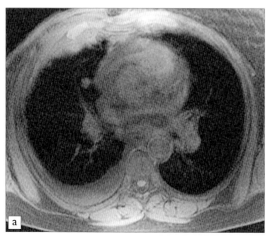

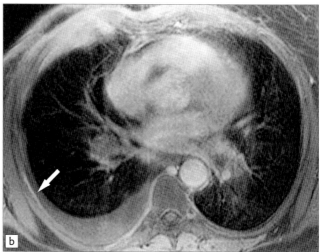

Figure 40.30. *A 41-year-old woman with metastatic breast cancer to the right chest wall and a malignant right pleural effusion. Fat-saturated pre- and postcontrast T1-weighted images (a and b) demonstrate high signal intensity in the right chest wall and pleural fluid. Postcontrast (b) image show enhancement of the pleura (arrow).*

Key points: pleural metastases

- Pleural metastases can manifest as effusions, pleural thickening, nodules or masses
- The most common malignancies that spread to the pleura are lung, breast and lymphoma
- More than 300 ml of pleural fluid is necessary for detection on an erect chest radiograph

- The majority of malignant exudative effusions are not associated with pleural thickening on CT
- Pleural nodules and circumferential or mediastinal pleural thickening are the most helpful CT features in distinguishing benign from malignant disease

Summary

- CT scanning is now routinely used in the screening and follow-up of patients with pulmonary metastatic disease; helical CT offers advantages over chest radiography in the detection of lung nodules

- HRCT gives exquisite detail of the lung parenchyma and enables the radiologist to localize tumour involvement more accurately and establish a more specific differential diagnosis based on the lung compartments involved

- The patterns of metastatic pulmonary disease vary between tumours, but solid nodules are most common. Other patterns, such as ground glass attenuation, branching configuration, calcification or cavitation, are identifiable on CT and can be specific for tumour types

- Reticular disease or involvement of the interstitium suggests lymphangitic and interstitial spread of tumour. A mixed parenchymal pattern including consolidation may also be seen with metastatic disease, most commonly in patients with bronchioloalveolar cell carcinoma or lymphoma

- Metastatic disease within the pleural space can manifest as effusions, pleural thickening or pleural nodules. The most common malignancies are adenocarcinomas from the lung, breast or from lymphoma

- Ultrasound and CT are more sensitive than chest radiography in identifying pleural effusions. Most malignant effusions show no other CT abnormality

- The presence of pleural nodules or circumferential pleural involvement is more indicative of malignancy

References

1. Vock P, Soucek M, Daepp M, Kalender W A. Lung: spiral volumetric CT with single-breath-hold technique. Radiology 1990; 176: 864–867

2. Remy-Jardin M, Remy J, Giraud F, Marquette C H. Pulmonary nodules: detection with thick-section spiral CT versus conventional CT. Radiology 1993; 187: 513–520

3. Diederich S, Lentschig M G, Winter F et al. Detection of pulmonary nodules with overlapping vs non-overlapping image reconstruction at spiral CT. Eur Radiol 1999; 9: 281–286

4. Rydberg J, Buckwalter K A, Caldemeyer K S et al. Multisection CT: scanning techniques and clinical applications. Radiographics 2000; 20: 1787–1806

5. Berland L L, Smith J K. Multidetector-array CT: once again, technology creates new opportunities. Radiology 1998; 209: 327–329

6. Waters D J, Coakley F V, Cohen M D et al. The detection of pulmonary metastases by helical CT: a clinicopathologic study in dogs. J Comput Assist Tomogr 1998; 22: 235–240

7. Ambrogi V, Paci M, Pompeo E, Mineo T C. Transxiphoid video-assisted pulmonary metastasectomy: relevance of helical computed tomography occult lesions. Ann Thorac Surg 2000; 70: 1847–1852

8. Margaritora S, Porziella V, D'Andrilli A et al. Pulmonary metastases: can accurate radiological evaluation avoid thoracotomic approach? Eur J Cardiothorac Surg 2002; 21: 1111–1114

9. Picci P, Vanel D, Briccoli A et al. Computed tomography of pulmonary metastases from osteosarcoma: the less poor technique. A study of 51 patients with histological correlation. Ann Oncol 2001; 12: 1601–1604

10. Patz E F, Lowe V J, Hoffman J M et al. Focal pulmonary abnormalities: evaluation with F-18 fluorodeoxyglucose PET scanning. Radiology 1993; 188: 487–490

11. Sazon D A, Santiago S M, Soo Hoo G W et al. Fluorodeoxyglucose-positron emission tomography in the detection and staging of lung cancer. Am J Respir Crit Care Med 1996; 153: 417–421

12. Pieterman R M, van Putten J W, Meuzelaar J J et al. Preoperative staging of non-small-cell lung cancer with positron-emission tomography. N Engl J Med 2000; 343: 254–261

13. Mawatari T, Watanabe A, Ohsawa H et al. Surgery for metastatic lung tumors at our department during the last 10 years. Kyobu Geka 2003; 56: 28–31 (in Japanese)

14. Watanabe M, Deguchi H, Sato M et al. Midterm results of thoracoscopic surgery for pulmonary metastases especially from colorectal cancers. J Laparoendosc Adv Surg Tech A 1998; 8: 195–200

15. Karnak I, Emin Senocak M, Kutluk T et al. Pulmonary metastases in children: an analysis of surgical spectrum. Eur J Pediatr Surg 2002; 12: 151–158

16. McCormack P M, Bains M S, Begg C B et al. Role of video-assisted thoracic surgery in the treatment of pulmonary metastases: results of a prospective trial. Ann Thorac Surg 1996; 62: 213–217

17. Benditt J O, Farber H W, Wright J, Karnad A B. Pulmonary hemorrhage with diffuse alveolar infiltrates in men with high-volume choriocarcinoma. Ann Intern Med 1988; 109: 674–675

18. Patel A M, Ryu J H. Angiosarcoma in the lung. Chest 1993; 103: 1531–1535

19. Hirakata K, Nakata H, Haratake J. Appearance of pulmonary metastases on high-resolution CT scans:

comparison with histopathologic findings from autopsy specimens. Am J Roentgenol 1993; 161: 37–43

20. Kim Y, Lee K S, Jung K J et al. Halo sign on high-resolution CT: findings in spectrum of pulmonary diseases with pathologic correlation. J Comput Assist Tomogr 1999; 23: 622–626

21. Bhagavan B S, Dorfman H D, Murthy M S, Eggleston J C. Intravascular bronchiolo-alveolar tumor (IVBAT): a low-grade sclerosing epithelioid angiosarcoma of lung. Am J Surg Pathol 1982; 6: 41–52

22. Johnson G L, Askin F B, Fishman E K. Thoracic involvement from osteosarcoma: typical and atypical CT manifestations. Am J Roentgenol 1997; 168: 347–349

23. Maile C W, Rodan B A, Godwin J D et al. Calcification in pulmonary metastases. Br J Radiol 1982; 55: 108–113

24. Ikezoe J, Johkoh T, Takeuchi N et al. CT findings of endobronchial metastasis. Acta Radiol 1991; 32: 455–460

25. Baumgartner W A, Mark J B. Metastatic malignancies from distant sites to the tracheobronchial tree. J Thorac Cardiovasc Surg 1980; 79: 499–503

26. Berg H K, Petrelli N J, Herrera L et al. Endobronchial metastasis from colorectal carcinoma. Dis Colon Rectum 1984; 27: 745–748

27. Mason A C, White C S. CT appearance of endobronchial non-Hodgkin lymphoma. J Comput Assist Tomogr 1994; 18: 559–561

28. Aquino S L, Gamsu G, Webb W R, Kee S T. Tree-in-bud pattern: frequency and significance on thin section CT. J Comput Assist Tomogr 1996; 20: 594–599

29. Shepard J A, Moore E H, Templeton P A, McLoud T C. Pulmonary intravascular tumor emboli: dilated and beaded peripheral pulmonary arteries at CT. Radiology 1993; 187: 797–801

30. Kang C H, Choi J A, Kim H R et al. Lung metastases manifesting as pulmonary infarction by mucin and tumor embolization: radiographic, high-resolution CT, and pathologic findings. J Comput Assist Tomogr 1999; 23: 644–646

31. Nelson E, Klein J S. Pulmonary infarction resulting from metastatic osteogenic sarcoma with pulmonary venous tumor thrombus. Am J Roentgenol 2000; 174: 531–533

32. Dodd G D, Boyle J J. Excavating pulmonary metasteses. Am J Roentgenol 1961; 85: 277–293

33. Chaudhuri M R. Cavitary pulmonary metastases. Thorax 1970; 25: 375–381

34. Shin M S, Shingleton H M, Partridge E E et al. Squamous cell carcinoma of the uterine cervix. Patterns of thoracic metastases. Invest Radiol 1995; 30: 724–729

35. Ohdama S, Akagawa S, Matsubara O, Yoshizawa Y. Primary diffuse alveolar septal amyloidosis with multiple cysts and calcification. Eur Respir J 1996; 9: 1569–1571

36. Essadki O, Chartrand-Lefebvre C, Finet J F, Grenier P. Cystic pulmonary metastasis simulating a diagnosis of histiocytosis X. J Radiol 1998; 79: 886–888

37. Thalinger A R, Rosenthal S N, Borg S, Arseneau J C. Cavitation of pulmonary metastases as a response to chemotherapy. Cancer 1980; 46: 1329–1332

38. Smevik B, Klepp O. The risk of spontaneous pneumothorax in patients with osteogenic sarcoma and testicular cancer. Cancer 1982; 49: 1734–1737

39. Stein M G, Mayo J, Muller N et al. Pulmonary lymphangitic spread of carcinoma: appearance on CT scans. Radiology 1987; 162: 371–375

40. Mathieson J R, Mayo J R, Staples C A, Muller N L. Chronic diffuse infiltrative lung disease: comparison of diagnostic accuracy of CT and chest radiography. Radiology 1989; 171: 111–116

41. Heyneman L E, Johkoh T, Ward S et al. Pulmonary leukemic infiltrates: high-resolution CT findings in 10 patients. Am J Roentgenol 2000; 174: 517–521

42. Dodd G D, Ledesma-Medina J, Baron R L, Fuhrman C R. Post-transplant lymphoproliferative disorder: intrathoracic manifestations. Radiology 1992; 184: 65–69

43. Ichikawa Y, Kinoshita M, Koga T et al. Lung cyst formation in lymphocytic interstitial pneumonia: CT features. J Comput Assist Tomogr 1994; 18: 745–748

44. Carignan S, Staples C A, Muller N L. Intrathoracic lymphoproliferative disorders in the immunocompromised patient: CT findings. Radiology 1995; 197: 53–58

45. Shahar J, Angelillo V A, Katz D, Moore J A. Recurrent cavitary nodules secondary to Hodgkin's disease. Chest 1987; 91: 273–274

46. Lee K S, Kim Y, Primack S L. Imaging of pulmonary lymphomas. Am J Roentgenol 1997; 168: 339–345

47. Berkman N, Breuer R, Kramer M R, Polliack A. Pulmonary involvement in lymphoma. Leuk Lymph 1996; 20: 229–237

48. Lewis E R, Caskey C I, Fishman E K. Lymphoma of the lung: CT findings in 31 patients. Am J Roentgenol 1991; 156: 711–714

49. Jang H J, Lee K S, Kwon O J et al. Bronchioloalveolar carcinoma: focal area of ground-glass attenuation at thin-section CT as an early sign. Radiology 1996; 199: 485–488

50. Aquino S L, Chiles C, Halford P. Distinction of consolidative bronchioloalveolar carcinoma from pneumonia: do CT criteria work? Am J Roentgenol 1998; 171: 359–363

51. Akira M, Atagi S, Kawahara M et al. High-resolution CT findings of diffuse bronchioloalveolar carcinoma in 38 patients. Am J Roentgenol 1999; 173: 1623–1629

52. Tan R T, Kuzo R S. High-resolution CT findings of mucinous bronchioloalveolar carcinoma: a case of pseudopulmonary alveolar proteinosis. Am J Roentgenol 1997; 168: 99–100

53. Wolff S D, Kuhlman J E, Fishman E K. Thoracic Kaposi sarcoma in AIDS: CT findings. J Comput Assist Tomogr 1993; 17: 60–62

54. Fentiman I S, Millis R, Sexton S, Hayward J L. Pleural effusion in breast cancer: a review of 105 cases. Cancer 1981; 47: 2087–2092

55. Sears D, Hajdu S I. The cytologic diagnosis of malignant neoplasms in pleural and peritoneal effusions. Acta Cytol 1987; 31: 85–97

56. van de Molengraft F J, Vooijs G P. Survival of patients with malignancy-associated effusions. Acta Cytol 1989; 33: 911–916

57. Marel M, Zrustova M, Stasny B, Light R W. The incidence of pleural effusion in a well-defined region. Epidemiologic study in central Bohemia. Chest 1993; 104: 1486–1489

58. Salyer W R, Eggleston J C, Erozan Y S. Efficacy of pleural needle biopsy and pleural fluid cytopathology in the diagnosis of malignant neoplasm involving the pleura. Chest 1975; 67: 536–539

59. Rabin C B, Coleman N S. Bilateral pleural effusion and significance in association with a heart of normal size. J Mt Sinai Hosp 1957; 24: 45–53

60. Monte S A, Ehya H, Lang W R. Positive effusion cytology as the initial presentation of malignancy. Acta Cytol 1987; 31: 448–452

61. Sahn S A. Pleural diseases related to metastatic malignancies. Eur Respir J 1997; 10: 1907–1913

62. Chernow B, Sahn S A. Carcinomatous involvement of the pleura: an analysis of 96 patients. Am J Med 1977; 63: 695–702

63. Rodriguez-Panadero F, Borderas Naranjo F, Lopez Mejias J. Pleural metastatic tumours and effusions. Frequency and pathogenic mechanisms in a post-mortem series. Eur Respir J 1989; 2: 366–369

64. Xaubet A, Diumenjo M C, Marin A et al. Characteristics and prognostic value of pleural effusions in non-Hodgkin's lymphomas. Eur J Respir Dis 1985; 66: 135–140

65. Castellino R A, Blank N, Hoppe R T, Cho C. Hodgkin disease: contributions of chest CT in the initial staging evaluation. Radiology 1986; 160: 603–605

66. McLoud T C, Flower C D. Imaging the pleura: sonography, CT, and MR imaging. Am J Roentgenol 1991; 156: 1145–1153

67. Moskowitz H, Platt RT, Schachar R, Mellins H. Roentgen visualization of minute pleural effusion. An experimental study to determine the minimum amount of pleural fluid visible on a radiograph. Radiology 1973; 109: 33–35

68. Eibenberger K L, Dock W I, Ammann M E et al. Quantification of pleural effusions: sonography versus radiography. Radiology 1994; 191: 681–684

69. Yang P C, Luh K T, Chang D B et al. Value of sonography in determining the nature of pleural effusion: analysis of 320 cases. Am J Roentgenol 1992; 159: 29–33

70. Akaogi E, Mitsui K, Onizuka M et al. Pleural dissemination in non-small cell lung cancer: results of radiological evaluation and surgical treatment. J Surg Oncol 1994; 57: 33–39

71. Aquino S L, Webb W R, Gushiken B J. Pleural exudates and transudates: diagnosis with contrast-enhanced CT. Radiology 1994; 192: 803–808

72. Arenas-Jimenez J, Alonso-Charterina S, Sanchez-Paya J et al. Evaluation of CT findings for diagnosis of pleural effusions. Eur Radiol 2000; 10: 681–690

73. Leung A N, Muller N L, Miller R R. CT in differential diagnosis of diffuse pleural disease. Am J Roentgenol 1990; 154: 487–492

74. Hierholzer J, Luo L, Bittner R C et al. MRI and CT in the differential diagnosis of pleural disease. Chest 2000; 118: 604–609

75. Gupta N C, Rogers J S, Graeber G M et al. Clinical role of F-18 fluorodeoxyglucose positron emission tomography imaging in patients with lung cancer and suspected malignant pleural effusion. Chest 2002; 122: 1918–1924

Chapter 41

Bone metastases

Daniel Vanel, Janet E Husband and Anwar R Padhani

Introduction

Bone is a complex composite tissue that has an important role in human physiology as it is the site of immunological, haematological and metabolic processes.[1,2] Evaluation of the bone marrow in patients with cancer may be useful for determining treatment and prognosis. Traditionally, bone marrow biopsy has been used to evaluate metastatic involvement, but this is prone to sampling errors and unguided biopsy may yield results that are not representative of changes in the rest of the bone marrow.[3] The purpose of imaging is to identify bone metastases, to determine the extent of disease, to evaluate complications such as spinal cord compression or fractures, and to monitor therapeutic response. Imaging may be undertaken for routine screening in those tumours which have a high incidence of bone metastases such as breast and prostate cancer, if and only if there are practical consequences.[4,5] It is also frequently employed in symptomatic patients presenting with pain or neurological deficit. Imaging studies complement clinical examination, serum tumour-marker estimations which may point to disseminated disease (e.g. prostate-specific antigen levels in prostate cancer) and trephine bone marrow biopsy.

Imaging studies are able to detect bone metastases non-invasively. These include:

- Radionuclide scintigraphy
- Plain radiography
- Computed tomography (CT)
- Magnetic resonance imaging (MR)
- Positron emission tomography (PET)

Radionuclide scintigraphy can provide a survey of bone marrow directly (using radiolabelled colloid or iron)[6] or the supporting bone (diphosphonate bone scan). The latter is the most commonly used radionuclide study for the assessment of bone but lacks anatomical detail and has low specificity. Detection of lesions by plain radiography requires the presence of bone destruction. Computed tomography also detects bone metastases by virtue of bone destruction and is more sensitive than plain radiography.

Magnetic resonance imaging is an important technique for evaluating the bone marrow because it has excellent spatial and contrast resolution, multiplanar imaging capability and the unique ability to separate haemopoietic (red) marrow from non-haemopoietic (yellow) marrow.[7] It also provides the opportunity to survey large volumes of bone marrow at a single examination.

2-[F-18]fluoro-2-deoxy-D-glucose positron emission tomography ([18]FDG PET) produces metabolic images, most often linked to glucose taken up by the tissues and, although a promising technique, is still under investigation for bone metastases.

Clinical features of bone metastases

Most bone metastases are asymptomatic. Symptoms occur when lesions reach a certain size, when destruction of trabecular bone leads to bone weakening and collapse, or when a fracture from a metastasis occurs in a long bone. Pain may also occur when a metastasis has broken through the cortex of a vertebra to produce a paravertebral soft tissue mass and may be associated with neurological deficit if there is compression of nerve roots or the spinal cord. Vertebral collapse causing spinal cord compression is seen in 5–10% of patients with vertebral body metastases. Vertebral instability occurs when the dorsal elements of vertebrae are also involved.

Treatment of bony metastatic disease depends on:

- The nature of the primary tumour
- The presence of soft tissue disease
- Complications
- The presence of other bony metastases

For example, treatment of a solitary bone metastasis in an asymptomatic patient with advanced local disease and other soft tissue metastases may not be indicated, whereas a patient with a solitary bone metastasis and no other evidence of disseminated malignancy may be given radiotherapy or chemotherapy depending upon the sensitivity of the primary tumour to different therapy regimens. Thus if a solitary metastasis is found within a vertebral body it is important to determine whether other lesions are present, as this will significantly alter management. Localized spinal cord compression may be treated with radiotherapy if there is a significant soft tissue component, alternatively surgical intervention with a laminectomy may prevent irreversible neurological damage.

Incidence

The most common focal bone marrow pathology in cancer patients is metastatic disease. Metastatic cancer to the skeletal bone occurs in 30–70% of all cancer patients.[8,9] Recently, with improved patient survival, the overall incidence of metastatic bone disease has increased. In 1950, Abrams[9] reported an incidence of 27% from 1,000 consecutive autopsy patients who died from epithelial cancers. The sites of the primary tumours most commonly associated with bony metastases were:

- Breast (73%)
- Lung (32%)
- Kidney (24%)

Other sites included:

- Rectum
- Pancreas
- Stomach
- Colon
- Ovary

Today, breast and prostate cancer are the most common causes of bone metastases. Overall, breast cancer is responsible for approximately 70% of all bone metastases in women and prostate cancer represents the primary site in 60% of bone metastases in men.[10]

Distribution

Bone involvement by cancer occurs most commonly by haematogenous spread although direct invasion of bone from tumour in adjacent soft tissues is not uncommon.[11,12] Over 90% of metastatic lesions are found in the distribution of the red marrow in adults (Fig. 41.1).[13] In a series of 2,001 cases, Clain[14] reported the percentage of patients with metastases to different sites as follows:

- Vertebrae (69%)
- Pelvis (41%)
- Femur, especially the proximal femora (25%)
- Skull (14%)

The upper extremity is much less commonly involved (10–15%).[9] For most cancers, the pattern of involvement is similar, although some tumours show a predilection for specific sites (e.g. pelvic bones in prostate and bladder cancer). Peripheral long bone metastases are most commonly seen in lung and breast cancer (Fig. 41.2).[15,16] Metastases expanding the bone are mainly seen in renal and thyroid cancer. Metastases usually involve multiple sites although approximately 10% are solitary, most frequently from renal or thyroid primary tumours.[17] It may be difficult

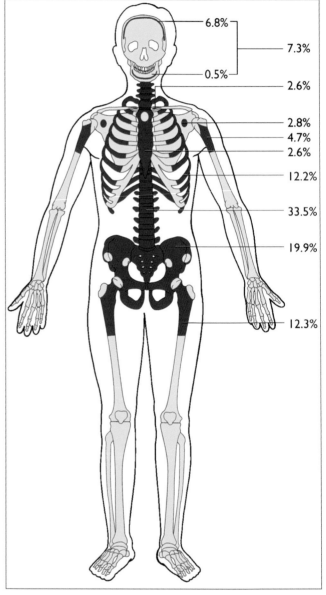

Figure 41.1. *Adult pattern of red and yellow marrow distribution with incidence of metastatic disease.*

on occasion to differentiate these metastases from a primary bone tumour. In general, metastatic deposits are small (1–3 cm); however, deposits in the pelvis are often very extensive by the time of diagnosis, and can mimic primary tumours.[18,19] Extra-osseous tumour extension into the adjacent soft tissues is rare in metastatic disease and is a useful distinguishing feature between primary and metastatic malignant lesions.

Metastases in long bones initially involve the metaphysis which is the site of residual red marrow. Less commonly, the mid-diaphysis is first affected. Primary cortical metastases are rare but have been reported in lung cancer[20] (Fig. 41.2) as well as in metastatic melanoma and sarcomas.[21]

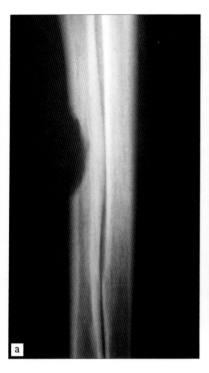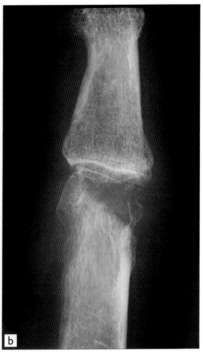

Figure 41.2. *Atypical bone metastases may suggest the primary tumour site. (a) Cortical and (b) distal metastases. Fifty percent of such lesions are from lung cancer.*

Pathophysiological features

The venous system is the main pathway for transport of cancer cells to the skeleton as bone does not contain lymphatic channels.[22] It is well established that the network of vertebral epidural and perivertebral veins plays a significant role in the transport of cancer cells to the vertebral bone marrow.[23–25] The system parallels, joins and bypasses the normal venous system and its presence, in part, explains the frequency of distribution of metastases within the vertebral column, pelvis and shoulder girdles. In addition, the increased susceptibility of the red marrow compared with yellow marrow is related to haemodynamic factors which contribute to tumour extravasation and hence to the development of metastases.[11]

Tumour cells may destroy bone directly or by the production of mediators that stimulate reabsorption by osteoclasts. Prostaglandins and other tumour-derived growth factors also appear to be important.[26,27] As metastatic lesions enlarge within the marrow, the surrounding bone undergoes osteoclastic (resorptive) and osteoblastic (depositional) activity. The level of these activities differs among tumour types and sometimes for the same tumour at different skeletal locations. The balance of these two processes determines the final radiographic appearance of lytic, sclerotic or mixed lesions.

Key points: general features

- Most bone metastases are asymptomatic

- Over 90% of metastases occur within the distribution of the red marrow

- Approximately 10% of metastases are solitary

- Extra-bony spread into the soft tissues is rare

- In long bones, metastases usually occur in the metaphysis

- Cortical bone metastases most frequently occur in lung cancer

- The network of vertebral, epidural and perivertebral veins plays a significant role in transport of cancer cells to the vertebral column

Imaging techniques for detection of metastases

Accurate assessment of bony metastases requires the combination of clinical evaluation, biochemical parameters and appropriate imaging studies. Radionuclide bone scans and plain radiographs remain key investigations but CT and MR have important supplementary roles and [18]FDG PET is evolving as a potentially useful new modality in this clinical setting. All these techniques have strengths and weaknesses which should be recognized so that they are used appropriately in a cost-effective manner.

Radionuclide scintigraphy

Bone may be imaged using Tc-99m-diphosphonate (MDP) scanning. The bone scan image reflects skeletal metabolic activity and the major factors affecting diphosphonate uptake by the skeleton are osteoblastic activity and, to a lesser extent, skeletal vascularity.[28] The MDP bone scan is an extremely useful imaging modality for the diagnosis and management of patients with skeletal metastases[29–31] and is used for detection and staging of cancer but is less useful for following the response of bony lesions to treatment. The major advantages of bone scans are excellent sensitivity for lesion detection and visualization of the whole skeleton. In general, bone scans will detect metastatic lesions before they are evident on plain radiographs. Despite high sensitivity, bone scans have low specificity and cannot distinguish benign from malignant causes of increased tracer uptake. Bone scans are reliable for the detection of metastases from the breast, prostate, lung and kidney. However, bone scans are less reliable for the diagnosis of round cell tumours, myeloma, lymphoma and the leukaemias.[12,32] Photopenic areas are observed with myeloma and aggressive metastatic lesions that have rapid lytic bony destruction, e.g. renal cancer. Overall, false negative results are uncommon. False positive results may occur from traumatic, infectious or metabolic causes as well as from benign bone tumours. Metastatic superscans may be seen in breast and prostate cancer (Fig. 41.3).

A common problem encountered with bone scans is that of the solitary lesion in a patient with known malignancy. This occurs in 5–8% of all patients.[29] The anatomical site is important; 80% of vertebral lesions compared with 18% of rib lesions prove to be metastatic.[29] If scintigraphy reveals a solitary lesion, plain radiographs, CT or MR may aid in the differential diagnosis (Fig. 41.4).

Radionuclide bone scans are relatively insensitive for evaluating treatment response but, in general, healing is indicated by a decrease in activity. However, in 10–15% of patients, a 'flare phenomenon' is seen in which increased bony uptake is due to stimulation of osteoblastic activity in response to treatment.[30,33] In rare cases, previously undetected lesions may become visible due to the same phenomenon, thus simulating progressive disease.

Key points: radionuclide scintigraphy

- ■ MDP scanning has excellent sensitivity in the detection of bone metastases and visualizes the whole skeleton

- ■ MDP bone scans are unreliable in myeloma, lymphoma and leukaemia

- ■ Osteoblastic metastases are more easily detected than osteolytic lesions

- ■ MDP bone scans are relatively insensitive for evaluating treatment response

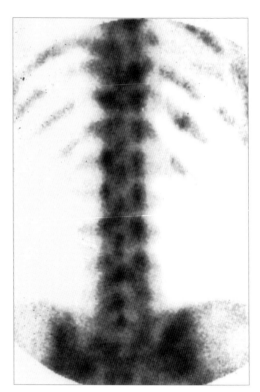

Figure 41.3. *Metastatic superscan. Posterior view of MDP bone scan in a patient with metastatic breast cancer. Multiple irregular focal areas of increased tracer uptake are seen and are characteristic of metastatic disease. There is minimal uptake of the tracer in the soft tissues and kidneys.*

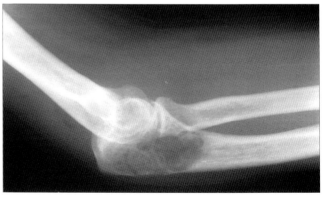

Figure 41.4. *Osteolytic metastasis. Well-defined lytic metastasis from breast cancer in the olecranon and proximal ulnar bone. There is predominant involvement of the medulla with thinning of the cortex. A pathological fracture is present. There is a small associated soft tissue mass.*

Plain radiography

Conventional plain radiographs provide important information about cortical and trabecular bone, but little information regarding the presence of lesions confined to the bone marrow. Radiographic sensitivity is dependent on the presence of bone destruction and the type and degree of host response. Considerable bone destruction must be present before a bone metastasis is evident radiographically and, indeed, it has been estimated that a 30–50% reduction in bone density is required to visualize a lesion in cancellous bone.[34] Plain radiographs are therefore an insensitive method of detecting metastatic bone disease but have the major advantage of high specificity.

On plain radiographs, bone metastases are seen as osteolytic, osteoblastic or less commonly mixed lesions (Table 41,1). Combinations of all three types may also be observed. Osteolytic metastases show three different appearances on plain radiographs which include:

- Moth-eaten appearance – multiple small- to medium-sized lesions coalescing to form larger defects
  - Ill-defined zone of transition
  - No sclerotic margins
  - No periosteal reaction
  - Soft tissue mass absent or small
  - Typically seen in breast cancer
- Diffuse infiltration – lesions infiltrating the whole bone
  - Ill-defined zone of transition
  - No sclerotic margins
  - No periosteal reaction
  - No soft tissue mass
  - Typically seen in neuroblastoma
- Large bubbly expansile lesions – may be solitary
  - Well-defined
  - Sharp zone of transition
  - May have sclerotic margin
  - Periosteal reaction sometimes seen
  - Soft tissue mass may be present
  - Typically seen in thyroid and renal cancer

Table 41.1. *Radiographic appearance of skeletal metastases*

Primary tumour	Radiographic appearance
Common primary cancer	
Breast	Lytic; also mixed; frequently blastic
Lung	Lytic; also mixed; occasionally blastic
Kidney	Invariably lytic
Thyroid	Invariably lytic
Prostate	Usually blastic; occasionally lytic
Head and neck	Usually lytic
Gastro-intestinal tract	
Oesophagus	Lytic or mixed
Stomach	Lytic or mixed; occasionally blastic
Colon	Lytic or mixed; infrequently blastic
Rectum	Lytic or mixed; infrequently blastic
Pancreas	Lytic or mixed; occasionally blastic
Liver	Lytic or mixed
Gallbladder	Lytic or mixed
Genito-urinary tract	
Urinary bladder	Lytic; infrequently blastic
Adrenal	Lytic
Reproductive system	
Uterine cervix	Lytic or mixed; occasionally blastic
Uterine corpus	Lytic
Skin	
Squamous and Basal cell carcinoma	Lytic
Malignant melanoma	Lytic
Carcinoid tumours	Bronchial and abdominal blastic; frequently mixed

Osteoblastic lesions are less common and are most frequently seen in patients with breast and prostate cancer.

Osteoblastic metastases (Fig. 41.5) may show any of the following features:

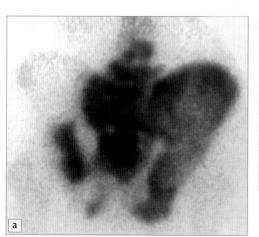
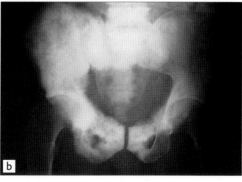

Figure 41.5. *Diffuse sclerotic metastases. (a) Posterior view of pelvis of MDP bone scan in a patient with metastatic prostate cancer. Marked tracer uptake is seen in the lower lumbar and sacral spine and both iliac bones. (b) Pelvic radiograph shows corresponding mottled sclerotic deposits with expansion of the bones and irregularity and poor definition of the cortical outlines.*

- Round discrete lesions of uniform high density
- Irregular lesions showing a mottled appearance due to varying degrees of sclerosis
- Diffuse large lesions of high density with poorly defined borders

The osteoblastic component of the metastasis represents a reaction of normal bone to the metastatic process and thus the degree and pattern of sclerosis varies among different tumours and in the same tumour at different sites. The degree of sclerosis is considered to indicate the rate of tumour growth and, hence, dense reactive sclerosis usually reflects slow tumour growth. In fast-growing tumours with a tendency to induce sclerosis, a mixed lytic and sclerotic pattern may be seen. Increasing sclerosis is also a sign of repair following treatment (Fig. 41.6).

Plain radiographs are primarily used to:

- Establish the diagnosis
- Determine the target volume for radiotherapy
- Assess treatment response
- Evaluate bones for structural integrity

Fractures may occur when >50% of the thickness of the cortex in a long bone is involved radiographically.[35] Prophylactic therapy at appropriate sites should be considered for lesions that are >2.5 cm in size, when >50% of the cortical bone is compromised and for pain.

Key points: plain radiographs

- ■ A 30–50% reduction in bone density is required before a lesion in cancellous bone will be visible on plain films

- ■ Osteolytic lesions are more difficult to identify than osteoblastic lesions

- ■ Fractures may occur when >50% of the thickness of the cortex of the long bone is involved radiographically

Computed tomography

Computed tomography continues to play an important role in the evaluation of vertebral metastases when dural compression is suspected and for distinguishing benign from malignant causes of vertebral collapse.[36] An important use of CT is to provide guidance for percutaneous bone biopsy and image-guided treatment (Fig. 41.7). Computed tomography not only demonstrates the most appropriate route for biopsy but also demonstrates the presence of an associated soft tissue mass, which may be easier to biopsy than the bone itself. If no soft tissue mass is seen, then CT may demonstrate areas of destruction of the cortex, again

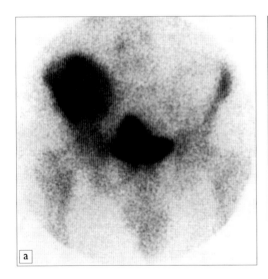

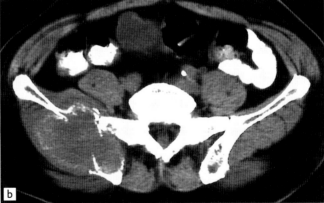

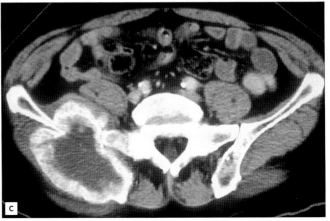

Figure 41.6. *Calcifying metastatic bladder cancer. (a) Tc-99m-diphosphonate bone scan of pelvis showing marked focal increased tracer uptake in the right iliac bone. (b) CT scan demonstrates a lytic lesion with a large soft tissue component with some matrix calcification in the soft tissue component. (c) CT scan 4 months after commencement of chemotherapy demonstrates marked calcification/ossification of the metastatic deposit, indicating response to therapy.*

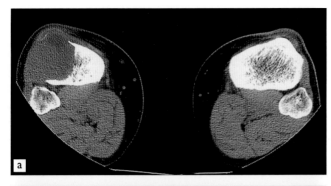

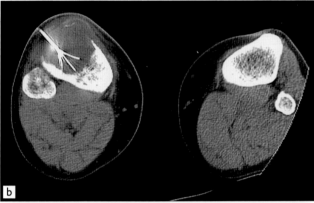

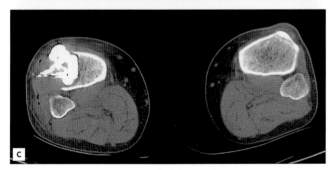

Figure 41.7. *Lytic painful tibial metastases from a malignant melanoma. (a) CT scan showing metastases. (b) CT scan showing local treatment using radiofrequency. (c) CT scan showing injected cement to relieve pain and strengthen bone.*

depicting the most suitable biopsy site. In summary, the role of CT in evaluating bone metastases is:

- Detection of bone metastases only if MR is not available, e.g. a solitary hot spot on a bone scan
- Preoperative planning for decompression for spinal metastases
- Distinction of benign from malignant vertebral collapse
- Guidance of percutaneous biopsy

Magnetic resonance imaging

Magnetic resonance imaging is ideally suited for the evaluation of bone marrow because the technique shows:

- Bone marrow and bone marrow disorders directly
- Excellent soft tissue contrast
- Good anatomical detail
- Multiplanar imaging capabilities[7,37,38]

Magnetic resonance imaging is highly sensitive for the detection of bone marrow metastases demonstrating lesions in the presence of normal radiographs and negative radionuclide bone scans.[39–43] Not uncommonly, MR demonstrates incidental bone marrow metastases in patients undergoing MR for primary tumour staging, e.g. prostate cancer. The opportunity to study the whole skeleton on a single MR examination in a reasonable time (around 20 min) makes MR even more efficient (Fig. 41.8).[44,45] The appearance of the bone marrow on MR is dependent on a number of factors including mineral, fat and water composition.

MR sequences

Fat and water distribution in bone marrow, indirect visualization of normal bone trabeculae, indirect evaluation of bone oedema and cell density and the study of vascularization can be ingeniously combined to enable good detection and characterization of lesions.

Fat and water

Normal marrow contains both fat and water (yellow marrow 80% fat, but also 15% water, and red marrow 40% fat

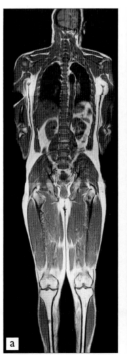
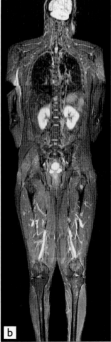

Figure 41.8. *MR examination of the whole skeleton. (a) T1-weighted spin-echo and (b) STIR images. The images combine four acquisitions. Total acquisition time: 20 min.*

and 40% water). In infiltrative disorders, fat disappears in a diffuse, disseminated or solitary way. Sequences displaying differences between fat and water signal are thus useful.

T1-weighted spin-echo sequences Fat has a shorter signal than water and the highest signal. Thus, fatty marrow containing 80% of fat exhibits a high signal intensity and any focal lesion showing a lower signal intensity is easy to detect. This explains why this sequence is very useful and usually the first used. Haematopoietic marrow, containing water but also fat, is hypointense to fat but hyperintense to normal muscles. A marrow signal that is hypointense to the muscles and discs in the spine is abnormal.

Chemical-shift imaging The difference in resonance frequency between water and fat protons can be used. It has no consequence on the contrast on conventional spin-echo sequences as the 180° pulse cancels the difference. Normally, the read-out gradient is centred on the echo, which appears symmetrically on the 90° pulse with respect to the 180° pulse. The signal intensity is thus proportional to the sum of water and fat protons (in-phase image). By shifting the read-out window, it is possible to obtain images in which contrast is related to the difference between the quantities of water and fat protons (opposed-phase images).

In gradient-echo sequences, the same phenomenon occurs, depending only on the echo time. If fat and water protons are in-phase, their signals are added; if they are opposed-phase, they are subtracted. If a lesion replaces normal marrow, fat can be obliterated and no subtraction will occur. The difference between the signal produced by normal marrow, which always contains water and fat, will be emphasized on opposed-phase sequences.

Fat-suppression techniques A 180° inversion pulse is used initially for short tau inversion recovery (STIR) sequence. The inversion time is chosen to cancel the signal of fat. This sequence can be obtained on any MR unit, but it is unfortunately time-consuming and only a limited number of slices can be acquired. This can be overcome by using fast STIR sequences. The main drawback of the STIR sequence is that it cancels every signal identical to fat, for example blood in haematoma or contrast-enhanced tissue.

The difference between fat and water proton frequency is also used for fat presaturation. A saturation pulse with a narrow band at the exact fat frequency is used before the usual pulse. A very homogeneous magnetic field is required, therefore this sequence is not effective on every unit.

Bone trabeculae
Because of the lack of mobile protons, trabecular bone yields no detectable signal, but creates magnetic field heterogeneities. These have minimal impact on spin-echo sequences, as their effect is cancelled by the 180° pulse but there may be a visible effect on gradient-echo sequences as field heterogeneity is not cancelled. If the TE is long enough, the signal can be decreased considerably because of the presence of normal trabeculae. This is particularly visible in the vertebrae, pelvic bones and the proximal ends of the long tubular bones. If bone trabeculae have been destroyed, the signal will be higher than in the preserved parts of the bone. Thus this provides an indirect technique for the diagnosis of a trabecular lysis (Fig. 41.9).[46]

Diffusion Diffusion imaging, using echo planar imaging (EPI), is well known in the assessment of brain lesions but the technique is more difficult to apply outside the brain because the signal is weak. However, single-shot spin-echo sequences are now available, opening the way to the use of diffusion imaging more widely. When multiple cellular walls prevent diffusion (e.g. when tumour cells are tightly packed), the signal is higher than in areas of oedema or necrosis, where diffusion readily occurs (Fig. 41.10).[47]

Contrast medium
After injection of gadolinium (Gd) chelates, changes in the signal of normal marrow are not visible on T1-weighted images and measurements display either no increase or only a limited (<10%) increase. Various pathologies, in contrast, usually exhibit a strong signal increase. The absence of uptake practically rules out involvement of the bone marrow. Uptake is usually evaluated on T1-weighted spin-echo sequences. A precontrast injection sequence is mandatory, as the enhanced signal intensity of the lesion may make it equal to the signal of fatty marrow, and thus render it invisible. This problem can be overcome by using T1-weighted sequences with fat presaturation.

Key points: magnetic resonance imaging

- MR visualizes large portions of the bone marrow directly and has excellent soft tissue contrast resolution and multiplanar capabilities
- A fast total body skeletal study is now available
- MR is highly sensitive in the detection of bone marrow metastases
- Both trabecular and cortical bone produce little or no signal due to the lack of mobile protons
- Bone marrow metastases are seen because they have longer T1 and T2 relaxation times than normal marrow
- Bone marrow metastases are well-demonstrated on T1- and T2-weighted images. Fast spin-echo T2-weighted sequences with fat presaturation often show metastases as very high signal intensity lesions
- Gradient-echo sequences are prone to susceptibility artefacts from trabecular bone
- Bone marrow metastases usually enhance following injection of intravenous (IV) contrast medium

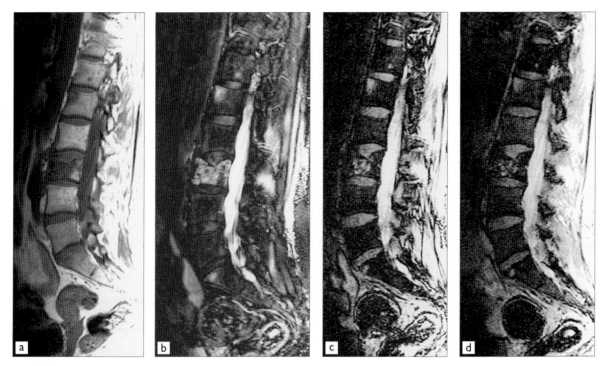

Figure 41.9. *Multiple bone metastases. Vertebral collapse of L3. (a) T1-weighted spin-echo, (b) T2-weighted fast spin-echo fat-saturation, (c) in-phase and (d) opposed-phase gradient-echo images. The collapsed vertebral body has a higher signal intensity than the normal ones on in-phase image because the trabeculae are destroyed, thus confirming a metastatic and not osteoporotic involvement. On the opposed-phase image, both the lack of trabeculae and non-subtraction of fat and water in the lesion contribute to the high signal intensity of the lesion.*

Metastatic disease

Several patterns of bony marrow involvement have been described using T1- and T2-weighted sequences. Metastatic lesions are typically focal with low signal on T1-weighted images and higher signal intensity (greater than marrow fat) on T2-weighted sequences (Fig. 41.11). On fast spin-echo T2-weighted fat-saturated sequences, lesions are often of very

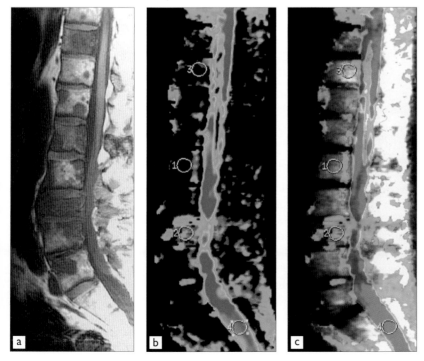

Figure 41.10. *Multiple metastases with collapse of L3. (a) T1-weighted spin-echo image. (b) The diffusion sequence allows mapping of diffusion on the whole image. (c) Superimposition of T1-weighted image and diffusion-weighted image.*

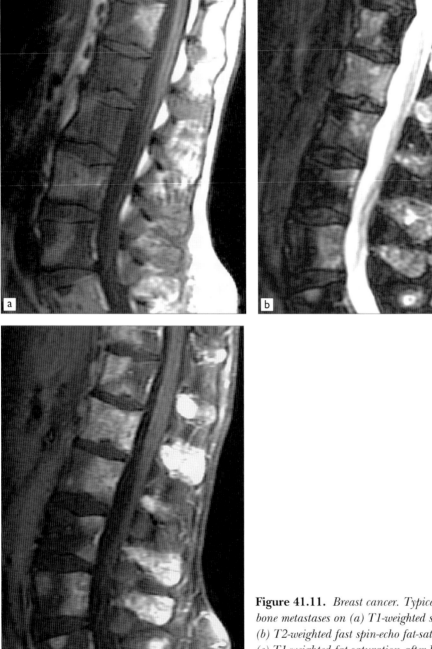

Figure 41.11. *Breast cancer. Typical pattern of bone metastases on (a) T1-weighted spin-echo, (b) T2-weighted fast spin-echo fat-saturation and (c) T1-weighted fat-saturation after IV contrast medium injection.*

high signal intensity, particularly lytic metastases such as those from the kidney, thyroid or bladder cancer. Sclerotic lesions are of low signal intensity on T1- and T2-weighted images, typically seen in metastases from prostate and breast cancer. A third pattern is a diffuse inhomogeneous low signal involving the whole bone. Rarely, a diffuse homogeneous low signal is seen on T1-weighted intensity images and homogeneous increased signal intensity is seen on T2-weighted images. This pattern can also be identified in lymphoma, leukaemia and other bone marrow-infiltrating disorders.[48]

Metastases enhance following injection of IV contrast material. The T1 shortening with the administration of Gd-DTPA produces a high signal intensity on T1-weighted images and metastases are therefore best shown on T1-weighted images with fat suppression (Fig. 41.11).[49] Studies using dynamic MR after the administration of Gd-DTPA demonstrate a sharper more rapid peak in enhancement for malignant lesions compared with benign masses.[50] When a potentially operable vertebral compression is discovered on an MR examination, the whole spine must be studied to rule out another level of compression, which could change patient management (Fig. 41.12). If no

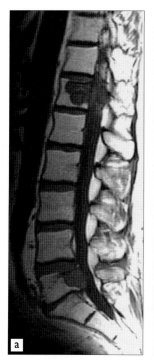
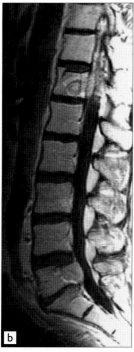

Figure 41.12. *Clinical spinal cord compression. (a) Sagittal T1-weighted images before IV contrast medium and (b) after contrast medium injection. Two levels of spinal cord compression are well seen: at T12 and L5. When an isolated level of compression is seen, and surgery is planned, a complete study of the whole spine must be performed to rule out another level of compression.*

abnormality is detected on an MR performed for a suspected cord compression, contrast medium must be used to detect leptomeningeal metastases (Fig. 41.13).[51]

The differentiation of metastatic or other malignant bone marrow processes from benign and traumatic conditions remains a problem. Non-malignant conditions that may be confused with neoplastic involvement include:

- Normal haemopoietic marrow
- Degenerative disc disease
- Fatty deposits
- Schmorl's nodes
- Osteomyelitis
- Primary bone tumours
- Compression fractures
- Bone islands
- Infarcts

Evaluation of vertebral collapse

The loss of vertebral height in a patient with a known malignancy poses a diagnostic problem as the distinction between malignant and osteoporotic vertebral collapse cannot always be made on standard radiographs. The clinical history, age and radiographic changes are important. A history of trauma and multiple areas of involvement in an elderly person suggest non-metastatic disease (Fig. 41.14). The location of the lesion is also important as a vertebral collapse in the upper thoracic spine is more likely to be malignant than post-traumatic.[52,53] On plain radiographs, uniform compression of the end-plates is more likely to be due to osteopenia or trauma, whereas irregularity is more commonly seen with metastases. Multiple levels of vertebral involvement, a soft tissue mass and destruction of pedicles

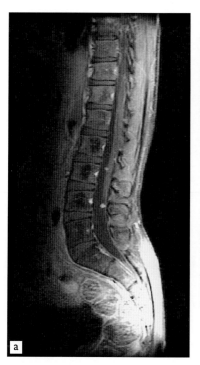
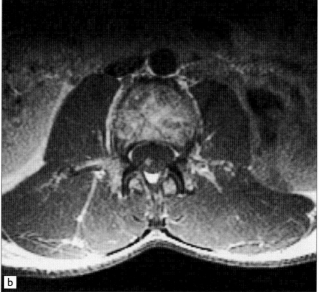

Figure 41.13. *Malignant melanoma: possible spinal cord compression. Normal examination without IV contrast medium. Leptomeningeal metastases are only visible after contrast medium injection. (a) Sagittal and (b) axial T1-weighted MR images with fat presaturation.*

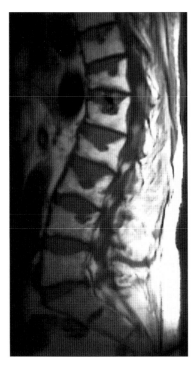

Figure 41.14.
Osteoporotic vertebral collapse of T11–L4 in a 65-year-old female patient. The marrow signal intensity on this T1-weighted spin-echo MR image is normal for a patient of this age with colon cancer. Note anterior wedging together with superior end-plate depression by disc bulges.

are more likely to indicate metastases. However, a paravertebral soft tissue mass can also be seen with trauma.

Both CT and MR can be used for distinguishing benign from malignant causes of acute vertebral collapse.[36] Computed tomography features suggesting benign vertebral collapse include:

- Cortical fractures
- Retropulsion of bone fragments into the spinal canal
- Fractures within cancellous bone
- Absence of bony destruction
- Thin diffuse paraspinal soft tissue mass

Malignant acute vertebral collapse is characterized by:

- Anterolateral or posterior cortical bone destruction
- Destruction of cancellous bone
- Destruction of pedicles
- Focal paraspinal soft tissue mass

Magnetic resonance imaging also provides important information on the nature of collapse. In benign vertebral collapse, the features depend on the age of the injury. In the acute setting, the vertebral marrow is oedematous with uniform loss of signal on T1-weighted images and an increased signal on T2-weighted and STIR sequences.[53–55] The absence of other focal lesions and of a soft tissue mass makes the diagnosis of a benign fracture more likely. When the collapse is longstanding, the marrow signal is similar to

that of normal vertebral bodies (Figs. 41.14 and 41.15). Bone marrow oedema following a benign fracture usually returns to normal or nearly normal signal intensity after 1–3 months. Involvement of the posterior elements of a vertebra is also more likely in malignant disease.

Magnetic resonance imaging features suggestive of malignant vertebral collapse include:

- Involvement of the posterior vertebral body and posterior elements
- Associated soft tissue mass
- Diffuse involvement of the whole vertebra
- Contrast enhancement of the abnormal area
- Multiple lesions

Direct signs bring a higher specificity in the analysis of vertebral collapse. They use diffusion and gradient-echo techniques (Fig. 41.10).[46,47] On diffusion-weighted sequences, protons diffuse readily in the free water of osteoporotic vertebral collapse, thus the signal intensity is reduced. Conversely, diffusion is limited by the walls of the tumour cells in metastatic vertebral collapse, thus a higher signal intensity is maintained.

On in-phase gradient-echo images, the lack of trabeculae in metastatic collapse allows a higher signal intensity, whereas the preserved trabeculae in osteoporotic collapse make the signal intensity low.

Key points: magnetic resonance findings

- The MR appearances in any bone reflect the relative composition of red and yellow marrow

- The vertebral body has a higher signal intensity than the intervertebral disc on T1-weighted images and this is a useful guide for detecting early infiltrative processes

- Osteolytic metastases have a low signal intensity on T1 weighting and a high signal intensity on T2 weighting

- Sclerotic metastases have a low signal intensity on both T1 and T2 weighting

- Normal marrow shows mild diffuse homogeneous enhancement after administration of IV contrast medium

- Metastases enhance following injection of IV contrast medium to a greater degree than normal marrow

- Metastases may have a similar appearance to a variety of benign lesions

- Abnormal signal intensity in the posterior aspect of the vertebral body extending into the posterior elements should suggest metastatic disease

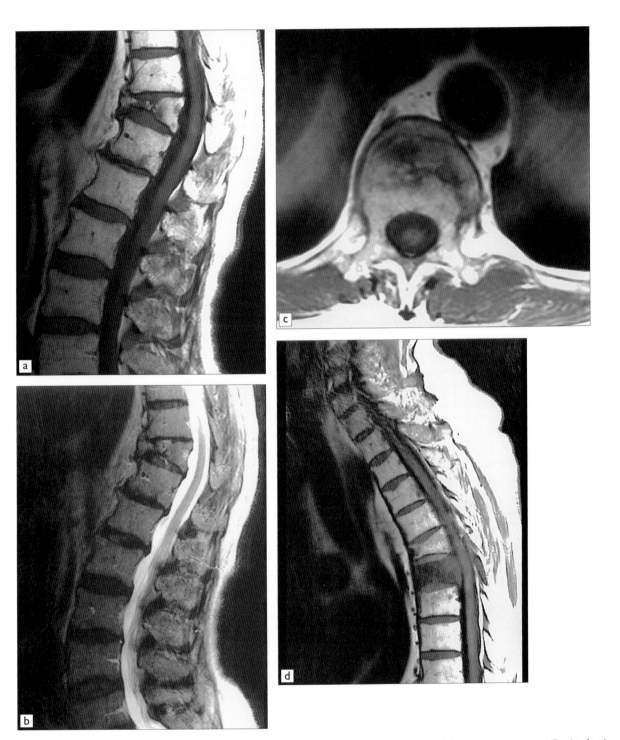

Figure 41.15. *Osteoporotic and vertebral collapse and metastatic disease in a patient with prostate cancer. (a) Sagittal spin-echo T1-weighted and (b) turbo spin-echo T2-weighted MR images through the lumbodorsal junction. Loss of vertebral height of T11 with anterior wedging is seen. (c) The axial T1-weighted image shows cortical fractures, the absence of bony destruction and preserved normal marrow signal characteristic of benign vertebral collapse. (d) Same patient at a higher level. The sagittal T1-weighted spin-echo image shows a uniform decreased signal intensity with expansion of the T7 vertebral body causing thecal compression. The posterior elements are involved (arrow).*

Comparison of imaging techniques

Several studies have now demonstrated that MR is more sensitive than radionuclide bone scanning for detecting bone marrow metastases. Jones et al.[56] reported a 7% yield of MR over MDP bone scans and plain radiographs in patients with primary breast cancer. Although MR may demonstrate metastases in the presence of negative bone scans, the converse is also occasionally true. Radionuclide scanning and MR are highly sensitive techniques but radionuclide scanning clearly lacks specificity. Magnetic resonance imaging also has limitations due to non-specificity of signal intensity patterns but morphological features outlined above may point to a malignant process. Plain radiographs are insensitive to the detection of metastases but are highly specific; a major role of plain radiography being to determine the nature of increased tracer uptake demonstrated on radionuclide bone scans. Plain radiographs may also yield metastatic bone disease in tumours in which radionuclide scanning has a low yield such as myeloma, renal carcinoma, lymphoma and some sarcomas. Computed tomography is a highly sensitive method of evaluating cortical and trabecular bone showing areas of early destruction not visible on plain radiographs. The technique has been shown to be more sensitive than plain radiography in evaluating patients with abnormal bone scans and provides complementary information to plain radiographs, particularly in areas where plain films are difficult to interpret, such as the sacrum and skull base.

Monitoring tumour response to treatment

Tumours in bone marrow respond to treatment with a reduction in size of tumour and a change in signal intensity. Changes in lesion size are best demonstrated on T1-weighted images but signal intensity changes are often better appreciated on T2-weighted or STIR images. When treatment is effective, a fatty halo may appear, marking a decrease in tumour size (Fig. 41.16). When, after radia-

tion therapy, the marrow becomes completely fatty, there are no lesions left. Most often, after radiation or chemotherapy, lesions are still visible. The differentiation between fibrosis and viable tumour is not possible, and imaging is not recommended to evaluate treatment effectiveness.

After spine surgery (Fig. 41.17), a medial sagittal MR image can be obtained, if surgical fixation is lateral (transpedicular) and titanium is used.

Conclusion

The accurate assessment of bone metastases in cancer patients requires a combined multidisciplinary approach of clinical and biochemical assessment in combination with imaging studies in patients with breast and prostate cancer in which the incidence of bone metastases is high. It has nevertheless been clearly proven that an earlier detection of metastases in breast cancer does not improve either survival or the quality of life of the patients.[4,5] In the same way, bone metastases from prostate cancer should be systematically detected only if their discovery changes the treatment. Between 20 and 30% of positive bone scans represent benign disease, including degenerative change. Thus, in patients with inconclusive radio-isotope scans, other methods of imaging with higher specificity are required such as plain radiographs. Plain radiographs will usually be undertaken first, followed by MR or CT, depending upon the availability of equipment. In patients with lung, renal or bladder cancer, the incidence of skeletal metastases is only about 10% in the absence of symptoms; routine screening with bone scintigraphy is not recom-

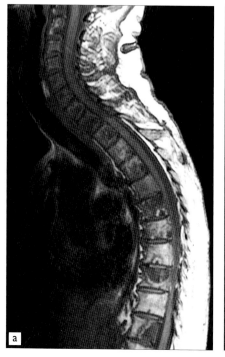
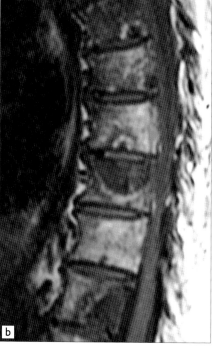

Figure 41.16. *Bone metastases. MR imaging examination after effective chemotherapy. (a) T1-weighted spin-echo image and (b) magnification image. Lesions are surrounded by a fatty halo indicating tumour regression.*

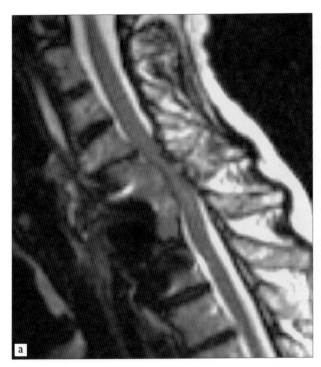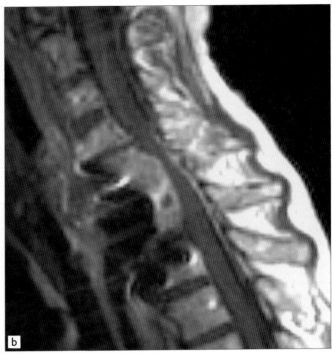

Figure 41.17. *Sagittal MR images post surgery. (a) T2 and (b) T1 fat-saturation after IV contrast medium injection. Despite the screws and the cement, spinal cord compression is well shown.*

mended. However, in patients with symptoms of pain, the yield of bone scintigraphy rises to between 75 and 85% and is therefore the initial investigation of choice.

In patients with a solitary bone lesion considered to represent a metastasis, biopsy is indicated in the absence of metastases elsewhere. This is best performed under fluoroscopic or CT guidance.

The use of CT is declining as it is only of value in certain well-defined circumstances. Conversely, the use of MR is increasing as it is able to evaluate a wide variety of neoplastic and non-neoplastic bone marrow diseases. MR imaging is the most sensitive method for evaluation of the bone marrow as it is able to visualize the individual marrow components directly. ¹⁸FDG PET may become a very useful technique, as it allows a global evaluation of the patient (Fig. 41.18).

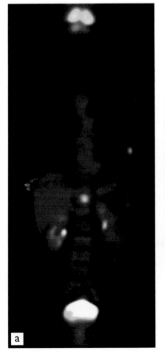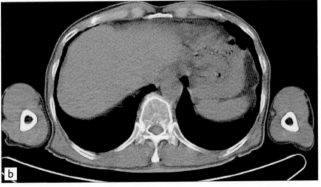

Figure 41.18a–b. *¹⁸FDG PET/CT evaluation on a patient with metastatic melanoma. (a) ¹⁸FDG PET image. There is a focus of high activity in a left rib, and the vertebral body of T11. (b) On CT the vertebral lesion is hardly visible (continued overleaf).*

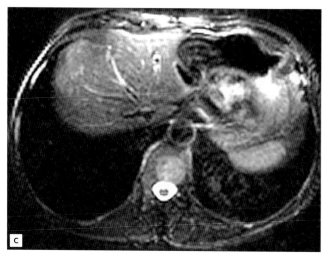

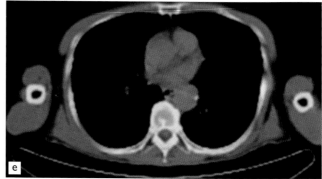

Figure 41.18c–e. *¹⁸FDG PET/CT evaluation on a patient with metastatic melanoma. (c) The lesion is well seen on the T2-weighted fast spin-echo MR image performed for a liver study. (d and e) Superimposition of CT and ¹⁸FDG PET. The rib lesion is only visible as a thickening of the soft tissues on CT.*

Summary

- Imaging plays a complementary role to clinical and biochemical evaluation in the detection of metastases

- Radionuclide bone scans are the initial investigation of choice in the majority of patients

- Screening with radionuclide studies for bone marrow metastases has a high yield in breast and prostate cancer, but should not be routinely undertaken

- Plain radiographs should be used to elucidate inconclusive radionuclide abnormalities

- CT has a role in detecting lesions at sites difficult to evaluate on plain radiographs

- CT is useful for guidance of percutaneous biopsy

- MR is the most sensitive technique currently available for the detection of bone metastases and is moderately specific

- CT and MR are both useful in the evaluation of the cause of vertebral collapse

- Response to treatment of bone marrow metastases is usually identified as a reduction in size of the lesion and a change in signal intensity

References

1. Vogler J B, Murphy W A. Bone marrow imaging. Radiology 1988; 168: 679–693

2. Ehman R L. MR imaging of medullary bone. Radiology 1988; 167: 867–868

3. Jones R J. The role of bone marrow imaging. Radiology 1992; 183: 321–322

4. Boccardo F, Bruzzi P, Cionini L, et al. Appropriateness of the use of clinical and radiologic examinations and laboratory tests in the follow-up of surgically-treated breast cancer patients. Results of the Working Group on the Clinical Aspects of Follow-up. Ann Oncol 1995; 6 (Suppl 2): 57–59

5. Roselli del Turco M, Palli D, Cariddi A et al. Intensive diagnostic follow-up after treatment of primary breast cancer. A randomized trial. National Research Council Project on Breast Cancer follow-up. JAMA 1994 ; 271: 1593–1597

6. Datz F L, Taylor A. The clinical use of radionuclide bone marrow imaging. Semin Nucl Med 1985; 15: 239–259

7. Porter B A, Sheilds A F, Olson D O. Magnetic resonance

imaging of bone marrow disorders. Radiol Clin North Am 1986; 24: 269–289

8. Silverberg E, Lubera J. Cancer statistics, 1987. CA Cancer J Clin 1987; 37: 2–19

9. Abrams H L, Spiro R, Goldstein N. Metastases in carcinoma. Analysis of 1000 autopsied cases. Cancer 1950; 2: 74–85

10. Napoli L D, Hansen H H, Muggia F M. The incidence of osseous involvement in lung cancer with special reference to the development of osteoblastic changes. Radiology 1973; 108: 17–21

11. Berrettoni B A, Carter J R. Mechanisms of cancer metastasis to bone. J Bone Joint Surg (Am) 1986; 68: 308–312

12. Galasko C S. Skeletal metastases. Clin Orthop 1986; 210: 18–30

13. Krishnamurthy G T, Tubis M, Hiss J et al. Distribution pattern of metastatic bone disease. A need for total body skeletal image. JAMA 1977; 237: 2504–2506

14. Clain A. Secondary malignant disease of bone. Br J Cancer 1965; 19: 15–29

15. Fragiadakis E G, Panayotopoulous G. Metastatic carcinoma of the hand. Hand 1972; 4: 268

16. Kerin R. Metastatic tumors of the hand. J Bone Joint Surg (Am) 1958; 40: 263

17. Willis R A. The Spread of Tumours in the Human Body. London: Butterworth, 1973; 229–250

18. Vilar J, Lezana A H, Pedrosa C S. Spiculated periosteal reaction in metastatic lesion of bone. Skeletal Radiol 1979; 3: 230

19. Wyche L D, De Santos L A. Spiculated periosteal reaction in metastatic disease resembling osteosarcoma. Orthopedics 1978; 1: 215

20. Deutsch A, Resnick D. Eccentric cortical metastases to the skeleton from bronchogenic carcinoma. Radiology 1980; 137: 49–52

21. Pagani J J, Libshitz H I. Imaging bone metastases. Radiol Clin North Am 1982; 20: 545–560

22. Malawer M M, Delaney T F. Treatment of metastatic cancer to bone. In: DeVita V T, Hellman S, Rosenberg S A (eds). Cancer Principles and Practice of Oncology. Philadelphia: Lippincott, 1993; 2225–2245

23. Batson O V. The function of the vertebral veins and their role in the spread of metastases. Ann Surg 1940; 112: 138–149

24. Dodds P R, Caride V J, Lytton B. The role of the vertebral veins in the dissemination of prostatic carcinoma. J Urol 1981; 126: 753–755

25. del-Regato J A. Pathways of metastatic spread of malignant tumors. Semin Oncol 1977; 4: 33–38

26. Galasko C S B. Mechanisms of lytic and blastic metastatic disease of bone. Clin Orthop 1982; 169: 20–27

27. Manishen W J, Sivananthan K, Orr F W. Resorbing bone stimulates tumour cell growth. A role for the host microenvironment in bone metastasis. Am J Pathol 1986; 123: 39–45

28. Francis M D, Fogelman I. 99mcTc-diphosphonate uptake mechanisms in bone. In: Fogelman I (ed). Bone Scanning in Clinical Practice. London: Springer-Verlag, 1987; 1–6

29. McNeil B J. Value of bone scanning in neoplastic disease. Semin Nucl Med 1984; 14: 277–286

30. Pollen J J, Witztum K F, Ashburn W L. The flare phenomenon of radionuclide bone scan in metastatic prostate cancer. Am J Roentgenol 1984; 142: 773–776

31. Hortobagyi G N, Libshitz H I, Seabold J E. Osseous metastases of breast cancer. Clinical, biochemical, radiographic and scintigraphic evaluation of response to therapy. Cancer 1984; 53: 577–582

32. Weaver G R, Sandler M P. Increased sensitivity of magnetic resonance imaging compared to radionuclide bone scintigraphy in the detection of lymphoma of the spine. Clin Nucl Med 1987; 12: 333–334

33. Janicek M J, Hayes D F, Kaplan W D. Healing flare in skeletal metastases from breast cancer. Radiology 1994; 192: 201–204

34. Edelstyn G A, Gillespie P J, Grebbell F S. The radiological demonstration of osseous metastases: experimental observations. Clin Radiol 1967; 18: 158–162

35. Fidler M. Incidence of fracture through metastases in long bones. Acta Orthopscond 1981; 52: 623–627

36. Laredo J D, Lakhdari K, Bellaiche L et al. Acute vertebral collapse: CT findings in benign and malignant non-traumatic cases. Radiology 1995; 194: 41–48

37. Ludwig H. Fruhwald F, Tscholakoff D et al. Magnetic resonance imaging of the spine in multiple myeloma. Lancet 1987; 2: 364–366

38. Ehman R L, Berquist T H, McLeod R A. MR imaging of the musculoskeletal system: a 5-year appraisal. Radiology 1988; 166: 313–320

39. Colman L K, Porter B A, Redmond J et al. Early diagnosis of spinal metastases by CT and MR studies. J Comput Assist Tomogr 1988; 12: 423–426

40. Ghanem N, Altehoefer C, Hogerle S et al. Comparative diagnostic value and therapeutic relevance of magnetic resonance imaging and bone marrow scintigraphy in patients with metastatic solid tumors of the axial skeleton. Eur J Radiol 2002; 43: 256–261

41. Traill Z C, Talbot D, Golding S et al. Magnetic resonance imaging versus radionuclide scintigraphy in screening for bone metastases. Clin Radiol 1999; 54: 448–451

42. Kattapuram S V, Khurana J S, Scott J A et al. Negative scintigraphy with positive magnetic resonance imaging in bone metastases. Skel Radiol 1990; 19: 113–116

43. Algra P R, Bloem J L, Tissing H et al. Detection of vertebral metastases: comparison between MR imaging and bone scintigraphy. RadioGraphics 1991; 11: 219–232

44. Eustace S, Tello R, DeCarvalho V et al. A comparison of whole-body turboSTIR MR imaging and planar 99mTc-methylene diphosphonate scintigraphy in the examination of patients with suspected skeletal metastases. Am J Roentgenol 1997; 169: 1655–1661

45. Lauenstein T C, Freudenberg L S, Goehde S C et al. Whole-body MRI using a rolling table platform for the detection of bone metastases. Eur Radiol 2002; 12: 2091–2099

46. Vanel D, Bittoun J, Tardivon A. MRI of bone metastases. Eur Radiol 1998; 8: 1345–1351

47. Baur A, Stabler A, Bruning R, et al. Diffusion-weighted MR imaging of bone marrow: differentiation of benign versus pathologic compression fractures. Radiology 1998; 207: 349–356

48. Thomsen C, Sorensen P G, Karle H et al. Prolonged bone marrow T1 relaxation in acute leukaemia: in vivo characterisation by magnetic resonance imaging. Magn Reson Imaging 1987; 5: 251–257

49. Stimac G K, Porter B A, Olson D O et al. Gadolinium-DTPA enhanced MR imaging of spinal neoplasms: preliminary investigation and comparison with unenhanced spin echo and STIR sequences. Am J Roentgenol 1988; 151: 1185–1192

50. Hawighorst H, Libicher M, Knopp M V et al. Evaluation of angiogenesis and perfusion of bone marrow lesions: role of semiquantitative and quantitative dynamic MRI. J Magn Reson Imaging 1999; 10: 286–294

51. Loughrey G J, Collins C D, Todd S M et al. Magnetic resonance imaging in the management of suspected spinal canal disease in patients with known malignancy. Clin Radiol 2000; 55: 849–855

52. Hayes C W, Jensen M E, Conway W F. Non-neoplastic lesions in vertebral bodies. Findings in magnetic resonance imaging. RadioGraphics 1989; 9: 883–901

53. Yuh W T, Zachar C K, Barloon T J et al. Vertebral compression fractures: distinction between benign and malignant causes with MR imaging. Radiology 1989; 172: 215–218

54. Baker L L, Goodman S, Perkash I et al. Benign versus pathological compression fractures of vertebral bodies: assessment with conventional spin-echo, chemical shift and STIR MR imaging. Radiology 1990; 174: 495–502

55. Berquist T H, Ehman R L, King B F et al. Value of MR imaging in differentiating benign from malignant soft tissue masses: study of 95 lesions. Am J Roentgenol 1990; 155: 251–255

56. Jones A L, Williams M P, Powles T J et al. Magnetic resonance imaging in the detection of skeletal metastases in patients with breast cancer. Br J Cancer 1990; 62: 296–298

Chapter 42

The liver

Philip J A Robinson

Introduction: Incidence and sources of liver metastases

Almost one half of all patients dying with malignant disease have metastatic tumours in the liver. The incidence of liver metastasis from various primary tumours, derived from autopsy series,[1–3] is shown below (Table 42.1). These data reflect end-stage disease, whereas clinical interest for imaging will focus on the detection of liver metastases at the time of initial presentation of the primary tumour, and also on the likelihood of development of liver metastases during follow-up. About 25–40% of patients with gastro-intestinal primary neoplasms and small cell lung cancers have liver metastases at the time of first clinical presentation but, with other common primary tumours, liver metastases are rarely found at initial staging. Different primary malignancies can be classified into high-, intermediate- and low-risk groups with reference to the likelihood of metachronous liver metastases developing after the initial presentation and treatment of the primary lesion (Table 42.2).

In considering the clinical management of patients who have or who are at risk of developing liver metastases, it is

Table 42.1. *Incidence of liver metastases from various primary tumours at autopsy*

Primary site	Patients with liver metastases (%)
Oesophagus	30–100
Stomach	38–100
Colorectal	40–100
Pancreas	50–73
Bile ducts and gall bladder	45–80
Small cell lung cancer	38–67
Breast	49–73
Melanoma	69
Ovary	48–68
Uterus	24–75
Renal cell cancer	40
Urothelial cancer	37–38
Thyroid	20
Prostate	9–74

Table 42.2. *Likelihood of developing liver metastases during follow-up according to site of primary tumour*

High-risk	Intermediate-risk	Low risk
Oesophagus	Breast	Prostate
Stomach	Melanoma	Renal cell
Large bowel	Ovary	Cervix
Carcinoids	Soft tissue sarcoma	Head/neck (squamous cell)
Pancreas	Testis	
Primary liver	Thyroid	
Gall bladder/biliary	Bone sarcoma	
Lung (small cell)		

important to take into account the progression of disease elsewhere. The presence of liver lesions becomes less significant if patients already have widespread metastatic disease in bones, lungs or central nervous system. Also, when multiple liver lesions are discovered in a patient under surveillance following treatment of a primary malignancy, it should not be assumed automatically that the liver lesions arise from the same pathology as the initial tumour, particularly if the combination is biologically unlikely. For example, liver metastases discovered during surveillance of a patient who has been successfully treated for prostatic cancer are more likely to arise from a second malignancy in the gastro-intestinal tract than from recurrence of prostate cancer.

Biology of metastatic liver tumours

The liver is a fertile ground for seeding of metastatic tumours. The reasons for this are not fully established but probably include the following:[4]

- The vast majority of liver metastases arrive via the bloodstream, and the liver receives about 25% of the cardiac output
- The dimensions of liver sinusoids are suitable for trapping small clumps of cells and gaps that exist in the subendothelial basement membrane, which in other organs provides a barrier to spread

- Continuous regeneration of liver cells is a normal phenomenon probably controlled by local humoral mechanisms that may also stimulate the growth of neoplastic cells once in situ
- Some tumours that commonly metastasize to the liver carry specific receptors for host endothelial cells

Routes of spread

Primary tumours arising in the lower oesophagus, stomach, small bowel, colon, rectum and pancreas metastasize via lymphatics to local nodes and via portal venous spread to the liver. Ovarian malignant tumours and some gastrointestinal and retroperitoneal neoplasms produce surface metastases on the liver by transperitoneal spread (Fig. 42.1). Hepatocellular carcinomas and cholangiocarcinomas tend to spread by seeding along portal veins and bile ducts. Liver metastases from tumours elsewhere arrive via the hepatic arterial route.

At the time of presentation or discovery, liver metastases from melanoma, testicular non-seminomatous germ cell tumours and carcinomas of lung, breast and kidney appear, typically, as numerous small deposits scattered throughout the liver. There is rarely any indication for local treatment of the liver lesions. Similarly, patients with surface metastasis from transperitoneal spread of abdominal and pelvic tumours are treated with chemotherapy, either systemic or intraperitoneal. However, patients with liver metastasis from gastro-intestinal primary tumours often have a small number of overt lesions at the time of diagnosis and more detailed imaging is required to assess the possibility of local or regional treatment.

Growth rates

Because all metastases start out as individual cells or as clumps of cells, it follows that there is a latent period of occult disease between the seeding and the time when the lesions become manifest on imaging or by clinical presentation. The duration of this latent period varies with:

- Site of the primary tumour
- Histological cell type
- Grade of malignancy
- Local extent of the primary tumour
- Presence of subpopulations of different cell types within the primary

In addition, tumour growth rates are affected by local factors, incompletely described and understood. Because surgical attempts to cure liver metastases have focused largely on patients with colorectal cancer, much more is known about the natural history of colorectal lesions than about other types of liver metastases. Surveillance studies after removal of colorectal primary tumours have shown that about one third of patients whose livers appear normal to visual inspection and palpation at the time of laparotomy for removal of the primary tumour, are harbouring occult metastases which become overt over the next 2 years.[5,6] Techniques for detecting occult disease at this stage have been piloted but have not yet reached widespread acceptance (see below). The size-doubling times for colorectal liver metastases in untreated patients vary widely from 30 days to 3 years, and with chemotherapy the rates of growth are even less predictable (Fig. 42.2).

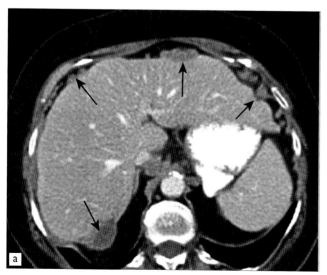
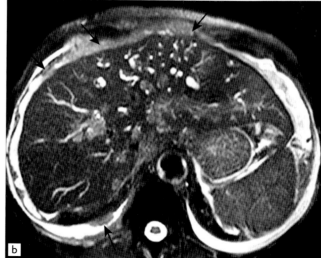

Figure 42.1. *Metastases on the liver surface in two patients with ovarian cancer. (a) On CT, low attenuation lesions of various sizes are scattered over the surface of the liver (arrows). (b) Magnetic resonance shows parenchymal lesions of intermediate signal intensity on T2, and surface lesions (arrows) highlighted by surrounding ascites and pleural fluid.*

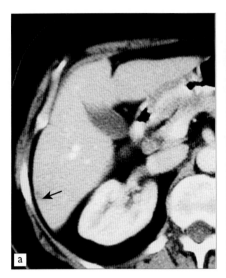
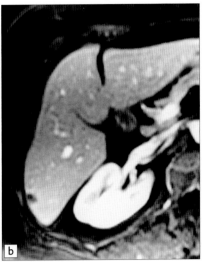
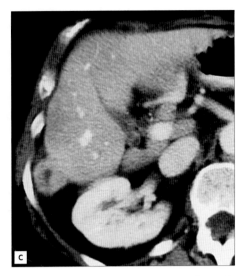

Figure 42.2. *Metastasis from colorectal cancer. (a) Initial CT shows small lesion of indeterminate character (arrow). (b) Gd-enhanced MR shows the lesion has an enhancing rim, indicative of metastasis. (c) CT 8 months later shows rapid growth of the lesion.*

Blood supply of liver metastases

Histopathological studies suggest that metastases develop from clumps of tumour cells which adhere to the endothelium of the presinusoidal arterioles, the terminal portal venules, or in the sinusoids themselves, then migrate into the adjacent spaces of Disse. For micrometastases up to about 100 µm diameter, surface diffusion probably provides sufficient nutrients for continuing growth. Further growth depends upon the development of a blood supply within the lesion and this is promoted by angiogenesis factors produced locally in response to the presence of the tumour. This neovascularity arises from the hepatic arterial circulation and rarely involves the portal venules. The blood supply of larger metastases is derived almost totally from the hepatic arterial route,[7–9] although with some lesions there is a portal venous supply to the tumour periphery,[10,11] which may develop further after hepatic artery ligation.[12] Shunting of blood between the arterial and portal elements is a recognized feature of the normal hepatic microvasculature, and is usually increased in cirrhosis. Recent experimental work suggests that even in those tumours with anatomically demonstrable portal venous branches, arterial inflow effectively replaces portal inflow via high pressure arterio-portal shunts around the tumour periphery.[13] This may account for the demonstrable change in arterial/portal flow ratio which occurs soon after the implantation of micrometastases in the liver.[14]

The vascular supply to liver metastases is of particular interest in relation to local treatment by chemo-embolization, arterial ligation or local infusion of chemotherapeutic or radioactive agents. In most types of liver disease there is

a relative increase in hepatic arterial inflow and a decrease in portal venous inflow to the liver. This phenomenon has been used to detect liver metastases at a stage when they are too small for detection by anatomic imaging methods. The arterial blood supply of tumours is also a major consideration in imaging techniques using intravenous (IV) contrast agents with computed tomography (CT), MR imaging and sonography.

Key points: biology of liver metastases

- The majority of tumours metastasize to the liver via the bloodstream

- There is a latent period between the seeding of a metastasis and the time it becomes manifest on imaging or clinical evaluation

- Metastases develop from clumps of cells which lodge in presinusoidal arterioles, terminal portal venules, sinusoids and spaces of Disse

- The growth of a metastasis depends on the development of neovascularity

- The blood supply of larger metastases is derived almost totally from the hepatic arterial route

- Arterio-portal shunts develop around the tumour periphery

- There is an increase in the hepatic arterial blood flow/portal venous blood flow ratio which develops soon after the implantation of micrometastases

Pathophysiology of liver metastases relevant for imaging

Physical characteristics

Imaging focal mass lesions within the liver depends on the demonstration of anatomical or physiological characteristics which are distinctly different from those of the surrounding liver tissue. With sonography, detection of lesions relies on microscopic structural differences that produce an increased or decreased number of reflective surfaces or an alteration in their architecture; these changes result in hyper- or hypoechogenicity, or heterogeneity, respectively. Most tumours have a greater water content than the surrounding liver, which accounts for their reduced attenuation on unenhanced CT, and for the typical MR findings of reduced signal intensity on T1-weighted and increased signal intensity on T2-weighted images. Other influential factors include fat or melanin within the tumour, matrix calcification and haemorrhage. Tumour necrosis, which occurs at a surprisingly early stage in some rapidly growing lesions, tends to produce a central area with fluid characteristics on imaging.

Contrast enhancement

Using CT, MR and sonography, rapid imaging techniques with intravascular contrast media show enhancement patterns that are unique to the liver owing to its dual vascular supply. When a bolus of contrast medium is injected intravenously, the hepatic arterial component arrives at the liver 6–15 seconds before the portal venous component, allowing the acquisition of images during consecutive phases of enhancement. These are described as:

- Early arterial phase – about 20–30 seconds after injection
- Late arterial phase – about 30–40 seconds after injection
- Sinusoidal or portal phase – about 60–70 seconds after injection
- Equilibrium phase – about 2–3 minutes after injection
- Delayed phase – from about 5 minutes after injection onwards

Lesions with homogeneously increased arterial flow relative to normal liver (many hepatocellular tumours and some metastases) are best seen during the arterial-dominant phase of enhancement (Fig. 42.3). Dynamic imaging using thin-section CT or MR shows that many metastases, which appear hypovascular in the portal phase of enhancement, also transiently exhibit a thin rim of arterial hypervascularity. Demonstration of this arterially enhancing rim helps to distinguish small metastases from cysts and benign malformations (Fig. 42.2). Arterial rim enhancement indicates a well-vascularized lesion with a necrotic centre. With some tumours, slow diffusion of contrast into the centre may be seen. Rim enhancement, which first appears on late-phase or delayed images, suggests the presence of a fibrous capsule, typically seen with hepatocellular carcinoma but also a feature of some metastatic tumours. A broad and ill-defined ring of transient or sustained enhancement may also be seen in liver tissue surrounding some metastases, probably a result of local oedema or inflammatory reaction.

Lesions with normal or sluggish flow but a large blood pool (e.g. vascular areas within hemangiomas, aneurysms and arterio-venous malformations) show rapid arterial phase enhancement which declines in parallel with that of the major vessels. The inflow of contrast medium from the portal venous supply to tumours is negligible so those

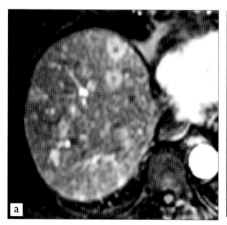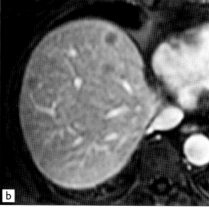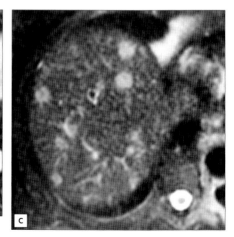

Figure 42.3. *Metastases from pancreatic islet cell tumour. Numerous hypervascular lesions, the larger ones with necrotic centres, are shown most effectively during (a) arterial phase of Gd-enhanced MR; (b) venous phase image and (c) T2-weighted image show the larger lesions but many of the small metastases are not visible.*

lesions which do not have increased arterial inflow become most conspicuous during the sinusoidal enhancement phase when the uptake of contrast by normal liver is at its peak. The majority of hypervascular tumours show a rapid washout of contrast and some become indistinguishable from adjacent liver in the later phases of enhancement. Where fibrous tissue forms a major component of a liver tumour (e.g. cholangiocarcinoma, central scars in focal nodular hyperplasia and in larger hemangiomas), enhancement is typically slow and prolonged, owing to diffusion of the contrast agent into the extracellular space of the tissue. These areas appear hypovascular on early images, but continue to enhance on delayed images when contrast is already washing out of other tissues.

Although metastases rarely spread along the main portal veins, local occlusion of portal branches is a common pathological finding. This accounts for the fairly common feature of wedge-shaped areas of arterial hyperperfusion that are shown on CT and MR as transient areas of hyperattenuation or increased signal intensity during the arterial-dominant phase of enhancement, often in association with liver tumours (see 'THADs' below).

Key points: contrast medium enhancement

- Following a bolus injection of IV contrast medium, the hepatic arterial component arrives at the liver 6–15 seconds before the portal venous component

- The phases of enhancement are early and late arterial, portal, equilibrium and delayed

- Lesions with a homogeneously increased arterial flow, relative to normal liver, are best seen in the arterial phase of enhancement, e.g. hepatocellular carcinoma and a minority of metastases

- Lesions that do not have an increased arterial flow are most conspicuous during the portal phase of enhancement when the uptake of contrast medium by normal liver is at its peak

- Rim enhancement of a liver tumour in the arterial phase indicates a well-vascularized lesion with a necrotic centre, and is frequently seen using thin-slice CT or MR

- A broad or ill-defined ring of enhancement may result from oedema/inflammation around the lesion

- In those tumours where fibrous tissue forms a major component, enhancement is slow and prolonged

- Metastases often produce occlusion of peripheral portal vein branches leading to wedge-shaped areas of arterial hyperperfusion on CT

Objectives of imaging

Two attributes of metastatic disease determine the applications of imaging – firstly, the presence or absence of liver metastasis has a major influence on the prognosis and treatment of patients with primary tumours, and secondly, improved surgical and other locoregional forms of treatment for liver tumours require precise preoperative imaging. In the context of metastatic disease, the primary objectives of imaging the liver are:

- Detecting the presence of liver lesions
- Characterizing known or suspected liver abnormalities
- Establishing the likely resectability of liver tumours
- Assessing disease progression or response to treatment

Detecting and characterizing liver metastases

Computed tomography

Dual-phase acquisition is recommended for patients in whom hepatocellular tumours or hypervascular metastases are suspected. A single-phase volume acquisition is usually adequate[15] for screening purposes and for primary tumours at sites that usually give rise to hypovascular liver lesions.

Single-phase volumetric computed tomography
Helical volume acquisition through the whole of the liver should be obtained in a single breath hold, and should be timed so as to capture the period of peak enhancement of liver parenchyma after a bolus injection of IV contrast. Normal liver tissue enhances maximally about 30–40 seconds after the end of bolus injection of contrast media, so the optimum interval from the start of injection varies with the rate and volume of contrast injected. Typically, effective enhancement is achieved with an injection rate of 5 ml/s, a volume of 1.5–2 ml/kg body weight and a delay of 60–70 seconds between start of injection and start of acquisition.

With multislice, multidetector CT,[16] beam collimation and reconstructed slice thickness are widely variable. For lesion detection, optimal slice thickness is probably about 2.5–3 mm,[17,18] as noise levels on thinner slices reduce the conspicuity of small solid lesions. The ratio of table speed to beam collimation (pitch) can be extended to 1.6–1.8 without significant loss of resolution.

Dual-phase computed tomography technique[19]
Consecutive volume acquisitions are timed so as to encompass arterial and portal venous or sinusoidal-phase enhancement. With multiphase imaging, timing of acquisition is critical. Arterial anatomy is best depicted with 'early arterial' phase images, obtained about 20–30 seconds from

the start of contrast injection, and thin-slice (1–1.5 mm) or overlapping reconstructions. Hypervascular tumours are best seen in the late arterial phase about 30–40 seconds after injection. Because the circulation time of individual patients varies considerably, accurate timing of arterial phase acquisitions is improved if the arrival time of a test bolus of a few ml of contrast is measured using sequential low-dose scans through the upper abdominal aorta before initiating the main contrast injection.

Other computed tomography techniques

Unenhanced images are not routinely necessary for lesion detection and characterization, except when focal fatty change is suspected. *Computed tomographic arteriography* (CTA) requires rapid sequential or volume acquisition after a bolus of contrast medium is delivered through a catheter placed in the hepatic artery.[20] The technique is invasive but sensitive for tumours with arterial hypervascularity. Its main application has been in detecting hepatocellular carcinoma in patients with cirrhosis, and so far there seems little place for this technique in dealing with metastatic liver disease.

Computed tomography with arterial portography (CTAP) produces intense and specific enhancement of the liver parenchyma by injection of contrast medium directly into the superior mesenteric or splenic arteries.[21] Because liver tumours receive their blood supply via the hepatic arterial route, portal inflow of contrast material enhances only the normal liver parenchyma and therefore tumour to liver differentiation is maximized (Fig. 42.4). Although this technique is highly sensitive for lesion detection, it requires the placement of an arterial catheter and it is also subject to

false positive results caused by focal perfusion anomalies.[22] Accessory or replaced right hepatic arteries arise from the superior mesenteric artery (SMA) in 15–20% of patients, and these reduce the sensitivity of CTAP in the affected parts of the liver. Placement of the catheter in the splenic artery is technically more difficult than SMA placement, owing to the relatively frequent occurrence of asymptomatic coeliac axis compression in older patients, but is thought by some users to give a more even distribution of contrast medium into the liver. Acquisition factors are similar to those used for IV bolus helical CT, using 75–100 ml contrast injected at 2–3 ml/s with a time delay of about 40 seconds before starting the volume acquisition. A second volume acquisition 2–3 minutes later is useful to aid discrimination between tumours and focal perfusion disturbances shown on the initial series.

Key points: computed tomography detection

- ■ Dual-phase CT is recommended for the detection of hepatocellular carcinoma and hypervascular liver metastases

- ■ Single-phase volumetric CT is adequate for detection of hypovascular liver lesions and for screening purposes

- ■ CTA is invasive; its main indication is for the detection of hepatocellular carcinoma in patients with cirrhosis

- ■ CTAP is highly sensitive for detecting liver lesions, although invasive and subject to false positive results

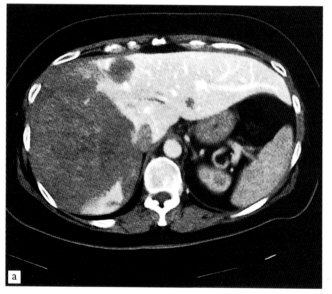 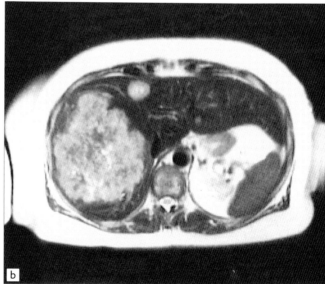

Figure 42.4. *Metastases from colorectal cancer. (a) CT with arterial portography shows three lesions, also demonstrated on (b) SPIO-enhanced T2-weighted MR. Note the disturbance of perfusion in liver tissue adjacent to the large tumour, which exaggerates the size of the lesion on CTAP.*

Appearances of liver metastases

Some small lesions are indistinguishable from normal liver on unenhanced CT but most larger lesions and a minority of small tumours show reduced attenuation. Calcification is not uncommon in larger lesions, particularly metastases from mucin-secreting tumours of the gastro-intestinal tract (Fig. 42.5). After chemotherapy, calcification is more common, particularly in slow-growing lesions, e.g. carcinoids, islet cell metastases. Small lesions are usually round and homogeneous, larger tumours often become irregular in shape and heterogeneous (Fig. 42.6). The unsharp margin, which is typical of most metastases, is explained by a combination of volume averaging with irregularity of the interface between tumour surface and adjacent liver. In the sinusoidal phase of contrast enhancement, the majority of

lesions are more conspicuous because they are hypovascular compared with adjacent liver.

Hypervascular tumours show a contrast medium blush during the arterial-dominant phase of enhancement which may persist into the sinusoidal phase. However, most hypervascular tumours show a fairly rapid washout of contrast and become hypoattenuating on delayed images. Hypervascular tumours with central necrosis produce a 'bull's eye' appearance with a peripheral ring of early enhancement. Primary tumours which commonly produce hypervascular liver metastases include:

- Islet cell tumours of the pancreas
- Carcinoids
- Phaeochromocytoma
- Melanoma
- Renal cell cancer

However, all of these tumours may also give rise to hypovascular liver metastases and attempts to correlate the histology of individual tumours with the imaging characteristics of their liver metastases have been unsuccessful. A small minority of liver secondaries from carcinomas of bronchus, breast, colorectal and other gastro-intestinal primaries also appear hypervascular. Whilst most metastases appear solid when small, cystic elements are common in larger lesions, and after chemotherapy lesions of any size may become cystic (Fig 42.7). The transcoelomic spread of ovarian tumours typically produces deposits on the peritoneal surfaces of the liver, usually associated with ascites (Fig. 42.1).

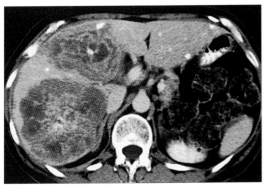

Figure 42.5. *Portal phase CT scan in a patient with metastases from mucin-secreting colorectal cancer. The large tumours contain some central calcification and several small surface lesions are densely calcified following chemotherapy. All the lesions shown here were successfully resected.*

Key points: appearance on CT

■ The majority of metastases have an ill-defined margin due to irregularity of interface between tumour and adjacent liver

■ The majority of metastases are more conspicuous in the sinusoidal (parenchymal) phase of contrast enhancement but often show a thin rim of enhancement in the arterial phase

■ Hypervascular metastases show a contrast blush during the arterial phase and most have a relatively rapid washout

Magnetic resonance

Optimum technique requires the usual trade-off between spatial resolution, contrast resolution and temporal resolution. Continuing advances in MR technology have impacted on each of these aspects. Phased-array surface coils provide improved signal-to-noise ratio, high-powered gradients with fast switching allow multislice or volume acquisitions covering the whole liver in a single breath hold and liver-specific pharmaceuticals provide improved con-

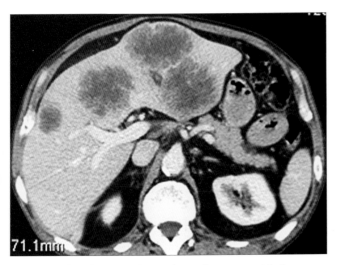

Figure 42.6. *Metastases from colorectal cancer – typical appearances on portal phase CT with multiple low attenuation lesions of irregular shape with heterogeneous structure.*

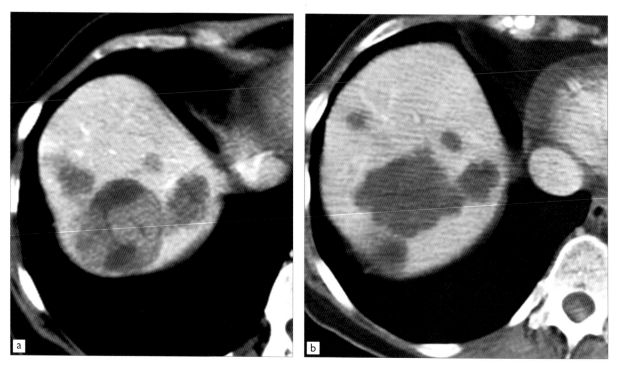

Figure 42.7. *Metastases from gastro-intestinal stromal tumour. (a) Initial CT shows multiple deposits of heterogeneous attenuation. (b) In the post-treatment CT, lesions show uniform attenuation of watery density.*

trast. The MR technique chosen will depend firstly on the hardware and the contrast agents available to the user, and secondly on the objective of the examination. The approach used in the author's department will be described below, but the reader should be aware that development in this field is rapid and the techniques described here will inevitably be overtaken.

Detection of lesions

The use of contrast agents

There is evidence that the use of superparamagnetic iron oxide (SPIO) contrast media offers the most sensitive method for detecting small liver lesions with MR.[23–27] Superparamagnetic iron oxide particles are of colloidal size (30–200 nm diameter). After IV injection, they are phagocytosed by the reticulo-endothelial cells of the liver, spleen and bone marrow. The major effect of SPIO is to cause shortening of T2*, producing a marked reduction in signal intensity on proton density and T2-weighted images which lasts for several hours after injection.[28] Because metastases show higher signal intensity than adjacent liver tissue on unenhanced T2 images, SPIO increases their conspicuity (Figs. 42.8 and 42.9). The magnitude of the SPIO effect increases with field strength, so for equivalent enhancement, smaller doses of SPIO are needed at higher field strengths. Gradient recalled echo (GRE) sequences are much more sensitive to the susceptibility effects produced by SPIO than are fast spin-echo sequences, so when using SPIO contrast agents T2*-weighted GRE techniques are

required.[29] Superparamagnetic iron oxide also has a transient T1-enhancing effect, again more marked at higher field strengths. Following injection of SPIO, normal liver produces virtually no signal intensity on T2-weighted images so it may be difficult to distinguish metastases close to the liver surface from lesions outside the liver, for example in the lung base. Non-contrast T1-weighted images will usually allow this distinction to be made by demonstrating the major anatomical landmarks.

Rivalling SPIO-enhanced T2-weighted imaging for the detection of small metastases is the use of three-dimensional T1-weighted sequences obtained dynamically after the bolus injection of extracellular gadolinium (Gd) chelates.[30] Another possible approach is to use hepatocyte-enhancing T1 contrast agents (gadobenate, gadoxetic acid and mangafodipir), which increase the conspicuity of tumours by selectively enhancing normal liver tissue.[31,32] Direct comparison of these T1 agents with SPIO-enhanced studies and with three-dimensional dynamic techniques has not yet demonstrated a clear advantage. However, in circumstances where the characterization or anatomic mapping of metastases is critical to surgical treatment, the combined use of SPIO and gadolinium enhancement may be helpful.[33]

Techniques for lesion characterization

Chemical-shift imaging

The detection of lesions within a fatty liver, and the differentiation of focal fatty change from tumour, is usually

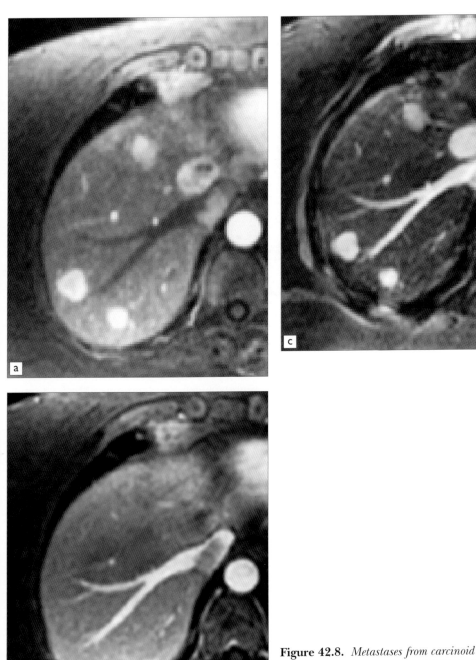

Figure 42.8. *Metastases from carcinoid tumour. Hypervascular tumours are well shown on (a) T1-weighted MR during the arterial phase of gadolinium enhancement, but are barely visible during (b) the venous phase; (c) SPIO-enhanced T2-weighted MR shows lesions and vessels as areas of high signal intensity.*

achieved by obtaining specific fat-sensitive MR sequences.[34] Because the resonant frequencies of fat and water protons are slightly different, tissues in which fat and water are mixed at a microscopic level will produce signals of two different frequencies. By selecting an appropriate TE, the signal intensity can be sampled at a time when the fat and water components are either in-phase or out-of-phase. The signal from fatty liver, whether focal or diffuse, is distinctly reduced on opposed-phase images compared with in-phase images.

T2-weighted imaging
Acquisitions with a long echo train (such as fast spin-echo T2 and HASTE sequences) are influenced by magnetization transfer effects, which occur to a much lesser extent in cysts and hemangiomas than in metastases. These benign lesions

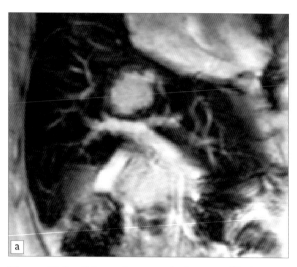 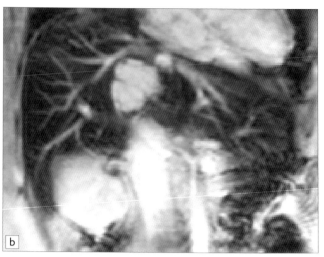

Figure 42.9. *Colorectal metastasis shown on SPIO-enhanced T2-weighted MR. (a) Right anterior oblique coronal slice through the porta hepatis shows the relation of the tumour to the portal vein branches. (b) A more posterior slice shows the position of the tumour relative to right and left hepatic veins.*

show bright signal intensity on such sequences whilst solid tumours appear less intense, so unenhanced images with heavy T2 weighting are helpful for discriminating between metastases and benign malformations. A similar distinction can be made by extending the TE of a fast spin-echo sequence to 160–180 ms, which increases the T2 weighting.[35]

Dynamic gadolinium-enhanced imaging

Extracellular gadolinium chelates produce shortening of T1, leading to increased signal intensity in the liver and its major vessels. For dynamic imaging after gadolinium, a rapid dynamic T1-weighted fat-suppressed three-dimensional volume sequence is used to give complete coverage of the liver in a single breath hold. A flip angle of 12–15° maintains the signal intensity from stationary tissues, whilst repetition time (TR) and echo time (TE) are minimized, typically to TR of 3.5–4.2 ms and TE of 1.3–1.9 ms.[30] The dynamic series should include baseline precontrast images, then sequential acquisitions in the arterial-dominant phase (0–20 seconds after injection), portal phase (30–50 seconds) and equilibrium phase (1–2 minutes). Using this technique, metastases can usually be differentiated from cysts, hemangiomas and other benign malformations. If the nature of the lesion is still doubtful, delayed images after 10 minutes may be helpful.

Liver-specific contrast media

Hepatocellular lesions, which contain functioning reticuloendothelial cells (focal nodular hyperplasia, some adenomas and some well-differentiated hepatomas), will take up SPIO whilst malignant lesions show very little or no uptake.[36] Specific chelates of gadolinium (gadoxetic acid, gadobenate) and manganese (mangafodipir), which are

actively taken up by hepatocytes, produce increased signal intensity on T1-weighted images, and so increase the conspicuity of liver lesions that contain no functioning hepatocytes. Results with these T1 agents have shown improved detection of metastases compared with unenhanced images,[37,38] but the incidence of adverse reactions is a little higher than with Gd-DTPA or SPIO.

Key points: magnetic resonance techniques

- Dynamic Gd-enhanced imaging in the arterial and equilibrium phases is a valuable technique for characterizing liver lesions

- Opposed-phase imaging can distinguish focal fatty liver from metastatic disease

- SPIO contrast studies are the most sensitive method for detecting small liver lesions on MR

- SPIO contrast agents are useful for characterizing lesions which contain functioning reticulo-endothelial cells (e.g. focal nodular hyperplasia)

Appearances of liver metastases

Unenhanced magnetic resonance images

Metastases from liposarcoma and from melanoma, which may contain fat and melanin, respectively, can be hyperintense on T1-weighted images, but in the absence of haemorrhage other metastatic deposits are hypointense on T1-weighted images. On T2 images, lesions which are calcified or contain altered blood may be hypointense, but almost all tumours are hyperintense. Tumour necrosis produces a central area of watery characteristics (bright on T2, low signal intensity on T1) so that metastases may be occasionally difficult to distinguish from abscesses.

Gadolinium-enhanced images

Most metastases are hypovascular compared with the surrounding liver so with extracellular gadolinium contrast agents they become more conspicuous on T1 images in the portal venous phase of enhancement. A complete ring of peripheral enhancement is commonly present in tumours with central necrosis, and is best seen in the arterial phase. The pattern of marked arterial phase enhancement with rapid fading of the initial blush is characteristic of hypervascular metastases (Figs. 42.8 and 42.10). Early washout of the contrast from the lesion on delayed images strongly indicates malignancy (Fig. 42.11).[39] Larger lesions are usually heterogeneous. Only very rarely do metastases take up liver-specific contrast agents.

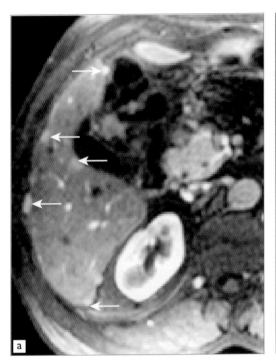 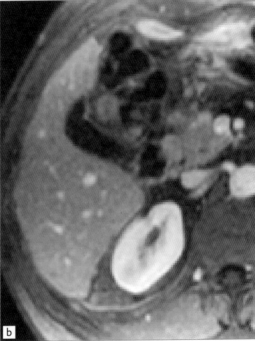

Figure 42.10.
Metastases from gastric cancer. (a) Arterial phase Gd-enhanced T1-weighted MR shows numerous parenchymal and surface lesions (arrows) which are not visible on (b) the venous phase.

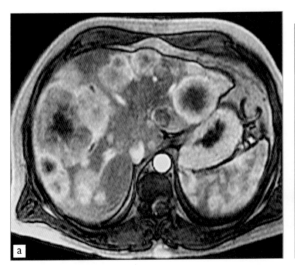 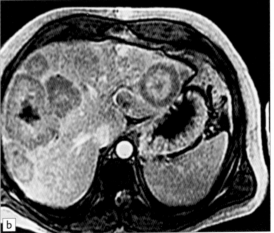

Figure 42.11. *Peripheral washout shown by metastases from gastrinoma. (a) Arterial phase Gd-enhanced T1-weighted MR shows multiple hypervascular lesions, the larger ones with hypointense centres. (b) In the equilibrium phase, the contrast has diffused into the necrotic centres of the large lesions but has also been washed out of the hypervascular periphery.*

Key points: appearance on magnetic resonance

- The majority of metastases are hypointense on T1-weighted images and hyperintense on T2-weighted images

- Signal intensity of metastases may be altered due to the presence of fat, melanin, calcification, altered blood and necrosis

- The majority of metastases show similar contrast enhancement patterns to those of CT, e.g. hypervascular metastases show marked arterial phase enhancement with a rapid washout

Sonography

Real-time and colour-flow Doppler

Real-time ultrasound with colour flow and power Doppler examination provides a rapid and non-invasive method for screening patients with suspected right upper quadrant disease. Sonography is ideal for exploring the biliary tract, major liver vessels and inferior vena cava as well as surveying the liver parenchyma and surrounding structures. The majority of liver lesions can be correctly characterized[40,41] and imaging guidance for biopsy is quicker and simpler with ultrasound than with CT or MR. Colour flow Doppler imaging is used to confirm the patency of major vessels and the direction of blood flow. Sonography is also most useful for detecting and monitoring local postoperative complications after hepato-biliary surgery.

Vascular contrast agents[42]

Contrast agents for sonography comprise air bubbles of about 1–10 μm in diameter surrounded by a thin shell of lipid or galactose with surfactant-like properties. The particles remain within the vascular compartment with a blood half-life of a few minutes. They produce markedly increased echogenicity within blood vessels. This improves the sensitivity for detection of vascular abnormalities, and assists in the differential diagnosis of tumour, but the role of these agents in routine diagnostic applications is still being explored.

Appearances of liver metastases

Liver metastases most often appear as areas of reduced (less often increased, or heterogeneous) echogenicity within the liver parenchyma (Fig. 42.12). The majority of lesions show

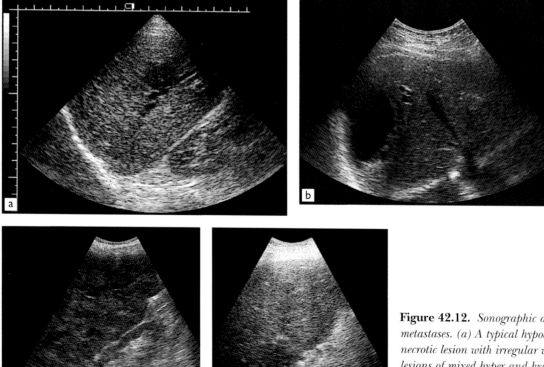

Figure 42.12. *Sonographic appearance of liver metastases. (a) A typical hypoechoic lesion; (b) large necrotic lesion with irregular wall; (c) multiple small lesions of mixed hyper and hypoechogenicity from lung cancer; (d) multiple small hypoechoic metastases from breast carcinoma (Courtesy of J Bates).*

less vascularity than surrounding liver with sonographic contrast agents (Fig. 42.13). Liver cysts are anechoic with increased through transmission and should be readily distinguishable from solid lesions. In patients with clear-cut metastatic liver lesions, the combination of sonography with guided biopsy may eliminate the need for further imaging. One limitation of sonography is that the exclusion value of a negative examination is influenced both by the size and shape of the patient and by the expertise of the operator. Obesity, high position of the liver under the costal margin, and a colon distended with gas all mitigate against confident exclusion of small liver lesions by sonography. For formal staging procedures, CT is preferred partly for this reason and partly for its better reproducibility on consecutive follow-up examinations for re-assessment of lesion size.

Intraoperative ultrasound

Direct application of the sonographic probe to the liver surface overcomes the problem of signal intensity loss in the soft tissues of the thoraco-abdominal wall, and also allows the use of a higher frequency probe (5–7.5 mHz), with a resulting improvement in spatial resolution. This technique will detect lesions down to about 2 mm in diameter and has been shown to be superior to preoperative imaging and visual examination and palpation of the liver at laparotomy.[43,44] In expert hands, the technique should add only 10–15 minutes to the operative procedure. Currently, intraoperative ultrasound (IOUS) is used for confirming the presence of small liver lesions shown on preoperative imaging, clarifying the nature of equivocal lesions detected preoperatively and any additional lesions detected at surgery, and excluding the presence of lesions from those segments which the surgeon plans to leave behind. Laparoscopic

ultrasonography has also been used to supplement non-invasive imaging in the detection of small liver lesions,[45] but its role is yet to be established.

Key points: metastases on ultrasound

- Liver metastases usually appear as lesions of low echogenicity on ultrasonography

- Power Doppler is sensitive to blood flow and helps to characterize liver lesions

- IV contrast agents improve the detection of liver lesions

- IOUS may identify lesions down to 2 mm in diameter

Nuclear medicine

Conventional scintigraphy no longer has a role in the detection of metastatic disease because the spatial resolution of sonography, CT and MR is much better. Dynamic flow scintigraphy has a potential application in the early detection of occult metastasis (see below).

Characterization of hepatocellular lesions

Technetium-labelled colloid is usually accumulated within areas of focal nodular hyperplasia, whereas malignant tumours and other hepatocellular lesions hardly ever contain sufficient functioning Kupffer cells to take up this agent. Technetium-99m-labelled iminodiacetic acid compounds are specifically extracted by hepatocytes and secreted into the bile. Benign hepatocellular lesions typically accumulate these agents, whereas the vast majority of

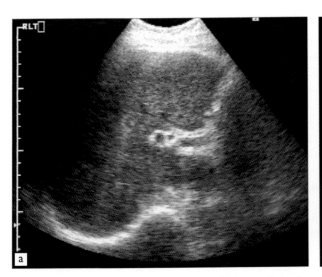
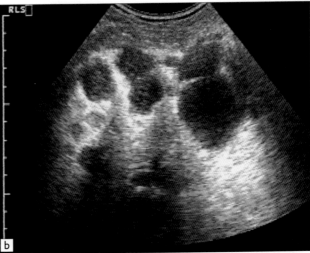

Figure 42.13. *(a) Colorectal metastases which are almost isoechoic with normal liver are very clearly shown as (b) areas of reduced echogenicity after a micro-bubble contrast agent (Courtesy of J Bates).*

hepatocellular carcinomas and all metastases show no uptake.

Somatostatin receptor imaging[46]

[111]Indium-labelled octreotide, a synthetic analogue of somatostatin, is typically concentrated in carcinoids, islet-cell tumours and in other lesions of neuroendocrine origin. Using single-photon emission tomography (SPECT), active lesions, including both liver metastases and primary tumours in the pancreas or bowel, may be detected down to about 1 cm in size (Fig. 42.14). Although the limited spatial resolution of scintigraphy means that this method will rarely detect liver lesions not visible on CT or MR, demonstration of the functional status of primary or secondary tumours may be useful in differential diagnosis and in planning treatment, for example by therapeutic doses of targeted radionuclides.

Immunoscintigraphy[47–49]

Numerous different monoclonal antibodies and antibody fragments have been evaluated for the detection of primary and secondary malignancies, including liver metastases. One major disadvantage is that most antibodies show some localization within normal liver tissue, so the recognition of abnormal accumulation in the target tumour is more difficult here than at other anatomic sites. The most useful contribution of these agents is in the distinction of residual or recurrent tumour from local scarring following surgery or radiation therapy to the primary site.

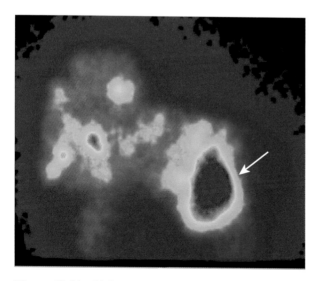

Figure 42.14. *Malignant islet cell tumour – pancreatic primary (arrow) and numerous liver metastases shown on somatostatin receptor scintigraphy.*

Positron emission tomography[50–52]

Using 2-[F-18]fluoro-2-deoxy-D-glucose ([18]FDG) positron emission tomography (PET) has been shown in early studies to be at least as accurate as CT and sonography in the local staging of tumours of the gastro-intestinal tract, and to be more sensitive and specific than CT in detecting local recurrence after treatment. Because [18]FDG accumulates in normal liver tissue, the value of [18]FDG PET in detecting liver metastases is less clear, but comparative studies have shown that it is as accurate as CT in detecting spread to the liver from colorectal and pancreatic primaries.

Key points: scintigraphy of metastases

- Conventional scintigraphy no longer plays a role in the detection of liver metastases

- Demonstration of uptake of Indium-labelled octreotide in liver metastases is useful in planning therapy

- [18]FDG PET is highly effective for detecting recurrent tumour at the primary site, and may be as accurate as CT in identifying liver metastases.

- The hepatic perfusion index (HPI) measures the ratio of the arterial to portal venous inflow of the liver

- Tc-99m-labelled colloid and duplex Doppler ultrasonography may reveal an elevated HPI in patients with occult metastatic disease

Early detection of liver metastases

Whereas large liver tumours may be amenable to loco-regional treatment by surgery, percutaneous ablation, embolization, intravascular perfusion chemotherapy etc, diffuse small lesions require systemic treatment, and the possibility of curative chemotherapy requires the earliest possible detection of metastatic disease. Tumours have mixed populations of cells, often with different degrees of sensitivity to chemotherapeutic agents, and populations of metastases may themselves be heterogeneous in terms of blood supply, local tissue responses, immune characteristics and other biological features. As an approximation, it is estimated that chemotherapeutic agents will penetrate lesions of 100 μm size, whereas with larger lesions the drug effectiveness may be compromised by its inability to reach the target cells. Current imaging technology is some way from detecting lesions of such a size, although 100 μm resolution is achievable with MR surface coils using a small field of view, and further developments will improve the resolution of liver imaging. Meanwhile, lesions smaller than 2–3 mm are regarded as 'occult' for imaging purposes and have only been demonstrated by innovative indirect methods described below.

Detecting occult metastases

Until recently, laparotomy has been used as the gold standard against which the sensitivity of imaging techniques were compared, but accumulating evidence shows that laparotomy itself substantially underestimates the incidence of micrometastases. A small series of autopsies performed within a month of initial surgery showed that 16% of patients with apparently normal livers were harbouring metastatic tumours.[53] When 150 livers containing metastases were examined at postmortem, in 11% of cases the liver looked and felt normal but contained deep-seated lesions on sectioning.[54] More recent follow-up studies on patients with colorectal cancer have shown that about one third of such patients, with no liver lesion detected at laparotomy, developed overt clinical or imaging evidence of liver metastasis within 2 years.[5,6] In colorectal cancer, surgical emphasis is placed upon Dukes' staging of the primary tumour, but it is now well established that survival is more closely related to the appearance of liver metastases than to primary tumour staging. With the possibility of adjuvant treatment for high-risk patients, the early detection of anatomically occult metastatic lesions appears to be an important goal, and physiological methods have been developed for this purpose.

Scintigraphic hepatic perfusion index

Technetium-99m-labelled colloidal particles pass freely through the pulmonary and intestinal capillaries but are almost totally extracted in their first passage through the liver. The hepatic arterial component of an intravenously administered bolus arrives about 8 seconds before the portal venous component so by monitoring the rate of arrival of the tracer in the liver over these separate periods, it is possible to measure the relative proportions of arterial and portal venous inflow, expressed as HPI. Having derived normal ranges from volunteers, Parkin et al.[55] found increased HPI in patients who harboured metastases at laparotomy. The same group also showed that patients in whom the liver appeared normal at the time of primary surgery, but later developed metastases during follow-up, also had abnormally elevated HPI on the preoperative studies.[5]

Doppler perfusion index

The same pathophysiology has been demonstrated using duplex colour Doppler sonography. Again, studying patients undergoing surgery for colorectal cancer, Leen et al.[56] showed abnormal Doppler perfusion indices in patients with surgically normal livers who subsequently developed overt metastatic disease.

Hepatic transit times

Blomley et al.[57] recently measured the arrival time in the hepatic veins of an IV bolus of an ultrasonic contrast agent and found that the transit was distinctly faster in patients with metastases than in controls.

In spite of initial success, these techniques have not become routine and their use remains developmental, partly because adjuvant treatment for patients with suspected occult disease has not yet been widely accepted in gastro-intestinal malignancy.

Detecting small lesions – physical limitations of imaging

For the purpose of discussion, 'small' lesions are defined as those of 2–15 mm diameter. Detecting metastases in this size range poses two questions – firstly, are any mass lesions present, and secondly, are they cysts, benign neoplasms or metastases.

Using MR or CT, the smallest size at which metastases can be detected in the liver depends upon the spatial resolution of the images and the difference in signal intensity or attenuation between the lesion and the adjacent liver tissue. Current MR and CT units can achieve resolution of the order of 1 mm within the plane of the section, so spatial resolution effectively depends upon slice thickness. Similarly, contrast resolution for large lesions is highly sensitive – signal intensity or attenuation differences of 5% can be detected. With small lesions, contrast is degraded by noise and spatial resolution is degraded by volume averaging. As an illustration, a 5 cm liver cyst shown on contrast-enhanced helical CT may exhibit a difference of 100 Hounsfield units (HU) between the watery fluid in the cyst and the enhanced liver tissue. A 2 mm cyst within a 5 mm slice would then show a maximum contrast of about 25 HU. Although the signal intensity relationships in MR are more complex, similar considerations apply – high-contrast lesions can be detected down to about one quarter of the slice thickness using optimum technique. Unfortunately, most small liver metastases have low intrinsic contrast and lesions of the same diameter as the slice thickness will often be invisible on unenhanced MR and CT. If we try to improve the detection of small lesions by using thinner slices the signal-to-noise ratio decreases, producing noisy images with lower contrast. In summary, CT and MR techniques for detecting liver metastases require a trade-off between speed of acquisition, spatial resolution and contrast discrimination.

The limitations of sonography include a few additional factors. Resolution of 1–2 mm along the axis of the beam is typical; resolution across the beam width is less. In effect, spatial resolution decreases with increasing depth in the patient so that the results and exclusion value of liver sonography are strongly influenced by the size and build of the patient, as well as by the expertise of the operator. As on CT and MR, small cysts and hemangiomas show greater contrast on sonography than small metastases. Whereas with MR and CT it is possible to obtain a volume acquisition of the whole liver during a single breath hold, sonography is performed by repeated sampling of individual sections so it is less easy to be sure that the whole liver volume has been examined. In individual cases, sonography may be superior to CT or MR in detecting small lesions but with a mixed population of patients and operators of different expertise, CT and MR are more reliable.

Distinguishing benign focal lesions from metastases

The widespread use of non-invasive liver imaging has revealed the presence of cysts, hemangiomas and focal fatty change in a significant proportion of patients with no symptoms of liver disease. When large, these lesions show typical features that allow their distinction from primary or secondary liver tumours, but with small masses this is more difficult. When small lesions are discovered incidentally during imaging for non-malignant disease, the likelihood of their being metastatic deposits is remote[58] and many patients with established primary tumours also harbour benign liver lesions.[59] However, small lesions appearing for the first time during surveillance after initial treatment of

malignant disease must be regarded with extreme suspicion, whatever their imaging appearance. Similarly, indeterminate lesions which become smaller or disappear during chemotherapy must be regarded as malignant.[60] In doubtful cases, multiple imaging methods may supplement each other to confirm a diagnosis.

Liver cysts

Liver cysts have a clear-cut margin representing a thin wall. The cyst contents are anechoic on sonography, show low attenuation on CT, low signal intensity on unenhanced T1-weighted MR and very high signal intensity on T2-weighted images, producing a 'light bulb' appearance (Fig. 42.15). With IV contrast medium, cysts show no enhancement on CT or MR. A minority of metastases contains a fluid component as a result of central necrosis, which is common in larger tumours but infrequent in lesions of less than 1.5 cm. When small tumours do exhibit central necrosis they usually have a characteristic enhancing rim of irregular thickness with rapid washout of contrast on delayed images. An exception to this is seen in some patients after chemotherapy in that small metastases may break down to produce cyst-like residues which can retain the potential for later malignant regrowth.

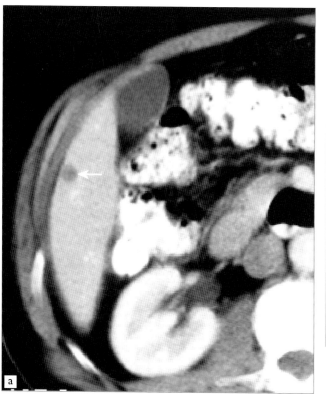
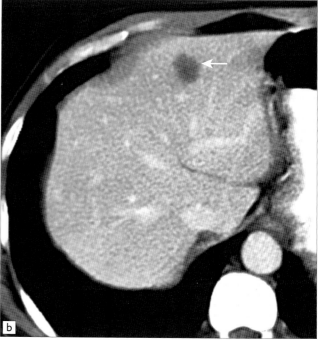

Figure 42.15a–b. *Coexistent benign cyst and metastasis from melanoma. (a) Portal phase CT shows a 1 cm lesion in segment 5 and (b) a larger lesion of similar appearance in segment 2 (arrows).*

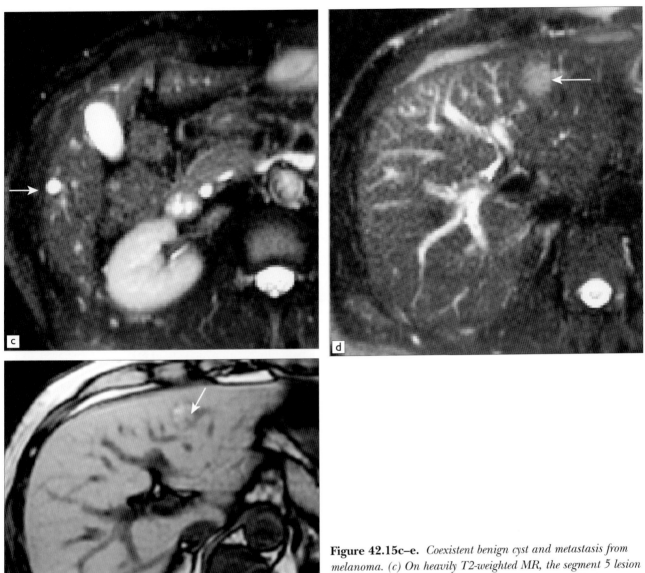

Figure 42.15c–e. *Coexistent benign cyst and metastasis from melanoma. (c) On heavily T2-weighted MR, the segment 5 lesion (arrow) shows intensely bright signal intensity typical of a cyst, whilst (d) the lesion in segment 2 (arrow) is only slightly hyperintense, typical of metastasis. (e) Unenhanced T1-weighted MR shows the segment 2 lesion to contain areas of high signal intensity (arrow), characteristic of melanoma.*

Hemangiomas

Hemangiomas are found in about 20% of autopsies[61] and are common in patients undergoing liver imaging for suspected metastatic disease. They are round or irregular in shape with clear-cut margins. Typical lesions are hyperechoic on sonography, with reduced attenuation on unenhanced CT, low signal intensity on unenhanced T1-weighted MR and bright signal intensity on T2 weighting. Their range of signal intensities overlaps with that of liver metastases but this overlap can be minimized or abolished by using very heavily T2-weighted acquisitions.[62] Using a longer TE, benign lesions remain bright whilst malignant lesions show a relative reduction in intensity. With large hemangiomas,

IV contrast medium produces a characteristic pattern of peripheral nodular enhancement on both CT and MR, with gradual enhancement of the centre of the lesion developing over a few minutes after injection. The lesions remain isointense with blood in the major vessels at all stages after contrast injection. Small hemangiomas may show uniform enhancement in the arterial dominant phase,[63] a similar appearance to that of hypervascular metastases,[64] but the latter usually show rapid washout of the contrast medium. Other atypical appearances of hemangiomas include the central dot sign (arterial phase enhancement with a small central vessel), and dense central fibrosis or hyalinization with lack of contrast enhancement in parts of the lesion.

Biliary microhamartomas (von Meyenburg complexes)[65,66]

Biliary microhamartomas share some imaging characteristics with cysts and hemangiomas – they appear bright on T2-weighted MR and have low attenuation on contrast–enhanced CT, although a thin rim of peripheral enhancement is not unusual. These malformations are often irregular or even angular in shape, and usually only a few mm in diameter.

Focal nodular hyperplasia[67]

With the widespread use of dual-phase CT, multiphase contrast-enhanced MR and the recent introduction of vascular contrast agents in sonography has come a realization that focal nodular hyperplasia (FNH) is not rare. Larger lesions typically show a rounded or lobulated shape with clear-cut margin, a mass effect displacing adjacent vessels and a central scar sometimes with radiating spokes towards the periphery. Their echogenicity, attenuation and signal intensity characteristics are little different to those of normal liver tissue. The lesions show marked arterial phase contrast enhancement, which usually fades rapidly to become iso-intense in the portal phase, although occasionally increased enhancement lasts for several minutes. Delayed enhancement of the central scar is characteristic. Lesions smaller than about 2 cm are often homogeneous with no central scar, but show the same enhancement characteristics. When found in patients with known malignancy, a confident diagnosis of FNH requires the demonstration of intact liver function within the lesion. The most effective method is to use SPIO enhancement. If the lesion shows substantial SPIO uptake (more than 40–50% of that taken up by the liver), it may be regarded as benign. Metastases do not take up SPIO, but well-differentiated hepatocellular cancers may take up just a little. Another approach is to use one of the hepatocellular MR contrast agents (mangafodipir, gadobenate, or gadoxetic acid). All of these agents are taken up by the functioning hepatocytes present in FNH lesions (and also in well-differentiated hepatocellular carcinoma), but because there is no biliary excretory pathway, the lesions retain the contrast for much longer than the normal liver, so becoming brighter on delayed T1-weighted images.

Focal fatty change[68,69]

Areas of focal fatty infiltration can be of any size but typically also show a clear-cut margin. Vascular architecture is preserved and there is no mass effect. However, nodular deposits of fatty change may resemble metastatic disease and nodular focal sparing within an otherwise diffuse fatty liver has also been described. Affected areas show locally increased echogenicity on sonography whilst with focal fatty sparing the reverse appearance is obtained. Fatty liver produces reduced attenuation on CT and is hypointense on opposed-phase T1-weighted gradient-echo images at MR. Contrast enhancement of liver tissue is usually uninflu-enced by the presence of fat but subtle differences in signal intensity or attenuation may be obscured with IV contrast medium. The most sensitive method for confirming focal fatty infiltration is to use in-phase/opposed-phase T1-weighted gradient-echo MR images (Fig. 42.16). Focal fatty change produces an appearance on CT and on opposed-phase T1-weighted MR which is similar to that associated with tumours, so detecting metastases in a fatty liver can be difficult. In-phase/opposed-phase MR will usually clarify these cases. Unenhanced images may show a rim of higher attenuation (CT) or signal intensity (opposed-phase MR) around a lesion which appears otherwise indistinguishable from the surrounding fatty liver parenchyma, probably resulting from focal fatty sparing surrounding the lesion.

Transient hepatic attenuation defects[70,71]

Arterial phase imaging often shows a wedge-shaped area of hyperperfusion in the area of liver immediately around and peripheral to a liver tumour. Characteristically, these areas become isointense with the remainder of the liver during the sinusoidal and later phases. Such transient hepatic attenuation defects (THADs) are believed to be caused by occlusion or compression of local portal vein branches by the tumour, so the detection of a THAD should stimulate a careful search of all images for an underlying focal lesion. However, occasionally THADs are seen in patients in whom no tumour can be found (Fig. 42.17) and probably result from local branch portal vein occlusions which may be transient. Around the periphery of segment 4, particularly just to the right of the falciform ligament anteriorly, and also anterior to the bifurcation of the portal vein, small areas of liver parenchyma may receive non-portal venous supply from the parabiliary venous plexus and from anomalous drainage of gastric, duodenal and pancreatic veins. This can produce small nodules of focal fatty change in these areas, or more commonly may result in small areas of altered enhancement after contrast. These normal variants need to be distinguished from small metastases.

Key points: benign lesions versus metastases

- Liver cysts have a clear-cut margin, are anechoic on sonography, show low attenuation on CT, low signal intensity on T1- and high signal intensity on T2-weighted MR

- A minority of metastases contains fluid and may be confused with cysts

- Hemangiomas are irregular in shape with clear-cut margins

- Typically hemangiomas are hyperechoic on sonography, low attenuation on CT and bright on T2-weighted MR

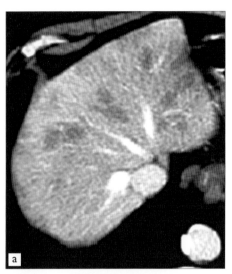

Figure 42.16. *Focal fatty change simulating metastases. (a) Portal phase CT shows multiple low attenuation lesions; (b) unenhanced opposed-phase T1-weighted MR shows the lesions as areas of reduced signal intensity, but the lesions are not visible on (c) unenhanced in-phase T1-weighted MR.*

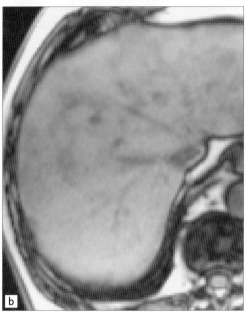

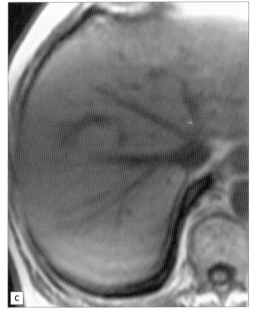

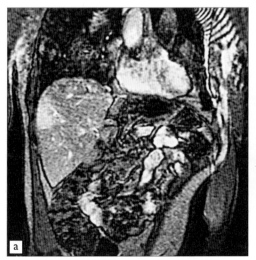

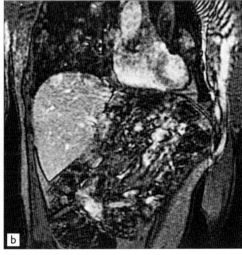

Figure 42.17. *Transient hepatic attenuation difference (THAD). (a) Coronal T1-weighted MR obtained 30 seconds and (b) 60 seconds after gadolinium injection showing a wedge-shaped area of arterial hyperenhancement which rapidly becomes isointense with adjacent liver – a THAD probably caused by segmental portal vein occlusion. No underlying tumour was found.*

- On CT and MR, characteristic enhancement patterns are observed in hemangioma

- Focal fatty change shows hyperechogenicity on sonography, low attenuation on CT and low signal intensity on opposed-phase T1-weighted MR

- Transient hepatic attenuation defects are wedge-shaped areas of hyperperfusion often due to occlusion or compression of portal vein branches adjacent to tumour but can occur in the absence of tumours

Strategies for imaging liver metastasis

Which imaging method for lesion detection?

Three factors explain the enormous variations in sensitivity, specificity and accuracy which have been recorded for various imaging techniques – firstly, different patient populations have been studied; secondly, imaging methods have been compared at different stages of technical development; and thirdly, the standards for verification of the true presence or absence of disease – gold standards – have been erratic. To command real credibility, comparative studies should fulfil the following criteria:

- If differing modalities are being compared, state of the art technology should be used in each case
- The gold standard should include histology wherever feasible, and surgical exploration with intraoperative ultrasound as a minimum standard
- In order to minimize the subjective effect of observer variation, multiple readers should be used
- To avoid variations in sensitivity and specificity, due to different 'decision thresholds', receiver operating characteristic (ROC) curve methodology should be used

Using surgery with intraoperative ultrasound as the reference standard for detection of lesions, SPIO-enhanced MR and CTAP both show 85–95% sensitivity in lesion detection.[23,72] Earlier studies showed that unenhanced MR is marginally superior to dynamic incremental CT in lesion detection and dynamic MR with gadolinium enhancement showed a little further improvement. SPIO-enhanced MR is even more sensitive[23–27] and the current comparison is among SPIO-MR, three-dimensional Gd-enhanced T1-weighted MR and thin-slice multidetector helical CT. In summary:

- SPIO-enhanced MR is probably the most sensitive non-invasive technique for detecting liver metastasis
- CTAP may be more sensitive than SPIO-MR, especially for lesions of less than 1 cm size, but is also prone to false positives, so accuracy is no better than SPIO-MR

- IOUS detects some additional lesions not seen on preoperative imaging

Preoperative assessment

Surgical interest for resection of liver metastases is focused on colorectal cancer. The reasons for this are:

- Colorectal cancer is common
- Complete excision of the primary tumour is achieved much more often than with gastric, oesophageal or pancreatic cancer
- With improved surgical techniques, metastatic disease is amenable to resection in an increasing proportion of cases (Fig. 42.18)
- Survival is clearly improved after successful resection

Survival in colorectal cancer is linked to local staging of the primary tumour at the time of surgery, but is even more strongly influenced by the presence or absence of liver

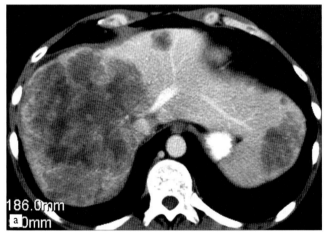

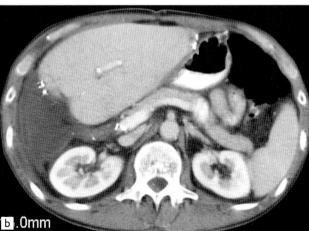

Figure 42.18. *(a) Extensive colorectal metastases involving both left and right lobes were successfully resected; (b) follow-up CT obtained 3 months after surgery shows regeneration of the small fraction of residual liver tissue.*

metastases. The median survival of untreated patients with clinically apparent liver metastasis is less than 12 months – even patients with one to three liver lesions have a 5-year survival of less than 10%.[73] Before the introduction of modern imaging methods, it was established that tumour resection in patients with metastases that are solitary or limited to a single segment or lobe substantially improves survival.[74] With improvements in preoperative imaging and advances in surgical technology, long-term survival rates of 40% have been achieved,[75] whilst the most recent results suggest 5-year survival rates of over 50%.[76] Surgical procedures for liver tumour resection are based on segmental anatomy (Fig. 42.19),[77] so the objectives for preoperative imaging are to:

- Demonstrate which liver segments are free of disease; up to 80% of liver tissue can be removed, so the minimum residue of normal liver required is about two segments
- Show the position of liver metastases with reference to segmental anatomy
- Demonstrate the relation of tumours to the main hepatic veins, the portal vein and its main divisions
- Exclude the presence of extrahepatic disease

Excluding the presence of metastases in those segments which the surgeon plans to leave behind requires three-dimensional Gd-enhanced T1-weighted MR, SPIO-MR, or

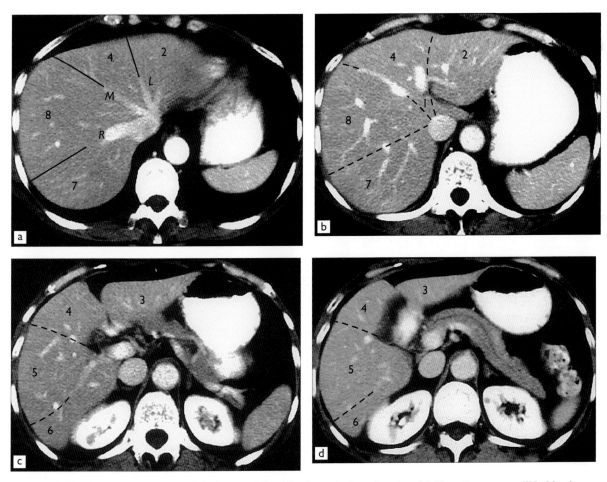

Figure 42.19. *Segmental anatomy of the liver is defined by the main hepatic veins, falciform ligament, gallbladder fossa and the plane of the main portal vein division (horizontal scisura). (a) Contrast-enhanced CT shows the left (L), middle (M) and right (R) hepatic veins at the superior aspect of the liver. (b) Inferior to this the caudate lobe (segment 1) lies between the inferior vena cava and the main portal vein. The left main portal vein separates segment 2 superiorly from segment 3 inferiorly, and similarly the right portal vein branch divides segments 5 and 6 inferiorly from segments 7 and 8 superiorly in the right lobe (a and b).*

CTAP, supplemented at the time of surgery by IOUS. Segmental localization and the demonstration of vascular anatomy can be achieved with multislice CT or Gd-enhanced MR with a combination of axial and coronal oblique imaging to give a complete demonstration of surgical anatomy. Right anterior oblique coronal views are usually the best for demonstrating the portal vein and its main divisions, inferior vena cava and right hepatic vein (Figs. 42.9 and 42.20). Middle and left hepatic veins may also be well shown by this approach but in some cases are better seen on transverse images. Exclusion of extrahepatic disease in patients with primary colorectal tumours requires helical CT of the chest and also CT of the lower abdomen and pelvis.

Imaging during follow-up

Although the majority of patients with apparently successful surgical clearance of liver metastases eventually develop late recurrence, few do so within a year.[78,79] For surveillance of asymptomatic patients, annual CT of thorax, abdomen and pelvis is suggested. Rising tumour markers or recurrent symptoms will require immediate re-imaging. In patients undergoing medical therapy for liver metastases, either sonography or CT can be used to monitor the progress of disease. For improved reproducibility of tumour size estimations, and because many patients either have or are at risk of extrahepatic disease, CT is preferred. Anatomic measurement of lesions to assess response to treatment is discussed in Chapter 5. For patients with large numbers of small lesions, individual measurements may be impractical and a useful alternative is to measure changes in the craniocaudal extent of the liver to give an indication of total tumour volume.

A practical approach

Imaging strategies must take into account the case-mix in the patient population and the resources available. The approach described below evolved in a large acute hospital, including major liver and oncology services, with modern imaging devices and a high throughput of patients.

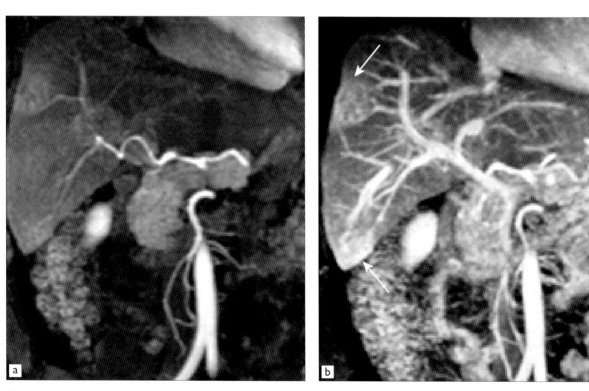

Figure 42.20. *(a) Hepatic vasculature shown on arterial phase and (b) portal phase Gd-enhanced T1-weighted MR obtained in the right coronal oblique plane; the relation of vessels to peripheral tumours (arrows) is shown.*

Summary

- For patients with clinical or biochemical evidence of liver disease, and those with signs or symptoms suggesting right upper quadrant pathology, sonography should be used first. This provides reliable assessment of the biliary tree and hepatic vasculature, and will detect, localize and characterize the majority of focal liver lesions

- In patients with unexpected or inconclusive sonographic results, and for baseline staging of patients with primary tumours, contrast-enhanced helical CT is recommended

- Single-phase acquisition is adequate for most patients but dual-phase imaging should be performed in patients suspected of harbouring hypervascular liver lesions

- Some liver lesions can be satisfactorily characterized by sonography or by CT, but in case of doubt MR should be performed using both T2-weighted imaging and

- dynamic Gd-enhanced T1 acquisitions. Benign hepatocellular lesions are best identified by the uptake of liver-specific contrast agents

- Patients who are candidates for surgical resection of liver tumours require SPIO-enhanced MR for maximum sensitivity in detecting lesions, and this can be combined with a Gd-enhanced coronal and axial series showing the relation of tumours to the hepatic and portal veins

- The more invasive procedure of CTAP can be reserved for patients who are unable to undergo MR, and those in whom MR is inconclusive

- Follow-up studies for patients undergoing chemotherapy can be regarded as restaging procedures. Single-phase helical CT will suffice

References

1. Willis R A. Secondary tumours of the liver. In: The Spread of Tumours in the Human Body, 3rd edn. London: Butterworth, 1973; 175–183

2. Cameron G R. The liver as a site and source of cancer. Br Med J 1954; Feb: 347–352

3. Okuda K, Kojiro M, Okuda H. Neoplasms of the liver. In: Schiff L, Schiff E R (eds). Diseases of the Liver, 7th edn. Philadelphia: J B Lippincott, 1993

4. Baker M E, Pelley R. Hepatic metastases: basic principles and implications for radiologists. Radiology 1995; 197: 329–337

5. Leveson S H, Wiggins P A, Giles G R et al. Deranged liver blood flow patterns in the detection of liver metastases. Br J Surg 1985; 72: 128–130

6. Finlay I G, McArdle C S. Occult hepatic metastases in colorectal carcinoma. Br J Surg 1986; 73: 732–735

7. Breedis C, Young G. Blood supply of neoplasms in the liver. Am J Pathol 1954; 30: 969–985

8. Ackerman N B, Lien W M, Kondi E S, Silverman N A. The blood supply of experimental liver metastases. 1. The distribution of hepatic artery and portal vein blood to 'small' and 'large' tumours. Surgery 1969; 66: 1067–1072

9. Lien W M, Ackerman N B. The blood supply of experimental liver metastases. II. A microcirculatory study of the normal and tumour vessels of the liver with the use of perfusion silicone rubber. Surgery 1970; 68: 334–340

10. Lin G, Hagerstrand I, Lunderquist A. Portal blood supply of liver metastases. Am J Roentgenol 1984; 143: 53–55

11. Haugeberg G, Strohmeyer T, Lierse W et al. The vascularisation of liver metastases. J Cancer Res Clin Oncol 1988; 114: 415–419

12. Nilsson L A V, Zettergren L. Effect of hepatic artery ligation on induced primary liver carcinoma in rats: preliminary report. Acta Pathol Microbiol Scand 1967; 71: 187–193

13. Kan Z, Ivancev K, Lunderquist A et al. In vivo microscopy of hepatic tumours in animal models: A dynamic investigation of blood supply to hepatic metastases. Radiology 1993; 187: 621–626

14. Nott D M, Grime J S, Yates J et al. Changes in the hepatic perfusion index during the growth and development of experimental hepatic micrometastases. Nucl Med Commun 1987; 8: 995–1000

15. Scott D J, Guthrie J A, Arnold P et al. Dual phase helical CT versus portal phase CT for the detection of colorectal liver metastases: correlation with intra-operative sonography, surgical and pathological findings. Clin Radiol 2001; 56: 235–242

16. Kopp A F, Heuschmid M, Claussen C D. Multidetector helical CT of the liver for tumor detection and characterization. Eur Radiol 2002; 12: 745–752

17. Weg N, Scheer M R, Gabor M P. Liver lesions: improved detection with dual-detector-array CT and routine 2.5-mm thin collimation. Radiology 1998; 209: 417–426

18. Haider M A, Amitai M M, Rappaport D C et al. Multi-detector row helical CT in pre-operative assessment of small (<1–5 cm) liver metastases: is thinner collimation better? Radiology 2002; 225: 137–142

19. Oliver J H, Baron R L. Helical biphasic contrast-enhanced CT of the liver: Technique, indications, interpretation and pitfalls. Radiology 1996; 201: 1–14

20. Inoue E, Fujita M, Hosomi N et al. Double phase CT arteriography of the whole liver in the evaluation of

hepatic tumours. J Comput Assist Tomogr 1998; 22: 64–68

21. Matsui O, Takashima T, Kadoya L et al. Liver metastases from colorectal cancers: Detection with CT during arterial portography. Radiology 1987; 165: 65–69

22. Soyer P, Lacheheb D, Levesque M. False positive diagnosis based on CT portography: correlation with pathological findings. Am J Roentgenol 1992;160: 285–289

23. Blakeborough A, Ward J, Wilson D et al. Hepatic lesion detection at MR imaging: a comparative study with four sequences. Radiology 1997; 203: 759–765

24. Oudkerk M, van den Heuvel A G, Wielpolski P A et al. Hepatic lesions: detection with ferumoxide-enhanced T1-weighted MR imaging. Radiology 1997; 203: 449–456

25. Ward J, Naik K S, Guthrie J A et al. Hepatic lesion detection: comparison of MR imaging after the administration of superparamagnetic iron oxide with dual-phase CT by using alternative free-response receiver operating characteristic analysis. Radiology 1999; 210: 459–466

26. Muller R D, Vogel K, Neumann K et al. SPIO-MR imaging versus double-phase spiral CT in detecting malignant lesions of the liver. Acta Radiol 1999; 40: 628–635

27. Del Frate C, Bazzochi M, Moertele K J et al. Detection of liver metastases: comparison of gadobenate dimeglumine-enhanced and ferumoxides-enhanced MR imaging examinations. Radiology 2002; 225: 766–772

28. Tanimoto A, Yuasa Y, Izutsu M et al. Time course of the liver enhancement by a novel MR contrast agent 'AMI 25'. Jap Pharmacol Ther 1994; 22: 713–724

29. Ward J, Guthrie J A, Wilson D et al. Colorectal hepatic metastases: detection with SPIO-enhanced breath-hold MR imaging: comparison of optimized sequences. Radiology 2003; 228(3): 709–718

30. Lee V S, Lavelle M T, Rofsky N M et al. Hepatic MR imaging with a dynamic contrast-enhanced isotropic volumetric interpolated breath-hold examination: feasibility, reproducibility, and technical quality. Radiology 2000; 215: 365–372

31. Helmberger T, Semelka R C. New contrast agents for imaging the liver. Magn Reson Imaging Clin N Am 2001; 9: 745–766

32. Oudkerk M, Torres C G, Song B et al. Characterization of liver lesions with mangafodipir trisodium-enhanced MR imaging: multicentre study comparing MR and dual-phase spiral CT. Radiology 2002; 223: 517–524

33. Ward J, Robinson P J. Combined use of MR contrast agents for evaluating liver disease. Magn Reson Imaging Clin N Am 2001; 9: 767–783

34. Mitchell D G, Kim I, Chang T S et al. Chemical-shift phase difference and suppression magnetic resonance imaging techniques in animals, phantoms, and humans: fatty liver. Invest Radiol 1991; 26: 1041–1052

35. McFarland E G, Mayo-Smith W W, Saini S et al. Hepatic haemangiomas and malignant tumours: Improved differentiation with heavily T2-weighted conventional spin-echo MR imaging. Radiology 1994; 193: 43–47

36. Ros P R, Freeny P C, Harms S E et al. Hepatic MR imaging with ferumoxides: a multicentre clinical trial of the safety and efficacy in the detection of focal hepatic lesions. Radiology 1995; 196: 481–488

37. Rosati G, Pirovano G, Spinazzi A. Interim results of phase II clinical testing of gadobenate dimeglumine. Invest Radiol 1994; 29 (Suppl.): S183–S185

38. Hamm B, Staks T, Muhler A et al. Phase I clinical evaluation of Gd-EOB-DTPA as a hepatobiliary MR contrast agent: safety, pharmacokinetics and MR imaging. Radiology 1995; 195: 785–792

39. Mahfouz A E, Hamm B, Wolf K J. Peripheral washout: a sign of malignancy on dynamic gadolinium-enhanced MR images of focal liver lesions. Radiology 1994; 190: 49–52

40. Reinhold C, Hammers L, Taylor C R et al. Characterisation of focal hepatic lesions with duplex sonography: findings in 198 patients. Am J Roentgenol 1995; 164: 1131–1135

41. Harvey C J, Albrecht T. Ultrasound of focal liver lesions. Eur Radiol 2001; 11: 1578–1593

42. Blomley M H, Albrecht T, Cosgrove D O et al. Improved imaging of liver metastases with stimulated acoustic emission in the late phase of enhancement with the US contrast agent SHU508a: early experience. Radiology 1999; 210: 409–416

43. Luck A J, Maddern G J. Intraoperative abdominal ultrasonography. Br J Surg 1999; 86: 5–16

44. Zacherl J, Scheuba C, Imhof M et al. Current value of intraoperative sonography during surgery for hepatic neoplasms. World J Surg 2002; 26: 550–554

45. Feld R I, Liu J B, Nazarian L et al. Laparoscopic liver sonography: Preliminary experience in liver metastases compared with CT portography. J Ultrasound Med 1996; 15: 289–295

46. Kwekkeboom D J, Krenning E P. Radiolabeled somatostatin analog scintigraphy in oncology: an overview. Eur Radiol 1997; 7: 1103–1109

47. Abdel-Nabi H, Doerr R J, Chan H-W et al. In-111-labelled monoclonal antibody immunoscintigraphy in colorectal carcinoma: safety, sensitivity and preliminary clinical results. Radiology 1990; 175: 163–171

48. Moffat F L, Pinsky C M, Hammershaimb L et al. Clinical utility of external immmunoscintigraphy with the IMMU-4 technetium-99m Fab' antibody fragment in patients undergoing surgery for carcinoma of the colon and rectum: results of a pivotal phase III trial. J Clin Oncol 1996; 14: 2295–2305

49. Lechner P, Lind P, Goldenberg D M. Can postoperative surveillance with serial CEA immunoscintigraphy detect resectable rectal cancer recurrence and potentially improve tumor-free survival? J Am Coll Surg 2000; 191: 511–518

50. Frolich A, Diederichs C G, Staib L et al. Detection of liver metastases from pancreatic cancer using FDG PET. J Nucl Med 1999; 40: 250–255

51. Nakamoto Y, Higashi T, Sakahara H et al. Contribution of PET in the diagnosis of liver metastases from pancreatic tumours. Clin Radiol 1999; 54: 248–252

52. Zhuang H, Sinha P, Pourdehnad M et al. The role of positron emission tomography with fluorine-18-deoxyglucose in identifying colorectal cancer metastases to liver. Nucl Med Commun 2000; 21: 793–798

53. Goligher J C. The operability of carcinoma of the rectum. Br Med J 1941; ii: 393–397

54. Ozarda A, Pickren J. The topographic distribution of liver metastases, its relation to surgical and isotope diagnosis. J Nucl Med 1962; 3: 149–152

55. Parkin A, Robinson P J, Baxter P et al. Liver perfusion scintigraphy: method, normal range, and laparotomy correlation in 100 patients. Nucl Med Commun 1983; 4: 395–402

56. Leen E, Angerson W J, Wotherspoon H et al. Detection of colorectal liver metastases: comparison of laparotomy, CT, US, and Doppler perfusion index and evaluation of postoperative follow-up results. Radiology 1995; 195: 113–116

57. Blomley M J, Albrecht T, Cosgrove D O et al. Liver vascular transit time analyzed with dynamic hepatic venography with bolus injections of a US contrast agent: early experience in seven patients with metastases. Radiology 1998; 209: 862–866

58. Jones E C, Chezmar J L, Nelson R C et al. The frequency and significance of small (<15 mm) hepatic lesions detected by CT. Am J Roentgenol 1992; 158: 535–539

59. Schwartz L H, Gandras E J, Colangelo S M et al. Prevalence and importance of small hepatic lesions found at CT in patients with cancer. Radiology 1999; 210: 71–74

60. Robinson P J, Arnold P, Wilson D. Characterising small 'indeterminate' lesions on computed tomography of the liver: a follow-up study. Br J Radiol 2003; 76: 866–874

61. Karhunen P J. Benign hepatic tumours and tumour-like conditions in man. J Clin Pathol 1986; 39: 183–188

62. McFarland E G, Mayo-Smith W W, Saini S et al. Hepatic haemangiomas and malignant tumours: improved differentiation with heavily T2-weighted conventional spin-echo MR imaging. Radiology 1994; 193: 43–47

63. Semelka R C, Brown E D, Ascher S L et al. Hepatic hemangiomas: a multi-institutional study of appearance on T2-weighted and serial gadolinium-enhanced gradient echo MR images. Radiology 1994; 192: 401–406

64. Larson R E, Semelka R C, Bagley A S et al. Hypervascular malignant liver lesions: comparison of various MR imaging pulse sequences and dynamic CT. Radiology 1994; 192: 393–399

65. Lev-Toaf A S, Back A M, Wechsler R J et al. The radiologic and pathologic spectrum of biliary hamartomas. Am J Roentgenol 1995; 165: 309–313

66. Lou T Y, Itai Y, Eguchi N et al. Von Meyenburg complexes of the liver: imaging findings. J Comput Assist Tomogr 1998; 22: 372–378

67. Robinson P J. Review: The characterization of liver tumours by MRI. Clin Radiol 1996; 51: 749–761

68. Yates C K, Steight R A. Focal fatty infiltration of the liver simulating metastatic disease. Radiology 1986; 159: 83–84

69. Tang-Barton P, Vas W, Weissman J et al. Focal fatty liver lesions in alcoholic liver disease: A broadened spectrum of CT appearances. Gastrointest Radiol 1985; 10: 133–137

70. Giovagnoni A, Terilli F, Ercolani P et al. MR imaging of hepatic masses: diagnostic significance of wedge-shaped areas of increased signal intensity surrounding the lesion. Am J Roentgenol 1994; 163: 1093–1097

71. Schlund J F, Semelka R C, Kettritz U et al. Transient increased segmental hepatic enhancement distal to portal vein obstruction on dynamic gadolinium-enhanced gradient echo MR images. J Mag Res Imag 1995; 4: 375–377

72. Seneterre E, Taourel P, Bouvier Y et al. Detection of hepatic metastases: ferumoxides-enhanced MR imaging versus unenhanced MR imaging and CT during arterial portography. Radiology 1996; 200: 785–792

73. Bengmark S, Halstrom L. The natural history of primary and secondary malignant tumours of the liver. Cancer 1969; 23: 198–202

74. Adson M A. The resection of hepatic metastases. Arch Surg 1989; 124: 1023–1024

75. Ruers T, Bleichrodt R P. Treatment of liver metastases, an update on the possibilities and results. Eur J Cancer 2002; 38: 1023–1033

76. Choti M A, Sitzmann J V, Tiburi M F et al. Trends in long-term survival following liver resection for hepatic colorectal metastases. Ann Surg 2002; 235: 759–766

77. Bismuth H. Surgical anatomy and anatomical surgery of the liver. World J Surg 1982; 6: 3–9

78. Sugihara K, Hojo K, Moriya Y et al. Pattern of recurrence after hepatic resection for colorectal metastases. J Surg 1993; 80: 1032–1035

79. Harned R K, Chezmar J L, Nelson R C. Recurrent tumour after resection of hepatic metastases from colorectal carcinoma: location and time of discovery as determined by CT. Am J Roentgenol 1994; 163: 93–97

Chapter 43

Metastatic effects on the nervous system

David MacVicar

Introduction

Neurological complications in the cancer patient are an increasingly common problem. A simplistic explanation for this is that patients survive longer with their tumour and therefore develop more metastases at all sites, but it is also possible that the central nervous system (CNS) is a genuine sanctuary site for malignant cells from common solid tumours treated with systemic chemotherapy, just as it is in leukaemia. A study of nearly 12,000 patients identified neurological complaints including altered mental state, headache, back pain and leg weakness in 15% of patients with a variety of tumours.[1] In small cell lung cancer, the incidence of neurological disorder caused by the disease is 29%,[2] and a report from the Johns Hopkins Cancer Centre identified neurological problems as the cause of 50% of unplanned hospital admissions, with changes in mental status, brain metastases and epidural spinal cord compression being the major problems.[3] The effects of metastatic disease on the nervous system can be severely disabling, with a catastrophic effect on the quality of life of a patient whose tumour may be eminently treatable. This is partly because the brain and spinal cord are enclosed in bone, and thus relatively small-volume disease can cause disproportionately severe symptoms. In addition, the CNS lacks lymphatics, making removal of oedema and biological detritus difficult, and the capacity for regeneration of nervous tissue after damage is very limited.

A further difficulty is the sometimes bewildering clinical presentation of neurological problems in the cancer patient. An apparently simple symptom such as leg weakness has a wide differential diagnosis in a patient with systemic cancer, including:

- Cerebral deposits
- Compression of the spinal cord or cauda equina
- Leptomeningeal metastatic disease
- The effects of therapy such as cytotoxic drugs or steroids
- General debility

The effects of cancer on the nervous system may be classified into:

- Metastatic or direct effects of cancer
- Mass lesions compressing or infiltrating nervous tissues.
- Indirect effects – non-metastatic or paraneoplastic syndromes

Paraneoplastic phenomena include vascular disorders, infections, metabolic effects, sequelae of treatment and the unusual but fascinating paraneoplastic syndromes. For the radiologist, a more useful approach is to classify by site in an attempt to narrow the area to be examined.

Once the area of greatest clinical suspicion has been identified, the majority of important differential diagnoses can be addressed using the most appropriate technique. The principal causes of neurological presentation in cancer patients according to site are listed in Table 43.1.

Brain

Clinical presentation

Brain metastases may arise from any primary systemic cancer, but the majority of brain metastases originate from:

- Carcinoma of lung (especially small cell and adenocarcinoma)
- Carcinoma of breast
- Melanoma

Less common primary sites include renal and gastro-intestinal tumours and non-seminomatous testicular tumours; a significant number of brain metastases develop from a primary source that remains unknown even at autopsy.[4] The following tumours rarely metastasize to the brain:

- Prostate
- Ovary
- Osteosarcoma
- Hodgkin's lymphoma

Most brain metastases, particularly those which arise from primary neoplasms other than the lung, occur at a late stage in dissemination of malignancy, and the presence of brain deposits is commonly associated with more widespread disease. Autopsy series have shown that

Table 43.1. *Major neurological problems (classified by site)*

Site	Differential diagnosis
Brain	Parenchymal metastasis
	Leptomeningeal metastasis
	Infection (meningitis, brain abscess)
	Radiation encephalopathy
	Cerebral haemorrhage or infarction
	Metabolic and toxic encephalopathy (e.g. following cytotoxic chemotherapy)
	Primary brain tumours
Cranial neuropathy	Parenchymal deposits (false localizing signs)
	Leptomeningeal metastases
	Bony lesions of skull base
Spinal cord and cauda equina	Epidural compression
	Leptomeningeal metastasis
	Intramedullary metastasis
	Epidural abscess or haematoma
	Radiation myelopathy
	Myelopathy following intrathecal chemotherapy
	Paraneoplastic myelopathy
Peripheral nerves and plexuses	Extrinsic compression by tumour mass
	Direct infiltration by tumour
	Drug toxicity
	Varicella zoster infection
	Radiation plexopathy
	Paraneoplastic neuropathy
Neuromuscular junction and muscle	Drugs
	Paraneoplastic disorders (Eaton–Lambert myasthenic syndrome, myasthenia gravis)
	Corticosteroid-induced myopathy
	Cachectic myopathy
	Paraneoplastic polymyositis or dermatomyositis

asymptomatic brain metastases are present in patients dying of disseminated cancer in as many as 30% of cases.

The commonest presenting symptoms are:

- Headache
- Focal weakness
- Mental disturbance
- Seizures

Unsteadiness of gait is a prominent presenting complaint when the tumour lies in the cerebellum or brain stem but may occasionally occur as a result of a large frontal lobe metastasis or hydrocephalus caused by obstruction of cerebrospinal fluid (CSF) pathways. Less common presenting symptoms are:

- Difficulty with speech
- Visual disturbance
- Sensory disturbance

Signs of visual field loss and sensory abnormalities may be elicited by neurological examination. Some physical signs are present in most, but not all, patients with brain metastases. The onset of symptoms is frequently insidious.

Pathophysiology of brain metastases
Metastasis is a complicated pathophysiological process which is not completely understood. For malignant cells to metastasize from, for example, breast to brain, they must first enter the bloodstream, then cross the pulmonary capillary bed to enter the arterial blood supply of the brain. The tumour embolus, if large enough, is likely to lodge in the watershed areas of the brain at the terminations of the major

end-arteries, and also in the grey/white junction where penetrating arterioles separate into capillary beds. This simple haemodynamic model should result in a predictable distribution of metastases within the brain, but there is clearly some variation in the distribution of metastases from certain tumours. The fertile soil hypothesis proposes that the host organ may synthesize and secrete factors which attract certain clones of circulating tumour cells and promote their growth.[5] Delattre et al. have drawn attention to the preferential distribution of metastatic lesions to watershed areas, but also noted that in patients with gastro-intestinal and pelvic tumours, there was predominant involvement of the posterior fossa, whereas with other tumours, the cerebral hemispheres were more likely to be involved.[6] It appears that infiltrating ductal carcinoma of the breast has a predilection to cause parenchymal brain metastases, whereas infiltrating lobular carcinoma is said to affect meningeal surfaces preferentially.[7] Melanoma frequently metastasizes to the grey matter, and experimental mouse melanoma lines have been developed which have specific predilection for brain parenchyma or the leptomeninges.[8] Although these preferential distributions are fascinating, in practice virtually any tumour can metastasize to any part of the brain or meninges, and variance with the expected pattern of distribution should not discourage the diagnosis of metastatic disease.

Imaging techniques

In 1972, the introduction of computed tomography (CT) by Hounsfield and Ambrose revolutionized the diagnosis of brain tumours. Over 30 years later it remains a viable method of establishing the presence of brain deposits. Ideally, CT scans should be performed before and after intravenous (IV) contrast administration, but if a patient has a known primary tumour and a clinical presentation strongly supporting a diagnosis of metastasis, little is lost by performing postcontrast scans only.

Although CT is sufficient for diagnosis in many cases, there is no doubt that magnetic resonance (MR) imaging is a more sensitive technique than contrast-enhanced CT scanning for the detection of metastases to the brain parenchyma.[9,10] A suitable protocol would include axial T2-weighted spin-echo and T1-weighted spin-echo images supplemented by gadolinium (Gd)-enhanced T1-weighted spin-echo sequences. A fluid attenuation inversion recovery (FLAIR) sequence is also useful for detecting metastatic oedema and small focal areas of ischaemic change. The use of the coronal plane should be considered, particularly if surgery is being contemplated, but the key factor is to ensure that the entire brain is covered. There is controversy over the dosage of gadolinium, particularly in the USA. Some authorities consider a dosage of 0.1 ml/kg body weight to be adequate, while others recommend a high-dose technique using three times this dose. Advocates of the high-dose technique point out the increased sensitivity as its chief advantage; in practical terms this is only important if local therapy is being considered for an ostensibly

solitary metastasis, and the cost implications of trebling the dose prevent routine use of this technique. Most European centres routinely administer an intermediate dose of gadolinium of 0.2 mg/kg body weight.[11–13]

Newer imaging methods involving inversion recovery, e.g. FLAIR or magnetization transfer, have been advocated as sensitive methods of detecting focal brain abnormalities. These methods are currently being evaluated, and are not available on every MR unit, but may result in a reduced utilization of contrast material in the future (Fig. 43.1).[14,15]

Other modalities are not useful; cerebral angiography is rarely helpful and plain radiographs and electroencephalography are obsolete. Isotope studies, including 2-[F-18]fluoro-2-deoxy-D-glucose positron emission tomography ([18]FDG PET) and single photon emission computed tomography (SPECT), lack the sensitivity and spatial resolution to challenge MR imaging as the investigation of choice.[16]

Screening for asymptomatic brain metastases

Cranial CT and MR imaging are only occasionally used as staging techniques at initial presentation of disease in a patient with no neurological symptoms.

One clinical situation in which the brain is staged routinely is where thoracotomy is being considered with curative intent for non-small cell lung cancer. Despite its rather disappointing sensitivity and specificity in diagnosis of lymph node involvement in the mediastinum, CT of the chest is still recommended for preoperative staging of lung cancer. This reflects the propensity of lung cancer to metastasize to the brain relatively early in the disease compared with other common malignancies. Many series, mostly using CT as the staging technique, have reported the incidence of asymptomatic brain metastases as ranging from 5 to 30% and many specialist centres now perform CT of the brain as part of the same investigation.[17,18]

In one series using CT, attention has been drawn to the variation of incidence of asymptomatic metastases at presentation, depending on histology and local tumour stage. In patients with Stage I and Stage II squamous cell carcinoma, no brain metastases were found, but in potentially resectable Stage III disease the incidence was 8%. For Stage III localized adenocarcinoma, the incidence was 23%; for Stage III large cell carcinoma, 57%. For Stage III non-small cell tumours of all histological types, the overall incidence of asymptomatic brain deposits was 17.5%, which is clearly relevant when considering such patients for surgery. In patients with small cell carcinoma and apparently limited disease, the incidence of asymptomatic brain deposits was 14%.[19] Although very few patients with small cell lung cancer are suitable for surgery, cranial irradiation can palliate, and some centres include brain scanning as a staging investigation for this disease.[20] If a policy of screening for asymptomatic brain metastases is to be pursued with any primary tumour, MR remains the most sensitive investigation. [18]FDG PET used as a 'whole-body' staging method has been

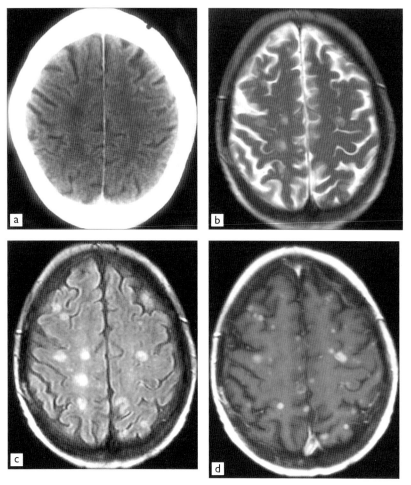

Figure 43.1. *Comparison of imaging techniques for small volume cerebral metastases. (a) Contrast-enhanced CT scan of a patient with known carcinoma of breast with clinical suspicion of brain metastases. The deep cerebral white matter shows possible abnormality of attenuation, but no focal mass lesion was identified and the investigation was reported as clear of cerebral deposits. (b) T2-weighted spin-echo MR sequence obtained 2 days later owing to persisting clinical suspicion of cerebral metastatic disease shows abnormality of signal in white matter and at grey/white junction. (c) Fluid attenuation inversion recovery (FLAIR) sequence shows multiple areas of abnormal signal. (d) Gadolinium-enhanced T1-weighted spin-echo sequence at the same slice shows multiple enhancing lesions characteristic of cerebral deposits in white and grey matter of both hemispheres. Gadolinium-enhanced MR is a reliable and sensitive method of detecting brain metastases and remains the gold standard imaging investigation in most centres.*

demonstrated to be less sensitive and specific for demonstration of brain metastases.[21] However, technical developments are being made which allow co-registration of anatomical images from MR and CT with [18]FDG PET studies.[22,23] Integrated [18]FDG PET–CT systems are now commercially available and this technique has the potential to become an important investigation in cancer imaging,[24] and can demonstrate brain metastases, but the place of hybrid cross-sectional and nuclear medicine instruments in clinical practice is currently under investigation.

Computed tomography or MR imaging of the brain are included as staging investigations in selected patients with non-seminomatous germ cell tumours of the testis (NSGCT). Asymptomatic brain metastases may be seen at presentation in patients with aggressive disseminated disease and are more common in patients with trophoblastic teratoma than with any other histological type.[25] Those patients considered at high risk will have grossly elevated serum tumour markers [human chorionic gonadotrophin (HCG) >20,000 IU] or multiple pulmonary metastases (more than 50). Asymptomatic brain deposits may also be seen at the time of large-volume pulmonary relapse following chemotherapy, and any patient being put forward for high-dose salvage chemotherapy for multiple relapses of non-seminomatous germ cell tumour should have a brain scan. If cerebral deposits are present, any residual mass following treatment is likely to contain differentiated tumour, and will be resected if accessible.

Notwithstanding these exceptions, and acknowledging that brain lesions may be the presenting symptom of unknown primaries, the majority of brain metastases present late in the natural history of the disease, and are usually associated with some symptomatology, however vague. Early diagnosis of asymptomatic brain lesions rarely influences the outcome of disease, and brain imaging is not recommended as a staging investigation in most clinical circumstances.[20]

General imaging features

The majority of metastases in the brain grow as spherical masses, displacing rather than destroying brain tissue. Some metastases are more irregular, and all create oedema in the surrounding white matter. The amount of oedema is extremely variable, and its extent is not a reliable sign in differential diagnosis of metastasis from other pathological entities. Brain metastases are usually solid, but if they grow rapidly, they may undergo central necrosis. 'Cystic' lesions occasionally occur, particularly from primary breast carcinoma and squamous cell carcinoma from any site. At a pathological level, metastatic brain tumours usually show extensive neovascularization, and are accompanied by breakdown of the blood–brain barrier. Some tumours, for example melanoma and NSGCT, have a tendency to be haemorrhagic. The typical appearance of a metastasis from a primary carcinoma on CT is a mass of similar attenuation to normal brain, associated with surrounding oedema and brisk enhancement following IV contrast injection. On MR, most metastatic lesions are masses with a signal intensity higher than that of normal brain on T2-weighted sequences and surrounded by very high signal intensity oedema. On T1-weighted sequences they are isointense with brain and show enhancement with Gd-DTPA (Fig. 43.2). Metastases are usually discrete masses but are not necessarily multiple. The maxim that not all metastases are multiple, and not all multiple lesions are metastases remains valid in clinical practice.

Differential diagnosis of brain metastases

In general, the diagnosis of brain metastasis in a patient known to have cancer presents few difficulties. The most difficult differential diagnosis is with primary tumours such as:

- Meningioma
- Pituitary adenoma
- Acoustic neuroma
- Glioma

Gliomas tend to be more diffuse in their growth pattern, but metastases in an appropriate anatomical situation may mimic meningioma and other primary tumours almost exactly. In one study, six of 54 patients with known cancer and solitary brain lesions did not have metastases on biopsy, and three of these had non-neoplastic lesions.[26] However, if the clinical history and appropriate imaging features, especially with multiple lesions, are present, the diagnosis of brain metastases can be established with reasonable certainty. Other clinical differential diagnoses include:

- Cerebral haemorrhage
- Cerebral embolus
- Abscess
- Viral infections
- Cytotoxic leuco-encephalopathy
- Radiation injury

Cerebral haemorrhage or embolus will have characteristic imaging features. Infections, particularly abscess formation, can cause problems of differential diagnosis, especially in patients with lymphoma and haematological malignancies (Fig. 43.3). Viral infections have a tendency to diffuse involvement of the brain without mass formation and often have a characteristic clinical syndrome. Examples are herpes simplex encephalitis (Fig. 43.4) and progressive multifocal leuco-encephalopathy (Fig. 43.5), which is thought to be a result of reactivation of papova virus infection during prolonged suppression of cellular immunity. Cytotoxic leuco-encephalopathy may be seen with drug regimens involving 5-fluorouracil and levamisole, or intrathecal methotrexate (Fig. 43.6).[27,28] Focal changes, detectable as high signal lesions in the deep cerebral white matter on MR imaging, have also been demonstrated with a variety of high-dose IV chemotherapy regimens, particularly those involving bone marrow transplantation. These lesions do not enhance with Gd-DTPA, and clinically present with non-specific problems such as headache and seizures. The changes are reversible, and should not be confused with metastases.[29] (These treatment complications are also discussed in Chapter 52.)

Radiation necrosis may be difficult to differentiate from recurrent brain metastases as it tends to enhance and may form ring lesions. However, it is rarely a problem at initial diagnosis of brain metastases. Occasionally, intercurrent

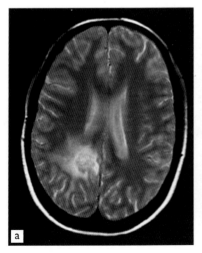
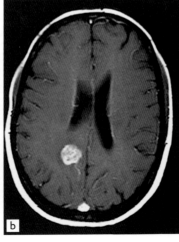

Figure 43.2. (a) T2-weighted MR image, axial plane. Typical appearance of cerebral metastatic disease. The tumour mass is of higher signal intensity than surrounding brain. Surrounding oedema returns high signal intensity. (b) T1-weighted MR image following Gd-DTPA shows an enhancing mass.

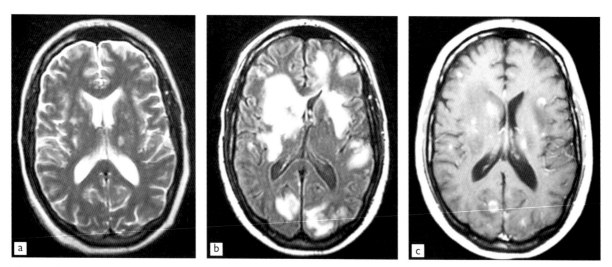

Figure 43.3. *Patient presenting with headache following bone marrow transplantation for acute myeloid leukaemia. (a) T2-weighted spin-echo sequence in axial plane shows vague areas of increased signal in white matter. These lesions did not enhance following gadolinium. (b) Follow-up imaging 3 weeks later; patient with increasing confusion. FLAIR imaging now shows mass lesions with surrounding high signal intensity due to oedema. (c) Following gadolinium, multiple enhancing lesions are seen. At biopsy, a diagnosis of cerebral toxoplasmosis was made.*

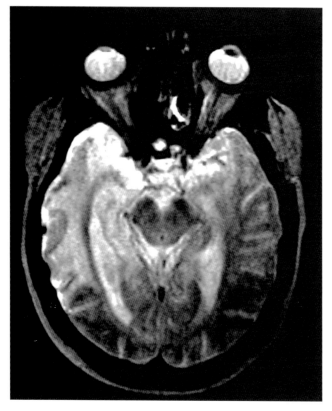

Figure 43.4. *T2-weighted MR image, axial plane. Herpes simplex encephalitis. There is diffuse high signal intensity in both temporal lobes. There is no discrete mass lesion, the abnormality affects grey and white matter, and is asymmetrical. The features are typical of herpes simplex encephalitis, and are unlikely to be confused with metastatic disease.*

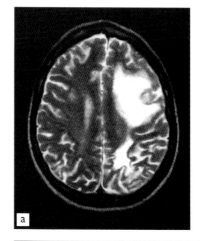

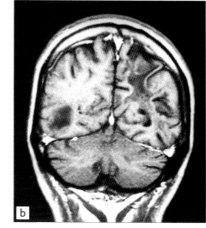

Figure 43.5. *(a) T2-weighted MR image, axial plane. Areas of diffuse grey and white matter abnormality are seen bilaterally. (b) T1-weighted MR image, coronal plane. Rather than mass effect, there is loss of substance within the grey and white matter. These appearances are typical of progressive multifocal leuco-encephalopathy, which may be seen following prolonged suppression of cellular immunity in patients on treatment for malignancy, particularly lymphoma.*

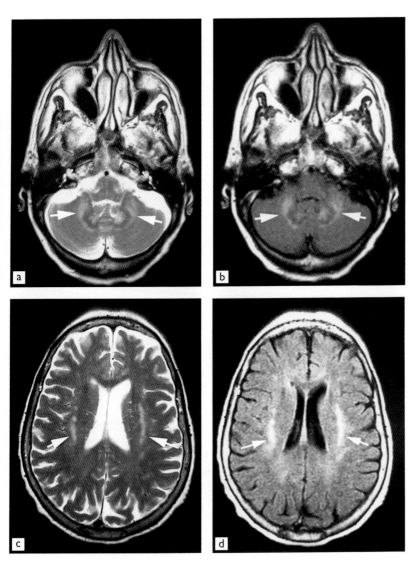

Figure 43.6. *T2-weighted and fluid attenuation inversion recovery (FLAIR) images through posterior fossa (a and b) and cerebral hemispheres (c and d), showing high signal in cerebellar and cerebral white matter (arrows). Changes are seen on both pulse sequences and are slightly more pronounced on FLAIR images. The patient was receiving intrathecal methotrexate and had developed non-specific neurological symptoms, including headache and a mild confusional state. The appearance is consistent with white matter change seen in association with intrathecal chemotherapy.*

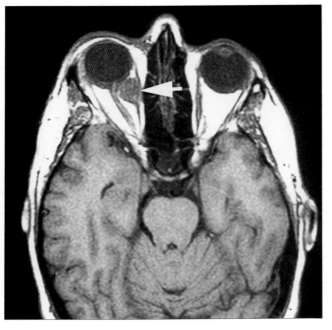

common diseases, such as multiple sclerosis, are seen in patients known to have cancer. In the absence of typical imaging features of metastatic disease, a review of the clinical features is of paramount importance, and will frequently influence image interpretation. For example, patients presenting with disturbance of eye movements or other cranial nerve symptoms and signs may have disease around the skull base or in the orbit rather than brain metastases (Fig. 43.7).

Figure 43.7. *T1-weighted axial MR. A patient with gaze paralysis interpreted as possible right 6th nerve palsy. A melanoma deposit is present in the right orbit (arrow).*

Key points: brain metastases

- Most brain metastases occur late in the natural history of malignant disease

- Gd-enhanced MR imaging is more sensitive than CT for detecting brain metastases

- Screening for brain metastases in non-small cell lung cancer prior to thoracotomy has shown that 5–30% of patients harbour asymptomatic brain metastases

- ^{18}FDG PET and ^{18}FDG PET–CT are evolving as staging modalities in non-small cell lung cancer and other solid tumours

- Screening for brain metastases is recommended in selected patients with non-seminomatous germ cell tumours of the testis

- The differential diagnosis of brain metastases includes primary brain tumours, cerebral haemorrhage, infection, cytotoxic leuco-enephalopathy and radiation injury

Imaging features of some common brain metastases

Metastases from all primary tumours may look identical, but some of the common causes have 'trademark' features, which if present, may increase confidence in diagnosis. Virtually all cancers are capable of metastasizing to the brain. Lung and breast are the commonest organs of origin, followed by malignant melanoma.

Bronchial tumours are the single commonest cause of metastatic deposits in the brain. Adenocarcinoma of the lung and squamous cell carcinoma typically metastasize to the grey/white junction, and both may produce ring-like enhancement on both CT and MR (Fig. 43.8). A small cell lung cancer may produce large masses, but frequently produces innumerable small metastases throughout the brain. These small lesions are best seen on enhanced T1-weighted MR imaging, emphasizing the increased sensitivity available with this technique (Figs. 43.9 and 43.10).

Carcinoma of the breast has a tendency to metastasize to the periphery of the brain. An association between breast cancer and meningioma has created considerable interest in the literature. Some authors report a higher incidence of meningioma in women with breast cancer, although this has been disputed.[30–32] Meningiomas have a relative lack of

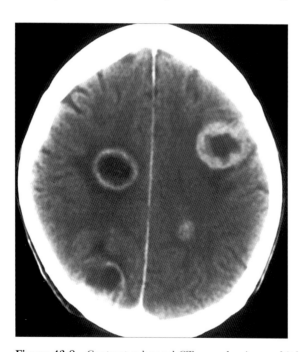

Figure 43.8. *Contrast-enhanced CT scan showing multiple ring-enhancing lesions, a typical appearance in metastatic squamous cell carcinoma of lung, but also seen with metastatic adenocarcinoma. (Reproduced with permission from MacVicar D, Neurological presentations in the cancer patient. Imaging 2000; 12: 115–120.)*

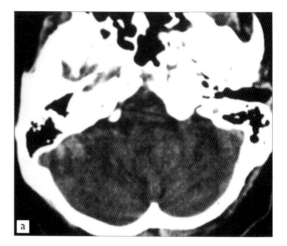

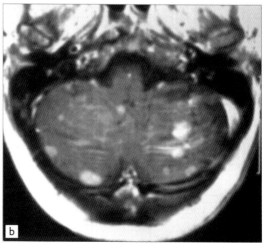

Figure 43.9. *Small cell lung cancer. (a) Contrast-enhanced CT scan through posterior fossa is equivocal. Individual metastases cannot be reliably identified. (b) T1-weighted MR image following gadolinium administration performed 2 days later. Multiple small lesions were scattered throughout the posterior fossa.*

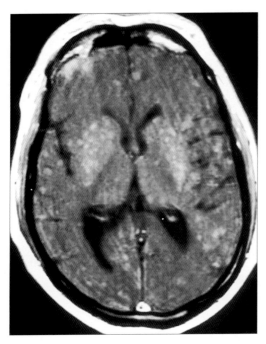

Figure 43.10. *Metastases from small cell carcinoma. Gadolinium-enhanced T1-weighted spin-echo MR shows multiple small enhancing lesions throughout the brain. (Reproduced with permission from MacVicar D, Neurological presentations in the cancer patient. Imaging 2000; 12: 115–120.)*

peritumoural oedema, and show homogeneous contrast enhancement and attachment to the dura. However, the practical problem is that metastases from breast carcinoma may mimic in every way the features of meningioma, and vice versa. Oncologists are naturally keen to establish the definitive diagnosis and consider surgery. An early follow-up scan is frequently helpful as it will establish the tempo of disease; a rapidly enlarging lesion, with or without new lesions, will confirm a diagnosis of metastatic disease and will avoid inappropriate craniotomy (Fig. 43.11). Breast carcinoma also has a tendency to metastasize to the pituitary gland where it can mimic an adenoma.

Metastases from malignant melanoma can exhibit some characteristic features. Like metastases from malignant testicular tumours and renal carcinoma, these tumours can be large and may have a prominent haemorrhagic component. The breakdown products of blood may have paramagnetic or superparamagnetic effects. In addition, melanin pigments have intrinsic paramagnetic properties as a result of their molecular structure.[33] This can result in melanoma deposits having a high signal intensity on unenhanced T1-weighted images and a low signal intensity on T2-weighted images owing to the paramagnetic effect of pigments on proton relaxation (Fig. 43.12).

Colon cancer deposits may also exhibit paramagnetic effects, with a high signal intensity on T1-weighted images and a low signal intensity on T2 weighting. This is presumed to be caused by mucinous macromolecules (Fig.

43.13). Very occasionally, a similar appearance is seen in metastases from mucinous adenocarcinomas of ovary, breast, stomach and pancreas.

Involvement of the brain by lymphoma is becoming more common, particularly in patients with human immunodeficiency virus (HIV) infection and other forms of immunosuppression (see chapter 30). Lymphoma deposits are typically of higher attenuation than normal brain on unenhanced CT images and show only slight contrast enhancement (Fig. 43.14). There is relatively little oedema, and the lesions are situated characteristically around the midline. On T2-weighted MR imaging, lesions are often hypointense compared with normal brain.

Intracranial meningeal disease

Cancer may reach the meninges by direct contact with tumour in brain or bone, or by haematogenous dissemination. Once contact is made with the CSF, tumour cells are likely to be shed and will float along CSF pathways to seed elsewhere in either a diffuse pattern or as multiple individual foci. Meningeal metastases are increasingly recognized, and are common in the leukaemias. They are sometimes seen in:

- Non-Hodgkin's lymphoma
- Breast carcinoma
- Lung carcinoma
- Malignant melanoma

Meningeal deposits have also been described in a wide variety of other tumours. The clinical presentation can be obscure, with non-specific symptoms, such as headache, mental change, nausea and vertigo predominating. It can be difficult to diagnose with imaging studies, particularly if diffuse. Meningeal metastases enhance with contrast medium, but can be demonstrated on CT only if gross. Magnetic resonance imaging with gadolinium enhancement is more reliable but false negative examinations may occur.[34–36] There are several causes of false positive results:

- Some meningeal enhancement can frequently be demonstrated in normal patients without meningeal disease
- Lumbar puncture with or without intrathecal chemotherapy can cause the meninges to enhance abnormally
- Previous surgery and radiation also result in diffuse abnormality for months or years

However, despite these difficulties, MR is the most useful imaging technique, as its multiplanar imaging capability allows the demonstration of meningeal masses around the calvarium and skull base more readily than CT (Figs. 43.15 and 43.16). A meningeal mass lesion in the appropriate clinical setting is adequate confirmation of diagnosis of

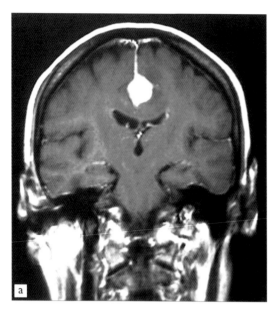

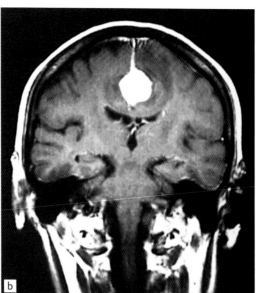

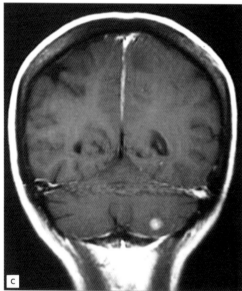

Figure 43.11. *Patient with carcinoma of breast, presenting with headaches: (a) T1-weighted spin-echo MR image following gadolinium administration, coronal plane. There is an enhancing mass apparently centred on the falx. The differential diagnosis lies between a deposit from carcinoma of the breast and a falx meningioma. (b and c) Rather than immediate craniotomy, a follow-up scan was obtained after a 4-week interval. This shows a clearly discernible enlargement of the falx lesion over a 4-week period, and further small lesions became detectable within the cerebellum during the interval. A diagnosis of cerebral metastatic disease was made.*

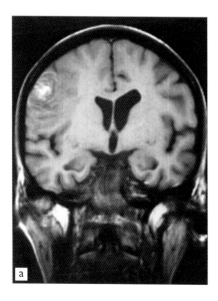

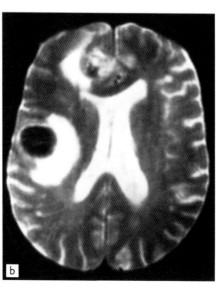

Figure 43.12. *(a) T1-weighted spin-echo MR image, coronal plane. A mass in the posterior frontal lobe returns signal hyperintense to surrounding brain. (b) T2-weighted spin-echo MR image, axial plane. The mass lesion is hypointense to normal brain. Surrounding oedema is present. The appearance is due to the paramagnetic effect of melanin within a deposit of metastatic melanotic melanoma.*

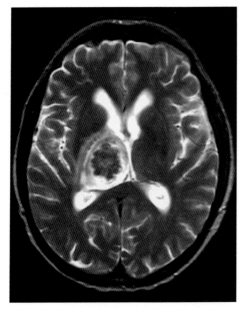

Figure 43.13. *T2-weighted spin-echo MR image, axial plane. Carcinoma of colon. Marked signal hypointensity is present in the central part of the deposit, which was not calcified on CT scanning. This appearance may be seen with mucinous adenocarcinoma deposits.*

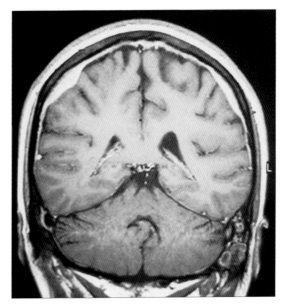

Figure 43.15. *There is asymmetrical thickening and enhancement of the dura around the calvarium consistent with metastatic infiltration, demonstrated on Gd-enhanced T1-weighted coronal imaging.*

meningeal disease. Nodular enhancement of the leptomeninges deep in the cerebral sulci is the most convincing manifestation of intracranial meningeal metastasis. An important clinical circumstance in which meningeal deposits may arise is following surgery for primary brain tumours. The appearance of the meningeal disease is similar to metastases from distant common solid tumours, but often more florid (Figs. 43.17 and 43.18). If imaging is negative, lumbar puncture may then be utilized to confirm positive malignant cytology in the CSF.[31,32]

A further advantage of the use of MR is its ability to demonstrate metastasis to the bones of the skull base. Cranial nerve abnormalities are not usually the presenting feature of meningeal disease, although subtle signs are frequently detectable. The main differential diagnosis is between involvement of the cranial nerves at the meningeal level or tumour deposits within bone. When seen, meningeal metastases are usually small, although occasionally they are large enough to mimic extrinsic tumours such as acoustic neuromas and meningiomas (Fig. 43.19). If skull base deposits are suspected as the cause of cranial neu-

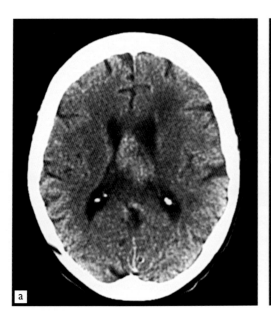

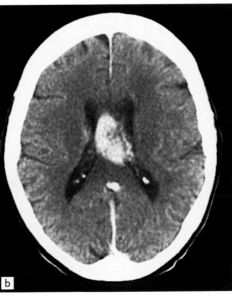

Figure 43.14. *(a and b) Pre- and postcontrast CT scan. There is a mass involving the corpus callosum associated with little oedema and of attenuation slightly higher than normal brain. Modest enhancement is present after IV contrast. The distribution and appearance are characteristic of lymphoma. The patient had suffered several relapses of non-Hodgkin's lymphoma before presenting with headache.*

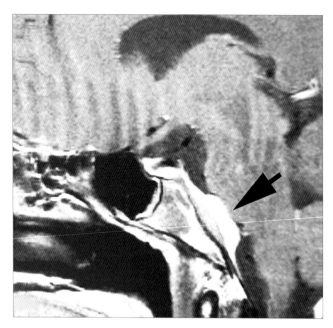

Figure 43.16. *Sagittal T1-weighted imaging demonstrates a plaque of lymphoma (arrow) involving the basal meninges.*

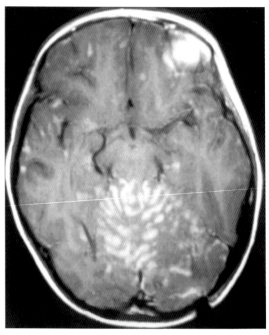

Figure 43.17. *T1-weighted spin-echo with gadolinium enhancement shows extensive abnormal enhancement of the tentorium and further enhancing lesions in the leptomeninges, for example in the right sylvian fissure. The patient had been previously treated for medulloblastoma, and the appearance represents recurrent meningeal disease. (Reproduced with permission from MacVicar D, Neurological presentations in the cancer patient. Imaging 2000; 12: 115–120.)*

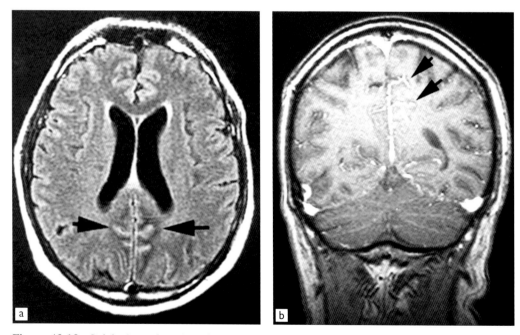

Figure 43.18. *Subtle signs of meningeal metastatic disease. (a) Axial MR using fluid attenuation inversion recovery (FLAIR) sequence shows localized abnormality of signal in the para-falcine meninges and adjacent grey matter (arrows). (b) Gadolinium-enhanced T1-weighted coronal images show nodular asymmetrical enhancement in the leptomeninges of the medial parietal lobes. Some enhancement of the dura may be seen under normal circumstances, but nodular enhancement deep in the sulci (arrows), which was seen at several sites in this patient, is sufficient to make the diagnosis of meningeal metastatic disease in appropriate clinical circumstances. This patient had presented with headache and had known pulmonary metastases from melanoma.*

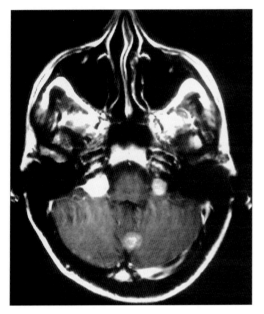

Figure 43.19. *T1-weighted spin-echo MR image following gadolinium, axial plane. Bilateral enhancing masses are present in the cerebello-pontine angles mimicking acoustic neuromas. There is a further lesion between the cerebellar hemispheres. Postmortem examination confirmed meningeal metastases from melanoma.*

ropathy, sequences such as short tau inversion recovery (STIR) are frequently useful in highlighting bony pathology.

Key points: cerebral meningeal metastases

■ Meningeal deposits are seen in the leukaemias, non-Hodgkin's lymphoma, breast cancer, lung cancer and malignant melanoma

■ The clinical features are often non-specific

■ Meningeal metastases enhance with contrast medium and are best demonstrated on MR imaging

■ Dural meningeal enhancement may be seen in normal patients

Spinal cord and cauda equina

Epidural spinal cord compression

While most symptomatic intracranial metastases involve the brain parenchyma, in the spinal canal most symptomatic tumours compress the spinal cord or cauda equina from the epidural space, while intramedullary and meningeal disease is more unusual.

Most epidural compression is caused by a tumour that has metastasized to the vertebral body; the most frequent cancers are:

- Carcinoma of breast
- Carcinoma of lung
- Carcinoma of prostate
- Multiple myeloma

In patients with systemic cancer, incidences of symptomatic spinal cord compression reported in the literature vary from 1 to 5%, and at autopsy approximately 5% of patients dying from cancer exhibit spinal cord or cauda equina compression.[37–40]

Clinical presentation

Pain is the earliest and most frequent presenting symptom of spinal cord compression. It is usually mild at first but becomes progressively more severe. However, absence of pain does not mean absence of cord compression. The pain may be of several types:

- Local
- Radicular
- Funicular

In most patients the initial pain is local and perceived as a steady ache at the site of the involved vertebral body. Compression of nerve roots within the spinal canal or within the exit foraminae generates radicular pain, which may precede local pain and is typically band-like if the lesion is in the thoracic region, and radiates to arms and legs in cervical and lumbar regions, respectively. Funicular pain is caused by compression of ascending (sensory) spinal cord tracts, causing symptoms that are apparently remote from the lesion and in a non-dermatomal distribution. For example, upper thoracic or cervical cord compression can cause funicular pain in the lower extremities, or band-like pain around the thorax and abdomen.

Following the prodrome of pain which may be prolonged, other symptoms and signs develop rapidly, including:

- Weakness
- Sensory loss
- Autonomic dysfunction

Weakness is the second most common finding. It usually results from damage to the corticospinal tracts. The weakness begins in the legs, regardless of the level of compression and is more marked proximally early in the course of development of symptoms. The patient usually complains of difficulty walking and climbing stairs, and this symptom should precipitate a sense of urgency in the investigative chain, as treatment at this stage may enable full recovery of power. In the early stages, typical signs of upper motor neurone weakness may be absent, with spasticity and hyper-reflexia developing later. If the onset of spinal cord compression is sudden and leads to complete paraplegia, most patients are flaccid with areflexia, as a result of distal spinal reflex inhibition.

Lower motor neurone weakness results from compression of the cauda equina, and is characterized by hypotonia, atrophy and areflexia. Dysfunction of anterior horn cells in the spinal cord may also be seen, possibly as a result of vascular abnormality rather than true mechanical compression. The presence of lower motor neurone weakness will mask upper motor neurone signs at a higher level, so it should be remembered that in the presence of cauda equina compression, which explains lower motor neurone signs in the legs, an additional level of true cord compression may also be present.

Sensory loss follows shortly after the development of weakness, and the level will rise to arrive at the true level of compression given time. However, at the time of imaging, the sensory level may be several segments below the compressive lesion. Sensory loss is rarely as profound or disabling as weakness. Autonomic dysfunction causes bladder and bowel dysfunction, and impotence in men in more than 50% of patients by the time of diagnosis of spinal cord or cauda equina compression. Bladder dysfunction predominates, with urinary retention being associated with sudden onset of compression, while urgency with incontinence is a relatively frequent complaint if symptoms are evolving slowly.

Key points: spinal cord compression

- Most tumours that compress the spinal cord are situated in the epidural space

- Pain is the earliest presenting feature and may be local, radicular or funicular

- In the early stages of spinal cord compression, upper motor neurone signs may initially be absent

- Lower motor neurone weakness will mask upper motor neurone signs from compression at a higher level

- The sensory level may initially be several segments below the true compressive lesion

- Bladder dysfunction is the predominant autonomic disturbance

Pathophysiology

The neurological presentation of spinal cord compression can be variable and occasionally confusing, and this is partly explained by consideration of the site of the epidural compressive lesion and its relationship with the blood supply of the cord and the site of motor and sensory tracts within the cord.

The advent of MR has clearly demonstrated that the vertebral body is involved more often than the posterior elements in patients with spinal cord compression, but all parts of the vertebra are susceptible. Some tumours, notably lymphoma, can invade the epidural space without involving the vertebrae. The dura is up to a millimetre thick and relatively resistant to penetration by tumour. Epidural tumours rarely breach the dura to invade the cord, but may interfere with the delicate blood supply. The cord receives its blood supply predominantly from the anterior spinal artery which forms an anastomotic chain running the length of the cord and breaking into cauda equina arteries in the lumbar region (Fig. 43.20). The anterior spinal artery is supplied by radicular arteries which are branches of the vertebral artery in the cervical region. In the thoracic region the anterior spinal artery is supplied via the anterior radicular arteries, which come off the dorsal branch of the posterior intercostal arteries, which in turn emanate directly from the aorta. The anatomy is variable and some major anterior radicular arteries, such as the artery of Adamkiewicz, are well known to angiographers. The blood supply of the cord is vulnerable where the anterior radicular artery penetrates the neural foramen and where the anterior spinal artery runs immediately behind the vertebral body. The anterior spinal artery may be occluded by a deposit in the vertebral body growing posteriorly on to the anterior aspect of the cord. At each segment the anterior spinal artery gives off branches supplying the anterior part of the cord that carries the anterior horn cells and major corticospinal pathways, and the damage resulting from ischaemia and infarction is responsible for clinically catastrophic power loss. A small volume of epidural disease at these critical sites can cause vascular compromise.

Some deposits grow from the posterior elements, compressing the cord from a lateral or posterior direction. Because the sensory tracts occupy a peripheral position in the lateral and posterior cord, sensory symptoms may predominate in this instance. A limited part of the cord's blood supply comes from the posterior radicular artery, which branches from the anterior radicular artery in the neural foramen to form a posterior anastomotic chain. If the direction of compression is from the lateral or posterior aspect, the major part of the blood supply to the cord, from the anterior spinal artery, is likely to be preserved.

Technique of examination with imaging

Given the potential complexity of the neurological presentation, an imaging technique must take account of the fact that the clinically relevant lesion may be some distance away from the site suggested by the neurological signs. Abnormalities may be present within the vertebral bone marrow, epidural soft tissue, or both. As a result of its versatility in imaging the whole spine and surrounding soft tissues, MR imaging has replaced myelography (with or without CT myelography) as the investigation of choice in

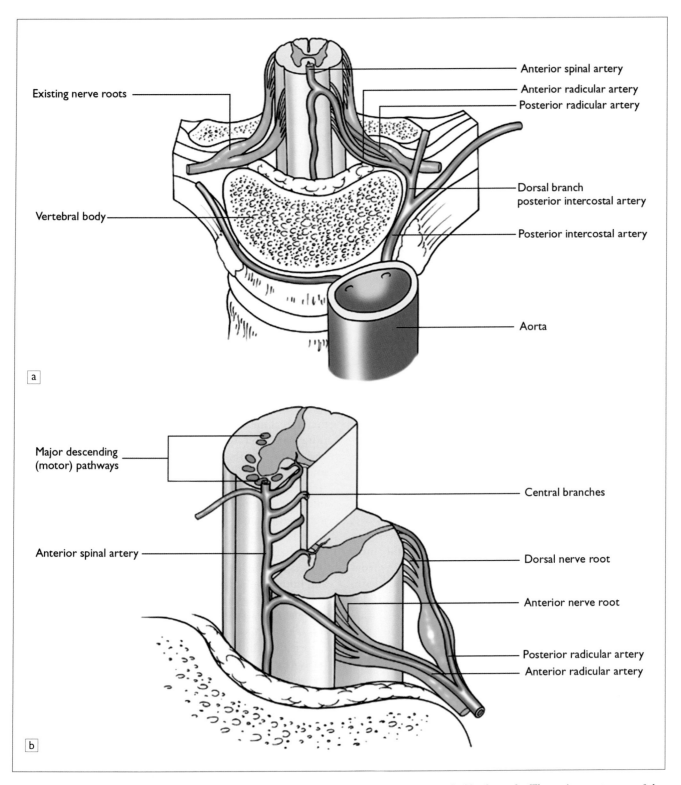

Figure 43.20. *(a and b) Schematic representation of spinal cord anatomy demonstrating the blood supply. The major component of the cord's blood supply comes via the anterior radicular artery, which emanates from the dorsal branch of the posterior intercostal artery. The anterior radicular artery runs through the neural foramen where a smaller posterior radicular artery comes off. The anterior radicular artery feeds the anterior spinal artery, which forms a single anastomotic chain running the length of the cord. From the anterior spinal artery, penetrating central branches supply the functionally crucial descending motor pathways. Some posterior and peripheral parts of the cord have some blood supply from a plexus of small pial vessels coming directly from the anterior and posterior radicular arteries. Interruption of the blood supply by compression of anterior radicular or anterior spinal arteries can cause infarction of the cord even in the absence of major mechanical compression.*

suspected spinal cord compression. Only when MR is contraindicated should other techniques be employed.

Plain radiographs remain a worthwhile investigation. If clinical signs point to a fairly definite level, many radiotherapists are prepared to commence steroids and plan an initial radiation field on a discrete bony abnormality if present. The sensitivity of plain radiographs in detecting lesions at other levels is low, and soft tissue extension can rarely be evaluated accurately. However, little is lost by obtaining plain radiographs while MR is scheduled at the earliest opportunity. Isotope studies are sensitive in detecting bony deposits, but less so than MR.[41] They are unlikely to be helpful in the acute management of spinal cord compression unless MR is unavailable.

If MR imaging is contraindicated, CT (without myelography) may demonstrate vertebral bone and soft tissue disease extending into the spinal canal and the relationship of tumour to the spinal cord. Multidetector CT permits reconstruction of images in the sagittal and coronal planes with superb image quality; thus the full extent of disease can be shown in detail for radiotherapy planning.

Myelography with water-soluble contrast agents should include the entire spine, with cervical as well as lumbar puncture if necessary. Subsequent CT scans (CT myelography) can identify paravertebral lesions growing into the spinal canal, and also bony lesions and herniated discs. For maximum information, CT myelography should be performed within a few hours, by the same radiologist or a radiologist with full access to the myelographic findings, so that all appropriate levels can be imaged.

The exact MR technique will depend on which sequences are available and how long the data acquisition takes but it is important to obtain a set of images of the entire spine. Levels of compression should be readily identifiable; most up-to-date scanners should be able to cover the spine from sacrum to foramen magnum in two sequences with a sufficient degree of overlap to identify levels confidently. If this is not possible, some form of skin marker will be necessary so that adequate overlap can be ensured and exact levels of compression accurately identified. A T1-weighted spin-echo sequence in the sagittal plane should be obtained initially. Contrast between normal marrow and metastatic deposits will normally allow detection of malignant infiltration of the vertebral bodies and posterior elements. If doubt exists, a high contrast sequence, for example STIR, a gradient-echo sequence with T2*-weighted or a T2-weighted spin-echo sequence may indicate the site of metastatic bony lesions. T2*-weighted gradient-echo or T2-weighted spin-echo sequences produce an excellent myelographic effect with high signal intensity CSF and a low signal intensity cord. Sagittal scans may be up to 4–5 mm thick, but the neural foraminae must be covered, if necessary by widening slice thickness, inserting interslice gaps or obtaining two blocks. After review of sagittal images, the radiologist should maintain a low threshold for obtaining sequences in orthogonal planes, as important lesions in the paravertebral region and intervertebral foraminae are easier to detect and interpret using the axial, or occasionally the coronal, plane. Gadolinium enhancement is not used routinely but, if the clinical presentation is suggestive of intramedullary or leptomeningeal disease, contrast-enhanced T1-weighted spin-echo sequences, initially in the sagittal plane, are mandatory.[34,35]

Typical imaging features and differential diagnosis

The differential diagnosis of myelopathy includes:

- Epidural cord compression
- Meningeal metastases
- Intramedullary deposits
- Glioma of the spinal cord
- Meningioma
- Neurofibroma
- Radiation myelopathy
- Postinfection transverse myelitis
- Bone abscess, e.g. TB
- Osteoporotic vertebral collapse

Most causes of myelopathy which may be confused clinically with epidural cord compression can be accurately diagnosed by MR imaging. In the patient with systemic cancer, meningeal metastases and intramedullary tumours are the principal differentials. Glioma of the cord, meningioma and neurofibroma are rare. Radiation myelopathy is unusual, and requires an appropriate history. Like postinfectious transverse myelitis, it will be seen as high signal intensity within the cord, which may enhance on T1-weighted sequence following IV gadolinium and shows little mass effect. Epidural haematoma usually has a precipitant such as recent lumbar puncture, epidural abscess should be associated with clinical signs of sepsis, and both should have recognizable morphological features and signal intensity characteristics to enable differential diagnosis. However, an infection involving bone, for example a tuberculous abscess or fungal infiltration, may be extremely difficult to differentiate from tumour. An osteoporotic acute vertebral collapse should be suspected if it is the solitary spinal lesion, particularly if the posterior elements of the vertebra are entirely normal and there is no evidence of a soft tissue mass. A herniated degenerative disc and malignant involvement of the spine may coexist, but the two are rarely confused.

Tumour tissue in the epidural space typically returns low signal intensity on T1-weighted sequences, intermediate to high signal intensity on T2-weighted spin-echo sequences, and high signal intensity on T2* and STIR images. When bony lesions are discrete and focal, they are easy to discern. When very extensive diffuse bony metastatic disease is present, epidural spread of disease can be more difficult to identify. Where there is gross disease, several levels of compression may be present, underlining the necessity to cover the whole spine (Fig. 43.21). In the presence of

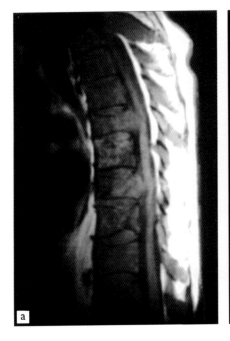
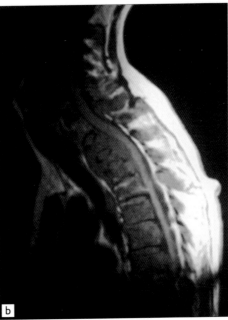

Figure 43.21. *(a and b) T1-weighted spin-echo MR image, sagittal plane. Extensive bony disease is present, metastatic from carcinoma of breast. Multiple levels of cord compression are identified in the lower thoracic region and cervico-thoracic junction. It is unlikely that all of these levels would have been demonstrated by myelography. Magnetic resonance imaging should include the whole spine, as discovery of a level in the lower thoracic region does not exclude higher levels of compression, particularly in the presence of extensive bony metastatic disease.*

diffuse disease, any subtle abnormality of cord morphology identified on the sagittal images should raise the index of suspicion, and orthogonal plane imaging should be performed, which may reveal lateral compression of the cord from expanded pedicles (Figs. 43.22 and 43.23). This type of compression is not infrequently seen in metastatic prostate and breast cancer.

Bony changes may be subtle or even absent. Soft tissue extension of tumour (in a 'dumb-bell' fashion) may occur with a variety of tumours:

- Lymphoma
- Neurofibroma
- Neuroblastoma
- Malignant thymoma
- Mesothelioma
- Lung cancer

Apart from the classical but uncommon neurofibroma and neuroblastoma, bronchial carcinoma can penetrate the

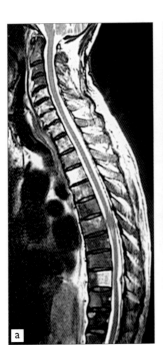
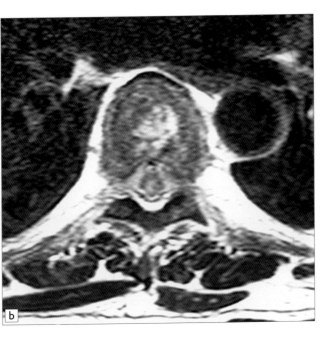

Figure 43.22. *Spinal cord compression as a result of metastases to the spine from prostate carcinoma. (a) T2-weighted sagittal image shows anatomical distortion of the spinal cord at T7. Any abnormality such as this should precipitate orthogonal plane imaging. (b) T2-weighted axial imaging through T7 shows epidural soft tissue surrounding the spinal cord, and some high signal centrally within the cord. Although the imaging changes are not gross, the clinical syndrome of cord compression at mid-thoracic level was clear, and it is likely that ischaemia or infarction of the cord was present.*

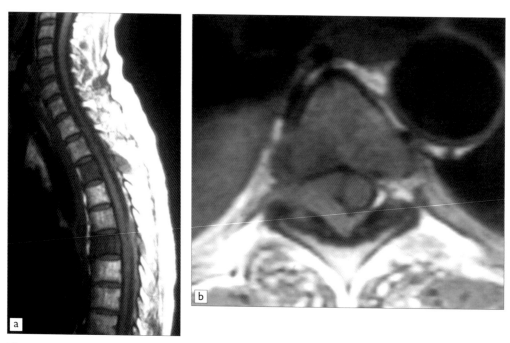

Figure 43.23. *(a) Sagittal T1-weighted MR image of spine. Low signal is returned from the vertebral body and posterior elements at T3 and T6 (metastatic disease from breast carcinoma). There is a plaque of soft tissue apparently lying posteriorly to the cord at T6. (b) Orthogonal plane imaging (axial T1-weighted sequence) at T6 shows soft tissue epidural disease compressing the cord from the right. In this patient, pain was the major presenting clinical feature, and weakness was present but not profound. A good clinical response to steroids and radiation therapy was obtained. (Reproduced with permission from MacVicar D, Neurological presentations in the cancer patient. Imaging 2000; 12: 115–120.)*

intervertebral foramen while causing little bony destruction, particularly in superior sulcus tumours. Malignant thymoma and mesothelioma may also compress the cord by soft tissue extension (Fig. 43.24).

One of the most important dumb-bell tumours is lymphoma in the posterior mediastinum, retrocrural region and retroperitoneum. The tendency of lymphoma to involve the epidural spaces has been recognized for many years.[42] The incidence of spinal cord compression by lymphoma reported in the literature varies between 1 and 7%. Epidural masses may be small and subtle (Fig. 43.25) but any symptomatology should be vigorously investigated, as early treatment should result in a favourable response to treatment in keeping with the overall prognosis of the disease. If paraplegia is allowed to develop, it is unlikely to recover.[43] In current practice it is most likely that a patient known to have lymphoma presenting with back pain and neurological symptoms will be referred for MR imaging. The same principles apply as for any tumour; the entire spine should be imaged, using orthogonal planes as necessary to elucidate soft tissue disease. In addition, when CT scans are performed as staging investigations for lymphoma, the epidural spaces should be an area subjected to special scrutiny as subtle signs, such as the obliteration of fat planes in the intervertebral foraminae, may give early warning of epidural space invasion and incipient neurological dysfunction (Fig. 43.25).

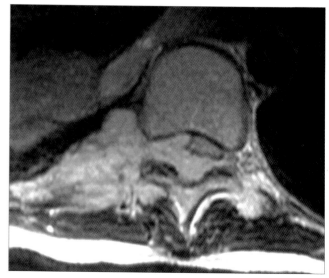

Figure 43.24. *Malignant thymoma. Axial MR in the thoracic region reveals a soft tissue mass involving pleura and chest wall to the right of the midline. Tumour penetrates the neural foramen in a 'dumb-bell' configuration and is displacing and compressing the spinal cord predominantly from a posterior and lateral direction. Pain was present, with relatively little power loss, indicating that the blood supply of the cord has not been significantly compromised by fairly marked anatomical displacement. (Reproduced with permission from MacVicar D, Neurological presentations in the cancer patient. Imaging 2000; 12: 115–120.)*

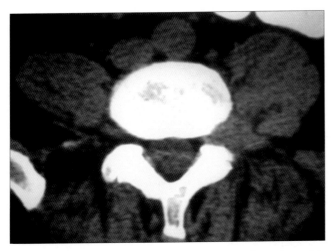

Figure 43.25. *Axial CT scan in lumbar region of a patient with non-Hodgkin's lymphoma and back pain radiating to the left leg. A small soft tissue mass lies behind the left psoas, extending into the neural foramen. This is a characteristic site and appearance for epidural lymphoma. Patients may present with prolonged back pain, and if this is neglected, compression of the spinal cord or cauda equina may develop and lead to permanent neurological damage. However, if detected promptly, epidural lymphoma will respond to treatment and prognosis is no worse than for lymphoma at any other site. Note that the fat planes in and around the neural foramen are obliterated on the affected side but preserved on the normal side. The intervertebral foraminae should be a 'check area' on staging CT scans performed for lymphoma. (Reproduced with permission from MacVicar D, Neurological presentations in the cancer patient. Imaging 2000; 12: 115–120.)*

Key points: magnetic resonance imaging features of spinal cord compression

- ■ MR imaging is the investigation of choice in suspected spinal cord compression

- ■ The entire spine should be evaluated as metastatic disease may produce multiple levels of compression

- ■ T2-weighted sequences provide an excellent 'myelographic' effect

- ■ Most causes of myelopathy that mimic spinal cord compression can be accurately diagnosed with MR

- ■ Lymphoma is the most common malignant tumour to invade the spinal canal through the intervertebral foraminae without any bony destruction

Spinal meningeal disease

As is the case with leptomeningeal disease in the cranial cavity, disease may spread to the meninges by:

- The haematogenous route
- Cerebrospinal fluid pathways
- Direct extension along peripheral nerves

The clinical presentation may be somewhat obscure. Symptoms can be divided into two broad categories, namely those caused by invasion of spinal nerve roots (i.e. neural dysfunction) and those caused by invasion of the leptomeninges alone (i.e. meningeal irritation).

Neural dysfunction is likely to result in a constellation of symptoms and signs that are anatomically remote owing to the selective involvement of individual nerve roots. If an isolated lumbar nerve root is involved, radicular pain will result, mimicking a herniated lumbar disc. However, there are usually some vague symptoms attributable to meningeal irritation such as back pain, neck pain or headache. When the referring clinician describes a neurological presentation which may be very vague or verging on the bizarre, it is important to consider the diagnosis of leptomeningeal disease, since the MR technique must involve T1-weighted sagittal sequences of the entire spine before and after IV Gd-DTPA administration. In contrast to the situation within the cranial cavity, any enhancement of the meninges in the spinal canal should be considered abnormal. Some tumours, notably carcinomas of lung and breast, produce enhancing masses within the meninges (Fig. 43.26). Leukaemia and lymphoma tend to result in plaques or sheets of enhancing tissue (Fig. 43.27). Melanoma, which frequently metastasizes to the meninges, may do either (Fig. 43.28). When present, the appearance of enhancing plaques or masses of tumour is sufficiently characteristic to allow confident diagnosis. However, MR is a distinctly insensitive technique, particularly in leukaemia and lymphoma. If MR imaging is negative, lumbar puncture can be used subsequently and may yield positive cytology.[34,35]

Primary brain tumours that have a tendency to seed spinal meninges via CSF spread include:

- Ependymoma
- Medulloblastoma
- Pinealoblastoma
- Intracranial germ cell tumours
- Intracranial primitive neuro-ectodermal tumours (PNET)

Magnetic resonance is frequently used as a staging technique, notwithstanding its relative lack of sensitivity. Changes may be subtle, and it is important to ensure coverage of the meninges in the neural foraminae. An enhancing mass is diagnostic of drop metastases, which are more commonly found at the time of recurrence following treatment for primary brain tumours, particularly in children (Fig. 43.29). Myelography is capable of detecting meningeal nodules but is now rarely used.

Intramedullary deposits

Tumour deposits are occasionally identified within the spinal cord. In these circumstances, clinical presentation is similar to meningeal disease, giving neurological symptoms and signs that cannot be unified to a single anatomical site.

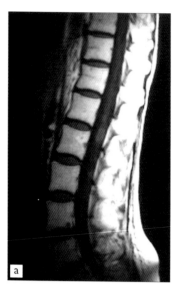
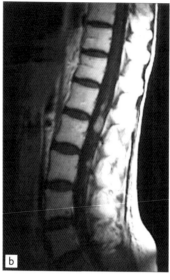

Figure 43.26. *(a and b) T1-weighted spin-echo MR images before and after IV Gd-DTPA. Meningeal deposits from carcinoma of the breast. Some thickening of the meninges is just discernible before contrast. After administration of gadolinium, enhancing masses on the meninges are clearly identifiable. This is the characteristic appearance of carcinoma metastatic to the meninges.*

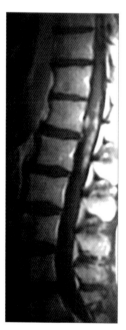

Figure 43.27. *T1-weighted spin-echo MR image following gadolinium administration. Meningeal spread of lymphoma. The tumour appears as an enhancing sheet of tissue in the lumbar meninges. The patient had presented with backache and leg weakness as the initial manifestation of non-Hodgkin's lymphoma. Biopsy at lumbar laminectomy confirmed the diagnosis. Staging CT scan revealed lymphadenopathy in mediastinum and retroperitoneum.*

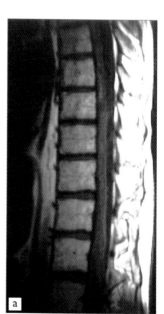
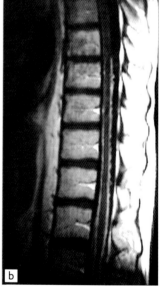

Figure 43.28. *(a and b) T1-weighted spin-echo MR images before and after Gd-DTPA, sagittal plane. Diffuse nodular enhancement extends throughout the thoracic meninges. The appearance is due to diffuse meningeal involvement by melanoma seen better following contrast injection (b).*

Carcinoma of breast and lung and malignant melanoma are once again the most frequent culprits. Metastases to the spinal cord are seen as enhancing masses on MR imaging following Gd-DTPA injection, and appear to have a predilection for the conus (Fig. 43.30). Small cell lung cancer may give multiple small enhancing lesions throughout the cord, of similar appearance to small cell deposits metastatic to the brain parenchyma (Fig. 43.31).

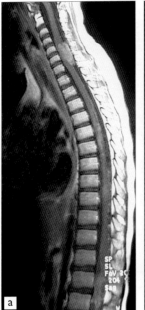
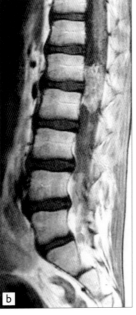

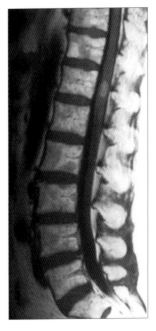

Figure 43.30. *Gadolinium-enhanced T1-weighted spin-echo MR sequence demonstrating an enhancing nodule in the conus in a patient with disseminated metastatic disease from carcinoma of the breast. (Reproduced with permission from MacVicar D, Neurological presentations in the cancer patient. Imaging 2000; 12: 115–120.)*

Figure 43.29. *(a and b) Contrast-enhanced T1-weighted sagittal images through whole spine demonstrating gross drop metastases in cervical and lumbar regions in a child aged 9, with recurrent ependymoma following treatment for an intracranial primary tumour.*

Key points: spinal meningeal and cord involvement

- Spinal meningeal disease is caused by invasion of spinal nerve roots or by haematogenous spread to the leptomeninges

- Patients frequently present with neurological features that do not point to a single specific site

- T1-weighted sagittal sequences of the entire spine before and after IV contrast medium are mandatory

- MR imaging is an insensitive technique and, if negative, lumbar puncture is indicated

- Primary brain tumours produce spinal seedlings

- Intramedullary metastases most frequently occur in breast and lung cancer and malignant melanoma

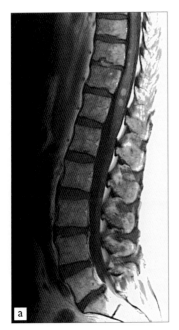
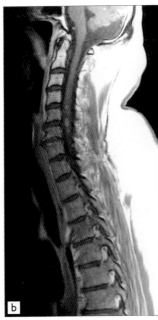

Figure 43.31. *(a and b) T1-weighted MR images following Gd-DTPA, sagittal plane. Very small enhancing lesions are identified within the cord. The intramedullary lesions were scattered through the spinal cord and brain, and were due to metastases from small cell carcinoma.*

Metastatic involvement of peripheral nerves and muscle

Major nerve plexuses

The two major areas of nerve plexus formation are the brachial plexus and the lumbosacral plexus. The brachial plexus is most commonly involved, by superior sulcus tumours invading directly, or by lymph nodes metastatic from breast carcinoma (see Chapter 25). Both of these pathologies usually invade the plexus from below, affecting those fibres that begin as C8 and T1 roots and end as the ulnar nerve. The primary symptom is pain, which may localize to the posterior aspect of the shoulder or around the elbow; this pain may sometimes lead the physician to instigate fruitless investigations of the bony and soft tissue structures of the shoulder and elbow. Paraesthesia and numbness are often present, particularly affecting the medial part of the hand. The differential diagnosis from radiation fibrosis of the brachial plexus can be difficult, and CT and MR can both be used to detect soft tissue masses in this region. Magnetic resonance, as a result of its multiplanar imaging capability and superior contrast resolution, has greater versatility but it may be impossible to discriminate between radiation fibrosis and infiltrative forms of tumour that do not present as a morphological mass.[44-47] Brachial plexopathy is further discussed in Chapter 25.

Tumours that frequently affect the lumbosacral plexus include carcinomas of rectum, cervix, bladder and prostate. The clinical presentation is dominated by pain, usually in a radicular distribution. Radiation damage to the lumbosacral plexus is less common than in the brachial plexus. Often, the crucial question is to establish whether the plexus is involved by a soft tissue mass or by bony involvement of the lumbosacral spine. Computed tomography is frequently adequate for detecting a soft tissue mass extending from the pelvic organs into the sacral plexus. However, in the absence of a soft tissue mass, MR is more sensitive for detecting malignant involvement of the sacrum (Figs. 43.32 and 43.33).

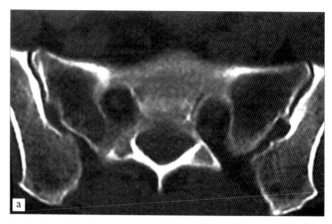

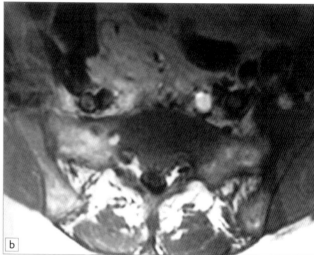

Figure 43.32. *This patient with a history of melanoma, presented with lower back pain radiating to the left leg. (a) CT scan with bony windows failed to reveal any explanation for the symptoms; (b) T1-weighted spin-echo MR image, axial plane. Involvement of the sacral marrow cavity and impingement on the nerve root is clearly demonstrated, owing to the high sensitivity of MR in detecting bony lesions.*

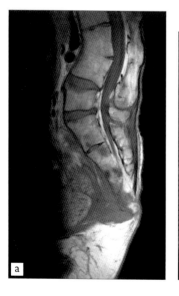

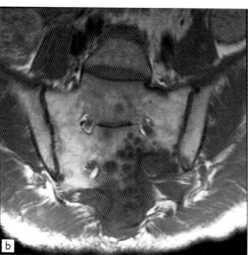

Figure 43.33. *The patient had a history of transitional cell carcinoma of the bladder treated by cystectomy. He presented with radicular pain. (a) T1-weighted spin-echo MR image, sagittal plane. There is a presacral soft tissue abnormality due to pelvic soft tissue recurrence; (b) T1-weighted spin-echo MR image, paracoronal plane. Bony invasion affecting the sacrum and involving the nerve roots is clearly demonstrated.*

Peripheral nerves

Peripheral neuropathy in a patient with systemic cancer is usually due to chemotherapy. Diffuse or focal involvement of nerves by tumour, resulting in a sensorimotor neuropathy, is rare and usually associated with lymphoma, leukaemia and other haematological malignancies.[48,49] Isolated mononeuropathies may result from invasion by adjacent tumour, particularly if a nerve is located at a point where it passes directly over a bone, or through a bony canal. The radial and ulnar nerves may be affected by bony metastatic disease around the elbow or within the axilla. The sciatic nerve is also vulnerable to involvement by bony or soft tissue tumour at several sites in the pelvis, and the obturator nerve may be compressed or invaded as it passes through the obturator canal. Imaging studies are only likely to be useful if there is a strong clinical indication that an individual nerve has been affected by metastatic disease; in these circumstances, cross-sectional techniques including MR, CT and ultrasound can give useful confirmation that there is a pathological mass in the vicinity of the affected nerve.

Key points: peripheral nerves

■ The brachial plexus is most commonly involved in breast and lung cancer by direct soft tissue invasion

■ The lumbosacral plexus is usually involved by direct extension of bone metastases, e.g. carcinoma of the prostate

Muscle

Soft tissue metastases involving muscles are unusual, but may occasionally be seen in lymphoma and leukaemia (chloroma).

Some solid tumours may also metastasize to the muscle:

- Malignant melanoma
- Lung cancer
- Rhabdomyosarcoma

Such lesions are usually obvious clinically, and cross-sectional imaging techniques can be used to determine the extent of the abnormality, but these lesions rarely have specific diagnostic features.

Conclusion

As is the case in non-malignant neurological disease, MR is assuming an increasingly central role in the investigation of the effects of metastatic disease on the CNS, although CT remains a valid and useful technique in many clinical circumstances. Interpretation of images of metastatic disease is often straightforward, but the radiologist must remain mindful of the protean manifestations of metastatic disease, and endeavour to ensure that the most appropriate imaging technique is used sooner rather than later.

Summary

■ Neurological disorders are an increasingly common problem in the cancer patient

■ The radiologist should focus on the clinical findings so that the most appropriate investigation is performed

■ Many metastases arise from cancers of the lung, breast and melanoma

■ Other primary sources of tumour include the kidneys and gastro-intestinal tract

■ In a significant number of patients the primary source is unknown

■ MR is the most sensitive imaging technique available for detecting brain metastases but screening is only undertaken in selected tumours (e.g. lung cancer preoperatively)

■ Symptomatic spinal cord compression is seen in 1–5% of patients with disseminated malignancy

■ Imaging of spinal cord compression should include the whole spine. Magnetic resonance is the preferred investigation

■ Spinal meningeal disease results in a wide range of neurological symptoms that cannot be unified to a single anatomical site

■ The brachial plexus is most commonly involved in breast cancer and apical lung cancer by direct soft tissue invasion

■ The lumbosacral plexus is usually involved as a result of direct extension of bone metastases

■ Peripheral neuropathy is usually due to chemotherapy but, occasionally, a bone metastasis may involve an adjacent nerve

■ Muscle deposits are unusual. They may be seen in lymphoma, leukaemia, melanoma, lung cancer and rhabdomyosarcoma

References

1. Clouston P D, de Angelis L M, Posner J B. The spectrum of neurologic disease in patients with systemic cancer. Ann Neurol 1992; 31: 268–273

2. Sculier J P, Feld R, Evans W K et al. Neurological disorders in patients with small cell lung cancer. Cancer 1987; 60: 2275–2283

3. Gilbert M R, Grossman S A. Incidence and nature of neurological problems in patients with solid tumours. Am J Med 1986; 81: 951–954

4. Eapen L, Vachet M, Catton G et al. Brain metastases with an unknown primary: a clinical perspective. J Neurooncol 1988; 6: 31–35

5. Nicholson G L. Organ specificity of tumour metastasis: role of preferential adhesion, invasion and growth of malignant cells at specific secondary sites. Cancer Metastasis Rev 1988; 7: 143–188

6. Delattre J-Y, Kroll G, Thaler H T et al. Distribution of brain metastases. Arch Neurol 1988; 45: 741–744

7. Smith D B, Howell A, Harris M et al. Carcinomatous meningitis associated with infiltrating lobular carcinoma of the breast. Eur J Surg Oncol 1985; 11: 33–36

8. Nicholson G L, Kawaguchi T, Kawaguchi M et al. Brain surface invasion and metastasis of murine malignant melanoma variants. J Neurooncol 1987; 4: 209–218

9. Sze G, Milano E, Johnson C et al. Detection of brain metastases: comparison of contrast-enhanced with unenhanced MR and enhanced CT. Am J Neuroradiol 1990; 11: 785–791

10. Cherryman G R, Olliff J F C, Golfieri R et al. A prospective comparison of Gadolinium-DTPA enhanced MRI and contrast-enhanced CT scanning in the detection of brain metastases arising from small cell lung cancer. Medicom. Contrast media in MRI. 1990

11. Sze G, Johnson C, Kawamura Y et al. Comparison of single- and triple-dose contrast material in the MR screening of brain metastases. Am J Neuroradiol 1998; 19: 821–828

12. Yuh W T C, Tall T E, Nguyen H D et al. The effect of contrast dose, imaging time and lesion size in the MR detection of intracerebral metastases. Am J Neuroradiol 1995; 16: 73–80

13. Black W C. High-dose MR in evaluation of brain metastases: will increased detection decrease costs? Am J Neuroradiol 1994; 15: 1062–1064

14. Boorstein J M, Wong K T, Grossman R I et al. Metastatic lesions of the brain imaging with magnetisation transfer. Radiology 1994; 191: 799–803

15. Okubo T, Hayashi N, Shirouzu I et al. Detection of brain metastases: comparison of Turbo FLAIR imaging, T2-weighted imaging and double dose gadolinium-enhanced MR imaging. Radiat Med 1998; 16: 273–281

16. Griffeth L K, Rich K M, Dehashiti F et al. Brain metastases from non-central nervous system tumours: evaluation with PET. Radiology 1993; 186: 37–44

17. Armstrong P, Vincent J N. Staging non-small cell lung cancer. Clin Radiol 1993; 48: 1–10

18. Whitehouse J M A (ed). Management of Lung Cancer. Current Clinical Practices. Standing Medical Advisory Committee of Department of Health: Working Group Report, 1994

19. Salbeck R, Grau H C, Artmann H. Cerebral tumour staging in patients with bronchial carcinoma by computed tomography. Cancer 1990; 66: 2007–2011

20. Royal College of Radiologists. The Use of Computed Tomography in the Initial Investigation of Common Malignancies. London: Royal College of Radiologists, 1994

21. Rohren E M, Provenzale J M, Barboriak D P et al. Screening for cerebral metastases with FDG-PET in patients undergoing whole body staging of non-central nervous system malignancy. Radiology 2003; 226: 181–187

22. Myers R. The application of PET-MR image registration in the brain. Br J Radiol 2002; 75: S31–35

23. Marsden P K, Strul D, Keevil S F et al. Simultaneous PET and NMR. Br J Radiol 2002; 75: S53–59

24. Steinert H C, von Schulthess G K. Initial clinical experience using a new integrated PET/CT system. Br J Radiol 2002; 75: S36–38

25. MacVicar D. Staging of testicular germ cell tumours. Clin Radiol 1993; 47: 149–158

26. Patchell R A, Tibbs P A, Walsh J W et al. A randomised trial of surgery in the treatment of single metastases to the brain. N Engl J Med 1993; 22: 495–500

27. Asato R, Akiyama Y, Ito M et al. Nuclear magnetic resonance abnormalities of the cerebral white matter in children with acute lymphoblastic leukaemia and malignant lymphoma during and after central nervous system prophylactic treatment with intrathecal methotrexate. Cancer 1992; 70: 1997–2004

28. Hook C C, Kimmel D W, Kvols L K et al. Multifocal inflammatory leuko-encephalopathy with 5-fluorouracil and levamisole. Ann Neurol 1992; 31: 262–267

29. Stemmer S M, Stears J C, Burton B S et al. White matter changes in patients with breast cancer treated with high-dose chemotherapy and autologous bone marrow support. Am J Neuroradiol 1994; 15: 1267–1273

30. Rubinstein A B, Schein M, Reichenthal E. The association of carcinoma of the breast with meningioma. Surg Gynaecol Obstet 1989; 169: 334–336

31. Smith F P, Slavik M, Macdonald J S. Association of breast cancer with meningioma: Report of two cases and review of the literature. Cancer 1978; 42: 1992–1994

32. Jacobs D H, Holmes F F, McFarlane N J. Meningiomas are not significantly associated with breast cancer. Arch Neurol 1992; 49: 753–756

33. Enochs W S, Hyslop W B, Bennett H F et al. Sources of the increased longitudinal relaxation rates observed in melanotic melanoma. An in vitro study of synthetic melanins. Invest Radiol 1989; 24: 794–804

34. Yousem D M, Patrone P M, Grossman R I.

Leptomeningeal metastases: MR evaluation. J Comput Assist Tomogr 1990; 14: 255–261

35. Collie D A, Brush J P, Lammie G A et al. Imaging features of leptomeningeal metastases. Clin Radiol 1999; 54: 765–771

36. Singh S K, Agris J M, Leeds N E et al. Intracranial leptomeningeal metastases: comparison of depiction at FLAIR and contrast enhanced MR imaging. Radiology 2000; 217: 50–53

37. Bansal S, Brady L W, Olsen A et al. The treatment of metastatic spinal cord tumours. J Am Med Assoc 1967; 202: 686–688

38. Hildebrand J. Lesions of the Nervous System in Cancer Patients. Monograph Series of the European Organisation for Research on Treatment of Cancer, Vol. 5. New York: Raven Press, 1978

39. Klein S L, Sanford R A, Muhlbauer M S. Paediatric spinal epidural metastases. J Neurosurg 1991; 74: 70–75

40. Barron K D, Hirano A, Araski S et al. Experiences with metastatic neoplasms involving the spinal cord. Neurology 1959; 9: 91–106

41. Jones A L, Williams M P, Powles T J et al. Magnetic resonance imaging in the detection of skeletal metastases in patients with breast cancer. Br J Cancer 1990; 62: 296–298

42. Murphy W T, Bilge N. Compression of the spinal cord in patients with malignant lymphoma. Radiology 1964; 82: 495–501

43. MacVicar D, Williams M P. CT scanning in epidural lymphoma. Clin Radiol 1991; 43: 95–102

44. Moore N R, Dixon A K, Wheeler T K. Axillary fibrosis or recurrent tumour. An MRI study in breast cancer. Clin Radiol 1990; 42: 42–46

45. Posniak H V, Olson M C, Dudiak C M. MR imaging of the brachial plexus. Am J Roentgenol 1993; 161: 373–379

46. Iyer R B, Fenstermacher M J, Libshitz H I. MR Imaging of the treated brachial plexus. Am J Roentgenol 1996; 167: 225–229

47. Qayyum A, MacVicar D, Padhani A R et al. Symptomatic brachial plexopathy following treatment for breast cancer: utility of MR imaging including surface coil techniques. Radiology 2000; 214: 837–842

48. Sumi S M, Farrell D F, Knauss T A. Lymphoma and leukaemia manifested by steroid responsive polyneuropathy. Arch Neurol 1983; 40: 577–582

49. McLeod J G. Peripheral neuropathy associated with lymphomas, leukaemias and polycythaemia vera. In: Dyck P J, Thomas P K (eds). Peripheral Neuropathy, Vol. 2, 3rd edn. Philadelphia: W B Saunders, 1993; 1591–1598

Chapter 44

Adrenal metastases

Rodney H Reznek and Anju Sahdev

Introduction

The routine use of cross-sectional imaging in the staging of intra-abdominal and extra-abdominal malignancy has shown that the adrenal gland is a frequent site of unexpected metastatic disease. Although modern computed tomography (CT) and MR can be expected to detect nodules exceeding 8–10 mm, autopsy studies show that many adrenal metastases go undetected due to their small size.

Demonstration of adrenal metastases almost always alters the patient's management by indicating that the patient has Stage IV disease. However, a major problem exists in the radiological demonstration of metastases; benign cortical adenomas are common and always have to be distinguished from metastases before assuming that the patient has metastatic disease.

Incidence

The adrenal glands are the fourth most common site of metastases after the lungs, liver and bone. Common sites of origin of adrenal metastases are listed in Table 44.1. At autopsy, adrenal metastases are found in up to 27% of patients dying of cancer.[1] Certain tumours show a higher incidence; around 30–40% of patients with breast and lung cancer have adrenal metastases.[2,3] Fifty percent of melanomas spread to the adrenal.[4] Adrenal metastases are found in gastro-intestinal tumours and renal tumours in between 10 and 20% of cases.[5,6]

Infiltration is usually within the normal cortex and/or medulla, but spread to adenomas has been reported.[7,8] Metastases are asymptomatic as a rule, but occasional cases of hypoadrenalism have been observed.[9]

Imaging, by cross-sectional techniques, will only detect metastases if there is a focal mass or distortion of the contour of the adrenal gland, but a normal-appearing gland does not exclude microscopic tumour infiltration.[10] One study of patients with small cell lung cancer and morphologically normal adrenal glands on CT found that 17% of the glands were positive for metastases on fine-needle aspiration.[11] This study was performed in 1983 but with modern CT techniques this phenomenon is unlikely to be as common.

The normal adrenal gland

An appreciation of the normal appearances of the adrenal gland is important if small abnormalities are to be observed. The adrenals are usually well visualized as an inverted Y or V shape against the surrounding retroperitoneal fat on both CT and MR. On ultrasound, identification of the normal adrenal gland is technically difficult; the gland is very small and its echotexture is similar to that of the surrounding tissues. Bowel gas can often obscure the gland, particularly on the left.

To date, normal measurements have referred almost entirely to the body of the adrenal gland. However, in view of the predominance of cortical tissue within the limbs, measurement of their size is important.[12] The maximum width of the body measured perpendicular to the long axis, at the junction of the adrenal body and limb, is 0.79 cm (SD 0.21) on the left and 0.6 cm (SD 0.2) on the right.[12] The thickness of the limbs of the right adrenal are slightly less than the left, measuring 0.14–0.49 cm, compared with 0.13–0.52 cm on the left. In practice, the normal adrenal limb should not measure over 5 mm.[12]

Imaging appearances of adrenal metastases

The radiological appearances of adrenal metastases are not specific. They can be large or small, unilateral or bilateral. Small adrenal metastases (<2 cm) are difficult to detect on ultrasound; however, large adrenal masses should be readily identifiable. Metastases are usually rounded or oval and poorly reflective. Ultrasound imaging will not differentiate between metastases and a benign adenoma.

Table 44.1. *Common sites of origin of adrenal metastases*

Breast
Lung
Melanoma
Gastro-intestinal
Kidney

On CT, metastases <3 cm in diameter are usually homogeneous. Larger lesions may show central necrosis or areas of haemorrhage (Fig. 44.1). They tend to be of inhomogeneous density and occasionally have a thick enhancing rim after intravenous (IV) contrast medium (Fig. 44.2).[13]

On MR they are typically hypointense compared to liver on T1-weighted images and relatively hyperintense on T2-weighted images (Figs. 44.1b and 44.1c). Some adrenal metastases are atypical and either iso- or hypointense relative to liver on T2-weighted images.[14,15]

In addition, some metastases have very long T2 relaxation times and can mimic phaeochromocytomas, although phaeochromocytomas can usually be differentiated on clinical grounds (Figs. 44.3 and 44.4). Thus, adrenal metastases often cannot be distinguished definitively from benign lesions such as an adenoma, haematoma, pseudocysts or inflammatory masses on the basis of morphology (Figs. 44.5a and 44.5b). As discussed below, CT attenuation and chemical-shift MR can be helpful in distinguishing between adenomas and metastases.

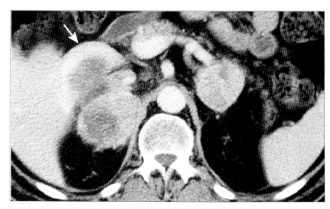

Figure 44.2. *Bilateral adrenal metastasis in a patient with lung cancer. The right adrenal metastasis demonstrates a thick, enhancing rim anteriorly after intravenous contrast medium administration (arrow).*

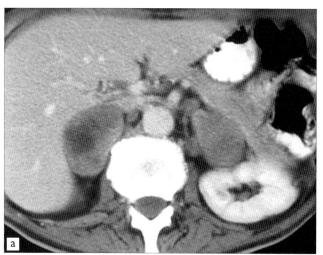

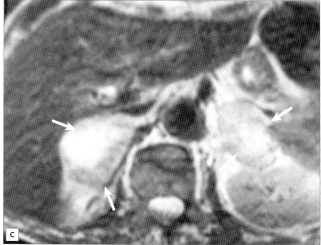

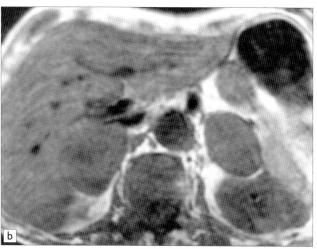

Figure 44.1. *Bilateral adrenal metastases in a patient with oat cell lung cancer. (a) CT scan performed after intravenous injection of contrast medium showing large bilateral adrenal masses enhancing only partially and inhomogeneously; (b) T1-weighted MR image showing masses of intermediate signal intensity; (c) T2-weighted image on the same patient showing typical inhomogeneous appearance of metastases with areas of very high signal intensity interspersed with areas of low signal intensity within large bilateral adrenal masses (arrows).*

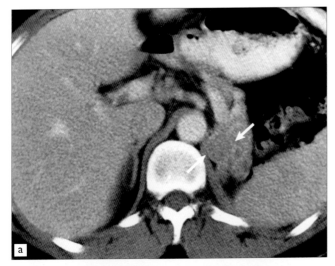

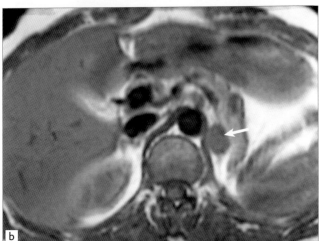

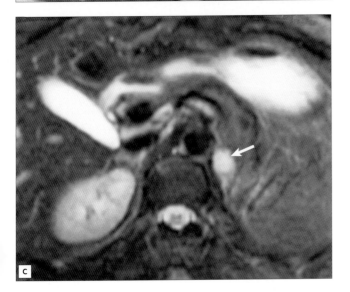

Figure 44.3. *Adrenal metastasis in a patient with carcinoma of the kidney. (a) Contrast-enhanced CT scan showing normal right adrenal and left adrenal metastasis (arrows); (b) T1-weighted MR image showing the mass to be of intermediate signal intensity (arrow); (c) T2-weighted MR image of the same mass showing signal mimicking a phaeochomocytoma (arrow).*

Differential diagnosis of an adrenal mass
(Table 44.2)

The differential diagnosis of a non-hyperfunctioning adrenal mass includes a benign cortical adenoma, adrenal cyst, adrenal carcinoma and a myelolipoma. Functioning adrenal masses such as phaeochromocytomas should also be considered, especially if there is an underlying syndrome such as von Hippel–Lindau, or multiple endocrine neoplasia (Figs. 44.6a, 44.6b and 44.6c). Some of these masses have specific imaging features that help in the diagnosis.

Table 44.2. *Differential diagnosis of adrenal metastases*

Unilateral	Bilateral
Adrenal adenoma	Bilateral adenoma
Adrenal cyst	Bilateral phaeochromocytoma
Adrenal carcinoma	Tuberculosis
Myelolipoma	
Phaeochromocytoma	

Adrenal cysts are rare and occur more commonly in women than men.[16] They have a similar appearance on imaging to cysts elsewhere in the body, although the presence of proteinaceous fluid, infectious debris or haemorrhage within a cyst will alter its appearance. *Primary adrenal carcinomas* are rare, highly malignant tumours. They are usually large (>6 cm) and are heterogeneous where there is necrosis and calcification.[17] However, 16% of tumours are <6 cm and on imaging are homogeneous, morphologically resembling a non-hyperfunctioning adenoma.[18]

Myelolipomas are composed of mature fat and haemopoietic tissue in varying proportions. The diagnosis is made by demonstrating the presence of fat within an adrenal mass. This can be accomplished with either CT or MR, although the presence of haemorrhage or infection can complicate the diagnosis.[19] Nevertheless, the use of narrow collimation on CT will usually allow demonstration of any fat that is present. On MR, the presence of fat is best demonstrated on T1-weighted images with and without fat suppression. The fat-containing area in a myelolipoma should be equal in signal intensity to that of subcutaneous and retroperitoneal fat on all pulse sequences.[20]

Evaluation of the adrenal masses in oncological patients

Influence on staging

Adrenal masses are frequently discovered during staging of patients with cancer. One autopsy study demonstrated the presence of microscopic and macroscopic adenomas in almost 65% of the population.[21] In most cancers, the pres-

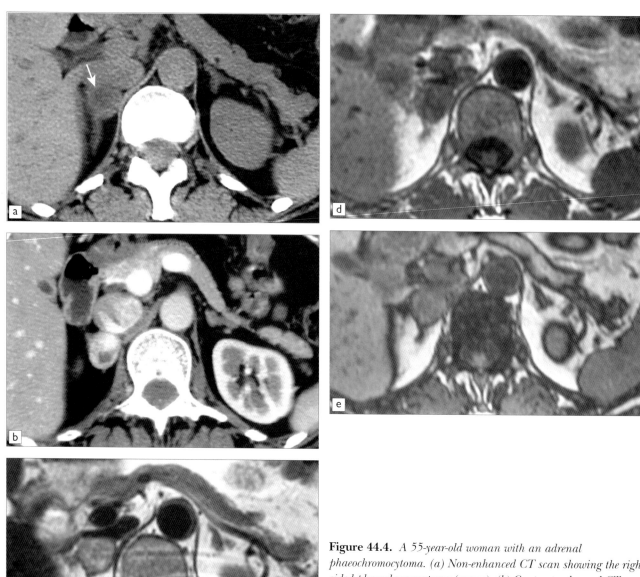

Figure 44.4. *A 55-year-old woman with an adrenal phaeochromocytoma. (a) Non-enhanced CT scan showing the right-sided phaeochromocytoma (arrow). (b) Contrast-enhanced CT scan acquired 60 seconds after contrast administration with the phaeochromocytoma demonstrating rim enhancement and central necrosis. (c) T2-weighted MR image showing the phaeochromocytoma as an intermediate/ high signal intensity mass. (d) In-phase chemical shift image and (e) out-of-phase chemical shift image showing no loss of signal intensity within the mass.*

ence of adrenal metastases, even as the sole site of distant spread, will render the tumour Stage IV (i.e. distant metastases). The exception is in renal cell carcinoma when the demonstration of ipsilateral adrenal involvement does not increase the stage of the disease from Robson Stage II, but involvement of the contralateral gland upgrades the staging to IV-B (Fig. 44.7).

However, not all adrenal masses are metastases, even in patients with known malignancy.[22] When an adrenal mass is the only finding suspicious of metastatic disease in an oncological patient, confirmation of its nature may be crucial in determining whether curative therapy of the primary

tumour is warranted. This dilemma occurs most commonly in patients with carcinoma of the lung, because confirmation of an isolated adrenal metastasis will preclude a thoracotomy or curative radiotherapy. However, non-functioning macroscopic adrenal adenomas are very common, with a prevalence at autopsy in the general population of approximately 3%.[23] Benign adrenal masses of at least 1 cm are found in 0.6–1.5% of the population during abdominal CT.[24,25] The number and size of these nodules increase with age (0.2% in patients younger than 30 years and 6.9 % in patients older than 70 years),[26] and they occur with increased frequency in obese, diabetic patients and elderly

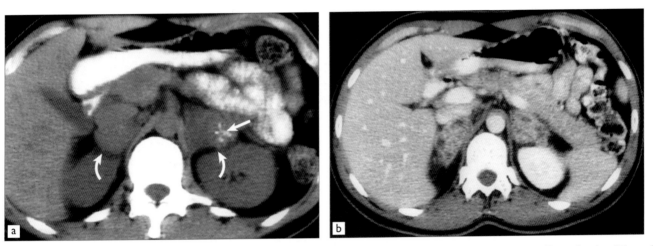

Figure 44.5. *Adrenal tuberculosis. (a) Computed tomography scan prior to intravenous injection of contrast medium showing bilateral adrenal masses (curved arrows). Typical punctate calcification is demonstrated in the left adrenal gland (small arrow). (b) Appearance following intravenous injection of contrast medium showing typical non-enhancing areas within the gland corresponding to multiple small caseating granulomata.*

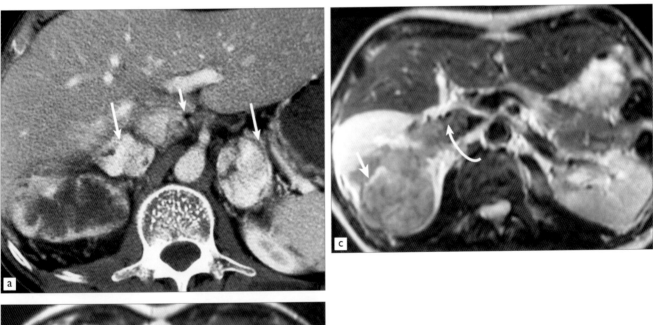

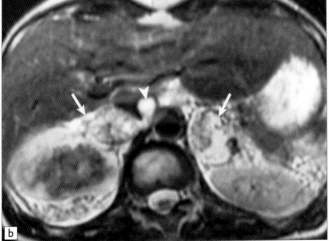

Figure 44.6. *Bilateral phaeochromocytomas and small paraganglioma in association with a right renal cancer in a patient with von Hippel–Lindau disease. (a) Computed tomography scan taken after injection of intravenous contrast medium showing large bilateral adrenal masses enhancing intensely (large arrows). A third smaller mass consistent with a paraganglioma can be seen lying just medial to the inferior vena cava (small arrow); (b) T2-weighted FSE MR sequence corresponding to CT scan showing the typical high signal intensity of the phaeochromocytomas bilaterally (arrows) and the high signal intensity of the small paraganglioma (arrowhead); (c) T2-weighted MR image of the large right renal carcinoma (arrow) infiltrating the right renal vein (curved arrow).*

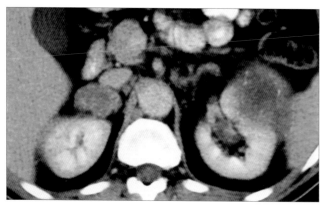

Figure 44.7. *Contrast-enhanced CT scan of a patient with a left-sided renal cell carcinoma and a contralateral homogeneous adrenal metastasis. The contralateral metastasis upgrades the renal cell carcinoma to a stage IV-B.*

women.[27] Even in patients with lung cancer, an adrenal mass is more likely to be an adenoma than a metastasis.[22]

When characterizing adrenal masses by non-invasive imaging the consequences of incorrectly characterizing a mass must be considered. In a patient with an extra-adrenal primary neoplasm it is unlikely that potentially curative treatment of the primary tumour would be withheld without biopsy confirmation of an adrenal lesion thought to be the sole site of metastatic spread. Non-invasive characterization of the adrenal mass as an adenoma, however, could result in a decrease in the number of percutaneous biopsies. Thus, the specificity for diagnosis of an adenoma needs to be very high, to ensure that a patient with adrenal metastases does not unnecessarily undergo curative resection of the primary tumour because of misdiagnosis of the adrenal lesion as an adenoma. The sensitivity is much less critical as the only consequence of a false negative diagnosis is that a percutaneous biopsy will be necessary to establish the diagnosis.

Adrenal masses >3 cm are malignant in 90–95% of cases, and 78–87% of lesions <3 cm are benign.[28,29] However, several studies have shown that the size alone is poor at discriminating between adenomas and non-adenomas.[30–32] Lee, using a threshold of 1.5 cm, found the specificity for the diagnosis of adenoma to be reasonably high (93%), but the sensitivity only 16%.[31] In the same series, using 2.5 cm as the size cut-off, the specificity was 79% and the sensitivity 84%.

The presence of bilateral masses does not confirm a diagnosis of metastases. Katz et al. showed that bilateral adrenal adenomas were almost as common as bilateral metastases even in patients with known malignant disease.[33] Other causes of bilateral masses such as phaeochromocytoma and tuberculosis also result in confusion (Figs. 44.5 and 44.6).

Computed tomography

Computed tomography is extensively used for the characterization of adrenal masses. Many studies have now con-

firmed the usefulness of attenuation value measurements at non-enhanced, enhanced and delayed enhanced CT in differentiating benign from malignant masses.[34–39] Computed tomography characterization uses two independent properties of adenomas, their intracellular lipid content and the rapid loss of attenuation value after IV contrast enhancement. The majority of adrenal adenomas are lipid-rich, thus lowering their unenhanced attenuation values (Fig. 44.8). Analysis of the CT literature shows that the optimal sensitivity (71%) and specificity (98%) for the diagnosis of adrenal adenomas results from choosing a threshold attenuation value of 10 Hounsfield units on non-enhanced CT.[34] There is a small subset of lipid-poor adenomas that cannot be characterized by non-enhanced CT alone (Fig. 44.9a). Metastatic adrenal masses are also lipid-poor. This group of lesions therefore requires additional workup to establish the diagnosis.

Standard contrast medium-enhanced attenuation values obtained 60 seconds after contrast injection or dynamic enhanced scans show too much overlap between adenomas and malignant lesions.[30] Enhanced attenuation values alone are therefore of limited value.

Attenuation values of less than 30–40 Hounsfield units, 10–15 minutes after contrast enhancement, are almost always adenomas.[37] In addition to the absolute delayed CT attenuation value, the percentage of washout of initial enhancement and the relative enhancement washout can be used to differentiate adenomas from malignant disease. These enhancement washout values are only applicable to relatively homogeneous masses without large areas of necrosis or haemorrhage. It has been demonstrated that washout of contrast from adenomas occurs much faster than from metastasis.[39] Both lipid-rich and lipid-poor adenomas behave similarly as this property of adenomas is independent of their lipid content.

The percentage of enhancement washout can be calculated thus:

$$\% \text{ Enhancement washout} = \frac{\substack{\text{Enhanced attenuation value} - \\ \text{delayed enhanced attenuation value}}}{\substack{\text{Enhanced attenuation value} - \\ \text{non-enhanced attenuation value}}} \times 100$$

At 15 minutes, if the percentage enhancement washout is 60% or higher, this has a sensitivity of 88% and a specificity of 96% for the diagnosis of an adenoma.[40]

However, the measurement of absolute contrast medium enhancement washout requires an unenhanced image. Frequently, in clinical practice, only postcontrast images are available. In these patients the percentage relative enhancement washout can be calculated.

$$\% \text{ Relative enhancement washout} = \frac{\substack{\text{Enhanced attenuation} \\ \text{value} - \text{delayed enhanced} \\ \text{attenuation value}}}{\substack{\text{Enhanced attenuation} \\ \text{value}}} \times 100$$

At 15 minutes if a relative enhancement washout of 40% or higher is achieved, this has a sensitivity of 96–100% and a

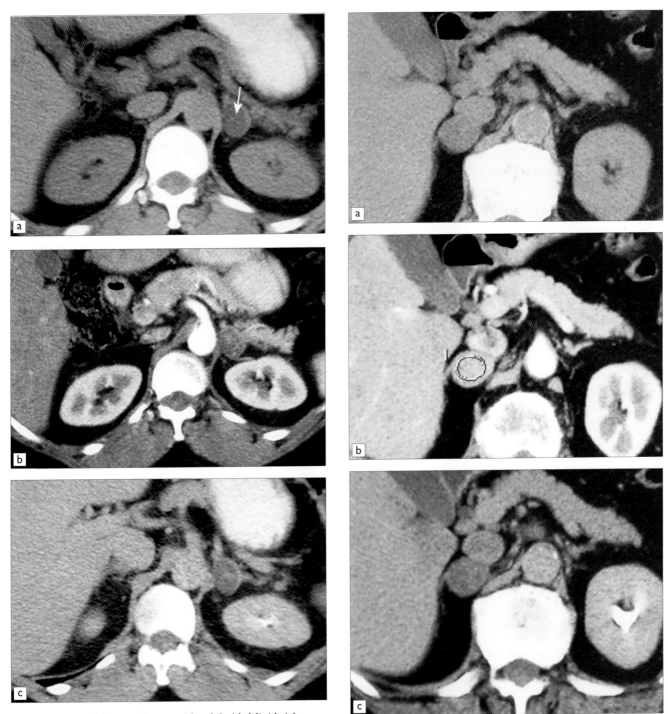

Figure 44.8. *A 59-year-old man with a left-sided lipid-rich adenoma. (a) Non-enhanced CT scan showing a low-density left adrenal mass measuring 1 Hounsfield unit (HU) (arrow). (b) On contrast-enhanced CT, 60 seconds after contrast administration, the Hounsfield measurement of the mass was 52 HU. (c) Delayed contrast enhancement, 15 minutes later, showed the density of the mass was 19 HU. The percentage washout of the mass is (52–19/52–1) × 100 = 65%. The mass is therefore an adenoma by washout criteria and non-enhanced CT attenuation value.*

Figure 44.9. *A 68-year-old woman with a lipid-poor adenoma. (a) Non-contrast enhanced CT scan showing the right adrenal mass which measured 15 Hounsfield units (HU). (b) After contrast administration, the mass measured 67 HU at 60 seconds and (c) 33 HU at 15 minutes. The percentage washout is (67–33/67–15) × 100 = 65%. The mass is therefore an adenoma by washout criteria.*

specificity of 100% for the diagnosis of an adenoma.[40,41] A combination of unenhanced CT and delayed enhanced CT correctly characterizes nearly all adrenal masses as adenomas or metastases.

Key points: adrenal computed tomography

- At non-enhanced CT, a homogeneous adrenal mass with a Hounsfield measurement of less than 10 will be an adenoma in 96% of cases

- At non-contrast-enhanced CT, an adrenal mass with a Hounsfield measurement greater than 10 may be a lipid-poor adenoma or other pathology and contrast-enhanced and 15-minutes delayed enhanced CT imaging is required

- If the absolute contrast medium enhancement washout is >60% and/or the relative enhancement washout is >40%, the mass is an adenoma

- If the absolute contrast medium enhancement washout is less than 60% and/or the relative enhancement washout is less than 40%, the mass must still be considered indeterminate

---

Magnetic resonance

A variety of MR protocols using different pulse sequences have been advocated in an attempt to distinguish between benign and metastatic lesions. Techniques include conventional spin-echo imaging, gadolinium (Gd)-enhanced imaging, chemical-shift and fat-saturation imaging.

Conventional spin-echo imaging

Early reports were enthusiastic that MR would allow differentiation of benign from malignant adrenal masses on the basis of signal intensity differences on T2-weighted spin-echo images. Metastases frequently possess a longer T2 and are of higher signal intensity on T2-weighted images than the surrounding normal adrenal gland. Adenomas are homogeneously iso- or hypointense compared to the normal adrenal gland.[14,42] Visual perception of signal intensity on T2-weighted images is problematic as most adrenal masses appear at least of moderately high signal intensity on fat-saturated T2-weighted images. This is because the suppression of fat leads to re-scaling of the signal intensities of abdominal organs. For similar reasons, most adrenal masses appear moderately low in signal intensity on spin-echo T2-weighted images because of the surrounding high fat signal intensity.[43] Several studies performed on middle-field strength magnets reported that adrenal-to-liver and adrenal-to-fat signal intensity ratios could distinguish benign from malignant masses. However, considerable overlap was seen in most of these studies, with up to 31% of lesions being indeterminate, based on their signal intensity characteristics.[14,44–47] The hepatic signal intensity may not be a reliable universal standard at high-field strengths; because of this some investigators have recommended the use of adrenal mass T2 calculations for differential diagnosis.[15,40] However, even with this method there is still overlap between benign and malignant masses. In addition, T2 measurements are prone to numerous machine-related errors and may vary on different MR machines. Thus, neither of these techniques has proved useful clinically.

Gadolinium-enhanced magnetic resonance

The accuracy of MR in differentiating benign from malignant masses can be improved by using IV gadolinium injection with gradient-echo imaging.[48–50] On MR images obtained after administration of gadolinium, adenomas show mild enhancement with quick washout, whereas malignant tumours and phaeochromocytomas show strong enhancement and slower washout. Uniform enhancement (capillary blush) on postgadolinium capillary phase images is common for adenomas, 70% in one series, but rare in other masses.[51] Adenomas also commonly demonstrate a thin rim of enhancement in the late phase of Gd-enhanced images.[52] Metastases frequently have heterogeneous enhancement. However, again there is considerable overlap in the characteristics of benign and malignant masses, limiting clinical applicability in distinguishing adenomatous from non-adenomatous masses.

Chemical-shift imaging

More recent attempts have been made to characterize adrenal masses with MR on the basis of fat content.[53–58] Benign non-functioning adenomas generally contain large lipid-laden cells, in contrast to malignant lesions which contain little or none. Chemical-shift imaging relies on the fact that protons in water molecules precess at a slightly different rate to the protons in lipid molecules in a magnetic field. As a result, water and fat protons cycle in and out of phase with respect to one another. By selecting an appropriate TE, one can acquire an in-phase and an out-of-phase image. The signal intensity of a pixel on an in-phase image is derived from the signal of water plus fat protons. On out-of-phase images the signal intensity is derived from the difference of the signal of water and fat protons. Therefore, adenomas lose signal intensity on out-of-phase images compared with in-phase images, whereas metastases remain unchanged (Figs. 44.10 and 44.11). The most accurate method for demonstrating that a mass is an adenoma is to show loss of signal intensity on out-of-phase images.

There are several ways of assessing the degree of loss of signal intensity. Quantitative analysis can be made using a variety of ratios, essentially comparing the loss of signal in the adrenal with that of liver, paraspinal muscle or spleen on in-phase and opposed-phase images. Fatty infiltration of the liver (particularly in oncology patients receiving chemotherapy) and iron overload make the liver an unreliable internal standard. Fatty infiltration may also affect

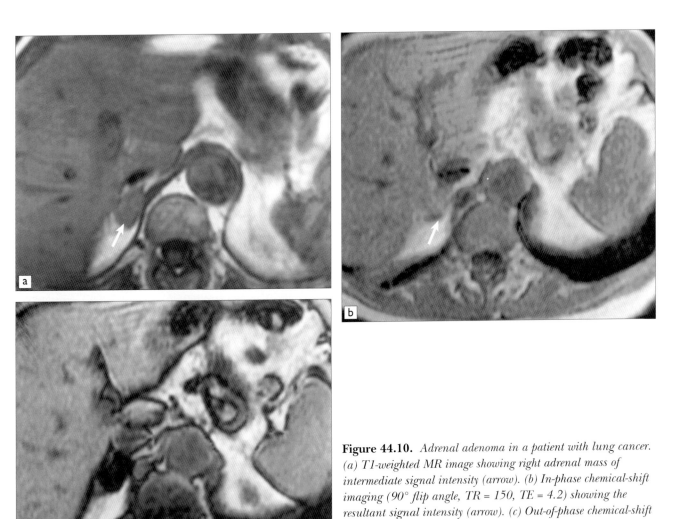

Figure 44.10. *Adrenal adenoma in a patient with lung cancer. (a) T1-weighted MR image showing right adrenal mass of intermediate signal intensity (arrow). (b) In-phase chemical-shift imaging (90° flip angle, TR = 150, TE = 4.2) showing the resultant signal intensity (arrow). (c) Out-of-phase chemical-shift imaging (90° flip angle, TR = 150, TE = 2.3) showing marked loss of signal intensity, indicating the presence of intracellular fluid.*

Figure 44.11. *Chemical-shift imaging to evaluate adrenal masses in patients with carcinoma. Adrenal metastases from a lung cancer. (a) In-phase chemical-shift imaging (90° flip angle, TR = 150, TE = 4.2) shows a left adrenal mass of intermediate signal intensity (arrow). (b) Out-of-phase imaging (90° flip angle, TR = 150, TE = 2.3) showing that there has been no loss of signal intensity and that the presence of intercellular fat has not been demonstrated.*

skeletal muscle to a lesser extent. The spleen has been shown to be the most reliable internal standard, although this may also be affected by iron overload.[56]

To calculate the adrenal lesion-to-spleen ratio (ASR) ROIs are used to acquire the signal intensity (SI) within the adrenal mass and the spleen from in-phase and out-of-phase images. The ASR reflects the percentage signal drop off within the adrenal lesion compared to the spleen and it can be calculated as follows:

$$ASR = \frac{\dfrac{SI \text{ lesion (out-of-phase)}}{SI \text{ spleen (out-of-phase)}}}{\dfrac{SI \text{ lesion (in-phase)}}{SI \text{ spleen (in-phase)}}} \times 100$$

ASR ratio of 70 or less has been shown to be 100% specific for adenomas but only 78% sensitive. Crucially, this threshold does not label any metastases as adenomas but adenomas may have higher ASR than 70.[59,60]

Simple visual assessment of relative signal intensity loss, in comparison with the reference organ, is just as accurate as quantitative methods, but quantitative methods may be useful in equivocal cases.[56,57] A signal intensity loss of greater than 20% is diagnostic of adenomas.[60] However, although specificities of 100% are reported, metastatic lesions from hepatocellular carcinomas, renal cell carcinomas and liposarcomas can contain lipid, and two cases of adrenocortical carcinomas containing microscopic amounts of fat showing areas of loss of signal intensity on chemical-shift imaging have been reported.[61] However, in these cases, signal loss was heterogeneous and not uniform. Conversely, it is probable that some functioning adenomas may contain insufficient lipid to result in loss of signal on out-of-phase imaging.[50,62] However, these would presumably be identified biochemically.

The combination of spin-echo signal characteristics, gadolinium enhancement and chemical-shift imaging is currently 85–90% accurate in distinguishing between adenomas and non-adenomas.[60,63]

Evidence from a histological study showed that both non-contrast CT alone and chemical-shift imaging rely on the same property of adenomas, their lipid content, and therefore both techniques have a high correlation.[59] Adenomas that were indeterminate on one technique were also indeterminate on the other.

Key points: magnetic resonance

■ Conventional spin-echo techniques and Gd-enhanced MR demonstrate overlap in the appearances of adenomas and malignant lesions

■ Chemical-shift imaging relies on the presence of intracellular lipid in adenomas and is the most accurate MR sequence for the diagnosis of an adenoma

Nuclear scintigraphy

Radiocholesterol agents [^{131}I-6-(beta)-iodomethyl-norcholesterol (NP-59) and 75-SE-selenomethyl-norcholesterol] are conveyed to the adrenal cortical tissue via low-density lipoprotein receptors. Their uptake is affected by adrenocorticotropic hormone (ACTH) and renin–angiotensin systems. Radiocholesterol scintigraphy can be used to identify functioning but not hypofunctioning adrenal masses in the adrenal cortex. This allows characterization of a mass as a benign functioning or a non-functioning lesion. Non-functioning lesions include malignant tumours and benign conditions such as haemorrhage and inflammatory lesions, resulting in an overlap between benign and malignant processes. In two studies the specificity of scintigraphy for the diagnosis of an adenoma was 100% even for masses as small as 1–2 cm in diameter.[64,65] The sensitivity was comparable to CT density and chemical-shift MR.

Whole-body positron emission tomography with 2-[F-18]fluoro-2-deoxy-D-glucose ([18]FDG PET) allows the recognition of malignant adrenal lesions. The contribution of [18]FDG PET has been well evaluated in large studies in relation to lung cancer.[66–68]

Using [18]FDG PET, these studies have shown a 100% sensitivity and specificity for the diagnosis of a malignant adrenal mass when CT or MR identify enlarged adrenal glands or a focal mass.[65,69] For the diagnosis of a malignant adrenal tumour, the positive predictive value (PPV) of [18]FDG PET was 100% and negative predictive value (NPV) to rule out malignancy was also 100%. Within these study populations, [18]FDG PET also has the ability to detect metastatic lesions in nonenlarged adrenal glands but the accuracy of this has not been fully evaluated.[66] [18]FDG PET also has the advantage of simultaneously detecting metastasis at other sites.

The routine use of [18]FDG PET is presently limited by availability and its high cost. Other PET radiopharmaceuticals such as 11-C-etiomidate and 11-C-metiomidate have been used to image the adrenals but require evaluation for routine clinical use.[70–72]

Key point: radionuclide imaging

■ Early studies indicate that [18]FDG PET has a 100% specificity and sensitivity for the diagnosis of a malignant adrenal mass

Percutaneous adrenal biopsy

With improved imaging and new techniques, such as contrast medium washout measurement on CT and chemical-shift MR, only a small percentage of adrenal masses cannot be accurately characterized and require percutaneous biopsy for diagnosis. In a study of 33 patients with known malignancy, 48% were characterized as benign on CT and chemical-shift MR. Forty-six percent were thought to be malignant. Only 5% were considered indeterminate on MR and CT and required biopsy for diagnosis.[60] Percutaneous CT-guided adrenal biopsy is a relatively safe procedure in patients with a known extra-adrenal malignancy. Silverman et al., in a study evaluating 101 percutaneous adrenal biopsies, showed the PPV for malignancy was 100%.[63] In the study by Harisinghani et al., 225 adrenal biopsies were evaluated.[73] For malignant disease, there were no false negative biopsies, giving an NPV of 100%. Adrenal biopsies can therefore safely exclude malignant disease. The reported accuracy ranges from 90 to 96%. One study showed accuracy was increased with the use of larger needles.[74]

Minor complications of adrenal biopsy include abdominal pain, haematuria, nausea and small pneumothoraces. Major complications, generally regarded as those requiring treatment, occur in 2.8–3.6% of cases and include pneumothoraces requiring intervention and haemorrhage, with isolated reports of adrenal abscesses, pancreatitis and seeding of metastases along the needle track.[63,74–76] The type of complication varies with the approach used but does not appear to be related to needle size.[74,76]

Non-metastatic adrenal enlargement

Diffuse adrenal enlargement without metastatic adrenal involvement has been demonstrated in patients with malignant disease, including lymphoma, not known to produce ectopic ACTH (Figs. 44.12 and 44.13). The glands enlarge uniformly with preservation of the normal shape of the adrenal gland and without CT evidence of focal or multifocal masses. It is thought to be due to adrenal hyperplasia and is not related either to the site of primary disease or the stage of disease.[77] These patients can be shown not to suppress serum cortisol levels on a low-dose dexamethasone-suppression test, indicating that they are biochemically Cushingoid. Nevertheless, the ACTH levels are low, indicating that this phenomenon is not due to ectopic ACTH but is mediated through some other factor.[78]

Summary

- The adrenal glands are a relatively frequent site of metastatic disease

- Demonstration of adrenal metastasis almost always indicates Stage IV disease

- Adrenal metastases have to be distinguished from other adrenal masses, particularly adenomas

- CT and MR have a high specificity for benign adrenal adenomas

- Whole-body [18]FDG PET has a high specificity for malignant adrenal masses

- When an adrenal mass remains indeterminate on non-invasive imaging, percutaneous adrenal biopsy may be required

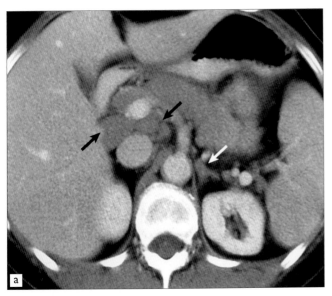
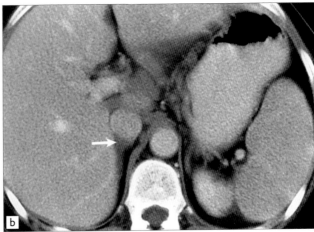

Figure 44.12. *Lymphadenopathy (black arrows in a) due to lymphoma with bilateral adrenal hyperplasia: of the (a) left (arrow) and (b) right adrenal gland (arrow). This patient failed to suppress on a low-dose dexamethasone-suppression test but the ACTH level was undetectable, indicating that the patient was biochemically Cushingoid and that this was not due to ectopic ACTH production.*

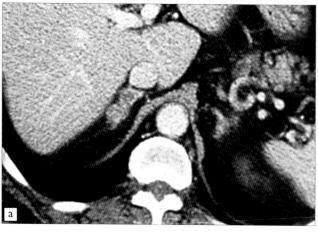

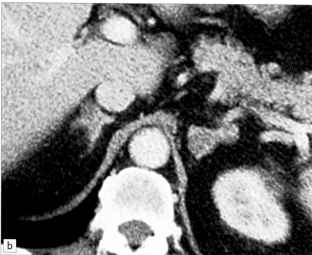

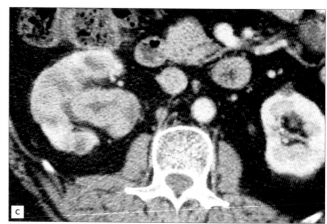

Figure 44.13. *Bilateral adrenal hyperplasia in a patient with transitional cell carcinoma of the right renal pelvis. (a and b) Contrast-enhanced CT scans showing bilateral nodular enlargement of the adrenal glands. (c) Contrast-enhanced CT scan showing the primary tumour expanding the right renal pelvis and extending into the proximal ureter and the renal cortex.*

References

1. Abrahams H L, Spiro R, Goldstein N. Metastases in carcinoma. Cancer 1950; 3: 74–85
2. Cho S Y, Choi H Y. Causes of death and metastatic patterns in patients with mammary cancer. Am J Clin Pathol 1986; 73: 232–234
3. Sahagian-Edwards A, Holland J F. Metastatic carcinoma of the adrenal glands with cortical hypofunction. Cancer 1954; 7: 1242–1245
4. Das Gupta T, Brasfield R. Metastatic melanoma. A clinicopathological study. Cancer 1964; 17: 1323–1339
5. Cedermark B J, Blumenson L E, Pickren J W et al. The significance of metastases to the adrenal glands in adenocarcinoma of the colon and rectum. Surg Gynaecol Obstet 1977; 144: 537–546
6. Campbell C M, Middleton R G, Rigby O F. Adrenal metastases in renal cell carcinoma. Urology 1983; 21: 403–405
7. Moriya T, Manabe T, Yamashita K, Arita S. Lung cancer metastases to adrenocortical adenomas. A chance occurrence or a predilected phenomenon? Arch Pathol Lab Med 1988; 112: 286–289
8. McMahon R F. Tumor to tumor metastases: bladder carcinoma metastasising to an adrenocortical adenoma. Br J Urol 1991; 67: 216–217
9. Travis W D, Oertel J E, Lack E E. Miscellaneous tumors and tumefaction lesions of the adrenal gland. In: Lack E E (ed). Pathology of the Adrenal Glands. New York: Churchill Livingstone, 1990; 351–378
10. Allard P, Yankaskas B C, Fletcher R H et al. Sensitivity and specificity of CT for the detection of adrenal metastatic lesions among 91 autopsied lung cancer patients. Cancer 1990; 66: 457–462
11. Pagani J J. Normal adrenal glands in small cell lung carcinoma: CT-guided biopsy. Am J Roentgenol 1983; 140: 949–951
12. Vincent J M, Morrison I D, Armstrong P, Reznek R H. The size of normal adrenal glands on computed tomography. Clin Radiol 1994; 49: 453–455
13. Gillams A, Roberts C M, Shaw P et al. The value of CT scanning and percutaneous fine needle aspiration of adrenal masses in biopsy-proven lung cancer. Clin Radiol 1992; 46: 18–22

14. Reinig J W, Doppman J L, Dwyer A J et al. Adrenal masses differentiated by MR. Radiology 1986; 158: 81–84
15. Kier R, McCarthy S. MR characterization of adrenal masses: field strength and pulse sequence considerations. Radiology 1989; 171: 671–674
16. Ghandur-Mnaymneh L, Slim M, Muakassa K. Adrenal cysts: pathogenesis and histological identification with a report of six cases. J Urol 1979; 122: 87–91
17. Dunnick N R, Heaston D, Halvorsen R et al. CT appearance of adrenal cortical carcinoma. J Comput Assist Tomogr 1982; 6: 978–982
18. Fishman E K, Deutch B M, Hartman D S et al. Primary adrenocortical carcinoma. CT evaluation with clinical correlation. Am J Roentgenol 1987; 148: 531–535
19. Manger W M, Gifford R W, Hoffman B B. Phaeochromocytoma: a clinical and experimental overview. Curr Probl Cancer 185; 9: 1–89
20. Cyran K M, Kenney P J, Mernel D S, Yacoub I. Adrenal myelolipoma. Am J Roentgenol 1996; 166: 395–400
21. Dobbie J W. Adenocortical nodular hyperplasia: the aging adrenal. J Pathol 1969; 99: 1
22. Oliver T W Jr, Bernardino M E, Miller J I et al. Isolated adrenal masses in non-small-cell bronchogenic carcinoma. Radiology 1984; 153: 217–218
23. Commons R R, Callaway C P. Adenomas of the adrenal cortex. Arch Intern Med 1984; 81: 37–41
24. Glazer H S, Weyman P J, Sagel S S et al. Non-functioning adrenal masses: incidental discovery on computed tomography. Am J Roentgenol 1982; 139: 81–85
25. Ambos M A, Bosniak M A, Lefleur R S, Mitty H A. Adrenal adenoma associated with renal cell carcinoma. Am J Roentgenol 1981; 136: 81–84
26. Doppman J L, Travis W D, Nieman L et al. Cushing syndrome due to primary pigmented nodular adreno cortical disease: findings at CT and MR imaging. Radiology 1989; 172: 415–420
27. Gross M D, Wilton G P, Shapiro B et al. Functional and scintigraphic evaluation of the silent adrenal mass. J Nucl Med 1987; 28: 1401–1407
28. Candel A G, Gattuso P, Reyes C V et al. Fine needle aspiration of adrenal masses in patients with extraadrenal malignancy. Surgery 1993; 114: 1132–1137
29. McGahan J P. Adrenal gland: MR imaging. Radiology 1988; 166: 284–285
30. Korobkin M, Brodeur F J, Yutzy G G et al. Differentiation of adrenal adenomas from nonadenomas using CT attenuation values. Am J Roentgenol 1996; 166: 531–536
31. Lee M J, Hahn P F, Papanicolaou N et al. Benign and malignant adrenal masses: CT distinction with attenuation coefficients, size, and observer analysis. Radiology 1991; 179: 415–418
32. van Erkel A R, van Gils A P G, Lequin M et al. CT and MR distinction of adenomas and nonadenomas of the adrenal gland. J Comput Assist Tomogr 1994; 18: 432–438
33. Katz R L, Shirkhoda A. Diagnostic approach to incidental adrenal nodules in the cancer patient. Cancer 1985; 55: 1995–2000
34. Boland G W L, Lee M J, Gazelle S G et al. Characterization of adrenal masses using enhanced CT: an analysis of the CT literature. Am J Roentgenol 1998;171: 201–204
35. Boland G W L, Hahn P F, Pena C, Mueller P R. Adrenal masses: characterization with delayed contrast-enhanced CT. Radiology 1997; 202: 693–696
36. Korobkin M, Brodeur F J, Francis I R et al. Delayed enhanced CT for the differentiation of benign from malignant masses. Radiology 1996; 200: 737–742
37. Szolar D H, Kammerhuber F. Quantitative CT evaluation of adrenal gland masses: a step forward in the differentiation between adenomas and nonadenomas? Radiology 1997; 202: 517–522
38. Korobkin M, Brodeur F J, Francis I R et al. CT time-attenuation washout curves of adrenal adenomas and nonadenomas. Am J Roentgenol 1998; 170: 747–752
39. Szolar D H, Kammerhuber F H. Adrenal adenomas and nonadenomas: assessment of washout at delayed contrast-enhanced CT. Radiology 1998; 207: 369–375.
40. Dunnick N R, Korobkin M. Imaging of adrenal incidentalomas: current status. Am J Roentgenol 2002; 179: 559–568
41. Pena C S, Boland G W L, Hahn P F et al. Characterization of indeterminate (lipid poor) adrenal masses: use of washout characteristics at contrast-enhanced CT. Radiology 2000; 217: 798–802
42. Baker M E, Blinder R, Spritzer C et al. MR evaluation of adrenal masses at 1.5T. Am J Roentgenol 1989; 153: 307–312
43. Semelka R C. Adrenal glands. Abdominal-pelvic MRI. New York: Wiley-Liss, 2002: 695–740
44. Chang A, Glazer H C, Lee J K T, Heiken J P. Adrenal gland MR imaging. Radiology 1987; 163: 123–128
45. Remer E M, Weinfeld R M, Glazer G M et al. Hyperfunctioning and nonhyperfunctioning benign adrenal cortical lesions: characterization and comparison with MR imaging. Radiology 1989; 171: 681–685
46. Glazer G M, Woolsey E J, Borrello J et al. Adrenal tissue characterization using MR imaging. Radiology 1986; 158: 73–79
47. Baker M E, Spritzer C, Blinder R et al. Benign adrenal lesions mimicking malignancy on MR imaging: report of two cases. Radiology 1987; 163: 669–671
48. Krestin G P, Steinbrich W, Friedman G. Adrenal masses: evaluation with fast gradient-echo MR imaging and Gd DTPA-enhanced dynamic studies. Radiology 1989; 171: 675–680
49. Krestin G P, Friedman G, Fischbach R et al. Evaluation of adrenal masses in oncologic patients: dynamic contrast-enhanced MR vs CT. J Comput Assist Tomogr 1991; 15: 104–110
50. Semelka R C, Shoenut J P, Lawrence P H et al. Evaluation of adrenal masses with gadolinium

enhancement and fat-suppressed MR imaging. J Magn Reson Imaging 1993; 3: 332–343

51. Chung J J, Semelka R C, Martin D R. Adrenal adenomas: characteristic postgadolinium capillary blush on dynamic MR imaging. J Magn Reson Imaging 2001;13: 242–248

52. Ichikawa T, Ohtomo K, Uchiyama G et al. Adrenal adenomas: characteristic hyperintense rim sign on fat-saturated spin-echo MR images. Radiology 1994; 193: 247–250

53. Mitchell D G, Crovello M, Matteucci T et al. Benign adrenocortical masses: diagnosis with chemical shift MR imaging. Radiology 1992; 185: 345–351

54. Tsushima Y, Ishizaka H, Matsumoto M. Adrenal masses: differentiation with chemical shift, fast low-angle shot MR imaging. Radiology 1993; 186: 705–709

55. Bilbey J H, McLoughlin R F, Kurkjian P S et al. MR imaging of adrenal masses: value of chemical-shift imaging for distinguishing adenomas from other tumors. Am J Roentgenol 1995; 164: 637–642

56. Mayo-Smith W W, Lee M J, McNicholas M M J et al. Characterization of adrenal masses (<5 cm) by use of chemical shift MR imaging: observer performance versus quantitative measures. Am J Roentgenol 1995; 165: 91–95

57. Korobkin M, Lombardi T J, Aisen A M et al. Characterization of adrenal masses with chemical shift and gadolinium-enhanced MR imaging. Radiology 1995; 197: 411–418

58. Schwartz L H, Panicek D M, Koutcher J A et al. Adrenal masses in patients with malignancy: prospective comparison of echo-planar, fast spin-echo, and chemical shift MR imaging. Radiology 1995; 197: 421–425

59. Korobkin M, Giordano T J, Brodeur F J et al. Adrenal adenomas: relationship between histologic lipid and CT and MR findings. Radiology.1996; 200: 743–747

60. Nicholas M M J, Lee M J, Mayo-Smith W W et al. An imaging algorithm for the differential diagnosis of adrenal adenomas and metastases. Am J Roentgenol 1995; 165: 1453–1459

61. Schlund J F, Kenney P J, Brown E D et al. Adrenocortical carcinoma: MR imaging appearance with current techniques. J MRI 1995; 5: 171–174

62. Tsushima Y. Different lipid contents between aldosterone-producing and nonhyperfunctioning adreno cortical adenomas: in vivo measurement using chemical shift MRI. J Clin Endocrin Metab 1994; 79: 1759–1762

63. Silverman S G, Mueler P R, Pinkney L P et al. Predictive value of image-guided adrenal biopsy: analysis of results of 101 biopsies. Radiology 1993; 187: 715–718

64. Kloss R T, Gross M D, Shapiro B et al. The diagnostic dilemma of small incidentally discovered adrenal masses: a role for 131-I-6[beta]-iodomethyl-norcholesterol(NP-59) scintigraphy. World J Surg 1997; 21: 36–40

65. Maurea S, Klain M, Mainolfi C et al. The diagnostic role of radionuclide imaging in evaluation of patients with nonhypersecreting adrenal masses. J Nucl Med 2001; 42: 884–892

66. Lowe V J, Naunheim K S. Current role of positron emission tomography in thoracic oncology. Thorax 1998; 53: 703–712

67. Erasmus J J, McAdams H P, Patz E F Jr. Non-small cell lung cancer: FDG-PET imaging. J Thorac Imag 1999; 14: 247–256

68. Erasmus J J, Patz E F Jr. Positron emission tomography imaging in the thorax. Clin Chest Med 1999; 20: 715–724

69. Yun M, Kim W, Alnafisi N et al. 18F-FDG PET in characterizing adrenal lesions detected on CT or MRI. J Nucl Med 2001; 42: 1797–1799

70. Bergstrom M, Bonasera T A, Lu L et al. In vitro and in vivo primate evaluation of C-11-etomidate and C-11-metomidate as potential tracers for PET imaging of the adrenal cortex and its tumors. J Nucl Med 1998; 39: 982–989

71. Bergstrom M, Juhlin C, Bonasera T A et al. PET imaging of adrenal cortical tumors with the 11beta-hydroxylase tracer 11C-metomidate. J Nucl Med 2000; 41: 275–282

72. Boland G W, Goldberg M A, Lee M J et al. Indeterminate adrenal masses in patients with cancer: evaluation at PET with 2-[F-18]-fluoro-2-deoxy-D-glucose. Radiology 1995; 194: 131–134

73. Harisinghani M G, Maher M M, Hahn P F et al. Predictive value of benign percutaneous adrenal biopsies in oncology patients. Clin Radiol 2002; 57: 898–901

74. Habscheid W, Pfeiffer M, Demmrich J, Muller H A. Metastases to the needle puncture track after ultrasound-guided fine needle adrenal biopsy. A rare complication? Dtsch Med Wochenschr 1990; 115: 212–215

75. Welch T J, Sheedy P F, Stephens D H et al. Percutaneous adrenal biopsy: review of a 10-year experience. Radiology 1994; 193: 341–344

76. Mody M K, Kazerooni E A, Korobkin M. Percutaneous CT-guided biopsy of adrenal masses: immediate and delayed complications. J Comput Assist Tomogr 1995; 19: 434–439

77. Vincent J M, Morrison I D, Armstrong P, Reznek R H. Computed tomography of diffuse, non-metastatic enlargement of the adrenal glands in patients with malignant disease. Clin Radiol 1994; 49: 456–460

78. Jenkins P J, Sohaib S A, Trainer P J et al. Adrenal enlargement and failure of suppression of circulating cortisol by dexamethasone in patients with malignancy. Br J Cancer 1999; 80: 1815–1819

Peritoneal metastases

Jeremiah C Healy and Rodney H Reznek

Introduction

The peritoneal cavity is the potential space between the visceral and parietal layers of the peritoneum. It consists of a main region, termed the greater sac, and a diverticulum, the omental bursa or lesser sac, situated behind the stomach. In early foetal life as the abdominal cavity divides into the retroperitoneum and peritoneum, the parietal peritoneum is reflected over the peritoneal organs to form a series of supporting ligaments, mesenteries and omenta. These peritoneal reflections act as a natural connecting pathway not only for the dissemination of intra-abdominal disease within the peritoneum, but also for extension of disease from the retroperitoneum to structures enveloped by peritoneum, via the subperitoneal space.[1]

The anatomy of the peritoneum can therefore be considered as a system of spaces and peritoneal reflections that can act as conduits for spread of metastatic disease, which is the most common malignant process involving the peritoneum (Fig. 45.1). Metastases are usually from intra-abdominal primary neoplasms, such as carcinoma of the stomach, colon, ovary or pancreas, or from intra-abdominal lymphoma.

Prior to the advent of CT, peritoneal metastases were not radiographically detectable until late in the disease, when they displaced adjacent organs, caused intestinal obstruction, or produced radiological signs due to massive ascites on plain films. CT can identify peritoneal metastases as small as a few millimetres in size and also identify very small volumes of ascites. This information is essential in staging tumours, assessing resectability, monitoring response, and identifying recurrence.

Imaging techniques

Computed tomography

Computed tomography is the best imaging procedure for the evaluation of patients with known or suspected peritoneal metastases. The use of intraperitoneal positive contrast and pneumoperitoneum with CT has been suggested to improve the detection of small peritoneal metastases but these techniques do not routinely opacify all the peritoneal recesses.[2–4] These methods are more interventional and time consuming and consequently are not widely used.

Barium studies

Barium studies provide only indirect signs of peritoneal and mesenteric disease and thus are not used initially. However, a barium study will occasionally reveal abnormalities related to peritoneal metastases that are not clearly demonstrated on CT.

Magnetic resonance imaging

Recent reports describe the use of MR imaging in identifying peritoneal implants.[5–7] MR of the peritoneum has been most successfully achieved using surface phased array or body coils. In addition to T1- and T2-weighted images, fat saturated T1-weighted sequences following intravenous gadolinium have been found to be most useful (Fig. 45.2e,f,g).[8,9] A recent report from the Radiological Diagnostic Oncology Group has shown that CT and MR are equally accurate in staging advanced ovarian cancer. MR is particularly good at showing peritoneal metastases on the surface of the liver that may have become invaginated within the liver (Fig. 45.3). At present, however, CT is more rapid, less prone to artefacts and more widely accessible as a staging tool for identifying peritoneal metastases. In addition, CT has superior spatial resolution to MR, and with the advent of multidetector CT, images can be reformatted in any plane without loss of resolution.

Ultrasound

Ultrasound will demonstrate superficial peritoneal and omental metastases as small as 2–3 mm in the presence of ascites. However, centrally located deposits, for example in the small mesentery, will not be visualized because of the acoustic impedance of bowel gas and fat.[10,11]

Scintigraphy

In oncological nuclear medicine, some attempts have been made to detect peritoneal metastases using tumour-specific monoclonal antibodies, but these techniques have limited use because of poor spatial resolution and the need for CT for anatomical location.[12] Positron emission tomography (PET) using 2-[F-18]fluoro-2-deoxy-D-glucose ([18]FDG) may be useful in detecting peritoneal metastases by demonstrating foci of increased uptake, thus facilitating their identification; however, low-volume peritoneal tumour 'seeding' is difficult to diagnose. In one study, [18]FDG-PET failed to show peritoneal lesions smaller than 1 cm.[13] Low-volume disease

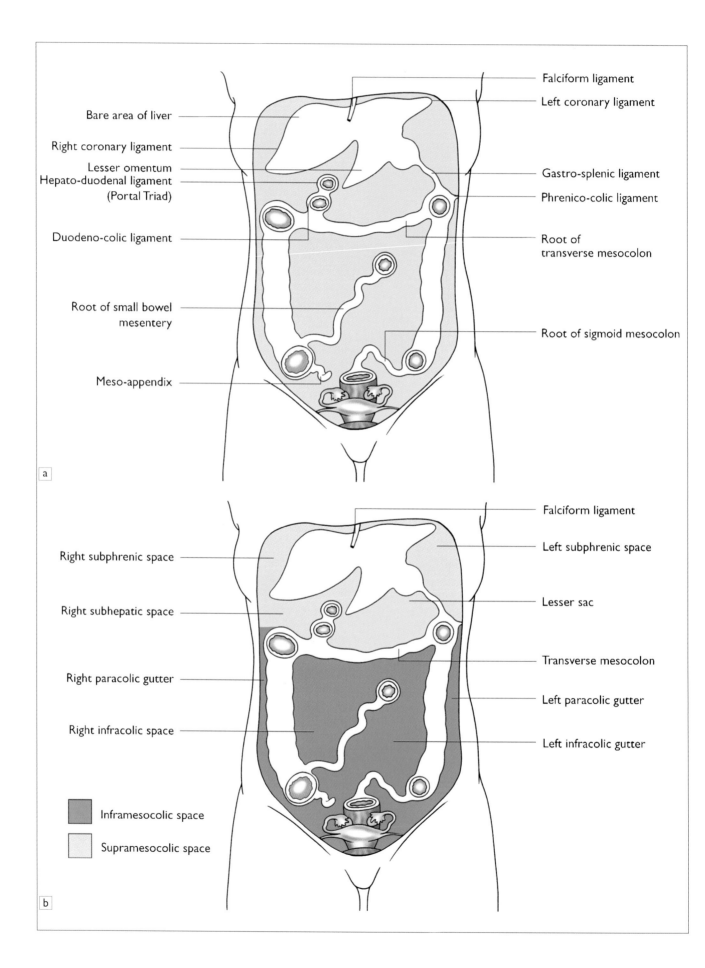

a

Falciform ligament

Left coronary ligament

Bare area of liver

Right coronary ligament

Lesser omentum
Hepato-duodenal ligament
(Portal Triad)

Gastro-splenic ligament

Phrenico-colic ligament

Duodeno-colic ligament

Root of
transverse mesocolon

Root of small bowel
mesentery

Root of sigmoid mesocolon

Meso-appendix

b

Falciform ligament

Left subphrenic space

Right subphrenic space

Right subhepatic space

Lesser sac

Transverse mesocolon

Right paracolic gutter

Left paracolic gutter

Right infracolic space

Left infracolic gutter

Inframesocolic space

Supramesocolic space

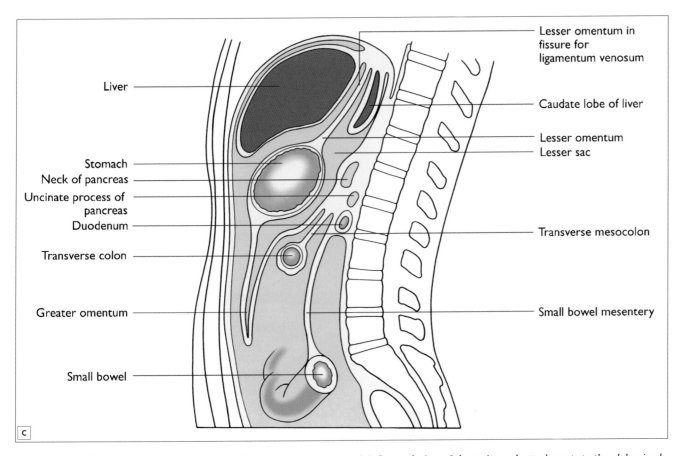

Figure 45.1. *Diagrammatic representation of the peritoneal anatomy. (a) Coronal view of the peritoneal attachments to the abdominal wall. (b) Coronal view of the posterior peritoneal spaces. (c) Mid-sagittal section through the upper abdomen to show the peritoneal spaces and mesenteries.*

is associated with patchy uptake, which may be attributed to normal uptake by bowel. It may be of value where conventional imaging modalities are inconclusive, especially in the context of colonic or ovarian recurrent cancer.[14] [18]FDG-PET also has limitations in detecting mucinous neoplasms (e.g. from colon or ovary) as they have low cellularity and do not display a hypermetabolic state of glucose.[15]

Key points: imaging techniques

- Although the overall sensitivity of CT in detecting peritoneal metastases is less than 50%, the specificity exceeds 85% and the sensitivity is much improved in peritoneal deposits greater than 1 cm

- CT can guide biopsy, reducing the need for laparoscopy, laparotomy and the need to identify the primary site of disease

- MR imaging has a similar sensitivity and specificity to CT for the detection of peritoneal metastases

- Although ultrasound can detect extremely small peritoneal deposits in the presence of ascites, centrally located deposits (e.g. in the small bowel mesentery) will usually be obscured

- [18]FDG-PET may be of value where conventional imaging modalities are inconclusive, especially in the context of colonic or ovarian recurrent cancer

- [18]FDG-PET has limitations in detecting mucinous neoplasms (e.g. from colon or ovary) as they have low cellularity and do not display a hypermetabolic state of glucose

Modes of spread and imaging appearances

Metastases spread throughout the peritoneum in four ways:

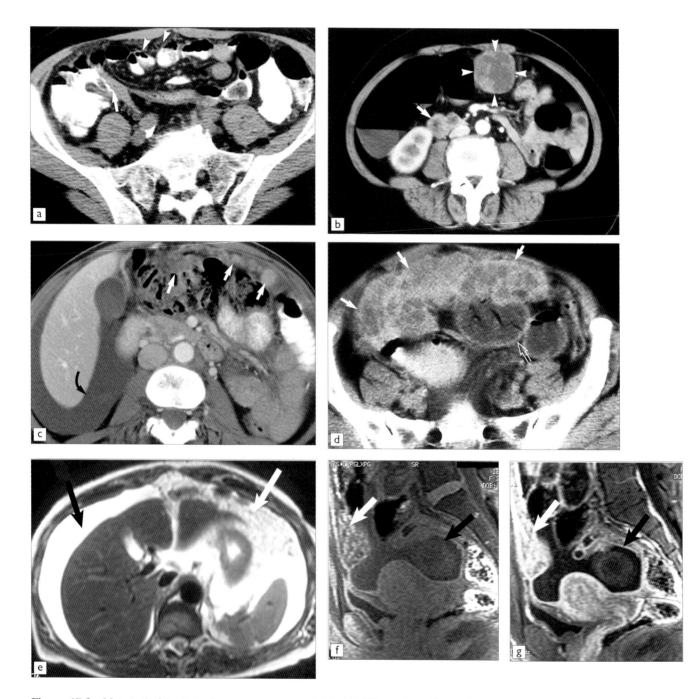

Figure 45.2. *Metastatic deposits in the greater omentum. (a) Axial CT scan in a 42-year-old male with a carcinoid tumour of the terminal ileum (arrow) showing minimal nodular and linear deposits in the greater omental fat (arrowheads). (b) Postcontrast axial CT scan in a 65-year-old female with carcinoma of the ovary showing a well-defined, round mass in the greater omentum, with fluid attenuation centrally (arrowheads). Note also precaval enlarged lymphadenopathy (arrow). (c) Postcontrast axial CT scan in a 49-year-old female with carcinoma of the ovary showing several nodular, ill-defined masses in the greater omentum anterior to the colon (white arrows). Note also the ascites surrounding the right lobe of the liver (black arrow). (d) Axial postcontrast CT scan in a 66-year-old female with adenocarcinoma of the bowel showing a bulky, 'cake-like', enhancing omental deposit (arrows). (e) Axial T2-weighted MR in a 62-year-old female patient with ovarian cancer showing extensive ascites in the upper abdomen (black arrow) and intermediate signal peritoneal metastases within the greater omentum (white arrow). (f) Sagittal T1-weighted MR with fat saturation in the same patient as (e) showing peritoneal metastases of intermediate signal intensity within the greater omentum (white arrow) with thickening of the visceral peritoneum (black arrow) surrounding ascites within the pelvis. (g) Sagittal T1-weighted MRI with fat saturation after intravenous gadolinium in the same patient as (e) and (f) showing marked enhancement of the peritoneal metastases within the greater omentum (white arrow) and enhancement of the peritoneal thickening elsewhere (black arrow) indicating metastatic disease.*

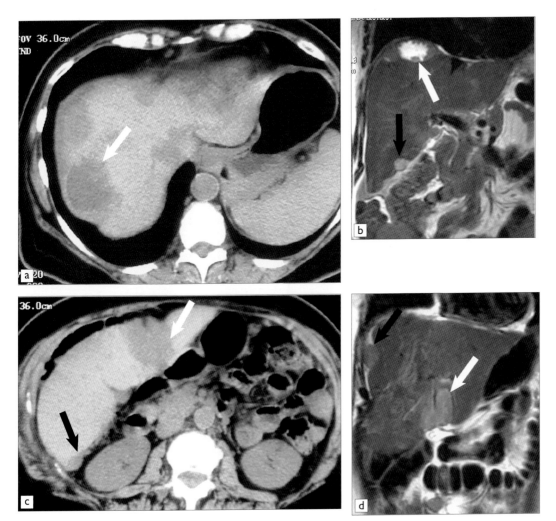

Figure 45.3. *Peritoneal metastases on the surface of the liver in a 64-year-old female with ovarian cancer. (a) Axial precontrast CT showing several low attenuation lesions in the liver. The largest lesion (white arrow) appears intrahepatic on the axial CT scan. (b) On coronal T2-weighted MR, this lesion is shown to lie on the superior surface of the liver. It appears predominantly cystic (white arrow) with surrounding intermediate soft tissue extending over the superior surface of the liver. In addition there is a further peritoneal deposit of intermediate signal intensity on the inferior surface of the right lobe (black arrow). (c) Axial precontrast CT in the same patient shows a low attenuation lesion within what appears to be the left lobe of the liver (white arrow). (d) On coronal T2-weighted MR, this lesion is shown to lie within the falciform ligament extending to the surface of the liver (white arrow). Note also a further peritoneal metastasis on the superior surface of the right lobe of the liver (black arrow).*

- Directly along peritoneal ligaments, mesenteries and omenta to non-contiguous structures
- Intraperitoneal seeding via the flow of ascitic fluid
- Lymphatic extension
- Embolic haematogenous spread[16]

Direct spread

Direct invasion from primary tumours to non-contiguous organs occurs along the peritoneal reflections (Figs. 45.1b and 45.1c). These include:

- Eight ligaments – the right and left coronary, falciform, hepatoduodenal, duodenocolic, gastrosplenic, splenorenal, and phrenicocolic ligaments
- Four mesenteries – the small bowel mesentery, the transverse mesocolon, the sigmoid mesocolon, and the mesoappendix
- Two omenta – the lesser and greater omentum[16,17]

Spread along these peritoneal reflections is commonly seen with malignant neoplasms of the stomach, colon, pancreas and ovary.

Appearances on CT

Carcinoma of the stomach often spreads directly into the left lobe of the liver via the lesser omentum, extending between the lesser curvature of the stomach and the liver (Figs. 45.1b and 45.1c, Fig 45.4).[18] CT shows loss of the fat plane between these two organs.[19] Direct spread from retroperitoneal tumours, such as carcinoma of the pancreas, into the liver can occur along the hepatoduodenal ligament, which is the free edge of the lesser omentum, extending from the junction of the first and second parts of the duodenum to the porta hepatis. The portal vein, hepatic artery and common bile duct are found within this ligament (Fig. 45.1b).[20,21] Biliary and hepatic malignancies can also spread in the reverse direction to the stomach and pancreas via the lesser omentum and hepatoduodenal ligaments. On CT these masses are often hypervascular and may have low attenuation centrally due to central necrosis.[22,23]

Neoplasms of the colon, stomach, and pancreas often use the transverse mesocolon and greater omentum as conduits for spread (Figs. 45.1b and 45.1c).

The transverse mesocolon suspends the transverse colon within the peritoneal cavity, passing anterior to the descending duodenum and pancreas (Figs. 45.1b and 45.1c). It is continuous in the left upper quadrant with the splenorenal and phrenicocolic ligaments (Fig. 45.1b). Direct invasion is well demonstrated on CT as increased density or discrete soft tissue masses in the fat of the transverse mesocolon. The right hand margin of the transverse mesocolon is thickened as the duodenocolic ligament providing a direct route for extension of colonic cancer from the hepatic flexure to the duodenum.[24,25]

The greater omentum extends from the greater curve of the stomach and suspends the transverse colon (Fig. 45.1c). On CT early involvement of the greater omentum produces increased density within the fat adjacent to the primary neoplasm (Fig. 45.2a). Subsequently, masses contiguous with the primary neoplasm may be seen extending into the greater omentum, producing 'omental caking', which separates the colon from the anterior abdominal wall (Figs. 45.2c and 45.2d). Spread of metastatic disease along the left hand margin of the greater omentum stops abruptly at the phrenicocolic ligament, extending from the splenic flexure to the diaphragm. It marks the point at which the mesenteric transverse colon becomes the extraperitoneal descending colon.

In the left upper quadrant the gastrosplenic ligament (Fig. 45.1b), continuous with the greater omentum, extends from the greater curve of the stomach to the spleen. It can be involved by extramural spread from gastric cancer and explains the association of splenic abscess with this, often seen on CT.[26]

Direct involvement of the small bowel mesentery is commonly seen in carcinoid (Fig. 45.5a,b), lymphoma, pancreatic, breast and colonic metastases.

The root of the small bowel mesentery is approximately 15 cm long, extending from the pancreas to the right iliac fossa (Figs. 45.1b and 45.1c). Spread from the retroperitoneum, via the subperitoneal space, to the small bowel is frequently seen in lymphoma. On CT, this produces soft tissue thickening within the mesenteric fat, perivascular encasement, and tethering of the bowel.

Appearances on barium studies

Direct invasion along the transverse mesocolon from pancreatic cancer produces tethering and pseudosacculation of the posterior–inferior margin of the colon on barium

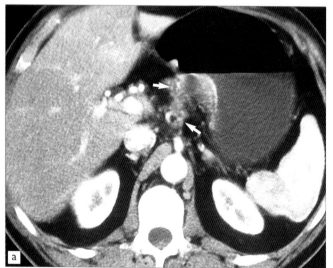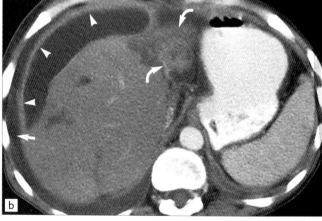

Figure 45.4. *Metastatic deposits in the lesser omentum. (a) Axial post-contrast CT scan in a 59-year-old male with gastric cancer showing extension of gastric cancer into the lesser omental fat (arrows). (b) Axial post-contrast CT scan in a 41-year-old female with carcinoma of the ovary, showing a large metastatic deposit in the lesser omentum (curved arrows). Note also ascites with marked uniform peritoneal thickening (arrowheads) and a right pleural effusion (straight arrow).*

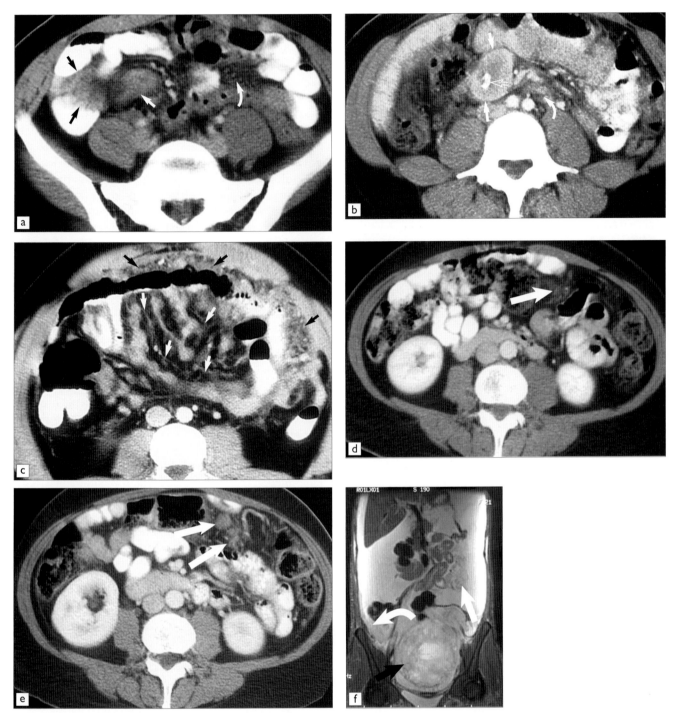

Figure 45.5. *Small bowel mesenteric deposits. (a) Postcontrast axial CT scan in a 28-year-old female with carcinoid tumour of the terminal ileum (straight black arrows). Note the large mesenteric mass at the root of the small bowel mesentery (straight white arrows) and linear soft tissue stranding in the small bowel mesenteric fat elsewhere (curved white arrows). (b) The same patient as in Figure 45.5a demonstrating a mesenteric deposit (straight arrows) containing calcification (open arrow). There are also ill-defined masses elsewhere within the mesenteric fat (curved arrow). (c) Axial postcontrast CT scan in a 70-year-old male with adenocarcinoma of the colon showing soft tissue thickening around the perivascular bundles (white arrows). In addition, note the ill-defined omental 'cake' in the greater omentum (black arrows). (d) Axial postcontrast CT scan in a 62-year-old female with ovarian cancer showing subtle increased attenuation in the small bowel mesentery suspicious for early, low volume peritoneal metastases (white arrow). (e) Same patient as in (d) 4 months later demonstrating disease progression with several mass-like peritoneal metastases in the small bowel mesentery at the site of previous minimal disease (arrow). (f) Coronal T2-weighted MR in a 56-year-old female with ovarian cancer showing high signal peritoneal metastatic disease in the small bowel mesentery suspending small bowel loops (white arrow). The ovarian cancer can be seen as a high signal mass in the pelvis (black arrow). Note also visceral peritoneal metastases in the right iliac fossa (white curved arrow).*

studies. This is because the transverse mesocolon inserts into the taenia mesocolica on the inferior margin of the colon. Direct spread of gastric cancer along the greater omentum causes similar appearances along the superior haustral margin of the transverse colon, as the greater omentum inserts superiorly into the taenia omentalis.[27]

Intraperitoneal seeding

Intraperitoneal fluid is constantly circulating throughout the abdomen influenced by gravity and negative intra-abdominal pressure, produced beneath the diaphragm during respiration. It allows transcoelomic dissemination of malignant cells: their deposition, fixation and growth are encouraged in particular sites due to relative stasis of ascitic fluid.[28]

The tumours that most commonly spread in this fashion include ovarian cancer in females and malignancies of the gastrointestinal tract in males, especially cancer of the stomach, colon and pancreas.

The sites most commonly involved by peritoneal seeding are (Fig. 45.1a):

- The pelvis, especially the pouch of Douglas
- The right lower quadrant at the inferior junction of the small bowel mesentery
- The superior aspect of the sigmoid mesocolon
- The right paracolic gutter[28]

Spread of deposits to the right subhepatic and subphrenic spaces is also frequently seen, especially in ovarian cancer. Almost 90% of patients with ovarian cancer have peritoneal implants at postmortem and 60–70% have ascites.[29,30]

CT and MR appearances

On CT, seeded metastases appear as nodular or plaque-like soft tissue masses in association with ascites. Intraperitoneal deposits as small as 5 mm can be identified, even in the presence of small amounts of ascites.[31–33] Rounded or oval low density deposits on the surface of the liver are frequently seen on CT in ovarian cancer, and these may appear partially cystic on MR (Figs. 45.3, 45.6).[34] MR is particularly sensitive for identifying peritoneal metastases on the surface of the liver, which may appear intrahepatic on CT (Fig. 45.3). These are generally of 0.5–1 cm diameter, located on the dorsomedial and dorsolateral parts of the right lobe of the liver and often associated with deposits in Morison's pouch (Figs. 45.3b and 45.6b). The parietal peritoneum may be diffusely involved producing smooth (Figs. 45.2f, 45.2g and 45.4b) or nodular thickening (Figs. 45.7a and 45.7c) on CT that often enhances (Figs. 45.7b).[35] Peritoneal calcification is also frequently seen on CT with serous cystadenocarcinoma of the ovary (especially after treatment) (Fig. 45.7c), carcinoid, and rarely with gastric carcinoma.[36–38] Calcification may also be seen diffusely along the peritoneum following successful treatment of ovarian cancer (Fig. 45.7d).

A distinctive CT appearance is produced by *pseudomyxoma peritonei*, resulting from the rupture of a mucinous cystadenocarcinoma or cystadenoma of the ovary or appendix (Figs. 45.8a and 45.8b). The gelatinous nature of the deposits produces a mantle of low-density material over the surface of the liver, causing scalloping of its margin, in association with cystic peritoneal collections (Fig. 45.8a). The walls of the cystic collections may contain calcification. The pressure of the gelatinous material prevents the bowel loops floating up towards the anterior abdominal wall, which may be a useful sign in differentiating pseudomyxoma peritonei from ascites (Fig. 45.8b).[39]

The *small bowel mesentery and greater omentum* are frequently involved by intraperitoneal seeding of metastases. Four patterns of involvement are described on CT: round masses (Fig. 45.2b), 'cake-like' masses (Figs. 45.2c, 45.2d

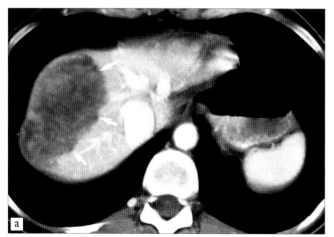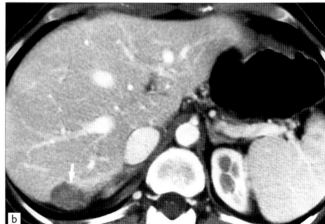

Figure 45.6. *Intraperitoneal seeding producing metastatic deposits on the surface of the liver in a 52-year-old female with carcinoma of the ovary. (a) Axial postcontrast CT scan shows a large, low density, ill-defined deposit on the superior surface of the liver (arrows). (b) This is associated with a low density cystic deposit in Morison's pouch (arrow).*

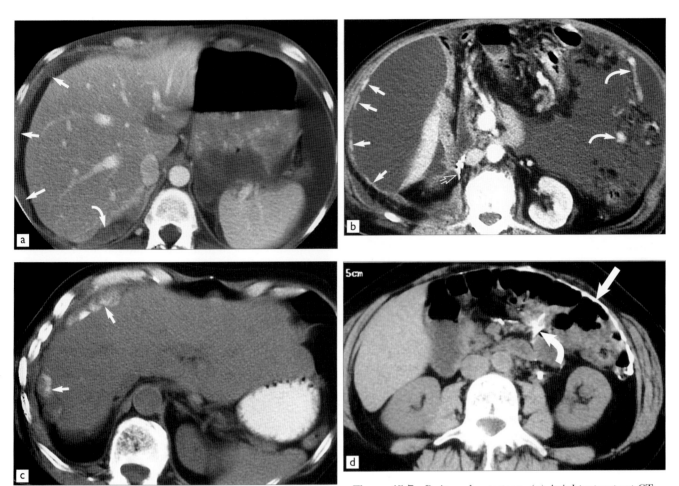

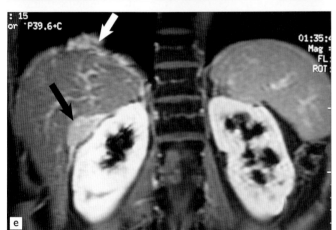

Figure 45.7. *Peritoneal metastases. (a) Axial postcontrast CT scan in a 49-year-old female with carcinoma of the ovary demonstrating nodular parietal peritoneal thickening (straight arrows) in association with a deposit in Morison's pouch (curved arrow) and ascites. (b) Axial postcontrast CT scan in the same patient as in Figure 45.2d. Note the clips from previous renal surgery (open arrow). Multiple enhancing peritoneal metastases are outlined by ascites (straight arrows). Note also enhancing deposits in the greater omental fat (curved arrows). (c) Axial CT scan in a 66-year-old female with carcinoma of the ovary showing calcified peritoneal metastases (arrows). (d) Axial CT in a 60-year-old female with treated ovarian cancer showing extensive calcification in the greater omentum (white straight arrow) and small bowel mesentery (white curved arrow) at the site of previous disease. (e) Coronal T2-weighted MRI scan in a 65-year-old female with ovarian cancer showing intermediate signal peritoneal metastases in the hepatorenal fossa (Morison's pouch) (black arrow) and on the superior surface of the liver (white arrow).*

and 45.2e), ill-defined masses (Figs. 45.5e and 45.5f), and stellate masses.[40] CT can pick up small volume disease as subtle increased attenuation within the mesenteric or omental fat (Figs. 45.5d and 45.5e). On MR, omental/mesenteric masses produce masses of intermediate signal intensity, which lower the high signal intensity of normal fat on T1- and T2-weighted images (Figs. 45.2e and 45.5f). These metastases may enhance markedly on T1-weighted images with fat saturation following intravenous gadolinium (Figs. 45.2f and 45.2g).

Irregular, 'cake-like' masses are seen most often with ovarian cancer.[41] Densely calcified omental 'cake' has been

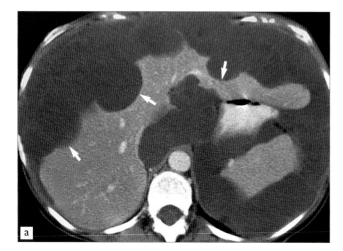

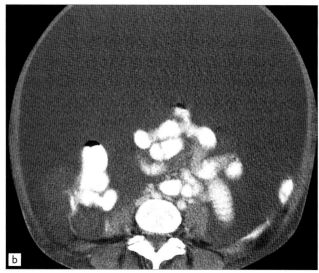

Figure 45.8. *Pseudomyxoma peritonei in mucinous cystadenocarcinoma of the appendix in a 44-year-old female. (a) Axial postcontrast CT scan shows low density deposits producing scalloping of the liver margin (arrows). (b) The pressure of the gelatinous material prevents bowel loops floating up towards the anterior abdominal wall.*

reported in metastatic serous cystadenocarcinoma.[42] The stellate pattern of mesenteric or omental mass is seen with pancreatic, colonic and breast cancer and results from diffuse infiltration, causing thickening and rigidity of the perivascular bundles (Fig. 45.5c). Widespread peritoneal metastases including omental infiltration are a rare consequence of retroperitoneal malignancy, such as renal cell carcinoma (Figs. 45.2d and 45.7b).[43]

Metastatic deposits to the ovaries from gastric or colonic primary tumours in association with ascites and other peritoneal deposits are a well-recognized entity. These tumours, known as '*Krukenberg*' tumours, are presumed to be a consequence of transcoelomic spread and are clearly visualized on CT.[44]

A recent report demonstrated the use of CT in guiding

peritoneal core biopsy, particularly from the greater omentum. Image-guided peritoneal biopsy provides sufficient tissue to identify the primary site and guide treatment in most patients without recourse to laparoscopy or laparotomy. It also limits the need for investigation to exclude primary tumours at other sites.[45]

Appearances on barium studies
Metastatic seeding in the pouch of Douglas produces a characteristic nodular mucosal impression on barium enema, with associated mucosal tethering on the ventral aspect of the rectosigmoid junction.

Metastatic seeding in the small bowel mesentery, especially in the right infracolic space, can produce separation of small bowel loops in a parallel configuration, known as 'palisading', on barium follow-through studies. Marked bowel angulation and mucosal tethering is also seen if the deposits stimulate a desmoplastic response, which is commonly seen with pancreatic carcinoma and mucin-secreting gastric carcinoma.

Lymphatic metastases
Lymphatic metastases play a minor role in the intraperitoneal dissemination of metastatic carcinoma but are very important in the spread of lymphoma to mesenteric lymph nodes. Almost 50% of patients with non-Hodgkin's lymphoma will have mesenteric nodes at presentation, compared to only 5% of patients with Hodgkin's disease.[46] On CT, mesenteric lymph node involvement in lymphoma produces round or oval masses in the mesenteric fat that may displace adjacent loops of bowel.[40] Large conglomerations of lymph nodes may surround the superior mesenteric artery and vein on CT and demonstrate the so-called 'sandwich sign' in which lymphomatous mesenteric masses are separated from retroperitoneal lymphadenopathy by an intact anterior pararenal fat plane.[40,47]

Embolic metastases
The abdomen is a common site for haematogenous metastases from both intra-abdominal and extra-abdominal primary tumours. The emboli spread via the mesenteric arteries to deposit on the antemesenteric border of the bowel in the smallest arterial branches, where they grow into mural nodules.

The tumours that most commonly metastasize embolically to bowel and the peritoneal reflections are melanoma, breast and lung cancer. These metastases often occur several years after treatment of the primary neoplasm. Occasionally bowel obstruction or intussusception, as a consequence of embolic metastases, may be the first manifestation of an occult malignancy.

CT appearances
On CT, embolic metastases may produce thickening of the bowel wall, which is often asymmetric with associated ulceration, and thickening of the adjacent bowel wall.[48] They

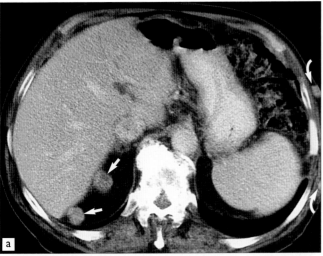

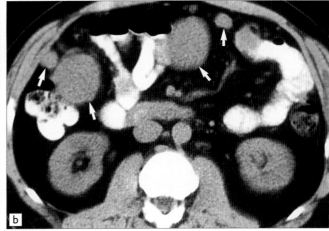

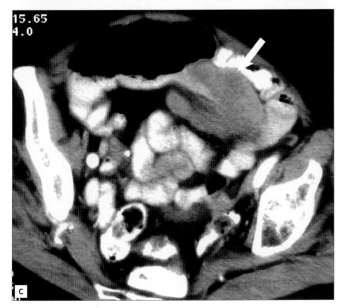

Figure 45.9. *Embolic metastases. (a) Postcontrast axial CT scan in a 60-year-old male with malignant melanoma showing well-defined embolic deposits in Morison's pouch (straight arrows). Note the subcutaneous melanomatous deposits in the left flank (curved arrows). (b) Axial CT scan in a 40-year-old male with leiomyosarcoma of the retroperitoneum showing multiple, well-defined, soft tissue masses adjacent to the bowel in the mesenteric fat (arrows). (c) Axial postcontrast CT in a 45-year-old male with malignant melanoma demonstrating a hypervascular serosal metastasis enveloping the small bowel (arrow) and causing small bowel obstruction.*

may also appear as well-defined round masses within the peritoneal fat (Figs. 45.9a and 45.9b). Embolic metastases to the stomach from breast cancer produce marked gastric wall thickening with almost complete obliteration of its lumen, an appearance that is indistinguishable from primary scirrhous gastric carcinoma or lymphoma.[49] Embolic metastases can envelop the serosal surface of the bowel, presenting with bowel obstruction (Fig. 45.9c).

Appearances on barium studies

On barium studies embolic metastases produce a 'bull's-eye' appearance due to their submucosal site. Their borders are usually well defined with central ulceration, and sometimes linear fissuring gives a 'spoke-wheel' pattern. They grow eccentrically with bulky extension into the lumen of the bowel. Larger lesions may undergo necrosis to produce apparent aneurysmal dilatation of the bowel.[50]

Embolic metastases to the stomach from breast produce a marked 'linitis plastica' appearance, with thickened and angulated gastric folds and diminished or absent peristalsis.

Key points: imaging techniques

- Malignant spread to the peritoneum occurs directly along peritoneal ligaments, mesenteries and omenta, through seeding via the flow of ascitic fluid, via lymphatic extension and haematogenously

- Seeding of cells most commonly occurs in the pelvis (especially the pouch of Douglas), at the inferior junction of the small bowel mesentery, the superior aspect of the sigmoid mesocolon, and the right paracolic gutter

■ Embolic metastases to bowel and peritoneal reflections occur most commonly in tumours arising in the breast and lung, and in malignant melanoma

■ Lymphatic spread plays only a small role in the spread of malignant disease to the peritoneum and its reflections

Accuracy of CT in identifying peritoneal metastases

The CT identification of peritoneal metastases has been correlated with second-look laparotomy. The specificity of CT for the diagnosis of peritoneal metastases is high, ranging from 85 to 87%; however its sensitivity is low, ranging from 42 to 47%.[51,52]

Laparoscopy has also demonstrated a significant incidence of peritoneal metastases in patients with a negative CT scan. Notably, if ascites is present but no peritoneal deposits are seen on CT, laparoscopy demonstrates deposits in 75% of cases.[53]

Spiral CT has greatly improved the sensitivity for detecting peritoneal metastases. A recent study using spiral CT has reported areas under the receiver operating characteristic (ROC) curve of 0.89–0.95 for the detection of peritoneal metastases.[54] Overall sensitivities ranged from 85 to 93%, specificities ranged from 78 to 91%, positive predictive value (PPV) was 88–95%, and negative predictive value (NPV) 78–88%. For implants less than 1 cm, the reader sensitivities were significantly lower, ranging from 25 to 50%.

Accuracy of MR in identifying peritoneal metastases

The Radiological Diagnostic Oncology Group has recently compared MR and CT in staging advanced ovarian cancer.[8] In their study, 62% (n = 73) of patients had Stage III or IV disease. Peritoneal metastases were found in 59% (n = 70) of these patients. MR and CT had similar areas under the ROC curves of 0.96 for the identification of peritoneal metastases. The sensitivity of MR was 95%, the specificity 80%.

CT depicted slightly more disease than MR in this study, but the differences were not statistically different. The very good results in this study probably related to the large size of the peritoneal implants: only 5 patients had implants less than 2 cm.

MR may be of value in distinguishing between intrahepatic and peritoneal lesions on the liver surface (Fig. 45.3). Also, it may be important to identify peritoneal deposits in evaluating primary tumours on MR. Particular examples of this are gynaecological malignancy or prostatic cancer.

Summary: peritoneal metastases

■ Dynamic factors affect the flow of peritoneal fluid, determining the eventual site of peritoneal metastases

■ A clear understanding of peritoneal anatomy is necessary for the identification of peritoneal metastatic disease, and will aid identification of the primary

■ Metastases disseminate throughout the peritoneum in four ways: direct spread along peritoneal ligaments, mesenteries and omenta; intraperitoneal seeding via the flow of ascitic fluid; lymphatic extension; and embolic haematogenous spread

■ Peritoneal metastases are usually from intra-abdominal primary neoplasms, such as carcinoma of the stomach, colon, ovary and pancreas, or from intra-abdominal lymphoma. The site and nature of the primary facilitate a particular direction and method of spread

■ Modern CT is quite sensitive and very specific in identifying peritoneal metastases greater than 1 cm.

However, the sensitivity and specificity are relatively poor for identifying smaller peritoneal metastases

■ The sensitivity and specificity of MR for identifying peritoneal metastases is similar to CT, but CT is much more accessible and cost effective. Multislice CT also offers greater spatial resolution and multiplanar reformatting

■ [18]FDG-PET may be of value where conventional imaging modalities are inconclusive, especially in the context of colonic or ovarian recurrent cancer

■ Despite its limitations, CT is the imaging procedure of choice for evaluating patients known to have or suspected of having peritoneal metastases. It is essential in staging tumours, assessing resectability, monitoring response, and identifying recurrence. It may also be used to guide biopsy, reducing the need for laparoscopy, laparotomy and investigations to identify the primary site

References

1. Oliphant M, Berne A S, Meyers M A. The subperitoneal space of the abdomen and pelvis: Planes of continuity. Am J Roentgenol 1996; 167: 1433–1439
2. Halvorsen R A, Panushka C, Oakley G J et al. Intraperitoneal contrast material improves the CT detection of peritoneal metastases. Am J Roentgenol 1991; 157: 37–40
3. Nelson R C, Chezmar J L, Hoel M J et al. Peritoneal carcinomatosis: preoperative CT with intraperitoneal contrast material. Radiology 1992; 182: 133–138
4. Caseiro-Alves F, Goncalo M, Abraul E et al. Induced pneumoperitoneum in CT evaluation of peritoneal carcinomatosis. Abdom Imaging 1995; 20: 52–55
5. Chou C K, Liu G C, Chen L T et al. MRI manifestations of peritoneal carcinomatosis. Gastrointest Radiol 1992; 17: 336–338
6. Chou C-K, Liu G-C, Su J-H et al. MRI demonstration of peritoneal implants. Abdom Imaging 1994; 19: 95
7. Tempany C M C, Zou K H, Silverman S G. Staging of advanced ovarian cancer: comparison of imaging modalities – Report from the Radiology Diagnostic Oncology Group. Radiology 2000; 215: 761–767
8. Kurtz A B, Tsimikas J V, Tempany C M C et al. Diagnosis and staging of ovarian cancer: comparative values of Doppler and conventional US, CT, and MR imaging correlated with surgery and histopathologic analysis – Report of the Radiology Diagnostic Oncology Group. Radiology 1999; 212: 19–27
9. Semelka R C, Lawrence P H, Shoenut J P et al. Primary ovarian cancer: prospective comparison of contrast enhanced CT and pre and post contrast, fat suppressed MR imaging, with histologic correlation. J Magn Reson Imaging 1993; 3: 99–106
10. Derchi L E, Solbiati L, Rizziatto G et al. Normal anatomy and pathologic changes of the small bowel mesentery: US appearance. Radiology 1987; 164: 649–652
11. Goerg C, Schwerk W-B. Malignant ascites: sonographic signs of peritoneal carcinomatosis. Eur J Cancer 1991; 27: 720–723
12. Carrasquillo J A, Sugarbaker P, Colcher D et al. Peritoneal carcinomatosis: imaging with intraperitoneal injection of I-131-labelled B72.3 monoclonal antibody. Radiology 1988; 167: 35–40
13. Fong Y, Saldinger P F, Akhurst T et al. Utility of F-FDG positron emission tomography scanning in selection of patients for resection of hepatic colorectal metastases. Am J Surg 1999; 178: 282
14. Nakamoto Y, Saga T, Ishimori T et al. Clinical value of positron emission tomography with FDG for recurrent ovarian cancer. Am J Roentgenol 2001; 176: 1449–1454
15. Berger K L, Nicholson S A, Dehdashti F, Siegel B A. FDG PET evaluation of mucinous neoplasms: correlation of FDG uptake with histopathologic features. Am J Roentgenol 2000; 174: 1005–1008
16. Meyers M A, Oliphant M, Berne M S et al. The peritoneal ligaments and mesenteries: pathways of intra-abdominal spread of disease. Annual oration. Radiology 1987; 163: 593–604
17. Oliphant M, Berne A, Meyers M A. Subperitoneal spread of intra-abdominal disease. In: Myers M A (ed). Computed Tomography of the Gastrointestinal Tract including the Peritoneal Cavity and Mesentery. New York: Springer Verlag, 1986: 95–137
18. Balfe D M, Mauro M A, Kooehler R E et al. Gastrohepatic ligament: normal and pathologic CT anatomy. Radiology 1984; 150: 485–490
19. Dehn C B, Reznek R H, Nockler I B et al. The preoperative assessment of advanced gastric cancer by computed tomography. Br J Surg 1984; 71: 413–417
20. Weinstein J B, Heiken J P, Lee J K T et al. High resolution CT of the porta hepatis and hepatoduodenal ligament. Radiographics 1986; 6: 55–73
21. Baker M E, Silverman P M, Halvorsen R A et al. Computed tomography of masses in periportal/hepatoduodenal ligament. J Comput Assist Tomogr 1987; 11: 258–263
22. Kim T K, Han J K, Chung J W et al. Intraperitoneal drop metastases from hepatocellular carcinoma: CT and angiographic findings. J Comput Assist Tomogr 1996; 20: 638–642
23. Ohtani T, Shirai Y, Tsukada K et al. Spread of gallbladder carcinoma: CT evaluation with pathologic correlation. Abdom Imaging 1996; 21: 195–201
24. Diamond R T, Greenberg H M, Boult I F. Direct metastatic spread of right colonic adenocarcinoma to duodenum: barium and computed tomography findings. Gastrointest Radiol 1981; 6: 339–341
25. McDaniel K P, Charnsangavej C, Du Brow R A et al. Pathways of nodal metastases in carcinomas of the caecum, ascending colon, and transverse colon. CT demonstration. Am J Roentgenol 1993; 160: 49–52
26. Chun C H, Raff M F, Conteras L et al. Splenic abscess. Medicine (Baltimore) 1980; 59: 50–65
27. Meyers M A, Volberg F, Katzen B et al. Haustral anatomy and physiology: a new look II. Roentgen interpretation of pathologic alterations. Radiology 1973; 108: 505–512
28. Meyers M A. Distribution of intraabdominal malignant seeding: dependency on dynamics of flow of ascitic fluid. Am J Roentgenol 1973; 119: 198–206
29. Bergman F. Carcinoma of the ovary: a clinicopathological study of 86 autopsied cases with special reference to mode of spread. Acta Obstet Gynaecol 1966; 45: 211–231
30. Dagnini G, Marin G, Caldironin M W et al. Laparoscopy in staging, follow-up, and re-staging ovarian carcinoma. Gastrointest Endosc 1987; 33: 80–83
31. Jeffrey R B Jr. CT demonstration of peritoneal implants. Am J Roentgenol 1980; 135: 323–326
32. Buy J-N, Moss A A, Ghossain M A et al. Peritoneal

implants from ovarian tumours: CT findings. Radiology 1988; 169: 691–694

33. Megibow A J, Bosniak M A, Ho A G et al. Accuracy of CT in detection of persistent or recurrent ovarian carcinoma: correlation with second look laparotomy. Radiology 1988; 166: 341–354

34. Triller J, Goldnirsch A, Reinhard J-P. Subcapsular liver metastases in ovarian cancer: computed tomography and surgical staging. Eur J Radiol 1985; 5: 261–266

35. Walkey M M, Friedman A C, Sohotra P et al. CT manifestations of peritoneal carcinomatosis. Am J Roentgenol 1988; 150: 1035–1041

36. Mitchell D G, Hill M C, Hill S et al. Serous carcinoma of the ovary: CT identification of metastatic calcified implants. Radiology 1986; 158: 649–652

37. Matsuoka K, Okuhira M, Nonaka T et al. Calcification of peritoneal carcinomatosis from gastric carcinoma: a CT demonstration. Eur J Radiol 1991; 13: 207–208

38. Woodard P K, Feldman J M, Paine S S, Baker M E. Midgut carcinoid tumours: CT findings and biochemical profiles. J Comput Assist Tomogr 1995; 19: 400–405

39. Seshul M B, Coulam C M. Pseudomyxoma peritonei: computed tomography and sonography. Am J Roentgenol 1981; 136: 803–806

40. Whitley N O, Bohlman M E, Baker L P. CT patterns of mesenteric disease. J Comput Assist Tomogr 1982; 6: 490–496

41. Cooper C, Jeffrey R B, Silverman P M et al. Computed tomography of omental pathology. J Comput Assist Tomogr 1986; 10: 62–66

42. Pandolfo I, Blandino A, Gaeta M et al. Calcified peritoneal metastases from papillary cystadenocarcinoma of the ovary: CT features. J Comput Assist Tomogr 1986; 10: 545–546

43. Tartar V M, Heiken J P, McClellan B L. Renal cell carcinoma presenting with diffuse peritoneal metastases: CT findings. J Comput Assist Tomogr 1991; 15: 450–453

44. Cho K C, Gold B M. Computed tomography of Krukenberg tumours. Am J Roentgenol 1985; 145: 285–288

45. Spencer J A, Swift S E, Wilkinson N et al. Peritoneal carcinomatosis: image-guided peritoneal core biopsy for tumour type and patient care. Radiology 2001; 221: 173–177

46. Goffinet D R, Castellino R A, Kim H et al. Staging laparotomies in unselected patients with non-Hodgkin's lymphoma. Cancer 1973; 32: 672–681

47. Mueller P R, Ferrucci J T Jr, Harbin W P et al. Appearance of lymphomatous involvement of the mesentery by ultrasonography and body computed tomography: the 'sandwich sign'. Radiology 1980; 134: 467–473

48. Kawashima A, Fishman E K, Kuhlman J E et al. CT of malignant melanoma: patterns of small bowel and mesenteric involvement. J Comput Assist Tomogr 1991; 15: 570–574

49. Caskey C I, Scatarige J C, Fishman E K. Distribution of metastases in breast carcinoma. CT evaluation of the abdomen. Clin Imaging 1991; 15: 166–171

50. Oddson T A, Rice R R P, Seiler H F et al. The spectrum of small bowel melanoma. Gastrointest Radiol 1978; 3: 419–423

51. Coakley F V, Choi P H, Gougoutos C A et al. Peritoneal metastases: detection with spiral CT in patients with ovarian cancer. Radiology 2002; 223: 495–499

52. Pectasides D, Kayianni H, Facou A et al. Correlation of abdominal computed tomography scanning and second look operation findings in ovarian cancer patients. Am J Clin Oncol 1991; 14: 457–462

53. De-Rosa V, Mangoni-di-Stefano M L, Brunetti A et al. Computed tomography and second-look surgery in ovarian cancer patients. Correlation, actual role and limitations of CT scan. Eur J Gynaecol Oncol 1995; 16: 123–129

54. Brady P G, Peebles M, Goldschmid S. Role of laparoscopy in the evaluation of patients with suspected hepatic or peritoneal malignancy. Gastrointest Endosc 1991; 37: 27–30

Chapter 46

Spleen

S A Aslam Sohaib and Rodney H Reznek

Introduction

The spleen is the largest collection of lymphoid tissue in the body and has important haematological and immunological functions. Metastatic disease in the spleen (i.e. secondary non-lymphoid tumours) is unusual and usually occurs late in the course of disseminated disease. This has to be distinguished from other splenic pathology as it has important prognostic implications.

Imaging techniques

Plain radiography is not routinely used in the evaluation of splenic pathology.

The spleen is readily visualized on ultrasound. The normal splenic parenchyma shows a homogeneous low-level echo pattern, which is generally of slightly lower reflectivity than hepatic parenchyma. Ultrasound is useful for detecting and characterizing focal lesions within the spleen as cystic or solid.

On non-enhanced CT, the normal spleen is homogeneous and has an attenuation of 35–55 HU, which is 5–10 HU less than that of liver.[1] The spleen is optimally evaluated with the use of intravenous contrast material. The spleen normally demonstrates heterogeneous enhancement immediately after bolus injection of contrast material. Only after a minute or more does the splenic parenchyma achieve uniform homogeneous enhancement.[2] This is thought to reflect the variable blood flow within different compartments of the spleen and should not be misinterpreted as pathology.[3]

On MR imaging, the normal splenic parenchyma is of lower signal intensity than liver and slightly greater signal than muscle on T1-weighted images. On T2-weighted images, the spleen shows higher signal intensity, appearing brighter than the liver. The signal intensities of normal splenic parenchyma and many pathologic processes are similar.[4] Consequently, the use of contrast-enhanced MR is important for evaluating the spleen. Intravenous gadolinium-based contrast agents are most commonly used. Images are acquired using a dynamic breath-hold T1-weighted spoiled gradient-echo sequence after an intravenous bolus injection of gadolinium. As in CT, the spleen shows heterogeneous enhancement on dynamic contrast-enhanced MR.[5]

More recently, superparamagnetic iron oxide particles have been used to evaluate the spleen. These particles are taken up by the reticuloendothelial system. They lower the signal intensity of the normal spleen and therefore increase the conspicuity of focal abnormalities in the spleen.[6]

Normal anatomy and variants

The shape and position of the normal spleen can vary considerably. Prominent lobes may mimic a mass lesion.[7,8] Ectopic splenic tissues of congenital origin give rise to an **accessory spleen** in 10–30% of the population.[9,10] They usually occur near the splenic hilum (75%) but may sometimes be found in its suspensory ligaments or in the tail of the pancreas and rarely elsewhere in the abdomen.[10] A single focus is found in 88% of cases.[11] Accessory spleens vary in size from a few millimetres to several centimetres in diameter. After splenectomy, an accessory spleen can hypertrophy markedly, causing a recurrence of problems in patients who have undergone splenectomy for hypersplenism. The typical accessory spleen has a smooth round or ovoid shape. Its blood supply is usually derived from the splenic artery with drainage into the splenic vein. When there is doubt, ^{99m}Tc-sulphur colloid or heat-denatured red cell scintigraphy is useful diagnostically to show functioning splenic tissue in areas of concern.[12]

Spleen size

The normal adult spleen measures approximately 12–15 cm in length, 4–8 cm in anteroposterior diameter and 3–4 cm in thickness.[3] However, the irregular shape and oblique orientation of spleen mean that these linear measurements are of limited use. Furthermore, splenic volume varies greatly from one individual to another. Normal in vivo adult splenic volume ranges from 107 to 314 cm³.[13] An assessment of splenic size can be made on imaging. On a plain film, vertical length measurement is the single best indicator of splenic size. A length greater than 11 cm is associated with a 70% probability of splenomegaly.[14] On ultrasound the long axis of the spleen is less than 12 cm in 95% of the population.[15,16] Measurement of the length and width of the spleen has been shown to correlate extremely well with in vivo measurements of splenic volume.[17] Ultrasound can be used to determine changes in spleen size with serial measurement.[15] Determination of splenic volume on CT using summation of cross-sectional areas is very accurate, with errors in the range of 3–5%.[18] However, this technique is cumbersome and, in practice, on CT or MR most observers judge splenic volume by subjective evaluation. Rounding of the normally crescentic shape, extension of the spleen anterior to the aorta or below the right hepatic lobe or rib cage are further clues to splenomegaly. On cross-sectional imaging a more accurate method for the assessment of the splenic volume is the splenic index, i.e. the product of the length, width and thickness.[19] The normal splenic index is between 120 and 480 cm^3.[19]

Splenomegaly

There are many causes of splenomegaly (Table 46.1), which occasionally may be related to neoplastic disorders such as lymphoma, leukaemia, primary benign or malignant tumours, and metastases. A clue to the underlying cause can sometimes be identified on imaging, e.g. abdominal lymph node enlargement may suggest lymphoma.

Splenic metastases

Metastases to the spleen are usually haematogenous. Transcoelomic spread to the spleen within the abdominal cavity is less frequent. Blood-borne spread usually results in parenchymal disease whilst peritoneal disease gives rise to surface disease.

It has been postulated that the relative infrequency of splenic metastases may be due to the lack of afferent splenic lymphatics, filtering of the blood in the lung and the liver, or anti-tumour activity due to the high concentration of lymphoid tissue.[20]

There are relatively few series reporting on splenic metastases, the incidence ranging from 0.3 to 10.3%.[20–28] Adenocarcinomas are the most common source of splenic metastases, accounting for almost 95% of cases.[20] Other tumours include melanoma and germ cell tumour. The primary carcinomas that most commonly spread to the spleen are:[20,22,28]

- Breast
- Lung
- Colorectal
- Ovary
- Gastric

The majority of carcinomas are adenocarcinomas; others include squamous cell, undifferentiated, and small cell cancer.

Isolated splenic metastasis, in the absence of metastases to other organs, is rare, found in only 5.3% of the cases at autopsy,[20] most frequently in ovarian carcinomas (Fig.

Table 46.1. *Causes of splenomegaly*

Neoplasms
Leukaemia/lymphoma
Metastases
Congestive
Portal hypertension
Cirrhosis
Cystic fibrosis
Splenic vein obstruction
Storage disease
Gaucher's disease
Niemann–Pick disease
Amyloidosis
Histiocytosis
Collagen vascular disease
Systemic lupus erythematosus
Rheumatoid/Felty's syndrome
Haemolytic anaemias
Haemoglobinopathies
Hereditary spherocytosis
Infections
Hepatitis
Malaria
Infectious mononucleosis
Tuberculosis
Typhoid
Extramedullary haematopoiesis
Myelofibrosis
Miscellaneous
Sarcoidosis
Porphyria

46.1). Other common primary sites that result in isolated splenic metastasis include colon and lung.

A higher frequency of splenic metastasis from ovarian cancer has been reported.[21] In this study of 321 patients, 10.3% of patients had splenic metastasis during the course of the disease with 5.3% at presentation. Splenic parenchymal metastases were present in 1.5% at presentation and in 3% during the course of disease. Disease on the splenic surface was more common, occurring in 5.3% at presentation and in 7.2% during the course of the disease. Parenchymal metastases were much less likely to respond to treatment than surface lesions but were more commonly a feature of

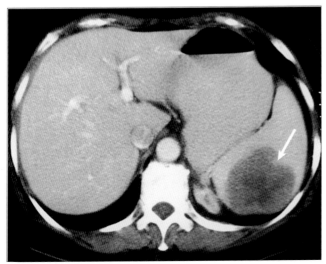

Figure 46.1. *Isolated splenic metastases in a patient with recurrent ovarian cancer. Contrast-enhanced CT showing a large solitary deposit (arrow).*

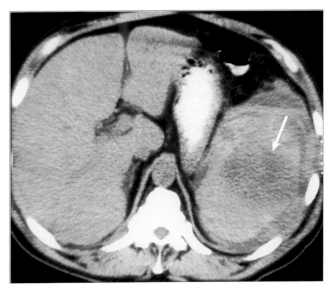

Figure 46.3. *Spontaneous splenic rupture in a patient with melanoma metastases to the spleen. Non-contrast-enhanced CT shows a low density melanoma metastasis (arrow) within the spleen which is surrounded by a perisplenic haematoma.*

relapsed disease.[21,29] The splenic metastases behaved similarly to liver metastases in ovarian cancer.[21] Ovarian cancer is the most common primary site in surgical series of patients undergoing splenectomies for metastases.[29]

Melanoma has the highest frequency of splenic involvement (Fig. 46.2) as up to 34% of melanoma patients show splenic metastases on autopsy series.[25] The risk of metastases increases with the depth of the melanoma lesions.[30]

Clinical features
Splenic metastases are more common in older patients, probably reflecting the age groups that have widely disseminated disease. Splenic deposits are usually asymptomatic. Symptoms usually include abdominal pain or an enlarging mass.[20] Spontaneous splenic rupture (Fig. 46.3) because of

metastatic carcinoma is rare. The symptomatic splenic lesions are larger and more frequently found in women and younger patients.[20]

Imaging characteristics
Splenic metastases involve the splenic capsule/surface or parenchyma. Metastases to the splenic serosa are predominantly from the ovary, but may be from other tumours that spread via a peritoneal route. Serosal metastases result in scalloping or indentation of the splenic surface (Fig. 46.4). Surface implants are usually well defined, biconvex and

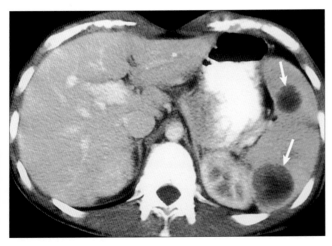

Figure 46.2. *Splenic metastases. Contrast-enhanced CT showing multiple deposits (arrowed) from malignant melanoma.*

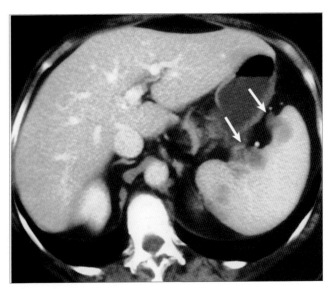

Figure 46.4. *Surface splenic metastases in a patient with ovarian cancer. Contrast-enhanced CT showing multiple deposits (arrowed) on the surface of the spleen.*

peripheral, and indent rather than replace the splenic parenchyma. Parenchymal lesions are most frequently multiple but may be solitary. They are often circular and partially or completely surrounded by spleen tissue. Splenic metastases, parenchymal or serosal, are usually hypoechoic on ultrasound and hypodense on CT (Figs. 46.1 and 46.4).

Metastases may be cystic in character. Such metastases usually arise from primary tumours of the ovary (Fig. 46.5), breast, endometrium, and from melanoma.

Calcification is uncommon but occurs in patients with primary mucinous adenocarcinoma (Fig. 46.6).

Key points: splenic metastases

- Splenic metastases are uncommon and usually occur as a part of disseminated disease

- Splenic involvement may either be due to surface disease from peritoneal spread of cancer or parenchymal disease from haematogenous spread

- Isolated splenic metastases are rare but typically occur in recurrent ovarian cancer

- Splenic metastases are usually asymptomatic, and are usually found at autopsy or at imaging

Other spleen lesions in oncology patients

Malignant lesions

Splenic lymphoma (Chapter 32) is the most common splenic malignancy. It is usually a manifestation of generalized lymphoma (Fig. 46.7) and therefore distinguished from metastatic disease to the spleen.

Other primary malignant tumours of the spleen are very rare. They include angiosarcoma, fibrosarcoma, leiomyosarcoma, malignant teratoma, and malignant fibrous histocytoma. **Splenic angiosarcoma** is the most common non-lymphoid primary malignant tumour of the spleen.[31] It is associated with exposure to Thorotrast (thorium dioxide),

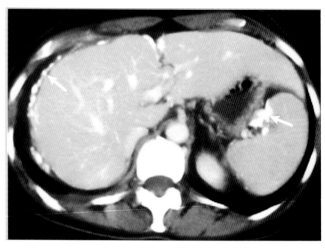

Figure 46.6. *Calcified splenic metastases in a patient with partly treated ovarian cancer. Contrast-enhanced CT showing multiple calcified peritoneal deposits (arrowed).*

used in the 1950s as an angiographic contrast medium. The prognosis is very poor (20% survive 6 months). Approximately 70% of all angiosarcomas metastasize to the liver and approximately 30% undergo spontaneous rupture.[32] Imaging reveals an enlarged spleen with a poorly defined mass and there may be areas of haemorrhage within it.

Key points: splenic malignancy

- Splenic lymphoma is the most common malignant disease to involve the spleen

- Other primary tumours of the spleen are extremely rare

Benign lesions

Splenic cysts

Non-neoplastic splenic cysts may be true (primary) cysts which possess a cellular lining or false (secondary) cysts which have no cellular lining. True cysts are either parasitic

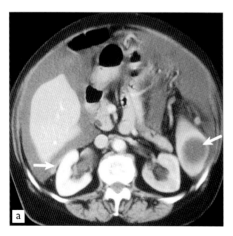
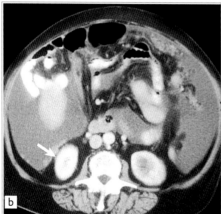

Figure 46.5. *Cystic splenic metastasis. Contrast-enhanced CT shows a cystic splenic metastasis (arrow) in a patient with advanced ovarian cancer. Peritoneal deposits and malignant ascites are also present.*

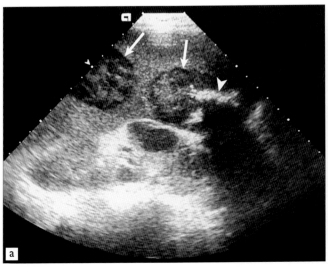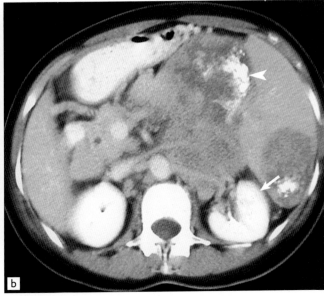

Figure 46.7. *High-grade non-Hodgkin's lymphoma involving the spleen. (a) Longitudinal ultrasound shows two large heterogeneous hypoechoic lesions (arrowed). The inferior lesion contains a central hyperechoic area (arrowhead) casting an acoustic shadow in keeping with calcification. (b) Contrast-enhanced CT shows the partly calcified splenic lesion (arrow) as well as bulky retroperitoneal calcified adenopathy (long arrowhead).*

(echinococcal) or non-parasitic (epithelial). True, non-parasitic, i.e. epithelial (also called epidermoid, mesothelial, or primary) cysts are congenital in origin. They are more common in females than males and are usually found in childhood or adolescence.[33] In 80% of cases congenital splenic cysts are unilocular and solitary. A false cyst, i.e. pseudocyst, is post-traumatic in origin and is thought to represent the final stage in the evolution of a splenic haematoma.

On CT and MR splenic cysts are well defined, of water density or signal, and show no enhancement after intravenous contrast. On ultrasound false cysts may contain internal echoes from debris and show echogenic foci with distal shadowing due to calcification in the wall. CT demonstrates cyst wall calcification in 14% of true cysts and 50% of false cysts[34] (Fig. 46.8). Cyst wall trabeculation or peripheral septation occurs in 86% of true cysts and 17% of false cysts. High attenuation cysts may occur in up to one third of false cysts.[34] On MR false cysts may have variable signal intensity on T1-weighted images, depending on the degree of proteinaceous material or haemorrhage present.

The differential diagnosis of a splenic cyst includes abscess (Fig. 46.9), acute haematoma, intrasplenic pancreatic pseudocyst, cystic neoplasm (lymphangioma or haemangioma), and cystic metastasis.

Haemangioma

Haemangioma is the most common primary benign neoplasm of the spleen occurring in 0.03% to 14% of cases at autopsy.[1] Splenic haemangiomas can be multiple and form part of a generalized angiomatosis as in Klippel–Trenaunay–Weber syndrome.[12] Most lesions are detected incidentally, but, in large haemangiomas, splenic rupture and anaemia, thrombocytopenia, and coagulopathy (Kasabach–Merritt syndrome) have been reported.[35]

The imaging characteristics of splenic haemangiomas range from solid to mixed to purely cystic lesions.[36] The ultrasound appearance is non-specific and may show cystic areas.[26] On CT, haemangioma may appear either solid or cystic, and may enhance in a similar pattern to hepatic haemangioma.[37] Some lesions are relatively avascular or show slow filling of contrast material.[37,38] The MR imaging appearance is also similar to hepatic haemangioma. The lesion with respect to the spleen is of low signal intensity or isointense on T1-weighted images with respect to the spleen and of high signal intensity on T2-weighted images. T2-weighted images may show heterogeneous signal intensity representing mixed solid and cystic components of the haemangioma.[39] T1-weighted images may show areas of high signal due to subacute haemorrhage or proteinaceous fluid.

Lymphangioma

Lymphangiomas can occur as single or multiple lesions, are usually asymptomatic, and are categorized as capillary, cavernous or cystic, depending on the size of the abnormal lymphatic channels.[40] In the spleen the cystic type is most common. On ultrasound lymphangioma appears as a hypoechoic mass, occasionally containing septation and debris.[41] CT shows multiple thin-walled, well-marginated cysts, often subcapsular in location. No enhancement is seen and the attenuation measurements vary from 15 to 35 HU.[42,43] On MR, lymphangiomas resemble cysts.[44]

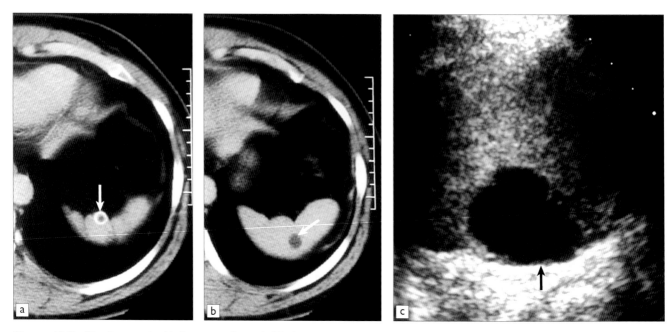

Figure 46.8. *Simple cysts. (a, b) Contrast-enhanced CT shows two simple cysts (arrows) within the spleen, one of which has a calcified wall. (c) Longitudinal ultrasound through the spleen in a different patient showing a subcapsular cyst (arrow).*

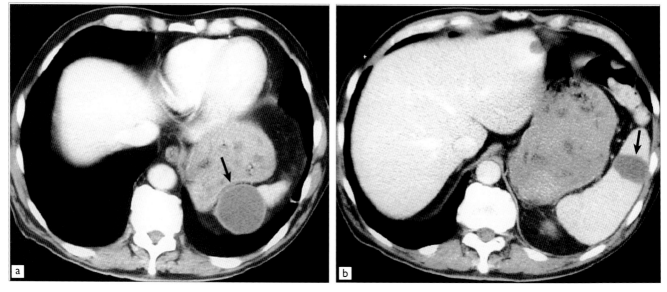

Figure 46.9. *Multiple splenic abscesses. (a, b) Contrast-enhanced CT shows two well-defined low density lesions (arrows) from splenic abscesses.*

Hamartoma

Splenic hamartomas (also called splenomas or nodular hyperplasia of the spleen) are rare benign lesions composed of an anomalous mixture of normal splenic elements with red pulp predominating.[9] Hamartomas occur singly or less commonly as multiple nodules. On ultrasound hamartomas are hyperechoic relative to the spleen and sometimes have a cystic component.[45] On CT they appear iso- or hypodense on the precontrast images with occasional lesions showing cystic components. On MR they are isointense on T1-weighted images and hyperintense on T2-weighted images.[41] On CT and MR, following injection of intravenous contrast material, they usually show slow enhancement and filling after intravenous contrast.[46]

Infection

Splenic infection, especially fungal infection, may arise as a consequence of immunosuppression from chemotherapy.[47] The most common pathogens are Candida, Aspergillus and Cryptococcus.[48] Fungal infection in the spleen is most likely to appear as a miliary or multifocal process. Hepatosplenic candidiasis may appear as multiple rounded areas of decreased attenuation, a so-called 'bull's-eye' lesion (hypoattenuating foci with a central core of higher attenuation), or as tiny 2–5 mm lesions of increased attenuation due to calcification. Calcification is seen in treated Candida microabscesses and lesions caused by other fungi, especially Histoplasma, mycobacteria (Fig. 46.10) and *Pneumocystis carinii*. Fungal abscesses in neutropenic patients are often small and not always detectable with any imaging modality.

Infarcts

Splenic infarcts may occur from mass lesions compressing splenic vasculature, e.g. pancreatic tumours (Fig. 46.11).

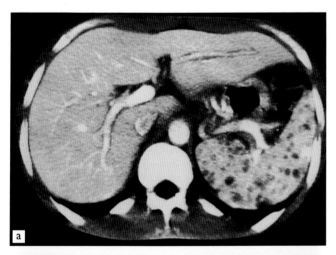

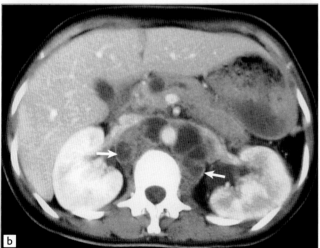

Figure 46.10. *Splenic tuberculosis. (a, b) Contrast-enhanced CT shows multiple small, enhancing lesions in the spleen. Note also the rim enhancement of the involved retroperitoneal nodes.*

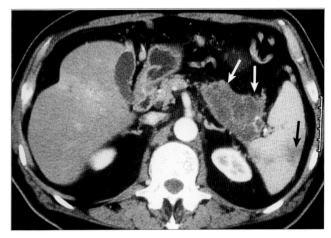

Figure 46.11. *Splenic infarct. Contrast-enhanced CT shows a tumour mass (arrows) in the tail of the pancreas causing occlusion to the splenic vein and a splenic infarct (black arrow).*

Splenic infarction may be diffuse or focal. On CT, infarcts typically appear as sharply marginated, low density wedge-shaped areas.[3,49] Occasionally, the infarct may be multiple, resulting in poorly defined hypodense lesions.[49] When the entire spleen is infarcted only rim enhancement of the capsule occurs from capsular vessels.[3] Splenic infarction can also be seen on MR: haemorrhagic infarcts have a high signal intensity on T1- and T2-weighted images.[50]

Key points: benign disease

- Non-neoplastic cysts of the spleen have the typical imaging appearances of cysts

- Haemangiomas are the most common benign primary tumour of the spleen and have similar imaging characteristics to haemangioma in the liver

- Focal splenic lesions in cancer patients may arise from other benign conditions such as infections and splenic infarcts

Diagnostic intervention

The diagnosis of splenic metastases is usually not difficult given the clinical setting. Rarely, where the diagnosis is uncertain, such as in an isolated splenic metastasis, patients usually undergo splenectomy. In other situations where a focal splenic abnormality is identified, and it is uncertain whether this is a metastasis or not, then either splenectomy or an image-guided biopsy may be performed. Percutaneous biopsy may be performed for cytological or histological diagnosis. A diagnostic rate of 55–90% has been reported.[51–54] The complication rate with fine-needle aspiration is low, but includes haemorrhage and pneumothorax.[51,52,55]

carcinoma: analysis of 1000 autopsied cases. Cancer 1950; 3: 74–85

29. Lee S S, Morgenstern L, Phillips E H et al. Splenectomy for splenic metastases: a changing clinical spectrum. Am Surg 2000; 66: 837–840

30. Shirkhoda A, Albin J. Malignant melanoma: correlating abdominal and pelvic CT with clinical staging. Radiology 1987; 165: 75–78

31. Chen K T, Bolles J C, Gilbert E F. Angiosarcoma of the spleen: a report of two cases and review of the literature. Arch Pathol Lab Med 1979; 103: 122–124

32. Mahony B, Jeffrey R B, Federle M P. Spontaneous rupture of hepatic and splenic angiosarcoma demonstrated by CT. Am J Roentgenol 1982; 138: 965–966

33. Younger K A, Hall C M, Conrad M R. Epidermoid cyst of the spleen: a case report and review of the literature. Splenic trauma: false-negative CT diagnosis in cases of delayed rupture [letter]. Br J Radiol 1990; 63: 652–653

34. Dawes L G, Malangoni M A. Cystic masses of the spleen. Am Surg 1986; 52: 333–336

35. Rolfes R J, Ros P R. The spleen: an integrated imaging approach. Crit Rev Diagn Imaging 1990; 30: 41–83

36. Duddy M J, Calder C J. Cystic haemangioma of the spleen: findings on ultrasound and computed tomography. Br J Radiol 1989; 62: 180–182

37. Ros P R, Moser R P J, Dachman A H et al. Hemangioma of the spleen: radiologic-pathologic correlation in ten cases. Radiology 1987; 162(1 Pt 1): 73–77

38. Moss C N, Van Dyke J A, Koehler R E, Smedberg C T. Multiple cavernous hemangiomas of the spleen: CT findings. J Comput Assist Tomogr 1986; 10: 338–340

39. Harris R D, Simpson W. MRI of splenic hemangioma associated with thrombocytopenia. Gastrointest Radiol 1989; 14: 308–310

40. Ferrozzi F, Bova D, Draghi F, Garlaschi G. CT findings in primary vascular tumors of the spleen. Am J Roentgenol 1996; 166: 1097–1101

41. Mortele K J, Mergo P J, Kunnen M, Ros P R. Tumoral pathology of the spleen. In: DeSchepper A M, Vanhoenacker F (eds). Medical Imaging of the Spleen. Berlin: Springer-Verlag, 2000: pp 101–122

42. Pyatt R S, Williams E D, Clark M, Gaskins R. Case report.

CT diagnosis of splenic cystic lymphangiomatosis. J Comput Assist Tomogr 1981; 5: 446–448

43. Pistoia F, Markowitz S K. Splenic lymphangiomatosis: CT diagnosis. Am J Roentgenol 1988; 150: 121–122

44. Ito K, Murata T, Nakanishi T. Cystic lymphangioma of the spleen: MR findings with pathologic correlation. Abdom Imaging 1995; 20: 82–84

45. Norowitz D G, Morehouse H T. Isodense splenic mass: hamartoma, a case report. Comput Med Imaging Graph 1989; 13: 347–350

46. Ohtomo K, Fukuda H, Mori K et al. CT and MR appearances of splenic hamartoma. J Comput Assist Tomogr 1992; 16: 425–428

47. Caslowitz P L, Labs J D, Fishman E K, Siegelman S S. The changing spectrum of splenic abscess. Clin Imaging 1989; 13: 201–207

48. Chew F S, Smith P L, Barboriak D. Candidal splenic abscesses [clinical conference]. Am J Roentgenol 1991; 156: 474

49. Balcar I, Seltzer S E, Davis S, Geller S. CT patterns of splenic infarction: a clinical and experimental study. Radiology 1984; 151: 723–729

50. Hess C F, Griebel J, Schmiedl U et al. Focal lesions of the spleen: preliminary results with fast MR imaging at 1.5 T. J Comput Assist Tomogr 1988; 12: 569–574

51. Civardi G, Vallisa D, Berte R et al. Ultrasound-guided fine needle biopsy of the spleen: high clinical efficacy and low risk in a multicenter Italian study. Am J Hematol 2001; 67: 93–99

52. Caraway N P, Fanning C V. Use of fine-needle aspiration biopsy in the evaluation of splenic lesions in a cancer center. Diagn Cytopathol 1997; 16: 312–316

53. Silverman J F, Geisinger K R, Raab S S, Stanley M W. Fine needle aspiration biopsy of the spleen in the evaluation of neoplastic disorders. Acta Cytol 1993; 37: 158–162

54. Kraus M D, Fleming M D, Vonderheide R H. The spleen as a diagnostic specimen: a review of 10 years' experience at two tertiary care institutions. Cancer 2001; 91: 2001–2009

55. Venkataramu N K, Gupta S, Sood B P et al. Ultrasound guided fine needle aspiration biopsy of splenic lesions. Br J Radiol 1999; 72: 953–956

Chapter 47

Malignant tumours of the skin

Guy J C Burkill and D Michael King

Introduction

Malignant tumours of the skin form a disparate group of cancers with a wide range of behaviours but collectively they are the most frequently occurring human malignancy.[1] Typically, these tumours are clinically obvious and radiology plays no role in their initial assessment. Increasingly, however, scintigraphy in the form of sentinel node localization and biopsy is employed for staging certain skin cancers and for planning their treatment.

Computed tomography (CT) remains the mainstay for the assessment of metastatic disease supplemented by ultrasound, magnetic resonance (MR) imaging and plain radiography. In common with other malignancies, 2-[F-18]fluoro-2-deoxy-D-glucose positron emission tomography ([18]FDG PET) is already beginning to play a pivotal role in the evaluation of distant spread.

Although the majority of cutaneous tumours are non-melanoma skin cancers (NMSC), this chapter is dominated by the imaging of melanoma, reflecting the greater importance of imaging in this malignancy.

Pathology

Cutaneous malignancies are categorized according to their cellular origin and have been summarized in Table 47.1.[2,3]

Epidemiology

Reliable epidemiological data, although sparse, are available for melanoma, basal cell carcinoma (BCC) and squamous cell carcinoma (SCC). Non-melanoma skin cancer (NMSC – BCC and SCC) is the most frequently occurring cancer in white populations and accounts for one third of all cancers in the USA. The reported ratio of BCC to SCC is 4 : 1.[4] In the UK, the 1998 age standardized incidence per 100,000 population was 232.7 for BCC and 33.8 for SCC.[5] Comparable figures for Australia are 3,253 for BCC and 2,087 for SCC.[6]

The incidence ratio of NMSC to malignant melanoma is approximately 20 : 1. Although melanoma accounts for 2% of all cancers in the UK, its incidence is increasing by

Table 47.1. *Classification of malignant tumours of the skin according to cellular origin*

Epidermal	Squamous cell carcinoma
	Keratoacanthoma
	Basal cell carcinoma
	Merkel cell carcinoma
	Paget's disease
Dermal	Dermatofibrosarcoma protuberans
	Malignant fibrous histiocytoma/atypical fibroxanthoma
Endothelial	Angiosarcoma
	Cutaneous Kaposi's sarcoma
Smooth muscle	Cutaneous leiomyosarcoma
Malignant appendageal tumours (cutaneous adnexal carcinomas)	Sweat gland carcinomas
	Malignant follicular tumours
	Sebaceous carcinoma
Melanocytes	Melanoma
Tumours of cellular immigrants to the skin	Primary cutaneous lymphomas
	Leukaemia cutis
	Mastocytosis
	Primary cutaneous Langerhans' cell histiocytosis
Metastases	

3–7% annually; this rate is higher than any other malignancy and, in the UK in 1998, there were approximately 57,700 new cases registered.[4,7] The cumulative lifetime risk for the development of malignant melanoma is 1 in 132 in the UK, 1 in 75 in the USA and 1 in 25 in Australia.[7–9]

Key points: epidemiology

■ Skin cancer is the most common human malignancy

■ BCC is the most common skin cancer

■ The incidence of melanoma is rising faster than any other malignancy

■ Cumulative lifetime risk of developing melanoma is currently 1 in 132 (UK) and 1 in 75 (USA)

Risk factors

There are a number of risk factors for the development of both NMSC and melanoma. Common to both groups of cancers is exposure to ultraviolet (UV) radiation, and burning of the skin before adolescence is of particular importance for fair- and freckled-skinned individuals.[7,10–13] In addition, those with a previous skin cancer are at higher risk of developing new tumours.[10] The use of sun beds clearly aggravates the UV factor and the Health and Safety Executive recommends that their use be restricted to fewer than 20 sessions per year.[7]

In SCC, additional risk factors include exposure to ionizing radiation and chemical carcinogens (e.g. soot, arsenic and polycyclic aromatic hydrocarbons). Risk factors also include chronically injured or scarred skin following burning or ulceration. Viruses such as human papillomavirus Types 6, 11 and 16 have also been implicated. Precancerous conditions include Bowen's disease ('intraepidermal SCC') and epidermodysplasia verruciformis.[12,13] Basal cell carcinomas may arise in the basal cell naevus syndrome (Gorlin's) and in organoid naevi.[11] The presence of numerous or atypical moles increases the chance of developing melanoma. An increased risk of melanoma exists for individuals with a family history of at least three affected relatives within the extended family. A number of genetic mutations are also associated with the development of melanoma, such as the loss of the tumour suppressor gene *p16INK4a* and a mutation of the oncogene *CDK4*.[7] However, routine genetic testing is not yet recommended.[14]

Immunosuppression is an important risk factor for skin cancers, which form the most common malignancy in organ transplant recipients demonstrating an increased incidence compared with the normal population of 65-fold for SCC, 10-fold for BCC, 3.4-fold for melanoma and 84-fold for Kaposi's sarcoma (KS).[15–17] Furthermore, skin

tumours in transplant recipients appear to be more aggressive, resulting in a higher mortality.[15,18–20]

Key points: risk factors

■ For NMSC and melanoma, sun exposure is the most important factor

■ Burning of the skin before adolescence is an important aetiological factor

■ Fair- and freckled-skin individuals are at greatest risk

■ For SCC there are a number of predisposing chemical carcinogens and viruses

■ There are premalignant lesions in both NMSC and melanoma

■ Genetic mutations have been implicated in melanoma

■ Immunosuppression is a risk factor for all skin malignancies

Staging

Staging classifications

TNM (tumour, node, metastases) staging for skin carcinomas is essentially pathological. T stage relates to tumour size up to T4, at which stage tumours invade deep extradermal structures (Table 47.2). Staging of the regional lymph nodes for each skin site is also defined in the TNM classifi-

Table 47.2. *TNM staging classification of skin carcinomas, 2002*[21]

Primary tumour

TX	Primary tumour cannot be assessed
T0	No evidence of primary tumour
Tis	Carcinoma *in situ*
T1	Tumour 2 cm or less in greatest dimension
T2	Tumour >2 cm ≤5 cm in greatest dimension
T3	Tumour >5 cm in greatest dimension
T4	Tumour invades deep extradermal structures, i.e. cartilage, skeletal muscle, or bone

Regional lymph nodes

NX	Regional lymph nodes cannot be assessed
N0	No regional lymph node metastasis
N1	Regional lymph node metastasis

Distant metastasis

MX	Distant metastasis cannot be assessed
M0	No distant metastasis
M1	Distant metastasis

cation, and staging as node-negative requires at least six tumour-free lymph nodes in the dissection specimen.[21]

The staging system for malignant melanoma is also based on histopathological findings and has recently been revised by the American Joint Committee on Cancer staging.[22] Major differences from the TNM classification include: assessment of ulceration within the T stage, inclusion of the number of metastatic lymph nodes and the distinction between micro- and macrometastases in the nodal staging. Site of distant metastases is also included and the serum lactate dehydrogenase level forms part of the M stage (Tables 47.3a and 47.3b).[22] There is no established staging system for Merkel cell cancer (MCC) but a simple system adopted by many is outlined in Table 47.4.[23]

For the purposes of clinical trial participation and subsequent evaluation there is a staging system for KS devised by the autoimmunodeficiency syndrome (AIDS) Clinical Trials Group (ACTG) which has recently been prospectively validated.[24] There are two main staging classifications for primary cutaneous lymphoma, namely those devised by the European Organization for Research and Treatment of Cancer (EORTC) and the revised European–American lymphoma (REAL) system. A more recent classification has been proposed by the World Health Organization (WHO).[25]

The staging of patients with rarer cutaneous malignancies is dictated by their behaviour as predicted by histological examination of biopsy material. Tumours that behave like BCCs require no further imaging. Those with behaviour similar to SCC require evaluation of the draining lymph node basin, initially by clinical examination with or without fine-needle aspiration cytology (FNAC). Patients with soft tissue sarcoma-like tumours exhibit a propensity for visceral spread and justify cross-sectional imaging.[26]

Local staging

Using probe frequencies of up to 60 MHz, ultrasound has been used to assess the thickness of primary cutaneous melanoma with good correlation with histological thickness, but this technique remains a research tool.[27–30]

Computed tomography may elegantly display local soft tissue extension of some skin tumours (Fig. 47.1), thus aiding preoperative planning of surgery but it has no role in the routine assessment of melanoma.

Table 47.3a. *AJCC Revised Version of the Melanoma TNM Classification*[22]

T Classification	Thickness	Ulceration status
T1	≤1.0mm	a. without ulceration and level II/III
		b. with ulceration or level IV/V
T2	1.01–2.0mm	a. without ulceration
		b. with ulceration
T3	2.01–4.0mm	a. without ulceration
		b. with ulceration
T4	>4.0mm	a. without ulceration
		b. with ulceration
N Classification	**No of metastatic nodes**	**Nodal metastatic mass**
N1	1 node	a. micrometastasis*
		b. macrometastasis†
N2	2–3 nodes	a. micrometastasis*
		b. macrometastasis†
		c. in transit met(s)/satellite(s) without metastatic nodes
N3	4 or more metastatic nodes, or matted nodes, or in transit met(s)/satellite(s) with metastatic node(s)	
M Classification	**Site**	**Serum lactate dehydrogenase**
M1a	Distant skin, subcutaneous, or nodal metastases	Normal
M1b	Lung metastases	Normal
M1c	All visceral metastases	Normal
	Any distant metastasis	Elevated

*Micrometastases are diagnosed after sentinel or elective lymphadenectomy.
†Macrometastases are defined as clinically detectable nodal metastases confirmed by therapeutic lymphadenectomy or when nodal metastasis exhibits gross extracapsular extension.

Table 47.3b. *Proposed stage groupings for cutaneous melanoma*[22]

	Clinical Staging*			Pathological Staging†		
	T	**N**	**M**	**T**	**N**	**M**
0	Tis	N0	M0	Tis	N0	M0
IA	T1a	N0	M0	T1a	N0	M0
IB	T1b	N0	M0	T1b	N0	M0
	T2a	N0	M0	T2a	N0	M0
IIA	T2b	N0	M0	T2b	N0	M0
	T3a	N0	M0	T3a	N0	M0
IIB	T3b	N0	M0	T3b	N0	M0
	T4a	N0	M0	T4a	N0	M0
IIC	T4b	N0	M0	T4b	N0	M0
III‡	Any T	N1	M0			
		N2				
		N3				
IIIA				T1–4a	N1a	M0
				T1–4a	N2a	M0
IIIB				T1–4b	N1a	M0
				T1–4b	N2a	M0
				T1–4a	N1b	M0
				T1–4a	N2b	M0
				T1–4a/b	N2c	M0
IIIC				T1–4b	N1b	M0
				T1–4b	N2b	M0
				Any T	N3	M0
IV	Any T	Any N	Any M1	Any T	Any N	Any M1

*Clinical staging includes microstaging of the primary melanoma and clinical/radiological evaluation for metastases. By convention, it should be used after complete excision of the primary with clinical assessment for regional and distant metastases.

†Pathologic staging includes microstaging of the primary melanoma and pathological information about the regional lymph nodes after partial or complete lymphadenectomy. Pathologic stage 0 or stage IA patients are the exception; they do not require pathologic evaluation of their lymph nodes.

‡There are no stage III subgroups for clinical staging.

Table 47.4. *Proposed staging system for Merkel cell carcinoma*[23]

Stage	
I	Localized disease
IA	≤2 cm
IB	>2 cm
II	Lymph node involvement
III	Distant metastases

Magnetic resonance imaging has also been used to evaluate skin lesions (Fig. 47.1) and, in melanoma, differences in the tumour-to-fat contrast ratio (%T/F contrast) on T2-weighted scanning allow the differentiation of primary malignant melanoma from benign pigmented lesions. Benign lesions demonstrate a positive signal ratio whilst a negative value is obtained in primary cutaneous melanoma. However, this technique is insufficiently accurate to avoid excision biopsy of clinically suspicious lesions and application in clinical practice is seldom justified.[31] Both MR and CT are able to detect perineural spread along the V and VII cranial nerves by NMSCs of the face and scalp. The features on imaging are enlargement or abnormal enhancement of the nerve, loss of the surrounding fat plane and enlargement or destruction of the neural foramen. These imaging findings can be used to plan radiotherapy and may help in predicting prognosis.[32]

Sentinel node localization

Although melanoma, SCC and MCC have a tendency towards orderly lymph node spread, elective dissection of the draining lymph node basin is not generally advocated.[10,12,33,34] Sentinel lymph node biopsy for planning therapeutic lymph node dissection is being used in selected patients, particularly those with clinical Stage II melanoma and, in some centres, in patients with MCC.[10,33–35] The technique of sentinel lymph node localization for biopsy initially used the intradermal injection of the vital dyes patent blue-violet and isosulfan blue intraoperatively. However, the blue dye technique fails to identify the sentinel node in approximately 20% of cases,[36,37] hence two further techniques have been introduced to aid the identification of the sentinel node; namely the gamma-detecting probe (GDP) technique and preoperative dynamic lymphoscintigraphy. These two methods both utilize intradermal injection of the same radiopharmaceutical but the GDP method employs a handheld gamma probe during surgery to identify the sentinel node. Both techniques are complementary and, when used in combination, result in over 95% of sentinel nodes being identified.[37–40] Dynamic lymphoscintigraphy provides the surgeon with a road map prior to surgery and is of particular value in cases of unpredictable lymphatic drainage and in the identification of in-transit lymph nodes lying between the primary tumour and the regional lymph node basin. [18]FDG PET is insufficiently sensitive to replace sentinel node biopsy for evaluating the draining nodal basin but is a useful adjunct to staging when the sentinel node contains metastasis and distant spread is suspected.[41,42]

Distant staging

It is clear that the use of routine chest radiography for screening patients with early-stage melanoma is not justified. A retrospective review of chest radiography in 876 asymptomatic patients with localized cutaneous melanoma found a true positive rate of just 0.1% for pulmonary metastases. Furthermore, 135 (15%) of patients had focal lesions unrelated to melanoma, necessitating further inves-

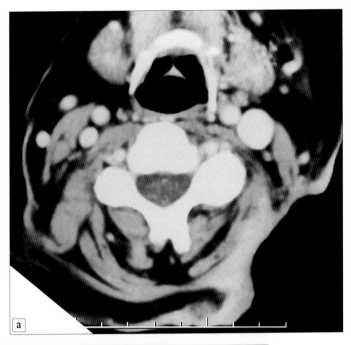

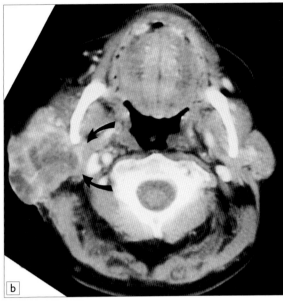

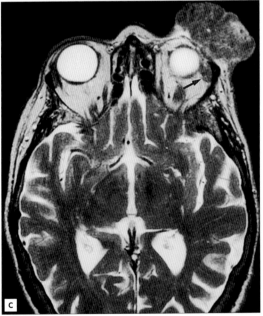

Figure 47.1. *Skin involvement. (a) CT scan of large, ulcerating, long-standing, basal cell carcinoma involving left posterior neck. Note uniform enhancement of 1 cm thick tissue in the base of the ulcer and the characteristic 'rolled edge'. (b) Contrast-enhanced CT showing a soft tissue mass centred on the right parotid gland involving the skin. Note heterogeneous enhancement and deep extension behind the mandible (arrows). (c) Axial T2-weighted MR of the brain at the level of the orbits, demonstrating a very large exophytic squamous cell carcinoma arising from the left eyelid. Posterior encroachment of tumour along the lateral aspect of the globe (arrow) precluded preservation of the globe.*

tigation.[43] Thus patients with Stage I or IIA melanomas need no imaging investigation,[10] but it is currently recommended that those with Stage IIB disease and above undergo chest radiography and liver ultrasound or contrast-enhanced CT of the chest, abdomen with or without the pelvis. The addition of a bone scintigram is dictated by symptoms.[10]

The rarity of MCC militates against the establishment of imaging algorithms. Most experience lies with CT, with some authorities recommending coverage of the chest, abdomen and pelvis to search for metastases after histological diagnosis.[44,45] Octreotide scanning has been successfully employed in the staging of MCC together with, more recently, [18]FDG PET.[45]

Key points: staging

- There are separate staging systems for NMSC, melanoma, MCC and KS

- Local staging is pathological

- Elective lymph node dissection is not recommended

- Sentinel node biopsy for lymph node staging has been used in SCC, melanoma and MCC but is not yet recommended for routine use

- Melanoma staged as IIB and above warrant imaging investigation for metastatic disease

Clinical features

Dermatological diagnosis is based on visual pattern recognition. Basal cell carcinoma is typically a smooth non-pigmented ulcerating nodule exhibiting a pearly appearance, telangiectasia and a rolled edge.

Melanoma assumes several forms. The nodular type typically presents as a brown/black nodule whilst the superficial spreading form appears as a flat, irregular plaque. A typical MCC is a <2cm red/violaceous dome-shaped nodule or indurated plaque on the head, neck or limbs. Larger tumours may ulcerate.[2]

Epidemiological descriptions of KS categorize the disease into four groups, namely:

- Classical KS, a slowly progressive cutaneous tumour of the lower limbs
- Endemic African KS
- Epidemic (AIDS-related) KS
- Iatrogenic or transplant-related KS.[24]

The clinical features and behaviour of cutaneous KS vary according to the epidemiology of the disease. The lesions themselves are typically red, purple or brown nodules, plaques or patches.[24] Recent years have seen a decline in the incidence of epidemic KS by 50% coinciding with the introduction of highly active antiretroviral therapy (HAART).[46]

Prognosis

Prognosis in all skin cancers is markedly improved by early detection and this particularly applies to melanoma. Generally, local recurrence rates and metastatic potential for most cutaneous malignancies are highly variable and depend on the prognostic factors that have been determined for each tumour type. For SCC and BCC, prognostic factors include tumour site, size, depth (SCC), marginal definition (BCC), histological type/differentiation, local recurrence and host immunocompetence.[11,12] Most patients with SCC have an excellent prognosis but 10-year survival is dramatically reduced to 20% by the presence of regional nodal metastases and to 10% when there is disseminated disease.[13]

Malignant melanoma confined to the epidermis is effectively curable and thin lesions carry a >98% 5-year survival rate.[47,48] Tumour thickness and ulceration are the most powerful predictors of survival in early-stage (I and II) disease. In Stage III melanoma, the number of metastatic nodes and the extent of their invasion, together with melanoma ulceration, best predict survival. Metastatic site determines the survival of Stage IV patients, with skin, subcutaneous and distant nodes being more favourable than lung and other visceral organ involvement.[49] Mean survival of patients with disseminated disease is 7–8 months.[48]

Merkel cell carcinoma is highly aggressive with a tendency for local and nodal recurrence, which exceeds that of malignant melanoma.[50,44] Survival is determined by the stage of disease at presentation. Those presenting with Stage III disease have a mean survival of eight months.[51] Aggressive tumours which metastasize widely include:

- Sebaceous carcinoma – metastasizes to lacrimal system as well as haematogenous and lymph node sites[52]
- Malignant sweat gland tumours – 5-year survival <30%[53]
- Malignant fibrous histiocytoma with muscle invasion spreads to lung, liver, lymph nodes and bone[2]
- Angiosarcomas metastasize widely, resulting in a 5-year survival rate of only 10%[2]
- Cutaneous leiomyosarcoma rarely metastasizes, in contrast to leiomyosarcoma of the subcutis, which disseminates in 30% of patients, usually to the lungs[2]
- African KS and epidemic KS usually have a poor prognosis. The prognosis in transplant-related KS is dependent on the degree of immunocompetence[24]

The survival of patients with primary cutaneous lymphoma is highly variable, being dependent on cell type and stage and has been detailed elsewhere.[54]

The behaviour of Langerhans' cell histiocytosis (LCH) is not uniform and there are reports of spontaneous regression in some cases, whereas highly aggressive forms may exhibit generalized cutaneous involvement, lymphadenopathy and pulmonary metastases.[55–57]

Key points: prognosis

- Prognosis is markedly improved by early detection
- NMSC prognosis is determined by site, size, depth, margin and histological differentiation
- Melanoma prognosis is most dependent on thickness and ulceration
- Survival in Stage IV melanoma is determined by site of metastasis

Treatment options

Treatment of primary skin tumours is typically surgical and generally includes a wide excision margin.[2,3,10–12] These recommended surgical margins for various tumours have been studied and recommendations published.[10–12,50,58–60]

A range of alternative surgical and non-surgical options are available for some cutaneous malignancies, e.g. BCCs and SCCs, and include curettage, cryosurgery, carbon dioxide laser surgery, radiotherapy, topical 5-fluorouracil and intralesional interferon. The choice of therapy depends on an assessment of tumour characteristics, patient perform-ance status and preference, as well as local expertise.[11,12]

Elective lymph node dissection is not routinely recom-mended in malignant melanoma and, ideally, sentinel node biopsy for staging Stage II disease should be con-ducted as part of a clinical trial. When draining nodes are deemed suspicious clinically or radiologically fine needle aspiration cytology, (FNAC) should be performed and repeated if necessary. Open biopsy should be considered where there is continuing strong suspicion despite negative cytology. Node-positive patients should be fully staged by imaging (see above) and should undergo nodal dissection in limited disease.[10]

Malignant melanoma is not chemosensitive and adju-vant therapies are not recommended outside the clinical trial setting. Suitable studies [e.g. alpha-interferon (IFN-α)] are currently actively recruiting those with Stage IIB dis-ease and over.[10]

Solitary local or regional recurrence is best treated sur-gically. When there are multiple locoregional sites of relapse, isolated limb perfusion with cytotoxic agents may be applied or carbon dioxide laser ablation might be con-sidered.[61] Isolated or limited metastases involving, for example, skin or brain, might be considered for resection. Radiotherapy to skin or bone metastases may offer short-term control and palliative radiotherapy for unresectable brain disease may be offered.[10]

No significant survival benefit has been shown from sys-temic chemotherapy (e.g. single-agent decarbazine) in metastatic disease, but such cases may be considered for enrolment into a clinical trial of novel therapies.[10]

For MCC, initial surgical excision forms the mainstay of treatment but in advanced disease both palliative radiother-apy and a number of chemotherapy regimens have been used. Unfortunately, treatment responses are seldom sus-tained[51] but responses to somatostatin have been reported.[35]

Key points: treatment

- Surgical resection is generally the treatment of choice
- There are recommended resection margins for the various skin tumours
- Trials for adjuvant treatment in high-risk malignant melanoma are ongoing
- Resection of limited malignant melanoma metastases should be considered

Surveillance

The merits of imaging in the follow-up programme of melanoma are dubious given that the majority (89–94%) of recurrences are detected by self-examination or by clinical assessment.

A 10-year review of Stage I malignant melanoma in a sin-gle practice found that just 10% of relapses were detected on chest radiography and abdominal ultrasound; CT con-ferred no benefit.[62] Unsurprisingly, there is a lack of con-sensus as to the best method of postoperative surveillance but the cornerstone of follow-up appears to comprise clinic visits, chest radiography, full blood count and liver function tests. More sophisticated radiological tests are rarely employed on a routine basis.[63,64]

Follow-up ultrasound of the melanoma resection site, lymphatic track and regional lymph node basin is more sen-sitive for the detection of recurrence than clinical examina-tion, being 89.2% and 71.4%, respectively. However, the two techniques have equal specificity (99.7%). Further studies are required to assess the impact of these data on survival.[65]

Key points: surveillance

- Self-examination and clinical examination detect most recurrences
- Recommendations for clinical surveillance are published
- Chest radiography detects few relapses
- Ultrasound of the melanoma resection site and nodal basin is more sensitive than clinical examination for detecting recurrence but survival data are awaited

Metastatic disease

Melanoma

Initially, malignant melanoma has a predictable pattern of spread with involvement of the regional lymph node basin, and this is the rationale for sentinel lymph node sampling in staging and initial surgical management. Once the tumour escapes the regional draining nodes it becomes far less predictable and has the potential to involve virtually any site within the body. This wide and random dissemina-tion potential has stimulated interest in [18]FDG PET in the identification of sites of metastatic melanoma but, to date, the use of CT remains predominant.

In descending order of frequency, the most common sites for metastases in malignant melanoma at autopsy are:

- Lymph nodes (74%)
- Lungs (71%)
- Soft tissues (68%)
- Liver (58%)
- Brain (55%)
- Bone (49%)
- Adrenal glands (47%)
- Gastro-intestinal tract (44%)[66]

Lymph nodes

On ultrasound, metastatic nodal disease is suspected when nodes are increased in size, show loss of their central echogenic hilum on grey scale and their hilar vessels on colour Doppler, and tend to be round rather than oval shape.[67] Computed tomography and MR rely on established size criteria (see Chapter 39) (Fig. 47.2). In our experience, splenic deposits are unusual in the absence of liver lesions. The size of splenic deposits and their characteristics on ultrasound and MR are variable. They are typically hypodense on CT (Fig. 47.3).[68]

Lung

Pulmonary metastases in melanoma usually number at least five (Fig. 47.4), although a single lung nodule in a melanoma patient is still more likely to be a metastasis than a primary bronchogenic carcinoma.[69,70] When deposits are few in number, or preferably solitary, and there has been a long disease-free interval of at least 36 months there is potential for prolonged remission following pulmonary metastasectomy.[71,72]

Skin and soft tissues

Not surprisingly the skin and subcutaneous tissues are the most frequent soft tissue site for metastatic melanoma and the lesions are usually clinically evident. The distribution of muscle metastases reflects the relative muscle mass, hence the lower limb is most frequently affected (Fig. 47.5).[73] Sonographic appearances of melanoma metastases in the skin and subcutaneous tissues are typically those of a well-defined, smooth-bordered, heterogeneous mass, hypoechoic to muscle. One third of deposits are isoechoic. Hyperechogenicity is a rare finding being seen in just 6% of patients. Over 70% of lesions demonstrate enhanced acoustic through transmission and internal arterial flow on colour Doppler.[74] On CT, skin, subcutaneous and muscle deposits are often well-defined and may show vascular enhancement (Figs. 47.5 and 47.6). On MR, the majority of soft tissue melanoma metastases have non-specific signal intensity characteristics.

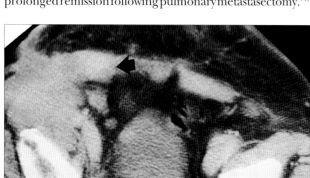

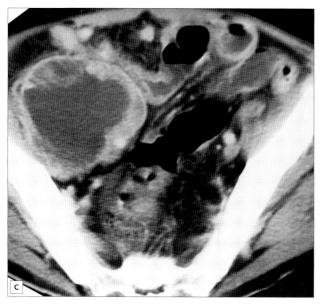

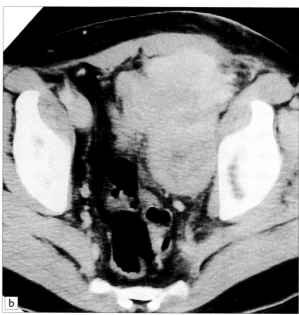

Figure 47.2. *Nodal metastases. (a) Extensive recurrent Merkel cell tumour in the right external iliac nodal chain. Note cutaneous scarring following previous excision and diffusely infiltrating tumour deep to the associated external iliac vessels and, medially, extension into the rectus abdominis muscle (arrow). (b and c) Large volume metastasis to pelvic lymph nodes from malignant melanoma. CT scans demonstrate the varying appearances ranging between solid enhancing tumour (b) and cystic degeneration (c). Both masses remain relatively well-defined.*

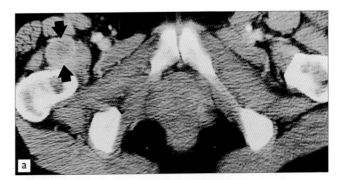

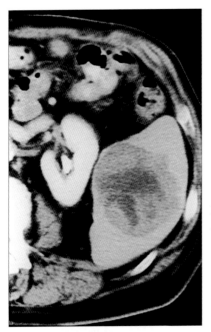

Figure 47.3. *Enhanced CT scan demonstrating a typical well-defined relatively non-enhancing melanoma metastasis in the spleen.*

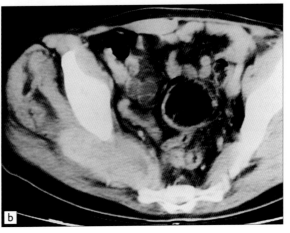

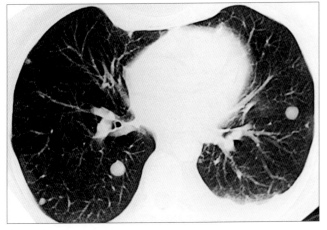

Figure 47.4. *CT scan showing multiple well-defined pulmonary metastases from melanoma.*

Figure 47.5. *Muscle metastases. (a) Well-defined enhancing melanomatous metastasis in the right ileo-psoas on CT (arrow). (b) CT scan showing an enhancing metastasis replacing the right pyriformis and extending through sciatic notch into overlying gluteal muscles. Note absence of bone erosion despite close application by soft tissue mass.*

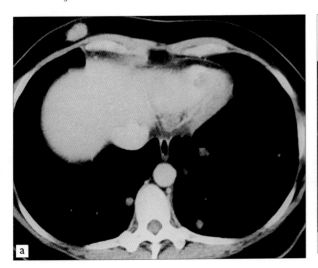

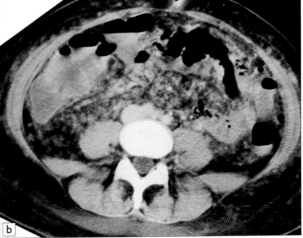

Figure 47.6. *Subcutaneous metastasis from melanoma. (a) A typical well-defined melanoma deposit in the subcutaneous fat anteriorly in the chest wall. Note metastases in the lungs. (b) Showers of metastases in the subcutaneous tissue, abdominal peritoneum and mesentery.*

Liver and biliary system

The majority of liver metastases from malignant melanoma are of low attenuation on CT when compared to the normal parenchyma (Fig. 47.7). Portal venous phase scanning alone fails to detect 14% of liver deposits but portal venous phase CT combined with either an unenhanced scan or an arterial phase scan shows improved conspicuity and both techniques have similar efficacy for the detection of liver metastases.[75] On MR, just 20–25% of liver deposits are hyperintense on T1-weighted images and hypo- or isointense on T2-weighted and short tau inversion recovery (STIR) images consistent with a paramagnetic effect of melanin. However, this signal pattern is not specific to melanin-containing deposits as it is also seen in other lesions such as focal fat deposits, intra-hepatic haemorrhage or haematoma and protein-containing lesions. Melanoma metastases are best demonstrated on fat-suppressed T1-weighted spin-echo or STIR images and there appears to be no advantage in using intravenous (IV) contrast medium.[76,77]

Melanoma accounts for more than half of all metastases to the gallbladder[78] (Fig. 47.8) and involvement of the gall-bladder is seen in up to 20% of melanoma deaths at autopsy.[66,79–81] Biliary involvement is usually clinically occult but, if symptomatic, is likely to mimic acute cholecystitis.[80–82] Gallbladder deposits can be single or multiple and they are typically non-shadowing hyperechoic masses on ultrasound, with a diameter greater than 1 cm. They are attached to the gallbladder wall and project into the lumen.[83,84]

Central nervous system

The antemortem detection rate for cerebral metastases to the brain is 6–10%, but they carry a grave prognosis, with a median survival of 4 months.[85,86] Cerebral metastases are typically multiple and supratentorial, although any intracranial site can be involved.[86] Peritumoural oedema, a nodular contour, uniform enhancement following IV contrast and high attenuation on unenhanced CT are characteristic features (Fig. 47.9).[87,88] The MR characteristics are highly variable, with only a quarter of lesions returning 'typical' melanotic signal of hyperintensity on T1-weighted images and hypointensity on T2-weighted images relative to the cortex (Fig. 47.10). On histological examination, such metastases tend to have a higher proportion of melanin-containing cells.[89] Intramedullary spinal metastases have similar imaging features to intracerebral deposits (Fig. 47.11).[90]

Gastro-intestinal tract

Melanoma is the most frequently implicated tumour in blood-borne metastases to the gastro-intestinal tract.[91] In the upper region, the tongue and tonsil are the prime sites[92] but distal to the hypopharynx in descending order of frequency are:

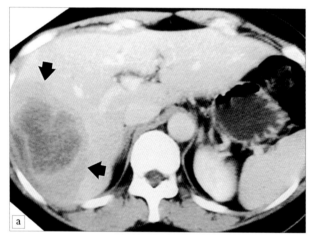

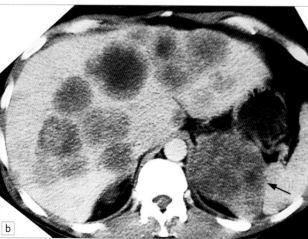

Figure 47.7. *Metastatic melanoma. (a and b) Hepatic CT in the portal venous phase of enhancement showing large hypoattenuating metastasis in the right lobe of the liver (arrows). In (b), note the large deposit in the left adrenal (arrow).*

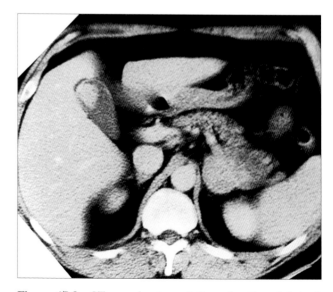

Figure 47.8. *CT scan showing soft tissue density nodule in the gallbladder, subsequently shown to be malignant melanoma when the patient developed obstructive jaundice associated with occluding tumour in the biliary tree.*

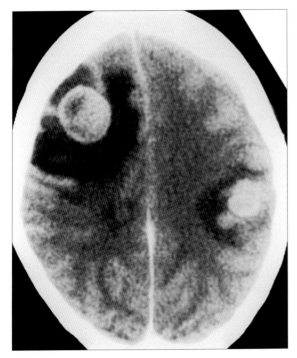

Figure 47.9. *Contrast-enhanced CT of the brain demonstrating typical avidly enhancing metastases from melanoma with associated surrounding oedema.*

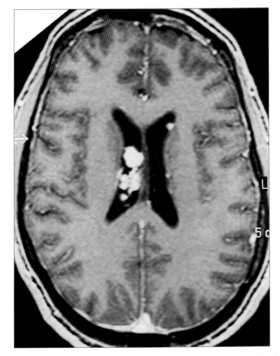

Figure 47.10. *Unenhanced T1-weighted axial MR showing high signal intensity choroidal metastases.*

- Small bowel
- Stomach (Fig. 47.12)
- Colon
- Rectum
- Oesophagus and anus[79]

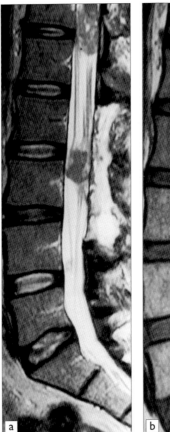
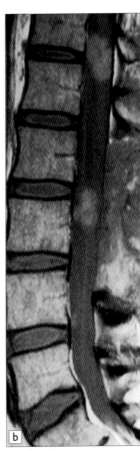

Figure 47.11. *Multiple leptomeningeal tumour nodules of melanoma within the spinal canal. (a) T2-weighted sagittal MR shows low signal intensity lesions, and (b) unenhanced T1-weighted image showing characteristic high signal intensity due to the paramagnetic features of melanin.*

Deposits within the small bowel often precipitate intussusception and small bowel obstruction. They are typically multiple and polypoid.[93] Endoscopy and contrast studies are the investigations of choice as CT has a sensitivity of only 60–70% for small bowel metastases (Fig. 47.13). Peritoneal deposits have variable appearances ranging from extensive studding to scattered larger nodules leading to large volume confluent disease (Fig. 47.6).[94]

Bone

Bone involvement is a late feature of melanoma, being detected in 0.8–6.9% of patients within clinical series, most of whom will have other sites of disease.[95–97] They are indistinguishable from other osteolytic metastases on imaging and pathological fracture occurs in nearly a quarter of patients whilst soft tissue invasion (12.5%), marginal sclerosis (12.5%) and osteoblastic deposits are atypical. Bone scintigraphy has a false negative rate of 15% in the spine, making MR the investigation of choice in the search for metastatic disease.[95,97]

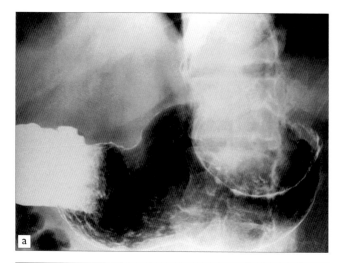

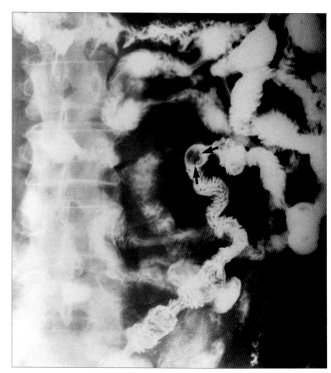

Figure 47.13. *A barium follow-through examination of a patient presenting with recurrent melanoma. A small polypoidal small bowel metastasis (arrows) was resected.*

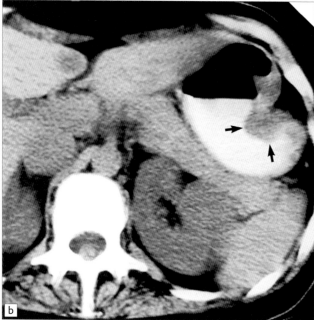

Figure 47.12. *Gastric metastases. (a) Large rounded melanoma deposit in the fundus of the stomach demonstrated on double contrast barium meal. (b) CT scan showing a metastasis from melanoma protruding into the stomach lumen contrast (arrows).*

Pancreas

The pancreas is an unusual site for metastases but up to 42% of patients with metastases will have multiple pancreatic deposits (Fig. 47.14). The imaging features are broadly similar to primary adenocarcinoma of the pancreas as compared with normal pancreatic parenchyma; these lesions are hypoechoic on ultrasound and of relatively low attenuation on CT. However, peri-pancreatic fat infiltration, duct obstruction and vascular invasion are seldom featured in melanoma metastases.[98]

Genito-urinary tract

The kidney is the most commonly involved site of metastatic disease in the urinary tract followed by the bladder and

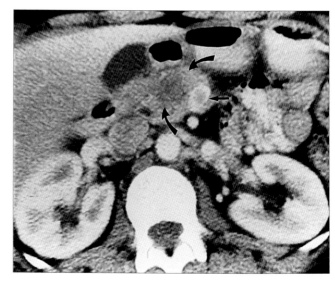

Figure 47.14. *CT scan of patient with pancreatic involvement by melanoma. Note that the low density tumour in the head of the pancreas (arrows) is associated with superior mesenteric vein thrombosis (straight arrow).*

urinary collecting system.[99] Melanoma metastasizing to the urethra has been described.[100] Renal metastases are typically small, multiple and cortical. Rarely, these lesions may manifest as a large parenchymal mass with similar appearances to those of renal cell carcinoma (Fig. 47.15).[99,101]

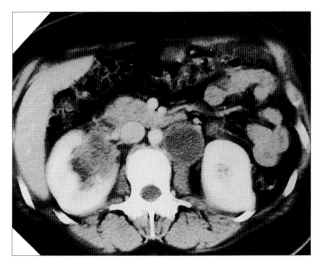

Figure 47.15. *CT scan demonstrating an irregular relatively non-enhancing mass in the hilum of the right kidney in a patient with widespread metastatic melanoma. A left para-aortic lymph node metastasis is also present.*

Collecting system, ureteric and bladder metastases (Fig. 47.16) are more likely to provoke symptoms than renal disease and this will therefore trigger investigation. The urographic findings of single or multiple smooth or irregular filling defects are clearly non-specific but, in the clinical context of malignant melanoma, the appearances should raise the suspicion of disseminated disease.[99,101–103]

The female genital tract is more frequently and extensively involved than the male genital tract.[104] The ovaries are the most frequently affected site presenting with uni- or bilateral involvement with large, smooth, lobulated solid or solid/cystic masses (Fig. 47.17). The imaging features tend to be non-specific on all modalities, including MR, as only a minority contain significant quantities of melanin.[105–107] Endometrial and placental metastases are rare (Fig. 47.18).[108]

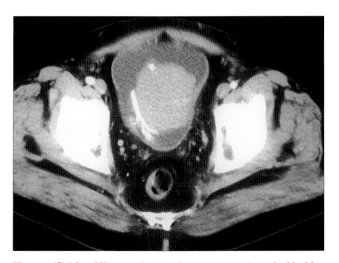

Figure 47.16. *CT scan showing large metastasis to the bladder. Note urinary stent in situ.*

The testis is more frequently involved than the penis and in itself is a rare antemortem diagnosis. The testicular mass is often suspected to be a primary testicular neoplasm

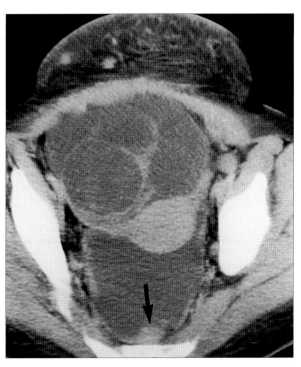

Figure 47.17. *Thick-walled multiloculate ovarian cyst in a patient with extensive metastatic melanoma. Note fluid and peritoneal plaques (arrow) in the Pouch of Douglas as well as subcutaneous deposits anteriorly.*

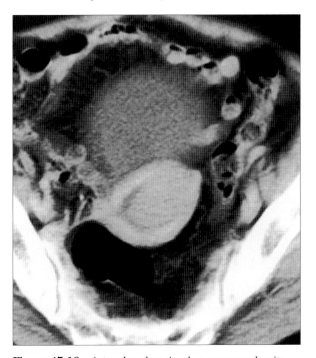

Figure 47.18. *A poorly enhancing homogeneous density melanomatous tumour expanding the endometrial cavity, demonstrated on CT and confirmed when continuous bleeding required hysterectomy.*

and a history of primary melanoma may be crucial in aiding diagnosis.[109,110] Melanoma metastasizing to the prostate has been reported.[111]

Endocrine system

The adrenal gland is the most frequently involved endocrine organ. In clinical studies, adrenal metastases have a mean diameter of 4 cm and are usually unilateral but at autopsy they are usually found to be bilateral.[66,76,112]

A new thyroid abnormality in a patient with disseminated malignancy has been reported as three times more likely to be due to a metastasis than a new primary tumour.[113] Metastases to the thyroid from several primary sites, including malignant melanoma, exhibit diminished activity on scintigraphy and are typically solid, homogeneous and hypoechoic on ultrasound, thus warranting FNAC. Thyroid function is almost invariably normal.[113–115]

One fifth of patients with cerebral metastases at autopsy also have disease involving the hypothalamus or pituitary gland.[104]

Breast

Indistinguishable from a primary breast lesion, melanoma metastasizing to the breast often presents as a solitary, painless mass in the upper outer quadrant requiring tissue sampling for definitive diagnosis (Fig. 47.19).[116] In a case report of bilateral breast metastases, MR showed that all five lesions had a high signal intensity on T1-weighted images and low signal intensity on T2-weighted images.[117] It is recommended that, even in the presence of more widespread visceral disease, resection of melanoma metastases should be performed in order to achieve local control.[117, 118]

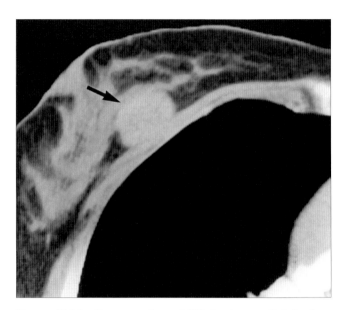

Figure 47.19. *Contrast-enhanced CT showing a well-defined ovoid enhancing melanoma deposit (arrow) deep within the tissue of the right breast.*

Cardiovascular system

Melanoma has a propensity for metastasizing to the heart, particularly the myocardium of the right-sided chambers.[119,120] The discrepancy between ante- and postmortem detection rates of 1% and approximately 50%, respectively, reflects the small size of these deposits and lack of symptoms. Tachycardia, dyspnoea and features of right heart failure in a patient with malignant melanoma should prompt echocardiography.[120,121] Cardiac MR is complementary to echocardiography; CT can also demonstrate large melanoma metastases (Fig. 47.20).[121,122]

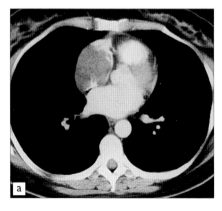

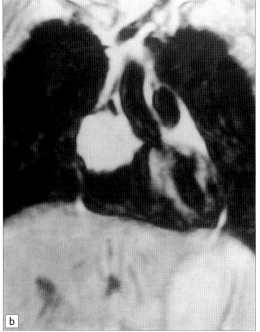

Figure 47.20. *Cardiac metastasis from melanoma. (a) Contrast-enhanced CT and (b) coronal MR demonstrating a large mass of melanoma which almost fills the right atrium.*

Key points: malignant melanoma metastases

- Initial predictable mode of spread to locoregional lymph nodes

- The majority of melanoma metastases on MR do not demonstrate high signal intensity on T1-weighted images

- Pulmonary metastasectomy may prolong survival in those with limited disease

- Skin is the most frequent site of metastatic disease

- Lower limbs are the most frequent site of muscle deposits

- 20–25% of liver metastases have a high signal intensity on T1-weighting and a low signal intensity on T2-weighting

- Melanoma accounts for >50% of all metastases to the gallbladder

- Brain metastases carry a very poor prognosis

- Malignant melanoma is the most frequent cause of metastases to the gastro-intestinal tract

- Bone involvement is a late feature of the disease

- Pancreatic deposits are uncommon and are multiple in 42%

- Renal involvement may mimic primary renal cell carcinoma

- Ovarian metastases are the most common manifestation of involvement of the genital tract

- Most adrenal metastases identified on imaging are large (>4 cm) unilateral lesions

- Breast metastases are usually solitary and non-specific

- Cardiac metastases are seldom detected during life

Squamous cell carcinoma

Although considerably more common than melanoma, SCC demonstrates a comparatively low propensity to metastasize and deposits are seen in only 2–3% of cases.[123–125] The majority of these will involve the locoregional lymph nodes and only 15% spread to more distant nodal sites.[13] Lymph node metastases frequently exhibit central low density and avid rim enhancement on contrast-enhanced CT. Although rare, haematogenous spread to distant sites, including lungs, liver, brain, skin and bone, have been reported. Pulmonary metastases are typically multiple and may cavitate.[126]

Basal cell carcinoma

Metastatic BCC is extremely rare, with a reported incidence of only 0.0028–0.55%.[127] The median time interval from primary diagnosis to metastatic disease is 9 years and the 5-year survival thereafter is just 10%.[128,129] The sites for metastatic disease in descending order of frequency are the lymph nodes, lungs, skin, liver and pleura. Deposits in the kidney, spleen, heart, adrenal glands, brain and bowel have also been reported.[128]

Merkel cell carcinoma

In common with malignant melanoma, once MCC has spread beyond the regional nodal basin it has a propensity for wide and unpredictable dissemination. There is a dearth of literature on the description of MCC metastases. Due to the propensity for head and neck involvement (>50% of cases), lymph node metastases in the neck, especially level 2, are a frequent finding.[35] Beyond the draining nodal basin any nodal group may be involved. Lymph node metastases are hyper- or iso-attenuating to muscle on contrast-enhanced CT.[45]

Subcutaneous and muscle deposits are described which once again show iso- or hyper-attenuation compared to muscle on contrast-enhanced CT.[45] Chest involvement can present as nodal disease, intrapulmonary nodules and masses or bone/chest wall invasion. In common with melanoma, both solid-organ and hollow visceral disease can occur in the abdomen and pelvis. The liver is a frequently targeted abdominal organ, with metastases typically demonstrating ring enhancement on contrast-enhanced CT.[35,45]

The central nervous system (CNS) is not a frequent metastatic site but neurological symptoms/signs will usually warrant MR examination, and deposits so discovered may show central necrosis.[35,130]

Owing to the neuro-endocrine origin of Merkel cells, assessment of recurrent and metastatic disease is amenable to somatostatin receptor scintigraphy (SRS) using indium-111-labelled octreotide. Although demonstrating good specificity in MCC, this technique lacks sensitivity, particularly in the skin and in organs that demonstrate physiological octreotide uptake, most notably the liver and spleen.[35,131] [18]FDG PET has been successfully used in the assessment of response of MCC to isolated limb perfusion in a single case.[132]

Kaposi's sarcoma

Kaposi's sarcoma is a multifocal neoplasm with each new visceral lesion developing de novo from the endothelial cells lining the lymphatics or blood vessels rather than representing metastases from mucocutaneous neoplasms.[133] In classical KS, skin lesions can regress whilst new lesions appear. The sites of involvement beyond the skin are numerous, including lymph nodes, bowel, liver, lungs, kidneys and spleen. Testicular and cerebral disease is rare. Visceral lesions are usually only seen in the presence of cutaneous disease.[133] The lymphadenopathic form of endemic African KS is an aggressive form involving the lymph nodes, and occasionally visceral organs, of children.[133]

Epidemic (AIDS-related) KS can affect the lymphatics

and viscera, e.g. lungs, liver, gastro-intestinal tract, spleen and kidneys, with mucocutaneous disease not being a prerequisite.[133] Chest radiographic findings in pulmonary KS include:

- Peribronchovascular opacities (86%)
- Lung nodules (71%)
- Pleural effusion (41%)
- Interlobular septal thickening (29%)
- Lymphadenopathy (29%)[134]

Computed tomography may also reveal patchy ground glass attenuation surrounding or separate from nodules, and dis-

tortion and nodularity of the fissures.[135] Iatrogenic or transplant-related KS is usually confined to the skin, with visceral involvement being atypical.[133]

Key points: metastatic disease

- SCC, melanoma and MCC predictably metastasize to the draining nodal basin

- Melanoma and MCC have a tendency to disseminated unpredictable spread beyond the regional lymph nodes

- SCC metastasizes in 2–3% and BCC very rarely

Summary

- Malignant tumours of the skin form a disparate group of cancers with a wide range of behaviours

- Skin cancer is the most common human malignancy

- Skin tumours are categorized according to cellular origin and the common forms divided into non-melanoma skin cancer and melanoma

- Staging is pathological

- Elective lymph node dissection is not recommended

- Nodal staging with FNAC or sentinel node biopsy should be considered in selected cases

- Surgical excision of the primary is generally the treatment of choice

- Surveillance largely relies on self-examination and clinical follow-up

- Metastasis of SCC, melanoma and MCC is initially to the regional lymph nodes

- Melanoma and MCC have a propensity to wide and unpredictable spread

- CT and, increasingly, [18]FDG PET form the basis for investigation of metastatic disease

References

1. Bruce A J, Brodland D G. Overview of skin cancer detection and prevention for the primary care physician. Mayo Clin Proc 2000; 75: 491–500
2. Brown M D. Recognition and management of unusual cutaneous tumors. Dermatol Clin 2000; 18: 543–552
3. Skidmore R A Jr, Flowers F P. Non-melanoma skin cancer. Med Clin North Am 1998; 82: 1309–1323
4. Diepgen T L, Mahler V. The epidemiology of skin cancer. Br J Dermatol 2002; 146 (Suppl. 61): 1–6
5. Holme S A, Malinovszky K, Roberts D L. Changing trends in non-melanoma skin cancer in South Wales, 1988–98. Br J Dermatol 2000; 143: 1224–1249
6. Buettner P G, Raasch B A. Incidence rates of skin cancer in Townsville, Australia. Int J Cancer 1998; 78: 587–593
7. CancerStats. Incidence – UK, September 2002. Cancer Research UK 2002
8. Wingo P A, Tong T, Bolden S. Cancer statistics. Cancer J Clin 1995; 45: 8–30
9. Rigel D S, Friedman R J, Kopf A W. The incidence of malignant melanoma in the United States: issues as we

approach the 21st century. J Am Acad Dermatol 1996; 34: 839–847
10. Roberts D L, Anstey A V, Barlow R J et al. The British Association of Dermatologists: The Melanoma Study Group. UK guidelines for the management of cutaneous melanoma. Br J Dermatol 2002; 146: 7–17
11. Telfer N R, Colver G B, Bowers P W. Guidelines for the management of basal cell carcinoma. British Association of Dermatologists. Br J Dermatol 1999; 141: 415–423
12. Motley R, Kersey P, Lawrence C. The British Association of Dermatologists: The British Association of Plastic Surgeons: The Royal College of Radiologists, Faculty of Clinical Oncology. Multiprofessional guidelines for the management of the patient with primary cutaneous squamous cell carcinoma. Br J Dermatol 2002; 146: 18–25
13. Murad A, Ratner D. Primary care: cutaneous squamous cell carcinoma. N Engl J Med 2001; 344: 975–983
14. Kefford R F, Newton Bishop J A, Bergman W, Tucker M A. Counselling and DNA testing for individuals

Summary

■ Early heterogeneous enhancement in the spleen should not be misinterpreted as pathology

■ The most common splenic malignancy is lymphoma. The spleen is involved as part of generalized lymphoma. An enlarged spleen is not a reliable indicator of lymphomatous involvement

■ Metastases to the spleen are uncommon. The primary tumours most commonly metastasizing to the spleen include those of breast, lung, ovary, and colorectum, and melanoma

■ Splenic metastases may be serosal from peritoneal spread of tumour or parenchymal from haematogenous metastases

References

1. Rabushka L S, Kawashima A, Fishman E K. Imaging of the spleen: CT with supplemental MR examination. Radiographics 1994; 14: 307–332
2. Glazer G M, Axel L, Goldberg H I, Moss A A. Dynamic CT of the normal spleen. Am J Roentgenol 1981; 137: 343–346
3. Warshauer D M, Koehler R E. Spleen. In: Lee J K, Sagel S S, Stanley R J, Heiken J P (eds). CT with MRI Correlation, 3rd edn. Philadelphia: Lippincott-Raven, 1998: 845–872
4. Hahn P F, Weissleder R, Stark D D et al. MR imaging of focal splenic tumors. Am J Roentgenol 1988; 150: 823–827
5. Semelka R C, Shoenut J P, Lawrence P H et al. Spleen: dynamic enhancement patterns on gradient-echo MR images enhanced with gadopentetate dimeglumine. Radiology 1992; 185: 479–482
6. Weissleder R, Hahn P F, Stark D D et al. Superparamagnetic iron oxide: enhanced detection of focal splenic tumors with MR imaging. Radiology 1988; 169: 399–403
7. Gooding G A. The ultrasonic and computed tomographic appearance of splenic lobulations: a consideration in the ultrasonic differential of masses adjacent to the left kidney. Radiology 1978; 126: 719–720
8. Piekarski J, Federle M P, Moss A A, London S S. Computed tomography of the spleen. Radiology 1980; 135: 683–689
9. Dachman A H, Friedman A C. Radiology of the Spleen. St Louis: Mosby-Year Book, 1993
10. Wadham B M, Adams P B, Johnson M A. Incidence and location of accessory spleens [letter]. N Engl J Med 1981; 304: 1111
11. Subramanyam B R, Balthazar E J, Horii S C. Sonography of the accessory spleen. Am J Roentgenol 1984; 143: 47–49
12. Freeman J L, Jafri S Z, Roberts J L et al. CT of congenital and acquired abnormalities of the spleen. Radiographics 1993; 13: 597–610
13. Prassopoulos P, Daskalogiannaki M, Raissaki M et al. Determination of normal splenic volume on computed tomography in relation to age, gender and body habitus. Eur Radiol 1997; 7: 246–248
14. Whitley J E, Maynard C D, Rhyne A L. A computer approach to the prediction of spleen weight from routine films. Radiology 1966; 86: 73–76
15. Dardenne A N. The spleen. In: Cosgrove D O, Meire H B, Dewbury K C D (eds). Clinical Ultrasound. Edinburgh: Churchill Livingstone, 1993: 353–365
16. Frank K, Linhart P, Kortsik C, Wohlenberg H. [Sonographic determination of spleen size: normal dimensions in adults with a healthy spleen]. [German]. Ultraschall Med 1986; 7: 134–137
17. Lamb P M, Lund A, Kanagasabay R R et al. Spleen size: how well do linear ultrasound measurements correlate with three-dimensional CT volume assessments? Br J Radiol 2002; 75: 573–577
18. Breiman R S, Beck J W, Korobkin M et al. Volume determinations using computed tomography. Am J Roentgenol 1982; 138: 329–333
19. Strijk S P, Wagener D J, Bogman M J et al. The spleen in Hodgkin disease: diagnostic value of CT. Radiology 1985; 154: 753–757
20. Lam K Y, Tang V. Metastatic tumors to the spleen: a 25-year clinicopathologic study. Arch Pathol Lab Med 2000; 124: 526–530
21. Spencer N J, Spencer J A, Perren T J, Lane G. CT appearances and prognostic significance of splenic metastasis in ovarian cancer. Clin Radiol 1998; 53: 417–421
22. Warren S, Davis A H. Studies of tumor metastasis: the metastases of carcinoma to the spleen. Am J Cancer 1934; 21: 517–533
23. Marymont J G J, Gross S. Patterns of metastatic cancer in the spleen. Am J Clin Pathol 1963; 40: 58–66
24. Nash D A Jr, Sampson C C. Secondary carcinoma of the spleen. Its incidence in 544 cases and a review of the literature. J Natl Med Assoc 1966; 58: 442–446
25. Berge T. Splenic metastases. Frequencies and patterns. Acta Pathol Microbiol Scand [A] 1974; 82: 499–506
26. Goerg C, Schwerk W B, Goerg K. Splenic lesions: sonographic patterns, follow-up, differential diagnosis. Eur J Radiol 1991; 13: 59–66
27. Siniluoto T, Paivansalo M, Lahde S. Ultrasonography of splenic metastases. Acta Radiol 1989; 30: 463–466
28. Abrams H L, Spiro R, Goldstein N. Metastases in

perceived to be genetically predisposed to melanoma: a consensus statement of the Melanoma Genetics Consortium. J Clin Oncol 1999; 17: 3245–3251

15. Berg D, Otley C C. Skin cancer in organ transplant recipients: epidemiology, pathogenesis, and management. J Am Acad Dermatol 2002; 47: 1–17

16. Jensen P, Hansen S, Moller B et al. Skin cancer in kidney and heart transplant recipients and different long-term immunosuppressive therapy regimens. J Am Acad Dermatol 1999; 40: 177–186

17. Hartevelt M M, Bavinck J N, Kootte A M et al. Incidence of skin cancer after renal transplantation in The Netherlands. Transplantation 1990; 49: 506–509

18. Penn I, First M R. Merkel's cell carcinoma in organ recipients: report of 41 cases. Transplantation 1999; 68: 1717–1721

19. Veness M J, Quinn D I, Ong C S et al. Aggressive cutaneous malignancies following cardiothoracic transplantation: the Australian experience. Cancer 1999; 85: 1758–1764

20. Penn I. Malignant melanoma in organ allograft recipients. Transplantation 1996; 61: 274–278

21. Sobin L H, Wittekind Ch (eds). TNM Classification of Malignant Tumours, 6th edn. San Francisco: Wiley-Liss, Inc., 2002

22. Greene F L, Page D L, Fleming I D et al (eds). American Joint Committee on Cancer (AJCC) Cancer Staging Handbook, 6th edn. Berlin: Springer, 2002

23. Yiengpruksawan A, Coit D G, Thaler H T et al. Merkel cell carcinoma. Prognosis and management. Arch Surg 1991; 126: 1514–1519

24. Aboulafia D M. Kaposi's sarcoma. Clin Dermatol 2001; 19: 269–283

25. Harris N L, Jaffe E S, Stein H et al. A revised European–American classification of lymphoid neoplasms: a proposal from the International Lymphoma Study Group. Blood 1994; 84: 1361–1392

26. Topping A, Wilson G R. Diagnosis and management of uncommon cutaneous cancers. Am J Clin Dermatol 2002; 3: 83–89

27. Shafir R, Itzchak Y, Heyman Z et al. Preoperative ultrasonic measurement of the thickness of cutaneous malignant melanoma. J Ultrasound Med 1984; 3: 205–208

28. Hoffman K, Jung J, el Gammal S, Altemeyer P. Malignant melanoma in 20 MHz B scan sonography. Dermatology 1992; 185: 49–55

29. Semple J L, Gupta A K, From L et al. Does high frequency ultrasound imaging play a role in the clinical management of cutaneous melanoma? Ann Plast Surg 1995; 34: 599–606

30. Shafir R. Does high frequency ultrasound imaging play a role in the clinical management of cutaneous melanoma? Ann Plast Surg 1996; 36: 599–560

31. Takahashi M, Kohda H. Diagnostic utility of magnetic resonance imaging in malignant melanoma. J Am Acad Dermatol 1992; 27: 51–54

32. Williams L S, Mancuso A A, Mendenhall W M.

Perineural spread of cutaneous squamous and basal cell carcinoma: CT and MR detection and its impact on patient management and prognosis. Int J Radiat Oncol Biol Phys 2001; 49: 1061–1069

33. Sian K U, Wagner J D, Sood R et al. Lymphoscintigraphy with sentinel lymph node biopsy in cutaneous Merkel cell carcinoma. Ann Plast Surg 1999; 42: 679–682

34. Hill A D, Brady M S, Coit D G. Intraoperative lymphatic mapping and sentinel lymph node biopsy for Merkel cell carcinoma. Br J Surg 1999; 86: 518–521

35. Nguyen B D, McCullough A E. Imaging of Merkel cell carcinoma. Radiographics 2002; 22: 367–376

36. Morton D L, Wen D-R, Wong J H et al. Technical details of intraoperative lymphatic mapping for early-stage melanoma. Arch Surg 1992; 127: 392–399

37. Gennari R, Bartolomei M, Testori A et al. Sentinel node localisation in primary melanoma: preoperative dynamic lymphoscintigraphy, intraoperative gamma probe and vital dye guidance. Surgery 2000; 127: 19–25

38. Alex J C, Weaver D L, Fairbank J T et al. Gamma-probe-guided lymph node localization in malignant melanoma. Surg Oncol 1993; 2: 303–308

39. Krag D N, Meijer S J, Weaver D L et al. Minimal access surgery for staging of malignant melanoma. Arch Surg 1995; 130: 654–658

40. Yudd A P, Kempf J S, Goydos J S et al. Use of sentinel node lymphoscintigraphy in malignant melanoma. Radiographics 1999; 19: 343–353

41. Acland K M, Healy C, Calonje E et al. Comparison of positron emission tomography scanning and sentinel node biopsy in the detection of micrometastases of primary cutaneous malignant melanoma. J Clin Oncol 2001; 19: 2674–2678

42. Schwimmer J, Essner R, Patel A et al. A review of the literature for whole-body FDG PET in the management of patients with melanoma. Q J Nucl Med 2000; 44: 153–167

43. Terhune M H, Swanson N, Johnson T M. Use of chest radiography in the initial evaluation of patients with localised melanoma. Arch Dermatol 1998; 134: 569–572

44. Medina-Franco H, Urist M M, Fiveash J et al. Multimodality treatment of Merkel cell carcinoma: case series and literature review of 1024 cases. Ann Surg Oncol 2001; 8: 204–208

45. Gollub M J, Gruen D R, Dershaw D D. Merkel cell carcinoma: CT findings in 12 patients. Am J Roentgenol 1996; 167: 617–620

46. Rabkin C S. AIDS and cancer in the era of highly active antiretroviral therapy (HAART). Eur J Cancer 2001; 37: 1316–1319

47. NIH Consensus Development Panel on Early Melanoma. Diagnosis and treatment of early melanoma. J Am Med Assoc 1992; 268: 1314–1319

48. Day C L Jr, Mihm M C Jr, Lew R A et al. Cutaneous malignant melanoma: prognostic guidelines for

physicians and patients. CA Cancer J Clin 1982; 32: 113–122

49. Balch C M, Soong S-J, Gershenwald J E et al. Prognostic factors analysis of 17,600 melanoma patients: validation of the American Joint Committee on Cancer melanoma staging system. J Clin Oncol 2001; 19: 3622–3634

50. Goessling W, McKee P H, Mayer R J. Merkel cell carcinoma. J Clin Oncol 2002; 20: 588–598

51. Smith D F, Messina J L, Perrott R et al. Clinical approach to neuroendocrine carcinoma of the skin (Merkel cell carcinoma). Cancer Control 2000; 7: 72–83

52. Nelson B R, Hamlet K R, Gillard M et al. Sebaceous carcinoma. J Am Acad Dermatol 1995; 33: 1–15

53. Gortler I, Koppl H, Stark G B, Horch R E. Metastatic malignant acrospiroma of the hand. Eur J Surg Oncol 2001; 27: 431–435

54. Gilliam A C, Wood G S. Primary cutaneous lymphomas other than mycosis fungoides. Semin Oncol 1999; 26: 290–306

55. Itoh H, Miyaguni H, Kataoka H et al. Primary cutaneous Langerhans' cell histiocytosis showing malignant phenotype in an elderly woman: report of a fatal case. J Cutan Pathol 2001; 28: 371–378

56. Aoki M, Aoki R, Akimoto M, Hara K. Primary cutaneous Langerhans' cell histiocytosis in an adult. Am J Dermatopathol 1998; 20: 281–284

57. Lichtenwald D J, Jakubovic H R, Rosenthal D. Primary cutaneous Langerhans' cell histiocytosis in an adult. Arch Dermatol 1991; 127: 1545–1548

58. Balch C M, Urist M M, Karakousis C P et al. Efficacy of 2-cm surgical margins for intermediate-thickness melanomas (1 to 4 mm). Results of a multi-institutional randomized surgical trial. Ann Surg 1993; 218: 262–267

59. Veronesi U, Cascinelli N, Adamus J et al. Thin Stage I primary cutaneous malignant melanoma. Comparison of excision with margins of 1 or 3 cm. N Engl J Med 1988; 318: 1159–1162

60. Heaton K M, Sussman J J, Gershenwald J E et al. Surgical margins and prognostic factors in patients with thick (>4 mm) primary melanoma. Ann Surg Oncol 1998; 5: 322–328

61. Hill S, Thomas J M. Use of the carbon dioxide laser to manage cutaneous metastases from malignant melanoma Br J Surg 1996; 83: 509–512

62. Basseres N, Grob J J, Richard M A et al. Cost-effectiveness of surveillance of Stage I melanoma. A retrospective appraisal based on a 10-year experience in a dermatology department in France. Dermatology 1995; 191: 199–203

63. Provost N, Marghoob A A, Kopf A W et al. Laboratory tests and imaging studies in patients with cutaneous malignant melanomas: a survey of experienced physicians. J Am Acad Dermatol 1997; 36: 711–720

64. Virgo K S, Chan D, Handler B S et al. Current practice of patient follow-up after potentially curative resection of cutaneous melanoma. Plast Reconstr Surg 2000; 106: 590–597

65. Blum A, Schlagenhauff B, Stroebel W et al. Ultrasound examination of regional lymph nodes significantly improves early detection of locoregional metastases during follow-up of patients with cutaneous melanoma. Cancer 2000; 88: 2534–2539

66. Patel J K, Didolkar M S, Pickren J W, Moore R H. Metastatic pattern of malignant melanoma. A study of 216 autopsy cases. Am J Surg 1978; 135: 807–810

67. Moehrle M, Blum A, Rassner G, Juenger M J. Lymph node metastases of cutaneous melanoma: diagnosis by B-scan and colour Doppler sonography. J Am Acad Dermatol 1999; 41: 703–709

68. Imada H, Nakata H, Horie A. Radiological significance of splenic metastases and its prevalence at autopsy. Nippon Igaku Hoshasen Gakkai Zasshi 1991; 51: 498–503

69. Krug B, Dietlein M, Groth W et al. Fluoro-18-fluorodeoxyglucose positron emission tomography (FDG-PET) in malignant melanoma. Acta Radiol 2000; 41: 446–452

70. Quint L E, Park C H, Iannettoni M D. Solitary pulmonary nodules in patients with extrapulmonary neoplasms. Radiology 2000; 217: 257–261

71. Pastorino U, Buyse M, Friedel G et al. Long-term results of lung metastasectomy: prognostic analysis based on 5206 cases. J Thorac Cardiovasc Surg 1997; 113: 37–49

72. Leo F, Cagini L, Rocmans P et al. Lung metastases from melanoma: when is surgical treatment warranted? Br J Cancer 2000; 83: 569–572

73. Damron T A, Heiner J. Distant soft tissue metastases: a series of 30 new patients and 91 cases from the literature. Ann Surg Oncol 2000; 7: 526–534

74. Nazarian L N, Alexander A A, Kurtz A B et al. Superficial melanoma metastases: appearances on grey-scale and colour Doppler sonography. Am J Roentgenol 1998; 170: 459–463

75. Blake S P, Weisinger K, Atkins M B, Raptopoulos V. Liver metastases from melanoma: detection with multiphasic contrast-enhanced CT. Radiology 1999; 213: 92–96

76. Premkumar A, Sanders L, Marincola F et al. Visceral metastases from melanoma: findings on MR imaging. Am J Roentgenol 1992; 158: 293–298

77. Smirniotopoulos J G, Lonergan G J, Abbott R M et al. Image interpretation session 1998. Radiographics 1999; 19: 205–233

78. Backman H. Metastases of malignant melanoma in the gastrointestinal tract. Geriatrics 1969; 24: 112–120

79. DasGupta T K, Brasfield R. Metastatic melanoma of the gastrointestinal tract. Arch Surg 1964; 88: 969–973

80. Meyer J E. Radiographic evaluation of metastatic melanoma. Cancer 1978; 42: 127–132

81. O'Connell J B, Whittemore D M, Russell J C et al. Malignant melanoma metastatic to the cystic and common bile ducts. Cancer 1984; 53: 184–186

82. McFadden P M, Krementz E T, McKinnon W M P et al. Metastatic melanoma of the gallbladder. Cancer 1979; 44: 1802–1808

83. Daunt N, King D M. Metastatic melanoma in the biliary tree. Br J Radiol 1982; 55: 873–874

84. Holloway B J, King D M. Ultrasound diagnosis of metastatic melanoma of the gallbladder. Br J Radiol 1997; 70: 1122–1125

85. Moon D, Maafs E, Peterson-Schaefer K. A review of 567 cases of brain metastases from malignant melanoma. Melanoma Res 1993; 3: 40

86. Sampson J H, Carter J H Jr, Friedman A H, Seigler H F. Demographics, prognosis, and therapy in 702 patients with brain metastases from malignant melanoma. J Neurosurg 1998; 88: 11–20

87. McGann G M, Platts A. Computed tomography of cranial metastatic malignant melanoma: features, early detection and unusual cases. Br J Radiol 1991; 64: 310–313

88. Reider-Groswasser I, Merimsky O, Karminsky N, Chaitchik S. Computed tomography features of cerebral spread of malignant melanoma. Am J Clin Oncol (CCT) 1996; 19: 49–53

89. Isiklar I, Leeds N E, Fuller G N, Kumar A J. Intracranial metastatic melanoma: correlation between MR imaging characteristics and melanin content. Am J Roentgenol 1995; 165: 1503–1512

90. Crasto S, Duca S, Davini O et al. MRI diagnosis of intramedullary metastases from extra-CNS tumours. Eur Radiol 1997: 7: 732–736

91. Reintgen D S, Thompson W, Garbutt J, Siegler H F. Radiologic, endoscopic, and surgical considerations of melanoma metastatic to the gastrointestinal tract. Surgery 1984; 95: 635–639

92. Sood S, Nair S B, Fenwick J D, Horgan K. Metastatic melanoma of the tonsil. J Laryngol Otol 1999; 113: 1036–1038

93. Schuchter L M, Green R, Fraker D. Primary and metastatic diseases in malignant melanoma of the gastrointestinal tract. Curr Opin Oncol 2000; 12: 181–185

94. Kawashima A, Fishman E K, Kuhlman J E, Schuchter L M. CT of malignant melanoma: patterns of small bowel and mesenteric involvement. J Comput Assist Tomogr 1991; 15: 570–574

95. Potepan P, Spagnoli I, Danesini G M et al. The radiodiagnosis of bone metastases from melanoma. Radiol Med (Torino) 1994; 87: 741–746

96. Stewart W R, Gelberman R H, Harrelson J M, Siegler H F. Skeletal metastases of melanoma. J Bone Joint Surg Am 1978; 60: 645–649

97. Gokaslan Z L, Aladag M A, Ellerhorst J A. Melanoma metastatic to the spine: a review of 133 cases. Melanoma Res 2000; 10: 78–80

98. Boudghene F P, Deslandes P M, LeBlanche A F, Bigot J M R. US and CT features of intrapancreatic metastases. J Comput Assist Tomogr 1994; 18: 905–910

99. Goldstein H M, Kaminsky S, Wallace S, Johnson D E. Urographic manifestations of metastatic melanoma. Am J Roentgenol 1974; 121: 801–805

100. Das Gupta T, Grabstald H. Melanoma of genitourinary tract. J Urol 1965; 93: 607–614

101. Spera J A, Pollack H M, Banner M P et al. Metastatic malignant melanoma mimicking renal cell carcinoma. J Urol 1984; 131: 740–742

102. Meyer J. Metastatic melanoma of the urinary bladder. Cancer 1974; 34: 1822–1824

103. Chin J L, Sales J L, Silver M M, Sweeney J P. Melanoma metastatic to the bladder and bowel: an unusual case. J Urol 1982; 127: 541–542

104. de la Monte S M, Moore G W, Hutchins G M. Patterned distribution of metastases from malignant melanoma in humans. Cancer Res 1983; 43: 3427–3433

105. Fitzgibbons P L, Martin S E, Simmons T J. Malignant melanoma metastatic to the ovary. Am J Surg Pathol 1987; 11: 959–964

106. Young R H, Scully R E. Malignant melanoma metastatic to the ovary: a clinicopathological analysis of 20 cases. Am J Surg Pathol 1991; 15: 849–860

107. Moselhi M, Spencer J, Lane G. Malignant melanoma metastatic to the ovary: presentation and radiological characteristics. Gynaecol Oncol 1998; 69: 165–168

108. Bauer R D, McCoy C P, Roberts D K, Fritz G. Malignant melanoma metastatic to the endometrium. Obstet Gynecol 1984; 63: 264–268

109. Richardson P G G, Millward M J, Shrimankar J J, Cantwell B M J. Metastatic melanoma to the testis simulating primary seminoma. Br J Urol 1992; 69: 663–665

110. Skarin A. Diagnostic dilemmas in oncology: melanoma metastatic to the testis. J Clin Oncol 2000; 18: 3187–3192

111. Zein T A, Huben R, Lane W et al. Secondary tumours of the prostate. J Urol 1985; 133: 615–616

112. Branum G D, Epstein R E, Leight G S, Seigler H F. The role of resection in the management of melanoma metastatic to the adrenal gland. Surgery 1991; 109: 127–131

113. Ahuja A T, King W, Metreweli C. Role of ultrasound in thyroid metastases. Clin Radiol 1994; 49: 627–629

114. Eftekhari F, Peuchot M. Thyroid metastases: combined role of ultrasonography and fine-needle aspiration biopsy. J Clin Ultrasound 1989; 17: 657–660

115. Ferrozzi F, Campodonico F, De Chiara F et al. Thyroid metastases: the echographic and computed tomographic aspects. Radiol Med (Torino) 1997; 94: 214–219

116. Toombs B D, Kalisher L. Metastatic disease to the breast: clinical, pathological and radiographic features. Am J Roentgenol 1977; 129: 673–676

117. Ho L W C, Wong K P, Chan J H M et al. MR appearance of metastatic melanotic melanoma in the breast. Clin Rad 2000, 55: 572–573

118. Plesnicar A, Kovac V. Breast metastases from cutaneous melanoma: a report of three cases. Tumori 2000; 86: 170–173

119. Klatt E C, Heitz D R. Cardiac metastases. Cancer 1990; 65: 1456–1459

120. Gibbs P, Cebon J S, Calafiore P, Robinson W A. Cardiac metastases from malignant melanoma. Cancer 1999; 85: 78–84

121. Savoia P, Fierro M T, Zaccagna A, Bernengo M G. Metastatic melanoma of the heart. J Surg Oncol 2000; 75: 203–207

122. Freedberg R S, Kronzon I, Rumancik W M, Liebskind D. The contribution of magnetic resonance imaging to the evaluation of intracardiac tumours diagnosed by echocardiography. Circulation 1988; 77: 96–103

123. Epstein E, Epstein N N, Bragg K, Linden G. Metastases from squamous cell carcinomas of the skin. Arch Dermatol 1968; 97: 245–249

124. Katz A D, Uraback F, Lilienfeld A M. The frequency and risk of metastases in squamous cell carcinoma of the skin. Cancer 1957; 10: 1162–1166

125. Moller R, Reymann F, Hou-Jensen K. Metastases in dermatological patients with squamous cell carcinoma. Arch Dermatol 1979; 115: 703–705

126. Johnson T M, Rowe D E, Nelson B R, Swanson N A. Squamous cell carcinoma of the skin (excluding lip and oral mucosa). J Am Acad Dermatol 1992; 26: 467–484

127. Lo J S, Snow S N, Reizner G T et al. Metastatic basal cell carcinoma: report of 12 cases and a review of the literature. J Am Acad Dermatol 1991; 24: 715–719

128. von Domarus H, Stevens P J. Metastatic basal cell carcinoma. J Am Acad Dermatol 1984; 10: 1043–1060

129. Farmer E R, Helwig E B. Metastatic basal cell carcinoma: a clinicopathologic study of 17 cases. Cancer 1980; 46: 748–757

130. Eggers S D Z, Salomao D R, Dinapoli R P, Vernino S. Paraneoplastic and metastatic neurological complications of Merkel cell carcinoma. Mayo Clin Proc 2001; 76: 327–330

131. Guitera-Rovel P, Lumbroso J, Gautier-Gougis M S et al. Indium-111 octreotide scintigraphy of Merkel cell carcinomas and their metastases. Ann Oncol 2001; 12: 807–811

132. Lampreave J L, Benard F, Alavi A et al. PET evaluation of therapeutic limb perfusion in Merkel's cell carcinoma. J Nucl Med 1998; 39: 2087–2090

133. Friedman-Kien A E, Saltzman B R. Clinical manifestations of classical, endemic African, and epidemic AIDS-associated Kaposi's sarcoma. J Am Acad Dermatol 1990; 22: 1237–1250

134. Haramati L B, Wong J. Intrathoracic Kaposi's sarcoma in women with AIDS. Chest 2000; 117: 410–414

135. Traill Z C, Miller R F, Shaw P J. CT appearances of intrathoracic Kaposi's sarcoma in patients with AIDS. Br J Radiol 1996; 69: 1104–1107

Chapter 48

Radiological investigation of carcinoma of unknown primary site

Christopher J Gallagher, Rodney H Reznek and Janet E Husband

Introduction

Cancer of unknown primary site is a common referral problem accounting for between 3 and 9% of all patients seen in most tertiary treatment centres.[1-3] In the USA, as estimated by the SEER statistics (Surveillance Epidemiology and End Results), 2% of cancers were registered as cancer of unknown primary site within the population as a whole. Of these cancers, adenocarcinoma comprised 55%, squamous carcinoma 14%, cancer undifferentiated 21% and 10% other specific diagnoses such as sarcoma, neuro-endocrine cancer and melanoma.[4]

Patients present with the symptoms of their metastases without a clinically apparent primary site. The frequency of the site of presentation of the metastases varies, in part due to differences in patient selection in the reported series. However, the most common sites of presentation (excluding head and neck) are as shown in Table 48.1.[1,2]

The *definition* of a (metastatic) cancer of unknown primary site has shifted over the years largely due to changes in histological and radiological investigations. Thus, in the earlier clinical series, most patients simply had a careful clinical history, physical examination and chest X-ray. However, in recent series, most patients have already undergone a computed tomography (CT) scan of chest, abdomen and pelvis and, if appropriate, bilateral mammography before referral for investigation of the unknown primary site. Nevertheless, even after postmortem examination, the primary site will remain unknown in approximately 15–20% of patients diagnosed as having cancer of unknown primary site.[5,6]

Diagnostic pathology has improved remarkably over the past several years. Increased routine use of electron microscopy, immunohistochemistry and molecular genetics are now contributing to a more precise diagnosis of neoplasms. In general, therefore, the term carcinoma of unknown origin is almost always a light microscopical diagnosis. The most common cause of a non-specific light microscopical diagnosis is an inadequate or poorly handled biopsy specimen. If possible, fine-needle aspiration (FNA) should not be relied upon as a definitive diagnostic procedure because the histological pattern is not preserved and the ability to perform special studies is limited. Several instances have been documented in which FNA has suggested a specific diagnosis, which was proved later to be incorrect on tissue biopsy.[7]

Histology

The most critical step in the assessment of any patient with cancer of unknown primary site is a review of the histological findings, from which three main groups can be derived:[8]

- Adenocarcinoma (50–60%)
- Squamous carcinoma (5%)
- Poorly differentiated tumours (35%)

Other malignancies include:

- Lymphoma (6%)
- Germ cell (1%)
- Melanoma, sarcoma, neuro-endocrine (1%)

The most common histological type is that of adenocarcinoma, comprising 50–60% of patients in all series. Immunohistochemistry can increasingly help identify likely primary sites, e.g. thyroid transcriptor factor (TTF-1) staining in metastatic lung cancer.[9] Squamous carcinomas are

Table 48.1. *Common sites of presentation of metastases*

Site	%
Lymph nodes	14–37
Thorax	28–30
Lung	28
Pleural	2–12
Liver	19–31
Adrenal	6
Abdomen pelvis (other)	15
Bone	16–28
CNS	8
Skin	2

present in 5% although perhaps under-represented by the exclusion of head and neck cancers from some series. Poorly differentiated cancers comprise an important group because these patients have the most highly treatable cancers. Careful histological and immunocytochemical review supplemented by molecular biology can identify chemotherapy-curable lymphoma in 6% and atypical germ cell tumours in 1%.[10]

Other specific histologies, such as melanoma, sarcoma and poorly differentiated neuro-endocrine tumours, are identified in a further 1% of cases.[11] It is not proposed in this chapter to discuss further the investigation of patients with specific histological types but rather to concentrate on patients with squamous cell tumours and adenocarcinomas.

Key points: histopathology

■ The most critical step in the evaluation of any patient presenting with the diagnosis of cancer of unknown primary site is a review of the histology

■ FNA should not be relied upon for a diagnosis and tissue should always be obtained

Squamous carcinoma of unknown origin

Most patients with squamous carcinoma of unknown primary origin present with cervical lymphadenopathy, although rarely inguinal nodal lymphadenopathy may be the first sign of disease which originates in the vulva or the penis.

Squamous carcinoma of cervical or supraclavicular nodes

Most malignant lymph node masses in the neck are metastatic and the majority (85%) arise from primary head and neck tumours,[12] especially when the upper or middle cervical lymph nodes are involved. When the lower cervical or supraclavicular lymph nodes are involved, a primary lung cancer should be suspected. The majority of primary sites are identified at routine clinical examination, with a further 16% being detected at panendoscopy and 4% by radiological investigation. This latter group usually comprises lung cancer presenting with enlarged nodes in the lower cervical region. However, between 3 and 9% have no identifiable primary site even after such a programme of investigation.

Patients identified as having head and neck primary tumours following investigation and treatment have a 20–30% 5-year survival rate, whereas those in whom the primary site is never discovered have a median survival of 1 year.[12]

Radiological examination including CT may be required for examination of:

- The paranasal sinuses
- Staging the extent of nodal enlargement
- Detection of mediastinal or lung disease prior to treatment

Patients without an identifiable primary tumour site and N1 disease (lymph nodes <3 cm on one side of the neck) have a better prognosis than those with N2 or N3 disease. However, series reporting the results of surgical resection alone have found that up to 40% of patients subsequently develop a primary site in the head and neck region. Therefore, most authors would now recommend the inclusion of radiotherapy in the primary treatment to include the naso-, hypo- and oropharynx as well as the contralateral neck nodes where there is a 15% likelihood of developing further deposits. This approach has led to up to 53% 5-year survival for these patients.[13,14]

Patients with low cervical and supraclavicular nodal involvement tend to have a worse prognosis because lung cancer is a frequent site of occult primary disease.

Squamous carcinoma involving inguinal lymph nodes

In most cases of inguinal lymph node involvement, the primary tumour is genital or anorectal in origin; primary sites most commonly include the vulva, vagina, cervix, penis or scrotum. In these cases imaging, particularly MR imaging, is useful for planning therapy.

Squamous carcinoma metastatic to other sites

Metastatic squamous carcinoma presenting in sites other than the cervical or inguinal nodes almost always represents spread from an occult primary lung cancer and therefore CT of the chest should be considered under these circumstances. Very rarely, the primary site may lie in the head and neck, oesophagus or anus.[7]

Key points: squamous cell carcinoma of unknown origin

■ Most patients with squamous cell carcinoma of unknown origin (SCUO) present with cervical lymphadenopathy, and 85% of these cases represent head and neck tumours

■ In SCUO in cervical lymph nodes, CT is usually required to identify paranasal sinus tumours, to detect lung cancer and to stage nodal disease

■ Patients with unilateral cervical nodal disease have a better prognosis than those with bilateral disease

Adenocarcinoma of unknown origin

Adenocarcinoma is the most frequent histology in cancers of unknown origin. In defining the plan of investigation, the likely incidence of the various primary diagnoses and the treatment options available following diagnosis need to be considered. Exhaustive investigation of patients with cancers of unknown primary site is often counterproductive because of the diminishing likelihood of identifying a primary site, the increasing expense of continuing investigation and discomfort to the patient with limited life expectancy.[2,3,6,15] Treatment options for this group of patients are also limited except in certain special circumstances (see below).

In series such as those reported by Le Chevalier and Nystrom, patients with adenocarcinoma of unknown primary site were subjected to postmortem examination and a primary site was identified in 82–84%.[5,6] The most common sites were:

- Lung (17–28%)
- Pancreas (11–27%)
- Liver (3–6%)
- Colorectal (4–6%)
- Gastric (3–5%)
- Renal (3–7%)
- Ovary (2%)
- Prostate (2–3%)
- Thyroid (1–3%)
- Adrenal (1–3%)
- Breast (1%)
- Parotid (<1%)

Clinical series have revealed a similar distribution of primary sites of cancer.[1,16]

Le Chevalier and Nystrom also compared postmortem findings with the investigations prior to death to define the investigational yield.[5,6] Their results revealed that primary tumour sites were identified prior to death by the following techniques:

- Chest radiography (12–24%)
- Intravenous urography (IVU) (6–9%)
- Barium enema (5–9%)
- Barium meal (4–6%)
- Thyroid scan (8%)

In other series, by contrast, with patients who did not undergo a postmortem, the primary site was identified in only 16% during life.[1,2] There have been few attempts to define the diagnostic performance of these conventional studies. One such study is summarized in Table 48.2, where the authors showed that the radiological investigations had a low sensitivity, low positive predictive value and variable specificity when correlated with postmortem findings.[6]

Key points: clinical presentation

- 3–9% of all referrals to an oncology unit are for investigation of a cancer of unknown primary site

- Adenocarcinoma is the most common histological type in this group of patients

- Poorly differentiated cancers (35%) are an extremely important group as they frequently represent those patients with the most treatable cancers

- Most patients with SCUO present with cervical lymphadenopathy and 85% of these cases arise from head and neck tumours

- In patients presenting with adenocarcinoma of unknown origin, postmortem studies show that the primary tumour most commonly arises in the lung or pancreas

Computed tomography and magnetic resonance

Overall, CT has proved to be the most successful technique for identifying the primary site in patients presenting with adenocarcinoma of unknown origin, showing up to 35–40% of all primary cancers discovered.[1,2,16,17] In the chest particularly, CT can show over 70% of all primary tumours. Abdomino-pelvic CT is also successful and, in one series, CT revealed 86% of all pancreatic cancers, 67% of ovarian primaries and 56% of renal primaries. At other sites, the investigational yield of CT was considerably less: 36% of colorectal primary tumours, 33% of hepatobiliary tumours and 20% of oesophageal cancers. In addition to detecting the primary site of malignancy, CT may detect other clinically unsuspected sites of metastasis in two thirds of patients examined.[17] However, it is not possible to estimate the sensitivity and specificity of these findings in most studies.

Table 48.2. *Test performance compared with postmortem findings*[7]

Test	Number performed	Sensitivity (%)	Specificity (%)	Positive predictive value (%)
Chest X-ray	302	69	63	38
Barium meal	150	75	92	30
Barium enema	105	71	96	55
Thyroid radio-iodine scan	45	57	76	31

Magnetic resonance has proved particularly advantageous in the pelvis[18] and in identifying occult breast cancers[19,20] in 50–86% of women with axillary lymph node metastases.

Positron emission tomography (Table 48.3)

The role of 2-[F-18]fluoro-2-deoxy-D-glucose positron emission tomography ([18]FDG PET) to detect occult primary carcinomas has been addressed in six small series of patients.[21–26] The majority of patients presented with cervical lymphadenopathy and, while some conclusions can be drawn about the use of [18]FDG PET in this group of patients, it is not possible to comment on the clinical usefulness of [18]FDG PET in the diagnosis of the more common visceral adenocarcinoma presentations. In these studies, on average, a potential primary site was identified in 49% of patients (24–71%), with confirmation from histology at biopsy or postmortem achieved in only half the cases. Caution should be exercised in interpreting these results as the number of patients included in each of these series is small (Table 48.3). Furthermore, false positive and false negative results for identifying the primary site were 20–25% and 14–25%, respectively. The primary sites were equally divided between the head and neck region and the lung, with most patients exhibiting squamous carcinoma histology, which reflects the selection of patients inherent in these series. It is extremely difficult to evaluate the performance of [18]FDG PET in patients presenting with head and neck adenocarcinoma of unknown primary site. However, extracting data for this from three studies showed a 24–45% detection rate, especially for adenocarcinoma of the lung and primary sites in the head and neck, including the thyroid gland.[24–26]

Changes in treatment as a result of information made available only from [18]FDG PET occurred in a small proportion of patients in most series, although the reported range is from 10 to 69%. As in other aspects of evaluating the role of [18]FDG PET in the detection of occult primary tumours, the significance of these results is difficult to assess in the light of the very few patients studied to date (see Table 48.3). An equal proportion of patients benefited from confirmation of localized disease in head and neck tumours who were therefore suitable for curative treatment, as did those found to have disseminated disease for whom palliative approaches were more appropriate.

Poorly differentiated carcinoma of unknown primary site (with or without features of adenocarcinoma)

There is a distinctive subgroup of patients with poorly differentiated carcinoma or adenocarcinoma of unknown primary site in whom the clinical characteristics differ from patients with well known adenocarcinomas.[7] The median age group of this group is younger than those with well-differentiated disease and they have a history of rapid progression of symptoms (<30 days) with evidence of rapid tumour growth.[27–29] Most important, from a radiological viewpoint, is that the metastases occur more commonly in the lymph nodes, mediastinum and retroperitoneum than in patients with well-differentiated adenocarcinoma.[7] It is important to identify this subset of patients as they may include a high proportion of germ cell tumours that may be more responsive to chemotherapy and potentially curable.[7] Indeed, Hainsworth and colleagues,[30] using a multivariate analysis, showed that several features independently predicted a favourable treatment outcome. These included:

- A tumour location in the retroperitoneum, or
- Lymph nodes, limited to one or two metastatic sites, and
- A younger age (<35 years)[30]

It is recommended, therefore, that CT of the chest and abdomen should be performed as an initial investigation in this group of patients.[31] However, further data are awaited before recommending the routine use of [18]FDG PET in this group.

Table 48.3. *Role of [18]FDG PET to detect occult primary carcinomas*

Author	Number patients	Primary site possible/confirmed	False positive/negative	Metastases	Treatment changed
Aasar	17	12/9	3/nd	0	2
Kole	29	7/nd	0/3	5	3
Jungelhulsing	27	7/nd	0/5	7	8
Bohulslavzki	53	27/20	6/0	nd	nd
Rades	42	27/20	nd	16	29
Lassen	20	13/9	nd	nd	4
Total	188	92/56 (49/30%)			46/133 (34%)

nd = not done.

<table>
<tr><td>

Key point: poorly differentiated carcinoma or adenocarcinoma of unknown origin

■ Young patients presenting with poorly differentiated carcinoma with mediastinal or retroperitoneal disease at one or two sites may have potentially curable disease

</td></tr>
</table>

Neuro-endocrine carcinoma of unknown primary site

The majority of adult patients who present with features of a primary neuro-endocrine tumour (NET) have a known primary site (see Chapter 31). However, patients increasingly present with NETs of unknown primary site.[4] These can be of three typical histological and clinical types:

- A well-differentiated or low-grade NET with an unknown primary site and indolent biological behaviour
- A poorly differentiated tumour on light microscopy but with neuro-endocrine features and aggressive behaviour
- A group usually initially termed 'poorly differentiated carcinoma' on light microscopy, but recognized as PNETs on immunoperoxidase staining. These too are aggressive tumours

The imaging investigation of these patients is considered in Chapter 31. The poorly differentiated NET's are paradoxically likely to achieve the greatest palliative benefit from chemotherapy.[11]

Treatment opportunities and radiological strategy

The investigational strategy for patients presenting with metastatic adenocarcinoma should aim to identify those primary tumours with the greatest treatment potential. At present there are a relatively limited number of cancers that are likely to present as a cancer of unknown origin and for which treatment is able to prolong life. These include:

- Breast
- Ovary
- Prostate

These cancers represent a small proportion (approximately 5–26%)[1-3] of the adenocarcinomas of unknown primary, but their treatment potential makes it important for them to be identified with a high degree of sensitivity. Before the use of newer cross-sectional imaging modalities and the

greater choice of chemotherapy agents, only 11–14% of radiologically detectable primary tumours were considered treatable.[1,2,15,16] This proportion has increased, with a greater number being detected in the better prognostic groups in recent years, but up-to-date data are now needed.

The overall median survival for all cancers of unknown primary site varies from 12 weeks[16,31] to 22 weeks.[1,6,15] In general, those patients with only limited nodal sites involved, a performance status of 0–2 and weight loss of <10% represent a better prognostic group, with a median survival up to 11–14 months irrespective of the primary site.[6,15,16] Those in whom a primary site is found at initial investigation may have a better prognosis than those in whom a primary tumour is not found. In some series, however, this is almost entirely due to the identification of patients with breast and ovarian primaries.

A selective policy of investigating and identifying the primary site of origin in patients with adenocarcinoma of unknown primary will avoid overinvestigation of patients with a poor prognosis while allowing the clinician to apply established tumour guidelines or experimental treatment protocols to palliate disease where appropriate. Finding the primary site often provides much psychological relief for patient and physician, although the practical benefit may be relatively small. Bearing these points in mind, a radiological strategy should be agreed by clinician and radiologist to reflect locally available diagnostic facilities and treatment strategies. The cost of investigating such patients always needs to be considered. In one series, the estimated cost of a limited assessment was U$3,350 per patient, 70% of which was accounted for by the cost of CT scanning.

There are special clinical situations in which well-defined guidelines for investigation can be recommended:

- In women presenting with isolated axillary lymph node metastases, a primary breast cancer may be found in 40–70% of cases. In one series, only half of these were mammographically detectable, the remainder being found only on pathological examination of the mastectomy specimen.[32] Recently, MR has been found to be a valuable adjunct to mammography and ultrasound in examination of these patients.[19,20] The prognosis for the group as a whole with breast cancer type treatment is similar to that of other women with Stage II breast cancer with a median survival of 5 years.[32]

  On considering these statistics, it is clear that a thorough search for a primary breast cancer is justified. Ultrasound, mammography and MR, if available, should be performed in this group of patients. If a primary tumour is found, then a thorough staging should be carried out as for patients presenting with a clinically diagnosed primary breast cancer.
- Women presenting with peritoneal carcinomatosis,

in particular those with papillary serous carcinoma on histological examination but no primary tumour within the ovary, are another group of potentially treatable patients with adenocarcinoma of unknown primary site.

These patients may either have primary peritoneal carcinomatosis,[33,34] or spread from a pre-invasive ovarian primary and respond to platinum-based chemotherapy. The prognosis is similar to that in other women with Stage III ovarian carcinoma with a median survival of 17–23 months.

Computed tomography is the initial investigation of choice, which should include the chest, abdomen and pelvis. The information provided by CT gives an excellent baseline for monitoring response to platinum-based chemotherapy. Magnetic resonance should be reserved for those cases where the ovaries cannot be satisfactorily identified on CT or ultrasound.

- Men with adenocarcinoma of unknown primary and an elevated serum or tumour biopsy prostate-specific antigen (PSA) level are usually found to have an unsuspected primary prostatic cancer and form another readily treatable group, with a clinical course similar to those presenting with prostatic cancer. Response to androgen deprivation is approximately 70% and median survival is 18–24 months.[35]

In such patients, transrectal ultrasound or MR of the prostate gland should be performed in an attempt to identify the primary tumour. If a tumour is shown, then a biopsy may be helpful in patients with only minimal elevation of PSA in the serum.

In patients suspected of harbouring an occult prostatic tumour, full staging with a plain chest radiograph, CT of the abdomen and pelvis to identify nodal disease and a technetium bone scan is recommended.

- Occasionally, patients present with liver metastases, which are discovered incidentally or as a result of symptoms due to increasing abdominal discomfort and/or weight loss. In such patients, the nature of the liver metastases may occasionally point to the site of origin. For example, calcification within metastases is seen most commonly in gastro-intestinal and ovarian tumours.

In patients with bowel symptoms suspected of harbouring a gastro-intestinal tumour, colonoscopy or barium studies are warranted, as the primary tumour may be excised to avoid obstruction either before or after chemotherapy with 5-fluorouracil-based treatment.

- Other treatable patients include those with multiple small-volume lung metastases due to thyroid carcinoma. This is a rare clinical situation, but response to treatment with radio-iodine, if the tumour is shown to be metabolically active, can be achieved in a high proportion of patients.

- For the majority of other patients, investigation and treatment will be primarily determined by their performance status and a realistic discussion of palliative options with the patient. Good prognosis patients may require further investigation with, for example, [18]FDG PET scans to identify primary sites in the lung, pancreas or colon, for which there are increasingly different choices of multiagent chemotherapy. If, after all efforts, no primary site has been identified, palliative chemotherapy treatment can achieve responses in 20–40% of selected patients, with median survivals of 9–10 months and 5–10% surviving to 5 years.[36]

Key points: imaging investigation

- Currently, in patients presenting with cancer of unknown primary site, treatment will significantly prolong life in only 11–14% of radiologically identified primary tumours

- Imaging strategies should always take into account the likelihood of identifying those patients who are most suitable for treatment and those with limited disease for whom chemotherapy will be appropriate palliation

- In general, a good prognosis group can be identified with only limited nodal sites of disease, good performance status (0–2) and weight loss <10%

- Special situations that warrant thorough imaging studies include a search for breast cancer in women with isolated axillary lymph node metastases, ovarian carcinoma in women with peritoneal carcinomatosis and prostate cancer in men with elevated serum PSA

Conclusion

Patients presenting with cancers of unknown origin represent a heterogeneous group in which the detection of the primary site is becoming increasingly relevant to clinical oncological practice. There are now several tumours that present with metastatic disease and that are treatable with specific drugs, provided the organ of origin is known. Although the cost of investigation is high, there are certain situations in which a thorough search for the primary site is justified. In the future, it is likely that these special situations, in which the primary tumour is treatable, will be expanded to a much wider range of malignancies.

Summary

- The radiological investigation of patients with cancer of unknown primary site should be tailored to provide information that is relevant to prognosis and treatment

- All patients should have a chest radiograph

- Women should also undergo bilateral mammography and examination of the pelvic organs by ultrasound

- Men should be screened for a prostatic primary by transrectal ultrasound if the PSA is elevated

- Further investigation, for example for thyroid carcinoma, by ultrasound or radio-iodine scanning can be reserved for those cases with the appropriate histology and or metastatic pattern

- Further investigation may require MR scans for breast and ovarian masses, [18]FDG PET scans for head and neck, lung and possibly other primaries, and radioisotope scans for thyroid and carcinoid tumours

- For good prognosis patients wishing to have palliative chemotherapy, CT scans and endoscopy to identify lung, pancreas, colon or stomach primaries are indicated to guide the choice of chemotherapy agents

- The sophisticated information which can be obtained by our increasingly sensitive imaging techniques is not yet matched by improvements in the prognosis for patients with the most commonly discovered primary tumour sites in the lung and pancreas

References

1. Kirsten F, Chi C H, Leary J A et al. Metastatic adeno- or undifferentiated carcinoma from an unknown primary site: natural history and guidelines for identification of treatable subsets. Q J Med 1987; 62: 143–161

2. Abbruzzese J L, Abbruzzese M C, Lenzi R et al. Analysis of a diagnostic strategy for patients with suspected tumors of unknown origin. J Clin Oncol 1995; 13: 2094–2103

3. Hamilton C S, Langlands A O. ACUPS (Adenocarcinoma of unknown primary sites): a clinical and cost–benefit analysis. Int J Radiat Oncol Biol Phys 1987; 13: 1497–1503

4. Muir C. Cancer of unknown primary site. Cancer 1995; 75: 353–356

5. Nystrom J S, Weiner J M, Wolf R M et al. Identifying the primary site in metastatic cancer of unknown origin. JAMA 1979; 241: 381–383

6. Le Chevalier T, Cvitkovic E, Caille P et al. Early metastatic cancer of unknown primary origin at presentation. A clinical study of 302 consecutive autopsied patients. Arch Intern Med 1988; 148: 2035–2039

7. Greco F A, Hainsworth J D. Cancer of unknown primary site. In: de Vita V T, Hellman S, Rosenberg S A (eds). Cancer: Principles and Practice of Oncology, 6th edn. Philadelphia: Lippincott Williams and Wilkins, 2001; 2537–2560

8. Hainsworth J D, Greco F A. Treatment of patients with cancer of an unknown primary site. N Engl J Med 1993; 329: 257–263

9. Srodon M, Westra W H. Immunohistochemical staining for thyroid transcription factor-1: a helpful aid in discerning primary site of tumor origin in patients with brain metastases. Hum Pathol 2002; 33: 642–645

10. Summersgill B, Goker H, Osin P et al. Establishing germ cell origin of undifferentiated tumors by identifying gain of 12p material using comparative genomic hybridization analysis of paraffin-embedded samples. Diagn Mol Pathol 1998; 7: 260–266

11. Moertel C G, Kvols L K, O'Connell M J, Rubin J. Treatment of neuroendocrine carcinomas with combined etoposide and cisplatin. Cancer 1991; 68: 227–232

12. Jones A S, Cook J A, Phillips D E, Roland N R. Squamous carcinoma presenting as an enlarged cervical lymph node. Cancer 1993; 72: 1756–1761

13. Colletier P J, Garden A S, Morrison W H et al. Postoperative radiation for squamous cell carcinoma metastatic to cervical lymph nodes from an unknown primary site: outcomes and patterns of failure. Head Neck 1998; 20: 674–681

14. Iganej S, Kagan R, Anderson P et al. Metastatic squamous cell carcinoma of the neck from an unknown primary: management options and patterns of relapse. Head Neck 2002; 24: 236–246

15. Stewart J F, Tattersall M H N, Woods R L, Fox R M. Unknown primary adenocarcinoma: incidence of over investigation and natural history. Br Med J 1979; 1: 1530–1533

16. Abbruzzese J L, Abbruzzese M C, Hess K R et al. Unknown primary carcinoma: natural history and prognostic factors in 657 consecutive patients. J Clin Oncol 1994; 12: 1272–1280

17. McMillan J H, Levine E, Stephens R. Computed tomography in the evaluation of metastatic adenocarcinoma from an unknown primary site. Radiology 1982; 143: 143–146

18. Kurtz A B, Tsimikas J V, Tempany C M et al. Diagnosis and staging of ovarian cancer, comparative values of doppler and conventional US, CT, and MRI imaging correlated with surgery and histopathologic analysis:

report of the Radiologic Diagnostic Oncology Group. Radiology 1999; 212: 19–27

19. Orel S G, Weinstein S P, Schnall M D et al. Breast MR imaging in patients with axillary node metastases and unknown primary malignancy. Radiology 1999; 212: 543–549

20. Olson J A Jr, Morris E A, Van Zee K J et al. Magnetic resonance imaging facilitates breast conservation for occult breast cancer. Ann Surg Oncol 2000; 7: 411–415

21. Aasar O S, Fischbein N J, Caputo G R et al. Metastatic head and neck cancer: role and usefulness of FDG PET in locating occult primary tumors. Radiology 1999; 210: 177–181

22. Jungehulsing M, Scheidhauer K, Damm M et al. 2[F]-fluoro-2-deoxy-D-glucose positron emission tomography is a sensitive tool for the detection of occult primary cancer (carcinoma of unknown primary syndrome) with head and neck lymph node manifestation. Otolaryngol Head Neck Surg 2000; 123: 294–301

23. Bohuslavizki K H, Klutmann S, Kroger S et al. FDG PET detection of unknown primary tumors. J Nucl Med 2000; 41: 816–822

24. Kole A C, Neiweg O E, Pruim J et al. Detection of unknown occult primary tumors using positron emission tomography. Cancer 1998; 82: 1160–1166

25. Lassen U, Daugaard G, Eigtved A et al. 18F-FDG whole-body positron emission tomography (PET) in patients with unknown primary tumours (UPT). Eur J Cancer 1999; 35: 1076–1082

26. Rades D, Kuhnel G, Wildfang I et al. Localised disease in cancer of unknown primary (CUP): the value of positron emission tomography (PET) for individual therapeutic management. Annal Oncol 2001; 12: 1605–1609

27. Nystrom J S, Weiner J M, Heffelfinger-Juttner J et al. Metastatic and histologic presentations in unknown primary cancer. Semin Oncol 1977; 4: 53–58

28. van der Gaast A, Verweij J, Henzen-Logmans S C et al. Carcinoma of unknown primary: identification of a treatable subset? Ann Oncol 1990; 1: 119–122

29. Greco F A, Vaughn W K, Hainsworth J D. Advanced poorly differentiated carcinoma of unknown primary site: recognition of a treatable syndrome. Ann Intern Med 1986; 104: 547–553

30. Hainsworth J D, Johnson D H, Greco F A. Cisplatin-based combination chemotherapy in the treatment of poorly differentiated carcinoma and poorly differentiated adenocarcinoma of unknown primary site: results of a 12-year expereince. J Clin Oncol 1992; 10: 912–922

31. Van de Wouw A J, Janssen-Heijnen M L, Coebergh J W, Hillen H F. Epidemiology of unknown primary tumours; incidence and population-based survival of 1285 patients in Southeast Netherlands, 1984–1992. Eur J Cancer 2002; 38: 409–413

32. Rosen P. Axillary lymph node metastases in patients with occult noninvasive breast carcinoma. Cancer 1980; 46: 1298–1306

33. Strand C M, Grosh W W, Baxter J et al. Peritoneal carcinomatosis of unknown primary site in women. Ann Int Med 1989; 111: 213–217

34. Ransom D T, Patel S R, Keeney G L et al. Papillary serous carcinoma of the peritoneum. Cancer 1990; 66: 1091–1094

35. CRC Cancer Fact Sheet. Prostate cancer. June 2002

36. Greco F A, Burris H A III, Litchy S et al. Gemcitabine, carboplatin and paclitaxel for patients with carcinoma of unknown primary site: a Minnie Pearl cancer research network study. J Clin Oncol 2002; 20: 1651–1656

Part VI

IMAGING AND TREATMENT

Chapter 49

Interventional imaging: general applications

Anthony J Lopez

Introduction

There have been major advances in interventional imaging over the last few decades which have radically altered the management of many malignancies. Minimally invasive therapy or 'pinhole surgery' has a wide application in the diagnosis, active management and palliation of malignant disease. Many of the developments reflect advances in technology, including the development of digital imaging, major progress in image guidance techniques such as computed tomography (CT), ultrasound and endoscopy, and an increase in the wide range of needles, guidewires, catheters, stents and other prostheses. Magnetic resonance imaging may offer an extended role in interventional management with the development of open-plan magnet configurations and MR-compatible equipment for intervention, and techniques such as radio-frequency ablation are now in common usage. Other techniques showing great promise include percutaneous vertebroplasty and 'interstial' techniques such as prostate brachytherapy. The development of formal multidisciplinary teams for each malignancy has recognized the

important role of a suitably trained radiologist to optimize diagnosis and therapeutic intervention.

Thoracic intervention

Biopsy techniques

Percutaneous, endoscopic and open techniques have enabled the radiologist to image and treat disease in the thorax directly or in a multidisciplinary capacity. Fine-needle aspiration biopsy (FNAB) is usually sufficient for diagnosis, provided adequate cellular material has been aspirated, especially with new cytological techniques, e.g. DNA cytofluorometry, immunocytochemistry and tumour marker characterization. A cytologist should be in attendance whenever possible. In primary lymphoreticular malignancies, however, larger pieces of tissue are usually desirable for diagnosis, subclassification and immunotyping,[1] necessitating the use of larger 'cutting' needles to obtain good tissue cores (Fig. 49.1). Localization of superficial lesions can often be achieved with palpation or ultra-

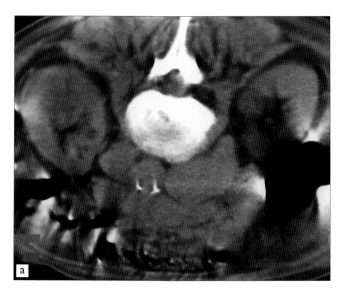
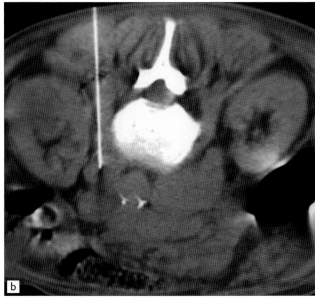

Figure 49.1. *CT-guided biopsy of lymph node in a patient with previously treated non-Hodgkin's lymphoma. (a) Bulky para-aortic lymphadenopathy (patient prone). (b) Tip of 18-gauge cutting needle in discrete left lateral para-aortic lymph node. Note presence of 'photon starvation artefact' confirming actual tip of needle.*

sound guidance using a free-hand technique. Significantly, image guidance has a more significant effect on results than sampling techniques.[2]

The most suitable indications for ultrasound guidance include pleural biopsy, rib lesions, subcutaneous deposits and peripheral lung lesions reaching a pleural surface. For deeper or poorly accessible lesions, e.g. pulmonary apices (Fig. 49.2), near the hila or diaphragms, either fluoroscopy or CT guidance is recommended,[3] especially when a tissue core is desirable where a co-axial technique may be useful.[4] For central and hilar lung lesions, bronchoscopy with transbronchial biopsy is usually safer and more appropriate, providing good tissue cores. Similarly, for oesophageal lesions, endoscopic biopsy is usually desirable unless the lesion is predominantly exophytic and not visible with the endoscope, requiring a percutaneous image-guided approach. Some complications of thoracic biopsy are suitably managed in the interventional suite, e.g. thoracocentesis or formal drainage for pneumo- or haemothorax and embolization for haemoptysis.

Image guidance has also been used for needle localization in the preoperative location of chest wall lesions as well as intrapulmonary nodules prior to thoracoscopic resection,[5] including the use of hooked wire markers similar to those used for breast localization procedures. A relatively new technique for biopsying mediastinal nodes for staging lung cancer is the use of endoscopic ultrasound (EUS) guidance with a multichannel scope introduced into the oesphagus. With this technique, accessible nodes can be biopsied using a fine needle, obviating invasive mediastinoscopy under general anaesthesia.

Key points: thoracic biopsy

■ FNAB is usually sufficient for diagnosis of malignancy if adequate cellular material has been obtained

■ Larger tissue cores are required to accurately classify primary lymphoreticular malignancies

■ Imaging guidance has a more significant effect on results than sampling techniques

■ CT-guided biopsy or EUS is recommended for lesions with poor accessibility

■ Transbronchial biopsy is safer and more appropriate for central and hilar lung lesions

Thoracic drainage procedures

Thoracic collections may occur as a complication of the malignancy (including malignant pleural and pericardial effusions), and following diagnostic or therapeutic interventional procedures. Examples are haemothorax following lung biopsy and biliary effusion following unexpected transpleural hepatic drainage procedures. Thoracic collections may also occur directly as a complication of treatment and include:

- Empyemas
- Parapneumonic and other pleural effusions
- Pulmonary and mediastinal abscesses

Percutaneous drainage can often be achieved using image guidance, particularly CT and ultrasound (Fig. 49.3). For pleural effusions, 7 French gauge (Fr) drainage catheters are usually effective except where the collection has become more organized and catheters up to 24 Fr (sometimes with intrapleural fibrinolysis) may be required. Ultrasound guidance is also particularly well suited to the drainage of malignant pericardial effusions using 'real-time'. Sclerotherapy of both pleural and pericardial collections in the absence of associated infection has been attempted, with variable results. The most commonly used agents are currently tetracycline, bleomycin and talc but not all agents have ever been licensed for such use!

Key point: ultrasound

■ Ultrasound guidance is particularly well suited to the drainage of malignant pleural and pericardial effusions

Venous access and related intervention

The rapid development of new chemotherapeutic agents and more intensive treatment regimens has been accompanied by an increase in requirements for central venous catheters, providing long-term access for chemotherapy, parenteral nutrition and other fluids, blood and related products, as well as a portal for the aspiration of blood samples. A wide range of catheters has been developed over the last 30 years, usually made of either silicone or polyurethane with one or more lumens, that may require

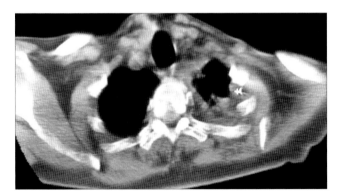

Figure 49.2. *CT-guided biopsy of right apical lung lesion. Small apical lesion with prominent adjacent bony structures limiting access for transaxial biopsy. Note tip of 21-gauge needle (scanned in short axis) within mass later confirmed as squamous cell carcinoma.*

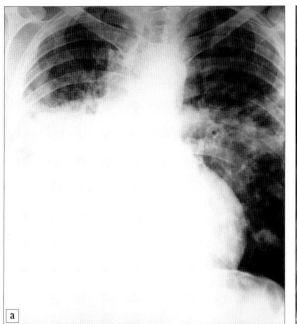
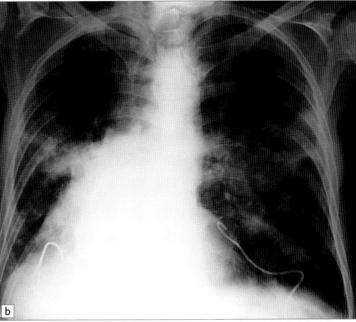

Figure 49.3. *Percutaneous drainage of malignant pleural and pericardial effusions in recurrent breast carcinoma. (a) Chest radiograph demonstrating massive pericardial and large right pleural effusions. Note also infective consolidation in left lung. (b) Two 7 Fr pigtail drainage catheters have been inserted using ultrasound-guidance with satisfactory postdrainage appearances. The acute pneumonia also responded to antibiotics with marked clinical improvement.*

subcutaneous tunnelling or implantation for port systems. Traditionally, venous access devices were inserted in theatre by surgical cutdown but most are currently inserted percutaneously by radiologists trained in interventional techniques using their expertise in image guidance and guidewire/catheter manipulation offering shorter procedure times, fewer complications and improved success rate compared with the surgical approach.[6] Furthermore, with such high demands for catheter insertion, the angiography suite has been shown to provide more flexibility than the rigid scheduling of theatre sessions while at the same time providing the necessary aseptic environment that is desirable.[7,8] There is, however, some debate on these issues and not all cancer centres utilize the services of radiology for central line insertion.

The preferred access routes are typically the internal jugular, subclavian or axillary veins, although in cases of difficulty the common femoral vein may be used. Translumbar and transhepatic vena caval puncture have also been described.[9] Dilated intercostal veins may even be used if there is associated central venous obstruction.[10]

The role of the radiologist in this field is expanding beyond that of insertion of central venous catheters and in many centres there is a requirement for radiologists to manage the complications associated with these devices. Assessment of such complications frequently requires diagnostic techniques such as direct catheter venograms, duplex sonography of *in situ* catheters and related veins, as well as peripheral venography (Fig. 49.4). Furthermore, where appropriate, thrombolysis of occluded catheters and veins can be performed as well as repositioning of misplaced or displaced catheters.

One of the commoner long-term complications associated with venous access systems is the development of catheter-related stenosis and thrombosis often requiring peripheral or central venous thrombolysis with or without venoplasty, endovascular stenting or superior vena cava (SVC) filtration.[11]

Central venous obstruction

Central venous obstruction may occur secondary to catheter-related stenosis or fibrosing mediastinitis in the treatment of malignant disease. A more sinister finding, however, is malignant venous obstruction typically seen in the SVC, either by direct tumour invasion, e.g. bronchial neoplasms, or by extrinsic compression from perihilar or paratracheal lymphadenopathy. Interventional techniques have been developed to provide palliation in these circumstances and self-expanding metallic stents are usually inserted following chemical or mechanical thrombolysis and angioplasty. It is also possible to perform a diagnostic core biopsy of such mediastinal tumours at the time of stenting.

When successful, this procedure is followed by almost immediate relief of the distressing symptoms (Fig. 49.5). In cases where there is obstruction of the central neck veins

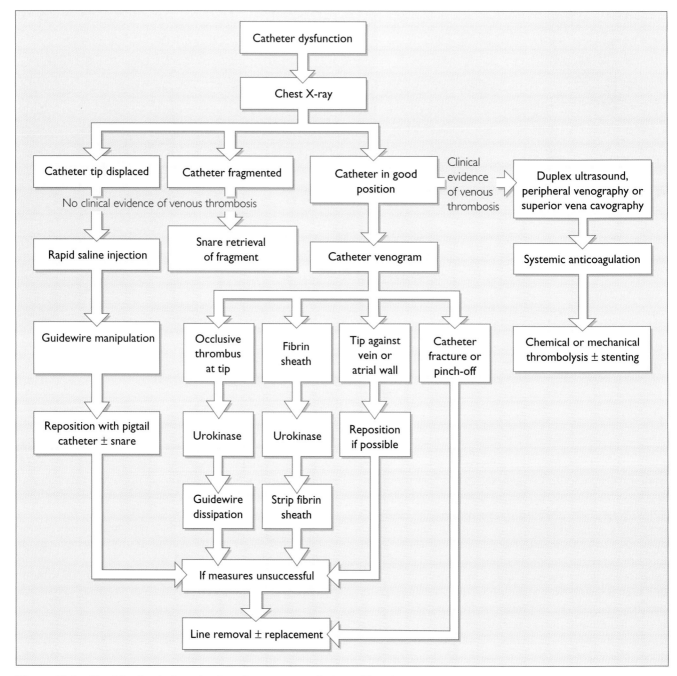

Figure 49.4. *Algorithm for the investigation of venous access device malfunction.*

bilaterally, as well as the SVC, relief of obstruction on one side alone often provides adequate palliation.[12] A metallic stent also provides an excellent visible localizer to optimize the target volume for palliative radiotherapy.

Similar techniques have been applied to the inferior vena cava (IVC) when obstructed secondary to large hepatic tumours or retroperitoneal nodal masses, with encouraging results.[13]

Key points: central line insertion

- ■ The interventional radiology suite is a suitable environment for the percutaneous insertion of central venous catheters and the management of catheter-related complications

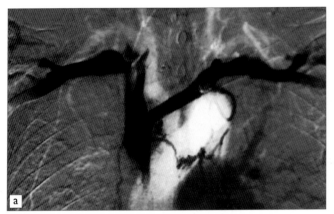
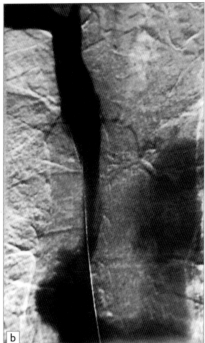

Figure 49.5. *Self-expanding metallic wall stent insertion (Schneider A G, Bülach, Switzerland) in superior vena cava (SVC) obstruction preceding palliative radiotherapy in bronchial carcinoma. (a) Superior vena cavagram demonstrating extrinsic compression of superior vena cava by tracheobronchial lymph nodes. (b) Repeat study following endovascular venoplasty and metallic stenting confirmed relief of SVC obstruction with good filling of right atrium and less prominent collaterals. There was immediate clinical improvement and further stent expansion occurred over the following week.*

- In the absence of conventional venous access sites, the transhepatic and translumbar routes may be useful

- In central venous obstruction, adequate palliation can be provided with stent insertion followed by chemical or mechanical thrombolysis and angioplasty

- New techniques allow biopsy of mediastinal tumour at the same time as stenting

Tracheobronchial stenting

One of the commonest malignancies in the Western world is bronchial carcinoma, which may be associated with obstruction of the major airways. Significant developments in stent technology and close working relationships between radiologists, thoracic surgeons and physicians have led to the introduction of self-expanding metallic stents of similar design to the venous stents already described (Fig. 49.6).[14] The stents are usually inserted under general anaesthesia using combined fluoroscopic and bronchoscopic guidance with stent insertion following balloon dilatation of the stricture (Fig. 49.7). This development has resulted in a reduction in morbidity associated with major airway obstruction from malignant disease.

Techniques for management of haemoptysis

Major haemoptysis in oncological patients is associated typically with bronchial malignancy, although it may result also from percutaneous and transbronchial biopsy techniques. Less frequently, haemoptysis occurs due to complications of treatment. For example, in immunosuppressed hosts,

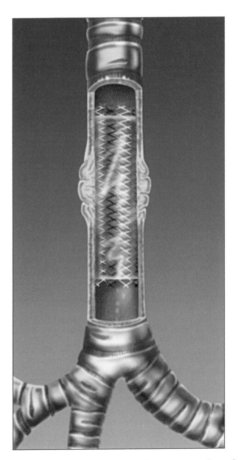

Figure 49.6. *Diagrammatic representation of a self-expanding uncovered metallic stent in situ across a malignant tracheal stricture.*

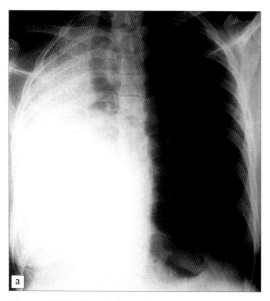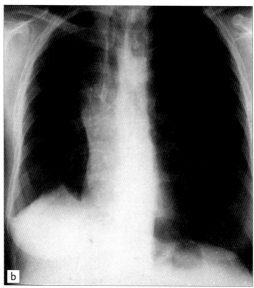

Figure 49.7. *Tracheobronchial stenting in a woman with recurrent squamous cell carcinoma (Reproduced from ref 14 with permission). (a) Chest radiograph immediately prior to stenting with complete collapse of right lung and ipsilateral mediastinal shift. (b) Chest radiograph 1 week after deployment of a 49 mm long, 8 mm diameter wall stent endoprosthesis (Schneider A G, Bülach, Switzerland) in the right main and intermediate bronchi showing complete expansion of remaining right lung (note patient has had a previous right upper lobectomy for a large cell carcinoma).*

haemoptysis may be due to tuberculosis or other pulmonary infections or may be seen in pneumonitis induced by radiotherapy.

Bronchial arteriography and embolization are well-recognized techniques used in the management of recurrent and significant haemoptysis (Fig. 49.8). The technique requires exquisite, preferably digital, imaging because anterior and posterior spinal arteries sometimes originate from the intercostal arteries and, in addition, bronchial to coronary artery communications are also well described. If such vessels are not appreciated, severe or even fatal consequences may ensue.

Key points: thoracic intervention

- Tracheobronchial stenting can palliate major airway obstruction

- Bronchial artery embolization may be required to palliate haemoptysis

Gastro-intestinal intervention

Biopsy techniques

Biopsy techniques have already been described in some detail in the previous section and the same general principles apply to the gastro-intestinal tract. Image guidance is particularly useful for obtaining the larger tissue cores required for lymph node histopathological examination to ensure accurate diagnosis, particularly if lymphoma is suspected (Fig 49.1). Empirically, enlarged para-aortic nodes should be biopsied in preference to paracaval nodes because haemorrhage from inadvertent injury of the IVC is much less likely to stop without intervention than haemorrhage from aortic injury.

Formerly, fluoroscopy was used from guidance of many procedures such as the biopsy of lymph nodes opacified at lymphography,[15] as well as biopsy of lesions in the opacified biliary tree (Fig. 49.9), gastro-intestinal tract and urinary tract. However, today, CT and ultrasound have superseded fluoroscopy as the standard methods for percutaneous image guidance.[16]

Remarkable developments have been made in endoluminal ultrasound and some lesions deep in the pelvis can now be biopsied using transrectal or transvaginal ultrasound guidance (Fig. 49.10). Certainly the transvaginal approach is the optimal method for the diagnostic aspiration of small ovarian cysts and the transrectal approach is now more commonly used for prostatic biopsy than the transurethral and transperineal methods, although the latter is preferred for brachytherapy. These endoluminal approaches may replace the transgluteal route for biopsy or abscess drainage.

Endoscopic ultrasound has been particularly useful for assessing the depth of tumour invasion in primary oesophageal carcinoma.[17] Regional lymph node metastases may also be detected but the specificity of the technique is limited as inflammatory nodes may mimic malignant lymphadenopathy. Endoscopic ultrasound-guided lymph node biopsy helps to overcome this constraint and can be used to

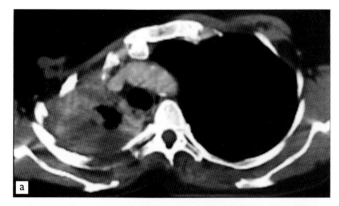

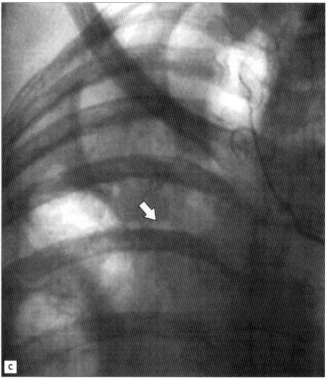

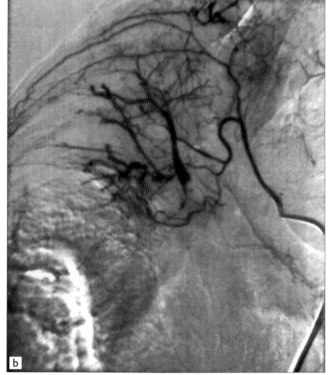

Figure 49.8. *Bronchial arteriography and embolization in a man with recurrent significant haemoptysis secondary to an apical adenocarcinoma arising in an old tuberculous scar and resistant to radiotherapy: (a) CT scan showing slightly necrotic and moderately enhancing right apical mass. Note lytic involvement of posterior end of adjacent rib. (b) Right bronchial arteriogram demonstrating hypervascular apical mass; (c) following successful embolization with polyvinyl alcohol and gelfoam, only staining of the embolized tumour (arrow) is demonstrated. Note preservation of the right superior intercostal artery with intercostal branches shown not to supply the tumour.*

diagnose and stage gastric and colorectal cancer as well as for localizing small pancreatic lesions.[18–20]

Radiologists are increasingly being requested to perform image-guided liver biopsy, which is clearly most appropriate when there are one or more focal hepatic lesions rather than diffuse disease. Standard percutaneous liver biopsy, however, may be contraindicated in patients with a significant or uncorrectable coagulopathy or bleeding diathesis. In such cases, morbidity and mortality can be reduced by using the transjugular approach for liver biopsy or by performing a plugged liver biopsy with embolization of the biopsy tract after removing the biopsy needle from the guiding sheath. A similar technique may be used to obtain a splenic core, advisable even when the bleeding and coagulation times are not prolonged (Fig. 49.11). A modification of the former technique is the use of the bioptome for percutaneous transcaval biopsy of tumours that have

invaded the IVC,[21] such as primary or secondary liver tumours and renal tumours. These techniques should be reserved for those situations when conventional methods are contraindicated or inappropriate.

Key points: gastro-intestinal biopsy

- Transrectal and transvaginal ultrasound are commonly employed for pelvic biopsy and drainage procedures

- EUS with biopsy is useful in the staging of oesophageal, gastric and colorectal malignancy

- If direct liver biopsy is contraindicated, a transjugular or percutaneous plugged approach should be considered

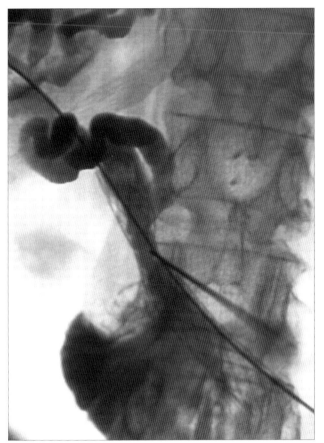

Figure 49.9. *Fluoroscopic biopsy of obstructive lesion subsequently shown to be cholangio-carcinoma. An 8.5 Fr metallic endoprosthesis has been inserted (Memotherm, Angiomed, Europe) via PTC to relieve the obstruction and the 21-gauge needle inserted into the tumour at the site of 'waisting'.*

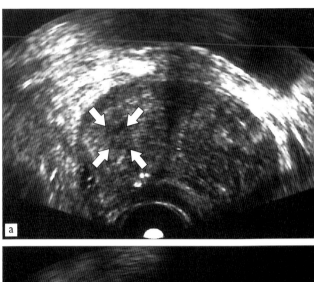

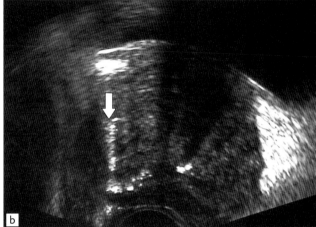

Figure 49.10. *Transrectal ultrasound-guided biopsy of prostatic lesion subsequently shown to be prostatic adenocarcinoma. (a) A 1.5 cm hypoechoic nodule (arrows) in peripheral zone of right mid gland (prostatic capsule intact). (b) Tip of 18-gauge needle within nodule (arrow) inserted using transrectal ultrasound guidance.*

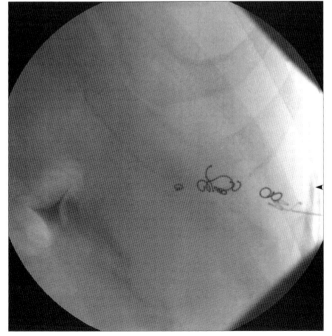

Figure 49.11. *Plugged splenic biopsy in patient with 'massive splenomegaly' and 'B' symptoms but no other abnormal appearances on CT. An 18-gauge biopsy needle was introduced through a sheath into the spleen. Following core biopsy (revealing diffuse lymphomatous infiltration), the track (shown not to communicate with a large vessel) has been plugged with alternating spongistan pledgets and 5-mm stainless steel coils. Note small linear area of contrast at splenic capsule (arrowhead) to show splenic edge ensuring coils remain within splenic parenchyma.*

Percutaneous drainage procedures

Abdominal ascites is a common finding in many gastro-intestinal and pelvic malignancies, particularly where there is peritoneal and/or omental seeding. Malignant ascites is distressing for the patient and can often be drained using a percutaneous technique without image guidance. In cases of difficulty, however, or loculation, ultrasound guidance using a free-hand technique is extremely useful for achieving complete drainage. If recurrent ascites becomes a problem, a formal peritoneo-venous shunt may be implanted under sedoanalgesia and local anaesthesia to obviate recurrent drainage and associated protein loss.

Abdominal fluid collections and abscesses may develop as a complication of treatment and, in the postoperative patient, subphrenic and pelvic collections are not uncommon. They are easily drained using ultrasound or CT for guidance. Pelvic abscess drainage is safer using the transrectal or transvaginal approach compared with the transgluteal route and is also considerably less painful for the patient.

Management of oesophageal and upper gastro-intestinal strictures

Malignant oesophageal strictures are typically due to primary oesophageal carcinoma and less frequently due to metastatic oesophageal lesions, nodal disease or local tumour invasion from bronchial neoplasms. Benign oesophageal strictures may also follow radiotherapy to the mediastinum, as a late complication. All these lesions can be managed effectively using either fluoroscopic or endoscopic techniques.

Traditionally, oesophageal strictures have been dilated using either rubber bougies (such as the Savary–Guillard type) or rigid metal dilators (Eder–Puestow type). Optimally, such dilatation, which can be up to 60 Fr, is performed endoscopically under fluoroscopic control, to reduce the risk of perforation and other complications. The endoscopic route also affords the possibility of performing diagnostic biopsy immediately after rigid or balloon dilatation, although this is better avoided. Alternatively, dilatation can be performed entirely fluoroscopically using a large balloon over a guidewire.

For malignant strictures, where staging using EUS or CT has indicated that primary surgical resection is impossible, stenting is advisable either using a self-expanding metallic stent (Figs. 49.12 and 49.13) or a rigid device (Fig. 49.14), both of which can be inserted directly under screening control or via endoscopy using fluoroscopic guidance.

In cases of tracheo-oesophageal fistula, similar techniques have been applied using a covered self-expanding metallic stent (uncovered for a short interval at either end to reduce 'migration'). These can be applied to the oesophagus up to just below the level of the cricopharyngeus muscle (Fig. 49.15). For higher lesions, covered stents have been inserted into the trachea, thereby successfully occluding the fistula.

One of the advantages of the expandable metallic stent is that it expands to a diameter of between 18 and 24 mm

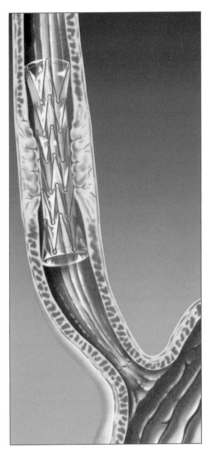

Figure 49.12. *Diagrammatic representation of a self-expanding covered metallic stent in situ across a distal malignant oesophageal stricture.*

despite delivery to the site on a relatively slim device. In cases of tumour overgrowth, laser therapy can be performed directly through the stent, or bougie of the stent can be performed using a balloon to shear off tumour from the mesh. Covered stents have been used in an attempt to reduce tumour in-growth and newer stents are being developed which are made of metal alloys of differing electro-chemical potentials, which create a current inhibiting tumour in-growth (personal communication) as well as newer 'drug-eluting' stents. It is also relatively simple to insert a further stent coaxially within the *in situ* stent. This is a useful manoeuvre if there is focal extrinsic compression or narrowing of the upper or lower ends either due to tumour recurrence or stent migration. An advantage of rigid stents over metallic stents is that they may be exchanged endoscopically as necessary.

Gastric outlet obstruction may occur as a complication of pyloric surgery, such as palliative bypass for pancreatic carcinoma, and is usually due to postoperative ischaemia. Other causes of gastric outlet obstruction include local tumour recurrence, invasive pancreatic malignancy and stomal malignancy following previous peptic ulcer surgery. The techniques of dilatation and stenting have been applied to the gastric outlet for malignant strictures with

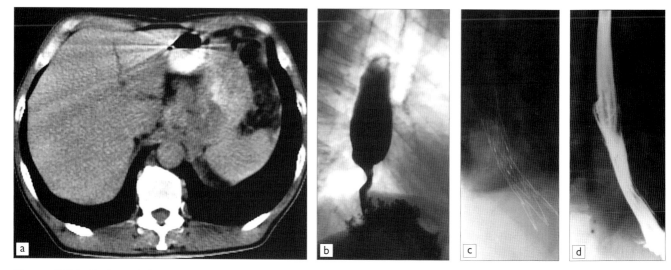

Figure 49.13. *Endoscopic insertion of self-expanding metallic endoprosthesis for unresectable adenocarcinoma of distal oesophagus involving cardia. (a) CT scan demonstrating bulky nodal disease along lesser curve and around coeliac axis. (b) Barium swallow showing tight malignant distal oesophageal stricture with 'shouldering' involving cardia. (c) A 12 cm long, 22 cm diameter Gianturco–Rösch covered metallic endoprosthesis (William Cook, Europe) has been inserted endoscopically across stricture ensuring distal 'funnel' end lies just within the stomach but adequately below the tumour margin. Note minor residual 'waisting' which subsequently disappeared without further dilatation. (d) Barium swallow (1 day post insertion) demonstrating widely patent stent with immediate relief of dysphagia.*

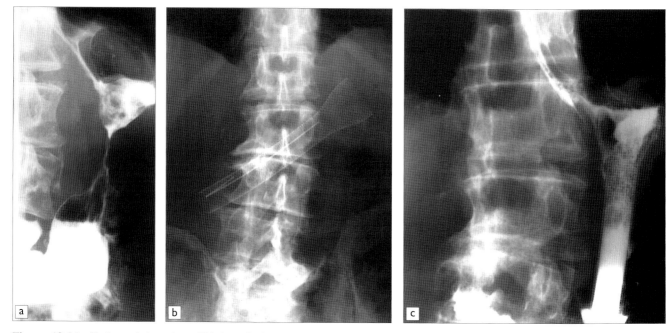

Figure 49.14. *Endoscopic insertion of Medoc tube for annular stenosing adenocarcinoma of stomach to palliate intractable emesis. (Reproduced with kind permission of Dr R A Frost.) (a) Spot film from upper gastro-intestinal series demonstrating tight gastric stricture. (b) A Medoc tube has been inserted endoscopically across stricture. (c) Relief of gastric obstruction demonstrated on barium meal.*

good palliation in some cases.[22] Although longer peroral delivery systems are being developed, gastrostomy may be required for stent insertion (Fig. 49.16). If stenting is unsuccessful, a double lumen gastro-enterostomy tube may be inserted with the distal lumen (for feeding) in the jejunum and the proximal lumen (for gastric drainage) in the gastric antrum.

Dilatation and stenting of lower gastro-intestinal tract strictures

Lower gastro-intestinal tract strictures can be managed in a similar manner to other gastro-intestinal lesions, either endoscopically, fluoroscopically or using a combined approach. In cases of benign postoperative stricture following resection of a malignant lesion, dilatation is usually suf-

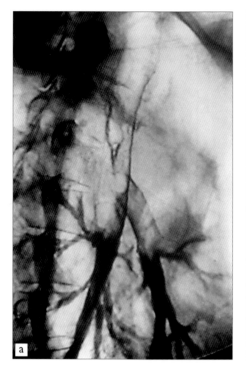
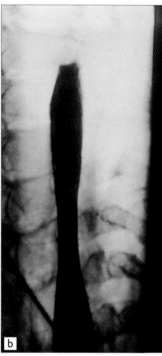

Figure 49.15. *Fluoroscopic insertion of covered metallic wall stent (Schneider A G, Bülach, Switzerland) for malignant tracheo-oesophageal fistula. (Reproduced with kind permission of Professor A. Adam). (a) Immediately following a contrast swallow, a bronchogram is demonstrated distal to a malignant tracheo-oesophageal fistula. (b) Following endoprosthesis insertion, the stented oesophagus is widely patent with minor residual 'waisting' only, but complete exclusion of the malignant fistula.*

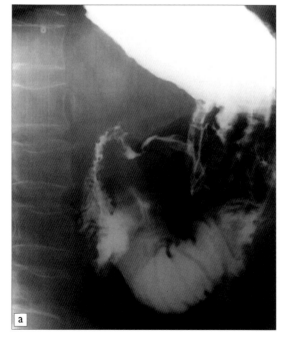

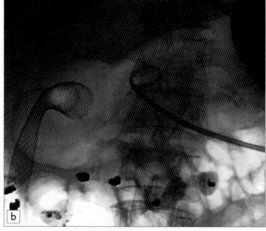

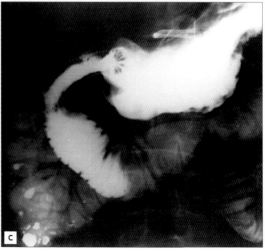

Figure 49.16. *Palliative stenting of malignant gastric outflow obstruction in advanced local pancreatic carcinoma. (a) Spot film from upper gastro-intestinal series demonstrating a tight irregular stricture involving proximal duodenum. (b) Following percutaneous gastropexy and gastrostomy, a 10 cm long, 20 mm diameter wall stent (Schneider A G, Bülach, Switzerland) has been deployed ensuring coverage of stricture; the proximal end lies across the pylorus 'flared' just within the stomach. (c) Spot film from upper gastro-intestinal series demonstrating widely patent stent in good position with immediate relief of gastric outflow obstruction.*

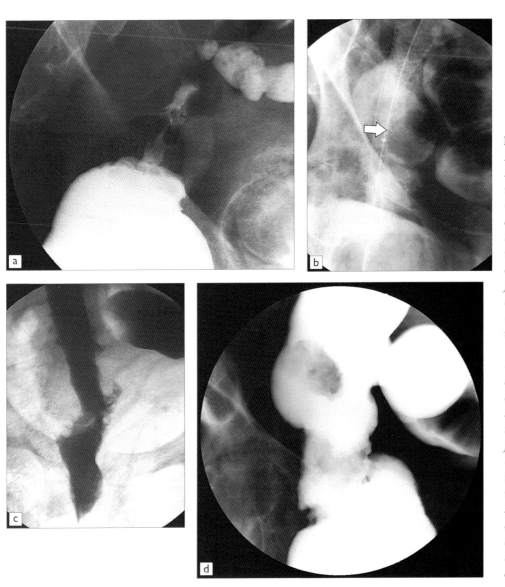

Figure 49.17. *Palliative stenting of malignant annular stenosing adenocarcinoma of rectosigmoid junction. (a) Oblique spot film from barium enema series demonstrating tight irregular stricture at rectosigmoid junction. (b) After crossing the stricture using fluoroscopic guidance, a 10 cm long 20 mm diameter Wall stent (Schneider) has been deployed with evidence of residual 'waisting' in mid-stent (arrow). (c) Frontal spot film from barium enema series demonstrating a widely patent stent with immediate relief of large bowel obstruction following stent deployment. (d) Five months following stent insertion and local palliative radiotherapy (patient refused surgery), the stricture was almost completely relieved and the stent passed with excellent luminal patency on contrast enema.*

ficient to achieve a good faecal passage with alleviation of obstruction. In the setting of acute large bowel obstruction secondary to a stenosing malignancy, the stricture may be crossed, dilated and stented accurately with metallic self-expanding stents to provide immediate relief of large bowel obstruction (Fig. 49.17). This may be a temporizing measure before proceeding to definitive surgery when the tumour and stent are removed, often with primary anastomosis rather than defunctioning colostomy.[23] Alternatively, where patients are not considered surgical candidates, the stent may provide adequate palliation. Any subsequent tumour overgrowth can be treated using endoscopic laser therapy.[24]

Insertion of gastrostomy and gastro-enterostomy feeding tubes

Nutritional support is essential in the overall management of patients with malignant disease, particularly those who are severely debilitated or unable to swallow. Tunnelled central venous catheters have been widely used for this pur-

pose, especially when there is a need for coexistent administration of intravenous chemotherapy, parenteral nutrition, blood and related products. The use of central venous lines for this purpose, however, is associated with significant morbidity and considerable expense. It is therefore desirable that enteric feeding support should be established via a nasogastric tube in the early stages and subsequently via a gastrostomy when appropriate. Gastrostomy feeding tubes can be inserted using a percutaneous/endoscopic approach or entirely percutaneously (with or without gastropexy) under fluoroscopic guidance, which has a reduced cost, as well as lower morbidity and mortality. Gastrostomy may also be performed for gastric drainage in patients with gastric outlet obstruction due to retroperitoneal or mesenteric malignancy.

In cases of gastric outlet obstruction or problems associated with the gastrostomy tube, including gastro-oesophageal reflux, aspiration or reflux along the stomal track, the gastrostomy can be converted to a gastro-enterostomy. This should be performed under fluoroscopic guidance to position the tube distal to the ligament of Treitz. In several institutions, primary transgastric jejunostomy has been adopted (Fig. 49.18). Surgical or laparoscopic gastrostomy usually requires general anaesthesia with risk of postoperative ileus, whereas radiological tube insertion is performed under sedoanalgesia using local anaesthesia. A further advantage of the percutaneous radiological approach is the ability to overcome pharyngeal or oesophageal strictures that can make the endoscopic approach extremely difficult. Several studies have shown that the percutaneous approach is less expensive and is associated with fewer minor and major complications than endoscopic or surgical gastrostomy.[25]

> ### Key points: gastro-intestinal strictures
>
> ■ Oesophageal strictures are dilated endoscopically and/or fluoroscopically with rigid bougies or balloons
>
> ■ Stents provide excellent palliation for malignant oesophageal strictures and/or fistulae
>
> ■ Metal stents may provide palliation for malignant gastric outflow obstruction and acute large bowel obstruction

> ■ External feeding should be established where appropriate if the gastro-intestinal tract is 'intact'

Management of obstructive jaundice

Obstructive jaundice with dilated extrahepatic and intrahepatic biliary ducts is easily demonstrated using ultrasound, CT or MR. The level of obstruction can often be determined as well as an indication of the likely nature of the underlying cause. In some cases, however, the obstructing lesion is not fully demonstrated using non-invasive techniques. Endoscopic retrograde cholangio-pancreatography (ERCP) and percutaneous transhepatic cholangiography (PTC) have been particularly useful in the further investigation of obstructive lesions as well as their interventional management (Fig. 49.19). The endoscopic method (ERCP) is preferred for low common bile duct lesions, while PTC is considered to have a high success and low complication rate for liver hilar lesions.

Percutaneous transhepatic cholangiography is now a readily available low-cost technique able to demonstrate the proximal level of obstruction (Fig. 49.19). With modern catheters and guidewires, the obstructive lesion can often be traversed and either an internal/external biliary drainage catheter left *in situ* or the obstruction can be stented *a priori* using plastic endoprostheses or self-expand-

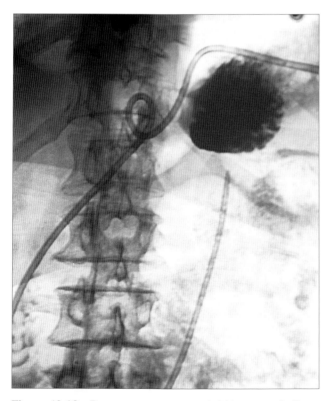

Figure 49.18. *Percutaneous transgastric jejunostomy feeding tube inserted for patient with advanced laryngeal malignancy where percutaneous endoscopic gastrostomy was precluded. Note the tip of the feeding tube at the duodenojejunal flexure and a self-retaining locking pigtail in the gastric antrum.*

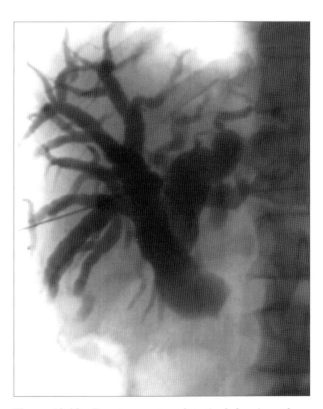

Figure 49.19. *Percutaneous transhepatic cholangiography demonstrating marked intra- and extrahepatic bile duct dilatation with malignant occlusion of common hepatic duct by cholangiocarcinoma.*

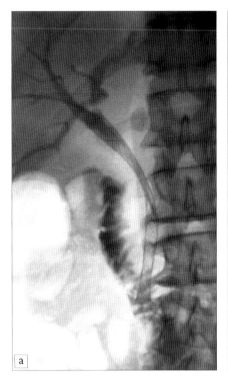
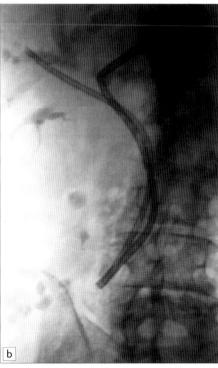

Figure 49.20. *Palliative stenting to relieve malignant obstructive jaundice. (a) Self-expanding metallic endoprosthesis (Memotherm, Angiomed, Europe) has been inserted following PTC and biliary drainage (same patient as Fig. 49.19.) Note a little residual 'waisting' but complete relief of biliary obstruction. (b) 'Kissing' plastic endoprostheses have been inserted to relieve malignant jaundice secondary to a Klatskin tumour. The right duct system was drained endoscopically with a 10.5 Fr Cotton–Leung stent and the left subsequently with a 12.5 Fr Carey–Coons stent following percutaneous left duct puncture.*

ing metallic stents (Fig. 49.20). Self-expanding metallic stents require a smaller transhepatic track for insertion yet provide a larger luminal diameter on full expansion compared to the plastic endoprosthesis (Fig. 49.21). Although they are considerably more expensive than plastic stents, these metallic stents have lower complication rates of haemorrhage, cholangitis and occlusion that lead to re-intervention.[26]

Although PTC and stenting can be performed as a primary one-step procedure, ERCP has become the procedure of choice in the initial invasive investigation of obstructive jaundice in our department as well as in many others. This strategy is adopted because strictures or occlusions are often traversed more easily using the retrograde approach and primary stenting (plastic or metallic) can be performed without the requirement for external drainage (Fig. 49.22).

Both techniques allow bile to be aspirated for cytological examination and brushings taken from a lesion suspected to be cholangiocarcinoma. However, the yield from the brush technique is often disappointing. Endoscopic retrograde cholangio-pancreatography has the advantage that tissue biopsy of lesions in the common bile duct, pancreatic duct and from the periampullary region can be performed although transcholedochal core biopsies can also be acquired percutaneously through a transhepatic sheath.

Endoscopic ultrasound, using the retrograde approach, is an excellent technique for imaging the distal common bile duct (and other upper gastro-intestinal lesions) and the development of new methods utilizing endobiliary probes, with or without cholangioscopy for diagnosis and staging of biliary tumours, may offer considerable potential in the evaluation of biliary tract tumours.

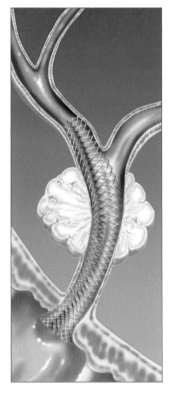

Figure 49.21. *Diagrammatic representation of a self-expanding uncovered metallic stent in situ across a malignant hilar biliary stricture.*

Biliary metallic stents can be redilated, restented or unblocked using the percutaneous transhepatic approach (Fig. 49.23). However, the retrograde approach by ERCP is probably the most desirable where possible, with removal of the occluded plastic biliary stent and exchange for a new stent as a one-stage procedure.

Iridium seeds have been implanted with good palliation

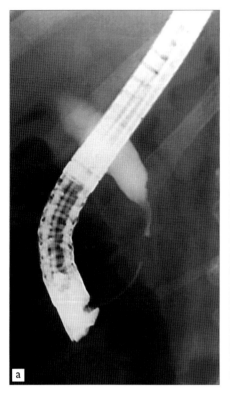

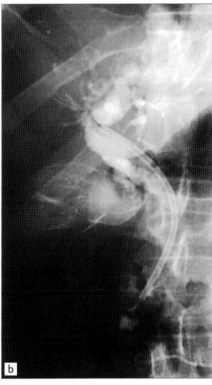

Figure 49.22. *Endoscopic relief of malignant obstructive jaundice secondary to carcinoma of head and pancreas. (a) ERCP demonstrating distal common bile duct stricture. (b) A 10.5 Fr Cotton–Leung plastic endoprosthesis has been inserted retrogradely to relieve biliary obstruction.*

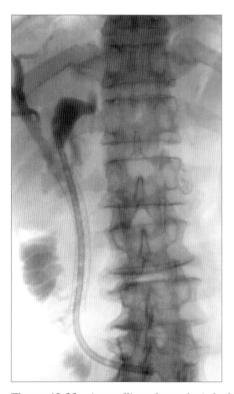

Figure 49.23. *A metallic endoprosthesis had been inserted 6 months previously to relieve obstruction secondary to cholangio-carcinoma. Following recurrent jaundice, a plastic stent was inserted at PTC as the patient had more advanced metastatic liver disease than at the time of primary stenting.*

in small cholangiocarcinomas using the nasobiliary, transhepatic and endoscopic routes for insertion.[27] In addition, in certain institutions, a superficial Roux loop marked with radio-opaque clips is used routinely for recurrent access to the biliary tree across a biliary-enteric anastomosis.[28]

Key points: obstructive jaundice

- Ultrasound, CT and MR cholangio-pancreatography are most useful for the initial non-invasive evaluation of biliary obstruction

- ERCP is the procedure of choice for low bile duct lesions

- ERCP enables stenting and biliary drainage to be performed as a one-step procedure

- PTC has a higher success and lower complication rate for hilar lesions than ERCP

- Metal stents have lower rates of haemorrhage, cholangitis, occlusion and re-intervention than plastic endoprostheses

Visceral arteriography and related intervention

Visceral arteriography has been shown to have an important role in the diagnostic and therapeutic management of patients with malignant disease. The coeliac axis, superior and inferior mesenteric arteries are usually catheterized via a common femoral artery approach. This technique is used for:

- Assessing the hepatic arterial supply to malignant lesions
- Detecting vascular involvement by infiltrative visceral malignancy (particularly pancreatic carcinoma)
- Identifying the site of bleeding in upper and lower gastro-intestinal malignancies prior to embolization

Although portal vein patency can be assessed using duplex sonography and CT (particularly spiral CT), elegant images of the superior mesenteric, splenic and portal vein and its branches can be imaged in real time using 'indirect' portography with the tip of the arterial catheter either in the superior mesenteric artery distal to any replaced hepatic arteries or in the splenic artery (Fig. 49.24). This principle

is also used to assess the portal venous supply to hepatic metastases using CT arterial portography (CTAP),[29] which has been shown to be one of the most sensitive methods for assessing small hepatic metastases (Fig. 49.25). Dual-phase scanning (arterial and portal) should be used with both conventional and spiral CT to differentiate hepatic lesions from perfusion anomalies.

Visceral arteriography may be combined with a number of ingenious biochemical methods to localize small gastro-intestinal tumours, particularly in the body and tail of the pancreas, avoiding direct transhepatic portal venous sampling. For example, calcium stimulation hepatic venous sampling has been used for the detection of occult insulinomas and other APUDomas.[30]

For hepatic metastases with a predominantly hepatic arterial supply and for primary hepatocellular carcinoma (HCC), visceral arteriography can be followed by hepatic

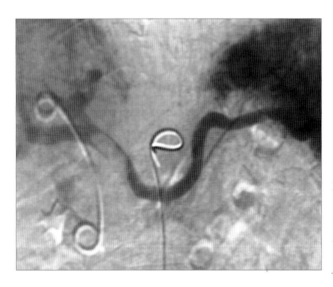

Figure 49.24. *Indirect splenoportogram demonstrating portal venous thrombosis secondary to malignant invasion. Note tip of Sidewinder II arterial catheter in proximal splenic artery and double pigtail-ended plastic endoprosthesis in situ. The latter had been inserted endoscopically for temporary relief of malignant jaundice from pancreatic carcinoma thought to be irresectable.*

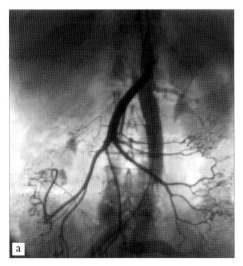
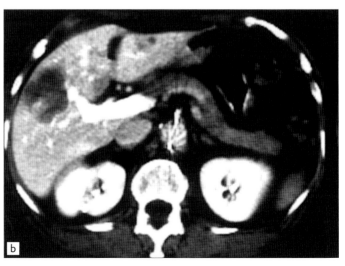

Figure 49.25. *CTAP demonstrating large metastasis in right lobe of liver and smaller lesions in left lobe. (a) Superior mesenteric arteriogram confirming conventional visceral arterial anatomy. (b) Dynamic CTAP image using conventional CT scanner showing excellent enhancement of portal vein with 'splaying' of vessels around large hepatic metastasis. The smaller lesions in the left lobe were confirmed as simple cysts on intraoperative ultrasound with aspiration and immediate cytology.*

chemoembolization using chemotherapeutic agents (e.g. 5-fluorouracil and epirubicin) combined with radio-opaque material, such as lipiodol, which has been shown to be taken up preferentially by the capillary circulation of hepatic tumours.[31] As well as providing high doses of chemotherapy locally, the lipiodol component of the preparation retained in the lesions is utilized as a marker of the tumour on subsequent CT examinations (Fig. 49.26). However, embolization of HCC should be avoided in patients with underlying cirrhosis where further hepatic failure may be precipitated. The principle of hepatic chemoembolization has been extended to percutaneous insertion of selectively placed catheters attached to implantable ports.[32] Unfortunately, the response to treatment of hepatic metastases is less than for primary HCC. More recently, embolic spheres containing beta-emitting agents have been used to selectively embolize hepatic tumours in this way (SIRT).[33]

Other indications for gastro-intestinal embolization in malignancy are for inoperable tumours and for bleeding caused by tumour or chemotherapeutic agents; for example, bleeding is a well-recognized complication of chemotherapy for gastric lymphoma. The technique is particularly suitable when endoscopic procedures have failed or are impractical.

The pancreas has a multiple arterial supply which therefore limits the effects of embolotherapy and, for this reason, the technique is rarely used for the treatment of pancreatic malignancy. In some cases, such as hypervascular APUDomas, superselective embolization has been used for symptomatic control of intractable pain, haemorrhage and hormone production. Splenic embolization is now rarely performed, although it has been recommended in the past for malignancies associated with marked splenomegaly such as lymphoma, the objective being to improve platelet function and achieve preoperative splenic devascularization prior to elective surgical splenectomy.[34]

Similarly, adrenal embolization is rarely performed but may help to palliate tumours or control hormone secretion. Either the three arteries supplying the adrenal or the single draining vein can be embolized. Deliberate 'obstruction' of the adrenal veins has been used to obliterate adrenal function as an alternative to bilateral surgical adrenalectomy in patients with advanced malignant disease.[35] In addition, wedged retrograde injection of contrast medium mixed with sclerosant liquids such as hypertonic dextrose and alcohol, have been used in the treatment of Cushing's syndrome and primary hyperaldosteronism from an adrenal adenoma.

Key points: visceral arteriography

- Visceral arteriography is used as a vehicle for indirect portography, CTAP, venous sampling and hepatic chemoembolization

- CTAP is one of the most sensitive methods for assessing small hepatic metastases

- HCC shows a greater response to hepatic chemoembolization than metastases

Percutaneous insertion of inferior vena cava filters and stents

A well-recognized indication for IVC filtration is recurrent pulmonary embolism despite optimal anticoagulation, or where there is significant risk of pulmonary embolism in patients who cannot be anticoagulated. Another indication is deep pelvic vein and ilio-femoral venous thrombosis due to local pelvic malignancy.

Contraindications to anticoagulant therapy in the oncology setting include:

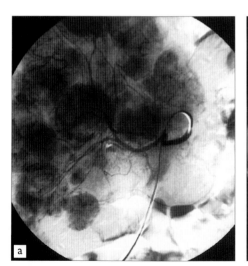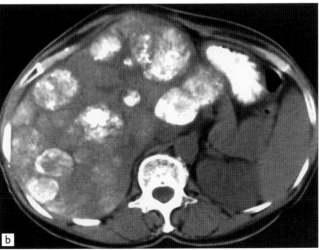

Figure 49.26. *Hepatic chemoembolization in a young woman with a resected colonic adenocarcinoma and multiple hepatic metastases. (a) Selective catheterization of common hepatic artery allows a mixture of lipiodol and 5-fluorouracil to be continuously injected. (b) A subsequent CT scan utilizes the retained lipiodol to help follow the progress of marker lesions.*

- Gastro-intestinal bleeding
- Recent major surgery
- Widespread metastatic disease
- Malignancy of the central nervous system (CNS)

A wide range of IVC filters have been designed including both permanent and temporary filters, the latter not usually being appropriate in patients with advanced local malignant disease unless they are inserted for a short period prior to surgical resection of tumour (Fig. 49.27). Although filters are usually inserted into the IVC in an infrarenal position, in patients with renal vein tumour invasion who are at risk of tumour emboli, the IVC filter may be placed in an infrahepatic suprarenal position in the IVC.

Brief mention has been given above to the use of IVC stenting which remains an uncommon procedure but may relieve inferior vena caval obstruction secondary to extrinsic compression, for example from paracaval nodal disease.[14]

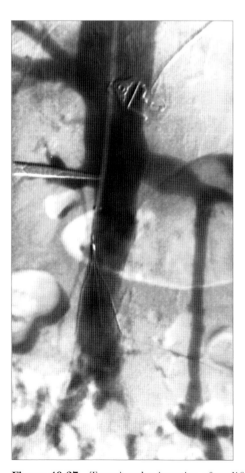

Figure 49.27. *Transjugular insertion of modified Günther Tulip IVC filter for temporary filtration prior to removal of large pelvic tumour. Note presence of thrombosis in iliac veins and preferential filling of left ascending lumbar vein. The filter was removed via the transjugular route seven days following tumour excision.*

Percutaneous neurolysis

An extensive network of neural tissue around the upper abdominal aorta constitutes the coeliac plexus. Direct invasion of the coeliac plexus and surrounding tissues results in considerable pain and, in some cases of visceral malignancy, the pain becomes intractable and unresponsive to conventional analgesia. Neurolytic coeliac plexus blockade is performed by injecting alcohol into the retroperitoneum near the coeliac plexus using a fine needle. The anterior, posterior translumbar and transaortic approaches under fluoroscopic or CT guidance may be used. The anterior approach is less commonly performed, contraindications including the presence of ascites, which introduces the risk of peritonitis, and an uncorrectable coagulopathy or bleeding diathesis.

Tumour ablation techniques

Most percutaneous ablation techniques have been directed towards isolated hepatic metastases using a wide range of destructive agents including:

- Absolute alcohol
- Cryotherapy
- Thermoablation
- Radio-frequency pulses

These and other techniques are described in greater detail in Chapter 50.

Ultrasound-guided percutaneous alcohol injection was first described by Sugiura et al. in 1983.[36] Similar techniques have been extended for use in renal, rectal and parathyroid tumours. Proponents of the technique have suggested that it is particularly suitable for lesions lacking hypervascularity and therefore unlikely to respond to transarterial chemoembolization. These tumours include adenomatous hyperplasia and atypical adenomatous hyperplasia, which are precursors of HCC. Both ultrasound and MR imaging have been used to guide fine needles for such interstitial therapy. One of the problems with liquid agents is the possibility of ethanol or microbubbles entering vessels (or bile ducts) or refluxing back along the needle tract. More recently, this has been obviated by the use of methods such as cryotherapy and thermoablation, high-intensity focused ultrasound and interstitial laser and radio-frequency pulses. Computed tomography guidance is used primarily for smaller lesions, either undetected by ultrasound or in those sites difficult for access such as under a diaphragmatic dome. Magnetic resonance has been extensively used to guide radio-frequency ablation.

Honda et al. have pioneered a technique of percutaneous hot saline injections which produce local heat-induced coagulation necrosis of the tumour, with the liquid returning to physiological saline on cooling.[37] Tabuse et al. reported the use of microwave tissue coagulation to prevent malignant seeding, bleeding and biliary leakage along the needle tract following liver biopsy.[38] More recently, Murakami et al. have applied these techniques to the treatment of HCC greater than 3 cm in diameter.[39] Microwaves produce larger volumes of coagulation necrosis than laser therapy during a shorter duration and the depth of microwave penetration can be limited.

Urinary tract intervention

Percutaneous nephrostomy and ureteric stent insertion

Percutaneous nephrostomy is one of the commonest procedures performed in oncological intervention. There are several indications in cancer management which include:

- Relief of urinary tract obstruction prior to ureteric stent insertion
- Provision of urinary diversion in cases of chemotherapy-related haemorrhagic cystitis
- Treatment of upper urinary tract fistulae prior to occlusion of the fistula whether with an embolic agent or by direct closure using a metal clip under percutaneous fluoroscopic guidance[40]

Variants to this procedure include percutaneous placement of large-bore rubber tubes to block the distal ureter accompanied by external drainage, and the use of endoluminal radio-frequency electric cautery to achieve permanent ureteral occlusion.[41,42] A modified occlusal nephro-ureteral catheter has been developed for severe haemorrhagic cystitis or bladder irritation from other causes such as tumour irradiation or chemotherapy.[43] More recently, radiologists have been asked to remove or exchange blocked indwelling ureteric stents and retrieve stent fragments which can also be performed fluoroscopically using a vascular snare (Fig. 49.28).

Following decompression of the dilated urinary tract with a percutaneous nephrostomy and diagnostic aspiration of urine for microbiological/cytological analysis, antegrade pyelography may demonstrate a ureteric stricture causing partial or complete obstruction (Fig. 49.29). It is usually possible to cross these lesions, even if the stricture is very tight, using appropriate guidewires and catheters. This

sometimes necessitates dilatation prior to insertion of a double pigtail ureteric stent so that the proximal pigtail can be positioned in the renal pelvis and the distal pigtail in the bladder (Fig. 49.30). Ureteric stenting is not only suitable for ureteric malignancies but it is also helpful for alleviation of obstruction secondary to malignant retroperitoneal masses and pelvic cancers, e.g. lymphadenopathy, cervical, bladder and prostate cancers as well as postradiation retroperitoneal fibrosis.

A major dilemma is whether to perform percutaneous nephrostomy and related intervention in patients with disseminated malignancy in whom relief of urinary tract obstruction may prolong life only for the patient to die from advanced local disease, often with distressing symptoms. However, if chemotherapy, radiotherapy or hormonal manipulation may be expected to provide good palliation then ureteric stenting is appropriate and easily performed.

Ureteric fistulae may result from radical pelvic surgery, pelvic malignancy or radiotherapy and, in such cases, ureteric stents may be inserted either retrogradely or antegradely. If a catheter and guidewire cannot be advanced across the fistula, consideration should be given to embolotherapy (*vide supra*). An alternative approach is medical nephrectomy by renal vascular embolization. Bilateral diversion of urinary flow may be required to assist healing to keep the patients dry for rectovesical or vesicovaginal fistulae.

Percutaneous and ureteroscopic tumour ablation

The traditional management of transitional cell carcinoma involving the upper urinary tract is nephro-ureterectomy with removal of a cuff of bladder surrounding the ipsilateral ureteral orifice. An alternative is endoscopic treatment of these tumours either by the antegrade approach via a percutaneous track to the renal pelvis or retrogradely at ureteroscopy. The indications for regional treatment using a minimally invasive approach are:

- Tumour involving a solitary kidney
- Bilateral synchronous tumours
- Renal insufficiency such that renal function will not be maintained by removal of one kidney
- Low-grade and low-stage lesions
- Transplanted kidneys when another organ is not available
- Benign upper-tract tumours including fibro-epithelial polyps
- Poor patient tolerance of a major surgical procedure

In a multidisciplinary setting, after the radiologist establishes a percutaneous approach, the urologist removes the tumour with a resectoscope, cold-cup biopsy forceps (with or without laser therapy), or by the placement of iridium (Ir-192) wires. Radiologists may also be asked to create percutaneous tracts to allow urologists to perform percutaneous cryotherapy to advanced renal cell carcinoma.

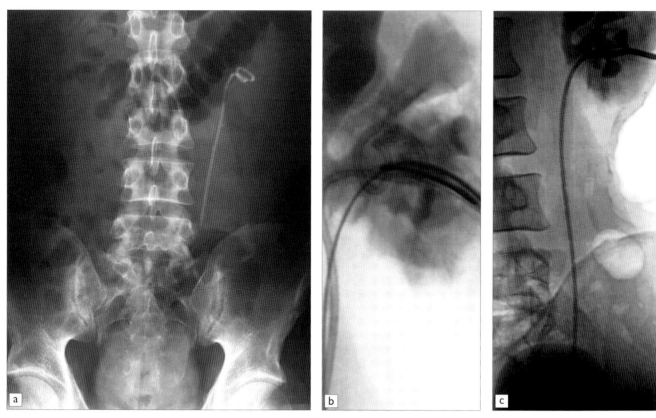

Figure 49.28. *Percutaneous retrieval of fragmented ureteric stent in patient with malignant distal ureteric stricture. (a) Plain abdominal radiograph demonstrating fragmented left ureteric stent following stent exchange at cystoscopy. (b) A percutaneous track has been created and the proximal end of the stent snared with a 'goose-neck' snare via an 8 Fr sheath (with the end cut at an angle to increase effective luminal diameter). (c) Following fragment extraction, the stricture has been crossed and a multiple side-hole drainage catheter left in situ prior to further definitive stenting.*

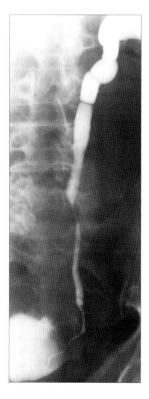

Figure 49.29. *Antegrade pyelography demonstrating tight irregular distal ureteric stricture. This examination was performed following percutaneous nephrostomy and drainage prior to ureteric stenting.*

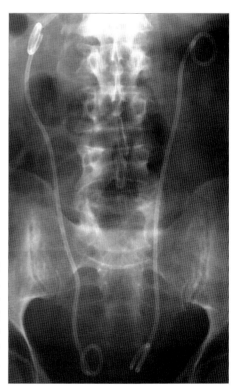

Figure 49.30. *Percutaneous insertion of bilateral double pigtailed ureteric stents in a woman with extensive para-aortic lymphadenopathy (Hodgkin's disease). Following bilateral nephrostomy and drainage the stents were inserted to relieve obstruction during chemotherapy and were subsequently removed fluoroscopically using a perurethral approach.*

Renal artery embolization

Renal cell carcinoma accounts for 3% of all malignancies. Surgical nephrectomy has been the conventional treatment for localized disease (Stages I–III). Tumours that are unresectable, due to a large tumour volume or evidence of local extension, can be downstaged to operable tumours by embolization. Embolization is not indicated for small tumours, oncocytomas or cancer of the renal pelvis. The aims of preoperative embolization are:

- Permanent blockage of capillary and precapillary arterioles by occlusion of the renal artery at or close to its division into segmental vessels but at a safe distance from the origin of the aorta (Fig. 49.31)
- Reduction of subsequent operative blood loss

An improved prognosis is noted in 3-year survival rates of Stage T3 tumours treated by preoperative arterial embolization. Reduced tumour cell dissemination during nephrectomy is assumed to be responsible for the increased survival rates. Embolization may also be used to palliate unresectable tumours and for managing complications associated with tumours such as pain and haematuria.

Key points: urinary tract intervention

■ Percutaneous nephrostomy enables stenting for urinary obstruction, allows urinary diversion and may help urinary fistulae to heal

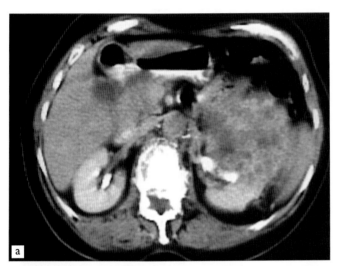

Figure 49.31. *Preoperative embolization of large renal cell carcinoma. (a) CT scan demonstrating a large tumour mass involving lower pole of left kidney and distorting left pelvicalyceal system. Note local invasion of perinephric fat. (b) Selective left renal arteriogram demonstrates large hypervascular tumour with marked neovascularity and some central necrosis. (c) Satisfactory appearances following selective embolization of tumour circulation with polyvinyl alcohol, gelfoam and two 4-mm platinum coils. Note residual staining of tumour capillary bed.*

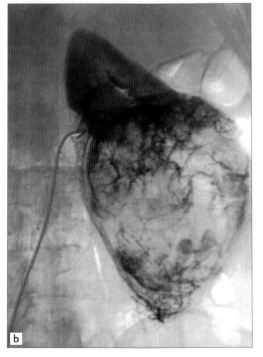

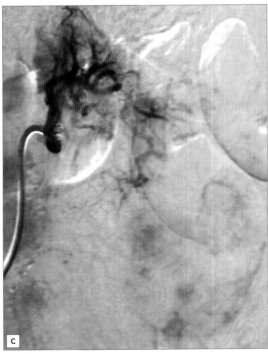

■ Medical nephrectomy may be required to aid healing of fistulae

■ Radiologists can create percutaneous tracks thus enabling endourological procedures to be performed

■ Renal and pelvic arterial embolization may be required as either a preoperative or palliative measure

Therapeutic pelvic embolization

The major indication for pelvic embolization is the treatment of pelvic malignancies, including bladder cancer, prostate cancer and gynaecological tumours. The commonest indications for therapeutic pelvic embolization include:

- Control of bleeding
- Palliation of pain
- Shrinkage of tumour
- Reduction of subsequent intraoperative blood loss in large vascular tumours

In addition, good palliation of intractable haemorrhage from the bladder, due to radiation cystitis, may be achieved by bilateral embolization of the anterior divisions of both internal iliac arteries.

Prostate brachytherapy

This relatively new technique is being increasingly used in the management of organ-confined prostate cancer. It is performed under general anaesthesia typically in a multidisciplinary environment in association with the urologist, radiotherapist and physicist. The procedure requires the ultrasound- and fluoroscopic-guided transperineal implantation of radio-iodine or other radioactive seeds into the peripheral zone of all segments of the prostate gland (Fig 49.32).[44]

Musculoskeletal intervention

Percutaneous skeletal biopsy

Percutaneous skeletal biopsy is a simple and safe procedure providing an effective alternative to open surgical biopsy. Needle biopsy is now much better accepted than previously as experience in interpretation of even small tissue samples has been gained.

Biopsy is usually performed using fluoroscopy or CT guidance with osteoblastic or sclerotic bone lesions biopsied using large-bore needles whilst osteolytic lesions can sometimes be managed with fine needles. If soft tissue masses are associated with destructive bone lesions, good cores can usually be obtained without the need to directly sample the associated destroyed bone (Fig. 49.33). Rib and extremity lesions are easily biopsied with either fine- or large-bore needles, according to the nature of the lesion.

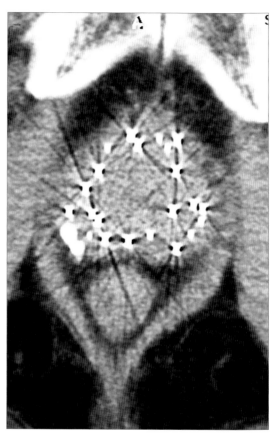

Figure 49.32. *Radio-iodine implants have been implanted into the peripheral zone of all segments of the prostate gland with organ-confined tumour and can be demonstrated on axial CT scan at follow-up.*

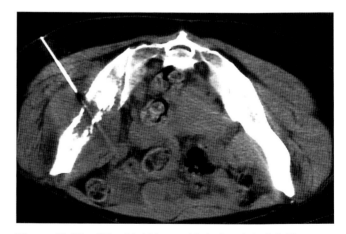

Figure 49.33. *CT-guided biopsy of lytic deposit in left ilium (patient prone). Note 'photon starvation artefact' demonstrating exact position of tip and confirming needle 'throw'. This technique will sample soft tissue masses as well as lytic bone deposits. Histology subsequently revealed metastatic renal cell adenocarcinoma.*

Thoracic and lumbar vertebral body lesions are best approached with the patient prone utilizing a posterolateral approach on the ipsilateral side of the lesion. Although fluoroscopic guidance alone can be used for biopsying the vertebral bodies of the lower cervical vertebrae (using a lateral approach), CT guidance is essential for biopsy of the upper cervical spine (using an anterior transpharyngeal or intra-oral approach) and the base of the skull and facial bones. Computed tomography guidance is also desirable for the posterolateral approach of thoracic lesions to avoid transgressing the pleural cavity. Bone biopsy is discussed further in Chapter 24.

Key points: musculoskeletal biopsy

- FNAB of the soft tissue mass adjacent to a bone lesion often provides adequate material for diagnosis

- Percutaneous vertebroplasty induces almost immediate pain relief

Percutaneous vertebroplasty

Percutaneous vertebroplasty, initially described for the treatment of 'malignant' vertebral haemangiomas, is also now commonly used in the management of vertebral metastases.[45] It involves the injection of acrylic cement directly into the vertebral lesion to achieve consolidation and direct embolization of the vertebra (Fig. 49.34). It provides almost immediate relief of pain compared to radiotherapy, which may take several weeks, and may be appropriate palliation when radiotherapy has been ineffective. This may help obviate further vertebral collapse and neurological compression.

Therapeutic ablation of lytic bone deposits in other sites is also easily performed particularly in the pelvis where lesions are more difficult to treat surgically than in the appendicular skeleton where prostheses may be inserted (Fig. 49.35).

Therapeutic embolization of bone and soft tissue tumours

The initial use of vascular embolization in the management of skeletal tumours was as a preoperative measure to reduce intraoperative blood loss in hypervascular tumours. This treatment has now been extended to palliative embolization, particularly when the tumour is inoperable and has failed to respond to radiotherapy (Fig. 49.36).

The commonest hypervascular tumours treated with preoperative embolization are giant cell tumours (particularly around the knee and distal radius) and metastatic renal adenocarcinoma; nasopharyngeal tumours and paragangliomas may also be treated in this way. Following

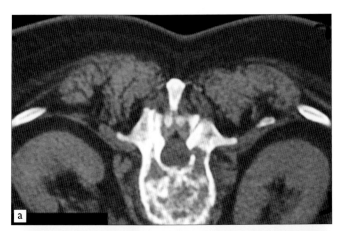

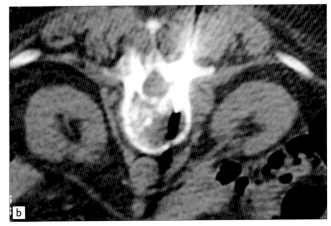

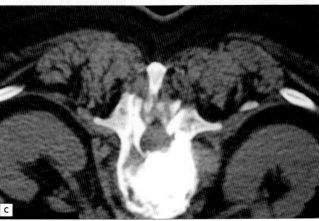

Figure 49.34. *Percutaneous vertebroplasty under image guidance in a patient with metastatic breast carcinoma. (a) Initial CT scan showing partial collapse associated with a spinal lytic metastatic deposit extending into the left pedicle. (b) Injection needle position confirmed on CT fluoroscopy. (c) Postvertebroplasty appearances confirming replacement of tumour in centrum and pedicle with radio-opaque acrylic cement providing symptom relief and reducing risk of further collapse and compromise of spinal canal.*

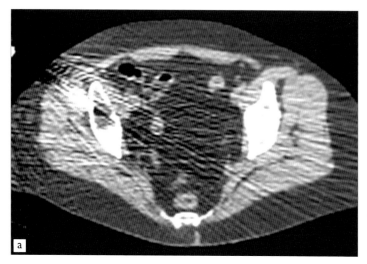

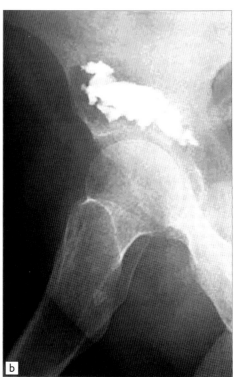

Figure 49.35. *Percutaneous acetabuloplasty under image guidance in a patient with metastatic renal cell carcinoma. (a) Large lytic deposit in right acetabulum on CT. (b) Plain radiograph showing six millilitres of cement has been injected to ablate the lytic tumour providing immediate symptom relief and reduce the risk of pathological fracture.*

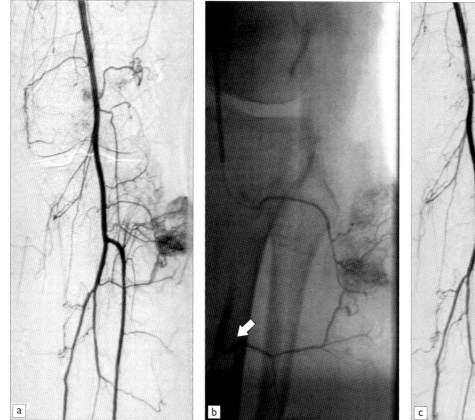

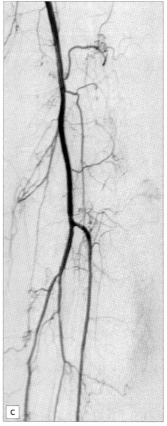

Figure 49.36. *Palliative embolization of recurrent soft tissue tumour mass (malignant melanoma). (a) Selective arteriogram demonstrating hypervascular tumour mass with multiple seeding vessels. (b) Superselective study revealing 'front' and 'back' door seeding supply. Note reflux into tibioperoneal trunk (arrowed) requiring both 'doors' to be 'closed' to prevent reflux of embolic material. (c) Tumour circulation has been excluded on final selective study with excellent palliation.*

embolization it may be desirable to transfer the patient from the interventional radiology suite to the operating theatre for immediate resection in order to minimize the 'postembolization syndrome'.

Giant cell tumours originating in the ilium are often advanced at presentation, precluding primary surgical resection. These tumours are usually insensitive to chemotherapy and irradiation carries the risk of sarcomatous transformation. Therefore, vascular embolization has a place in the multidisciplinary management of these tumours; for example, in unresectable giant cell tumours and aneurysmal bone cysts after other therapeutic methods have failed or are considered inappropriate.

Other oncological intervention

Breast intervention

Following improvements in mammography and ultrasound, as well as the development of specialized needles for localization and biopsy, breast intervention has become an integral part of breast cancer management. Such techniques are particularly important in the localization of mammographic abnormalities where reliable differentiation between benign and malignant lesions cannot be established with certainty. Biopsy and localization are also essential for possibly malignant yet non-palpable lesions.

Complex cysts are quite reasonably treated with caution, and aspiration biopsy should be considered regardless of patient symptomatology or mammographic appearance. Ultrasound is particularly useful for guidance using a free-hand technique to perform breast cyst aspiration and can characterize lesions as simple cysts, complex cysts, fibrosis, areas of fibrocystic disease or solid lesions. Patients with persistent nipple discharge in the absence of a palpable lesion or one that has been demonstrated on ultrasound or mammography may undergo galactography. This procedure outlines the involved duct unit and may be helpful in identifying small early intraductal carcinomas, benign papillomas, papillomatosis or papillary carcinomas. To facilitate surgical excision, the involved duct can be marked with a permanent dye, such as methylene blue.

Both fine-needle (22 gauge) and large-core breast biopsy (14–18 gauge with a 2 cm throw) can be performed using mammographic or ultrasound guidance under local anaesthesia. With ultrasound guidance, a free-hand technique is usually used and FNAB alone may be sufficient if a cytologist is in attendance. Approximately 80% of impalpable breast lesions are visible on ultrasound. Biopsy and wire localization under ultrasound guidance avoids the discomfort of breast compression, waiting for films to be processed and repositioning of wires. The remaining 20% of lesions (mainly microcalcifications and some architectural distortions) require mammographic guidance. Traditionally, conventional mammography has been used for localization although, more recently, stereotactic mammography has

provided exquisite accuracy. Some manufacturers provide stereotactic equipment that can accommodate both aspiration needles and automated biopsy guns for large-bore needles.

Needle localization of breast lesions has been used to reduce the amount of tissue excised at surgery. Hookwires have traditionally been used with either standard mammography units (with or without a fenestrated compression plate) or with stereotactic mammography. Once orthogonal or stereotactic views have confirmed that the tip of the needle is within the lesion (or close by), the hookwire can be deployed prior to transfer of the patient to theatre. Stereotactic mammography guidance for wire placement has a theoretical accuracy of within 1 mm. Ultrasound can also be used for accurate placement of wires, using the free-hand technique in particular.

Tumour localization using venous sampling

The use of transhepatic portal venous sampling and hepatic venous sampling following stimulation has been described above in the detection of occult APUDomas. In fact, venous sampling techniques can be applied to the detection of occult tumours in many other areas where perhaps cross-sectional imaging has failed to demonstrate the lesion adequately. This technique has been particularly useful in the detection of tumours causing increased hormone production, including parathyroid adenomas, Conn's tumours, phaeochromocytomas and pituitary tumours. The latter involves sampling the inferior petrosal venous sinuses and jugular veins, the sensitivity of the technique being increased by simultaneous stimulation of the appropriate releasing factor. Such intervention helps in the differentiation of pituitary-dependent Cushing's syndrome from ectopic adrenocorticotrophic hormone syndrome.

Parathyroid tumour ablation

In over 85% of cases, the cause for primary hyperparathyroidism is a solitary adenoma, with the remaining cases being mainly due to parathyroid glandular hyperplasia. Less than 1% of cases are caused by parathyroid carcinoma. Surgical excision has a success rate of approximately 95% in experienced hands but, where the risks of surgery are excessive or in cases of failed surgery, parathyroid venous sampling may be performed for tumour localization.

In view of the difficulties encountered in operating on a previously explored neck, which may be extensively scarred, parathyroid arteriography and angiographic ablation may be considered. Once the lesion has been identified on arteriography, a single end-holed catheter is wedged into the feeding vessel and multiple boluses of dense contrast material are injected to achieve intense parenchymal staining of the gland. This is followed by occlusion of the main feeding vessel with gelfoam or coils. In these difficult patients this technique has met with some considerable success with few complications.[46] Even if the procedure is unsuccessful, the technique will have localized the lesion elegantly for a further surgical attempt at excision.

Solbiati et al. performed parathyroid tumour ablation under sonographic guidance by percutaneous injection of absolute alcohol into the tumours.[47] Indications included high surgical risk, refusal of operation and recurrence after previous subtotal resection. The presence of all lesions was first confirmed on FNAB.

Percutaneous retrieval techniques

With the large number of intravascular catheters used for chemotherapy, the increasing usage of biliary and ureteric stents and the use of coils for palliative tumour embolization, there has been an increased requirement for the retrieval of displaced or misplaced fragments and a number of ingenious, yet well-established, techniques have been developed which include:

- Wire-loop snares
- Fragment graspers
- Dormia baskets
- Deflector wires

Minimally invasive techniques to achieve such extraction are particularly important in patients with malignancy who are often extremely ill and may have coagulopathy. In such patients, major surgery (for example, thoracotomy) is particularly undesirable.

Intraoperative ultrasound

Intraoperative ultrasound has been used to biopsy a number of lesions, for example liver, pancreas, kidney, brain and spinal cord.[48] In our institution we routinely localize hepatic metastases to segmental level prior to resection, using a dedicated operative probe that not only demonstrates the lesions but allows accurate anatomical mapping. More recently, image-guided ablation of small hepatic lesions has been performed at the time of surgical resection of larger lesions.

Locoregional chemotherapy

Selective infusion of intra-arterial chemotherapy may reduce the side-effects of systemic chemotherapy while increasing the local concentration of drug in an attempt to achieve the best tumour response. The most common example is hepatic chemoembolization described above. Other examples of chemo-infusion therapy include locoregional intra-arterial chemotherapy of local chest wall recurrence in breast carcinoma via the internal mammary artery, isolated limb perfusion in malignant melanoma and chemo-infusion therapy of advanced primary transitional cell carcinoma of the bladder (T3 and T4 bladder carcinomas) with or without simultaneous radiotherapy, and infusion of sarcomas, bone and cerebral tumours.

Interventional imaging of neurological tumours

Interventional CT, MR imaging and positron emission tomography (PET) techniques have been used to provide stereotactic guidance for the biopsy of image-proven tumours.[49] The technique has been extended to both CT-guided stereotactic interstitial brachytherapy, a technique in which radioactive sources have been implanted into unresectable brain tumours, and CT-guided stereotactic surgery when deep-seated intracerebral neoplasms can be vaporized using a stereotactically directed CO_2 laser ('Gamma knife' therapy).

Following presurgical evaluation of the vascular supply to intra- and extracranial vascular tumours, e.g. haemangiomas, meningiomas, glomus tumours and haemangioblastomas, preoperative embolization may be performed using particulate emboli in patients of poor operative risk.

Key points: other applications

- Galactography may help identify early intraductal carcinoma, papillomatosis or papillary carcinoma

- Stereotactic biopsy and localization provide pin-point accuracy for mammographically visible lesions

- Ultrasound guidance avoids uncomfortable breast compression, waiting for film processing and repositioning of wires

- Venous sampling techniques may help to localize occult tumours

- Parathyroid tumour ablation may be useful for the scarred, previously explored, neck

- Minimally invasive techniques may be employed to retrieve misplaced or displaced fragments and coils

Summary

- Fine-needle aspiration biopsy (FNAB) is usually sufficient for the initial diagnosis of malignancy, provided adequate cellular material has been obtained

- Tissue cores are required for the accurate classification of lymphoma

- In the chest, ultrasound guidance is well suited for the drainage of malignant effusions and other collections

- The interventional imaging suite is becoming increasingly used for percutaneous insertion of central venous catheters and for the management of ensuing complications

- In lung cancer, interventional techniques, such as bronchoscopic tracheobronchial stenting and bronchial artery embolization, have a useful role in patient management

- In the gastro-intestinal tract, endoscopic ultrasound (EUS) is becoming increasingly used for staging primary tumours, for biopsy of tumour and lymph nodes, and for drainage of fluid collections and abscesses

- Liver biopsy should be carried out using the transjugular approach or by performing a plugged liver biopsy in the presence of uncorrectable coagulopathy

- Endoscopic and fluoroscopic techniques (dilatation/stents) provide palliation for oesophageal strictures, fistulae, gastric outlet obstruction and large bowel obstruction. Gastrostomy feeding tubes can also be inserted using the percutaneous/endoscopic approach

- In the management of obstructive jaundice, both endoscopic retrograde cholangio-pancreatography (ERCP) and percutaneous transhepatic cholangiography (PTC) are useful for diagnosis; ERCP is the procedure of choice for low bile duct lesions, whereas PTC has a higher success and lower complication rate for hilar lesions

- Visceral arteriography is used as a vehicle for indirect portography, CT arterial portography (CTAP), venous sampling and hepatic chemoembolization

- Inferior vena caval infiltration is indicated for recurrent pulmonary embolism or in patients at high risk of pulmonary embolism who cannot be anticoagulated

- Image-guided tumour ablation techniques are mostly used for hepatic malignant lesions and include cryo- and thermoablation, high-intensity focused ultrasound and interstitial laser and radio-frequency pulses

- Renal and urinary tract interventional procedures include nephrostomy, ureteric stenting, ureteroscopic tumour ablation and renal arterial embolization

- Renal arterial embolization may be used for unresectable tumours in an attempt to downstage disease prior to surgery. It may also be used as a palliative procedure for pain and/or haematuria

- Therapeutic embolization for pelvic and musculoskeletal tumours may be preoperative or palliative measures

- Percutaneous vertebroplasty may be useful in the management of spinal metastatic pain

- Venous sampling techniques are useful for localizing occult tumours that are biochemically active

- Percutaneous retrieval techniques may be required for fragmented catheters, stents and misplaced coils

- Interventional CT, MR imaging and PET scanning are being developed to provide stereotactic guidance for biopsy, interstitial brachytherapy and surgery

References

1. Husband J E, Golding S J. The role of computed tomography-guided needle biopsy in an oncology service. Clin Radiol 1983; 34: 255–260

2. Anderson T, Eriksson B, Lindgren PG et al. Percutaneous ultrasonography-guided cutting biopsy from liver metastases of endocrine gastro-intestinal tumours. Ann Surg 1987; 206: 728–732

3. Van Sonnenberg E, Casola G, Ho M et al. Difficult thoracic lesions: CT guided biopsy experience in 150 cases. Radiology 1988; 167: 457–461

4. Haaga J R, Reich N E, Havrilla T R et al. Interventional CT scanning. Radiol Clin North Am 1977; 15: 449–456

5. Templeton P A, Krasna M. Needle/wire lung nodule localization for thorascopic resection. Chest 1993; 104: 953–958

6. Robertson L J, Mauro M A, Jacques P F. Radiologic placement of Hickman catheters. Radiology 1989; 170: 1007–1009

7. Page A C, Evans R A, Kaczmarshi R et al. The insertion of chronic indwelling central venous catheters (Hickman lines) in interventional radiology suites. Clin Radiol 1990; 42: 105–109

8. Adam A. Insertion of long-term central venous catheter: time for a new look. Br Med J 1995; 311: 341–342

9. Azizkhan R G, Taylor L A, Jaques P F et al. Percutaneous translumbar and transhepatic inferior

vena caval catheters for prolonged vascular access in children. J Pediat Surg 1992; 27: 165–169

10. Kaufman J A, Crenshaw W B, Kuter I et al. Percutaneous placement of a central venous access device. Am J Roentgenol 1995; 164: 459–460

11. Nadkani S, Macdonald S, Cleveland T J et al. Placement of a retrievable Günther tulip filter in the superior vena cava for upper extremity deep venous thrombosis. Cardiovasc Intervent Radiol 2002; 25: 524–526

12. Gaines P A, Belli A M, Anderson P B et al. Superior vena caval obstruction managed by the Gianturco Z Stent. Clin Radiol 1994; 49: 202–208

13. Furui S, Sawada, S, Kuramoto K et al. Gianturco stent placement in malignant caval obstruction: analysis of factors for predicting the outcome. Radiology 1995; 195: 147–152

14. Tan B S, Watkinson A F, Dussek J E et al. Metallic endoprosthesis for malignant tracheo-bronchial obstruction: initial experience. Cardiovasc Intervent Radiol 1996; 19: 91–96

15. Gothlin J H. Post-lymphographic percutaneous fine-needle aspiration biopsy of lymph nodes guided by fluoroscopy. Radiology 1976; 120: 205–207

16. Ho C S, McLoughlin M J, McHattie J D et al. Percutaneous fine-needle aspiration biopsy of the pancreas following endoscopic retrograde cholangiography. Radiology 1977; 125: 351–353

17. Botet J F, Lightdale C J, Zauber A G et al. Pre-operative staging of oesophageal cancer. Radiology 1991; 181: 419–425

18. Ziegler K, Sanft C, Zimmer T et al. Comparison of computed tomography, endosonography and intra-operative assessment in TN staging of gastric carcinoma. Gut 1993; 34: 604–610

19. Tio T, Coene P, Van Delden O et al. Colorectal carcinoma: Pre-operative TNM classification with endosonography. Radiology 1991; 179: 165–170

20. Müller F, Meyenberger C, Bertschinger P et al. Pancreatic tumours: evaluation with endoscopic US, CT and MR imaging. Radiology 1994; 190: 745–751

21. Jackson J E, Adam A. Percutaneous transcaval tumour biopsy using a 'road map' technique. Clin Radiol 1991; 44: 195–196

22. Iguchi H, Kimora Y, Yanada J et al. Treatment of a malignant stricture after oesophagojejunostomy by a self-expanding metallic stent. Cardiovasc Intervent Radiol 1993; 16: 102–104

23. Tejero E, Mainar A, Fernandez L et al. New procedure for the treatment of colorectal neoplastic obstructions. Dis Colon Rectum 1994; 37: 1158–1159

24. Rey J-F, Romancyk T, Grett M. Metal stents for palliation of rectal carcinoma: a preliminary report on 12 patients. Endoscopy 1995; 27: 501–504

25. Wollman B, D'Agostino H B, Walus-Wigle J R et al. Radiologic, endoscopic and surgical gastrostomy: an institutional evaluation and meta-analysis of the literature. Radiology 1995; 197: 699–704

26. Adam A, Chetty N, Roddie M et al. Self-expandable stainless steel endoprostheses for the treatment of malignant bile duct obstruction. Am J Roentgenol 1991; 156: 321–325

27. Fletcher M S, Brinkley D, Dawson J L et al. Treatment of high bile duct carcinoma by internal radiotherapy with iridium-192 wires. Lancet 1981; ii: 172–174

28. Hutson D G, Russell E, Schiffe E et al. Balloon dilatation of biliary strictures through a choledochojejunocutaneous fistula. Ann Surg 1984; 199: 637–644

29. Reduanly R D, Chezmar J L. CT arterial portography: technique, indications and applications. Clin Radiol 1997; 52: 256–268

30. O'Shea D, Rohrer-Theurs A W, Lynn J A et al. Localization of insulinomas by selective intra-arterial calcium injection. J Clin Endocrinol Metab 1996; 81: 1623–1627

31. Raoul J L, Bourguet P, Bretagne J F et al. Hepatic artery injection of I-131-labelled Lipiodol. Part I: Biodistribution study results in patients with hepatocellular carcinoma and liver metastases. Radiology 1988; 168: 541–545

32. Arai Y. Required basic procedures of hepatic arterial infusion chemotherapy for interventional radiologists. Jap J Clin Radiol 1993; 38: 1497–1508

33. Gray B, Van Hazel G, Hope M et al. Randomised trial of SIR-Spheres® plus chemotherapy vs chemotherapy alone for treating patients with liver metastases from primary large bowel cancer. Ann Oncol 2001; 12: 1711–1720

34. Wholey M H, Chamorro H A, Rao G et al. Splenic infarction and spontaneous rupture after therapeutic embolization. Cardiovasc Radiol 1978; 1: 249–253

35. Jahlonski R D, Meaney T F, Schumacher C P. Transcatheter adrenal ablation for metastatic carcinoma of the breast. Cleveland Clin Quart 1977; 44: 57–63

36. Sugiura N, Takara K, Ohto M et al. Percutaneous intratumoral injection of ethanol under ultrasound imaging for treatment of small hepatocellular carcinoma. Acta Hepatol Japonica 1983; 24: 920–924

37. Honda N, Guo Q, Uchida H et al. Percutaneous hot saline injection therapy for hepatic tumours: an alternative to percutaneous ethanol injection therapy. Radiology 1994; 190: 53–57

38. Tabuse Y, Tabuse K, Mori K et al. Percutaneous microwave tissue coagulation in liver biopsy: experimental and clinical studies. Arch Jpn Chit 1986; 55: 381–392

39. Murakami R, Yoshimatsu S, Yamashita Y et al. Treatment of hepatocellular carcinoma: value of percutaneous microwave coagulation. Am J Roentgenol 1995; 164: 1159–1164

40. Lund A, Rysavy J A, Hunter D W et al. Percutaneous occlusion of the ureter: a new approach for relief of urinary tract fistulae. Semin Intervent Radiol 1984; 1: 92–98

41. Castaneda F, Moradian G P, Epstein D H et al. A new technique for complete temporary occlusion of the ureter. Am J Roentgenol 1989; 153: 81–82

42. Kopecky K U, Sutton G P, Bihrle R et al. Percutaneous transrenal endoluminal radio-frequency electrocautery for occlusion: Case report. Radiology 1989; 170: 1047–1048

43. Bush W, Mayo M. Catheter modification for transrenal temporary total ureteral obstruction: the 'occlusive' nephroureteral catheter. Urology 1994; 43: 729–733

44. Langley S E M, Laing R W. Prostate brachytherapy has come of age: a review of the technique and results. Br J Urol Int 2002; 89: 241–249

45. Weill A, Chiras J, Simon J M et al. Spinal metastases: indications for and results of percutaneous injection of acrylic surgical cement. Radiology 1996; 199: 241–247

46. Miller D L, Doppman J L, Change R et al. Angiographic ablation of parathyroid adenomas: lessons from a 10-year experience. Radiology 1987; 165: 601–607

47. Solbiati L, Giangrande A, De Pra L et al. Percutaneous ethanol injection of parathyroid tumours under US guidance: treatment for secondary hyperparathyroidism. Radiology 1985; 155: 607–610

48. Machi J, Sigel B, Kurohisi T et al. Operative ultrasound guidance for various surgical procedures. Ultrasound Med Biol 1990; 16: 37–42

49. Quinones-Molina R, Alaminos A, Molina H. Computer-assisted CT-guided stereotactic biopsy and brachytherapy of brain tumours. Stereotactic Functional Neurosurg 1994; 63: 52–55

Chapter 50

Interventional imaging: tumour ablation

Alice R Gillams

Introduction

Image-guided tumour ablation is a rapidly expanding field. Ten years ago there were a handful of pioneering centres; today hundreds of centres are practising tumour ablation. Technical innovations and new applications are frequently reported with over 100 papers published in 2002. Whilst it is accepted that ablation can be an effective therapy, there are still several unanswered questions and techniques are constantly being refined. It remains difficult to achieve large (>5 cm) areas of confluent necrosis and further modifications are needed. Accurate tumour control and assessment of treatment effect remain a contentious issue. The optimal relationship between local ablation and systemic therapy is not known. Patient selection and the role of ablation relative to other therapies need to be studied.

Technical aspects

Energy sources can be grouped into four major categories:

- Those employing thermal energy, either heating or cooling
- Direct injection therapies
- Photodynamic therapy (PDT)
- Ionizing radiation

Thermal energy

With all the heating techniques the aim is to raise the temperature of the tissue to be destroyed to between 60°C and 100°C. This is to produce coagulative necrosis yet avoid charring and vaporization of tissue. There are five thermal techniques: radio-frequency (RF), laser, microwave, cryotherapy and high-intensity focused ultrasound (HIFU).[1] A summary of their characteristics is shown in Table 50.1.

Radio-frequency

In the late 19th century, d'Arsonval, a physicist, reported the use of alternating RF to generate heat in biological tissue.[2] Radio-frequency current induces ionic agitation, which in turn, results in heating. Radio-frequency has been used for many years to perform electrocautery in the oper-

Table 50.1. *Comparison of thermal ablation techniques*

Technique	Efficacy	Implementation	Cost
RF	+++	++	++
Laser	++	+	+++
Microwave	+	++	++
Cryotherapy	+++	+/−	+++
HIFU	+/−	+/−	?

ating room or to produce discrete, focal lesions that interrupt aberrant cardiac conduction pathways. Initial electrodes were unipolar of low power, <50 W, and were not internally cooled. Bipolar electrodes are effective in producing small, discrete lesions but have limited usefulness in the treatment of tumours.[3] More recent RF technology has introduced arrays of electrodes that are activated simultaneously, internally water-cooled electrodes, high-power generators <200 W and simultaneous perfusion of the tissue with saline.[4–9] Most experience has been gained with two multi-electrode designs, a water-cooled cluster of three parallel 17 G electrodes (Tyco Healthcare, USA) and an expanding electrode design (Fig. 50.1). The expanding electrodes are introduced collapsed within a hollow (14–15 G) needle. Once correctly positioned, multiple prongs or tines are deployed resulting in a final configuration that resembles a grappling hook (RITA Medical Systems, CA, USA) or an umbrella (Radiotherapeutics, CA, USA).[10] A comparison of water-cooled, triple cluster electrodes and

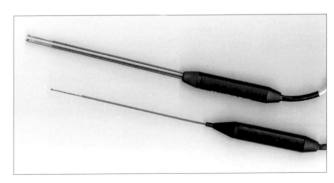

Figure 50.1. *An example of a RF electrode. An internally cooled straight needle design – both a single and a cluster of three electrodes.*

the expandable, multi-tined electrodes showed that larger volumes of necrosis were produced using the water-cooled design.[11] Since then, there have been modifications to the expandable electrode design, including an increase in the number of active tines, the use of higher power generators and combination with saline perfusion technology. New technological developments include the development of an MR-compatible, water-cooled electrode and new electrode designs, a two-tine expandable electrode developed for very small lesions and a bendable shaft expandable electrode to facilitate scanning within a gantry after electrode positioning.

Laser

Both neodymium yttrium aluminium garnet (Nd:YAG λ 1064 nm) and solid-state lasers (λ 805 nm) have been used successfully in tumour ablation. Photon absorption and heat conduction produce hyperthermia and coagulative necrosis. Laser energy is delivered through flexible, thin fibres 400–600 μm in diameter. Fibre morphology can be varied depending on the area to be treated. A point source from a bare-tip fibre will produce a sphere of necrosis, whereas a diffuser fibre will produce an elliptical ablation. Recent technological improvements have included an increase in laser power <40 W and the addition of water-cooling. Although more expensive to set up and support than RF, laser ablations are a little more predictable. Laser energy is deposited around the fibre tip, whereas RF pathways and therefore energy deposition vary, are more complex and less predictable.

Microwave

Microwaves (2,450 MHz) cause rotation and vibration of water molecules thus producing heat. The equipment consists of a generator and a monopolar needle electrode which is introduced through a 14 G access needle. Multiple percutaneous electrodes are generally required. Each microwave application produces a discrete focus of necrosis; for example a single treatment for 120 s at 60 W provides approximately 1.6 cm of necrosis. For this reason, microwave ablation has most often been used for the treatment of small (<3 cm) hepatocellular carcinoma (HCC).

Cryotherapy

Cryotherapy uses repetitive freezing and thawing of tissue to produce necrosis. Irreversible tissue destruction occurs at temperatures below 20–30°C. Liquid nitrogen and argon gas are used as coolants. Traditional cryotherapy probes have been large, requiring laparotomy access for the treatment of liver tumours. Recent advances have seen the development of percutaneous cryotherapy probes of <2.5 mm in diameter. Cryoprobes of different sizes and shapes are available to map the morphology of the area to be treated. The development of the ice ball can be monitored using ultrasound or MR guidance with an accuracy of 1–5 mm. Most cryotherapy has been applied to tumours of the liver and prostate.

High-intensity focused ultrasound

High-intensity focused ultrasound uses frequencies of 0.8–3.2 MHz and focal peak intensities of 5,000–20,000 W/cm^2.[12] The basic mechanism is heat-induced coagulative necrosis. Pathological studies demonstrate particular damage to vessels, including tumour microvasculature.[13] High-intensity focused ultrasound has the advantage of being a trackless technique, performed without anaesthesia and with no risk of tumour seeding. A clear acoustic path from skin to the tissue to be ablated is required. The technique has been available since the 1940s but improvements in imaging and in HIFU technology, e.g. variable focusing and electronic beam steering, have renewed interest in the technique. The main problem is the limited amount of necrosis that can be achieved per unit time. Most work has been performed in the prostate using transrectal devices.

Key points: thermal energy

■ Five thermal techniques exist: radio-frequency (RF), laser, microwave, cryotherapy and high-intensity focused ultrasound (HIFU)

■ Laser tumour ablations are more predictable than RF

■ Microwave ablations have most often been used for HCC <3 cm

■ Although HIFU is a trackless technique, without anaesthesia and no risk of seeding, only a limited amount of necrosis can be achieved per unit time

Direct injection therapies

Ethanol, acetic acid and gel-stabilized chemotherapeutic agents have all been used to ablate tumours with variable success. Gene therapy is hypothesized as the therapy of tomorrow.

Percutaneous ethanol injection

Percutaneous ethanol injection (PEI) was one of the first effective ablative techniques to be widely adopted for the treatment of small HCCs. Ethanol causes dehydration and, subsequently, necrosis.[14] Under ultrasound guidance, a fine needle (21–22 G) is introduced into the tumour and 95–100% ethanol injected. To achieve complete ablation, the ethanol must reach all parts of the tumour; however, ethanol spreads unevenly and the needle needs to be repositioned accordingly. Ethanol can reflux along the needle tract and cause pain; this limits the amount that can be injected at any one time in the conscious patient. Percutaneous ethanol injection is, therefore, either performed as a multistage, outpatient technique under conscious sedation or as a single-stage procedure under general anaesthesia. Percutaneous ethanol injection is most effective in encapsulated HCC and of little benefit in infiltrating HCC or in metastases. The scirrhous nature of liver metastases restricts the amount of ethanol that can be injected, often leading to extravasation and thus incomplete necrosis. Thermal techniques are therefore preferred for the treatment of metastases. In HCC, thermal techniques provide more necrosis in less time and in fewer sessions. Percutaneous ethanol injection still has a role in the treatment of HCC not amenable to RF, e.g. exophytic lesions, which can rupture with disastrous consequences during heating.

Key points: direct injection therapy

- PEI is of value in encapsulated rather than infiltrating HCC, but its role lies in tumours not amenable to RF, which produces more necrosis in less time

- PEI is of little benefit in liver metastases as their scirrhous nature limits the quantity of injected ethanol

Photodynamic therapy (PDT)

Principles
The combination of a photosensitizing agent and light of the appropriate wavelength in the presence of oxygen produces cell death. This is the basis of PDT. The cytotoxic intermediaries are thought to be short-lived free oxygen radicals. The development of second-generation photosensitizing agents has rekindled interest in PDT.[15–19] A literature search will reveal papers on multiple and diverse applications, e.g. photoangioplasty, treatment of dysplastic and early tumours, or palliation of advanced obstructing tumours in the lung and gastro-intestinal tract, treatment at surgery of the peritoneal surface in advanced ovarian carcinoma and open PDT for recurrent pituitary adenomas, to name just a few. Traditionally, PDT has been successfully applied to accessible tissue, e.g. skin, bladder, lung and gastro-intestinal tract.[20–25] *Interstitial PDT* is a new innovation requiring the introduction of a light source deep into the tissue to be treated. It was originally hoped that photosensitizing agents with selective tumour uptake could be developed. However, currently available agents exhibit only minimal selectivity. Therefore, image guidance is required to ensure exact delivery of light so that effective tumour ablation is achieved whilst minimizing collateral damage. Optimal tissue penetration is achieved with light of wavelengths 650–800 nm.[26,27]

Photosensitizing agents
There are a number of different porphyrin-based photosensitizing agents which vary in administration, tissue uptake, optimal wavelength, duration for which the patient remains photosensitized and effectiveness. In the gastro-intestinal tract, oral 5-amino laevulinic acid (5-ALA) works well for superficial treatments with a short duration of photosensitivity. The optimal wavelength for 5-ALA is 635 nm, i.e. outside the range for optimal tissue penetration. Recently, meso-tetra-hydro-phenylchlorin (mTHPC), which reacts to red light optimally of λ 652 nm, has become available for trials.

The interstitial technique
Using image guidance, 19 G hollow needles are inserted into the tumour. Laser fibres are introduced through the needles such that the tip protrudes 5–10 mm beyond the needle and light of the appropriate wavelength can be delivered. Lasers are a good light source as they deliver monochromatic, coherent light. Optimal positioning depends on the photosensitizing agent, energy and wavelength of light and tissue. For example, using mTHPC at a dose of 0.15 mg/kg administered intravenously 3 days prior to treatment and 20 J of red laser light (λ 652 nm), a sphere of necrosis 9 mm (range 7–11) in diameter was produced in pancreatic tumours.[28] To obtain large areas of confluent necrosis, multiple (up to eight) fibres are positioned, spaced appropriately. Diffuser fibres of 2–4 cm length can also be used in appropriate target tissues, e.g. central cholangiocarcinoma. Free oxygen radicals are short-lived and undetectable by imaging; therefore, it is not possible to monitor the effect of treatment during the procedure. Maximal necrosis occurs some time after the treatment, e.g. using mTHPC, maximal necrosis is seen at 72 hours. Contrast-enhanced techniques, either computed tomography (CT) or MR, can be used to show the extent of necrosis produced. Treatments are usually performed under conscious sedation and local anaesthesia. A drawback of mTHPC is that photosensitivity lasts 6–10 weeks and, therefore, appropriate measures are required to avoid direct sunlight during this period.

Key points: photodynamic therapy

- With interstitial PDT, a light source is introduced deep into the tumour under imaging guidance

- PDT requires administration of a photosensitizing agent, which is usually porphyrin-based and has only minimal tissue selectivity

Ionizing radiation
Image-guided procedures include radioactive seed implantation in the prostate and transhepatic biliary access for cholangiocarcinoma. Although over 20 years old in concept, improvements in seeds, three-dimensional ultrasound guidance and radiotherapy planning have increased the use of this technique as a treatment for T1 and T2 stage prostate cancer. Brachytherapy delivers conventional doses of radiotherapy over a period of months.

Applications to specific organs

Liver tumours

Choice of technique

More clinical experience has been gained in the treatment of liver tumours than in any other area. The liver is a relatively forgiving organ with substantial reserve and an ability to regenerate. Most techniques, including all the thermal techniques and PDT, have been tried in the liver. Today, PEI has been replaced by laser or RF ablation in most centres. Although both of these latter techniques are effective, currently RF is the preferred technique and the one most widely practised. Laser has the advantage of being more MR-compatible, permitting direct MR monitoring.[29] Magnetic resonance-compatible RF electrodes are being developed, but the application of RF current and image acquisition are incompatible and have to be alternated. Comparisons of laser and RF suggest that larger volumes of ablation and, in particular, the ablation of a margin of normal liver has been easier and quicker to achieve with RF.[30] Cryoablation, whilst effective, carries a higher complication rate. Animal work has shown that whereas cryoablation results in acute lung injury, RF does not.[31] Comparisons of laparoscopic RF with cryoablation have shown a lower complication rate with RF.[32] One study reported a 40.7% complication rate with cryotherapy as compared to 3.3% with RF.[33] Comparisons of percutaneous cryotherapy and RF have shown a higher complete ablation rate with RF.[34] Microwave has been used, particularly in China, and a few centres have performed PDT. High-intensity focused ultrasound is still experimental. *RF is currently, therefore, the preferred technique for liver tumour ablation.*

Pathological validation of RF
The efficacy of RF has been validated in at least two cohorts of patients who subsequently underwent surgical resection.[35,36] Pathological specimens resected immediately after ablation showed irreversible cell damage with an absence of enzymatic activity. Coagulative necrosis developed later and was consistently demonstrated on specimens resected 3–7 days after thermal ablation.

Definitions of success in liver tumour ablation

The aim is complete tumour ablation with a margin of apparently normal tissue without collateral damage. Treatment efficacy is improved by intraprocedural imaging assessment. Hepatocellular carcinoma can be assessed with contrast-enhanced ultrasound.[37] In all tumours, treatment efficacy can be assessed by dynamic contrast-enhanced CT or MR. Complete ablation is defined as the absence of visible tumour on imaging so that there is an absence of enhancement following intravenous (IV) injection of contrast medium. Despite the appearance of complete ablation, recurrence adjacent to the ablated area can occur, particularly where blood flowing in adjacent vessels results

in tissue cooling and protects microscopic quantities of tumour. Wide variations in early reported recurrence rates reflect different definitions and assessment techniques. The accepted definition is any evidence of hypo- or hypervascular tumour adjacent to or within the ablation zone, with or without an increase in the size of the lesion. In patients with colorectal metastases, new tumours develop in the liver at a distance to the ablated site in 57%.[38] For HCC, the 5-year recurrence rate in the liver following successful resection varies from 67.6 to 100%.[39–43] Therefore, an important aspect of ablation is careful, structured imaging follow-up with dynamic contrast-enhanced CT or MR to detect new lesions and recurrence, such that further ablation can be offered as appropriate.

> ### Key points: liver tumour ablation – choice of technique and assessing efficacy
>
> - RF ablation is currently the preferred technique for liver tumour ablation and its effect has been histologically validated
>
> - Recurrence is defined as evidence of hypo- or hypervascular tumour adjacent to or within the ablation zone *with or without* an increase in the size of the lesion

Liver metastases

Colorectal

Limited colorectal liver metastases are the most commonly treated metastatic lesion. The liver is often the first and only site for metastases. There is good evidence that most patients will succumb from their liver metastases and, therefore, local control can improve life expectancy. This has been the reasoning behind hepatic resection. Surgical resection is the accepted first-line treatment for patients with resectable disease. Five-year survival figures range from 25 to 39%.[44] Traditionally, most patients (80–90%) are not candidates for surgical resection due to the extent or distribution of disease, or concurrent medical disability.[45] Although historical chemotherapy results have been disappointing, recent results are better. Irinotecan has resulted in the first significant improvement in survival to a median 17.4 months and 1-year survival of 69%.[46] Improved response rates have been achieved with Oxaliplatin, 53% as compared to 28% with 5-fluorouracil (5-FU) and folinic acid.[47] There are data showing that down-staging with neoadjuvant chemotherapy followed by ablation or resection is useful.[48,49]

Between 1993 and 1995 we performed laser thermal ablation and reported a median survival of 27 months.[50] More recent results with RF show a median of 34 months and 3-year survival of 36% from the time of thermal ablation (Fig. 50.2).[51,52] Thirty-six percent survival at 3 years in

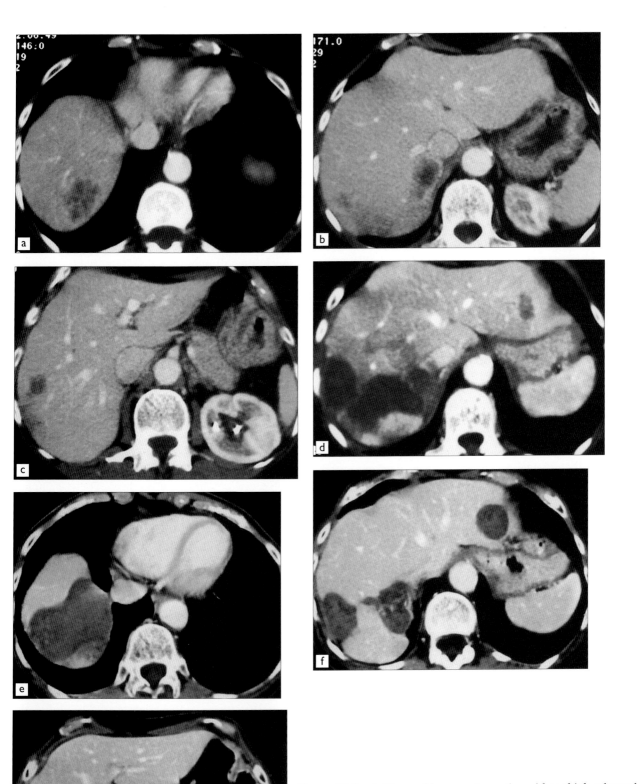

Figure 50.2. *A 61-year-old woman presenting with multiple colorectal liver metastases. (a–c) Initial CT scans performed in 1999 show four metastases, including one lesion adjacent to the cava. These were treated with RF ablation. (d) On follow-up in 2000, a fifth metastasis developed in the left lobe. There is also some recurrence adjacent to the cava. Further RF ablation was performed and followed by systemic chemotherapy. (e–g) CT scans performed in October 2002 showing areas of ablation without evidence of tumour recurrence. This patient is tumour-free 3 years after presentation with inoperable liver metastases.*

inoperable patients compares reasonably well with 3-year survival of 42–44% for patients undergoing resection for operable disease.[53,54] Other thermal ablation groups have reported similar survival results.[38,55]

Patient selection

Our current recommendation is to accept patients with five metastases or less, each with a maximum diameter not exceeding 5 cm, but we are also studying RF ablation in patients with as many as nine tumours with a maximum diameter of no more than 4.5 cm.

Where the distribution of disease is not amenable to surgery, the use of a combination of RF and resection can be considered. For those with concurrent disability, RF ablation is a much less invasive alternative than surgery and has lower complication rates. Other applications for RF ablation include patients with limited liver disease who have insufficient residual liver to allow resection, usually posthemihepatectomy patients with new metastases in the residual lobe.

Radio-frequency ablation, like surgery, is most effective in small tumours. The ideal RF candidate is often the ideal surgical candidate. Retrospective comparisons of RF and repeat hepatic resection show similar survival benefits.[56] At our institution, a retrospective comparison of RF and surgery in solitary metastases showed a similar survival rate. However, until we have prospective trials comparing the two treatments, surgery will remain the first-line treatment for those who are suitable. Radio-frequency can be performed either concurrently or sequentially to chemotherapy, and can be repeated if new lesions or recurrence occurs. If the patient develops more extensive disease, such that RF can no longer be performed, then chemotherapy should be considered.

From the preceding discussion it becomes clear that patients with colorectal liver metastases may undergo resection, RF ablation and chemotherapy at different times during the course of their disease. Ideally, these patients should be able to move smoothly between the specialties and receive the treatment appropriate to their disease status. This is often best achieved by regular multidisciplinary meetings and management by consensus. Randomized, controlled trials are now in process. The European CLOCC trial aims to compare the effect of ablation in conjunction with systemic chemotherapy with systemic chemotherapy alone in patients with inoperable colorectal metastases.

Key points: colorectal liver metastases

- Surgical resection remains the first-line treatment for patients with resectable disease

- In disease not amenable to surgery, or in patients who have undergone surgery, RF ablation is used to good effect

- 3-year survival following RF ablation in inoperable patients compares well with survival following resection

Neuroendocrine

The treatment options for these patients are limited. Few patients are eligible for surgery and the alternatives produce symptomatic improvement but have less impact on tumour load.[57] Aggressive cytoreduction followed by octreotide analogues can be the best way to achieve prolonged symptom control.[58] Radio-frequency can be used to reduce hormone secretion and/or to reduce tumour load. Siperstein et al. successfully treated 15 patients with laparoscopic RF ablation.[59] Our experience in 17 patients showed benefit in 11, local control of tumour volume in seven and relief or reduction in hormone-related symptoms in four of six with secreting tumours.[60] Theoretically, a reduction in tumour load could eventually translate into a survival benefit but much longer follow-up will be required to establish any improvement in survival.

Non-colorectal, non-neuroendocrine including breast

Isolated liver metastases are an uncommon occurrence in breast cancer. Some surgeons will perform hepatic resection for limited liver metastases. A 22% 5-year survival postresection has been reported.[61] Radio-frequency has been performed to good effect; Livraghi reported on 24 patients of whom 10 were free of disease at a mean follow-up of 10 months.[62] Our experience in 11 patients suggests that breast metastases are easier to destroy than colorectal metastases with thermal techniques. Recurrence following ablation is unusual and those who do succumb often die of disseminated disease outside of the liver. There is limited experience of RF in other non-colorectal, non-neuroendocrine metastases, but good surgical results have been reported when there has been an interval of more than 2 years between the primary and the development of detectable metastatic disease.[63] Therefore, RF could be considered in these patients if they are not candidates for surgery.

Hepatocellular carcinoma

Unlike liver metastases, local ablative therapy is well established in HCC. Historically, ablation was performed using pure ethanol. Trials of PEI and liver resection suggest a comparable survival. In one trial, Childs Pugh Class A patients had a 3-year survival of 71% following PEI compared to 79% following surgery, and Childs Pugh Class B patients had a 3-year survival of 41% and 40%, respectively.[64] Radio-frequency has been compared to PEI in a randomized trial setting and shown to have a higher complete ablation rate in fewer treatment sessions but also a higher complication rate.[65] Microwave therapy has been used but again comparative studies suggest that RF is more efficacious.[66] Encapsulated HCC is generally easier to destroy than metastases as the heat is contained and amplified within the lesion, a phenomenon known as the 'oven effect'. Several centres use laser effectively in the treatment of HCC and, to date, there has been no comparison of laser and RF in HCC.[67] Current recommendations for RF in HCC are Childs Pugh Class A or B cirrhosis and no more than three lesions, no larger than 4.5 cm (Fig. 50.3).[68] Screening programmes for the detection of early HCC in patients with hepatitis C or B are not widespread and, therefore, many patients present with large tumours. Although the survival advantage of transarterial chemoembolization (TACE) alone remains controversial, the combination of selective TACE and thermal ablation has been explored with some success in this cohort.[69,70] Different techniques have been used, e.g. laser followed weeks later by TACE, or balloon occlusion of the hepatic artery during RF followed by selective catheterization of the tumour-feeding vessels and chemoembolization immediately afterwards. It is not yet known what the optimal sequence and timing of the two therapies will be.

Key point: hepatocellular carcinoma ablation

■ Current recommendations for RF ablation in HCC are Childs Pugh Class A or B cirrhosis and no more than three lesions no larger than 4.5 cm

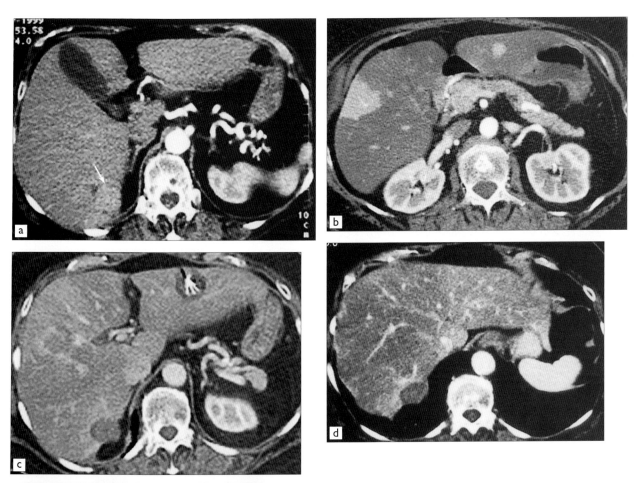

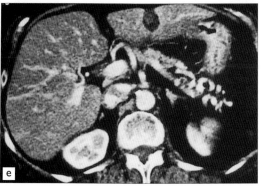

Figure 50.3. *HCC treated with RF. A 78-year-old woman with a previous colorectal primary. (a) Initial scans performed in November 1999 showing a solitary hypervascular tumour in the postero-medial aspect of the right lobe (arrow). The AFP was normal and therefore this lesion was biopsied. Histology showed HCC. This was treated with RF. (b) During follow-up a new hypervascular lesion develops in the left lobe. There is also a wedge-shaped perfusion anomaly in the right lobe. (c) CT scan performed immediately after RF ablation showing an expandable electrode with surrounding low attenuation necrosis. (d, e) CT scans performed in October 2002 showing complete ablation with no active tumour. This patient is tumour-free 3 years after her original ablation.*

Complications

The complication rate following ablation varies from 2 to 10% and the mortality is less than 0.8%.[71,72] Needle puncture or thermal injury can result in:

- Subcapsular haematoma
- Occlusion or thrombosis of hepatic veins or portal vein branches
- Bile duct strictures
- Injury to adjacent viscera such as stomach, duodenum, gall bladder, colon (manifested as perforation or fistula formation) or the lung or pleura (pneumothorax or pleural effusions)

Complication rates will increase with increasing numbers of punctures, larger volumes of necrosis, more advanced Child Pugh class and treatment of lesions close to the diaphragm, into the liver hilum, close to vessels or viscera. The worst morbidity is associated with infection of necrotic-ablated metastases, and the major aetiological factor for this is the presence of a biliary endoprosthesis or a previous bilio-enteric anastomosis.

Approach – percutaneous, laparoscopic or open?

Radio-frequency ablation can be performed using image guidance and a percutaneous approach,[73–76] laparoscopic guidance,[59,77,78] or at open laparotomy.[79–81] At open laparotomy, RF ablation can be combined with liver resection, i.e. resection of one area of the liver and ablation of another. If a patient is undergoing laparotomy for some other surgical procedure then it is reasonable to perform RF at the same time. With this exception it is difficult to justify the added morbidity, invasiveness and expense of a laparotomy compared to a percutaneous procedure. The laparoscopic approach has been used when tumour is adherent to structures that would be damaged by thermal ablation, e.g. tumour adherent to stomach, colon or duodenum. Some centres prefer the laparoscopic approach where there is poor tumour visualization transcutaneously and also for large HCCs requiring multiple punctures.[82,83] Radio-frequency ablation will most commonly be performed in the radiology department, but there is a subgroup of patients who will benefit from open or laparoscopic RF.

Thermal ablation and blood flow manipulation

Normal liver responds to thermal injury with an increase in perfusion. Using CT we have quantified this effect in a group of 32 patients.[84] There was a mean 3.3-fold increase in hepatic arterial flow adjacent to the ablated area. Tissue perfusion has a direct impact on the volume of necrosis that can be produced. This has been confirmed using pharmacological manipulation where, for example, a halothane-induced reduction in blood flow of 46% resulted in a 50% increase in the diameter of the ablation.[85] Several groups have explored vascular occlusion as a method for increasing the volume of necrosis.[86,87] Vascular occlusion, either portal venous, hepatic arterial or both, have been shown to be beneficial in animal models with increases in measured temperature at the treatment site and increases in the size of ablation.[88,89] Surgeons have the option of clamping the vascular pedicle during RF ablation, and percutaneous balloon occlusion is also effective. Although vascular occlusion increases the volume of ablation, it also removes the protective effect of blood flow and, as a result, there is an associated increase in bile duct injury. An alternative approach, favoured by our group, is the use of hypotensive general anaesthesia, similar to that used at hepatic resection, i.e. maintenance of a systolic pressure of approximately 80 mmHg.

Key points: ablation techniques

- Ablation techniques have been successfully applied to both primary and secondary tumours

- The number and size of tumours that can be ablated varies with the technique and primary pathology

- Percutaneous techniques have a lower morbidity and complication rate than intraoperative techniques

- Retrospective analysis suggests that ablation improves patient survival in both colorectal liver metastases and HCC

- Ablation can be used in conjunction with other therapies to good effect

- Randomized controlled trials of chemotherapy and ablation versus chemotherapy alone and resection versus ablation are underway

Pancreas

Endoscopic ultrasound-guided RF has been performed in pigs[90,91] but, in general, thermal methods of tumour destruction have not been widely researched in pancreatic cancer. We performed animal experiments and a Phase I clinical project in the early 1990s. Although our early experiments in dog pancreas over 10 years ago resulted in a high incidence of pancreatitis, this was not seen in eight human subjects. We have recently completed a Phase I study of PDT in patients with small-volume pancreatic ductal adenocarcinoma.

Our rationale for this treatment was that the median survival for a patient with pancreatic adenocarcinoma is 5 months, and for those with operable disease the median is 18–20 months. However, most patients present with inoperable disease. The most common cause for inoperability is vascular invasion, which occurs early on in the disease despite a relatively small tumour load. Alternatives to surgery include chemotherapy and/or radiotherapy. Currently, Gemcitabine is the best chemotherapeutic option, offering symptomatic relief and a small increment in survival. External beam radiotherapy in combination with chemotherapy also produces a modest improvement in survival. Given the lack of good alternative therapies, we evaluated PDT in a pilot study.[92–94]

We studied the use of interstitial PDT in the treatment of 16 patients with localized but inoperable pancreatic adenocarcinoma.[28] Biliary stents were always positioned prior to PDT. Three to five days after administration of IV mTHPC, up to eight percutaneous hollow needles were positioned within the tumour (Fig. 50.4). Then, 20 J of red light were delivered at each treatment station. Treatment was performed at multiple stations to produce confluent necrosis. Median total light energy delivered was 240 J (range 40–480 J).

The median volume of necrosis as measured on contrast-enhanced CT was 36 cc (range 9–60 cc). Endoscopic evaluation of the duodenum showed haemorrhagic necrosis, which healed rapidly over 4–6 weeks. The median survival was 12.5 months (range 6–34 months). There were six complications: haemorrhage in two patients, needle track seeding in one and the subsequent development of fibrous duodenal strictures in three. The results of this pilot study suggest that necrosis can be produced in pancreatic cancer; further studies are being planned to see if this will influence the course of the disease.

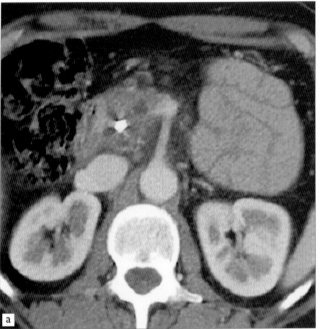

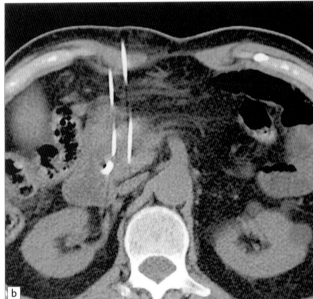

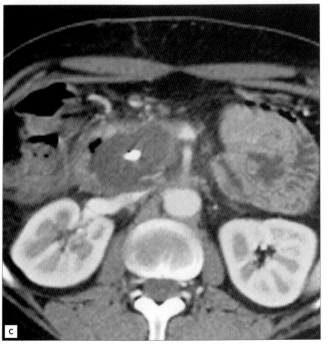

Figure 50.4. *Pancreatic PDT. (a) CT scan showing an irregular, low attenuation mass lesion in the head of the pancreas with a bile duct stent in situ. Biopsies showed adenocarcinoma. (b) Axial CT scan performed during treatment showing multiple needles positioned through the anterior abdominal wall into the pancreatic tumour. (c) Axial contrast enhanced CT scan performed 3 days after PDT. There is a large confluent area of absent enhancement consistent with necrosis in the head of the pancreas.*

Head and neck

The thyroid and parathyroid

Ultrasound-guided ethanol injection and laser[95] have been used to ablate thyroid tissue. Ethanol injection is also used in parathyroid adenomas and, more recently, to ablate lymph node metastases from papillary thyroid carcinoma. These are frequently numerous, very small and would require extensive block dissection of the neck. Conventional surgical techniques often fail to find some of the smaller lesions. Ultrasound visualization of papillary metastases is exquisite with state-of-the-art equipment and it is simple to inject very small quantities of ethanol through a 25 G needle into tumours as small as 5 mm in diameter. The major effect of injected ethanol is to sclerose the vascular endothelium, and perfusion through a tumour disappears immediately. Any residual blood flow detected by colour Doppler indicates viable tumour that can be re-treated.[96]

Adenocarcinoma metastases to the neck are more difficult to deal with. They are typically infiltrative, extremely hard and relatively avascular. Ethanol directly injected into these tumours will freely spill into the surrounding tissues. Thermal methods need to be used with great caution.[97] Myelin presents a major problem. It melts at a slightly lower temperature than fat and is, therefore, very easily damaged. Once melted, the damage is irreversible and neurological deficit ensues.

This explains why we have been exploring new methods of tissue destruction such as PDT for areas where nerve damage can be critical.

Palliation with photodynamic therapy in head and neck cancer

Therapeutic options for recurrent head and neck cancer are limited. Surface illumination for mucosal PDT has been applied to dysplasia and localized carcinoma in the oropharynx, as well as for recurrent head and neck cancer when other therapeutic options have been exhausted. One group treated 51 patients with a range of different head and neck primaries and reported both symptomatic benefit and improvements in tumour control.[98] In our unit, patients are treated using ultrasound or MR guidance, and with a similar technique to that used in the prostate and pancreas. Particular care is required to avoid damage to major vessels.[99] Follow-up imaging has revealed confluent areas of necrosis at the treatment site. Again, we found PDT was useful both to relieve symptoms and reduce disease extent. Photodynamic therapy does not normally affect nerves.

The breast

The aim of surgery to the breast in breast cancer is to obtain local control of a systemic disease. Extent or type of surgery performed does not affect the ultimate outcome. This is determined by the systemic spread of the disease.

However, the extent of local surgery is determined by the spread of tumour within the breast. Most screen-detected cancers are small and show little evidence of spread. A major goal in the management of breast cancer is to reduce the psychological and physical trauma of biopsy and surgery, and in particular, to compress the duration of the process from suspicion, screening and diagnosis to therapy as much as possible.

With combinations of digital stereotactic mammography, ultrasound, vacuum large-core biopsy and ablative technology, it is, in theory, possible to detect, diagnose and treat in rapid succession. The main limitation to developing this at the present time is in the delays necessary to obtain definitive histology. This will change over the next few years as reliable 'instantaneous' markers for malignant tissue will reach clinical application.

We have performed over 100 ablations of malignant breast cancer using a thermal laser technique immediately prior to conventional surgical resection. Although this has been a Phase I study with no attempt to destroy the whole cancer, we have achieved complete tumour destruction in nearly 40% of cases.[100] A thermal model for the treatment of breast cancer was recently constructed.[101] Radio-frequency, laser and cryotherapy techniques have also been recently applied to the breast.[102–105] Photodynamic therapy has been used for the treatment of superficial, locally recurrent breast cancer.[106–108]

Over the past few years, we have been trying a new method. Radiosurgery is a method developed by the Photoelectron Corporation in Boston. They have manufactured a battery-powered electron gun, which fires low kilovoltage electrons down an evacuated needle to a tungsten target to generate soft X-rays. The delivery system is only 3 mm in diameter and is small enough to be combined with stereotactic mammography, ultrasound or MR.

The advantages of radiosurgery are:

- Energy deposition is precisely known and its distribution within tissue can be calculated using radiotherapy planning methods
- Biological effects of ionizing radiation are well understood
- Effects of X-irradiation are reproducible and have some selectivity between tissue types

Radiotherapy in the breast is used for two reasons: first, to sterilize the margins of a resected tumour to avoid a local recurrence; second, to suppress multifocal disease elsewhere in the breast. Radiosurgery cannot only destroy residual tumour tissue in situ but can also act as a local boost to external beam radiotherapy. The radiosurgery needle is sufficiently small to be guided into position by ultrasound. There is no immediate treatment effect that can be recognized by imaging techniques.

Key points: breast cancer ablative therapy

- RF, laser and cryotherapy techniques have all been applied in the treatment of breast cancer

- PDT has been used for the treatment of superficial, locally recurrent, breast cancer

The prostate

The introduction of PSA screening has resulted in the earlier detection of small tumours, yet the best treatment for localized prostate cancer remains controversial. Reported long-term cure rates are 19–46% for radiotherapy and 40–75% for radical prostatectomy. These results are achieved at the expense of significant complications. Urinary incontinence and impotence occur in <40% and <60% of patients following radical prostatectomy, and <7% and <66%, respectively, after radiotherapy.[109–111]

Prostate cancer is an example of field change and is frequently multifocal at presentation. Successful ablation will often require treatment of the whole gland. Enthusiasm for cryotherapy has varied over time and reports of high complications have led many centres to abandon this technique.[112] Yet other centres have reported 5-year results that are competitive to established treatments while emphasizing the need for substantial training and meticulous technique.[113]

The 20-year old technique of radioactive seed implantation is now very popular in the USA. This has been revived through persistent development of better ultrasound control, three-dimensional planning of the irradiation and new isotopes. Despite this, both brachytherapy and external beam radiotherapy have a significant local failure rate (10–15% within 18 months for DXR) and there is a great need for a method to treat these recurrences. Salvage radical prostatectomy carries a much higher complication rate than de novo radical prostatectomy.

Thermal ablation

We have treated 14 patients who had relapsed after external beam radiotherapy with laser delivered under ultrasound guidance via the transperineal route. Significant reductions in PSA were seen in 60%. No major complications occurred, although expected worsening in impotence and incontinence was seen in some patients.[114] The prostate is very sensitive to heat and all procedures had to be performed under general anaesthetic. As with the pancreas, a painless method to achieve the same tissue destruction led to both animal and clinical trials with PDT.

Prostate PDT

We have studied the feasibility of using PDT in the treatment of recurrent prostate cancer following radiotherapy in 11 patients who have declined salvage prostatectomy.

Image-guidance options were a combination of transrectal ultrasound and fluoroscopy or MR (Fig. 50.5). A transperineal approach was used and multiple needles positioned. The initial light dose of 20 J per treatment station proved ineffective, with no fall in PSA and only small areas of necrosis visible on imaging. The dose was subsequently increased to 50–75 J. With the higher dose, a reduction in PSA levels was seen in seven of 11 patients, although only one had persistently lowered values after treatment. Biopsies performed after treatment showed complete absence of tumour in four patients. Two patients developed incontinence and two of four who were potent prior to the procedure became impotent. Sigmoidoscopy to assess rectal damage revealed minor mucosal erythema in two patients only.[115] Photodynamic therapy is capable of producing a large volume of necrosis within the prostate. We are now planning a second Phase I trial where our aim will be to ablate the entire gland.

Lung tumours

Early reports of CT-guided thermal ablation suggest that small <3.5 cm tumours can be treated with a low complication rate. Both inoperable primary and limited numbers (usually fewer than three per lung) of metastatic tumours have been treated. Computed tomography fluoroscopy, whilst not essential, can facilitate electrode placement as small, scirrhous lung lesions can be difficult to penetrate with a large calibre needle.[116–120] With larger lesions, as in the liver, RF is preferable to laser. There are relatively few complications, even in the treatment of patients with emphysema. Given the dwell time for treatment (20–30 minutes) and the calibre of RF electrodes (14–17 G), the pneumothorax rate is not that high, of the order of 40%, with 14% requiring temporary intercostal drainage. Other potential complications include infection, haemorrhage and bronchopleural fistulae.

Computed tomography scans performed during treatment often demonstrate oedema with or without pulmonary contusion. Post-treatment CT scans will commonly show pleural effusions, reaction or thickening (Fig. 50.6). There is often some associated consolidation and cavitation of the lesion. Importantly, cavitation does not necessarily denote infection. Over time, successfully treated lesions shrink in size to a scar. Future studies are likely to explore combination therapies of ablation and radiotherapy, and/or chemotherapy.

Photodynamic therapy has been extensively explored in lung malignancy both via the endoscopic and percutaneous route.[121–124]

Tumours of the kidney

Nephron-sparing surgery presents a challenge to the surgeon. Many small renal tumours are indeterminate or histology and may be of no clinical significance. Multiple renal tumours are not rare and can be difficult to resect without complication.

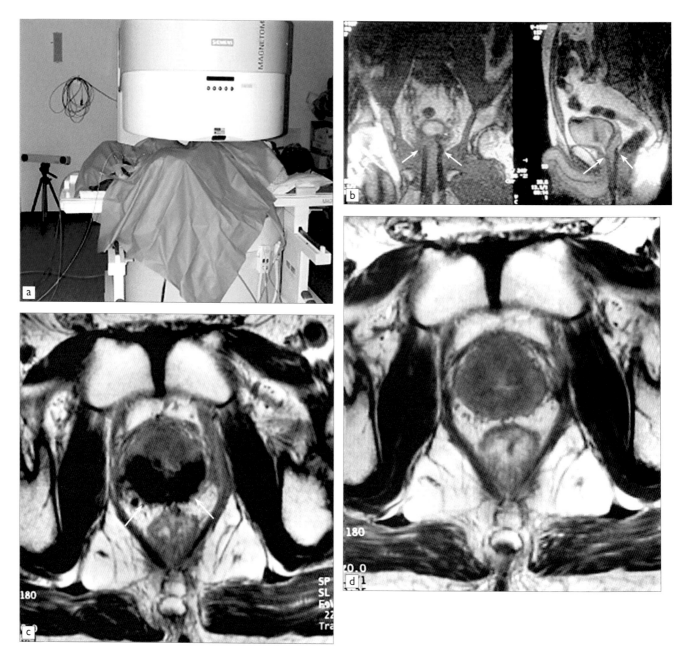

Figure 50.5. *Prostate photodynamic therapy. (a) Patient set-up during MR-guided transperineal photodynamic therapy in an open (0.2T) MR. (b) Intraprocedural coronal and sagittal images showing the needle positions (arrows). (c) Post-procedural contrast-enhanced T1-weighted axial image performed at 1.5 T showing absent enhancement in the peripheral zone posteriorly (arrows). Compare to (d), the pretreatment contrast-enhanced axial T1-weighted image.*

Renal tumours up to 3 cm in diameter can be destroyed in situ by laser or RF techniques with virtually no damage to the surrounding normal renal tissue. Following a number of promising early reports,[125–129] a few small series have been published.[130,131] One series of 21 patients, most of whom had von Hippel–Lindau disease, showed complete absence of tumour enhancement on contrast-enhanced CT in 79% with only four minor complications.[131]

Abdominal and pelvic nodes or local recurrence

Where nodal recurrence has occurred despite maximal radiotherapy treatment, local ablative techniques can be effective.[132] The main problem is the potential for collateral damage to either adjacent bowel loops or neural injury. For most thermal techniques, a distance of 1 cm is required from the area to be ablated and any important local structure. Some centres advocate the positioning of a thermo-

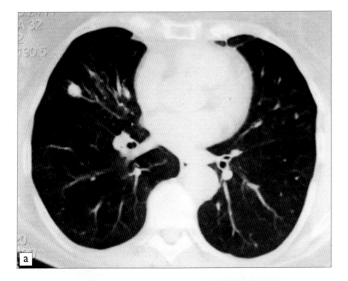

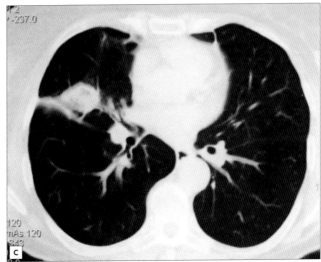

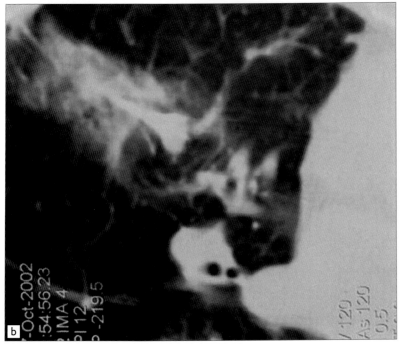

Figure 50.6. *Lung ablation. (a) Pretreatment CT scan of a small metastasis in the right middle lobe in a patient with treated colorectal liver metastases, chronic bronchitis and emphysema. (b) Magnified view of the right middle lobe. CT scan during treatment showing the expandable electrode around the metastasis. There is some associated pulmonary contusion which was not clinically significant. (c) Follow-up CT scan at 1 month showing a large area of ablation with some associated pleural thickening.*

couple at the interface with the structure to be protected so that treatment can be discontinued if temperatures rise unacceptably.

Gynaecological malignancy

In the majority of cases, the first-line approach to pelvic tumours is surgical. Radiotherapy is usually the next therapeutic option. Many patients with recurrent pelvic tumours will experience multiple surgical procedures and will have reached their maximum tolerance of radiotherapy. Effective therapeutic options do not remain. Both RF and laser techniques can be very effective in this circumstance. Collateral damage is the main problem; the tumour destruction is relatively easy.[133]

Bone tumours

Primary bone tumours will be treated by chemotherapy, radiotherapy and surgery. However, if aggressive therapy is delivered at an early stage, recurrence can be very difficult to treat. Treatment by RF ablation may be curative, but is more likely to form part of a palliative treatment regimen. Either CT or MR are the usual guidance methods (Fig. 50.7).

Radio-frequency ablation has been advocated in the symptomatic palliation of bone metastases following radiotherapy.[134] Initial results suggest that ablation can produce significant reductions in pain levels and analgesic requirements. Only limited numbers of metastases can be treated. It is important to select patients with a clearly defined and

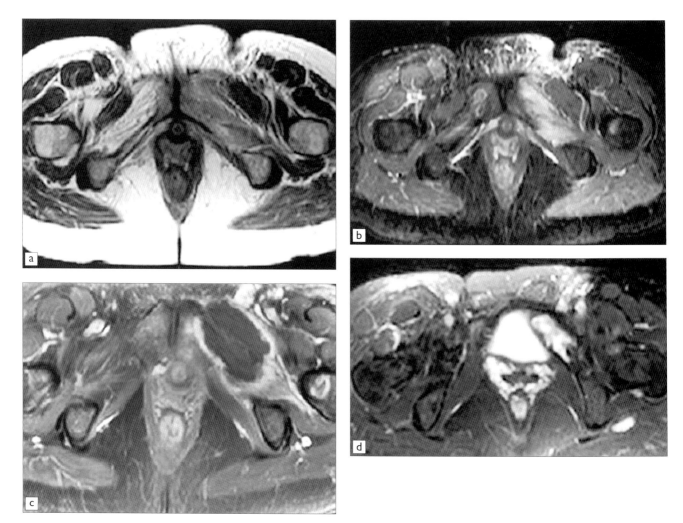

Figure 50.7. *Bone tumour ablation. Recurrent biopsy-proven chondrosarcoma in a patient who had already undergone multiple surgical procedures and radiotherapy such that further radiotherapy or surgery were not feasible. This was treated with ultrasound and MR-guided RF ablation. (a) Gadolinium-enhanced axial T1-weighted image showing a mildly enhancing mass next to the left inferior pubic ramus. (b) Axial inversion recovery sequence showing the tumour as indistinct high signal intensity. (c) Immediate postablation: gadolinium-enhanced fat-suppressed, T1-weighted image showing an area of absent enhancement that embraces the original tumour. There is a surrounding inflammatory reaction seen as enhancement at the periphery. (d) Axial inversion recovery image at follow-up showing the area of necrosis has reduced in size and become well defined. This patient has had no further recurrence in 3 years.*

understood dominant site of bone pain. The exact mechanism of action is not understood. The aetiology of bone pain in metastases is complex, with a variety of tumoural effects (release of chemical mediators, bone destruction, pressure effects, fractures, stretching of the periosteum) contributing to pain. It is thought to be more important to ablate the tumour–bone interface than to debulk the tumour.

Combination therapy and chemoprevention

The great promise of ablation, namely its focality and minimal invasiveness, is also its limitation. Local ablative techniques need to be used carefully, preferably within the context of multidisciplinary meeting and consensus. It is important to recognize the need for more extensive treatment in those cancers that arise within field change (e.g. the prostate), and also to combine ablation with systemic therapies for those cancers that are part of a systemic process. There is also a role for chemoprevention in conjunction with local ablation, for example, in HCC. Immunopreventions such as interferon (IFN) and glycyrrhizin have been used to suppress the development of HCC. Interferon prevents HCC in two groups, in those with long-term elimination of the hepatitis C virus (15–35% of patients) and in those with a sustained normalization of serum transaminases (an additional 10%). Interferon has been shown to reduce recurrence after surgery.[135] Glycyrrhizin, on the other hand, has no antiviral activity but acts by reducing liver inflammation as indicated by suppressed transaminases.[136]

The chemopreventative agent polyprenoic acid, an acyclic retinoid, induces the disappearance of serum lectin-reactive alpha-fetoprotein (AFP), suggesting a clonal deletion of minute premalignant cells. It has been shown to reduce the incidence of recurrent or new HCC post curative resection to 27% versus 49% at 38 months. Finally, another technique that had more modest success in reducing the incidence of recurrence postresection, was a single dose of intra-arterial ^{131}I lipiodol. This resulted in a recurrence rate of 28.5% versus 59% at a median follow-up of 34.6 months.[137] In future, a combination of immuno- and chemo-preventions will be explored.

Summary

- There are multiple different technologies available for tumour ablation and the technology continues to improve

- The preferred technique and guidance will vary with the area treated

- The current preferred technique for liver tumours is RF ablation

- There are multiple applications for ablation ranging from symptomatic palliation in bone metastases to complete ablation of liver tumours

- Initial experience has been gained in inoperable tumours but retrospective evidence suggests ablation may supplant resection for small liver tumours

- Prospective randomized controlled trials are in process and the results are expected to be good

- Ablation will form one part of the oncologic therapeutic armamentarium. Local therapy is usually combined with systemic therapy. The role of ablation within oncologic therapy needs to be established. This will be an area of active study in the next few years

References

1. Dodd G, Soulen M, Kane R et al. Minimally invasive treatment of malignant hepatic tumors: at the threshold of a major breakthrough. Radiographics 2000; 20: 9–27

2. d'Arsonval M A. Action physiologique des courants alternatifs. CR Soc Biol 1891; 43: 283–293

3. Curley S, Davidson B, Fleming R et al. Laparoscopically guided bipolar radiofrequency ablation of areas of porcine liver. Surg Endosc 1997; 11: 729–733

4. Lorentzen T. A cooled-needle electrode for radiofrequency tissue ablation: thermodynamic aspects of improved performance compared with conventional needle design. Acad Radiol 1996; 3: 556–563

5. Goldberg S N, Gazelle G S, Dawson S L et al. Tissue ablation with radiofrequency using multiprobe arrays. Acad Radiol 1995; 2: 670–674

6. Miao Y, Ni Y, Yu J, Marchal G. A comparative study on validation of a novel cooled-wet electrode for radiofrequency liver ablation. Invest Radiol 2000; 35: 438–444

7. Miao Y, Ni Y, Mulier S et al. Ex vivo experiment on radiofrequency liver ablation with saline infusion through a screw-tip cannulated electrode. J Surg Res 1997; 71: 19–24

8. Livraghi T, Goldberg N, Monti F et al. Saline-enhanced radio-frequency tissue ablation in the treatment of liver metastases. Radiology 1997; 202: 205–210

9. Goldberg S N, Ahmed M, Gazelle G S et al. Radio-frequency thermal ablation with NaCl solution injection: effect of electrical conductivity on tissue heating and coagulation – phantom and porcine liver study. Radiology 2001; 219: 157–165

10. McGahan J P, Dodd G D. Radiofrequency ablation of the liver. Current status. Am J Roentgenol 2001; 176: 3–16

11. de Baere T, Denys A, Johns Wood B et al. Radiofrequency liver ablation: experimental comparative study of water-cooled versus expandable systems. Am J Roentgenol 2001; 176: 187–192

12. ter Haar G. High intensity ultrasound. Semin Laparosc Surg 2001; 8: 77–89

13. Wu F, Chen W, Bai J et al. Pathological changes in human malignant carcinoma treated with high-intensity focused ultrasound. Ultrasound Med Biol 2001; 27: 1099–1106

14. Livraghi T. Percutaneous ethanol injection in the treatment of hepatocellular carcinoma in cirrhosis. Hepatogastroenterology 2001; 48: 20–24

15. Moore J V, West C M L, Whitehurst C. The biology of photodynamic therapy. Phys Med Biol 1997; 42: 913–935

16. Dougherty T J. Photodynamic therapy (PDT) of malignant tumors. Crit Rev Oncol Hematol 1984; 2: 83–116

17. Keller S M. Photodynamic therapy. Biology and clinical application. Chest Surg Clin N Am 1995; 5: 121–137

18. Li J H, Guo Z H, Jin M L et al. Photodynamic therapy in the treatment of malignant tumours: an analysis of 540 cases. J Photochem Photobiol B 1990; 6: 149–155

19. McCaughan J S Jr. Photodynamic therapy: a review. Drugs Aging 1999; 15: 49–68

20. Koren H, Alth G, Schenk G M, Jindra R H. Photodynamic therapy: an alternative pathway in the treatment of recurrent breast cancer. Int J Radiat Oncol Biol Phys 1994; 28: 463–466

21. Patelli M, Lazzari Agli L, Poletti V, Falcone F. Photodynamic laser therapy for the treatment of early-stage bronchogenic carcinoma. Monaldi Arch Chest Dis 1999; 4: 315–318

22. Furuse K, Fukuoka M, Kato H et al. A prospective phase II study on photodynamic therapy with photofrin II for centrally located early-stage lung cancer. The Japan Lung Cancer Photodynamic Therapy Study Group. J Clin Oncol 1993; 11: 1852–1857

23. Karanov S, Kostadinov D, Shopova M, Kurtev P. Photodynamic therapy in lung and gastrointestinal cancers. J Photochem Photobiol B 1990; 6: 175–181

24. Chang S C, Bown S G. Photodynamic therapy: applications in bladder cancer and other malignancies. J Formos Med Assoc 1997; 96: 853–863

25. Puolakkainen P, Schroder T. Photodynamic therapy of gastrointestinal tumors: a review. Dig Dis 1992; 10: 53–60

26. Fielding D I, Buonaccorsi G A, MacRobert A J et al. Fine-needle interstitial photodynamic therapy of the lung parenchyma: photosensitizer distribution and morphologic effects of treatment. Chest 1999; 115: 502–510

27. Hornung R, Jentsch B, Crompton N E et al. In vitro effects and localisation of the photosensitizers m-THPC and m-THPC MD on carcinoma cells of the human breast (MCF-7) and Chinese hamster fibroblasts (V-79). Lasers Surg Med 1997; 20: 443–450

28. Vogl T, Muller P, Hammerstingl R et al. Malignant liver tumors treated with MR imaging-guided laser-induced thermotherapy: technique and prospective results. Radiology 1995; 196: 257–265

29. Lees W R, Gillams A. Comparison of the effectiveness of cooled tip radiofrequency and interstitial laser photocoagulation in liver tumour ablation. Radiology 1999; 213P: 123

30. Chapman W C, Debelak J P, Wright Pinson C et al. Hepatic cryoblation, but not radiofrequency ablation, results in lung inflammation. Ann Surg 2000; 231: 752–761

31. Bilchik A J, Wood T F, Allegra D et al. Cryosurgical ablation and radiofrequency ablation for unresectable hepatic malignant neoplasms. Arch Surg 2000; 135: 657–664

32. Pearson A S, Izzo F, Fleming R Y et al. Intraoperative radiofrequency ablation or cryoablation for hepatic malignancies: a proposed algorithm. Am J Surg 1999; 178: 592–599

33. Adam R, Hagopian E, Linhares M et al. A comparison of percutaneous cryosurgery and percutaneous radiofrequency for unresectable hepatic malignancies. Arch Surg. 2002; 137: 1332–1339

34. Scudamore C H, Lee S I, Patterson E J et al. Radiofrequency ablation followed by resection of malignant liver tumors. Am J Surg 1999; 177: 411–417

35. Goldberg S N, Gazelle G S, Compton C C et al. Treatment of intrahepatic malignancy with radiofrequency ablation: radiologic–pathologic correlation. Cancer 2000; 88: 2452–2463

36. Cioni D, Lencioni R, Rossi S et al. Radiofrequency thermal ablation of hepatocellular carcinoma: using contrast-enhanced harmonic power Doppler sonography to assess treatment outcome. Am J Roentgenol 2001; 177: 783–788

37. Solbiati L, Livraghi T, Goldberg S N et al. Percutaneous radio-frequency ablation of hepatic metastases from colorectal cancer: long-term results in 117 patients. Radiology 2001; 221: 159–166

38. Izumi N, Asahina Y, Noguchi O et al. Risk factors for distant recurrence of hepatocellular carcinoma in the liver after complete coagulation by microwave or radiofrequency. Cancer 2001; 91: 949–956

39. Ikeda K, Saitoh S, Tsubota A et al. Risk factors for intrahepatic recurrence in human small hepatocellular carcinoma. Gastroenterology 1995; 108: 768–775

40. Adachi E, Maeda T, Matsumata T et al. Risk factors for intrahepatic recurrence in human small hepatocellular carcinoma. Gastroenterology 1995; 108: 768–775

41. Nagashima I, Hamada C, Naruse K et al. Surgical resection for small hepatocellular carcinoma. Surgery 1996; 199: 40–45

42. Belghiti J, Panis Y, Frges O et al. Intrahepatic recurrence after resection of hepatocellular carcinoma complicating cirrhosis. Ann Surg 1991; 214: 114–117

43. Fong Y, Cohen A M, Fortner J G et al. Liver resection for colorectal metastases. J Clin Oncol 1997; 15: 938–994

44. Steele G, Ravikumar T. Resection of hepatic metastases from colorectal cancer. Ann Surg 1989; 210: 127–138

45. Douillard J Y. V303 Study Group. Irintoecan and high-dose fluorouracil/leucovorin for metastatic colorectal cancer. Oncology 2000; 14: 51–55

46. Giacchetti S, Perpoint B, Zidani R et al. Phase III multicenter trial of oxaliplatin added to chronomodulated fluorouracil–leucovorin as first-line treatment of metastatic colorectal cancer. J Clin Oncol 2000; 18: 136–147

47. Bismuth H, Adam R, Levi F et al. Resection of nonresectable liver metastases from colorectal cancer after neoadjuvant chemotherapy. Ann Surg 1996; 224: 509–522

48. Shankar A, Leonard P, Renaut A J et al. Neoadjuvant therapy improves respectability rates for colorectal cancer. Ann R Coll Surg Engl 2001; 83: 85–88

49. Gillams A, Lees W R. Survival after percutaneous, image-guided thermal ablation of hepatic metastases from colorectal cancer. Dis Colon Rectum 2000; 43: 656–661

50. Gillams A, Lees W R. Image-guided ablation of colorectal liver metastases: time for a randomized

controlled trial versus hepatic resection. Radiology 1999; 213P: 212

51. Gillams A. Thermal ablation of liver metastases. Abdom Imag 2001; 26: 361–368

52. Jenkins L T, Millikan K W, Bines S D et al. Hepatic resection for metastatic colorectal cancer. Am Surg 1997; 63: 605–610

53. Nordlinger B, Guiguet M, Vaillant C et al. Surgical resection of colorectal carcinoma metastases to the liver. Cancer 1996; 77: 1254–1262

54. Vogl T, Muller P, Mack M et al. Liver metastases: interventional therapeutic techniques and results, state of the art. Eur Radiol 1999; 9: 675–684

55. Elias D, de Baere T, Smayra T et al. Percutaneous radiofrequency thermoablation as an alternative to surgery for treatment of liver tumour recurrence after hepatectomy. Br J Surg 2002; 89: 752–756

56. Clouse M E, Perry L, Stuart K, Tokes K R. Hepatic arterial chemoembolization for metastatic neuroendocrine tumours. Digestion 1994; 55: 92–97

57. Chung M H, Pisegna J, Spirt M et al. Hepatic cytoreduction followed by a novel long-acting somatostatin analogue: a paradigm for intractable neuroendocrine tumors metastatic to the liver. Surgery 2001; 130: 954–962

58. Siperstein A, Rogers S, Hansen P, Gitomirsky A. Laparoscopic thermal ablation of hepatic neuroendocrine tumor metastases. Surgery 1997; 122: 1147–1155

59. Gillams A R, Lees W R. Thermal ablation of neuroendocrine liver metastases Eur Radiol 2001; 11: 340.

60. Selzner M, Morse M, Vredenburgh J et al. Liver metastases from breast cancer: long-term survival after curative resection. Surgery 2000; 127: 383–389

61. Livraghi T, Goldberg N, Solbiati L et al. Percutaneous radio-frequency ablation of liver metastases from breast cancer: initial experience in 24 patients. Radiology 2001; 220: 145–149

62. Laurent C, Rullier E, Feyler A et al. Resection of non-colorectal and non-neuroendocrine liver metastases: late metastases are the only chance of cure. World J Surg 2001; 25: 1532–1536

63. Livraghi T, Bolondi L, Buscarini L et al. No treatment, resection and ethanol injection in hepatocellular carcinoma: a retrospective analysis of survival in 391 patients with cirrhosis. Italian Cooperative HCC Study Group. J Hepatol 1995; 22: 522–526

64. Livraghi T, Goldberg S N, Lazzaroni S et al. Small heptocellular carcinoma: treatment with radiofrequency ablation versus ethanol injection. Radiology 1999; 210: 655–661

65. Shibata T, Iimuro Y, Yamamoto Y et al. Small HCC: comparison of radio-frequency ablation and percutaneous microwave coagulation therapy. Radiology 2002; 223: 331–337

66. Pacella C M, Bizzarri G, Magnolfi F et al. Laser thermal ablation in the treatment of small HCC; results in 74 patients. Radiology 2001; 221: 712–720

67. Livraghi T, Goldberg S N, Lazzaroni S et al. Hepatocellular carcinoma: radio-frequency ablation of medium and large lesions. Radiology 2000: 214: 761–768

68. Pacella C M, Bizzarri G, Cecconi O et al. Hepatocellular carcinoma: long-term results of combined treatment with laser thermal ablation and transcatheter arterial chemoembolization. Radiology 2001: 219: 669–678

69. Lencioni R, Cioni D, Donati F, Bartolozzi C. Combination of interventional therapies in hepatocellular carcinoma. Hepatogastroenterology 2001; 48: 8–14

70. Mulier S, Mulier P, Ni Y et al. Complications of radiofrequency coagulation of liver tumours. Br J Surg 2002; 89: 1206–1222

71. Rhim H, Dodd G D. Radiofrequency thermal ablation of liver tumours. J Clin Ultrasound 1999; 27: 221–229

72. Solbiati L, Ierace T, Goldberg S et al. Percutaneous US-guided radio-frequency tissue ablation of liver metastases: treatment and follow-up in 16 patients. Radiology 1997; 202: 195–203

73. Solbiati L, Goldberg S N, Ierace T et al. Hepatic metastases: percutaneous radio-frequency ablation with cooled-tip electrodes. Radiology 1997; 205: 367–373

74. Rossi S, Stasi M, Carini E et al. Percutaneous RF interstitial thermal ablation in the treatment of hepatic cancer. Am J Roentgenol 1996 167: 759–768

75. Lencioni R, Goletti O, Armilotta N et al. Radio-frequency thermal ablation of liver metastases with cooled tip electrode needle: results of a pilot clinical trial. Eur Radiol 1998; 8: 1205–1211

76. Cuschieri A, Bracken J, Boni L. Initial experience with laparoscopic ultrasound-guided radiofrequency thermal ablation of hepatic tumours. Endoscopy 1999; 31: 318–321

77. Siperstein A, Garland A, Engle K et al. Local recurrence after laparoscopic radiofrequency thermal ablation of hepatic tumours. Ann Surg Oncol 2000; 7: 106–113

78. Curley S A, Izzo F, Delrio P et al. Radiofrequency ablation of unresectable primary and metastatic hepatic malignancies: results in 123 patients. Ann Surg 1999; 230: 1–8

79. Jiao L, Hansen P, Havlik R et al. Clinical short-term results of radiofrequency ablation in primary or secondary liver tumors. Am J Surg 1999; 177: 303–306

80. Wood T F, Rose D M, Chung M et al. Radiofrequency ablation of 231 unresectable hepatic tumors: indications, limitations and complications. Ann Surg Oncol 2000; 7: 593–600

81. Montorsi M, Santambrogio R, Bianchi P et al. Radiofrequency interstitial thermal ablation of hepatocellular carcinoma in liver cirrhosis. Role of the laparoscopic approach. Surg Endosc 2001; 15: 141–145

82. Podnos Y D, Henry G, Ortiz J A et al. Laparoscopic

ultrasound with radiofrequency ablation in cirrhotic patients with hepatocellular carcinoma: technique and technical considerations. Am Surg 2001; 67: 1181–1184

83. Gillams A R, Lees W R. Thermal ablation-induced changes in hepatic arterial perfusion. Radiology 1999; 213P: 382

84. Goldberg S, Hahn P, Halpern E et al. Radio-frequency tissue ablation: effect of pharmacological modulation of blood flow on coagulation diameter. Radiology 1998; 209: 761–767

85. Patterson E J, Scudamore C H, Owen D A et al. Radiofrequency ablation of porcine liver in vivo: effects of blood flow and treatment time on lesion size. Ann Surg 1998; 227: 559–565

86. Goldberg S N, Hahn P F, Tanabe K K et al. Percutaneous radiofrequency tissue ablation: does perfusion-mediated tissue cooling limit coagulation necrosis? J Vasc Interv Radiol 1998; 9: 101–111

87. de Baere T, Bessoud B, Dromain C et al. Percutaneous radiofrequency ablation of hepatic tumors during temporary venous occlusion. Am J Roentgenol 2002; 178: 53–59

88. Denys A, Portier F, Lamarre A, Wicky S. Hepatic vascular occlusions and radiofrequency liver ablation: from animal experiment to clinical observation? Am J Roentgenol 2001; 177: 1215–1216

89. Lees W R, Gillams A R, Schumillian C. Hypotensive anaesthesia improves the effectiveness of radiofrequency ablation in the liver. Radiology 2000; 217: 228

90. Goldberg S N, Mallery S, Gazelle G S, Brugge W. EUS-guided RF ablation in the pancreas: results in a porcine model. Gastrointest Endosc 1999; 50: 392–401

91. Livingston E H, Welton M L, Reber H A. Surgical treatment of pancreatic cancer. The United States Experience. Int J Pancreatol 1991; 9: 153–157

92. Warshaw A L, Fernandez-del Castillo C. Pancreatic carcinoma. N Engl J Med 1992; 326: 455–465

93. Burris H, Moore M J, Andersen J et al. Improvements in survival and clinical benefit with gemcitabine as first-line therapy for patients with advanced pancreas cancer: a randomised trial. J Clin Oncol 1997; 15: 2403–2413

94. Bown S, Rogowska A, Whitelaw D et al. Photodynamic therapy for cancer of the pancreas. Gut 2002; 50: 549–557.

95. Pacella C M, Bizzari G, Guiglemi R et al. Thyroid tissue: US-guided percutaneous interstitial laser ablation – a feasibility study. Radiology. 2000; 217: 673–677

96. Lagalla R, Caruso G, Finazzo M. Monitoring treatment response with color and power Doppler. Eur J Radiol 1998; 27(Suppl 2): S149–S156

97. Bockmuhl U, Knobber D, Vogl T, Mack M. Use of MR-controlled laser-induced thermotherapy in recurrent squamous epithelial carcinoma of the head-neck area. Laryngorhinootologie 1996; 75: 597–601

98. Vogl T, Mack MG, Muller P et al. Recurrent nasopharyngeal tumors: preliminary clinical results with interventional MR imaging-controlled laser-induced thermotherapy. Radiology 1995; 196: 725–733

99. Chang C J, Fisher D M, Chen Y R. Intralesional photocoagulation of vascular anomalies of the tongue. Br J Plast Surg 1999; 52: 178–181

100. Harries S, Amin Z, Smith M et al. Interstitial laser photocoagulation as a treatment for breast cancer. Br J Surg 1994; 81: 1617–1619

101. Robinson D S, Parel J M, Denham D B et al. Interstitial laser hyperthermia model development for minimally invasive therapy of breast carcinoma. J Am Coll Surg 1998; 186: 284–292

102. Jeffrey S S, Birdwell R L, Ikeda D M et al. Radiofrequency ablation of breast cancer: first report of an emerging technology. Arch Surg 1999; 134: 1064–1068

103. Bohm T, Hilger I, Muller W et al. Saline-enhanced radiofrequency ablation of breast tissue: an in vitro feasibility study. Invest Radiol 2000; 35: 149–157

104. Pfleiderer S, Freesmeyer M, Marx C et al. Cryotherapy of breast cancer under ultrasound guidance: initial results and limitations. Eur Radiol 2002; 12: 3009–3014

105. Dowlatshahi K, Francescatti D, Bloom K. Laser therapy for small breast cancers. Am J Surg 2002; 184: 359–363

106. Allison R, Mang T, Hewson G et al. Photodynamic therapy for chest wall progression from breast carcinoma is an underutilized treatment modality. Cancer 2001; 91: 1–8

107. Schuh M, Nseyo U O, Potter W R et al. Photodynamic therapy for palliation of locally recurrent breast carcinoma. J Clin Oncol 1987; 5: 1766–1770

108. Taber S W, Fingar V H, Wieman T J. Photodynamic therapy for palliation of chest wall recurrence in patients with breast cancer. J Surg Oncol 1998; 68: 209–214

109. Carlson K, Nitti V. Prevention and management of incontinence following radical prostatectomy. Urol Clin North Am 2001; 28: 595–612

110. McCullough A. Prevention and management of erectile dysfunction following radical prostatectomy. Urol Clin North Am 2001; 28: 613–627

111. D-Amico D, Coleman C. Role of interstitial radiotherapy in the management of clinically organ-confined prostate cancer: the jury is still out. J Clin Oncol 1996; 14: 304–315

112. Aus G, Pileblad E, Hugosson J. Cryosurgical ablation of the prostate: 5-year follow-up of a prospective study. Eur Urol 2002; 42: 133–138

113. Donnelly B, Saliken J, Ernst D et al. Prospective trial of cryosurgical ablation of the prostate: 5-year results. Urology 2002; 60: 645–649

114. Amin Z, Lees W R, Bown S G. Interstitial laser photocoagulation for the treatment of prostatic cancer. Br J Radiol 1993; 66: 1044–1048

115. Nathan T, Whitelaw D, Chang S et al. Photodynamic therapy for prostate cancer recurrence after radiotherapy: a Phase I study. J Urol 2002; 168: 1427–1432

116. Dupuy D E, Zagoria R J, Akerly W et al. Percutaneous radiofrequency ablation of malignancies in the lung. Am J Roentgenol 2000, 174: 57–59

117. Brookes J A, Lees W R, Bown S G. Interstitial laser photocoagulation for the treatment of lung cancer. Am J Roentgenol 1997; 168: 357–358

118. Brenner M, Shankel T, Waite T A et al. Animal model for thoracoscopic laser ablation of emphysematous pulmonary bullae. Lasers Surg Med 1996; 18: 191–196

119. Dupuy D E, Zagoria R J, Akerley W et al. Percutaneous radiofrequency ablation of malignancies in the lung. Am J Roentgenol 2000; 174: 57–59

120. Fielding D I, Buonaccorsi G, Hanby A et al. Interstitial laser photocoagulation of normal lung parenchyma in rats. Thorax 1998; 53: 692–697

121. Lam S. Photodynamic therapy of lung cancer. Semin Oncol 1994; 21: 15–19

122. McCaughan J S Jr. Survival after photodynamic therapy to non-pulmonary metastatic endobronchial tumors. Lasers Surg Med 1999; 24: 194–201

123. Ost D. Photodynamic therapy in lung cancer. Oncology (Huntingt) 2000; 14: 379–386, discussion 391–392

124. Pass H I, Pogrebniak H. Photodynamic therapy for thoracic malignancies. Semin Surg Oncol 1992; 8: 217–225

125. Gervais D A, McGovern F J, Wood B J et al. Radiofrequency ablation of renal cell carcinoma: early clinical experience. Radiology 2000; 217: 665–672

126. Gill I S, Hsu T H, Fox R L et al. Laparoscopic and percutaneous radiofrequency ablation of the kidney: acute and chronic porcine study. Urology 2000; 56: 197–200

127. Hall W H, McGahan J P, Link D P et al. Combined embolization and percutaneous radiofrequency ablation of a solid renal tumor. Am J Roentgenol 2000; 174: 1592–1594

128. Patel V R, Leveillee R J, Hoey M F et al. Radiofrequency ablation of rabbit kidney using liquid electrode: acute and chronic observations. J Endourol 2000;14: 155–159

129. Polascik T J, Hamper U, Lee B R et al. Ablation of renal tumors in a rabbit model with interstitial saline-augmented radiofrequency energy: preliminary report of a new technology. Urology 1999; 53: 465–472

130. Ogan K, Jacomides L, Dolmatch B et al. Percutaneous radio-frequency ablation of renal tumors: technique, limitations and morbidity. Urology 2002; 60: 954–958

131. Pavlovich C, McClellan W, Choyke P et al. Percutaneous radiofrequency ablation of small renal tumours: initial results. J Urol 2002; 167: 10–15

132. Mack M, Straub R, Eichler K et al. MR-guided laser-induced thermotherapy in recurrent extra-hepatic abdominal tumours. Eur Radiol 2001; 11: 2041–2046

133. Krimbacher E, Zeimet A G, Marth C, Kostron H. Photodynamic therapy for recurrent gynecologic malignancy: a report on four cases. Arch Gynecol Obstet 1999; 262: 193–197

134. Callstrom M, Charboneau J, Goetz M et al. Painful metastases involving bone: feasibility of percutaneous CT- and US-guided radio-frequency ablation. Radiology 2002; 224: 87–97

135. Ikeda K, Arase Y, Saitoh S et al. Interferon-beta prevents recurrence of hepatocellular carcinoma after complete resection or ablation of the primary tumor. A prospective randomized study of hepatitis C virus-related liver cancer. Hepatology 2000; 32: 228–232

136. Okuno M, Kojima S, Moriwaki H. Chemoprevention of hepatocellular carcinoma: concept progress and perspectives. J Gastroenterol Hepatol 2001; 16: 1329–1355

137. Lau W Y, Leung T W T, Ho S et al. Adjuvant intra-arterial iodine-131-labelled lipiodol for resectable hepatocellular carcinoma: a prospective randomised trial. Lancet 1999; 353: 797–801

Chapter 51

Imaging for radiotherapy treatment planning

H Jane Dobbs and Ann Barrett

Introduction

Conformal radiotherapy (CFRT) allows shaping of the radiation beam both geometrically and with modulation of the fluence of the beam, a technique known as intensity modulated radiation therapy (IMRT). This dramatic advance in the delivery of radiotherapy means that the volume of tissue treated is no longer a cube or rectangular box but a three-dimensional volume containing macroscopic tumour with a surrounding margin shaped to the individual patient's cancer. Studies such as those by Robinson et al.[1] and Crosby et al.[2] have shown that the volume of tissue irradiated is reduced by around 30–50% using CFRT compared with standard planning techniques.

Randomized trials of pelvic radiotherapy for prostate cancer[3,4] have shown reduction in normal tissue toxicity with CFRT as compared to conventional treatment (Table 51.1).[4] Intensity modulated radiation therapy affords the possibility of producing concave treatment shapes to avoid adjacent critical normal structures, a facility not possible with conventional planning techniques. This type of treatment is likely to reduce morbidity at anatomical sites such as the head and neck (avoiding spinal cord, eyes or salivary glands), thyroid (avoiding spinal cord), prostate (avoiding rectum) (Fig. 51.1) and paediatric tumours where reduction of dose to normal tissues is critical. A large Phase II study has also shown reduction in biochemical markers consistent with improved local control of prostate cancer with dose escalation and CFRT, where increased radiation doses have been given to a smaller but more focused target volume (Table 51.2).[5] These and other Phase II studies and randomized trials are 'proof of principle' of the value of three-dimensional CFRT.

However, achieving the potential for progress depends very much on having an excellent, dedicated multidisciplinary team that includes a radiologist committed to cancer

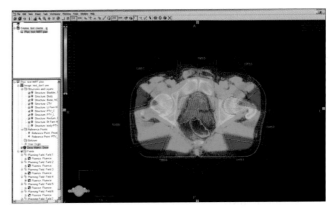

Figure 51.1. *Conformal plan for treatment of cancer of the prostate showing concave posterior border avoiding the rectum. (Courtesy of J Tomes, Norfolk & Norwich University Hospital NHS Trust.)*

imaging as well as an oncologist, physicist, planning technician and therapy radiographer to ensure that these technological advances are used accurately. Three-dimensional imaging with computed tomography (CT) and magnetic resonance (MR) imaging has provided more accurate visualization of tumours and normal organs for planning CFRT. 2-[F-18]fluoro-2-deoxy-D-glucose positron emission tomography ([18]FDG PET), single-photon emission CT (SPECT) and MR with dynamic scanning can create a map of biological function in addition to the anatomical images obtained with CT. Image registration tools are now available to combine all this diagnostic information in a format that can be used to focus and plan radiotherapy delivery. Multileaf collimators (MLC) made up of many individual leaves of 1 cm or less can be positioned at varying places within the beam to produce an irregularly shaped field (Fig. 51.2). In addition, patterns of MLC leaves can be

Table 51.1. *Randomized study of late toxicity using conformal versus conventional radiotherapy for prostate cancer*

Radiation proctitis and bleeding	Conformal radiotherapy (*n*=114)	Conventional radiotherapy (*n*=111)
RTOG Grade 1	37%	56% (*P*=0.004)
RTOG Grade 2	5%	15% (*P*=0.01)

Reproduced with permission from Dearnaley et al.[4]

Table 51.2. *Tumour control using conformal radiotherapy and dose escalation for prostate cancer in 1,100 patients (median follow-up 5 years)*

Prognostic group	PSA relapse-free survival rate	
	Radiation dose >75 Gy	Radiation dose <70 Gy
Favourable risk	90%	77% (P=0.05)
Intermediate risk	70%	50% (P=0.001)
High risk	47%	21% (P=0.002)

Reproduced with permission from Zelefsky et al.[5]

moved with different speeds to create a two-dimensional intensity-modulated beam. Electronic portal imaging devices record the geometry of the radiotherapy field delivered and these images can be compared electronically with the original field design to verify that delivery of treatment is accurate. Computerized verification systems enable on-line correction of the patient's position or millimetre changes in positioning of the radiation beam on a daily treatment basis according to an agreed action level of variance. Improved outcomes depend on appropriate expertise in the use of these technological developments at each stage of treatment planning and delivery.

Key points: introduction

■ CFRT allows shaping of the radiation beam both geometrically and with modulation of intensity (IMRT)

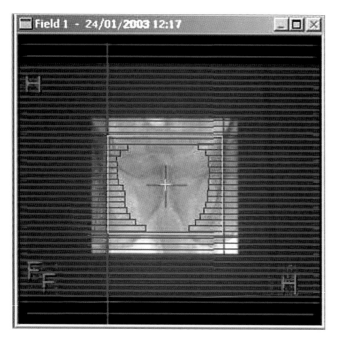

Figure 51.2. *Irregularly shaped field for treatment of prostate cancer obtained using multi-leaved collimation. (Courtesy of J Tomes, Norfolk & Norwich University Hospital NHS Trust.)*

■ CFRT reduces volume of tissue irradiated by 30–50%

■ CFRT permits reduction in normal tissue toxicity

■ MLCs can produce an irregularly shaped field

■ MLCs can move at different speeds producing a two-dimensional intensity-modulated beam

■ Electronic portal imaging devices record the geometry of the radiotherapy field delivered

Target volume

With this increase in sophisticated technology available to deliver radiotherapy conformally has come an urgent need to define the three-dimensional tumour and target volumes more accurately. A 'target' volume is defined so that both macroscopic and potential microscopic tumour spread are included in the volume that will receive a radical dose of radiation fractionated over up to 40 treatments during a 6- to 8-week period. The International Commission on Radiation Units and Measurements (ICRU) have published Report 50,[6] which provides internationally accepted definitions of tumour and target volumes, and Report 62,[7] which gives more detailed information about margin determination. This standardization of nomenclature enables comparisons to be made among radiotherapy treatments given in different centres around the world.

ICRU Report 50 first defines the gross tumour volume (GTV) as the palpable or visible extent of tumour representing macroscopic disease seen on clinical examination or optimal imaging. The GTV contains the maximum concentration of tumour cells, although there may be central necrosis where clonogenic cell numbers are reduced. Around the macroscopic or imaged tumour there may be a zone of direct local microscopic spread and a margin is therefore added around the GTV to create the clinical target volume (CTV). These microscopic extensions cannot be seen on cross-sectional imaging but new data are becoming available using functional studies and biological imaging which may provide more information about this tumour–normal tissue interface in the future. At the moment, this margin is the most controversial one in compiling the final target volume because data on which to base it are lacking for many tumour sites. The margin varies according to the clinician's experience and interpretation of the histological features of any particular tumour and what is known about its likely behaviour. Information from historical histopathological specimens removed at surgery or postmortem examination is used, as well as individual tumour parameters such as:

- Grade of tumour (which correlates with invasiveness and growth rate)
- Vascular and lymphatic permeation
- Histological subtype
- Knowledge of tumour-specific spread patterns

This zone around the GTV is assumed to have decreasing malignant cell density towards the periphery. For tumours such as those in the central nervous system (CNS), surrounding oedema may also contain tumour cells. Following chemotherapy, some tumours appear to shrink down to their point of origin, whereas others may leave nests of cells within a fibrotic matrix (e.g. Ewing's sarcoma), making the definition of target volume after chemotherapy difficult. Where the original tumour has been removed at surgery, the postoperative CTV may require localization using preoperative scans that have been co-registered with postoperative CT planning scans.

If radiotherapy is planned to lymph node areas in addition, there may be two CTVs, one for the primary tumour and one for the lymph node volume. The CTV is susceptible to a number of variabilities and uncertainties both during a radiotherapy treatment (intra-fraction) and from day to day during a prolonged course of treatment (inter-fraction). These uncertainties may be related to organ movement caused by:

- Respiration
- Cardiac motion
- Swallowing
- Displacement of organs such as the prostate with bladder and rectal filling

Uncertainties may also result from variations in the position of the patient on the treatment couch but this can be reduced by improved patient immobilization systems. A margin is therefore created around the CTV to define the planning target volume (PTV) which accounts for all these geometrical uncertainties. This final PTV becomes the daily target volume to which the radical dose of irradiation is given in order to cure the tumour (Fig. 51.3).

Image segmentation, or delineation of the tumour and adjacent normal organs, can be a time-consuming task and requires training in cross-sectional imaging[8] and the expert advice of a radiologist specializing in cancer imaging. Ideally, multidisciplinary sessions should be held specifi-

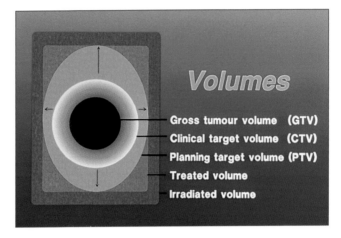

Figure 51.3. *ICRU target volumes (from reference 6 with permission). Note the treatment volume is smaller than the total irradiated volume.*

cally for target volume delineation of patients undergoing radiotherapy treatment planning attended by a radiologist, oncologist and treatment planning staff.[9]

It is clear that with the ability to deliver high precision radiotherapy using sophisticated technology there is an even greater requirement for precise definition of the GTV. In defining the margins of the PTV, accurate measurements of uncertainties need to be as small as possible to maximize tumour dose. To avoid risk of a geographical miss, it is possible to take a portal image of the location of the beam with respect to bony anatomy at each treatment visit and make direct comparison with the planned situation, which is documented on a digitally reconstructed radiograph (DRR) (Fig. 51.4). By verifying the location of the bony anatomy relative to the beam, uncertainties due to patient positioning and set-up errors can be identified, measured and corrected.

The degree of organ and patient movement varies in different parts of the body (Table 51.3).[10–13] For example, organ motion of the prostate can be measured by repeat CT scans or by implanting markers into the prostate and using portal images to monitor their position. Reduction of prostate motion can be achieved by ensuring constant bladder volume using detailed CT scan protocols, which restrict the volume of oral contrast given. Precise external patient set-up with immobilization protocols has also been shown to influence internal prostate motion.[14]

Table 51.4[11,14,15] shows results from the Netherlands Cancer Institute of measured data in three dimensions for prostate irradiation uncertainties. They are used to define the total error by adding the standard deviations in quadrature. The margin chosen around the CTV using these data is then a compromise between one that, if large, will increase risk of complications and one which, if too small, will risk a geographical miss.

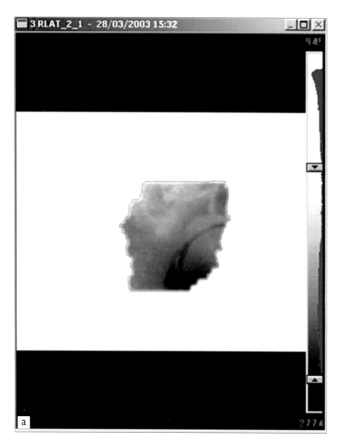

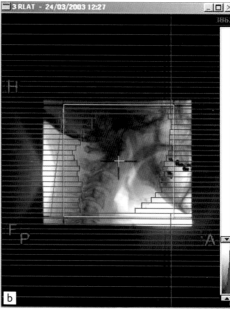

Figure 51.4. *Comparison of portal image (a) of treatment beam for cancer of the tonsil with DRR (b). (Courtesy of J Tomes, Norfolk & Norwich University Hospital NHS Trust.)*

Key points: target volume

■ A 'target' volume is defined so that both macroscopic and potential microscopic tumour spread are included in the volume that will receive a radical dose of radiation

■ The ICRU provides standard nomenclature for defining tumour and target volumes

■ The GTV is the palpable or visible extent of tumour representing macroscopic disease seen on clinical examination or optimal imaging

■ The CTV includes the GTV and a zone of direct local microscopic spread

■ The PTV includes the CTV and the GTV and represents an additional margin to take account of uncertainties in reproducibility of positioning etc.

A radiologist's role in gross tumour volume definition

The oncologist needs to know:

• Site of the tumour within the patient according to fixed reproducible coordinates
• Three-dimensional measurements of tumour size
• Details of the edge of the tumour where it forms a clear boundary with adjacent normal tissue
• Details of adjacent anatomy where no clear boundary exists
• Information regarding functional tumour activity and its relationship to anatomical imaging of the tumour

Although tumours are classified according to recognized staging systems such as the TNM system (discussed in Chapter 3), these rarely give guidelines on choice of optimal imaging modality to define the T stage for each primary site. Many studies have shown that the variability in delineating tumour and target volumes among different clinical observers can be very high. These include studies of tumours such as lung,[16,17] breast,[18,19] prostate cancer[20] and brain tumours.[21] 'Doctor's delineation error'[22] can be reduced by improving accuracy of GTV and CTV delineation and to achieve this requires the expertise of a fully trained radiologist working with an oncologist. However, the most effective way to obtain this collaboration has not yet been defined.

The radiologist must understand clearly the concepts of GTV and CTV. In some cases, delineating the GTV may be straightforward if there is a clear-cut density gradient between GTV and surrounding tissues. However, in many situations, it is well known that microscopic tumour spread

Table 51.3. *Set-up errors for different treatment sites*

Region	Direction	Systematic population error (1 SD, mm)	Random population error (1 SD, mm)	Reference
Head and neck	cc	3.6	2.1	Weltens et al.[10]
	ap	3.6	2.1	
Prostate	ml	2.3	2.1	Bel et al.[11]
	cc	2.2	2.0	
	ap	2.7	2.0	
Lung	ml	2.1	2.9	Vijlbrief et al.[12]
	cc	2.5	2.9	
	ap	1.8	2.2	
Breast	cc	4.1	3.7	Mitine et al.[13]
	ap	3.5	2	

ml = medial-lateral; cc = cranial-caudal; ap = anterior-posterior.

Table 51.4. *Geometric uncertainties in delineating the PTV for prostate cancer*

Type of error	Reference	Systematic errors (1 SD, mm)			Random errors (1 SD, mm)		
		LR	SI	AP	LR	SI	AP
Target volume delineation	Rasch et al.[15]	1.7	2–3.5*	2			
Organ motion	Van Herk et al.[14]	0.9	1.7	2.7	0.9	1.7	2.7
Set-up error	Bel et al.[11]	2.6	2.4	2.4	2.0	1.8	1.7
Total error		3.2	3.6–4.5*	4.1	2.2	2.5	3.2
Average LR, SI, AP				3.9			2.6

LR = left-right, SI = superior-inferior, AP = anterior-posterior.
*Due to large uncertainty in target volume delineation near the apex and seminal vesicles.

into surrounding oedema (brain tumours), fat (kidney) or bladder (prostate) may occur and that a single line drawn around visualized tumour may be somewhat arbitrary. Separation of GTV from CTV may then be difficult and knowledge of clinical tumour behaviour and treatment considerations may become important. In such cases, dialogue between the two specialists in front of the images may produce a more satisfactory outcome than if each works independently. In other cases, sparing normal tissues may be critical and lead to modifications in CTV. Joint discussion might be valuable when such decisions have to be taken, balancing the need to include all tumour within the target volume with the risk of high doses to surrounding normal organs.

Decisions about choice of target volumes must also be audited to help determine what margins are appropriate for different clinical situations. This can only be done jointly with the radiologist, relating GTV delineations to patterns of local relapse.

Other issues requiring debate are whether consulta-tion with remote viewing of images via PACS is as effective as the two specialists working together in the same place, and whether clinical oncologists need special training in radiological anatomy to collaborate effectively with radiologists in this task. Problems may arise if radiological specialization proceeds along image modality lines (i.e. in CT, MR, [18]FDG PET) while clinical oncologists specialize more and more in particular tumour types and require information from all types of images. More work is needed to define the best scanning modalities and protocols for each tumour type and stage, and state-of-the-art guidelines related to these issues are clearly required. There is a potential for considerable increase in workload for radiologists as their input is essential for optimal target volume definition in all patients with cancer. Such an increase might be offset by integration of staging and treatment planning for some tumour types, profiting from the major advances in speed of capturing images with multidetector CT and the use of image registration techniques.

Key point: radiologist's role

■ As the radiotherapy PTV becomes more sophisticated it is increasingly important for the radiologist and radiotherapist to work closely together

Treatment planning issues

To deliver high-precision CFRT accurately on a daily basis, attention has to be focused on basic requirements such as immobilization of the patient. If the patient and the organ containing the tumour move from day to day during the fractionated course of radiotherapy, a geographical miss may occur. Systematic and random set-up errors can be measured and often reduced with good immobilization protocols.[23]

Immobilization systems using skin tattoos or fiducial markers, lasers and devices such as perspex shells, vacuum bags and poles, pads and ankle stops to secure limbs are hence of prime importance in progressing to very high-precision therapy. As radiotherapy has progressed from delivery of 'fields' to precise 'target volumes', the use of CT-compatible immobilization systems to ensure accurate reproducibility of the patient's parameters between planning and treatment has increased. For breast radiotherapy, for example, new style CT-compatible breast boards have been developed which have the advantage of a variable wedge angle but also a comfortable support for the arms elevated and secured above the head to permit access into the CT scanner aperture (Fig. 51.5). It is important that CT scans taken for radiotherapy treatment planning are done under identical conditions to those for delivery of the subsequent radiotherapy to minimize geometrical uncertainties. External landmarks used for setting up the patient on the therapy unit and immobilization devices are all needed for the therapy CT scan which uses a system of lasers to align the patient. Protocols for CT scanning of different anatomical areas for planning should be drawn up jointly between the radiologist and oncologist. The use of contrast media should be discussed because an excessive volume of oral contrast medium given to patients with, for example bladder tumours, may cause a urinary diuresis, with unnecessary enlargement of the bladder after voluntary micturition. Patients with bladder tumours are irradiated immediately after micturition to empty the bladder as much as possible and to minimize the target volume. If the bladder is over-distended, the PTV will be unnecessarily large and the side-effects of radiotherapy on the bowel will increase. Small slice thickness and slice interval (2–3 mm) are essential for CT scanning for three-dimensional visualization of the tumour and construction of DRRs with which to compare electronic portal imaging on the therapy unit.

Studies are underway to deliver radiotherapy using suspended respiration. Treatment may be 'gated' to a particular part of the respiratory cycle,[24] or an active breathing control (ABC) device with a valve can be used.[25] These methods are being evaluated to try to reduce the large margin currently necessary to encompass lung tumours, especially in the periphery, that move with respiration[26] and also in the use of breast IMRT (Fig. 51.6).

Magnetic resonance imaging provides excellent soft tissue characterization of tumours and, for many sites, such as the CNS, prostate, rectum, cervix and soft tissue sarcomas, is the imaging modality of choice.[27] However, MR is not yet used directly for radiotherapy planning because of geometric distortions and lack of electron density information for dosimetry. Image registration tools are being developed to match the improved tumour definition obtained with MR and other imaging modalities with the geometric accuracy and electron density dosimetric capabilities of CT (Fig. 51.7).[28,29] Co-registration of images is a vital development in

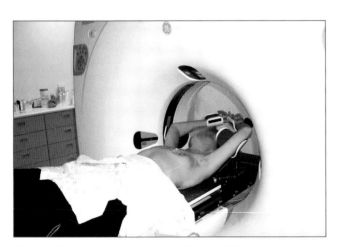

Figure 51.5. *Breast board compatible with CT scanner access. (Courtesy of J Tomes, Norfolk & Norwich University Hospital NHS Trust.)*

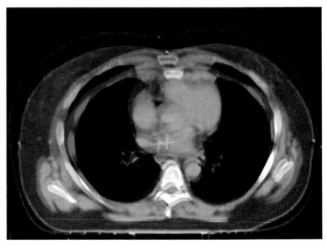

Figure 51.6. *Changes in contour and internal organs associated with respiration. (Courtesy of J Tomes, Norfolk & Norwich University Hospital NHS Trust.)*

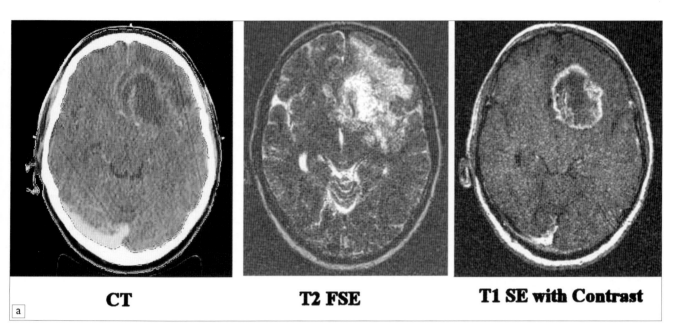

CT **T2 FSE** **T1 SE with Contrast**

a

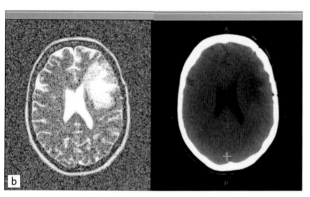

b

Figure 51.7. *Image registration. (a) Separate images obtained by CT and MR (b) are fused to allow optimal tumour definition for treatment planning. (Courtesy of J Tomes, Norfolk & Norwich University Hospital NHS Trust.)*

order to ensure that all diagnostic information from [18]FDG PET, SPECT, MR spectroscopy, dynamic contrast-enhanced MR, etc. can be reformatted or co-registered with the CT-based planning image to improve accuracy of the GTV.[15,30] In addition, if the tumour has been surgically removed or treated with chemotherapy, the original imaging performed at diagnosis may provide important information about the site and size of the tumour which is relevant to subsequent radiotherapy.[31] Integration of the post-treatment planning CT scan with the pretreatment CT, MR or [18]FDG PET scan improves delineation of the CTV. [18]FDG PET–CT scanners are now available and can provide functional information about tumours such as lymphomas[32] and lung cancer,[33] in addition to the anatomical map from CT, all displayed in a combined image. The ability to perform a CT scan under radiotherapy planning conditions combined with [18]FDG

PET data promises great potential for increasing the accuracy of GTV delineation for selected tumour sites.

For radiologists, the scope and possibilities of new imaging modalities have increased rapidly in recent years, improving both anatomical and functional understanding of tumours. Similarly, for clinical oncologists, technological developments in radiotherapy delivery have greatly enhanced the likelihood of local cure with reduced side-effects to normal tissues. However, to achieve the full potential of these advances, both specialties need to come together in closer collaboration, not only in local clinical practice but also in research and educational initiatives. Activities that encourage dialogue, working more closely together and joint development of protocols will help to ensure that new technology is used for optimal patient care.

Key points: target volume issues

- CT scans for radiotherapy planning must be performed under conditions identical to those for delivering therapy

- CT-compatible immobilization systems to ensure accurate reproducibility of the patient's parameters between planning and treatment should be used

- Systematic and random set-up errors can be measured and often reduced with good immobilization protocols

- Lasers are used for CT for alignment purposes

- MR is not yet used directly for radiotherapy planning

- Co-registration of images from different modalities is crucial for accurate target volume definition

- ^{18}FDG PET–CT scanners will provide more precise delineation of the PTV

Summary

- Conformal radiotherapy (CFRT) allows shaping of the radiation beam

- CFRT reduces volume of tissue irradiated by 30–50% and permits reduction in normal tissue toxicity

- Multileaf collimators (MLC) can produce an irregularly shaped field and a two-dimensional intensity modulated beam

- Electronic portal imaging devices record the geometry of the radiotherapy field delivered

- The gross tumour volume (GTV) is the palpable or visible extent of tumour representing macroscopic disease seen on clinical examination or optimal imaging

- The clinical target volume (CTV) includes the GTV and a zone of direct local microscopic spread

- The planned target volume (PTV) includes the CTV and the GTV

- Individual tumour parameters used to define the CTV include grade of tumour, vascular and lymphatic permeation and histological subtype

- Historical surgical or postmortem examination information is also used to define the PTV

- CT scans for radiotherapy planning must be performed under identical conditions to those for delivering therapy

- CT-compatible immobilization systems to ensure accurate reproducibility of the patient's parameters between planning and treatment should be used

- Systematic and random set-up errors can be measured and often reduced with good immobilization protocols

- Lasers are used for CT for alignment purposes for radiotherapy planning scans

- MR is not yet used directly for radiotherapy planning

- Co-registration of images from different modalities is crucial for accurate target volume definition

- ^{18}FDG PET–CT scanners will provide more precise delineation of the PTV

References

1. Robinson M H, Bidmead A M, Harmer C L. Value of conformal planning in the radiotherapy of soft tissue sarcoma. Clin Oncol 1992; 4: 290–293

2. Crosby T D, Melcher A A, Wetherall S et al. A comparison of two planning techniques for radiotherapy of high-grade astrocytomas. Clin Oncol 1998; 10: 392–398

3. Koper P, Stroom J, van Putten W et al. Acute morbidity reduction using 3D CRT for prostate cancer: a randomised study. Int J Radiat Oncol Biol Phys 1999; 43: 727–734

4. Dearnaley D, Khoo V, Norman A et al. Comparison of radiation side-effects of conformal and conventional radiotherapy in prostate cancer: a randomised trial. Lancet 1999; 353: 267–272

5. Zelefsky M J, Fuks Z, Hunt M et al. High-dose radiation delivered by intensity-modulated conformal radiotherapy improves the outcome of localized prostate cancer. J Urol 2001; 166: 876–881

6. ICRU (International Commission of Radiation Units and Measurements). Prescribing, Recording and Reporting Photon Beam Therapy. ICRU Report 50, Bethesda, MD, 1993. ISBN: 091 339 4483

7. ICRU (International Commission of Radiation Units and Measurements). Prescribing, Recording and Reporting Photon Beam Therapy. (Supplement to

ICRU Report 50). ICRU Report 62, Bethesda, MD, USA, 1999

8. Sundar S, Symonds R P. Diagnostic radiology for radiotherapist: the case for structured training in cross-sectional imaging (CT and MRI). Clin Oncol 2002; 14: 413–414

9. Royal College of Radiologists. Development and Implementation of Conformal Radiotherapy in the UK. London: Royal College of Radiologists, 2002

10. Weltens C, Kesteloot K, Vandevelde G, Van den Bogaert W. Comparison of plastic and Orfit masks for patient head fixation during radiotherapy: precision and costs. Int J Radiat Oncol Biol Phys 1995; 33: 499–507

11. Bel A, Vos P H, Rodrigus P T et al. High-precision prostate cancer irradiation by clinical application of an off-line patient set up verification procedure, using portal imaging. Int J Radiat Oncol Biol Phys 1996; 35: 321–332

12. Vijlbrief R, Belderbos J, de Goede J et al. Development and evaluation of a verification procedure for set up corrections of lung cancer patients. Proceedings of the 5th International Workshop on Electronic Portal Imaging. Phoenix, AZ, USA, 1998

13. Mitine C, Dutreix A, Van der Schueren E. Tangential breast irradiation: influence of technique of set up on transfer errors and reproducibility. Radiother Oncol 1991; 22: 308–310

14. Van Herk M, Bruce A, Kroes A P et al. Quantification of organ motion during conformal radiotherapy of the prostate by three-dimensional image registration. Int J Radiat Oncol Biol Phys 1995; 33: 1311–1320

15. Rasch C, Barillot I, Remeijer P et al. Definition of the prostate in CT and MRI; a multiobserver study. Int J Radiat Oncol Biol Phys 1999; 43: 57–66

16. Van de Steene J, Linthout N, de Mey J et al. Definition of gross tumour volume in lung cancer: inter-observer variability. Radiother Oncol 2002; 62: 37–49

17. Giraud P, Elles S, Helfre S et al. Conformal radiotherapy for lung cancer: different delineation of the gross tumour volume (GTV) by radiologists and radiation oncologists. Radiother Oncol 2002; 62: 27–36

18. Hurkmans C W, Borger J H, Pieters B R et al. Variability in target volume delineation on CT scans of the breast. Int J Radiat Oncol Biol Phys 2001; 50: 1366–1372

19. Pitkanen M A, Holli K A, Ojala A T, Laippala P. Variability in planning target volume delineation. Acta Oncol 2001; 40: 50–55

20. Fiorino C, Reni M, Bolognesi A et al. Intra- and inter-observer variability in contouring prostate and seminal vesicles: implications for conformal radiotherapy

treatment planning. Radiother Oncol 1998; 3: 207–212

21. Jansen E P M, Dewit L G H, Van Herk M, Bartelink H. Target volumes in radiotherapy for high-grade malignant glioma of the brain. Radiother Oncol 2000; 56: 151–156

22. BIR Joint Working Party. Geometric Uncertainties in Radiotherapy: defining the Planning Target Volume. London: British Institute of Radiology, 2003

23. Hurkmans C W, Remeijer P, Lebesque J V, Mijnheer B J. Set-up verification using portal imaging: review of current clinical practice. Radiother Oncol 2001; 58: 105–120

24. Ford E C, Mageras G S, Yorke E et al. Evaluation of respiratory movement during gated radiotherapy using film and electronic portal imaging. Int J Radiat Oncol Biol Phys 2002; 52: 522–531

25. Wong J W, Sharpe M B, Jaffray D A et al. The use of active breathing control (ABC) to reduce margin for breathing motion. Int J Radiat Oncol Biol Phys 1999; 44: 911–919

26. Ekberg L, Holmberg O, Wittgren L et al. What margins should be added to the clinical target volume in radiotherapy treatment planning for lung cancer? Radiother Oncol 1998; 48: 71–77

27. Royal College of Radiologists. A Guide to the Practical Use of MRI in Oncology. London: Royal College of Radiologists, 1999

28. Van Herk M, Kooy H M. Automatic three-dimensional correlation of CT–CT, CT–MRI and CT–SPECT using chamfer matching. Med Phys 1994; 21: 1163–1178

29. Studholme C, Hill D L G, Hawkes D J. Automated 3D registration of MR and PET brain images by multi-resolution optimisation of voxel similarity measures. Med Phys 1997; 24: 1

30. Caldwell C B, Mah K, Ung Y C et al. Observer variation in contouring gross tumour volume in patients with poorly defined non-small-cell lung tumours on CT: the impact of 18-FDG-hybrid PET fusion. Int J Radiat Oncol Biol Phys 2001; 51: 923–931

31. Rosenman J G, Miller E P, Tracton G, Cullip T J. Image registration: an essential part of radiation therapy treatment planning. Int J Radiat Oncol Biol Phys 1998; 40: 197–205

32. O'Doherty M J, Macdonald E A, Barrington S F et al. Positron emission tomography in the management of lymphomas. Clin Oncol 2002; 14: 415–426

33. Kalff V, Hicks R, MacManus M et al. Clinical impact of 18-Fluorodeoxy glucose positron emission tomography in patients with non-small-cell lung cancer: a prospective study. J Clin Oncol 2001; 19: 111–118

Chapter 52

Radiological manifestations of acute complications of treatment

John Spencer, Janet E Husband, Louise Wilkinson, David MacVicar

Introduction

Acute complications of treatment in the cancer patient typically occur within days or weeks of initiation of therapy but may be seen up to 3 months. Next to occur are sub-acute or early delayed complications. However, there is variation in susceptibility among individuals and there may be some overlap of the acute and early delayed effects in the first few weeks to months following treatment. Radiological manifestations are often non-specific and thus the clinical context and temporal relationship to induction of therapy are important considerations. Good communication between the radiologist and the oncologist is vital for the early recognition and accurate diagnosis of complications related to treatment. The role of the radiologist is to help clinical colleagues to make a distinction between the effects of the cancer and the effects of treatment so that ineffective or toxic therapies can be discontinued.

In this chapter, acute and early delayed complications, mainly related to chemotherapy, will be discussed concentrating on those processes that are likely to be encountered by the radiologist. Emphasis is placed upon complications whose recognition may spare the patient unnecessary harm or require specific changes in management. Complications of therapy which may mimic disease are highlighted. Historically, these complications have been seen most commonly with treatment of haematological malignancies, but with more intensive chemotherapy for solid tumours these are increasingly seen in general oncology. For convenience, complications are discussed by anatomic site: the chest, the abdomen and pelvis, and the brain and spine.

The complications associated with radiotherapy have been covered in detail elsewhere (see Chapters 53, 54 and 55). Late delayed complications related to chemotherapy are mentioned in other chapters as appropriate.

The chest

A variety of complications of treatment are seen. These relate to:

- Intravenous lines and catheters
- Drug reactions
- Opportunistic infections

Intravenous lines and catheters

Long-term intravenous catheters are increasingly used for infusion of chemotherapy of haematological malignancies and solid tumours, particularly as part of a high-dose regimen which results in marked marrow toxicity. These are increasingly inserted under image guidance in the radiology department using either ultrasound and/or fluoroscopic guidance. The side and site of central venous access varies with local practice and the needs of the individual patient.[1] Options for access may be limited by previous therapy, e.g. avoiding the side of previous breast surgery.

Immediate complications of insertion

The rate of complication varies among series but is up to 5% at the time of insertion.[2] The immediate complications of catheter insertion reflect malposition or trauma to adjacent structures and include:

- Pneumothorax
- Arterial puncture
- Trauma to adjacent structures
- Venous malposition
- Failure of placement

The tip of the catheter should lie in a large central vein able to accommodate the necessary flow rate and of sufficient size that positioning of the catheter will not cause flow disturbance or promote thrombosis.[3] The right subclavian vein is the favoured route of access because left-sided catheters are associated more commonly with erosion of the superior vena cava (SVC).[4] This manifests as mediastinal widening and pleural effusion within 1–7 days of catheter placement.[4] The optimal position of the central venous catheter tip is in the SVC. The distal catheter should be parallel to the vessel wall to avoid erosion by local pressure effects of the tip. A curve or other deformity at the tip of the catheter may indicate that the catheter tip is abutting the wall of the vessel.[5]

At the time of insertion, the catheter may be misdirected into any of the central veins.[6] With image guidance it is usually possible to recognize and remedy this problem. A detailed knowledge of the central veins (Fig. 52.1) and their anomalies is important for recognition of these complications. When there is doubt, contrast medium injection via the catheter under the image guidance may clarify the situation. Inadvertent arterial puncture with local bleeding may result in an apical extrapleural or mediastinal collection. Thus, problems with central venous catheterization may mimic disease progression. Local trauma at the time of insertion may uncommonly result in damage to the brachial plexus or in phrenic nerve injury with elevation of the diaphragm on subsequent radiographs. Catheters can be accidentally placed in the pleural space or subsequently migrate causing drugs or fluid to be infused intrapleurally (Fig. 52.2). Fragmentation of the catheter may be caused at the time of insertion, resulting in embolic fragments that can be removed by percutaneous techniques.[1] These are usually recognized during insertion but occasionally the postinsertion radiograph may reveal an unsuspected lost guidewire or fragment.

Key points: catheter insertion

- The right subclavian vein is the favoured route of access because left-sided catheters more commonly erode the SVC

- Local trauma at the time of insertion includes pneumothorax, arterial puncture and, rarely, brachial plexopathy or phrenic nerve injury

Complications of an established catheter: flow problems

Once the catheter is in place and immediate complications have been excluded, the most common early problem is of poor flow or inability to aspirate blood. This usually reflects an intrathoracic complication but another problem to consider is positional flow problem due to kinking of the catheter in the chest wall.[7] Complications with poor catheter flow or aspiration include:

- Occlusion or kinking of the catheter[7]
- Migration of the tip into a smaller vein (Fig. 52.3)
- Erosion into the mediastinum or pleural space (Fig. 52.2)
- Formation of fibrin sheath or crystallization (Fig. 52.4)
- Thrombosis of the vein (Figs. 52.5 and 52.6)

Migration, malposition, fibrin sheath, crystallization
An initial chest radiograph should be obtained following line placement, and follow-up films obtained in the event of malfunction to establish any change in the course or posi-

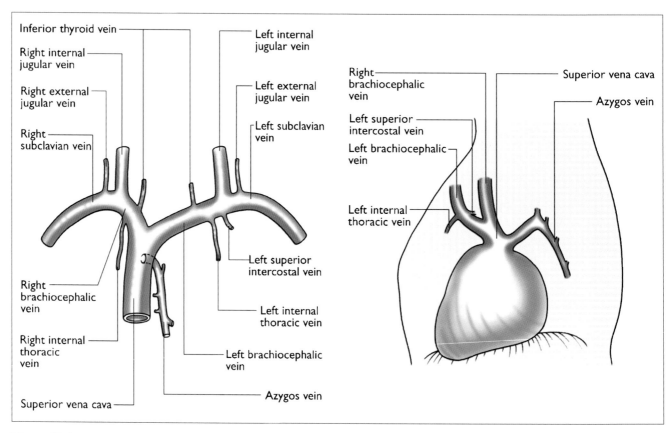

Figure 52.1. *Anatomy of the thoracic veins on the frontal and lateral radiographs.*

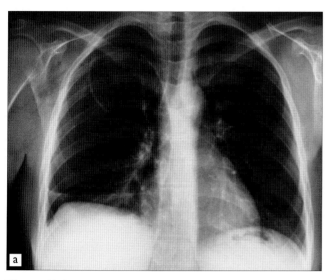 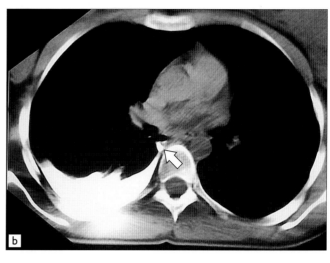

Figure 52.2. *(a) Chest radiograph shows a Hickman line in an apparently satisfactory position but a hydropneumothorax and surgical emphysema suggest that the pleura has been breached. There was a subpulmonic effusion following administration of fluids through the catheter. (b) Following administration of contrast (for a staging CT investigation) contrast has entered the pleural space. The catheter position (arrow) is shown behind the right main stem bronchus, presumably within the pleural space.*

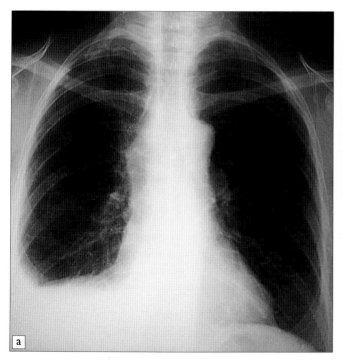 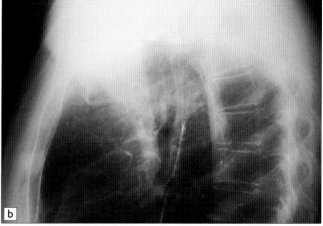

Figure 52.3. *Chest radiography in a patient with known oesophageal carcinoma undergoing chemotherapy with suspected catheter dysfunction. The PA film (a) shows the Hickman line entering the left subclavian vein crossing the mediastinum and with its tip possibly in the azygos vein. (b) The lateral film confirms this.*

tion or other complication. A lateral radiograph is valuable to demonstrate some malpositions (Fig. 52.3). With malposition it may be possible to resite the tip by catheter manipulation. Fibrin sheaths form around the tip of the majority of indwelling catheters and this complication should be considered if the catheter can be flushed but not aspirated. They are usually otherwise asymptomatic but may detach

and cause pulmonary embolism when the catheter is removed. Fibrin sheaths may be demonstrated by venography, or by a linogram (Fig. 52.4).[8] Occasionally, the line may be occluded due to crystallization of the infusion fluid. Occlusion by calcium carbonite crystals, during infusion of 5-fluorouracil (5-FU) and leucovorin through a single lumen, has been described.[9]

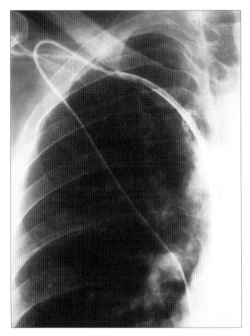

Figure 52.4. *Contrast injected through the catheter demonstrates a fibrin sheath around the intravascular component of the catheter.*

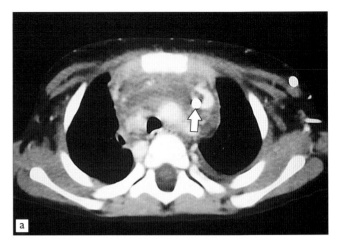

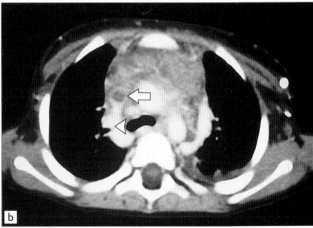

Figure 52.6. *CT scan in a 2-year-old child demonstrating (a) the tip of the catheter (arrow) adjacent to a distended superior intercostal vein and no contrast in the left brachiocephalic vein and (b) at a lower level showing the SVC with central thrombus (arrow) and peripheral contrast enhancement via a distended azygos vein (arrowhead).*

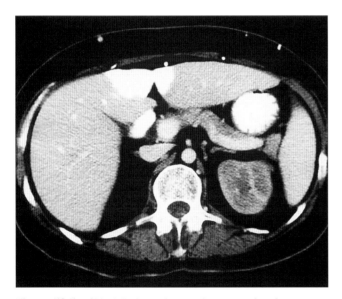

Figure 52.5. *CT of the liver showing hypervascular changes around the falciform ligament in keeping with intrahepatic shunts. Collateral vessels are seen in the abdominal wall. Chest CT showed an unsuspected thrombosis of the SVC.*

Mural thrombosis

Mural thrombosis is related to a number of factors, including the duration of catheter placement, sepsis, low cardiac output, hypercoagulability and compression related to disease progression.[10] It usually results in catheter malfunction and may progress to occlusion of the vessel. Pulmonary embolism is another concern and probably under-recog-

nized. Thrombosis may be asymptomatic and detected during routine reassessment. There are established pathways of venous collateral flow in the abdomen and sometimes it is only the recognition of such clues that alert to the possibility of venous thrombosis in the central veins, which may not have been included in the examination field. These include venous collaterals around the liver surface and intrahepatic shunts (Fig. 52.5).[11,12]

Thrombosis of the subclavian, axillary and jugular veins may be demonstrated on Doppler ultrasound scanning and this should be the first investigation in cooperative patients. The technique requires skill and flexibility but has the great strength of being able to be performed at the bedside in sick patients.[13] Even when thrombus cannot be directly visualized, accessory signs, including damped or diminished cardiac pulsatility or respiratory phasicity, accurately predict thrombosis or occlusion shown by venography.[14] Another useful sign is impaired augmentation of flow in more central veins during compression of the arm. Ultrasound assessment of the more central veins is limited. Alternatives include conventional contrast venography, computed tomography (CT) and magnetic resonance (MR) imaging. The former techniques are preferred because conventional venography may require bilateral simultaneous upper limb injections to demonstrate all the central veins.

Occlusion of the SVC (superior vena cava syndrome) is characterized by congestion and oedema of the upper extremities and head with engorged superficial veins. The chest radiograph shows superior mediastinal widening and there may be prominence of the left superior intercostal vein (aortic nipple) and azygos arch as collateral venous channels dilate.[15,16] Computed tomography with intravenous (IV) contrast medium (Fig. 52.6) is valuable and demonstrates the:

- Presence of occlusion
- Site of occlusion
- Presence of collateral vessels in the chest and abdomen (Fig. 52.5)
- Extent of thrombus (Fig. 52.6)
- Increased density of the mediastinal fat

A variety of MR techniques have been described to assess the central circulation, initially time-of-flight venography.[17] Currently, most researchers use breath-hold acquisition three-dimensional gadolinium (Gd)-enhanced MR venography sequences which can assess patency of the larger thoracic veins and demonstrate occlusion, stenoses, thrombosis or compression.[18,19] There are a number of pitfalls in the performance, and interpretation of these studies which can be critically dependent on the timing of the acquisition relative to the variable arrival of the contrast bolus. Some patients are unable to cooperate with the breathing requirements of the study. Other disadvantages include the cost and availability of MR and difficulties related to imaging critically ill patients. The technique is best regarded as a problem-solving tool.

Complications of the established catheter: sepsis

Reported rates of catheter-related sepsis vary and differ among oncology patients and others requiring long-term catheters, such as haemodialysis patients. In adults, the rates vary from 4 to 24%.[1,20] In children, a recent series of 100% technically successful implantations resulted in a 14% rate of catheter-related sepsis.[21] Infection is more common in neutropenic patients, in patients less than 2 years old and in patients with external catheters rather than implanted ports.

It is important to distinguish between systemic sepsis and superficial infection at the exit site of an external catheter or in the subcutaneous tunnel. Exit site infections in the absence of septicaemia require local wound care only. Tunnel or pocket infections with local cellulitis and pus formation are often only satisfactorily treated by removal of the catheter.[22] Catheter removal for sepsis occurred in 14 and

18% of two recent series.[1,21] However, infection of the catheter does not always result in septicaemia, and a concurrent septicaemia is not necessarily related to catheter infection. Catheter infection is confidently diagnosed by culture of the catheter tip but this requires its removal. Catheter-related septicaemia may be also be diagnosed without removing the device when simultaneous cultures show a five-fold greater number of colony-forming units from the line compared with simultaneous peripheral blood samples or when the line culture becomes positive at least 2 hours before a simultaneous peripheral sample.[23] Line removal is necessary with infection by *Staphylococcus aureus*, Gram-negative bacilli and Candida, but a local and systemic antimicrobial therapy may be used when no alternative access is possible.[24]

Evidence of multifocal septic emboli on the chest radiograph may be the first indication of line infection. Areas of confluent air-space shadowing, often cavitating, suggest staphylococcal infection. Cross-sectional imaging may also show induration around the catheter, thickening of the vessel wall, intraluminal air and thrombosis.[4]

Key points: catheter complications

- Occlusion of an established catheter may be due to kinking, malposition, fibrin sheaths or the development of thrombosis

- Fibrin sheaths develop in the majority of indwelling catheters and may detach, producing pulmonary emboli

- Thrombosis of the subclavian, axillary and jugular veins may be demonstrated on Doppler ultrasonography

- SVC occlusion is best assessed by CT but may be suggested on plain radiographs by mediastinal widening

- CT demonstrates the presence, site and extent of occlusion as well as presence of collaterals which may be seen in and around the liver in unsuspected cases at abdominal CT

- MR using breath-hold Gd-enhanced techniques demonstrates the great veins but is best reserved as a problem-solving tool

- Catheter-related sepsis rates vary but may lead to catheter removal in 15–20% of patients

Drug reactions

Chemotherapeutic agents are toxic and their administration may be limited by these adverse effects. There are various mechanisms of pulmonary toxicity, which may be idiosyncratic or dose-related. Four patterns of drug reaction are seen:[25]

- Interstitial pneumonitis/pulmonary fibrosis
- Diffuse alveolar damage

- Organizing pneumonia
- Hypersensitivity reaction

In some instances it is the combination of chemotherapeutic agents or their use in association with radiotherapy that results in harm. Vincristine and vinblastine do not cause pulmonary complications when used alone but result in pulmonary oedema, occasionally progressing to fibrosis, when used in combination with mitomycin C.[26] Pulmonary fibrosis associated with cytotoxic drugs is usually irreversible and may be fatal; it is therefore important to recognize drug-related changes as early as possible.

The plain chest radiograph is the simplest method of identifying pulmonary disease in symptomatic and asymptomatic patients, but other imaging modalities, such as high-resolution CT (HRCT), may also be necessary for accurate assessment of the pulmonary changes. Even with HRCT the patterns of drug reaction, infective and other considerations overlap. The value of HRCT beyond establishing a specific diagnosis is in guiding biopsy site and method, open or transbronchial, based on distribution and in providing an objective and reproducible modality for monitoring progress.[25] Drug-related pulmonary change is most easily classified according to the radiological patterns:[26,27]

- Diffuse air-space shadowing, e.g.
    Cytosine arabinoside and fludarabine
    Interleukin-2 (IL-2)
    Fluid loading prior to therapy
    Etoposide (haemorrhagic)
- Diffuse interstitial disease, e.g.
    Bleomycin
    Methotrexate
    Carmustine
    Busulphan
    Cyclophosphamide
    Procarbazine
    Mitomycin
    Gemcitabine
    Irinotecan
    Doxetaxel
- Multiple pulmonary nodules, e.g.
    Bleomycin
    Cyclosporin

Diffuse air-space shadowing

Many chemotherapy regimens involve prehydration, e.g. with high-dose melphalan, cisplatin, ifosfamide, which may cause transient fluid overload and pulmonary oedema. In other instances this is a toxic effect resulting in increased pulmonary capillary permeability. Pulmonary oedema caused by cytosine arabinoside (Ara-C) was presumed to be a major cause of death in one series of patients who had

received the agent.[28] Dyspnoea occurs within a month after the onset of treatment and the chest radiograph initially shows a diffuse (occasionally basal) interstitial and alveolar pattern. This resolves following withdrawal of the drug. Interleukin-2 may cause a capillary-leak syndrome within the first week of treatment, which also resolves after the drug is withdrawn. Radiographic signs of pulmonary oedema range from mild interstitial change to widespread confluent air-space shadowing.[29] A more aggressive, potentially fatal reaction causes symptoms of shock within 24 hours of administration of the drug.[30] Another agent which may cause an acute reaction is procarbazine. This rare hypersensitivity reaction occurs within hours of administration of the drug. Radiographic findings include interstitial opacities, pleural effusion and alveolar infiltrates.

Diffuse interstitial opacities; pulmonary nodules

Diffuse interstitial disease is the pattern most commonly associated with chemotherapy drug reactions. The risk is also increased by pre-existing lung disease and smoking.[31] Severe alveolar wall damage may progress to pulmonary fibrosis, but is occasionally due to a hypersensitivity reaction (e.g. methotrexate).[27] The main differential diagnoses are infection and tumour progression, leading to lymphangitis carcinomatosis.

Bleomycin toxicity is well-described and illustrates most aspects of this type of treatment complication. Pulmonary fibrosis secondary to bleomycin toxicity occurs in 2–3% of patients receiving bleomycin, and is fatal in approximately 1%.[32] Lung disease may be exacerbated by concomitant treatment with radiotherapy or oxygen. Initially, the effects are reversible if the drug is withdrawn, and patients should be monitored regularly with pulmonary function tests and chest radiographs.[32] The radiographic features of bleomycin toxicity include a diffuse bibasal infiltrate which may be linear or nodular, and which appears 6–12 weeks after treatment is commenced.[33] Small pleural effusions may be present. High-resolution CT will identify these changes when the chest radiograph is apparently normal and is superior in detection and diagnosis.[34] In the early stages, pleurally based nodules are seen predominantly posteriorly at the lung bases. This progresses to coarse reticular shadowing extending towards the hila (Fig. 52.7). In advanced disease, confluent irregular opacities are seen throughout the lung with relative sparing of the apices.[35] As with other causes of fibrosis there may be pneumothorax but also pneumomediastinum (Fig. 52.7). High-resolution CT may show a variety of patterns in drug-induced disease, including ground glass opacities, consolidation, interlobular septal thickening and centrilobular nodularity. However, there may be poor concordance between the HRCT interpretation and lung pathology. Further, the pattern, distribution and extent of HRCT abnormality may have limited prognostic value.[25]

Pulmonary nodules may be seen alone or in combination with other interstitial changes. Rarely, bleomycin toxi-

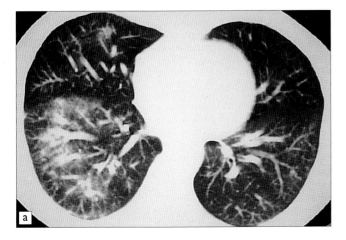

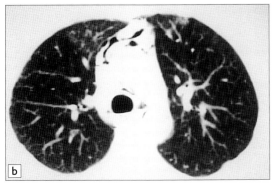

Figure 52.7. *High-resolution axial CT scan (a) of the lungs in early bleomycin toxicity showing a peripheral, bibasal interstitial infiltrate extending towards the hila. A more cranial section (b) in the same patient demonstrating a pneumomediastinum.*

city may cause multiple discrete nodules simulating metastases.[36]

There is a bewildering array of new chemotherapeutic agents and it is hard for the radiologist to keep abreast of their complications. However, these follow predictable patterns and it is thus important to raise the possibility of such drug reactions when they are encountered.[37,38]

Opportunistic infections of the lung

Patients with haematological malignancies, undergoing bone marrow transplantation (BMT) and with neutropenia related to chemotherapy may be severely immunocompromised and, in these patients, lung infections are potentially lethal. Opportunistic organisms are more common than community-acquired infections in this group of patients. The plain chest radiograph is the first investigation of a patient with pulmonary symptoms or pyrexia. Abnormalities revealed may be classified by the radiographic patterns recognizing some overlap in appearances. The differential diagnosis of infection on an abnormal radiograph includes:

- Progression of the underlying disease
- Drug reaction
- Radiation changes
- Non-specific interstitial pneumonitis

Given the overlap in radiographic appearances, even when assessed by HRCT, the clinical context must be considered. At different times during and after therapy certain complications are more likely. Thus, following BMT in the first few weeks, the acute neutropenic phase, fungal infections such as angioinvasive aspergillosis are a prime consideration but alveolar haemorrhage, pulmonary oedema from fluid challenges and drug reactions can produce similar radiographic findings. In the early phase from 3 to 14 weeks, concern is for cytomegalovirus (CMV) and Pneumocystis infection. Later in the disease course non-infective pneumonias and graft versus host disease (GVHD) predominate.[39]

Plain chest film patterns of opportunistic infection are detailed below:

Lobar or segmental consolidation:

- Bacterial
    Gram-negative organisms
    Gram-positive organisms
    Legionella pneumophila
- Mycobacterial disease

Pulmonary nodules and cavities +/− consolidation:

- Bacterial
    Septic infarcts (*S. aureus*)
    Nocardia
    Legionella micdedii

- Fungal
    Aspergillus
    Cryptococcus
    Mucormycosis
    Candida

Diffuse infective lung disease:

- *Pneumocystis carinii*
- Cytomegalovirus
- Herpes virus

Lobar or segmental consolidation

A variety of organisms produce focal or patchy consolidation which may be lobar or segmental. This may progress to cavitation with, for example, staphylococcal and Klebsiella infections. There may be small pleural effusions but empyema is rare. Tuberculous mycobacterial infection is relatively uncommon compared with bacterial infection and usually represents reactivation of disease.[40] The radiograph shows apical disease with or without cavitation (Fig. 52.8).[40] Atypical mycobacteria such as *Mycobacterium avium-intracellulare* complex (MAC), *M. kansasii* and *M. chelonae* should also be considered. Computed tomography cannot provide a bacteriological diagnosis but is valuable in defining equivocal lesions, planning diagnostic interventions, evaluating complications and monitoring therapy.[41] Radiographic signs suggesting atypical mycobacteria include an increased extent of cavitation with thinner walls and less dense surrounding consolidation than seen in tuberculous infection, anterior/apical segment disease rather than apico/posterior disease and marked pleural reaction over the involved lung.[42]

Pulmonary nodules and cavities

The infecting organisms are usually fungi or yeasts such as Aspergillus, Cryptococcus and Candida. Bacteria such as *S. aureus* and the transitional bacterium Nocardia, tuberculosis and toxoplasmosis should also be considered in the differential diagnosis. Invasive aspergillosis causes a severe necrotizing pneumonia. The chest radiograph shows multiple nodular opacities and areas of consolidation which are usually peripheral and may contain an 'air-crescent' sign (Fig. 52.9). This sign is often a reflection of a recovering neutrophil count.[39] Computed tomography shows single or multiple nodules which have a blurred edge of ground glass opacification due to peripheral haemorrhagic infarction.[38,43] These imaging features are also seen in patients with mucormycosis and cryptococcosis.[44,45] An alternative infective consideration is septic embolization related to long-term venous catheters.

Diffuse infective lung disease

In many patients with *Pneumocystis carinii* pneumonia (PCP) the initial chest radiograph is normal. Subsequently, there

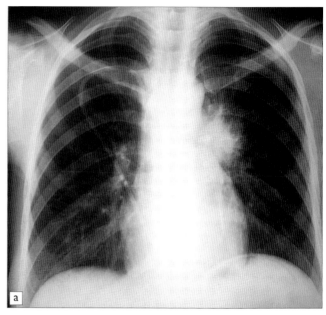

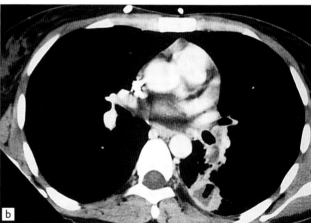

Figure 52.8. *Intercurrent infection with Mycobacterium tuberculosis in a patient on chemotherapy for acute lymphoblastic leukaemia. Chest radiograph shows a left hilar mass (a). CT scan demonstrates a cavitating lesion in the apical segment of the left lower lobe which was associated with left hilar and subcarinal lymphadenopathy (b).*

is a diffuse, bilateral, symmetrical perihilar infiltrate that may represent interstitial or air-space shadowing.[46] In patients receiving prophylactic pentamidine aerosol treatment, the distribution may be predominantly in the upper lobes. Pleural effusions and lymphadenopathy are rare. *Pneumocystis carinii* pneumonia may spare areas of irradiated lung.[47] Rarely, the cystic changes that are well described in autoimmunodeficiency syndrome (AIDS) patients are seen in other immunocompromised patients. The cystic lesions tend to be subpleural and predominantly of upper lobe distribution.[48]

Computed tomography is useful in the symptomatic patient with suspected PCP and an apparently normal chest

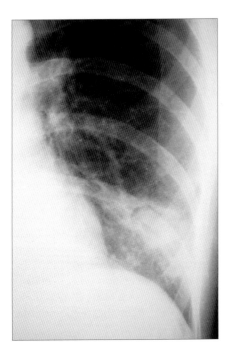

Figure 52.9. *Chest radiograph showing invasive aspergillosis in the left lower lobe. The cavitating nodule has a hazy edge and demonstrates the 'air-crescent' sign.*

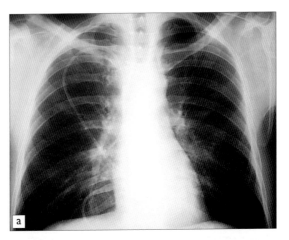

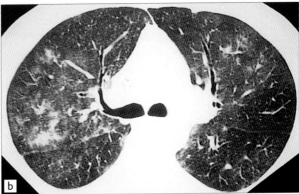

Figure 52.10. *Interstitial pneumonitis caused by CMV infection: (a) Chest radiograph shows a subtle perihilar infiltrate; (b) high-resolution CT demonstrates soft tissue opacities and ground glass opacification.*

radiograph. The CT findings cover a spectrum of abnormalities, from diffuse to patchy ground glass shadowing and there may be thickening of the interlobular septa. Interstitial fibrosis and cystic lesions are also well demonstrated.[46]

Atypical patterns occur in 5% of cases and include:[49]

- Lobar consolidation
- Multiple nodules
- Miliary patterns
- Endobronchial lesions
- Pleural effusions

Cytomegalovirus pneumonia is difficult to distinguish radiologically from other infective agents and gives a wide variety of radiographic appearances. It reflects reactivation of latent virus. The appearances on plain film include consolidation, linear interstitial infiltrate and ground glass shadowing. This is predominantly in the lower zone, and usually bilateral (Fig. 52.10). Small nodules have also been described,[50] and there may be associated pleural effusions, pneumothorax and pneumomediastinum.[51] Other viral pneumonias in the immunocompromised patient include herpes simplex virus, respiratory syncytial virus and measles. The radiographic appearances are non-specific.

Other causes of pulmonary disease in the immunocompromised patient

Pulmonary haemorrhage

Pulmonary haemorrhage occurs most commonly in patients with leukaemia. Rapid-onset diffuse and patchy airspace shadowing with perihilar and basal predominance is seen in the acute phase. Computed tomography shows ground glass opacification and sometimes frank consolidation.[52] If pulmonary haemorrhage is recurrent, then chest radiography in the later stages may also show interstitial changes and CT demonstrates a fine reticulo-nodular pattern.

Non-specific interstitial pneumonitis; graft versus host disease

These are more commonly late effects and, after BMT, are a consideration more than 100 days after therapy.[39] Bronchiolitis obliterans with organizing pneumonia (BOOP) and chronic GVHD may result and there is overlap in appearance between infective and non-infective pneumonias. Occasionally, even following lung biopsy, it is impossible to isolate an organism in some immunocompromised patients with an interstitial pneumonia. Histology is most likely to show non-specific interstitial pneumonitis.[53]

The pathological findings of pulmonary GVHD are non-specific and other disease entities such as cryptogenic organizing pneumonia and non-specific interstitial pneumonitis may coexist. The radiograph shows interstitial changes that may progress to fibrosis.[54]

Acute effects of treatment on the heart

Cyclophosphamide may cause an acute haemorrhagic pancarditis when the dose exceeds 100 mg/kg/week. This results in pericardial effusion, mural thickening and endocardial, myocardial and epicardial haemorrhage. Echocardiography demonstrates abnormal diastolic function, small pericardial effusions and occasionally a restrictive cardiomyopathy.[26]

Key points: pulmonary infections

- Lung infections in immunocompromised patients are potentially lethal

- Lobar or segmental consolidation is frequently seen in bacterial infection as well as tuberculous and non-tuberculous microbacterial infections

- Pulmonary nodules which may cavitate are frequently seen in fungal infection, particularly aspergillosis and cryptoccocosis

- Diffuse infective lung disease is the characteristic of *Pneumocystis carinii* and CMV pneumonia but may be seen with non-infective conditions

The abdomen and pelvis

A variety of drug-related complications affect the gastro-intestinal system. Most are predictable and self-limiting and result from bowel irritation with nausea, vomiting and diarrhoea. Opiates and other drugs result in disordered gut motility in the cancer patient with either diarrhoea or fecal impaction. More serious complications may result from direct toxicity on the affected organ or be secondary to myelosuppression with its attendant risks of bleeding and infection. A few require specific investigation and treatment and occasionally these are life-threatening. It is important to recognize that cancer patients are still at risk from general surgical conditions and, in the setting of an acute abdomen, the radiologist is required to consider these conditions as well as treatment-related complications. Acute complications are divided into:

- Surgical emergencies
- Severe infections
- Drug toxicity in specific organs

Acute complications of radiotherapy and postsurgical complications are discussed in Chapter 55.

Surgical emergencies

Cancer patients may develop common surgical conditions of the abdomen and pelvis and some therapies increase the likelihood of these. Treatment with both corticos-teroids and non-steroidal anti-inflammatory drugs may result in intestinal perforation. Disordered coagulation may result in either bleeding or thrombosis of the vascular pedicle. A number of more specific treatment-related conditions result in acute intestinal inflammation and these include infectious and non-infectious colitis including neutropenic colitis (typhlitis), other severe infections and GVHD.

There is a considerable overlap in the clinical and imaging features of these conditions. Symptoms such as diarrhoea and vomiting may be expected side-effects of treatment as well as early symptoms of more serious complications. The severity of pain and tenderness may be reduced by analgesia and corticosteroid medication masking clinical features. Some patients do not have specific gastro-intestinal symptoms, merely generalized constitutional symptoms and fever and thus investigation is for pyrexia of unknown origin. Given the paucity of specific clinical pointers the radiologist has a key role in the diagnosis and management of complications.

Plain abdominal radiographs are useful to assess alternative conditions such as bowel obstruction and pseudo-obstruction and to exclude pneumoperitoneum. It may be difficult to obtain satisfactory horizontal beam films of the chest and abdomen in the sick cancer patient who cannot travel to the radiology department. Plain radiographic signs of gastro-intestinal complications of therapy include:

- Ileus, particularly affecting the caecum
- Wall thickening, irregularity and mucosal islands (Fig. 52.11)
- Pneumatosis intestinalis (Fig. 52.12)
- Pneumoperitoneum, localized or generalized

Computed tomography is increasingly used as experience of imaging the acute abdomen increases. Additionally, CT offers the therapeutic intervention of aspiration or drainage of fluid collections. Computed tomography demonstrates the layers of the bowel wall as well as its surrounding fat, the peritoneal cavity, mesenteric vascular pedicle and solid organs. Intravenous contrast is valuable to show bowel wall vascularity and this may be better shown without administration of oral contrast, which is often poorly tolerated by these patients. When there is genuine concern for body wall or intestinal haemorrhage, preliminary unenhanced CT should be performed.[55] With inflammatory complications, CT findings in both the small and large bowel, of increasing severity, are:[56]

- Mucosal hyperaemia
- Wall thickening and oedema (the 'halo' sign)
- Dilatation or luminal narrowing
- Perienteric stranding and mesenteric oedema
- Localized or free intraperitoneal fluid
- Para-enteric abscess
- Localized or free pneumoperitoneum

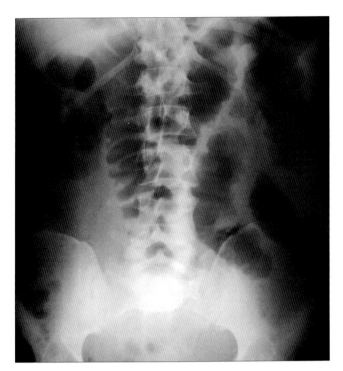

Figure 52.11. *Plain abdominal radiograph showing small bowel wall and fold thickening with thumbprinting, suggesting either intestinal ischaemia or haemorrhage. Venous ischaemia and intramural haemorrhage was found at surgery in this leukaemic patient with mesenteric vein thrombosis.*

Neutropenic colitis and typhlitis

This is a necrotizing inflammatory process originally decribed after chemotherapy for leukaemia[57] and childhood tumours but is increasingly recognized in treatment of lymphoma, AIDS[58] and solid tumours as regimens become more intensive. A wide variety of chemotherapeutic agents have been implicated. Neutropenia is defined as <1000 cells/mm[3]. It is believed that mucosal injury from the chemotherapy initiates the process which may be limited to mucosal inflammation or progress through transmural inflammation to perforation with overgrowth by a variety of organisms. Gram-negative bowel organisms are common pathogens but Gram-positive organisms, viruses and fungi are recognized.

There are three forms of neutropenic colitis but the right colon is predominantly involved. In the commonest form of typhlitis, the caecum is involved and dilates (in Greek a typhlon is a blind-ended sac). Another form also involves the terminal ileum, and in a third there is more generalized bowel ulceration. Patients present with right iliac fossa pain suggestive of appendicitis and, if untreated, may progress rapidly to perforation. Computed tomography is performed to assess alternative diagnoses such as appendicitis (Fig. 52.13) and to look for perforation and abscess formation. In typhlitis limited to the caecum, CT may show distension, circumferential wall thickening with a halo sign of wall oedema. Surgeons are wary of operating. Computed tomography may allow aspiration and drainage of any collection. Imaging findings overlap with other conditions but the finding of pneumatosis intestinalis with gas in the bowel wall is suggestive of typhlitis (Fig. 52.14).

Pseudomembranous colitis

Pseudomembranous colitis is classically associated with antibiotic use and is due to toxin production by *Clostridium difficile*. It is increasingly seen in cancer patients where the association with antibiotic use is more speculative. Rather than the distal or pancolitis seen in earlier reports it is now recognized to be predominantly right sided in 30–40% of

Figure 52.12. *Plain abdominal radiograph showing pneumatosis intestinalis in a 2-year-old leukaemic patient. The situation resolved without surgery and at follow-up CT the bowel appeared unremarkable.*

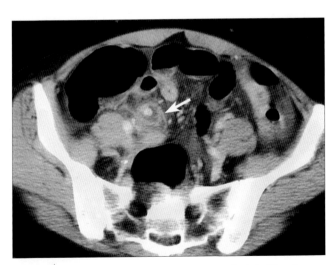

Figure 52.13. *CT of a leukaemic patient with right iliac fossa pain and caecal dilatation showing a thick-walled appendix postero-medial to this containing an appendicolith (arrowed) not visible on the abdominal radiograph. Surgery followed CT and imminent appendix rupture was found.*

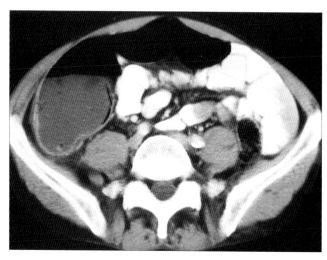

Figure 52.14. *CT of another leukaemic patient with right iliac fossa pain. In this case there is caecal dilatation, wall thickening and pneumatosis in its medial wall in keeping with typhlitis. The case was managed conservatively.*

cases. Stool culture, toxin analysis and proctosigmoidoscopy are usually diagnostic. Plain films show mucosal oedema and irregularity with thumbprinting. There may be progressive dilatation leading to mucosal destruction and perforation. It is now uncommon to perform contrast studies of the bowel but these show a non-specific colitis. If complications are suspected and the diagnosis remains uncertain, CT may be useful. There may be few symptoms and occasionally the diagnosis only comes to light on staging CT studies (Fig. 52.15). Computed tomography shows bowel wall thickening and mucosal hyperaemia which may

spare the rectum. In more severe cases there is marked thickening of the haustra, usually exceeding a centimetre but up to 3 cm, a helpful discriminator as this degree of thickening is rare in other colitides.[59-61]

Graft versus host disease

Graft versus host disease occurs in patients following BMT and represents an immunological response by donor lymphocytes against host tissues. Acute GVHD occurs within the first 100 days after transplant, causing a skin rash, severe mucosal inflammation and diarrhoea. Chronic GVHD may occur as early as 45–50 days after transplantation, with a skin rash resembling scleroderma. Severe mucosal inflammation is followed by fibrosis and stricture formation. The oesophagus is principally affected, less commonly the small and large bowel.[58,61] Plain radiographic findings are non-specific and include air–fluid levels, bowel wall and mucosal fold thickening, dilatation of bowel loops but occasionally a gasless abdomen.[62] Barium studies confirm the mucosal thickening and flattening, causing 'ribbon bowel', and a rapid transit time. In severe cases, prolonged coating of the bowel wall is seen as barium fills ulcers in the wall and may even be incorporated.[63] Both the colon and small bowel may be simultaneously involved although the ileocolic region is most prone to attack. Computed tomography findings are non-specific and show a spectrum of inflammatory changes.[64] With small bowel involvement, the length affected acts as a clue to the diagnosis but the clinical context is the key indicator (Fig. 52.16).[65]

Pneumatosis intestinalis

Pneumatosis intestinalis is an uncommon condition that is not well understood. Its clinical significance is variable. In some cases it is merely a reversible radiological fascination of no clinical significance (Fig. 52.12). However, GVHD,

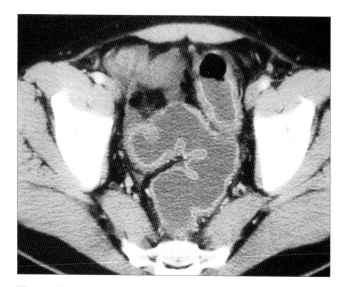

Figure 52.15. *CT of the pelvis in an outpatient showing pseudomembranous colitis with colonic mucosal hyperaemia and wall oedema. The patient had attributed symptoms to the chemotherapy.*

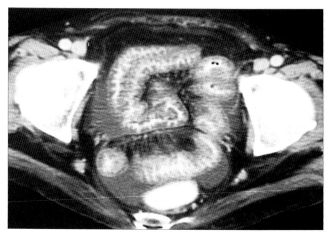

Figure 52.16. *CT of the pelvis showing diffuse small bowel thickening and some free fluid. The length of involvement in this bone marrow transplant patient suggests the diagnosis of graft versus host disease.*

CMV or other infections and typhlitis can all be complicated by pneumatosis and it may herald severe complications.[58] Pneumatosis is predominantly right-sided and is a poor prognostic indicator in the context of systemic infection and/or shock.[66]

Other complications resulting in an acute abdomen

Haemorrhage may occur at a variety of sites in thrombocytopenic patients, including the body wall musculature, notably the iliopsoas and rectus compartments, the bowel, the peritoneal cavity and within pre-existing lesions (Fig. 52.17), especially those undergoing rapid necrosis. Bleeding at any of these sites may result in acute abdominal symptoms. Plain film findings are typically normal unless mural haemorrhage results in intestinal obstruction but there may be wall thickening (Fig. 52.11). The distinction from intestinal ischaemia is difficult with enhanced CT. A short segment with greater than one centimetre of wall thickening favours haemorrhage.[67]

Response to some chemotherapies may lead to bowel complications. As well as bleeding into lesions there may be cystic enlargement or loculation of ascites leading to compression or obstruction.[68] Tumour lysis within bowel may lead directly to perforation or fistulation into adjacent involved solid organs.[69] This is seen with lymphoma (especially high-grade) and other chemosensitive tumours such as gastro-intestinal stromal tumours (Fig. 52.18).

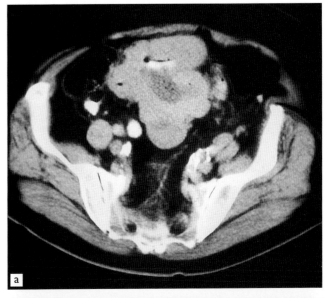

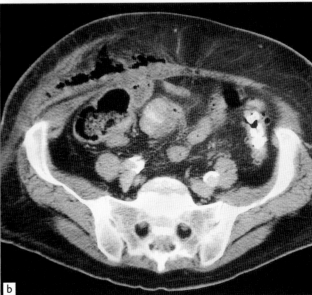

Figure 52.18. *Perforation of a gastro-intestinal stromal tumour. (a) CT at diagnosis showing a thick-walled loop of small bowel and (b) during chemotherapy showing virtually complete resolution of the mass but loculated gas and fluid anterior to the mass and within the abdominal wall. An enterocutaneous fistula was found at surgery.*

Severe infections

Candida albicans

Disseminated candidiasis may be seen in the severely immunocompromised patient and can affect almost any site but with few specific radiological features. In the gut it may cause mucosal erosion and ulceration. A highly suggestive appearance in the oesophagus is multiple pseudodiverticula. Abscess formation is common and these may be multiple microabscesses in the liver, spleen and kidneys (Fig. 52.19). Ultrasound and CT have been used tradition-

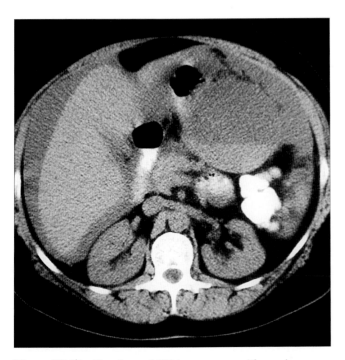

Figure 52.17. *Unenhanced CT in a woman with ovarian cancer presenting with acute epigastric pain showing layering out of acute haemorrhage within a cystic lesion in the lesser sac.*

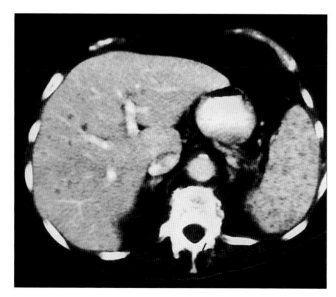

Figure 52.19. *CT of candidiasis with microabscesses in the liver and spleen.*

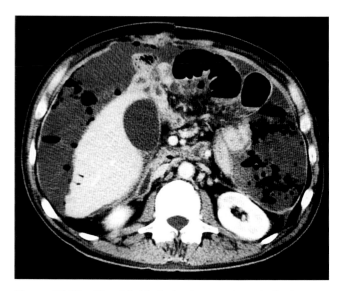

Figure 52.20. *Clostridial infection in a patient who had recently undergone gastric surgery for obstructing locally recurrent tumour whilst on chemotherapy. There are multiple tiny gas bubbles within the ascitic fluid as well as peripheral portal venous gas.*

ally to demonstrate visceral lesions that are typically less than 1 cm in size. The frequency of involvement is liver, spleen and then kidneys, and most patients have haematological malignancy.[70] Larger lesions cause a typical bull's eye appearance.[71] In suspected cases, MR may show more lesions but their appearances are not unique and both other infections such as tuberculosis and GVHD may mimic these.[72]

Cytomegalovirus

Abdominal radiographs in patients with CMV infection reveal bowel wall thickening, dilated bowel and fluid levels. Pneumatosis intestinalis may occur.[51] Patients who have undergone whole-body irradiation, and BMT with whole-body irradiation, are at risk for CMV infection and thus it can be difficult to distinguish this from GVHD in these patients.

Clostridial infection

As well as the toxic colitis which may result from intestinal Clostridial infection there are other severe and often fatal forms of invasive Clostridial infection including gas gangrene. Patients undergoing chemotherapy, particularly with leukaemia, are susceptible and again it is thought that mucosal injury allows invasion by normal gut pathogens. Recognition of gas formation within serosal cavities and tissue planes is crucial in suggesting the diagnosis and CT may be diagnostic well before clinical or radiographic signs are apparent. Here the radiologist has a key role in suggesting the diagnosis in the peritonitic or septic cancer patient (Fig. 52.20).[73] Soft tissue abscesses in neutropenic patients also result from *S. aureus* and Gram-negative bacteria but gas formation suggests Clostridial infection.

Drug toxicity in specific organs

Gastro-intestinal tract

Although many cancer patients have gastro-intestinal symptoms, there are few radiological manifestations. Complications are due to disordered motility, malabsorption, inflammation and ischaemia. 5-Fluorouracil causes gut toxicity and a clinical picture which mimics inflammatory bowel disease. Ischaemic colitis has been described with cisplatin and 5-FU.[74] Recently, docetaxel-based chemotherapy for metastatic breast cancer has been associated with a severe colitis, with some suggestion of exacerbation when in combination with vinorelbine.[75] Vincristine causes a neuropathy that may result in a chronic ileus with dilated, air-filled small bowel loops on the plain film.

Liver

Fatty infiltration, with increased echogenicity on ultrasonography and decreased attenuation on CT, is the most common manifestation and may be due to a variety of chemotherapies and corticosteroids.[76] Several drugs cause hepatic veno-occlusive disease, resulting in a clinical Budd–Chiari syndrome characterized by hepatomegaly and ascites.[76] Characteristic findings are a mosaic pattern within the liver which is well shown by contrast-enhanced CT or MR. The latter has the advantage of direct imaging along the plane of the hepatic veins.[77]

Pancreas

Acute pancreatitis may occur secondary to high-dose steroid therapy but it has also been described in patients receiving chemotherapy, notably L-asparaginase.[78]

Pancreatitis is usually diagnosed on clinical and biochemical features, but in more severe cases ultrasound and contrast-enhanced CT may be useful to assess the extent of the condition, including the degree of necrosis and complications such as pseudocyst and abscess formation. Both allow aspiration and drainage of complicated fluid collections. About 2% of children with acute lymphoblastic leuakaemia develop pancreatitis that is haemorrhagic. Ultrasound is the key imaging study in children.[78]

Urinary tract

Patients may present with acute renal failure due to nephrotoxic chemotherapy agents but urinary tract obstruction must be excluded. In any patient with deteriorating renal function, ultrasound is the investigation of choice to distinguish parenchymal disease from vascular disease and obstruction. Cytotoxic agents may cause non-opaque renal calculi, and treatment of myeloproliferative disorders can result in a uric acid nephropathy. Treatment of AIDS patients with protease inhibitors such as indivar also results in radiolucent stones, which may result in severe renal colic.[79] Computed tomography is valuable in confirming secondary signs of ureteric obstruction and excluding other causes of obstruction.

Key points: abdomino-pelvic complications

- Gastro-intestinal complications of chemotherapy include disordered motility, malabsorption inflammation and ischaemia. Most are predictable, self-limiting and require no imaging

- Bleeding diatheses may result in mural haemorrhage

- Neutropenic colitis (typhlitis) is an inflammatory transmural process causing thickening of the bowel wall around the caecum and terminal ileum

- Immunocompromised patients are susceptible to gut infection with Candida, CMV and Clostridium, including pseudomembranous colitis

- GVHD may affect the whole gastro-intestinal tract and is typically associated with skin changes

- Plain radiological signs of the above conditions are usually non-specific but pneumatosis intestinalis may indicate serious complications

- CT directly shows the bowel wall changes, perienteric inflammation and local or free perforation. It may allow abscess drainage

- The liver may show fatty infiltration as a response to many agents

- Acute pancreatitis has been described with L-asparaginase therapy in 2% of leukaemic children

- Cystic or haemorrhagic enlargement of lesions may result in bowel compromise

- Tumour lysis within bowel tumours, notably high-grade lymphoma, may result in perforation or fistulation

- Urinary tract complications of drug treatment include acute renal failure, renal calculi, which can be radiolucent in AIDS patients receiving protease inhibitors, and haemorrhagic cystitis

The central nervous system

In the central nervous system, complications of treatment for conditions such as leukaemia are more common than manifestations of the primary disease.[80] Simple and predictable complications of corticosteroid therapy, craniospinal radiotherapy and chemotherapy such as white matter changes and atrophy may be reversible. When atrophy is persistent after combination therapy this is usually the result of radiation damage. Myelosuppressive therapies lead to increased risks of infection and bleeding. Complications to be discussed are:

- Thrombosis and haemorrhage
- Drug-related toxicity
- Infectious complications

In a cancer patient with new cranial symptoms, the main concern is to exclude metastatic disease and brain CT should be the first investigation. With new spinal symptoms, MR is valuable in distinguishing between an intrinsic cord abnormality caused by tumour or myelitis (Fig. 52.21) and the various causes of spinal cord or cauda equina compression, including complications such as epidural infection or haemorrhage.

Thrombosis and haemorrhage

Patients with thrombocytopenia and other bleeding diatheses may develop intracranial or intraspinal haemorrhage. This may be intra-axial or affect any of the dural layers. Haemorrhage may complicate pre-existing primary tumours and metastases, leading to sudden deterioration. A particular concern is complications in patients undergoing lumbar puncture or other spinal interventions including intrathecal therapies.

Patients with cancer may also have an increased tendency to thrombosis leading to cerebral venous thrombosis. This diagnosis remains elusive unless suspected, especially as the haemorrhage and/or infarction resulting from this may give a ready explanation for symptoms whilst overshadowing the cause. Contrast-enhanced CT is valuable in investigation of this entity by showing the 'delta' sign but MR venography is the investigation of choice where available

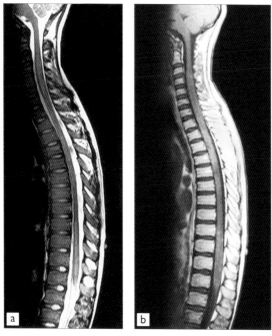

Figure 52.21. *MR of a 4-year-old leukaemic boy with previous craniospinal irradition and intrathecal chemotherapy presenting with a paraparesis. (a) A sagittal T2-weighted image of the spinal cord shows patchy high signal intensity, particularly in the conus and cervical region and (b) a post-gadolinium T1-weighted image showing no enhancement. CSF examination showed no leukaemic cells and a diagnosis of myelitis was made.*

(Fig. 52.22). Unenhanced CT is often the initial study and findings of venous thrombosis may be subtle, including a non-arterial territory distribution of infarcts, especially if bilateral and haemorrhagic. The presence of hyperdensity along the line of venous sinuses should alert to the diagnosis (Fig. 52.22).

Some chemotherapeutic agents such as L-asparaginase used in treatment of leukaemia may result in a disseminated intravascular coagulopathy with either bleeding or thrombotic sequelae including cerebral venous thrombosis.[81,82] Intra-axial bleeding is more common than extra-axial. Up to 2% of leukaemic patients treated with L-asparaginase develop haemorrhagic or non-haemorrhagic infarcts.[83]

Drug-related toxicity

A variety of drugs may be directly neurotoxic but the majority of these do not cause changes that can be identified radiologically (Table 52.1). The most common abnormality to be identified is craniospinal white matter change (leuco-encephalopathy).[84] The neurotoxic effects of chemotherapy may be potentiated by radiotherapy.[85] Drugs that cause leuco-encephalopathy include methotrexate, 5-FU, cytarabine and cyclosporin A.[86] The probable mechanism of chemotherapeutic toxicity is vascular injury, causing endothelial thickening, with eventual infarction and necro-

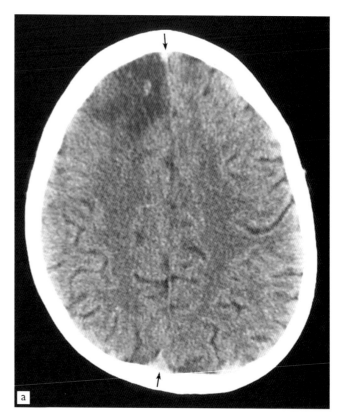

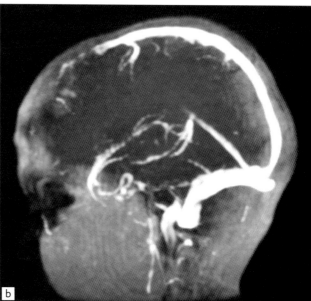

Figure 52.22. *A 9-year-old leukaemic patient presenting with a fit. (a) An unenhanced CT showing non-arterial territory infarction in the right frontal lobe with a petechial haemorrhage. High density is noted in the sagittal sinus (arrowed) and (b) MR venography confirming occlusion of the anterior end of the sagittal sinus.*

sis.[85] The other mechanism in leuco-encephalopathy is (re)activation of viral particles as seen with progressive multifocal leuco-encephalopathy (PML). These complications are discussed in Chapter 57.

Table 52.1. *Drugs causing neurotoxicity*

Drug	Toxicity
Vincristine	Peripheral neuropathy
Cisplatin	Peripheral neuropathy, encephalopathy
Cytarabine	Cerebellar dysfunction
Ifosfamide	Personality change, cerebellar dysfunction, cranial nerve lesions
5-Fluorouracil	Cerebellar dysfunction
Methotrexate	Focal neurological defects

With severe and established cases, focal or diffuse white matter low attenuation is seen with CT.[87] With MR there is high signal intensity on T2-weighted images.[84] Magnetic resonance usually reveals a greater burden of white matter lesions, especially with sequences using fluid-attenuated inversion recovery (FLAIR) sequence. There may be marginal enhancement with contrast media on either modality. A more aggressive focal or diffuse necrotizing leuco-encephalopathy with associated demyelination and necrosis is described as a later complication occurring after weeks or months of treatment. This is typically seen in treatment of leukaemia and is more common with combinations of intravenous and intrathecal methotrexate and radiotherapy. It may be reversed if intrathecal infusion of methotrexate is discontinued.[88] MR imaging reveals patchy involvement of the periventricular white matter and centrum semiovale, which becomes confluent. The subcortical U-fibres, corpus callosum, brain stem and cerebellum are spared. Enhancement and mass effect are only seen in the most severe cases mimicking tumour infiltration. Treatment of colonic cancer with 5-FU and levamisole may cause acute demyelination, with multifocal enhancing white matter lesions on MR.[89] It may preferentially affect the cerebellum causing ataxia.

There are also spinal effects of intrathecal therapies, resulting in a myelitis (Fig. 52.21) or radiculopathy. An anterior lumbosacral radiculopathy has been described with intrathecal methotrexate therapy. This entity is not well understood but may reflect gravitational dose-dependent toxicity on the nerve roots.[90] If the diagnosis is considered, intravenous injection of contrast medium is needed as root enhancement on MR may be the only abnormal finding in an examination performed to exclude an epidural haematoma.

Infectious complications

Neutropenic patients are predisposed to many infections of the central nervous system (CNS), including fungal and yeast infections, particularly aspergillosis, cryptococcus and candida. The risk is related to the degree of neutropenia. Fungi are a particular risk with neutrophil counts sustained for more than 2 weeks of less than 100/mm³.[82,91] Broad-spectrum antibiotic therapy also compounds this risk. Bacterial meningitis with *Haemophilus influenzae* and *S. pneumoniae* may occur in splenectomized patients.[92]

Infection of the meninges and brain may result from direct spread of aggressive infection in the paranasal sinuses and these should always be carefully inspected on CT and MR sections of the face and skull base, looking for bony changes on appropriate window settings (Fig. 52.23).[93] Complex sinus disease may also encroach into the orbit and there may be involvement of venous sinuses. In such cases the role of the radiologist is to alert to such complications, to look for abscess formation and, importantly, to consider the safety of lumbar puncture for microbiological assessment. In immunocompromised patients there may not be the immune response to infection seen in competent hosts and thus contrast enhancement may be reduced making distinction of masses and abscesses from infarcts more difficult.

It is not possible to provide a microbiological diagnosis on the basis of imaging features but a few key signs may be valuable in guiding antibiotic, antifungal or antiviral therapies. Aspergillosis[82,93] invades vascular structures with haemorrhagic infarction as well as abscess formation. Pulmonary or sinus infection is usually coincident. Cryptococcus[94] results in a meningitis with extension into the basal perforating substances with enhancing lesions in the midbrain and basal ganglia. Other organisms to consider with a basal meningitis are Listeria[86,95] and Tuberculosis,[86] which may show marked meningeal enhancement and lead to hydrocephalus. Cytomegalovirus infection affects the periventricular region with a nodular rim of subependymal enhancement. Many agents may result in an encephalitis but herpes simplex virus[86] preferentially attacks the temporal lobes. Changes are often asymmetric.

Progressive multifocal leuco-encephalopathy

Progressive multifocal leuco-encephalopathy has been described in patients treated with immunosuppressive agents, although recently it has been more commonly associated with AIDS. It is a demyelinating disease that results from reactivation of latent papovavirus. MR imaging shows asymmetric, patchy, non-enhancing lesions of the peripheral white matter which progress to large confluent lesions involving the deep white matter. The brain stem and cerebellum are affected in approximately one third of patients. Haemorrhage and peripheral enhancement occur rarely. Typically, the disease affects the cerebral hemispheres but, more recently, selective involvement of the brain stem is recognized.[96]

Conclusions

Most acute complications of treatment are predictable and self-limiting, well-recognized by experienced clini-

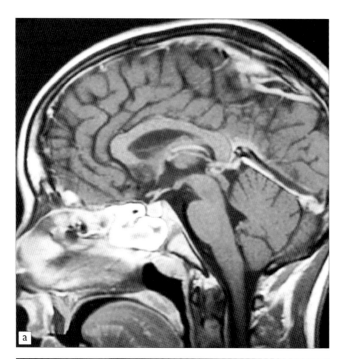

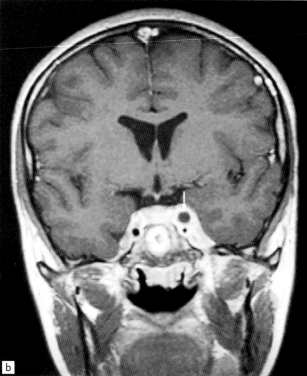

Figure 52.23. *MR of complicated sinus infection: a 14-year-old patient undergoing high-dose chemotherapy for soft tissue sarcoma presenting with left-sided ophthalmoplegia. (a) A T1-weighted midline sagittal section shows enhancing material in the sphenoid sinus and (b) a coronal section shows a septic thrombosis of the left cavernous sinus (arrowed) compressing the carotid artery below it.*

cians and require no involvement of the radiologist. With more serious symptoms the role of the radiologist is to help clinical colleagues to make a distinction between the effects of the cancer and those of its treatment so that ineffective or toxic agents can be discontinued. The radiologist may be able to provide support for diagnoses with appropriate aspiration and drainage of infected fluid collections as well as offering a variety of other palliative interventions. In the 'asymptomatic' patient, it is important to be alert to the possibility of complications that may have arisen between clinic visits. When a patient attends for re-staging CT prior to clinical reassessment, the radiologist may be the first physician to encounter the problem.

There is a bewildering array of new agents available to the oncologist and a tendency for treatment later into the natural history of the cancer. The radiologist cannot be expected to keep abreast of all their complications but these mainly follow patterns recognized with standard therapies. Good communication between the radiologist and the oncologist is vital for the early recognition and accurate diagnosis of complications related to treatment and is facilitated by involvement in regular multidisciplinary meetings.

Key points: CNS complications

- MR is the most sensitive imaging modality to identify the neurotoxic effects of cancer treatment

- MR venography shows venous sinus thrombosis, which is a complication of L-asparaginase therapy for leukaemia

- Spinal MR helps to distinguish between tumour, myelitis, epidural infection or haematoma, which may particularly complicate intrathecal therapies

- Necrotizing leuco-encephalopathy is usually seen in combination therapy with intravenous or intrathecal methotrexate and radiotherapy for the treatment of leukaemia

- Acute demyelination may be seen following treatment with other drugs such as 5-FU

- Immunocompromised patients are susceptible to CNS infection producing meningitis and encephalitis and this may spread from the paranasal sinuses

- PML is most commonly associated with AIDS and is associated with papovavirus infection

Summary

- Intravenous catheter-related complications include malposition, occlusion and sepsis

- Pneumothorax is the most common complication of insertion of an indwelling catheter

- CT is currently the method of choice for demonstrating superior vena caval thrombosis

- Doppler ultrasonography may show thrombus within the subclavian, internal jugular and axillary veins either directly or using accessory signs of damped flow or phasicity

- Catheter-related sepsis occurs in up to 20% of patients but if superficial may not require removal of the line

- Pulmonary fibrosis is the most common manifestation of lung toxicity due to chemotherapy and is seen most frequently with bleomycin

- Opportunistic infection of the lungs in immuno-compromised patients is an important potentially lethal condition

- GVHD following BMT affects the oesophagus and small bowel but is usually suggested by associated skin changes

- Neutropenic colitis (typhlitis) represents an inflammatory process involving the caecum and terminal ileum

- Pneumatosis intestinalis is seen in GVHD, CMV infection and typhlitis

- CT directly shows the bowel wall changes, perienteric inflammation and local or free perforation. It may allow abscess drainage

- Abdominal complications of drug treatment include gut toxicity, fatty infiltration of the liver, pancreatitis, acute renal failure, renal calculi and haemorrhagic cystitis

- A variety of drugs are neurotoxic but the majority do not produce changes visible on imaging

- MR is the most sensitive technique for identifying white matter abnormalities in the brain related to treatment

- MR venography shows venous sinus thrombosis which is a complication of L-asparaginase therapy for leukaemia

- The white matter effects of chemotherapy are often potentiated by radiotherapy, e.g. intravenous methotrexate and radiotherapy for treatment of acute leukaemia

- CNS infection is an important complication of treatment in immunocompromised patients

- Reactivation of papovavirus is implicated in the development of progressive multifocal leuco-encephalopathy. This is particularly common in AIDS

References

1. Denny D F Jr. Placement and management of long-term central venous access catheters and ports. Am J Roentgenol 1993; 161: 385–393

2. O'Neill V J, Jeffrey Evans T R, Preston J et al. A retrospective analysis of Hickman line-associated complications in patients with solid tumours undergoing infusional chemotherapy. Acta Oncol 1999; 38: 1103–1107

3. Aronchick J M, Miller W T Jr. Tubes and lines in the intensive care setting. Semin Roentgenol 1997; XXXII: 102–116

4. Duntley P, Siever J, Korwes M L et al. Vascular erosion by central venous catheters: clinical features and outcome. Chest 1992; 101: 1633–1638

5. Tocino I M, Watanabe A. Impending catheter perforation of superior vena cava: radiographic recognition. Am J Roentgenol 1986; 160: 467–471

6. Wechsler R J, Steiner R M, Kinori I. Monitoring the monitors: the radiology of thoracic catheters, wires and tubes. Semin Roentgenol 1988; 23: 61–84

7. Krutchen A E, Bjarnason H, Stackhouse D J et al. The mechanisms of positional dysfunction of subclavian venous catheters. Radiology 1996; 200: 159–163

8. Crain M R, Horton M G, Mewissen M W. Fibrin sheaths complicating central venous catheters. Am J Roentgenol 1998; 171: 341–346

9. Ardalan B, Flores M R. A new complication of chemotherapy administered by a permanent indwelling catheter. Cancer 1995; 75: 2165–2168

10. Hill S L, Berry R E. Subclavian vein thrombosis: a continuing challenge. Surgery 1993; 104: 561–567

11. Bashist B, Parisi A, Frager D H et al. Abdominal CT findings when the superior vena cava, brachiocephalic vein, or subclavian vein is obstructed. Am J Roentgenol 1996; 167: 1457–1463

12. Cihangiroglu M, Lin B H, Dachman A H. Collateral pathways in superior vena caval obstruction as seen on CT. J Comput Assist Tomogr 2001; 25: 1–8

13. Nazarian G K, Foshager M C. Color Doppler sonography of the thoracic inlet veins. Radiographics 1995; 15: 1357–1371

14. Patel M C, Berman L H, Moss H A et al. Subclavian and internal jugular veins at Doppler US: abnormal cardiac

pulsatility and respiratory phasicity as a predictor of complete central occlusion. Radiology 1999; 211: 579–583

15. Carter M M, Tarr R W, Mazer M J et al. The 'aortic nipple' as a sign of impending superior vena caval syndrome. Chest 1985; 87: 775–777

16. Brown G, Husband J E. Mediastinal widening: a valuable radiographic sign of superior vena cava thrombosis. Clin Radiol 1993; 47: 415–420

17. Finn J P, Zisk J H, Edelman R R et al. Central venous occlusion: MR angiography. Radiology 1993; 187: 245–251

18. Thornton M J, Ryan R, Varghese J C et al. A three-dimensional gadolinium-enhanced MR venography technique for imaging central veins. Am J Roentgenol 1999; 173: 999–1003

19. Oxtoby J W, Widjaja E, Gibson K M et al. 3D gadolinium-enhanced MRI venography: evaluation of the central chest veins and impact on patient management. Clin Radiol 2001; 56: 887–894

20. Yip D, Funaki B. Subcutaneous chest ports via the internal jugular vein. A retrospective study of 117 oncology patients. Acta Radiol 2002; 43: 371–375

21. Lorenz J M, Kunaki B, Van Ha T et al. Radiologic placement of implantable chest ports in paediatric patients. Am J Roentgenol 2001: 176: 991–994

22. Press O W, Ramsey P G, Larson E B et al. Hickman catheter infections in patients with malignancies. Medicine (Baltimore) 1984; 63: 189–200

23. Raad I I, Hanna H A. Intravascular catheter-related infections: new horizons and recent advances. Arch Intern Med 2002; 162: 871–878

24. Hachem R, Raad I I. Prevention and management of long-term catheter related infections in cancer patients. Cancer Invest 2002; 20: 1105–1113

25. Cleverley J R, Screaton N J, Hiorns M P et al. Drug-induced lung disease: high-resolution CT and histological findings. Clin Radiol 2002; 57: 292–299

26. Stoker D E. Pulmonary toxicity. In: DeVita V T, Hellmann S, Rosenberg S A (eds). Cancer: Principles and Practice of Oncology, 4th edn. Philadelphia: JB Lippincott, 1993

27. Aronchick J M, Gefter W B. Drug-induced pulmonary disorders. Semin Roentgenol 1995; XXX: 18–34

28. Haupt H M, Hutchins G M, Moore G W. Ara-C lung: noncardiogenic pulmonary edema complicating cytosine arabinoside therapy of leukemia. Am J Med 1981; 70: 256–261

29. Conant E F, Fox K R, Miller W T. Pulmonary edema as a complication of interleukin-2 therapy. Am J Roentgenol 1989; 152: 749–752

30. Comis R L. Bleomycin: Current status and new developments. In: Carter S K, Umezawa H, Crooke S T (eds). Bleomycin Pulmonary Toxicity. New York: Academic Press, 1978

31. Kreisman H, Wolkove N. Pulmonary toxicity of antineoplastic therapy. Semin Oncol 1992; 19: 508–512

32. Mills P, Husband J E. Computed tomography of

33. Horowitz A L, Freidman M, Smith J et al. The pulmonary changes of bleomycin toxicity. Radiology 1973; 106: 65–68

34. Padley S P G, Adler B, Hansell D M et al. High-resolution computed tomography of drug-induced lung disease. Clin Radiol 1992; 46: 232–236

35. Bellamy E A, Husband J E, Blaquiere R M et al. Bleomycin-related lung damage: CT evidence. Radiology 1985; 156: 155–158

36. Glasier C M, Siegel M J. Multiple pulmonary nodules: an unusual manifestation of bleomycin toxicity. Am J Roentgenol 1981; 137: 155–156

37. Bioselle P M, Morrin M M, Huberman M S. Gemcitabine pulmonary toxicity: CT features. J Comput Assist Tomogr 2000; 24: 977–980

38. Read W L, Mortimer J E, Picus J. Severe interstitial pneumonitis associated with doxetaxel administration. Cancer 2002; 94: 847–853

39. Worthy S A, Flint J D, Muller N L. Pulmonary complications after bone marrow transplantation: high-resolution CT and pathologic correlation. Radiographics 1997; 17: 1359–1371

40. Davis S D, Yankelevitz D F, Williams T et al. Pulmonary tuberculosis in immunocompromised hosts: epidemiological, clinical and radiological assessment. Semin Roentgenol 1993; XXVIII: 119–130

41. Goo J M, Im J G. CT of tuberculosis and nontuberculous mycobacterial infections. Radiol Clin North Am 2002; 40: 73–87

42. McLoud T C. Pulmonary infections in the immunocompromised host. Radiol Clin North Am 1989; 27: 1059–1066

43. Hruban R H, Meziane M A, Zerhouni E A et al. Radiologic–pathologic correlation of the CT halo sign in invasive pulmonary aspergillosis. J Comput Assist Tomogr 1987; 11: 534–536

44. McLoud T C, Naidich D P. Thoracic disease in the immunocompromised patient. Radiol Clin North Am 1992; 30: 525–554

45. Zinck S E, Leung A N, Frost M et al. Pulmonary cryptococcosis: CT and pathologic findings. J Comput Assist Tomogr 2002; 26: 330–334

46. Kuhlman J E. Pneumocystis infections: the radiologist's perspective. Radiology 1996; 198: 623–635

47. Panicek D M, Groskin S A, Cheung C T et al. Atypical distribution of *Pneumocystis carinii* infiltrates during radiation therapy. Radiology 1987; 163: 689–690

48. Ferre C, Baguena F, Podzamczer D et al. Lung cavitation associated with *Pneumocystis carinii* in the acquired immune deficiency syndrome: a report of six cases and review of the literature. Eur Resp J 1994; 7: 134–139

49. Kennedy C A, Goetz M B. Atypical roentgenographic manifestations of *Pneumocystis carinii* pneumonia. Arch Inter Med 1992; 152: 1390–1398

50. Kang E Y, Patz E F, Muller N L. Cytomegalovirus

pneumonia in transplant patients: CT findings. J Comput Assist Tomogr 1996; 20: 295–299

51. Olliff J F C, Williams M P. Radiological appearances of cytomegalovirus infections. Clin Radiol 1989; 40: 463–467

52. Cheah F K, Sheppard M N, Hansell D M. Computed tomography of diffuse pulmonary haemorrhage with pathological correlation. Clin Radiol 1993; 48: 89–93

53. Park J S, Lee K S, Kim J S et al. Nonspecific interstitial pneumonia with fibrosis: radiographic and CT findings in seven patients. Radiology 1995; 195: 645–648

54. Winer-Muram H T, Gurney J W et al. Pulmonary complications after bone marrow transplantation. Radiol Clin North Am 1996; 34: 97–117

55. Lane M J, Katz D S, Mindelzun R E et al. Spontaneous intramural small bowel haemorrhage: importance of non-contrast CT. Clin Radiol 1997; 52: 378–380

56. Macari M, Balthazar E J. CT of bowel wall thickening: significance and pitfalls of interpretation. Am J Roentgenol 2001; 176: 1105–1116

57. Wagner M L, Rosenberg H S, Fernbach D J et al. Typhlitis: a complication of leukemia in childhood. Am J Roentgenol 1970; 109: 341–350

58. Jones B, Wall S D. Gastrointestinal disease in the immunocompromised host. Radiologic Clin North Am 1992; 30: 555–577

59. Fishman E K, Kavuru M, Jones B et al. Pseudomembranous colitis: CT evaluation of 26 cases. Radiology 1991; 180: 57–60

60. Kawamoto S, Horton K M, Fishman E K. Pseudomembranous colitis: spectrum of imaging findings with clinical and pathologic correlation. Radiographics 1999; 19: 887–897

61. Horton K M, Corl F M, Fishman E K. CT evaluation of the colon: inflammatory disease. Radiographics 2000; 20: 399–418

62. Jones B, Cramer S S, Saral R et al. Gastrointestinal inflammation after bone marrow transplantation: graft-versus-host disease or opportunistic infection? Am J Roentgenol 1988; 150: 277–281

63. Belli A M, Williams M P. Graft versus host disease: findings on plain abdominal radiography. Clin Radiol 1988; 39: 262–264

64. Jones B, Fishman E K, Cramer S S et al. Computed tomography of gastrointestinal inflammation after bone marrow transplantation. Am J Roentgenol 1986; 146: 691–695

65. Horton K M, Corl F M, Fishman E K. CT of non-neoplastic diseases of the small bowel: spectrum of disease. J Comput Assist Tomogr 1999; 23: 417–428

66. Day D L, Ramsey N K C, Letourneau J G. Pneumatosis intestinalis after bone marrow transplantation. Am J Roentgenol 1988; 151: 85–87

67. Macari M, Chandarana H, Balthazar E et al. Intestinal ischemia versus intramural haemorrhage: CT evaluation. Am J Roentgenol 2003; 180: 177–184

68. Spencer J A, Crosse B A, Mannion R A et al. Gastroduodenal obstruction from ovarian cancer:

imaging features and clinical outcome. Clin Radiol 2000; 55: 264–272

69. Scott J, Spencer J A, MacLennan K A. Choledochoduodenal fistula complicating non-Hodgkin's lymphoma of the duodenum during chemotherapy. Clin Radiol. 2001; 56: 508–510

70. Shirkhoda A. CT findings in hepatosplenic and renal candidiasis. J Comput Assist Tomogr 1987; 11: 795–798

71. Haron E, Feld R, Tuffnell P et al. Hepatic candidiasis: an increasing problem in immunocompromised patients. Am J Med 1987; 83: 17–26

72. Semelka R C, Kelekis N L, Sallah S et al. Hepatosplenic fungal disease: diagnostic accuracy and spectrum of appearances on MR imaging. Am J Roentgenol 1997; 169: 1311–1316

73. Spencer J A, Elliot L. Clostridial infection of the abdomen: CT findings in two successfully treated patients. Am J Roentgenol 1996; 166: 1094–1096

74. Zilling T L, Ahren B. Ischaemic pancolitis. A serious complication of chemotherapy in a previously irradiated patient. Acta Chirurgica Scand 1989; 155: 77–79

75. Ibrahim N K, Sahin A A, Dubrow R A et al. Colitis associated with docetaxel-based chemotherapy in patients with metastatic breast cancer. Lancet 2000; 355: 281–283

76. Gatenby R A. The radiology of drug-induced disorders in the gastrointestinal tract. Semin Roentgenol 1995; XXX: 62–76

77. Ward J, Spencer J A, Guthrie J A et al. Liver transplantation: dynamic contrast-enhanced magnetic resonance imaging of the hepatic vasculature. Clin Radiol 1996; 51: 191–197

78. Sahu S, Saika S, Pai S K, Advani S H. L-Asparaginase (Leunase) induced pancreatitis in childhood acute lymphoblastic leukemia. Pediatr Hematol Oncol. 1998; 15: 533–538

79. Kohan A D, Armenkas N A, Fracchia J A. Indivar urolithiasis: an emerging cause of renal colic in patients with human immunodeficiency virus. J Urol 1999; 161: 1765–1768

80. Vazquez E, Lucaya J, Castellote A et al. Neuroimaging in pediatric leukaemia and lymphoma: differential diagnosis. Radiographics 2002; 22: 1411–1428

81. Ginsberg L E, Leeds L N. Neuroradiology of leukaemia. Am J Roentgenol 1995; 165: 525–534

82. Chen C, Zimmerman R A, Faro S et al. Childhood leukaemia: CNS abnormalities during and after treatment. Am J Neuroradiol 1996; 17: 295–310

83. Ho C L, Chen C Y, Chen Y C et al. Cerebral dural sinus thrombosis in acute lymphoblastic leukaemia with early diagnosis by fast fluid-attenuated inversion recovery (FLAIR) image: a case report and a review of the literature. Ann Hematol 2000; 79: 90–94

84. Packer R J, Zimmerman R A, Bilaniuc L T. Magnetic resonance imaging in the evaluation of treatment-related central nervous system damage. Cancer 1988; 61: 928–930

85. Paakko E, Vainionpaa L, Lanning M et al. White matter

changes in children treated for acute lymphoblastic leukaemia. Cancer 1992; 70: 2728–2733

86. Osborn A G. Diagnostic neuroradiology. St Louis, MO: Mosby, 1994

87. Pagani J J, Libshitz H I, Wallace S et al. Central nervous system leukaemia and lymphoma: computed tomographic manifestations. Am J Roentgenol 1981; 137: 1195–1201

88. Asato R, Akiyama Y, Ito M et al. Nuclear magnetic resonance abnormalities of the cerebral white matter in children with acute lymphoblastic leukaemia and malignant lymphoma during and after central nervous system prophylactic treatment with intrathecal methotrexate. Cancer 1992; 70: 1997–2004

89. Hook C C, Kimmel D W, Kvols L K et al. Multifocal inflammatory leukoencephalopathy with 5-fluorouracil and levamisole. Ann Neurol 1992; 31: 262–267

90. Koh S, Nelson M, Kovanlikaya A et al. Anterior lumbosacral radiculopathy after intrathecal methotrexate treatment. Pediatr Neurol 1999; 21: 576–578

91. Parisi M T, Fahmy J L, Kaminsky C K et al. Complications of cancer therapy in children: a radiologists guide. Radiographics 1999; 19: 283–297

92. Davenport C, Dillon W P, Sze G. Neuroradiology of the immunosuppressed state. Radiol Clin North Am 1992; 30: 611–637

93. Ashdown B C, Tien R D, Felsberg G J. Aspergillosis of the brain and paranasal sinuses in immunocompromised patients: CT and MR imaging findings. Am J Roentgenol 1994; 162: 155–159

94. Mathews V P, Alo P L, Glass J D et al. AIDS-related CNS cryptococcus: radiologic–pathologic correlation. Am J Neuroradiol 1992; 13: 1477–1486

95. Patchell R A, White C, Clark A W et al. Neurologic complications of bone marrow transplantation. Neurology 1985; 35: 300–306

96. Kastrup O, Maschke M, Diener H C, Wanke I. Progressive multifocal leukoencephalopathy limited to the brain stem. Neuroradiology. 2002; 44: 227–229

Part VII

EFFECTS OF TREATMENT ON NORMAL TISSUE

Chapter 53

Effects of treatment on normal tissue: thorax

Revathy B Iyer, Evelyne M Loyer, Reginald F Munden and Herman I Libshitz

Introduction

Radiotherapy and/or chemotherapy affect all tissues of the thorax. The evidence of these effects and the timing of their appearance vary from organ to organ. Radiation change is almost always seen in the lungs within weeks of completion of therapy. It is usually far less obvious in bone and takes years to be seen on conventional radiographs.

The details of the radiotherapy, including the volume and shape of the area treated, dose, time from completion of therapy, possible effects of other treatment, including chemotherapy, and the variability of human response are all factors that influence the appearance of radiotherapy change. The changes secondary to chemotherapy are usually dose-related. The radiotherapy changes described are for radiotherapy given with linear accelerators or Co-60 at 180–200 cGy/day with treatment given 5 days a week. The advent of three-dimensional conformal radiotherapy allows target volumes that minimize dose to normal structures and findings of radiation injury to the lung after such therapy will also be described.

Lung

Radiologists define radiation pneumonitis as evidence of acute radiotherapy changes in the lungs regardless of the clinical findings. Clinicians require that cough, fever and/or shortness of breath accompany the radiographic changes.[1] It has long been recognized that the radiographic changes of radiation pneumonitis are not necessarily accompanied by symptoms.[2]

Radiation pneumonitis is usually evident 6–8 weeks following completion of 3,500–4,000 cGy radiotherapy. It is generally not apparent below 3,000 cGy, variably seen between 3,000 and 3,500 cGy and almost always evident at doses over 4,000 cGy. For each 1,000 cGy over 4,000 cGy, it presents a week earlier following completion of therapy.

Radiation pneumonitis is most extensive about 3–4 months following completion of radiotherapy. From this point, the changes gradually organize, contract and evolve into radiation fibrosis. There are no pathognomonic histological findings of radiation pneumonitis.[3] The histological appearance of radiation pneumonitis is that of diffuse alveolar damage.[4] Similarly, the histological appearance of radi-

ation fibrosis is that of organizing diffuse, alveolar disease or end-stage fibrosis. This lack of histological specificity can result in difficulty in separating radiation effects from toxic effects of chemotherapeutic agents and/or infectious agents.

Key points: radiation pneumonitis

- Radiographic changes of radiation pneumonitis are not necessarily accompanied by symptoms

- Radiation pneumonitis is usually evident 6–8 weeks following completion of 3,000–4,000 cGy radiotherapy

- Radiation pneumonitis is most extensive about 3–4 months following completion of therapy

- On plain film, the fibrotic changes usually become stable 9–12 months following completion of therapy

Plain film findings

Radiation pneumonitis, when extensive, has sharp, well-defined areas of consolidation with borders that conform to the radiation portals, not anatomic boundaries.[5–7] Less extensive radiation pneumonitis may present as patchy consolidation in the irradiated fields (Fig. 53.1), or when early or minimal in extent, indistinctness of vessels. Familiarity with standard portals and the availability of prior radiographs facilitates identification of minimal changes. Reports of radiation change outside the radiation field are usually the result of oblique, rotational or misplaced fields.[8] A possible humoral cause is under investigation.[9]

Our experience indicates that radiation fibrosis or evidence of contraction secondary to fibrosis is seen in virtually all patients who received therapeutic doses of radiotherapy. Fibrosis usually presents as strand-like densities with volume loss.

When extensive, there is significant volume loss with bronchiectatic changes within it. While the fibrosis is usually obvious, it can be subtle (Fig. 53.2). The less obvious findings include minimal pleural thickening, slight elevation of one or both hila or the minor fissure, slight medial retraction of upper lobe pulmonary vessels, minimal tenting or elevation of a hemidiaphragm and minor blunting of cardiophrenic angles. The fibrotic changes usually become stable 9–12 months following completion of therapy (Fig.

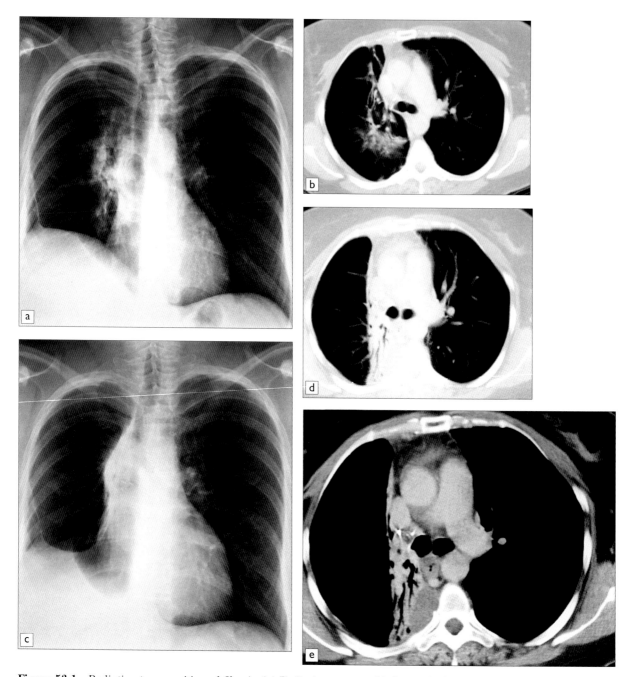

Figure 53.1. *Radiation pneumonitis and fibrosis. (a) Radiation pneumonitis is seen in the right lung 6 weeks following 6,000 cGy. A right upper lobectomy had also been performed for bronchogenic carcinoma. (b) CT scan at the same time as (a) showing patchy consolidation in the right lung. (c) Radiation fibrosis is present in the right lung 8 months following; (d) CT scan at the same time as (c) showing solid consolidation on lung windows. The sharp margin of the radiation changes is evident. (e) Same CT scan as (d) on soft tissue windows showing the bronchiectatic changes to better advantage. A small loculated pleural effusion is present medially (arrow).*

53.1). Any alteration in stable radiation fibrosis suggests either superinfection or recurrent disease.

The combined effect of radiotherapy and chemotherapy on normal lung is difficult to evaluate. Combined ther-

apy regimens are quite variable and chemotherapy has been given before, during and after radiotherapy. Empiric observation and small animal experimentation[10] has shown that the use of drugs that enhance the effects of radiation

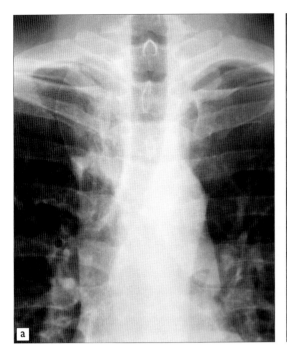

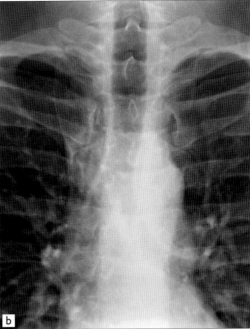

Figure 53.2. *Subtle changes of radiotherapy. (a) Baseline prior to radiotherapy for Hodgkin's disease. (b) Twelve months following radiotherapy there is slight retraction of the azygous fissure medially and slight medial contracture of the upper lobe vessels bilaterally as well as minimal elevation of the left hilum.*

cause greater radiation damage and a shorter time to the onset of radiation pneumonitis. The radiation-enhancing drugs include:

- Actinomycin D
- Adriamycin
- Bleomycin
- Cyclophosphamide
- Mitomycin C
- Vincristine[10]

There is disagreement regarding the effect of methotrexate.[10, 11]

Bleomycin, busulphan and methotrexate are recognized to cause pulmonary parenchymal injury independent of associated radiotherapy.[12] Bleomycin is used in the treatment of squamous cell carcinoma, lymphoma and testicular carcinoma. The toxicity is related to accumulation of drugs in the lung and is directly related to the cumulative dose administered.[12] The use of concomitant radiation, other chemotherapy, or oxygen therapy compounds the pulmonary toxicity. The early changes on chest radiography include a reticulonodular interstitial pattern, which is initially seen in the basal segments. Lung injury may be progressive, resulting in alveolar damage and eventual pulmonary fibrosis.[13] Gallium-67 is known to accumulate in damaged lung and is helpful in identifying bleomycin toxicity.[14] Busulphan used to treat leukaemia may also cause interstitial lung damage, resulting in a reticular pattern on conventional radiographs.[13] Methotrexate is also used in the treatment of leukaemia and other malignancies. A hypersensitivity reaction may occur resulting in alveolar infiltrates. Mediastinal adenopathy may also occur. The diffuse alveolar damage may result in fibrosis.[13]

Computed tomography and magnetic resonance findings

Computed tomography (CT), with its greater sensitivity to minimal differences in radiographic density, can identify radiation pneumonitis earlier than conventional radiographs.[15,16] It is also presumed that it can demonstrate radiation pneumonitis at lower radiotherapeutic doses than conventional radiographs. A dose-related effect with greater changes at higher doses has been described with CT.[17]

There have been four patterns of radiation change described at CT after conventional radiotherapy:[15]

- Homogeneous consolidation
- Patchy consolidation
- Discrete consolidation
- Solid consolidation

Homogeneous consolidation is thought to be a diffuse, minimal or early radiation pneumonitis that uniformly involves the irradiated lung. The appearance is similar to that of ground glass consolidation described in thin-section CT with vessels seen through the consolidation that uniformly affects the treated portions of the lungs. It may be seen within 2–3 weeks of completion of therapy. Patchy consolidation (Fig. 53.1) is thought to be the CT analogue of radiation pneumonitis on plain films. The consolidation is contained within the irradiated lung but does not involve the treated area uniformly. Discrete consolidation is defined by the irradiated field with well-demarcated borders but does not involve it uniformly (Fig. 53.3). Traction changes may be seen at the boundary of the treated lung. It is felt to represent fibrotic changes in treated lung with

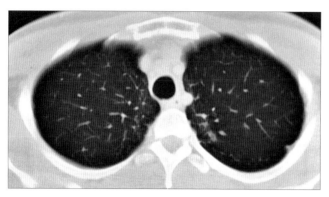

Figure 53.3. *Discrete consolidation is seen in the paramediastinal portions of both lungs 8 years following radiotherapy to the mediastinum for Hodgkin's disease (4,000 cGy). The irradiated volume is well defined with traction changes at the periphery of the field.*

areas of relative sparing. It is usually seen in the 3,500–4,000 cGy range as used in the therapy of Hodgkin's disease rather than in the higher doses used in treating lung cancer. Solid consolidation, which is generally seen at doses of 5,000 cGy and higher, more uniformly involves the treated lung causing consolidation and volume loss (Fig. 53.1). Bronchiectatic changes are seen within the area of volume loss in this pattern. It is the CT analogue of a dense radiation fibrosis.

Conventional radiotherapy results in the delivery of higher doses of radiation to surrounding tissues than to the primary tumour because of attenuation of the radiation. As more normal lung is included in the treatment, there is an increased risk of side-effects.[18] Three-dimensional conformal radiation therapy is used by radiation therapists to limit the amount of radiation injury to the lung and surrounding tissues. This technique uses multiple smaller beams of radiation aimed at the tumour so that large areas of surrounding tissues are not irradiated. This ensures that the entire target volume is adequately treated, while minimizing dose to normal structures.

Treatment planning for three-dimensional conformal radiation is accomplished using three-dimensional images of the patient. Computer software determines the best orientations of the radiation beams that will deliver therapeutic dosages to the tumour while at the same time limiting the dosage of radiation to the surrounding tissues. Each beam will have a portion of the total amount of radiation delivered. The radiation from these multiple ports is additive at the tumour and ensures that the entire tumour volume is adequately treated, allowing higher dosages of radiation to be delivered to the tumour without increasing injury to the surrounding tissues. This technique also potentially improves local tumour control and decreases toxicity from injury to normal structures.[19,20]

Three-dimensional radiation therapy is well suited to patients who are not surgical candidates because of pre-existing cardiac disease or who do not have adequate pulmonary reserve to tolerate lobectomy or standard radiation therapy. It is particularly useful in those patients with Stage I disease who cannot tolerate standard treatment; the radiation therapist can offer these patients treatment with curative intent.

However, this complex distribution of radiation dose to the tumour and surrounding lung tissue manifests as patterns of lung injury that are different than those reported after conventional radiotherapy. With less radiation of the surrounding tissue, the majority of radiation-induced injury is at the tumour site. Three patterns have been described as a result of three-dimensional conformal radiation therapy: mass-like, modified conventional and scar-like.[21] Mass-like opacities occur when the radiation fibrosis forms a mass appearance immediately surrounding the tumour. Modified conventional patterns occur when the radiation fibrosis looks like conventional radiation fibrosis, but the extent is limited to the lobe involved with tumour. The lung in the same plane as the tumour, but located peripherally, is not involved as in conventional fibrosis. Scar-like patterns occur when only a thin band of 1 cm or less of fibrosis remains after treatment (Fig 53.4). This thin band forms a scar-like appearance and one may not know a tumour existed without prior studies.

The oedema and inflammatory change of radiation pneumonitis are seen on MR imaging as increased signal intensity on T2-weighted images and low signal intensity on T1-weighted images.[22] Radiation fibrosis would be expected to demonstrate low signal intensity at both T1- and T2-weighted images. Unfortunately, increased signal intensity on T2-weighted images[23] and contrast enhancement[24] may be seen in irradiated lung at a time when fibrosis would be expected. These non-specific signal intensity changes have made MR evaluation of recurrent disease in irradiated patients problematic.

Other imaging findings

Other less common complications include:

- Hyperlucency of an irradiated lung[25]
- Spontaneous pneumothorax[26]
- Pleural effusions secondary to radiotherapy[27]
- Calcification in lymph nodes[28]

Effusions are usually small and more frequently seen with CT (Fig. 53.5). They are indistinguishable from malignant pleural effusions. They usually develop within 6 months of therapy and may resolve spontaneously.[27] Rapid increase or reaccumulation after thoracocentesis speaks for a malignant origin. If cytological examination is negative, prolonged follow-up may be necessary.

Calcification may occur in lymph nodes following therapy for lymphoma.[28] This is more frequent in Hodgkin's disease and far more common following radiotherapy than in patients treated only with chemotherapy. The calcifica-

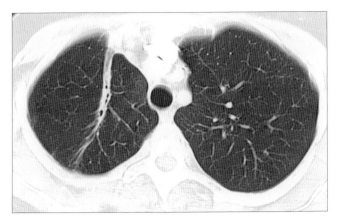

Figure 53.4. *Scar like pattern of three-dimensional conformal radiation therapy. CT of a patient treated for squamous cell carcinoma shows a linear band of radiation fibrosis at the site of original tumour.*

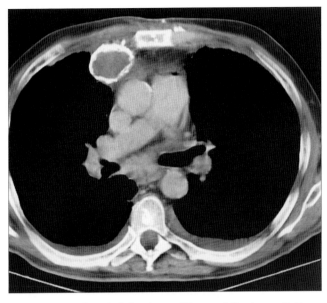

Figure 53.6. *Calcified thymic cyst 30 years following radiation therapy in a patient treated for Hodgkin's disease. The subcarinal adenopathy and small bilateral pleural effusions are related to a current non-small cell lung cancer.*

tion begins about a year after therapy and gradually gets denser over years. Cystic changes that may calcify have been described in the thymus in patients irradiated for Hodgkin's disease (Fig. 53.6).[29] Very rarely, malignant pleural mesotheliomas may develop after radiotherapy.[30]

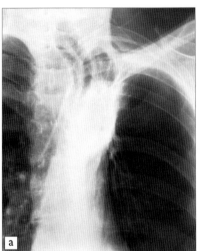

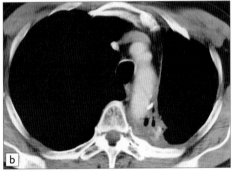

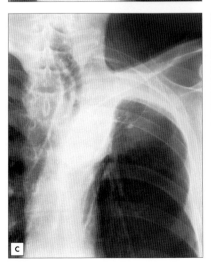

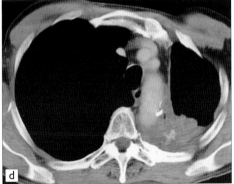

Figure 53.5. *Recurrent lung cancer following radiotherapy. (a) Close-up of left upper chest showing radiation change 9 months following radiotherapy. (b) CT scan at the same time as (a) showing solid consolidation. (c) Mass is now seen 3 months following (a) in the left upper chest and the air-containing lung above the aortic knob has been obliterated. (d) CT scan at the same time as (c) showing mass and filling in of bronchiectatic changes.*

Key points: imaging findings of pneumonitis

■ Ground glass consolidation can be seen on CT within 2–3 weeks after completion of therapy

■ Bronchiectatic changes may be seen within areas of volume loss

■ Three-dimensional conformal radiotherapy results in radiation-induced injury that is usually localized in the tumour site

■ Less common findings include hypotranslucency of the irradiated lung and even a spontaneous pneumothorax

Evaluation of treated areas

Identification of residual or recurrent malignancy in the thorax may be made more difficult by the superimposition of radiation changes in the areas of concern. In these cases, CT most often provides adequate visualization of pulmonary parenchymal masses and/or the mediastinum following radiotherapy (see also Chapter 7, Lung Cancer). In irradiated lymphoma, a residual mediastinal mass need not represent viable disease and in patients who have been appropriately treated, further therapy is not warranted.[31,32] Enlarging nodes or mass does speak for recurrence. By comparison, a residual mass in bronchogenic carcinoma generally represents residual disease.

Awareness of the timing of radiation change is most helpful in identifying recurrent disease. Routine follow-up studies at 2- to 3-month intervals following completion of radiotherapy aids in making these observations. Features that should suggest recurrent disease include:

• Alteration in stable contours of radiation fibrosis (Fig. 53.5)

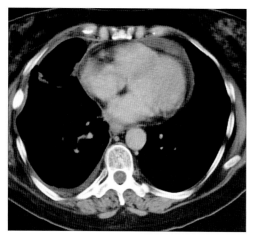

Figure 53.7. *Small right pleural effusion and eccentric small pericardial effusion 8 months following radiotherapy to a non-small cell bronchogenic carcinoma centrally in the right lung.*

• Failure of contracture of an area of radiation pneumonitis when expected 4 months or more after completion of therapy

• Absence of air-containing ectatic bronchi in an area of solid consolidation at CT, especially if ectatic bronchi were present previously.[33] The filling in of radiation therapy-induced ectatic bronchi may be the first sign of recurrence, or may be seen along with other signs of recurrence, and is a reliable CT sign of locally recurrent lung cancer[34]

Infection can usually be distinguished from radiation pneumonitis both by knowledge of the field size and shape, and the date of completion of therapy. However, it is virtually impossible to exclude superimposed infection in an area of radiation pneumonitis with imaging. Further bronchial ectasia or tissue destruction in a treated area suggests superinfection. Recurrent malignancy causing distal pneumonia may be confusing.

Key point: evaluation of treated areas

■ Awareness of the timing of radiation change, knowledge of the field size and shape and the date of completion of therapy, are essential for radiological identification of superinfection or of residual or recurrent malignant disease

Heart

The spectrum of radiation-induced heart disease includes:

• Acute and chronic pericarditis
• Coronary artery disease
• Valvular dysfunction
• Cardiomyopathy
• Conduction abnormalities

Radiation-induced heart disease, particularly ichaemic disease, is more frequent and of greater clinical significance than had been previously thought.[35,36] Evaluation of myocardial perfusion of asymptomatic long-term survivors, primarily patients treated for Hodgkin's disease, has shown a high incidence of subclinical myocardial lesions.[37]

Pericardial disease

Fajardo et al. have described thickening of the pericardium with fibrosis, fibrin deposition and protein-rich pericardial effusions. Myocardial fibrosis also occurs but, unlike the focal fibrosis seen after infarction, it has a patchy involvement that follows the collagen framework of the myocardium.[38]

The incidence of pericarditis is related to the dose, fraction size, volume irradiated and technique. Below 4,000 cGy, the incidence is quite low. At 4,000 cGy, it ranges from 2 to 6%[39–42] and has been reported to be as high as 20% at 4,500 cGy.[42] Cosset reported an incidence of 4.1% at 3,500–3,700 cGy that rose to 10.4% at 4,100–4,300 cGy.[41] Moderate-sized mediastinal fields have a 1% incidence of pericardial disease that rises to 17% when the fields are larger with treatment of extensive disease.[40] Techniques previously used with only anterior fields gave a 50% greater dose to the pericardium than the dose delivered to the mid-plane.[43] The dose relationship of coronary artery disease has not yet been demonstrated.[41]

Radiation pericarditis generally presents 6–9 months after therapy and the majority of cases will occur within 12–18 months of therapy, but it may appear many years after radiotherapy. Acute and chronic pericarditis is seen with equal frequency. Both are indistinguishable clinically from other causes of pericarditis.[44]

Symmetrical increase in the size of the cardiac silhouette is the typical appearance of radiation-induced pericardial effusion. Eccentric effusions may occur, presumably because of adhesions in the treated area of the pericardium, that prevent uniform distribution of the fluid (Fig. 53.7).[45] Small pericardial effusions or pericardial thickening are more easily identified with cross-sectional imaging techniques, ultrasound, CT or MR. Far higher incidences of pericardial effusion will be found with these techniques. In a series of breast cancer patients treated with radiotherapy, Ikäheimo found that 33% had pericardial effusions on ultrasound examination.[46]

Evidence of radiation change in the lungs, either pneumonitis or fibrosis depending on the timing following therapy, is almost always present and can raise the possibility of radiation as the cause of pericardial disease. The major differential consideration is malignant pericardial effusion, which may be suggested by nodularity of the pericardium or mediastinal adenopathy. Cytological evaluation of pericardial fluid is necessary for a definitive diagnosis and is not always positive even in malignant disease. Exclusion of a pericardial effusion as the cause of cardiac enlargement in a patient whose heart has been irradiated raises the question of cardiomyopathy or ischaemic heart disease.

Key points: pericardial disease

- The incidence of pericardial disease is related to the dose, fraction size, volume irradiated and technique – below 4,000 cGy the incidence is low

- Radiation pericarditis generally presents 6–9 months after therapy and the majority occur within 12–18 months after therapy

- Evidence of radiation change in the lungs is almost always present in association with pericardial disease

Myocardial disease

Myocardial abnormalities, particularly ischaemic in aetiology, can result from radiation. The development of cardiomyopathy may also result from the use of chemotherapeutic agents. At a total cumulative dose of 550 mg/m² of doxorubicin, 1–2% of patients have overt congestive heart failure.[47] Non-invasive diagnostic modalities, such as echocardiography and radionuclide cineangiogram, as well as invasive tests, such as endomyocardial biopsy, aid to assess risk-status of individuals receiving doxorubicin chemotherapy.

Using these techniques, some degree of cardiac injury is demonstrated in more than 50% of asymptomatic patients treated with doxorubicin.[47] While the total dose is the most significant factor contributing to the development of cardiomyopathy, other factors associated with an increased cardiotoxicity are:

- Age
- Pre-existing cardiac disease
- Mediastinal irradiation
- Concomitant administration of cyclophosphamide, actinomycin D and mitomycin C[47]

Stenosis, thrombosis and aneurysms in vessels such as the aorta, carotid and subclavian arteries have been associated with radiation.[48]

Key points: myocardial disease

- A high incidence of ischaemic heart disease and impaired myocardial perfusion is induced by radiotherapy, especially in the treatment of Hodgkin's disease

- Chemotherapy with doxorubicin results in some degree of myocardial disease in 50% of asymptomatic patients

Oesophagus

Radiation-induced injury to the oesophagus may be a limiting factor in therapy of thoracic neoplasms. Doses that result in radiation injury are of the order of 4,500 cGy and higher.[49] Chemotherapeutic agents such as adriamycin exacerbate these effects.

The abnormalities seen on oesophograms following radiotherapy include:

- Abnormal peristalsis
- Mucosal oedema
- Stricture (Fig. 53.8)
- Ulceration and fistula formation
- Oesophageal dysmotility which is the earliest and most common change

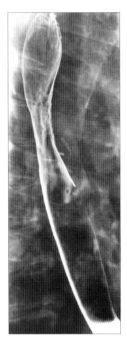

Figure 53.8. *Barium swallow shows slight narrowing of the mid-oesophagus with mucosal irregularity in a patient irradiated 3 months earlier for lung carcinoma. Endoscopy demonstrated oesophagitis.*

These, generally, occur within 4–12 weeks after completion of therapy. Focal segments with either decreased peristalsis or aperistalsis are seen and correspond to the portals used.[48] A serrated appearance of the oesophageal mucosa is seen when mucosal oedema is present.[50] Marked oesophagitis is usually seen endoscopically.

Cross-sectional imaging may demonstrate thickening of the oesophagus and mucosal enhancement corresponding to the inflammatory changes (Fig. 53.9). The differential diagnosis includes other causes of oesophagitis in the absence of an appropriate history.

Oesophageal strictures corresponding to the portals

used are not infrequent and in general develop 4–8 months following therapy.[49] Barium swallow shows narrowing, usually with smoothly tapered margins, although ulceration may also occur. Development of fistulae between the oesophagus and tracheobronchial tree is uncommon and is likely to be related to extrinsic tumour involvement of the oesophageal wall, with resultant erosion and fistula formation following therapy.[49] Radiation-induced strictures may be indistinguishable radiographically from those caused by other injury such as ingestion of caustic material or prolonged nasogastric intubation. Oesophageal cancers that respond to radiotherapy also frequently result in stricture formation.

A rare but well-described complication of therapeutic irradiation is carcinoma of the oesophagus. Squamous cell carcinoma is most common. The mean latency period is 14 years.[51]

Patients with malignancies may also develop infectious oesophagitis as a result of immune compromise due to cytotoxic and/or immunosuppressive drugs, or the malignancy itself. The most common pathogen in such patients is *Candida albicans*, normal flora in the pharynx that grows in the oesophagus as a result of the altered immunity. Clinical signs include odynophagia and dysphagia. The appearance on double-contrast oesophagrams is usually characteristic.[52] Mucosal plaques are seen which are generally diffuse and in severe cases a shaggy, irregular contour of the oesophagus results. Candida oesophagitis can result in stricture and tracheo-oesophageal fistula formation.[53] Herpes simplex virus also may cause oesophagitis in cancer patients. Discrete superficial ulcers can be seen with oesophagrams.[53]

Key points: oesophageal disease

■ Abnormalities within the oesophagus generally occur within 4–12 weeks after completion of radiotherapy

■ Oesophageal strictures generally develop 4–8 months following radiotherapy and are radiographically indistinguishable from those caused by other injury

■ Carcinoma of the oesophagus is a rare but well-described complication of radiotherapy, occurring usually about 14 years after radiation

■ Immune compromise due to cytotoxic or immunosuppressive drugs can result in infectious oesophagitis most commonly due to *Candida albicans*

Bone

A detailed account of changes to the bone marrow following radiotherapy is given in Chapter 54. The radiographic changes in adult bone following radiotherapy follow a temporal pattern. There is a latent period of 12 months or more during which no change is evident on conventional

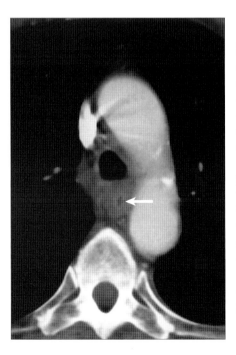

Figure 53.9. *CT scan of the chest demonstrates thickened oesophageal wall and mucosal enhancement (arrow) in a patient who received radiotherapy 4 months earlier for small cell carcinoma of the lung. The patient developed progressive dysphagia and odynophagia.*

radiographs.[54] Following this, some degree of demineralization may be seen. With progression, small lytic areas are seen through the cortex with thickening of the remaining trabeculae. This pattern usually develops 2–3 years or more following radiotherapy. These changes can be likened to multiple small foci of aseptic necrosis that are slowly progressive.[55]

Should the radiotherapy changes continue to progress, the lytic areas can reach 1–2 cm in size and may be similar to metastatic disease. It generally takes at least 5 years for the more pronounced changes to occur and in most patients metastatic disease will have developed earlier in the course of disease. The extent of the changes is generally much less with current megavoltage therapy than is seen with orthovoltage irradiation.[54] The presence of similar changes affecting adjacent bones in the irradiated field point to the correct diagnosis.[56] Absence of recurrent mass in the soft tissues with CT or MR speaks against local recurrence or soft tissue sarcoma.

Spontaneous fractures and aseptic necrosis can occur. Radiation-induced fractures may heal quite slowly, taking months to years to heal (Fig. 53.10). Non-union is not uncommon. Abnormal callus formation may be seen. Resorption of fracture fragments may occur. Despite the

decreased incidence with current therapy techniques, the changes still occur and long-term survivors from the orthovoltage era remain at risk. Bones subjected to muscular pull or constant weight-bearing tend to fracture more frequently. Radiation-induced fractures may be asymptomatic in non-weight-bearing bones.[57]

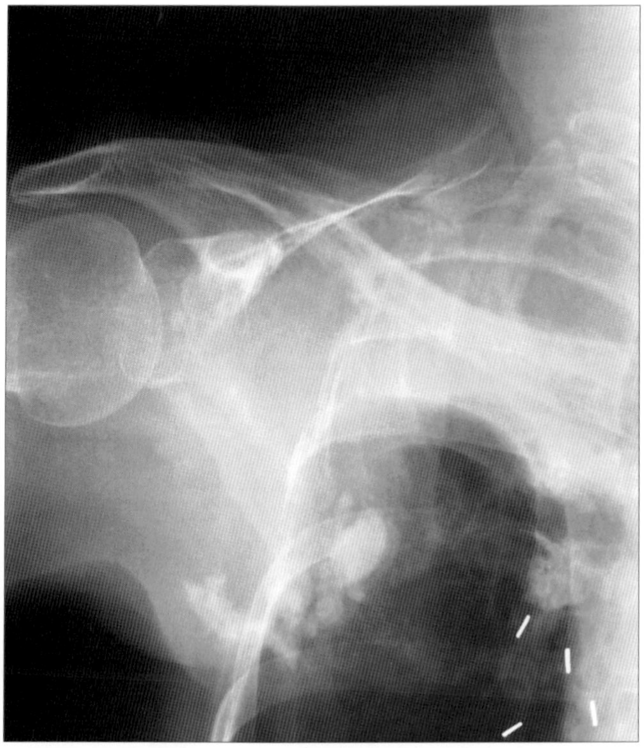

Rib fractures are far less common following megavoltage than orthovoltage irradiation[54] and more frequent when higher doses per fraction are used.[58] The current incidence of rib fractures is slightly less than 2%.[59] The fractures may be quite subtle and generally involve the anterior aspects of the ribs included in tangential fields of the chest wall. The abnormal callus at the fractures may simulate a radiation-induced sarcoma. Radiation brachial plexopathy may accentuate demineralization about a treated shoulder joint and may also result in the appearance of a neuropathic-like shoulder joint superimposed on the radiation change (Fig. 53.11). Radiation-induced ulcers of the chest wall may also develop (Fig. 53.12).

Radiation change in the adult spine is not generally obvious on conventional radiographs. However, therapeutic levels of radiotherapy cause conversion of haematopoietic bone marrow to fatty marrow. This is seen at MR as increased signal intensity on T1-weighted images.[60] The transformation begins as early as 2 weeks into a course of radiotherapy at a dose of approximately 1,600 cGy.[61]

The effects of therapeutic irradiation on growing bone are far more dramatic than those seen in adult bone because of associated growth impairment (Fig. 53.13). In the spine these changes in progressive order of severity include:

Figure 53.10. *Extensive chest wall changes, following postoperative radiation therapy for breast cancer 20 years earlier, are present. Multiple rib fractures with resorption, abnormal callus formation and dystrophic calcifications are present. The metallic clips are from coronary artery surgery. Radiation fibrosis is present in the upper right lung.*

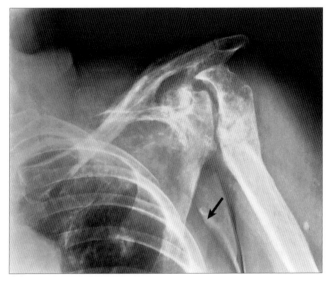

Figure 53.11. *Marked destruction of the left shoulder joint due in part to a radiation-induced brachial plexopathy 16 years following postoperative radiotherapy for breast cancer. Vascular calcification is seen (arrow). Rib and lung changes are also present.*

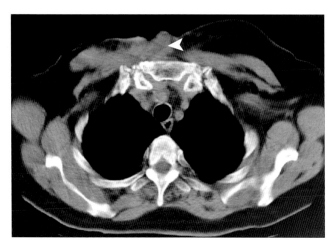

Figure 53.12. *Chest wall ulcer and radiation-induced soft tissue sarcoma. Twenty years earlier, this woman underwent subcutaneous mastectomies and radiotherapy for a right breast cancer. The soft tissue fullness beneath the skin ulcer (arrowhead) proved to be a malignant fibrous histiocytoma rather than inflammation related to the ulcer.*

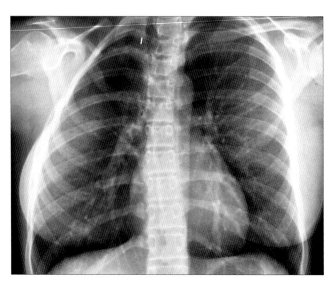

Figure 53.13. *Marked asymmetry is seen in the upper right thorax of this 17-year-old female who received postoperative radiotherapy at aged 3 years for a rhabdomyosarcoma. The clavicle spontaneously fractured and resorbed nearly completely several years before.*

- Growth arrest lines
- End-plate irregularity
- Anterior beaking
- Asymmetry of vertebral development[62]

Significant scoliosis or kyphosis following radiotherapy is rare using modern techniques, but minor scoliotic changes are commonly seen.[63]

Postradiation sarcomas

Postradiation sarcomas are an infrequent, but well-recognized complication of radiotherapy. They are estimated to occur in approximately 0.1% or fewer patients who receive radiotherapy and survive 5 years.[64,65] Postradiation sarcomas may occur in either bone or soft tissue. Osteosarcoma is more frequent in bone (Fig. 53.14) and malignant fibrous histiocytoma (Fig. 53.12) more common in soft tissue.[66–69] Review of Finnish data indicates soft tissue sarcomas are more common than osseous sarcomas.[66] In a review by Sheppard and Libshitz, 83% of postradiation sarcomas probably arose in bone, with 63% representing osteosarcoma.[67]

Postradiation sarcomas more commonly occur around the shoulder girdle and pelvis because of the more frequent use of radiotherapy in malignancies in these regions and better survival of patients with those malignancies. A higher incidence in women reflects the malignancies treated more often with radiotherapy.[68] Most postradiation sarcomas are now related to radiation for soft tissue neoplasms, particularly breast cancer, lymphoma and genitourinary cancer.[67]

A long latent period, averaging 10–15 years, is usually present between irradiation and the development of the sarcoma. However, postradiation sarcomas have developed as soon as 2–3 years following therapy, and as long as 45–55 years after treatment.[66–71]

The appearance of soft tissue sarcomas caused by radiotherapy is not different from the spontaneously developing sarcomas except that evidence of radiotherapy may be seen in adjacent bone or other tissues. They may get quite large if clinically silent.

With conventional radiographs postradiation sarcomas, arising in bone, most frequently present as an area of bony destruction.[55] A soft tissue mass may be evident but is better appreciated with CT or MR. Tumour matrix may be seen.

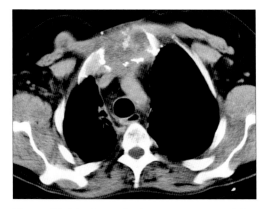

Figure 53.14. *Postradiation osteosarcoma of the sternum showing mass and bony destruction. The sarcoma developed 12 years after mediastinal irradiation at 3,600 cGy for metastases of a testicular seminoma.*

An expansile area in a previously irradiated bone suggests the development of sarcoma. Similarly, an area of lucency that is larger than the background pattern of radiation change is suspect.

At CT, a soft tissue mass and bony destruction are the most common findings.[70] A soft tissue density, rather than fat, in the marrow cavity of irradiated bones may be the earliest indicator that a sarcoma has developed.

The occasional late metastatic lesion may mimic a postradiation sarcoma. Infection that has developed in a treated bone may also mimic postradiation sarcoma. Biopsy may be necessary to make the distinction. The absence of a soft tissue mass is helpful in distinguishing between extensive benign radiation change and a postradiation sarcoma.

Radiation-induced osteochondromas (cartilaginous exostoses) may occur in children until growth stops. The incidence is about 12%.[72] Most are small and asymptomatic. Occasionally, the size and/or location cause symptoms. The appearance is that of the spontaneous osteochondromas and the same concerns apply.

Key points: radiation-induced bone disease

- Bone demineralization results only after 12 months following radiotherapy

- Small lytic areas are seen only 2–3 years following radiotherapy and larger lytic areas 1–2 cm in size occur only after 5 years

- Radiation-induced fractures may take months or years to heal

- Radiation-induced sarcomas occur in about 0.1% of patients who receive radiotherapy

- A latent period of 10–15 years usually exists between radiotherapy and the development of a sarcoma, but have developed within 2–3 years or as late as 45–55 years after treatment

- Radiation-induced osteochondromas may occur in children until growth stops

Summary

- Radiation pneumonitis is evident 6–8 weeks following completion of radiotherapy, and is most extensive 3–4 months after radiotherapy

- Radiation pulmonary fibrosis usually becomes stable 9–12 months after completion of therapy; any alteration thereafter suggests infection or recurrence

- Drugs that enhance radiation effect cause greater radiation damage and a shorter time to onset of radiation pneumonitis

- Bleomycin, busulphan and methotrexate cause pulmonary parenchymal damage independent of radiotherapy

- Identification of recurrent or residual malignant disease is made difficult by the presence of radiation change,

usually requires CT and an awareness of the timing of radiation change and follow-up at 2- to 3-monthly intervals

- Radiation-induced heart disease includes pericarditis, coronary artery disease, valvular dysfunction, cardiomyopathy and conduction abnormalities

- Chemotherapeutic agents, particularly doxorubicin, can result in cardiomyopathy

- Radiation injury to the oesophagus can result in oedema, dysmotility, stricture, ulceration and fistula formation or carcinoma

- Postradiation sarcomas occur after a long latent period, many more commonly in soft tissue than in bone

References

1. Maasilta P. Radiation-induced lung injury. From the chest physician's point of view. Lung Cancer 1991; 7: 367–384
2. Chu F C, Phillips R, Nickson J J et al. Pneumonitis following radiation therapy of the breast by tangential technique. Radiology 1955; 64: 642–653
3. Fajardo L F. Respiratory system. In: Pathology of Radiation Injury. New York: Masson Publishing, 1982; 34–46
4. Katzenstein A A, Astin F B. Surgical Pathology of Non-Neoplastic Lung Disease, 2nd edn. Philadelphia: W B Saunders, 1990; 9–57
5. Libshitz H I, Brosof A B, Southard M E. The radiographic appearance of the chest following extended field radiation therapy for Hodgkin's disease. Cancer 1973; 32: 206–215
6. Libshitz H I, North L B. Lung. In: Libshitz H I (ed). Diagnostic Roentgenology of Radiotherapy Change. Baltimore: Williams & Wilkins, 1979; 33–46
7. Libshitz H I. Radiation changes in the lung. Semin Roentgenol 1993; 28: 303–320
8. Wechsler R J, Ayyangar K, Steiner R M et al. The

development of distant pulmonary infiltrates following thoracic irradiation: the role of computed tomography with dosimetric reconstruction in diagnosis. Comput J Imag Graph 1990; 14: 43–51

9. Morgan G W, Briet S N. Radiation and the lung: a re-evaluation of the mechanisms mediating pulmonary injury. Int J Radiat Oncol Biol Phys 1995; 31: 361–368

10. Von der Maase H. Experimental drug-radiation interactions in critical normal tissues. In: Hill B T, Bellamy S A (eds). Antitumor Drug–Radiation Interactions. Boca Raton, FL: CRC Press, Inc, 1990; 191–205

11. Phillips T L. Effects of chemotherapy and irradiation on normal tissues. In: Meyer J L, Vaeth J M (eds). Radiotherapy/Chemotherapy Interactions in Cancer Therapy. Frontiers in Radiation Therapy in Oncology. Basel: Karger, 1992; 26: 45–54

12. Cooper J A, White D A, Matthay R A. Drug-induced pulmonary disease. Part I: Cytotoxic drugs. Am Rev Respir Dis 1986; 133: 321–340

13. Morrison D A, Goldman A L. Radiographic patterns of drug-induced lung disease. Radiology 1979; 131: 299–304

14. Richman S D, Levenson S M, Bunn P A et al. [67]Ga accumulation in pulmonary lesions associated with bleomycin toxicity. Cancer 1975; 36: 1966–1972

15. Libshitz H I, Shuman L S. Radiation-induced pulmonary change: CT findings. J Comput Assist Tomogr 1984; 8: 15–19

16. Ikezoe J, Takashima S, Morimoto S et al. CT appearance of acute radiation-induced injury in the lung. Am J Roentgenol 1988; 150: 765–770

17. Mah K, Poon P Y, van Dyk J et al. Assessment of acute radiation-induced pulmonary changes using computed topography. J Comput Assist Tomogr 1986; 10: 736–743

18. Graham M V, Purdy J A, Emami B et al. Clinical dose-volume histogram analysis for pneumonitis after 3D treatment for non-small cell lung cancer (NSCLC). Int J Radiat Oncol Biol Phys 1999; 45: 323–329

19. Armstrong J G. Three-dimensional conformal radiotherapy. Precision treatment of lung cancer. Chest Surg Clin North Am 1994; 4: 29–43

20. Graham M V, Matthews J W, Harms W B et al. Three-dimensional radiation treatment planning study for patients with carcinoma of the lung. Int J Radiat Oncol Biol Phys 1994; 29: 1105–1117

21. Koenig T R, Munden R F, Erasmus J J et al. Radiation injury of the lung after three-dimensional conformal radiation therapy. Am J Roentgenol 2002; 178: 1383–1388

22. Davis S D, Yankelevits D F, Henschke C I. Radiation effects on the lung: clinical features, pathology and imaging findings. Am J Roentgenol 1992; 159: 1157–1164

23. Glazer H S, Lee J K T, Levitt R G et al. Radiation fibrosis: differentiation from recurrent tumor by MR imaging. Radiology 1985; 156: 721–726

24. Werthmuller W C, Schiebler M L, Whaley R A et al. Gadolinium-DTPA enhancement of lung radiation fibrosis. J Comput Assist Tomogr 1989; 13: 946–948

25. Wencel M L, Sitrin R G. Unilateral lung hyperlucency after mediastinal irradiation. Am Rev Respir Dis 1988; 137: 955–957

26. Twiford T W, Zornoza J, Libshitz H I. Recurrent spontaneous pneumothorax after radiation therapy to the thorax. Chest 1978; 73: 388–389

27. Bachman A L, Macken K. Pleural effusions following supervoltage radiation for breast carcinoma. Radiology 1959; 72: 699–709

28. Brereton H D, Johnson R E. Calcification in mediastinal lymph nodes after radiation therapy of Hodgkin's disease. Radiology 1974; 112: 705–707

29. Kim H C, Nosher J, Haas A et al. Cystic degeneration of thymic Hodgkin's disease following radiation therapy. Cancer 1985; 55: 354–356

30. Shannon V R, Nesbitt J C, Libshitz H I. Malignant pleural mesothelioma after radiation therapy for breast cancer. Cancer 1995; 76: 437–441

31. Jochelson M, Mauch P, Balikian J et al. The significance of the residual mediastinal mass in treated Hodgkin's disease. J Clin Oncol 1985; 3: 637–640

32. Radford J A, Cowan R A, Flanagan M et al. The significance of residual mediastinal abnormality on the chest radiograph following treatment for Hodgkin's disease. J Clin Oncol 1988; 6: 940–946

33. Bourgouin P, Cousineau G, Lemire P et al. Differentiation of radiation-induced fibrosis from recurrent pulmonary neoplasm by CT. J Can Assoc Radiol 1987; 38: 23–26

34. Libshitz H I, Sheppard D G. Filling in of radiation therapy-induced bronchiectatic change: a reliable sign of locally recurrent lung cancer. Radiology 1999; 210: 25–27

35. Cosset J M, Henry-Amar M, Meerwaldt J H. Long-term toxicity of early stages of Hodgkin's disease: the EORTC experience. Ann Oncol 1991; 2: 77–82

36. Boivin J, Hutchison G B, Lubin J H et al. Coronary artery disease mortality in patients treated for Hodgkin's disease. Cancer 1992; 69: 1241–1247

37. Pierga J Y, Maunoury C, Valette H et al. Follow-up thallium-201 scintigraphy after mantle field radiotherapy for Hodgkin's disease. Int J Radiat Oncol Biol Phys 1993; 25: 871–876

38. Fajardo L F, Berthrong M. Radiation injury in surgical pathology. Am J Surg Pathol 1978; 2: 159–199

39. Tarbell N J, Thompson L, Mauch P. Thoracic irradiation in Hodgkin's disease: disease control and long-term complications. Int J Radiat Oncol Biol Phys 1990; 18: 275–281

40. Cosset J M, Henry-Amar M, Ozanne F et al. Les péricardites radiques: études des cas observés dans une série de 160 maladies de Hodgkin irradiées en mantelet a l'Institut Gustave-Roussy, de 1976 à 1980. J Eur Radiother 1984; 5: 297–308

41. Cosset J M, Henry-Amar M, Pellae-Cosset B et al. Pericarditis and myocardial infarctions after Hodgkin's

disease therapy. Int J Radiat Oncol Biol Phys 1991; 21: 447–449

42. Dana M, Colombel P, Bayle-Weisgerber C et al. Les péricardites après irradiation du médiastin par grands champs pour la maladie de Hodgkin. J Radiol Electrol 1978; 59: 335–341

43. Kinsella T J, Fraass B A, Glatstein E. Late effects of radiation therapy in the treatment of Hodgkin's disease. Cancer Treat Rep 1982; 66: 991–1001

44. Loyer E M, Delpassand E S. Radiation-induced heart disease: imaging features. Semin Roentgenol 1993; 28: 321–332

45. Green B, Zornoza J, Ricks J P. Eccentric pericardial effusion after radiation therapy of left breast carcinoma. Am J Roentgenol 1977; 128: 27–30

46. Ikäheimo M J, Niemal K O, Linnaluoto M M et al. Early cardiac changes related to radiation therapy. Am J Cardiol 1985; 56: 943–946

47. Gerling B, Gottdiener J, Borer J S. Cardiovascular complications of the treatment of Hodgkin's disease. In: Lacher M J, Redman J R (eds). Hodgkin's Disease: The Consequences of Survival. Philadelphia: Lea & Febiger, 1990; 267–295

48. Benson E P. Radiation injury to large arteries: three further examples with prolonged asymptomatic intervals. Radiology 1973; 106: 195–197

49. Lepke R A, Libshitz H I. Radiation-induced injury of the esophagus. Radiology 1983; 148: 375–378

50. DuBrow R A. Radiation changes in the hollow viscera. Semin Roentgenol 1994; 29: 38–52

51. Ogino T, Kato H, Tsukiyama I et al. Radiation-induced carcinoma of the esophagus. Acta Oncol 1992; 31: 475–479

52. Levine M S, Macones A J, Laufer I. Candida esophagitis: accuracy of radiographic diagnosis. Radiology 1985; 154: 581–587

53. Yee J, Wall S D. Infectious esophagitis. Radiol Clin North Am 1994; 32: 1135–1145

54. Howland W J, Loeffler R K, Starchman D E et al. Post-irradiation atrophic changes of bone and related complications. Radiology 1975; 117: 677–685

55. Libshitz H I. Radiation changes in the bone. Semin Roentgenol 1994; 29: 15–37

56. de Santos L A, Libshitz H I. Adult bone. In: Libshitz H I (ed). Diagnostic Roentgenology of Radiotherapy Change. Baltimore: Williams and Wilkins, 1979; 137–150

57. Dalinka M K, Neustafler L M. Radiation changes. In: Resnick D, Niwayama G (eds). Diagnosis of Bone and Joint Disorders. Philadelphia: Saunders, 1988; 3024–3056

58. Overgaard M. Spontaneous radiation-induced rib fractures in breast cancer patients treated with post mastectomy irradiation: a clinical radiobiological analysis of the influence of fraction size and dose–response relationships on late bone damage. Acta Oncol 1988; 27: 117–122

59. Pierce S M, Recht A, Lingos T L et al. Long-term radiation complications following conservative surgery (CS) and radiation therapy (RT) in patients with early stage breast cancer. Int J Radiat Oncol Biol Phys 1992; 23: 915–932

60. Ramsey R G, Zacharias C E. MR imaging of the spine after radiation therapy: easily recognizable effects. Am J Roentgenol 1985; 144: 1131–1135

61. Yankelevitz D F, Henschke C I, Knapp P H et al. Effect of radiation therapy on thoracic and lumbar bone marrow: evaluation with MR imaging. Am J Roentgenol 1991; 157: 87–92

62. Neuhauser E B, Wittenborg M H, Berman C Z et al. Irradiation effects of roentgen therapy on the growing spine. Radiology 1952; 59: 637–650

63. Heaston D K, Libshitz H I, Chan R C. Skeletal effects of megavoltage irradiation in survivors of Wilms' tumor. Am J Roentgenol 1979; 133: 389–395

64. Taghian A, de Vathaire F, Terrier P et al. Long-term risk of sarcoma following radiation treatment for breast cancer. Int J Radiat Oncol Biol Phys 1991; 21: 361–367

65. Tountas A S, Fornasier V L, Harwood A R et al. Postirradiation sarcoma of bone: a perspective. Cancer 1979; 43: 182–187

66. Wiklund T A, Blomqvist G P, R?ty J et al. Post irradiation sarcoma: analysis of a nationwide cancer registry material. Cancer 1991; 68: 524–531

67. Sheppard D G, Libshitz H I. Post-radiation sarcomas: a review of the clinical and imaging features in 63 cases. Clin Radiol 2001; 56: 22–29

68. Huvos A G, Woodard H Q, Cahan V G et al. Postradiation osteogenic sarcoma of bone and soft tissues: a clinicopathologic study of 66 patients. Cancer 1985; 55: 1244–1255

69. Laskin W B, Silberman T A, Enzinger F M. Postradiation soft tissue sarcomas: an analysis of 53 cases. Cancer 1988; 62: 2330–2340

70. Lorigan J G, Libshitz H I, Peuchot M. Radiation-induced sarcoma of bone: CT findings in 19 cases. Am J Roentgenol 1989; 153: 791–794

71. Weatherby R P, Dahlin D C, Ivins J C. Postradiation sarcoma of bone: review of 78 Mayo Clinic cases. Mayo Clin Proc 1981; 56: 294–306

72. Libshitz H I, Cohen M A. Radiation-induced osteochondromas. Radiology 1982; 142: 643–647

Chapter 54

Effects of treatment on normal tissue: bone and bone marrow

Lia A Moulopoulos

Introduction

As early as in 1926, Ewing reported osseous changes that he believed were related to radiation-induced vascular damage.[1] He introduced the term 'radiation osteitis' to describe these radiation-induced abnormalities. Since that time, many other investigators have described changes related to the effect of radiation on bone and have introduced many terms, such as osteonecrosis and radionecrosis.

Howland and his colleagues suggested that, because atrophy is the main event that takes place in the irradiated bone, the term 'atrophic changes' more accurately defines the expected, uncomplicated postradiation bony changes.[2] All other superimposed conditions, such as fractures, infection and aseptic necrosis can be considered complications of radiation therapy. The number of complications of radiation therapy that affect the osseous skeleton has been reduced, but not eliminated, since the advent of megavoltage therapy.

Pathophysiology of treatment-related osseous changes

The effect of radiation therapy on the bones has been documented by pathological studies.[3–5] The changes that occur in irradiated bone are due to destruction of the cellular bony matrix and the fine vasculature that supplies the bone. Radiation therapy induces an immediate inflammatory reaction in the bone marrow. All cellular elements die early in the postradiation period and, as early as the first week of therapy, the marrow becomes hypocellular accompanied by oedema and haemorrhage. Endarteritis occurs later in the postradiation period and is responsible for the late postradiation manifestations observed on radiographic examinations. Destruction of the microvasculature of the bone prevents the migration of haematopoietic elements from contiguous healthy bone marrow. Vascular compromise leads to bone necrosis. Necrotic bone is gradually removed by 'creeping substitution' and new bone is deposited over a period of years.

The development and the severity of postradiation changes of the bones depends on:

- Dose
- Fractionation
- Field size
- Type of radiation treatment

Regeneration of the bone marrow is possible if the microvasculature of the affected bone has not been completely obliterated. However, histological studies have not shown recovery of haematopoietic marrow with doses greater than 3,000–4,000 cGy.[5,6] Magnetic resonance (MR) imaging and radionuclide studies have shown similar results.[7–11]

The changes that occur in the bone marrow after chemotherapy have been studied on serial bone marrow specimens from patients with acute myeloid leukaemia.[12] Immediately after initiation of chemotherapy, depletion of the cellular elements takes place and the bone marrow becomes oedematous. The vascular sinuses dilate and large, unilocular adipocytes (structured fat), which are produced by multilocular precursor fat cells, appear in the irradiated marrow. It is only within these areas of structured fat that foci of regenerating haematopoietic marrow appear after the first week of treatment, suggesting a potential role of structured fat in the proliferation of stem cells (Fig. 54.1).

Imaging findings

Postradiation atrophic changes

Local demineralization and osteopenia is the earliest and, most often, the only postradiation change on conventional bone radiographs, together with coarsening of the bony trabecula and thickening of the cortex of the long bones; changes that have been likened to Pagetoid bone.[2] Such changes occur a year after radiation therapy and may become more pronounced with time. Later, both sclerotic and lytic foci representing dead and resorbed bone, respectively, may appear (Fig. 54.2). Postradiation atrophic changes are more obvious on computed tomography (CT) scans. Occasionally, lytic foci grow and simulate primary or secondary malignant bone tumours. Appearances that sup-

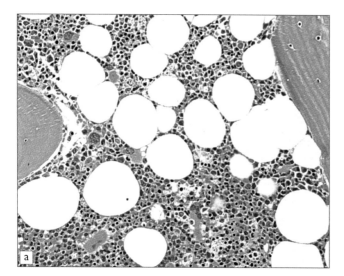

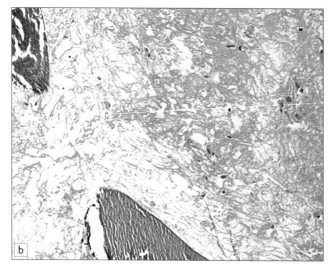

Figure 54.1. *(a) Bone marrow showing fatty change and fibrosis following chemotherapy. (b) Normal cellular bone marrow for comparison.*

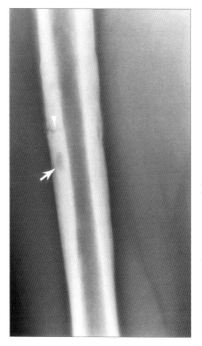

Figure 54.2. *Cortical lucency (arrow) and insufficiency fracture (arrowhead). Antero-posterior radiograph of the femur of a patient with soft tissue sarcoma who received 7,000 cGy 5 years ago. (Courtesy of H I Libshitz.)*

port the diagnosis of postradiation lytic change rather than neoplasm include:

- Localization to the radiation portals
- Absence of an extra-osseous mass
- Absence of a periosteal reaction
- A sharp transition zone to the uninvolved bone
- Slow growth of the lesion[13–15]

Computed tomography scans should be obtained if review of conventional bone radiographs poses the question of malignancy. If findings are equivocal on CT scans, MR studies may help in the detection of extra-osseous or bone marrow involvement.

Postradiation complications

Fractures

The irradiated, atrophic bone is brittle and may fracture, even under physiological stress such as muscular contractions, particularly in weight-bearing bones. The first radiation-induced fracture was described in the femoral neck, in 1927.[16] Since the introduction of megavoltage therapy, radiation-induced fractures are seen less often. They are infrequently observed earlier than 2 or 3 years after therapy.[15] They may be discovered incidentally on routine imaging studies or the patient may present with pain, particularly when weight-bearing bones are involved. Radiation-induced fractures heal more slowly than fractures of healthy bone. Formation of abnormal, exuberant callus, non-union of the osseous fragments or bony resorption may occur.

Radiation-induced insufficiency fractures of the pelvis occur earlier than fractures in other parts of the skeleton (Figs. 54.3 and 54.4).[15] After treatment with pelvic radiation, the sacrum loses its elasticity and may fracture under the stress of normal activity. A 34–89% incidence of sacral insufficiency fractures has been reported in patients treated with radiotherapy for cervical cancer.[17,18] Fractures of the pubic rami and subcapital fractures of the femoral head may also occur in such patients. In postmenopausal women, osteoporosis increases the probability of insufficiency fractures of irradiated bones. On conventional radiographs, findings may be absent or very subtle.[19] An H-shaped appearance of increased uptake on radionuclide studies is characteristic of sacral insufficiency fractures, which course vertically in the sacral alae.[20,21] The horizontal bar of the 'H' corresponds to a third transverse fracture of

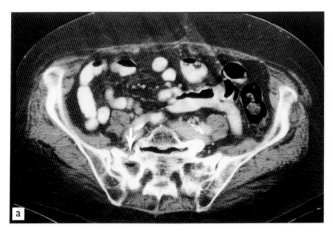
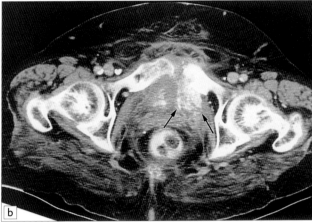

Figure 54.3. *Insufficiency fractures of the pelvis. CT scans of the pelvis of a 66-year-old woman who was treated with radiotherapy for vaginal cancer 2 years previously. In (a), the arrow points to a fracture of the right sacral wing. (b) Note healed insufficiency fracture of the left pubic bone and extra-osseous calcifications (arrows).*

the sacrum that need not necessarily be identified on radiographs.

In patients with known malignancies, it may be difficult to differentiate sacral insufficiency fractures, especially unilateral ones, from metastatic disease with conventional radiographs and radionuclide scans alone. CT or MR imaging can provide a definitive diagnosis in most cases. On T1-weighted MR images of sacral insufficiency fractures, the expected bright signal intensity of irradiated marrow is replaced by decreased signal intensity produced by the presence of free water in the oedematous marrow.[22] The water, and consequently the decreased signal intensity, extends well beyond the margins of the fracture (Fig. 54.5). MR imaging studies may demonstrate sacral insufficiency

fractures well before any changes appear on CT images because of the higher contrast resolution and capability for multiplanar image acquisition.

In patients who receive radiation therapy for breast cancer, rib fractures may occur. The incidence of this complication is about 1.8% but may be even higher when radiation doses exceed 5,000 cGy and if chemotherapy is administered as well.[23,24]

Avascular necrosis

Radiation therapy and steroids are known causes of avascular necrosis. Avascular necrosis develops several years after radiation treatment (Fig. 54.6). Before the introduction of MR imaging, radionuclide examination was the procedure of choice for the diagnosis of avascular necrosis. With this modality, however, false negative radionuclide scans of 18% have been reported.[25] In another study, radionuclide studies failed to detect 10% of cases of avascular necrosis which were positive on MR studies.[26]

The presence of the double-line sign on T2-weighted MR images is characteristic of avascular necrosis (Fig. 54.7). This consists of an outer dark line, which is produced by reactive sclerosis at the interface of the lesion with the healthy marrow, and a bright inner line, which corresponds to areas of hyperaemia and inflammation at the periphery of the ischaemic marrow.[26] Changes of early avascular necrosis may be accompanied by bone marrow oedema and joint effusion, both of which have been associated with transient bone pain even in the absence of collapse.[27] Recognition of the presence of avascular necrosis before the occurrence of a subchondral fracture is important for the success of conservative treatment. Magnetic resonance studies can detect avascular necrosis within days of the vascular insult. MR imaging has also been shown to identify those patients at particular risk for

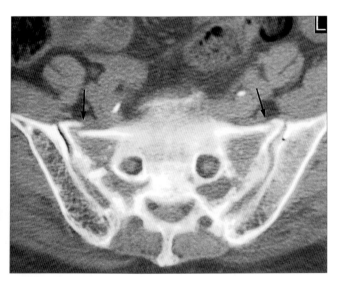

Figure 54.4. *Bilateral insufficiency fractures (arrows) on CT scan of the pelvis of a 60-year-old woman who underwent radiotherapy of the pelvis for colon cancer 1 year previously. The patient presented with severe back pain and a positive bone scan (not shown).*

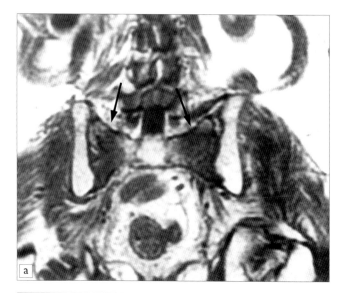

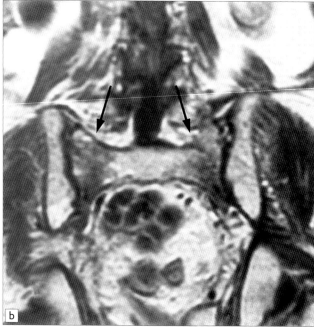

Figure 54.5. *Bilateral insufficiency fractures of the sacrum. T1-weighted (a) and enhanced T1-weighted (b) coronal MR of the sacrum in a 70-year-old woman who was treated with radiotherapy for cervical cancer 1 year previously. Note oedematous marrow (arrows) with faint enhancement in (b).*

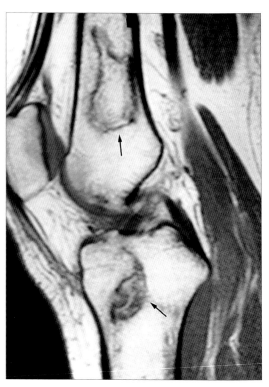

Figure 54.6. *T1-weighted sagittal MR of the knee shows bone infarcts (arrows) of the femoral and tibial metaphysis of a 26-year-old woman treated for Hodgkin's lymphoma 10 years ago.*

Key points: fractures and aseptic necrosis

- Radiation-induced fractures occur earlier in the pelvis than in other parts of the skeleton

- Sacral insufficiency fractures may be difficult to distinguish from metastases on conventional radiographs and radionuclide scans

- MR is the most sensitive and most specific technique in the detection of aseptic necrosis

Effects of radiation on the growing skeleton

The effect of radiation on the osseous skeleton depends on the type of bone involved, the dosage and, in particular, the patient's age at the time of therapy. The younger the child at the time of radiation therapy, the more pronounced the radiation-induced osseous changes because of the impairment of bone growth. The epiphysis, which is radiosensitive, may show signs of radiation-induced changes with doses as low as 400 cGy. Widening of the epiphyseal plate, and irregularity and sclerosis of the metaphysis are common findings in the growing skeleton which is exposed to radiation.[15] They may appear quite early after therapy and may resemble the osseous changes observed in rickets. In

developing avascular necrosis when exposed to known predisposing factors. In a study of patients treated with chemotherapy for testicular tumours, asymptomatic avascular necrosis was detected in 9% of patients with MR imaging.[28] The presence of a sealed-off epiphyseal scar in the femoral head has been associated with an increased risk for avascular necrosis.[29] Magnetic resonance imaging can also reliably assess the location and the extent of the necrotic bone relative to the weight-bearing area, factors that influence the course of avascular necrosis and affect the management of the patient.[30]

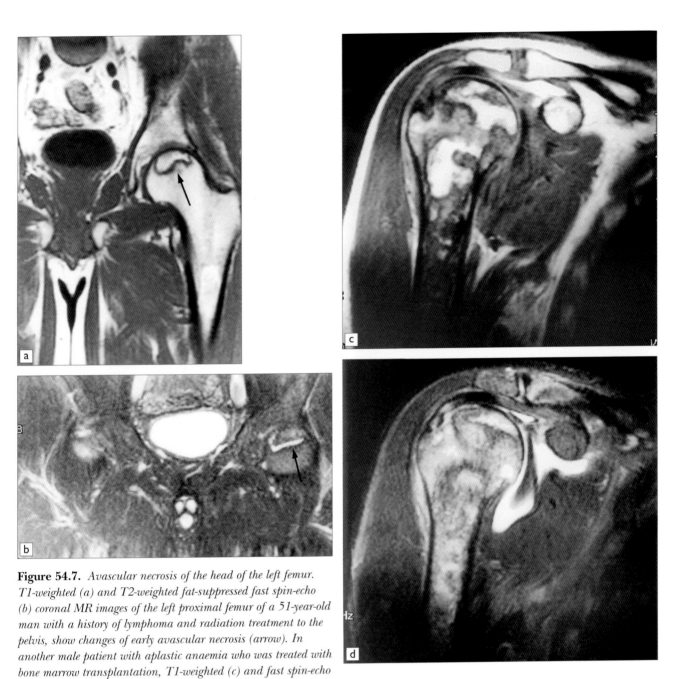

Figure 54.7. *Avascular necrosis of the head of the left femur. T1-weighted (a) and T2-weighted fat-suppressed fast spin-echo (b) coronal MR images of the left proximal femur of a 51-year-old man with a history of lymphoma and radiation treatment to the pelvis, show changes of early avascular necrosis (arrow). In another male patient with aplastic anaemia who was treated with bone marrow transplantation, T1-weighted (c) and fast spin-echo T2-weighted fat-suppressed (d) coronal MR images of the right shoulder show advanced avascular necrosis of the humeral head.*

the diaphyses, changes are minimal and include narrowing of the shaft and some degree of osteopenia.

Slipped capital femoral epiphysis and, less frequently, slipped capital humeral epiphysis represent a serious complication which occurs 1–7 years after treatment and at an earlier age than their idiopathic counterpart.[15,31,32] Administration of chemotherapy increases the possibility of epiphyseal slippage. Slipped epiphysis may be accompanied by avascular necrosis of the femoral or humeral head.[33] Because of the late manifestation of postradiation epiphyseal injuries, it is obvious that long-term follow-up is warranted for patients with a history of radiation therapy.

Radiation-induced changes of the growing spine are more pronounced in patients treated before the age of 6 years or at puberty, both being periods of increased skeletal growth.[33] Growth arrest lines, which are dense lines parallel to the vertebral end-plates, are a common manifestation of growth arrest related to prior radiotherapy. They appear within a year from therapy with doses greater than 1,000 cGy and may actually cause a 'bone within bone' appearance. Doses greater than 2,000 cGy are associated with more pronounced changes of growth disturbance that become apparent within 5 years of completion of therapy.[34] Such changes include short vertebral bodies, irregularity of the end-plates and, less frequently, contour abnormalities, which may resemble changes observed in mucopolysaccha-ridoses (Fig. 54.8).[35] Mild scoliosis, concave to the irradi-ated side, is a common complication when the spine is included in the radiation field. With the advent of mega-voltage therapy, it is unusual for scolioses greater than 5° to occur, because of more even distribution of the radiation beam to the vertebrae.[33,34] Kyphosis may accompany scolio-sis but it is extremely rare for it to occur alone.

Osteochondroma is the only benign tumour associated with a history of radiotherapy. While the incidence of spontaneous osteochondromas is less than 1%, the inci-dence of osteochondromas developing within a previously irradiated field has been reported to be up to 12%.[36] The tumours occur in patients who received radiotherapy during childhood and, histologically, they do not differ from those that occur spontaneously. They appear at an average of 8 years after radiotherapy and should be treated according to the same guidelines as those that occur spon-taneously.[35]

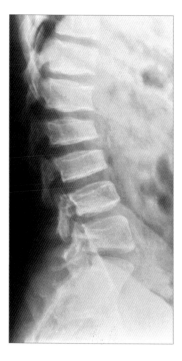

Figure 54.8. *Loss of vertebral body height and irregularities of vertebral end-plates. Lateral radiograph of the lumbar spine of a 17-year-old man who received radiation therapy for Wilms' tumour at the age of 2 years. (Courtesy of HI Libshitz.)*

Key points: effects of radiotherapy on the growing skeleton

■ In children, epiphyseal changes can occur with doses as low as 400 cGy

■ Slipped epiphyses occur 1–7 years after radiation and warrant long-term follow-up

■ Spinal changes are more pronounced in patients treated before age 6 or at puberty, both periods of increased skeletal growth

■ Osteochondromas occur in the irradiated field in about 12% of patients

■ Osteochondromas develop approximately 8 years after radiotherapy

Effects of chemotherapy on the growing skeleton

Paediatric oncology patients may suffer from complications related to the effect of certain chemotherapeutic agents on the growing skeleton.[37] Prolonged administration of steroids may cause diffuse osteopenia and fractures, partic-ularly in the spine. Avascular necrosis is a well-known com-plication of long-term steroid treatment. Methotrexate osteopathy is a rare syndrome, which was first described as a complication of maintenance treatment for children with acute lymphoblastic leukaemia.[38] It is also known to occur in 9% of children with osteosarcoma who receive high doses of methotrexate and it has been reported in children under 3 years of age who were treated for brain tumours.[39,40] Methotrexate osteopathy is manifested by:[41]

- Severe lower extremity bone pain
- Osteopenia
- Dense provisional zones of calcification
- Metaphyseal insufficiency fractures

Both steroids and methotrexate may directly inhibit skele-tal growth. Ifosfamide is an alkylating agent used in chil-dren for the treatment of soft tissue and bone sarcomas. It has a known nephrotoxic effect and it may cause hypophos-phataemic rickets.[42] A single case of periosteal new bone formation along the ulnar shafts was reported in a 4-year-old boy with neuroblastoma, who was treated with 13-cis-retinoic acid, a vitamin A analogue.[43]

Key points: effects of chemotherapy on the growing skeleton

■ Prolonged steroid therapy may induce osteopenia and fractures, especially in the spine

■ Methotrexate osteopathy may develop in children on maintenance therapy for acute lymphoblastic leukaemia

■ Ifosfamide is nephrotoxic and may induce hypophosphataemic rickets

Effects of radiation on the bone marrow

MR imaging has provided a means of recording *in vivo* the changes that occur in the irradiated bone marrow. Immediately after initiation of radiotherapy, the signal intensity of the bone marrow on T1-weighted MR images decreases. This drop in the signal intensity of the marrow reflects an increase in free water that occurs because of oedema and necrosis of the marrow. Early short tau inversion recovery (STIR) images show areas of increased signal intensity with a peak at 9 days.[44] As early as 2 weeks into therapy, and with doses as low as 800 cGy, the signal intensity of the bone marrow on T1-weighted MR imaging begins to rise as the number of adipocytes within the irradiated bone marrow grows (Fig. 54.9).[8,9,44] Conversion of the irradiated red marrow to fatty marrow is completed before the end and about 6–8 weeks after the start of radiation therapy in 90% of patients.[45] This 'bright' marrow is due to the short T1 value of adipose tissue and it is sharply delineated from bone marrow outside the radiation portals. Regeneration of the haematopoietic elements of the bone marrow has been reported to occur with doses lower than 3,000 cGy, 2–23 years after radiotherapy.[10] With higher doses, however, conversion to fatty marrow appears to be irreversible.[7,9,10] Blomlie et al. reported changes on MR of non-irradiated bone marrow as well, during radiation therapy.[45] These changes consist of an increase in fatty marrow and, according to the authors' conclusions, they are probably due to an indirect effect of radiation therapy rather than to scattered radiation. More recently, a significant, gradual decrease in contrast enhancement of non-irradi-ated bone marrow during and after the end of radiation therapy was observed with dynamic MR, and was considered to be suggestive of the effect of low radiation doses on the microvasculature of bone marrow outside the radiation portals.[46]

Effects of chemotherapy on magnetic resonance images of the bone marrow

During the first days after the administration of chemotherapy regimens, a drop in the signal intensity of the bone marrow is observed on spinal T1-weighted MR images together with increased brightness on T2-weighted images. The changes that occur in the bone marrow immediately after initiation of chemotherapy reflect the increase in free water in the congested bone marrow and vary, depending on the effect of chemotherapy on the bone marrow.[12] Later, an increase in fatty signal intensity is observed on MR of the bone marrow. When haematopoietic recovery occurs, about 3–4 weeks into chemotherapy, the marrow becomes dark again on T1-weighted MR images because of the presence of regenerating red marrow (Fig. 54.10). At this stage, differentiation of regenerating red marrow from malignant infiltration of the marrow may be difficult. Absence of a marked increase in signal intensity on T2-weighted images, and faint or no enhancement on enhanced T1-weighted images, favour the presence of red marrow recovery. Also, the signal intensity of haematopoietic bone marrow will drop on out-of-phase gradient recalled echo MR images but it will show no change on out-of-phase gradient-echo images of bone

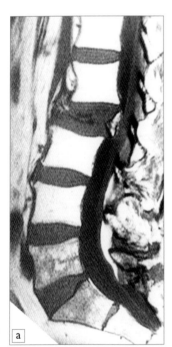
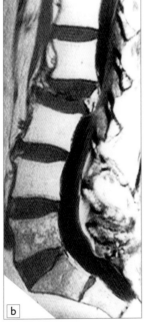

Figure 54.9. *Postradiation MR changes of the spine. Sagittal T1-weighted (a) and enhanced T1-weighted (b) MR images of the lumbosacral spine of a 56-year-old man who received radiotherapy for Ewing's tumour at L2. Note high signal intensity of postradiation change (T12–L4) which is sharply delineated from red marrow outside the radiation field; there is no perceptible enhancement of the intact red marrow or of the affected, compressed L2 vertebra.*

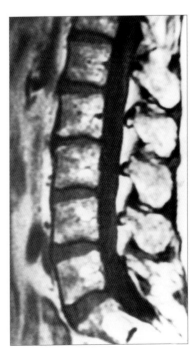

Figure 54.10.
Postchemotherapy changes of the spine. T1-weighted sagittal MR of the lumbar spine shows islands of regenerating red marrow in a 50-year-old man who is receiving chemotherapy for melanoma.

marrow, which is infiltrated by malignant cells (Figs. 54.11 and 54.12).[47,48]

Reconversion of fatty to red marrow occurs in the opposite direction to marrow conversion, that is, from the axonal skeleton to the periphery. When there is an increased need for additional haematopoiesis, red marrow will appear in the proximal metaphyses of the femur and humerus. In extreme cases, red marrow may appear at other parts of the peripheral skeleton, which are occupied by fatty marrow in healthy adults.

Changes related to increased haematopoiesis are accentuated on MR images of the bone marrow when growth factors are administered during chemotherapy.[49] Fletcher et al. reported changes of reconversion in the femoral diaphyses of children receiving haematopoietic growth factors in addition to chemotherapy for musculoskeletal tumours.[50] No such changes were observed in children who did not receive growth factors. Haematopoietic activity induced by growth factors may be asymmetric and it may simulate malignant dissemination to the bone marrow.[51] Awareness of the treatment regimens is necessary for the accurate interpretation of post-therapy MR images.

Magnetic resonance imaging has also been applied to the evaluation of bone marrow after transplantation. Patients who have undergone stem cell transplantation are currently assessed with serial bone marrow biopsies and aspirations. Prospective MR studies are being carried out in an attempt to introduce a potential non-invasive means of following the changes that occur in the marrow of these patients. Stevens and his colleagues reported a characteristic band pattern, which was present on T1-weighted images of all but one of 15 patients who received bone marrow transplants.[44] This band pattern consisted of a bright central zone of fatty marrow and a peripheral dark zone of haematopoietic cells. This band-like distribution of red and fatty marrow in the vertebral body may be explained by the pattern of vascular flow into the vertebra, which in turn determines the distribution of the proliferating blood cells.

Magnetic resonance imaging is the most accurate imaging modality for the evaluation of large volumes of bone marrow and provides information complementary to the bone marrow biopsy. Detailed knowledge of the expected changes in the bone marrow under different conditions and close collaboration between the radiologist and the clinician is important if complex bone marrow changes are to be interpreted correctly and appropriate action taken.

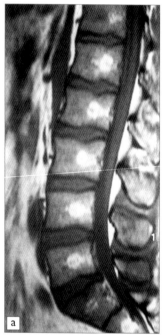
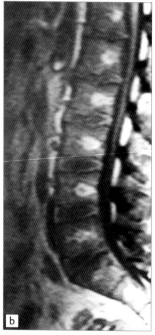
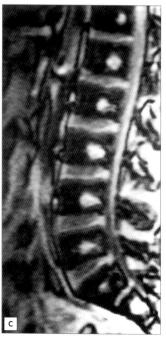

Figure 54.11. *T1-weighted (a), in-phase T1-weighted turbo field-echo (b) and out-of-phase T1-weighted turbo field-echo (c) sagittal MR image of the lumbosacral spine of a 25-year-old healthy individual. Note drop of signal intensity of red marrow on the out-of-phase image (c) relative to the in-phase image (b) because of coexistence of water and fat protons.*

Key points: bone marrow changes following treatment

■ Changes in the bone marrow can be seen on T1-weighted MR images immediately after initiation of radiotherapy due to an increase in free water

■ Within 2 weeks of the start of radiotherapy, fat starts to replace the red marrow; these changes can be irreversible with high doses

■ Chemotherapy results in an increase in water within the bone marrow within days; within a week, there is an increase in fat; about 3–4 weeks later, regenerating marrow appears. All these changes can be monitored on MR images

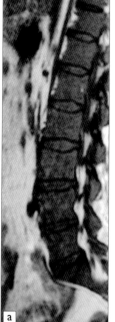
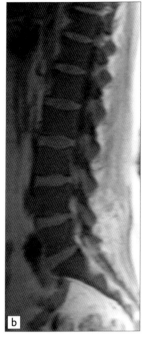
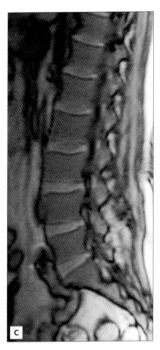

Figure 54.12. *T1-weighted (a), in-phase T1-weighted turbo field-echo (b) and out-of-phase T1-weighted turbo field-echo (c) sagittal MR of the lumbosacral spine in a 54-year-old woman with diffuse large cell lymphoma. Note absence of signal intensity drop of abnormal marrow on out-of-phase image (c).*

Summary

- Radiation therapy results in an immediate inflammatory reaction and hypocellularity in the bone marrow. Endarteritis occurs later and results in bone necrosis

- Local demineralization is the earliest, most often the only radiographic change following radiotherapy. Lytic foci may grow and simulate neoplastic lesions

- Radiation-induced fractures are seldom seen less than 2–3 years after therapy, are most common in the pelvis and are best detected on MR

- Avascular necrosis occurs years after radiation treatment. It is important to recognize its presence before the development of subchondral fractures

- In the growing skeleton subjected to radiotherapy, slipped epiphysis is a serious complication and is made more likely by the addition of chemotherapy

- Both radiotherapy and chemotherapy produce serial changes in the bone marrow that can be monitored on MR images

- Within 2 weeks of the start of radiotherapy, fat starts to replace the red marrow

- Chemotherapy results in an increase in water within the bone marrow within days

References

1. Ewing J. Radiation osteitis. Acta Radiol 1926; 5: 399–412

2. Howland W J, Loeffler R K, Starchman D E, Johnson R G. Post-irradiation atrophic changes of bone and related complications. Radiology 1975; 117: 677–685

3. Rubin P, Gasarett G W. Clinical Radiation Pathology, Vol. II. Philadelphia: Saunders, 1968; 557–608

4. Fajardo L F. Locomotive system. In: Pathology of Radiation Injury. New York, NY: Masson, 1982; 176–186

5. Knospe W H, Blom J, Crosby W H. Regeneration of locally irradiated bone marrow. I. Dose-dependent, long-term changes in the rat, with particular emphasis upon vascular and stromal reaction. Blood 1966; 28: 398–415

6. Sykes M P, Chu F C H, Savel H et al. Long-term effects of therapeutic irradiation upon bone marrow. Cancer 1946; 17: 1144–1148

7. Kauczor H U, Dietl B, Brix G et al. Fatty replacement of bone marrow after radiation therapy for Hodgkin's disease: quantification with chemical shift imaging. J Magn Res Imaging 1993; 3: 575–580

8. Remedios P A, Colletti P M, Raval J K. Magnetic resonance imaging of bone after radiation. Magn Reson Imaging 1988; 6: 301–304

9. Yankelevitz D F, Henschke C I, Knapp P H et al. Effect of radiation therapy in thoracic and lumbar marrow: evaluation with MR imaging. Am J Roentgenol 1991; 157: 87–92

10. Casamassima F, Ruggiero C, Caramella D et al. Hematopoietic bone marrow recovery: MRI evaluation. Blood 1989; 73: 1677–1681

11. Sacks E L, Goris M L, Glatstein E et al. Bone marrow regeneration following large field radiation: influence of volume, age, dose, and time. Cancer 1978; 42: 1057–1065

12. Islam A, Catovsky D, Galton D. Histological study of bone marrow regeneration following chemotherapy for acute myeloid leukemia and chronic granulocytic leukemia in blast transformation. Br J Hematol 1980; 45: 535–540

13. de Santos L A, Libshitz H I. Adult bone. In: Libshitz H I (ed). Diagnostic Radiology of Radiotherapy Change. Baltimore, MD: Williams and Wilkins, 1979; 137–150

14. Paling M R, Herdt J R. Radiation osteitis: a problem of recognition. Radiology 1980; 137: 339–342

15. Libshitz H I. Radiation changes in bone. Semin Roentgenol 1994; 29: 15–37

16. Baensch W. Knochenschädigung nach Röntgenbestrahlung. Fortschr Geb Roentgenstr 1927; 36: 1245–1247

17. Abe H, Nakamura M, Takahashi S et al. Radiation-induced insufficiency fractures of the pelvis: evaluation with ^{99m}Tc-methylenediphosphonate scintigraphy. Am J Roentgenol 1990; 158: 599–602

18. Blomlie V, Rofstad E K, Talle K et al. Incidence of radiation-induced insufficiency feactures of the female pelvis: evaluation with MR imaging. Am J Roentgenol 1996; 167: 1205–1210

19. Lundin B, Bjorkholm E, Lundell M, Jacobsson H. Insufficiency fractures of the sacrum after radiotherapy for gynecological malignancy. Acta Oncol 1990; 29: 211–215

20. Ries T. Detection of osteoporotic sacral fractures with radionuclides. Radiology 1983; 146: 783–785

21. Cooper K L, Beabout J W, Swee R G. Insufficiency fractures of the sacrum. Radiology 1985; 156: 15–20

22. Blomlie V, Lien H H, Iversen T et al. Radiation-induced insufficiency fractures of the sacrum: evaluation with MR imaging. Radiology 1993; 188: 241–244

23. Pierce S M, Recht A, Lingos T I et al. Long-term radiation complications following conservative surgery (CS) and radiation therapy (RT) in patients with early stage breast cancer. Int J Radiat Oncol Biol Phys 1992; 23: 915–923

24. Iyer R, Libshitz H I. Late sequelae after radiation therapy for breast cancer: imaging findings. Am J Roentgenol 1997; 168: 1335–1338

25. Bieber E, Hungerford D S, Lennox D W. Factors in diagnosis of avascular necrosis of the femoral head. Adv Orhop Surg 1985; 9: 93–96

26. Mitchell D G, Rao V M, Dalinka M K et al. Femoral head avascular necrosis: correlation of MR imaging radiographic staging, radionuclide imaging, and clinical findings. Radiology 1987; 162: 709–715

27. Koo K H, Ahn I O, Kim R et al. Bone marrow edema and associated pain in early stage osteonecrosis of the femoral head: prospective study with serial MR images. Radiology 1999; 213: 715–722

28. Cook A M, Dzik-Jurasz A S, Padhani A R et al. The prevalence of avascular necrosis in patients treated with chemotherapy for testicular tumours. Br J Cancer 2001; 85: 1624–1626

29. Jiang C C, Shih T T F. Epiphyseal scar of the femoral head: risk factor of osteonecrosis. Radiology 1994; 191: 409–412

30. Lafforgue P, Dahan E, Chagnaud C et al. Early-stage avascular necrosis of the femoral head: MR imaging for prognosis in 31 cases with at least 2 years of follow-up. Radiology 1993; 187: 199–204

31. Dickerman J D, Newberg A H, Moreland M D. Slipped capital femoral epiphysis (SCFE) following pelvic irradiation for rhabdomyosarcoma. Cancer 1979; 44: 480–482

32. Edeiken B S, Libshitz H I, Cohen M A. Slipped proximal humeral epiphysis: a complication of radiotherapy to the shoulder in children. Skel Radiol 1982; 9: 123–125

33. Probert J C, Parker B R. The effects of radiation therapy on bone growth. Radiology 1975; 114: 155–162

34. Heaston D K, Libshitz H I, Chan R C. Skeletal effects of megavoltage irradiation in survivors of Wilms' tumor. Am J Roentgenol 1979; 133: 389–395

35. Riseborough E J, Grabias S L, Burton R, Jaffe N. Skeletal alterations following irradiation for Wilms' tumor. J Bone Joint Surg [Am] 1976; 58: 526–536

36. Libshitz H I, Cohen M A. Radiation-induced osteochondromas. Radiology 1982; 142: 643–647

37. Roebuck D J. Skeletal complications in pediatric oncology patients. Radiographics 1999; 19: 873–875

38. Ragab H, Frech R S, Vietti T J. Osteoporotic fractures secondary to methotrexate therapy for acute leukemia in remission. Cancer 1970; 25: 580–585

39. Ecklund K, Laor T, Goorin A M et al. Methotrexate osteopathy in patients with osteosarcoma. Radiology 1997; 202: 543–547

40. Meister B, Gassner I, Streif W et al. Methotrexate osteopathy in infants with tumors of the central nervous system. Med Pediatr Oncol 1994; 23: 493–496

41. Schwartz A M, Leonidas J C. Methotrexate osteopathy. Skel Radiol 1984; 11: 13–16

42. Skinner R, Pearson A D J, Price L et al. Hypophosphatemic rickets after ifosfamide treatment in children. Br Med J 1989; 298: 1560–1561

43. Grissom L E, Griffin G C, Mandell G A. Hypervitaminosis A as a complication of treatment for neuroblastoma. Pediatr Radiol 1996; 26: 200–202

44. Stevens S K, Moore S G, Kaplan I D. Early and late bone-marrow changes after irradiation: MR evaluation. Am J Roentgenol 1990; 154: 745–750

45. Blomlie V, Rofstad E K, Skjonsberg A et al. Female pelvic bone marrow: serial MR imaging before, during and after radiation therapy. Radiology 1995; 194: 537–543

46. Otake S, Mayr N, Ueda T et al. Radiation-induced changes in MR signal intensity and contrast

enhancement of lumbosacral vertebrae: do changes occur only inside the radiation therapy field? Radiology 2002; 222: 179–183

47. Disler D G, McCauley T R, Ratner L M et al. In-phase and out-of-phase MR imaging of bone marrow: prediction of neoplasia based on the detection of coexistent fat and water. Am J Roentgenol 1997; 169: 1439–1447

48. Zampa V, Cosottini M, Michelassi C et al. Value of opposed-phase gradient-echo technique in distinguishing benign and malignant vertebral lesions. Eur Radiol 2002; 12: 1811–1818

49. Saadat-Arab M, Troufleua P, Stines J et al. MR imaging findings of bone marrow reconversion induced by growth factors in three patients. J Radiol 2002; 83: 147–152

50. Fletcher B D, Eall J E, Hanna S L. Effect of hematopoietic growth factors on MR images of the bone marrow in children undergoing chemotherapy. Radiology 1993; 189: 745–751

51. Ryan S P, Weinberger E, White K S et al. MR imaging of bone marrow in children with osteosarcoma: effect of granulocyte colony-stimulating factor. Am J Roentgenol 1995; 165: 915–920

Chapter 55

Abdomen and pelvis

Paul A Hulse, Bernadette M Carrington and M Ben Taylor

Introduction

Patients with abdomino-pelvic malignancy are principally treated with surgery, radiotherapy and chemotherapy, either alone or in combination. Each mode of therapy produces specific and non-specific post-treatment appearances. Awareness of the pathophysiological processes inducing post-therapy changes and expected time following treatment for their development enables them to be differentiated from other important pathology such as recurrent tumour or infection.

Following surgery, the imaging findings are typical and predictable. Tissue trauma and changes in blood supply induce inflammatory changes, usually leading to fibrosis. In the absence of postoperative infection, and with a few exceptions such as anastomotic stricture, adhesions and hernias, late effects are unusual.

Late effects are common after radiotherapy and are being increasingly recognized following chemotherapy. Different organs have different tolerances to radiotherapy and chemotherapy, so that the concept of threshold dose above which toxic effects are more likely to occur is important.

Plain radiography and contrast studies are often sufficient to demonstrate changes in the bones and hollow organs. Cross-sectional imaging, using computed tomography (CT), MR imaging and ultrasound, provides a more complete picture and can demonstrate subclinical tissue damage by displaying intra-organ anatomy and connective tissue changes.

It is very important for the radiologist to have a record of the patient's previous treatment, such as details of surgery including the operation note, the radiotherapy dose and fields, and prescribed chemotherapy.

Radiation and chemotherapy injury

Radiation affects those tissues with the most rapid cell turnover. Disruption of intracellular DNA prevents cellular replication and results in depletion in stem cell populations. Local cytokine and chemokine release causes inflammation and early tissue damage. Subsequently, damage to microvasculature develops resulting in ischaemia, tissue necrosis and fibrosis. Chemotherapy also affects tissues with rapid cell turnover, resulting in parenchymal cell depletion, but damage to microvasculature and fibro-connective tissue is absent.[1]

Radiation and drugs administered concurrently can act additively or synergistically to produce late tissue injury. When administered consecutively, they can each reveal pre-existing subclinical therapeutic damage. The term 'recall reaction' has been used to describe this phenomenon, but this is inappropriate as these therapeutic modalities act in different ways. In addition, they may aggravate the effects of infection, trauma and other physical stresses.

Organs and tissues have been accorded tolerance doses of radiation. The minimum tolerance dose ($TD_{5/5}$) and maximum tolerance dose ($TD_{50/5}$) are defined by severe life-threatening complications occurring within 5 years of treatment, in 5% and 50% of treated populations, respectively. For example, the ovary has a $TD_{5/5}$ to $TD_{50/5}$ of 2–6 Gy and the gastro-intestinal tract has a $TD_{5/5}$ to $TD_{50/5}$ of 2–10 Gy for a single dose. The tissue or organ with the lowest tolerance dose determines dose limits in a particular body area.[2]

As well as the total radiation dose, the following treatment factors affect the risk of radiation damage:

- Size, number and frequency of radiation fractions
- Volume of irradiated tissue
- Duration of treatment
- Method of radiation delivery (e.g. brachytherapy)
- Combination with chemotherapy and/or surgery
- Use of biological response modifiers (e.g. hypothermia radio-sensitizers, radio-protectors)

Patient factors increasing the risk of radiation injury are:

- Hypertension, atherosclerosis and diabetes mellitus[3,4]
- Pelvic inflammatory disease and infection[5,6]
- Adhesions from prior surgery causing prolonged radiation exposure to immobile small bowel fixed in the treatment field[7]

Key points: radiation and chemotherapy injury

- Knowledge of treatment details helps differentiate post-therapy changes from recurrent tumour and infection
- Radiation and chemotherapy initially affects tissues with the most rapid cell turnover

- Late effects are most common after radiotherapy and are due to ischaemia, tissue necrosis and fibrosis

- Treatment and patient factors influence radiation injury

- Radiation damages multiple organs and body systems in the abdomen and pelvis

Classification of treatment injury

Adverse effects following treatment are categorized as:

- Acute (occurring in the first 3 months)
- Subacute (occurring from 3 months to one year)
- Chronic (occurring later than 1 year)

There is considerable overlap between the groups; for example, acute effects characterized clinically and pathologically can occur after a delay of several months. Patients with severe acute radiation reactions are more likely to progress to serious chronic radiation damage. In 15–30% of patients,[8] multiple organs are involved, resulting in increased morbidity and mortality.

There have been many systems devised for scoring the clinical severity of treatment injury. The LENT/SOMA (Late Effects Normal Tissues/Subjective Objective Medical Management Analytic) system, agreed in 1995 by the RTOG (Radiation Therapy Oncology Group) and EORTC (European Organization Treatment of Cancer),[9] allows a comprehensive record of subjective and objective clinical side-effects, but does not usually include imaging findings.

Treatment effect versus residual/recurrent tumour

A major problem in oncological practice is the distinction between residual or recurrent tumour and treatment effect, particularly radiotherapy-induced changes. Cross-sectional imaging relies on failure of tumour resolution, the appearance of a new mass, or evidence of metastases to identify malignant disease. More infiltrative tumour recurrence can be particularly difficult to identify. Magnetic resonance has the advantage of identifying persistent or new abnormal signal intensity within an organ and can sometimes differentiate between tumour and fibrosis. Tumour usually demonstrates intermediate signal intensity on T1-weighted images, intermediate- to high-signal intensity on T2-weighted images and enhancement after intravenous (IV) contrast.[10,11] Fibrosis returns low signal intensity on both T1- and T2-weighted images and shows little or no enhancement after IV contrast injection. However, there is considerable overlap between tumour and fibrosis so that desmoplastic tumours (for example, breast, carcinoid and rectal tumours) may have similar signal intensity characteristics to fibrosis. Radiation therapy effect, with oedema and inflammation in the acute phase and capillary neovascularity in the chronic phase, may have MR features indistinguishable from tumour.[12]

When diagnostic difficulty occurs there are several man-

agement options. It may be necessary to adopt a wait-and-watch approach, rescanning the patient at regular intervals to identify disease outside the treatment field or the appearance of a mass lesion. Dynamic contrast-enhanced MR has been used to differentiate between recurrent tumour and radiation therapy effect in bladder cancer, with tumour enhancing earlier and to a greater degree.[13] Non-dynamic contrast-enhanced imaging is usually unhelpful in differentiating between recurrent tumour and treatment effect.[14] In some cases, percutaneous image-guided biopsy may be valuable.

Other options include 2-[F-18]fluoro-2-deoxy-D-glucose positron emission tomography ([18]FDG PET) imaging and radiolabelled antibodies to tumour markers such as carcinoembryonic antigen (CEA) and prostate-specific antigen (PSA). [18]FDG PET has been used to investigate patients for disease recurrence with varying success but should not be used fewer than 4 months after radiation therapy to minimize false positive results from radiation-induced inflammatory change. In recurrent rectal cancer, it has been shown to identify recurrence sites and predict for disease resectability better than anti-CEA scanning[15] (Fig. 55.1). In prostate cancer, [18]FDG PET and CT performed similarly in the detection of distant metastases, but were superior to PSA radionuclide imaging.[16] The results in small numbers of patients with recurrent ovarian cancer indicate that combined [18]FDG PET–CT imaging may be valuable in identifying sites of relapse[17] (Fig. 55.1).

Key points: treatment effect versus residual/recurrent tumour

- Differentiation can be made using CT and MR, but infiltrative tumours cause difficulties. T2-weighted MR is more specific than CT

- Contrast-enhanced MR is valuable but can cause confusion

- Alternative strategies are interval imaging, image-guided biopsy, radiolabelled antibody imaging and [18]FDG PET

For ease of reference, discussion in this chapter has been divided into the effects of surgery, chemotherapy and radiotherapy on the hepato-spleno-pancreatico-biliary, gastro-intestinal, genito-urinary and musculoskeletal systems. However, late effects, particularly following radiotherapy, are seldom limited to one organ or body system.

Hepato-spleno-pancreatico-biliary system

Surgical change

Hepatic resection is most commonly performed for hepatocellular carcinoma or colorectal metastases. Hepatic resection may be anatomical (conforming to Couinaud's system

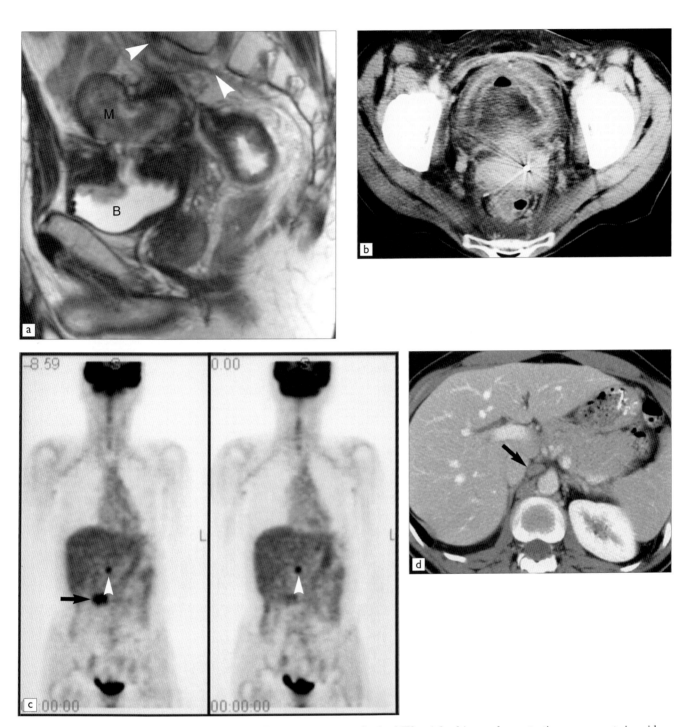

Figure 55.1. *Recurrent pelvic tumour. (a) Sigmoid cancer recurrence. Sagittal T2-weighted image demonstrating a recurrent sigmoid tumour mass (M), which has fistulated into the bladder (B) and extended postero-superiorly to the sacral promontory (arrowheads). (b) Infiltrative recurrence on CT. Transaxial CT image of the pelvis in a patient presumed to have severe radiation change affecting the bladder, rectum and adjacent pelvic connective tissues. A small locule of air is present within the bladder from a vesico-enteric fistula. However, at surgery, there was diffuse malignant infiltration of the pelvic organs. (c and d)* ¹⁸*FDG PET in recurrent colorectal cancer. (c) Coronal* ¹⁸*FDG PET image (maximum intensity projection) of a patient who had a persistently raised CEA, treated for caecal carcinoma. The examination reveals two areas of increased activity, one in the mid abdomen, localized to the bowel or mesentery (arrow) on transaxial images, and the other in the retroperitoneum (arrowhead). (d) Transaxial contrast-enhanced CT image demonstrating a small coeliac axis node (arrow) which was the site of the retroperitoneal second lymph node metastasis.*

of segmental anatomy) or non-anatomical (wedge resection). Metallic surgical clips are usually seen at the resection margin at CT. Perihepatic fluid collections are commonly seen immediately following surgery, but usually resolve within the first month. Postoperative complications include hepatic failure, perihepatic abscess and biliary leak. In the months following resection, the remaining liver regenerates and may recover to its original volume, making the previous resection difficult to appreciate; so attention should be paid to the portal and hepatic venous anatomy (Fig. 55.2). The liver is the most common site of recurrence and, if this is isolated, further surgery may be possible.[18]

Local tumour ablation is increasingly being used in the treatment of malignant liver tumours (see also Chapter 50). Cryotherapy (the use of low temperature to destroy tumour) is usually performed at laparotomy and may be used alone or as an adjunct to surgery. Radio-frequency ablation (RFA) is usually performed percutaneously under imaging guidance. Cryotherapy and RFA both produce a rounded non-enhancing defect on CT or MR. A thin, enhancing hyperaemic halo is commonly seen soon after ablation, which subsides over the first 3 months. Local tumour recurrence is diagnosed when there is nodular or irregular enhancement at the margin of the ablated area.[19–21]

Following pancreato-duodenectomy (Whipple's procedure), radiology is valuable in the identification and percutaneous drainage of abdominal abscesses. These may occur within the retroperitoneum or throughout the peritoneal cavity, therefore postoperative CT should include the entire abdomen and pelvis. The bile ducts are susceptible to damage at the time of surgery, which may lead to biloma, hepatic abscess or biliary stricture.[22]

Splenectomy may be necessary to achieve full surgical clearance of a gastric tumour, pancreatic tail or other retroperitoneal mass. Occasionally, splenectomy is performed for symptom control in patients with haematological malignancy. Following splenectomy, adjacent structures will prolapse into the subphrenic space and may be mistaken for tumour. The pancreatic tail, unopacified stomach or small bowel are most commonly misidentified.

Patients who undergo upper abdominal surgery for malignancy are at risk of portal venous system thrombosis; the risk following splenectomy is around 10%. Thrombosis may be recognized at postoperative CT or ultrasound; it is usually managed conservatively with anticoagulation and complications are rare.[23]

Chemotherapy change

A large number of chemotherapy agents may induce elevation of liver enzymes, which is commonly associated with hepatic steatosis. Radiologists should be aware of the appearance of focal fat deposition and focal fatty sparing to avoid erroneous diagnosis of metastasis. Focal fat deposition commonly occurs adjacent to the falciform ligament or anterior to the porta hepatis and is typically visible as a well-demarcated hyperechoic region on ultrasound and as an area of low density on CT, with a Hounsfield value close to that of water. Focal fat may occur in other areas of the liver and is recognized by its geographical margins and absence of mass effect (Fig. 55.3).[24,25] Areas of normal liver within an otherwise diffusely fatty liver are seen on ultrasound as hypoechoic lesions within a generally hyperechoic liver. These areas are commonly rounded and may easily be mistaken for tumour. When such a lesion is seen at a typical site (adjacent to the gallbladder or anterior to the porta hepatis), focal fatty sparing must be considered (Fig. 55.4).[26,27] Diagnosis is often difficult on ultrasound or CT, and MR may

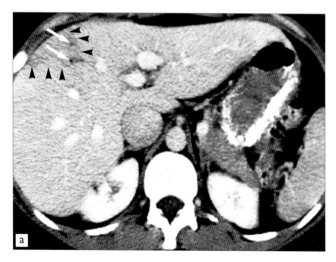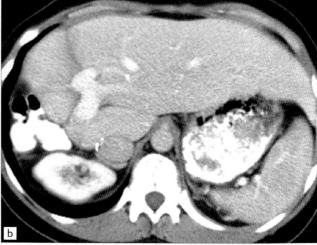

Figure 55.2. *(a) Transaxial contrast-enhanced CT image of the liver in a patient with colorectal carcinoma. There is a small metastasis centrally within Segment VIII (not visible), causing a wedge-shaped peripheral perfusion defect (arrowheads) and localized dilatation of the biliary radicals (arrows). (b) Transaxial CT image of the same patient following right hemihepatectomy, showing marked hypertrophy of the caudate lobe (Segment I) and Segments II and III.*

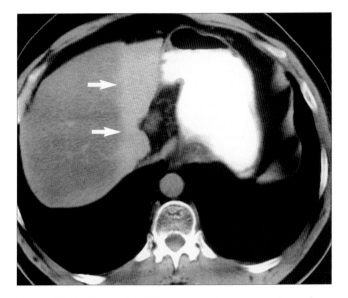

Figure 55.6. *Transaxial CT image of a patient several months following radiotherapy for a lymphomatous nodal mass. There is a clear, straight line of demarcation (arrows) between the irradiated liver and the hypodense, unirradiated liver. The unirradiated liver shows evidence of fatty infiltration. The straight line represents the right lateral edge of the treatment field and is the hallmark of previous radiotherapy.*

doses, in the region of 35–40 Gy, may result in splenic fibrosis and atrophy.[42,43]

Pancreas

The pathological changes in the irradiated pancreas are similar to those of chronic pancreatitis, resulting in necrosis and fibrosis. The acinar epithelium is more radiosensitive than the islet cells. Imaging features are non-specific and similar to chronic pancreatitis.[44,45]

Key points: liver, spleen and pancreas

- Characteristic findings occur following hepatic surgery or local therapy

- Hepatic fatty change and focal fatty sparing cause confusion on ultrasound and CT; MR may be required to confirm the diagnosis

- Hepatic VOD usually occurs in the first 20 days following BMT and myeloablative therapy; hepatic GVHD presents later

- Following splenectomy, unopacified bowel, pancreatic tail and stomach can be confused with tumour

- Changes in the irradiated pancreas cannot be differentiated from recurrent tumour without biopsy

Gastro-intestinal system

Surgical change

Early postoperative complications include anastomotic leak, abscess formation, bowel obstruction, haematoma, wound infection and pancreatitis.

Computed tomography is the investigation of choice in the evaluation of abdominal abscess, pneumo-peritoneum and anastomotic leak. Use of oral contrast is unnecessary in high-grade small bowel obstruction, but is of value in diagnosing anastomotic leak. Computed tomography helps to distinguish mechanical bowel obstruction from postoperative ileus; a transition point between proximal dilated and distal collapsed bowel should be sought.[46]

In the upper abdomen, gastric surgery often results in anatomical changes, which cause difficulty in follow-up imaging. Local recurrence of gastric carcinoma may be subtle and manifest as localized bowel wall thickening or nodular peritoneal thickening. Adjacent loops of bowel may become obstructed due to tumour infiltration, and biliary obstruction may develop due to porta hepatis or peripancreatic nodes.[47]

In the pelvis, the radiological appearance following abdomino-perineal resection (APR) for rectal or anal carcinoma causes particular difficulty. Following APR in the male, the bladder, seminal vesicles and prostate are retracted posteriorly into the rectal bed. Fibrosis in the presacral space may surround and tether the seminal vesicles. The vesicles are often indistinct on CT and may be difficult to distinguish from fibrosis or recurrent tumour; however, they are usually well seen on T2-weighted MR (Figs. 55.7 and 55.8). In the female, the uterus and ovaries prolapse posteriorly into the presacral space and can easily be mistaken for a soft tissue mass on CT (Fig. 55.9). On MR, the uterus and ovaries are more readily identified.

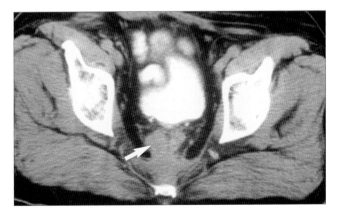

Figure 55.7. *Transaxial CT image of the pelvis in a patient who has had a previous APR and perioperative radiotherapy. The seminal vesicles (right vesicle arrowed) are retracted posteromedially and there is a large presacral soft tissue mass. The mass was unchanged in appearance over several years and is due to post-treatment fibrosis.*

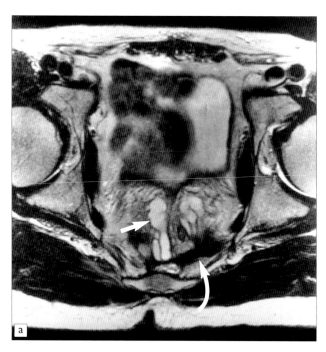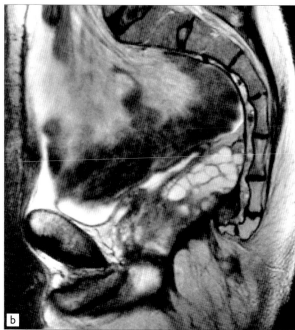

Figure 55.8. *(a) Transaxial and (b) sagittal T2-weighted MR images of the pelvis in a patient who had has a previous APR. The seminal vesicles (right vesicle arrowed) have been retracted posteromedially by a band of fibrous tissue (curved arrow). (b) The base of the prostate is seen to be displaced posteroinferiorly, with the prostate and seminal vesicles being fixed to the pelvic floor. Note the bladder is also being distorted. These T2-weighted images enable discrimination between anatomical structures, bands of fibrosis and/or soft tissue 'masses'.*

Presacral fibrosis varies in appearance on CT or MR from thin band-like strands to a rounded mass, making differentiation from recurrent tumour difficult. Magnetic resonance morphology and signal characteristics can help in

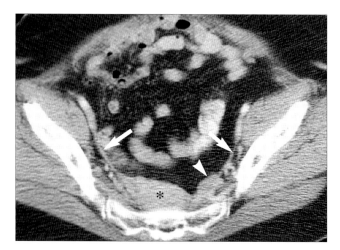

Figure 55.9. *Transaxial contrast-enhanced CT image of the pelvis in a female patient who has undergone previous APR. There is an apparent soft tissue mass with a smooth lobulated contour in the presacral space due to uterus (*) and the left ovary (arrowhead). Close inspection shows the round ligaments (arrows) extending from the mass, anteriorly along the pelvic walls. The uterus (*) and ovaries have prolapsed posteriorly following surgery.*

making this distinction, as tumour is more commonly of high signal intensity on T2-weighted images. However, fibrosis can also show high signal intensity on T2-weighted images, particularly following radiotherapy.[10] Dynamic contrast-enhanced MR is more accurate than non-enhanced imaging, with early enhancement suggesting tumour.[48–50] Invasion of adjacent structures can also be difficult to assess, as presacral fibrosis often involves the piriformis and levator ani muscles; however, sacral invasion indicates tumour. In practice, follow-up imaging and sometimes biopsy is necessary for confident diagnosis.

Radioimmunoscintigraphy using monoclonal antibodies directed against CEA has a similar sensitivity to CT for detection of local recurrence. The accuracy of the technique is improved by combining it with anatomical imaging.[51]

[18]FDG PET has a high specificity and is superior to CT in identifying local recurrence (Fig. 55.10). However, false positive results do occur as a result of inflammation from recent surgery or radiotherapy, so [18]FDG PET should not be performed for 4 months after surgery or radiotherapy.[52–56]

Chemotherapy change

Chemotherapy effects on bowel mainly occur in the early phase following treatment. These include typhlitis (neutropenic enterocolitis), GVHD and pseudomembranous colitis and are discussed in Chapter 52.

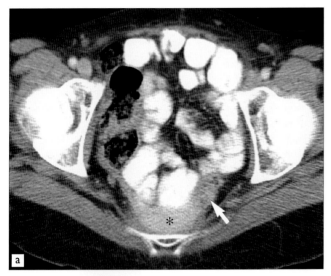

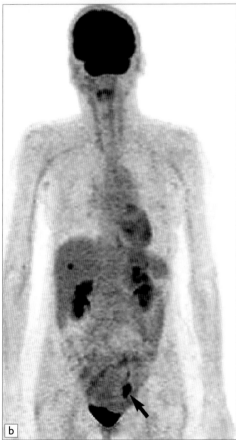

Figure 55.10. *(a) Transaxial contrast-enhanced CT image of a female patient who had undergone APR for anal carcinoma. The presacral mass (*) and left posterior pelvic soft tissue mass (arrow) were initially interpreted as being due to the uterus and left ovary. (b) Coronal* [18]*FDG PET image of the same patient shows a focus of increased activity in the left pelvis corresponding to the left pelvic mass, which is in fact recurrent tumour. A further focus is seen in the liver, this was not visible on CT but was presumed to represent a small metastasis.*

Radiation therapy change

Although the small bowel is more radiosensitive than the large bowel, radiation damage is seen more commonly in the rectum and distal sigmoid colon. This is because the pelvis is commonly irradiated for carcinomas of the cervix, rectum, bladder and prostate. The rectum and sigmoid are relatively fixed within the pelvis and therefore receive the largest dose. Conversely, the small bowel is mobile on a long mesentery with active peristalsis and receives a lower dose. However, adhesions from previous surgery can fix small bowel loops in the pelvis and make radiation damage more likely. Occasionally, surgical measures are taken to move the small bowel out of the radiotherapy field by packing the pelvis with either omentum or an absorbable synthetic mesh.

Stomach and duodenum

Damage to the stomach and duodenum most commonly occurs as a result of radiotherapy for retroperitoneal lymph node metastases or pancreatic carcinoma. Initial changes affect the mucosa, causing ulceration indistinguishable from benign peptic ulcer disease on barium studies. Chronic changes result in fibrosis of the stomach wall, causing narrowing and rigidity of the gastric lumen, often with gastric outlet obstruction. The gastric wall may be indurated on barium studies, making differentiation from gastric carcinoma difficult. Changes in the duodenum include ulceration, thickened mucosal folds and strictures.[41,57]

Chronic changes are manifest on CT as deformity of the stomach, with wall thickening and inflammatory stranding into the adjacent fat.

Small bowel

Radiation damage to the small bowel most commonly occurs following radiotherapy for cervical and prostatic carcinoma. The pelvic small bowel loops and terminal ileum are particularly affected. In the early phase following radiotherapy there may be acute small bowel obstruction due to oedema, which usually resolves spontaneously. Late effects present with chronic abdominal pain, diarrhoea and, less commonly, malabsorption. There may be recurrent attacks of subacute small bowel obstruction, rarely progressing to complete obstruction. On barium studies, one of the earliest changes of radiation damage is fixity of the small bowel loops within the pelvis, which is easily overlooked unless the bowel is palpated and compressed at fluoroscopy. Mucosal changes include thickening of the valvulae conniventes and nodular filling defects ('thumbprinting') due to submucosal oedema. Mucosal ulceration, which may be evident microscopically, is rarely seen radiologically. The bowel loops may be separated due to wall thickening and are commonly fixed and angulated. On fluoroscopy, the bowel shows reduced peristalsis with pooling of barium within the loops. Small bowel strictures and fistulae are late features, which may be difficult to demonstrate.[58–60] These radiological features are not specific for radiation damage and are particularly difficult to distinguish from Crohn's disease.

The role of CT in a previously irradiated patient with small bowel obstruction is to identify whether there is a single site or multiple sites of obstruction, to determine the anatomical level(s) and to identify whether obstruction is due to recurrent tumour. If a transition point between proximal dilated and distal collapsed bowel can be identified with no evidence of tumour, then the main differential diagnosis lies between radiation stricture and postoperative adhesions. Bowel wall thickening and mucosal abnormalities are pointers towards radiation damage, but often these conditions cannot be distinguished (Figs. 55.11 and 55.12).[46] Computed tomography is also useful in identifying fistulae, particularly if gas or oral contrast medium is identified outside the bowel.

Colon and rectum

Following pelvic radiotherapy, damage to the large bowel is usually confined to the rectum and sigmoid colon. Double-contrast barium enema (DCBE) is usually performed to assess the extent and severity of the disease. The earliest sign of DCBE is bowel spasm. Established disease most commonly manifests as a long smooth stricture with tapered margins involving the mid or distal sigmoid or proximal rectum. There may be shorter segments of more severe stenosis within the affected area and there may be multiple strictures (Fig. 55.13).[60] Characteristically, the mucosa is smooth and featureless, but ulceration and mucosal

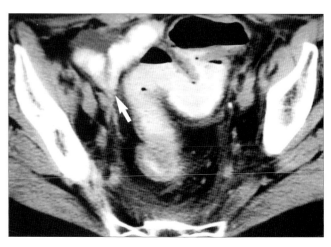

Figure 55.12. *Transaxial CT image of the pelvis in a female patient who has had previous radiotherapy. The distal ileal loop in the right iliac fossa is tethered, causing an acute angulation (arrow) in the loop. The valvulae conniventes are irregularly thickened and there is a small amount of ascites lying anterior to the loop. The sigmoid colon is abnormal, being dilated with an irregularly thickened wall. In addition, there is soft tissue stranding in the pelvic fat and a presacral soft tissue band. All these findings are due to previous radiotherapy.*

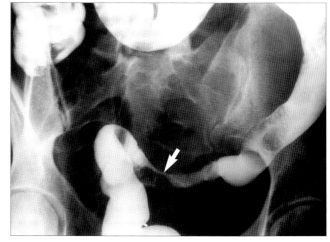

Figure 55.13. *Barium enema demonstrating a variable calibre stricture in the sigmoid colon. Overall, there is a long segmental stricture, within which there is a short-segment, very tight, stricture (arrow). This area of the sigmoid colon received a greater dose than the more proximal sigmoid stricture.*

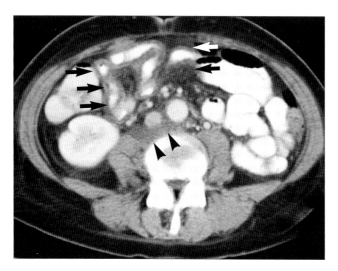

Figure 55.11. *Transaxial contrast-enhanced CT image of the mid-abdomen of a patient who has received radiotherapy to the para-aortic region for retroperitoneal lymphoma (arrowheads). The small bowel loops in the central abdomen are thick-walled with narrowing of the lumen and abnormal angulation. The adjacent mesentery shows linear stranding. The area of abnormal bowel has clearly defined linear margins, corresponding to the radiotherapy field (arrows).*

oedema may occur, producing a 'cobblestone' pattern. More rarely, there may be deep ulceration with the development of sinus tracts, pericolic or perirectal collections, or fistulae. Lateral views of the rectum often show widening of the presacral space.

Changes seen on CT include thickening of the rectal wall, increased attenuation of the perirectal fat and thickening of the perirectal fascia, resulting in widening of the presacral space (Fig. 55.14). In addition, presacral fibrosis may develop and can mimic a soft-tissue mass.[61,62]

The earliest changes of radiotherapy on MR are of increased signal intensity of the submucosa and inner (circular) muscle layer on T2-weighted images (Fig. 55.22f). Initially, the outer muscle layer retains its normal low signal intensity. As the radiation damage progresses, there is thickening of the rectal wall (greater than 6 mm), high signal intensity within the outer muscle layer and loss of differentiation of the rectal wall layers. There is high signal intensity on T2-weighted images within the perirectal fat, due to oedema, and thickening of the perirectal fascia to greater than 3 mm.[63] If IV gadolinium (Gd) is administered, there is non-specific enhancement of the rectal wall.

In severe radiation bowel disease, there is necrosis and breakdown of the bowel wall due to ischaemia, which can result in the development of sinus tracts or fistulae. Fistulation most commonly occurs between the rectum and vagina, but fistulae to the bladder, between loops of small and large bowel, and to skin may occur. Complex fistulae, involving the rectum, vagina and bladder are not uncommon, particularly in patients treated for cervical carcinoma. Contrast studies of the rectum, using either barium or water-soluble iodinated contrast, are sensitive for detection of rectovaginal or colovesical fistula (Fig. 55.15). Magnetic resonance is highly accurate in demonstrating pelvic fistulae.[64–66] These are normally well seen on spin-echo T2-weighted images, particularly if thin sections and a phased-array surface coil are employed (Fig. 55.16). Fat-suppressed T2-weighted and short tau inversion recovery (STIR) sequences have a higher sensitivity, but demonstrate the pelvic anatomy less well. Magnetic resonance has the added advantage of demonstrating extraluminal pelvic collections and recurrent tumour, which commonly coexist with radiation damage. Knowledge of the fistulous anatomy

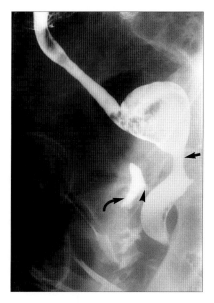

Figure 55.15. *Lateral view from a barium enema in a patient previously treated with pelvic radiotherapy for carcinoma of the cervix. The left hemicolon has been defunctioned and an antegrade barium enema performed via a Foley catheter. There is a radiation stricture in the rectum (arrow) and a fistula between the rectum and vagina. Contrast is present in the vagina (curved arrow) and a small fistulous tract (arrowhead) can be identified.*

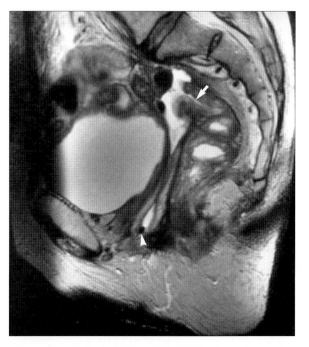

Figure 55.16. *Sagittal T2-weighted MR of a patient with recurrent cervical tumour on the left side of the pelvis involving the bladder and pelvic sidewall. The recurrent tumour is associated with a cavity containing fluid and air and there is a fistulous tract between the rectosigmoid junction through the recurrent tumour to the vault of the vagina. The communication with the large bowel is clearly seen (arrow). The vagina is clearly defined with a small amount of air being present at the introitus (arrowhead).*

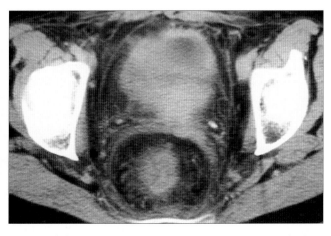

Figure 55.14. *Transaxial CT of the pelvis in a patient who has received pelvic radiotherapy. There is extensive soft tissue stranding in the perirectal space, together with thickening of the perirectal fascia. Oedema is present in the anterior abdominal wall and there is a general increase in density of the pelvic fat.*

and likely sites of recurrence assists the surgeon in planning examination under anaesthesia (EUA) and biopsy, and in deciding whether surgery is likely to be of value.

Key points: gastro-intestinal system

- ■ Radiation injury is most commonly seen in the rectum, sigmoid colon and pelvic small bowel

- ■ Acute bowel reaction to radiotherapy is frequently reversible

- ■ Chronic radiation damage is irreversible

- ■ Barium study features in the small bowel are non-specific with mucosal abnormalities, angulated fixed loops and strictures; in the large bowel, smooth tapered strictures are characteristic

- ■ Pelvic irradiation causes widening of the presacral space and thickening of the perirectal fascia

- ■ MR is sensitive for detection of early radiation changes in the bowel wall and is valuable in the investigation of pelvic fistulae

Genito-urinary system

The genito-urinary system is variably affected by cancer therapy, with the kidney and testis particularly susceptible and the ureters relatively resistant.

Surgical change

Standard genito-urinary surgical procedures and their complications are usually recognizable on cross-sectional imaging. Problems in postsurgical imaging usually occur in the following instances:

- When an organ has been partially resected, for example, following partial nephrectomy, partial cystectomy with bladder augmentation and subtotal hysterectomy (Fig. 55.17)
- When there are postsurgical complications simulating masses; for example, lymphoceles[67,68] and pelvic haematoma, which may be within the central pelvis, arise in the retracted spermatic cord after orchidectomy or in the round ligament after hysterectomy[69] (Fig. 55.18)
- When there is unusual postsurgical anatomy; for example, as part of a modified radical hysterectomy the ovaries can be transposed, usually into the iliac fossae, and may be mistaken for tumour masses.[70] Bladder surgery can entail hitching the bladder to the retroperitoneum or the formation of flaps for reimplantation of the ureters. The flaps can simulate a tumour mass (Fig. 55.19)

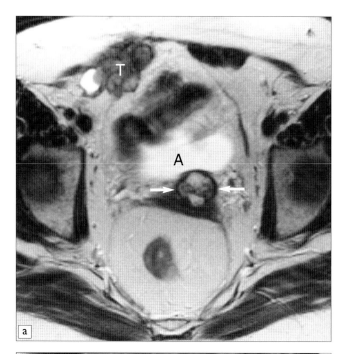

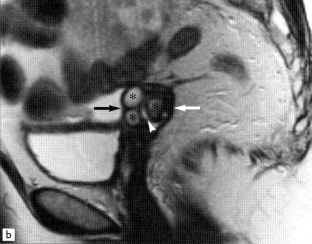

Figure 55.17. *Partial organ resection. Subtotal hysterectomy. (a) Transaxial and (b) sagittal T2-weighted MR images demonstrating an apparent mass in the central pelvis (arrows) in a patient with ovarian cancer and an anterior abdominal wall tumour recurrence (T). In (b) the mass is shown to be the retained cervix with a clearly visualized endocervical canal (arrowhead) and multiple Nabothian cysts (*). A – ascites. It is important to be aware of the exact surgical procedure performed in patients with pelvic cancer.*

- When there is significant inflammatory change and fibrosis. For example, the posthysterectomy vaginal vault is oversewn to give a 'bow tie' appearance with a flattened central portion and bulbous lateral margins representing the sutured fornices. The appearances may be confused with residual tumour. After radical prostatectomy, the prostate bed may be

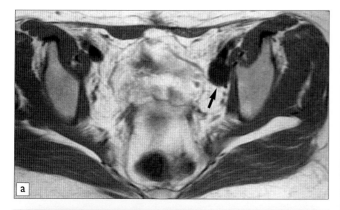

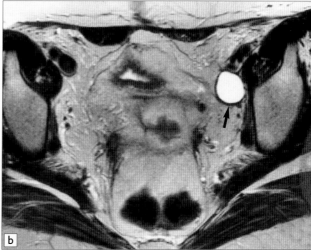

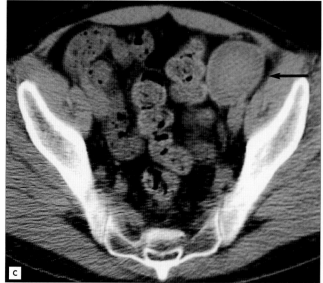

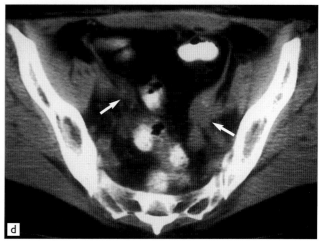

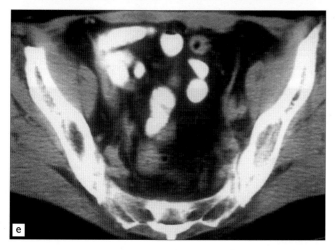

Figure 55.18. *Complications of the surgical procedure. (a and b) lymphocele. Transaxial (a) T1-weighted and (b) T2-weighted images in a patient postradical hysterectomy for cervical cancer demonstrating a left pelvic sidewall lymphocele (arrow) which is unilocular and of fluid signal intensity. (c) Postorchidectomy pelvic haematoma. Transaxial non-contrast-enhanced CT image demonstrating a left pelvic sidewall haematoma (arrow) secondary to bleeding from the retracted spermatic cord. Note the slight increase in attenuation in the centre of the haematoma due to increased electron density of the retracted clot. (d) Round ligament haematoma. Transaxial CT image of the pelvis demonstrating bilateral sidewall masses (arrows) continuous with the round ligaments in the early postoperative period. (e) These have almost completely resolved on a follow-up examination performed 6 months later.*

difficult to evaluate because of extensive postsurgical fibrosis at the anastomotic site between the bladder base and membranous urethra. This may be the site of postsurgical urethral stricture (Fig. 55.20)

Chemotherapy change

Chemotherapy has a direct toxic effect on the genito-urinary system, particularly the kidneys and the bladder.

Nephrotoxicity may be acute or chronic. The acute form is reversible and manifests as rapid-onset renal failure. Imaging is usually performed to exclude renal obstruction. Ultrasound may demonstrate enlarged kidneys with increased cortical echogenicity and lack of corticomedullary differentiation. Chronic nephrotoxicity ultimately results in atrophic kidneys with loss of cortical substance. Chemotoxicity on the bladder mucosa is most marked in cyclophosphamide- and ifosfamide-induced

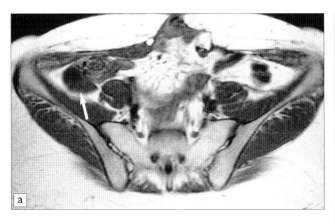
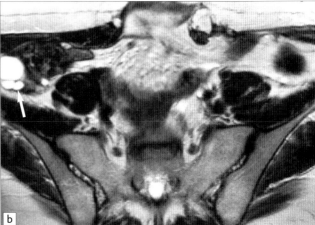

Figure 55.19. *Unusual postsurgical anatomy. Ovarian transposition. Transaxial (a) T1-weighted and (b) T2-weighted MR images showing a transposed ovary (arrow) in the right iliac fossa.*

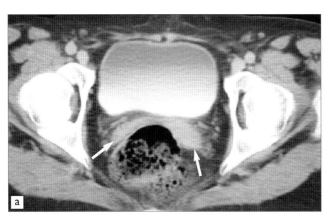
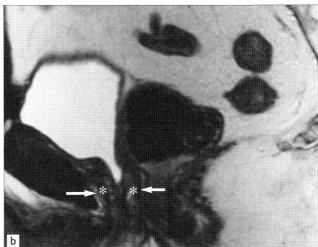
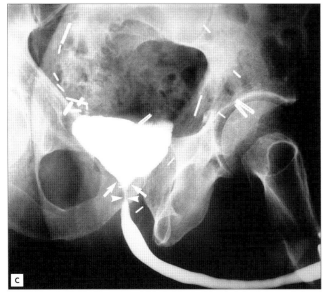

Figure 55.20. *Normal postoperative scarring. (a) Vaginal appearances after hysterectomy. Transaxial CT image demonstrating the normal appearance of the posthysterectomy vaginal vault. The central portion is apposed with rather bulbous but symmetrical oversewn fornices (arrows). (b) After prostatectomy. Sagittal T2-weighted MR demonstrating the anastomosis (arrows) between the bladder base and the membranous urethra. There is a thick rind of low signal intensity surgical scarring (*) present. (c) Postprostatectomy stricture. Micturating cystourethrogram in a patient who has undergone radical prostatectomy. The bladder base (arrows) is low lying behind the symphysis pubis due to its anastomosis with the membranous urethra. There is a mild stricture at the anastomotic site (arrowheads). Multiple surgical clips are present in the pelvis from lymph node dissection performed during the prostatectomy.*

haemorrhagic cystitis,[71] which produce a thickened bladder wall with intravesical clots. Intravesical chemotherapy directly affects the bladder wall and ultimately produces a contracted fibrosed bladder (Fig. 55.21).

Chemotherapy has an adverse effect on fertility, although there are usually no overt imaging findings in the male. In women, the ovaries may atrophy with reduction or absence of follicles.

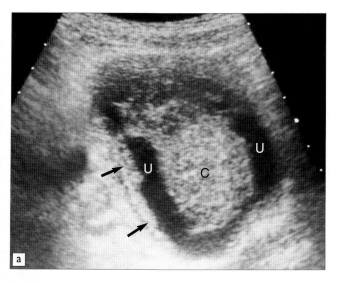

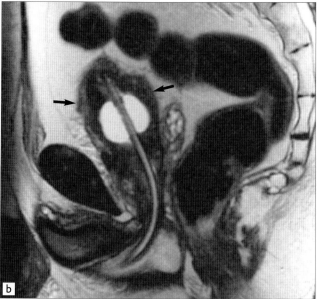

Figure 55.21. *Chemotherapy effects. (a) Haemorrhagic cystitis. Longitudinal ultrasound image demonstrating a thickened bladder wall (arrows) with a small amount of urine (U) identified in the periphery and a large central hyperechoic clot (C). (b) Bladder fibrosis after intravesical chemotherapy. Sagittal T2-weighted MR demonstrating that the wall of the bladder is irregular, thickened and of uniform low signal intensity (arrows). The patient is catheterized because of intolerable frequency arising from the reduced bladder capacity.*

Indirect effects of chemotherapy stem from neutropenia and thrombocytopenia. In the genito-urinary tract, infections most commonly affect the kidneys or bladder; and thrombocytopenia may cause haematuria.

Radiation therapy change

Bladder

The bladder is the most radiation-sensitive organ in the urinary tract.[72] Radiation bladder injury occurs in up to 20% of patients, half of whom go on to suffer severe long-term effects. In the acute phase, mucosal oedema, haemorrhage and necrosis may cause cystitis and haematuria. Subsequent fibrosis results in a small volume, non-distensible bladder producing symptoms of frequency and incontinence. Mucosal telangiectasia and ulceration may cause trouble-some haematuria.

Ultrasound, CT and MR all demonstrate radiation-induced acute changes and more chronic bladder wall thickening (Fig. 55.22). Adjacent perivesical fibrosis can be identified on CT and MR. In addition, MR can identify a spectrum of radiation change corresponding to the severity of clinical symptoms. The earliest abnormality is high-signal intensity of the mucosa on T1- and T2-weighted images, probably reflecting haemorrhage and oedema. Initially, this may be localized to the posterior wall and trigone,[63] but eventually the entire bladder mucosa may become involved. More severe radiation effect causes T2-weighted high-signal intensity of the outer bladder wall, increased radial diameter of the wall and poor distensibility. Intravenous Gd-DTPA injection may reveal enhancement of the bladder mucosa and patchy or diffuse enhancement of the outer wall, sometimes with variations in signal intensity between different layers of the bladder wall to give a banded or lamellated appearance.[12] This enhancement may persist for several years. With extreme radiation toxicity, fistula formation occurs between the bladder and the vagina or bowel.

Kidney

The kidney is radiosensitive and is often the dose-limiting organ during treatment of abdominal malignancies, with the risk of nephrotoxicity increased by prior or concurrent chemotherapy. Radiation-induced nephropathy appears from months to years after treatment, with an inverse relationship between the interval and the renal dose.[73] Radiation nephropathy will not develop providing one normally functioning kidney is excluded from the radiation field, but malignant hypertension may occur secondary to renin overproduction by the irradiated kidney. Ultimately, radiation nephrotoxicity results in small, poorly functioning, non-obstructed kidneys.

Ureter

Radiation-induced ureteric injury is uncommon, occurring in fewer than 5% of those sustaining complications from radiotherapy.[74] There are two types of injury: stricture formation and vesico-ureteric reflux. Stricture formation may remain clinically silent but cause insidious renal failure. It occurs most frequently in the distal ureter immediately above the vesico-ureteric junction.[60] Occasionally, high

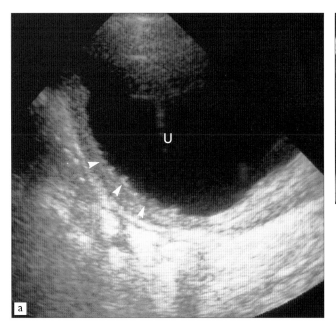

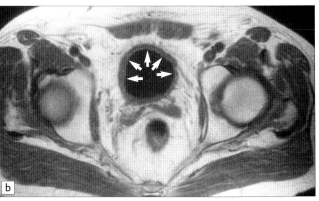

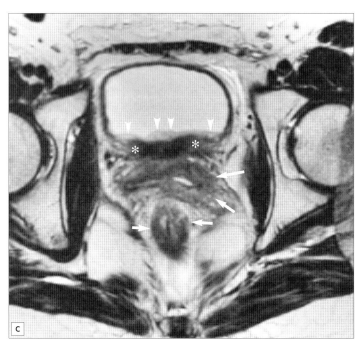

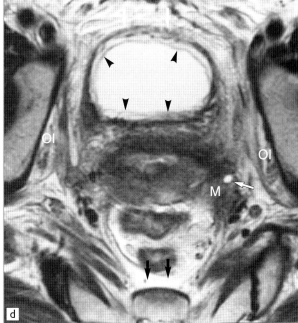

strictures occur where the pelvic ureters cross anterior to the iliac vessels.[60] Radiation strictures typically have a smoothly tapering distal margin but the appearances are non-specific and may be seen in patients with tumour recurrence. In some patients, strictures are adequately visualized on intravenous urography, but in others it may be necessary to perform antegrade pyelography. Isotope renography and glomerular filtration rate are valuable as sequential studies will often reveal deterioration in renal performance before clinical or biochemical abnormalities occur.

Vesico-ureteric reflux may occur secondary to distortion of the vesico-ureteric junction by bladder wall fibrosis. This predisposes the patient to infection and reflux nephropathy.

Prostate and seminal vesicles

Radiotherapy affects the prostate and seminal vesicles in a similar fashion to any other irradiated organ. It is the long-term fibrotic effect that becomes apparent on imaging, with atrophy of the prostate and seminal vesicles. On MR, the peripheral zone of the prostate becomes of uniformly low signal intensity on T2-weighted images[12] (Fig. 55.23), making the diagnosis of recurrent tumour difficult, as most prostate tumours are also of low/intermediate signal inten-

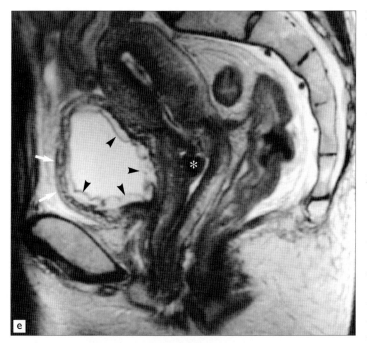

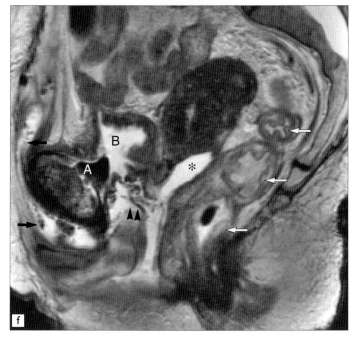

Figure 55.22. *Radiation therapy effect on the bladder. (a) Mucosal thickening. Longitudinal ultrasound scan demonstrating diffuse mucosal thickening of the bladder (arrowheads) in the acute phase after radiotherapy treatment. Urine (U). (b) Acute radiotherapy change with haemorrhage. Transaxial T1-weighted MR demonstrating a fine high signal intensity rind (arrows) on the inner margins of the bladder wall. This is due to haemorrhage within the mucosa. (c) Acute radiation change in the central pelvis. Transaxial T2-weighted MR demonstrating radiotherapy change in a patient treated for cancer of the cervix. The posterior bladder wall demonstrates high signal mucosal thickening (arrowheads) as well as intermediate to low signal intensity thickening of the muscle layer (asterisk). Note that the anterior bladder wall retains its normal low signal intensity muscle layer. The vaginal vault is also abnormal with mucosal and submucosal thickening particularly on the left (long arrows). The anterior portion of the rectum demostrates high signal intensity of the wall due to inclusion in the field (short arrows). Severe radiation change in the pelvis. (d) Transaxial and (e) sagittal T2-weighted MR demonstrating severe acute radiation change. The mucosa of the bladder is markedly thickened (arrowheads), the muscle layer is thickened and demonstrates abnormal high signal intensity with some preservation of portions of the low signal intensity muscle to give a lamellated appearance particularly anteriorly (white arrows). The posterior bladder wall is retracted towards the cervix in (e). The vagina and rectum demonstrate abnormal high signal intensity mural thickening due to the radiation therapy effect. There is a marker seed within the anterior lip of the cervix (asterisk). More generalized changes are seen with oedema in the presacral space (black arrows in d), generalized increase in stranding within the pelvic fat and abnormal high signal intensity of the obturator internus muscles (OI) due to an oedematous reaction. An abnormal intermediate to low signal intensity mass (M) is seen around the lateral margin of the uterus enveloping the distal left ureter (open arrow in d), this represents incomplete resolution of tumour. (f) Severe radiation change with fistula formation and abscess. Sagittal T2-weighted MR in a patient treated with radiation therapy for carcinoma of the cervix. The vagina is fluid-filled (*) and there is a fistula (arrowheads) communicating with the bladder (B) and a large retropubic abscess cavity (A). The abscess extends to the prepubic space (arrows). Note the abnormal signal intensity within the recto-anus (white arrow) due to treatment effect.*

sity on T2-weighted images. The seminal vesicles shrink and demonstrate uniform low signal intensity on T2-weighted sequences.[12]

Urethra

The male urethra is sensitive to radiotherapy, especially after prior transurethral resection of the prostate.[75] In severe cases, stricture formation occurs, usually in the pro-static or membranous portion of the urethra. This complication occurs more frequently after prostate brachytherapy unless the radiation dose is restricted in the periurethral region.

Testis

The adult male testis is an extremely radiosensitive organ; a dose of as little as 0.15 Gy can cause a significant drop in the

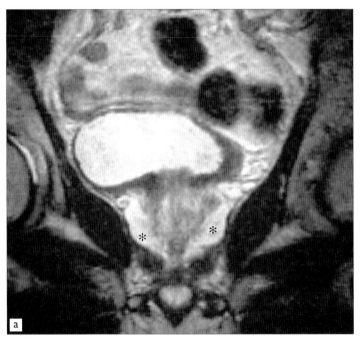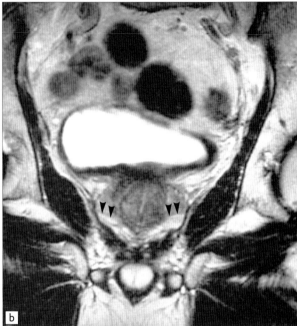

Figure 55.23. *Radiation therapy effect on the prostate. (a and b) Coronal T2-weighted MR images (a) before treatment and (b) after treatment for a bladder tumour. The normal high signal intensity of the peripheral zone is apparent in (a) (*) but in (b) there is a well demarcated low signal intensity component to the superior aspect of the peripheral zone bilaterally (arrowheads) which corresponds to the inferior aspect of the radiotherapy field used to treat the bladder.*

sperm count.[76] Consequently, treatment fields are designed to keep testicular doses to an absolute minimum consistent with adequate tumour coverage. When testicular exposure is inevitable, sperm banking should be considered. There is no recognizable imaging finding apart from atrophy and this is not invariably present even with severe azoospermia.

Uterus

In women of childbearing age, radiotherapy effect on the uterus results in atrophy, best appreciated on T2-weighted MR, where the normal zonal anatomy is lost and the myometrium becomes of uniform low signal intensity with a slit-like endometrium[77] (Fig. 55.24). Rarely, radiation-induced cervical stenosis produces hydro- or haemato-metria with increase in uterine size.[78]

Vagina

The vagina demonstrates low-signal intensity of its wall in the chronic phase after radiotherapy, although in the first 3 months after treatment, high-signal intensity may be seen within the vaginal submucosa on T2-weighted images (Fig. 55.22c) and there may be enhancement after IV Gd-DTPA injection.

Ovary

After radiation therapy, the ovaries shrink, lose their follicular cysts and eventually become fibrotic (Fig. 55.25). The effect of radiation on ovarian function depends on the radiation dose and the age of the patient. Relatively small doses

Key points : genito-urinary system

- Lymphoceles are common following radical lymph node dissection and are readily recognized as unilocular, thin-walled, fluid-filled lesions

- Chemotherapy is often nephrotoxic; ultrasound is useful for excluding renal obstruction

- The kidney is radiosensitive and is often the dose-limiting organ during treatment of abdominal malignancy

- The bladder is the most radiation-sensitive organ in the urinary tract, bladder injury occurring in up to 20% of patients following pelvic radiation

- Radiation induces fibrosis of bladder wall, which becomes thickened

- The gynaecological organs, prostate and seminal vesicles show fibrosis and atrophy following radiotherapy

- Radiation fibrosis and tumour may have indistinguishable features on MR, even following contrast enhancement

- Semiquantitative dynamic contrast-enhanced MR may improve specificity of MR indication of recurrence

- [18]FDG PET and monoclonal antibody imaging have a role in the distinction of radiation damage and tumour recurrence

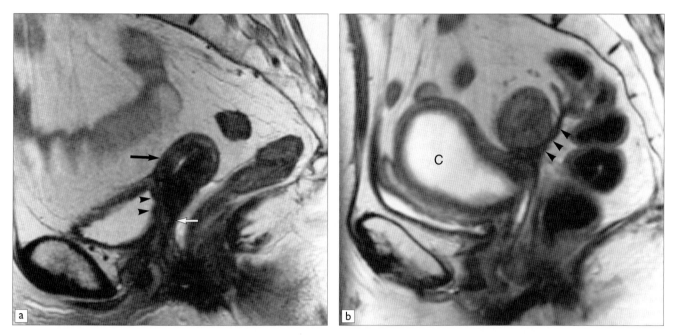

Figure 55.24. *Radiation effect on the uterus. Sagittal T2-weighted MR demonstrates (a) a small low signal intensity uterus (arrow) with loss of its junctional anatomy. The upper vagina (white arrow) is of similar low signal intensity and the posterior wall of the bladder is tethered to the uterus and upper vagina (arrowheads). (b) Hydrometria in a patient treated for carcinoma of the cervix. The uterine cavity (C) is distended and filled with high signal intensity material due to a radiation-induced stenosis of the cervix. Note band-like signal intensity extending from the posterior vaginal fornix along the line of the peritoneal reflection (arrowheads). This is not a typical radiotherapy finding and may have occurred secondary to previous inflammation or surgery, or represent the fibrotic residuum of tumour infiltration.*

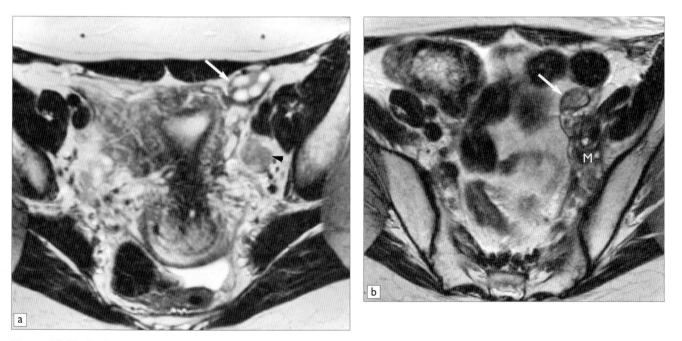

Figure 55.25. *Radiation effect on the ovary. Transaxial T2-weighted MR (a) before and (b) 18 months after radiotherapy for cervical cancer. The normal left ovary (arrow) is well seen in (a). After radiotherapy, the ovary (arrow in b) has decreased in size and signal intensity with atrophy of the ovarian follicles. Also note the left obturator lymph node metastasis (arrowhead in a). On follow-up there is an ill-defined mass (M) on the left pelvic sidewall. This was confirmed to be residual/recurrent tumour.*

can induce the menopause in middle-aged women, whereas young women require a higher total exposure to induce ovarian failure.

Premenarchal girls treated with high doses to the abdomen (in the order of 20–30 Gy) will experience premature ovarian failure[79] and the uterus may remain of infantile proportions. In the long-term, radiotherapy causes decreased distensibility of the uterus and abdomino-pelvic connective tissue, which probably contribute to the high incidence of miscarriage and premature birth.

Musculoskeletal system

Of the cancer treatment modalities, radiation therapy is principally responsible for treatment-induced injury of the normal musculoskeletal tissues, nerves and blood vessels of the abdomen and pelvis. Chemotherapy and corticosteroids can also have deleterious effects.

Bone

After therapeutic radiation there is damage to the cellular elements of bone marrow and to cortical and trabecular bone.

Understanding the normal pattern of conversion of haemopoietic (red) to fatty (yellow) marrow with ageing is key to the interpretation of MR after chemoradiotherapy. Conversion happens in an orderly pattern from distal to proximal, from the appendicular to the axial skeleton and from the diaphyses towards the metaphyses of the long bones.[80]

Appearances in the pelvic bones can cause confusion. Marrow conversion occurs later than in the long bones and haemopoietic marrow is more patchily distributed. Concentrations of fatty marrow are found around the sacro-iliac joints, acetabulae and symphysis pubis.[81–83] The normally bilateral and symmetrical appearance helps differentiate islands of haemopoietic tissue from tumour infiltration on T1-weighted images (Figs. 55.26 and 55.27).

Changes on MR of the lumbar spine and sacrum may be seen as early as the second week after radiotherapy, when STIR images demonstrate an increase in signal intensity of the bone marrow due to oedema and cell necrosis.[84] In addition, there is an early transient increase in contrast-enhancement following Gd-DTPA at 2 weeks after radiotherapy, followed by a progressive decrease in contrast enhancement after 4 weeks.[85] Subsequently, the signal intensity of the marrow on T1-weighted MR gradually increases as the haemopoietic marrow is replaced by fat. The bright appearance of irradiated lumbar vertebrae is irreversible when doses exceed 30Gy.[86] For lower doses, marrow regeneration may occur 1 year after radiotherapy.[87]

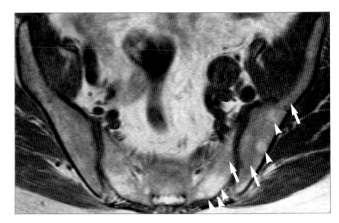

Figure 55.26. *Transaxial T1-weighted MR of pelvic bones showing normal patchy but symmetrical distribution of haemopoietic (arrows) and fatty (arrowheads) marrow.*

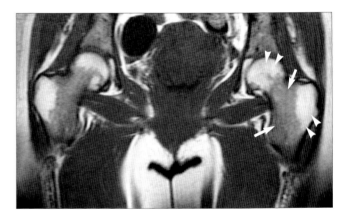

Figure 55.27. *Coronal T1-weighted MR of proximal femora showing normal, but strikingly symmetrical, distribution of haemopoietic (arrows) and fatty (arrowheads) marrow.*

The boundary of these changes normally corresponds closely with the radiation field,[88] although minor changes can be detected outside the field attributable to low-dose scattered radiation.[85]

When therapeutic radiation is followed by high-dose chemotherapy and bone marrow or stem cell transplantation, differentiating regenerating haemopoietic marrow from metastatic disease in the pelvis and lumbar spine using conventional MR sequences can be problematical. Both have heterogeneous intermediate signal intensity on T1-weighted images and increased signal intensity on T2-weighted images. Metastatic disease replaces the various marrow constituents but regenerating marrow does not, leaving some fatty elements. This phenomenon can be exploited using opposed-phase gradient-echo imaging when the fat elements of regenerating marrow have lower signal intensity than metastatic disease on out-of-phase imaging.[89]

Following radiotherapy, there is progressive ischaemia that affects the cortical and trabecular bone, rendering it vulnerable to fracture, infection and impaired healing. The appearances on plain radiographs reflect the initial resorption of dead bone and necrotic tissue followed by the deposition of new bone on unresorbed trabeculae, a process described as 'creeping substitution'.[90] A similar mixed lytic and sclerotic appearance is also seen on CT, but the superior contrast resolution of CT allows more subtle change to be appreciated, particularly in the pelvic bones. As a rule, postradiation atrophy can be differentiated from infiltrative metastatic disease by noting the absence of abnormality outside the radiation field, the lack of a radiographically recognizable periosteal reaction[91] and the time-delay before the development of an abnormality, as metastases tend to occur earlier in the course of the disease.

Insufficiency fractures of the sacrum, and less commonly the pubis, occur in patients irradiated for gynaecological malignancy in whom postmenopausal osteoporosis steroid therapy and other metabolic bone diseases may be additional risk factors[92,93] (see Chapter 54).

Subcapital fractures of the femoral neck previously occurred in approximately 2% of patients receiving pelvic radiation.[94] However, with the abandonment of lateral radiation fields, the change from ortho-voltage to super-voltage or mega-voltage treatment, and shielding of the femoral neck, these are now seldom seen.

Vertebral bodies that have their osseous matrix replaced by malignant tissue can collapse following chemotherapy or radiotherapy, as tumour resolves leaving little supporting bony substrate.[95] Differentiating between benign post-treatment collapse, osteoporotic collapse and collapse due to malignant disease is very difficult using plain radiography or CT, so that MR is the modality of choice. Findings supporting malignant fractures on MR are:

- Abnormality involving the entire vertebra
- Extension to the pedicles
- A bulging vertebral contour
- An epidural mass
- A cervical or lumbosacral location[96]
- Inhomogeneous enhancement following IV contrast[97]

Osteomyelitis is most likely to occur in the pelvis where radiation damage to pelvic bowel loops and surgical intervention increase the risk. The symphysis pubis is most commonly affected and there are usually symmetrical lytic and sclerotic changes in the pubic bones. On CT, an associated pelvic abscess is usually seen and a soft tissue mass, fistulae and gas in the symphysis pubis itself are possible additional findings.[98]

Avascular necrosis (AVN) occurs as a complication of chemotherapy,[99] radiotherapy, or corticosteroid therapy, either alone or in combination. Weight-bearing and trauma are possible additional risk factors accounting for the higher incidence in the femoral than humeral head.[100] Early diagnosis is critical to allow surgical intervention and modifica-

tion of therapy. Magnetic resonance is the modality of choice in demonstrating AVN as it is more sensitive than plain radiographs or radioisotope scans[101,102] and has the ability to identify any associated joint effusion or cartilage abnormality. Initially, on T1-weighted images there are diffuse areas of reduced signal intensity in the high signal intensity fatty marrow of the femoral head. Subsequently, low signal intensity bands or lines occur within the antero-superior aspect of the femoral head on both T1- and T2-weighted images. On T2-weighted images, an additional band of high signal intensity representing the interface between normal and infarcted marrow is seen (double line sign)[101] (Fig. 55.28). Progressive bone necrosis appears as high signal intensity on T2-weighted images and low signal intensity on T1-weighted images, and subsequent fibrosis as low signal intensity on both T1-weighted and T2-weighted images. Radiographically, the first sign of AVN is a patchy increase in the density of the femoral head followed by development of a subchondral lucency, mirroring the MR appearances. The joint space is usually preserved, but may be reduced if there is eventual collapse and fragmentation of the femoral head.

Radiotherapy may produce changes in and around joints: for example, the sacro-iliac joints may be wide and irregular following radiotherapy. Plain radiography shows sclerosis of the adjacent joint surfaces, often in a bilateral and symmetrical pattern resembling osteitis codensans illi.[103] Similar sclerotic changes in the pubis resemble osteitis pubis.

Skeletal muscle

Injury to skeletal muscle in the radiation field results from vascular damage and may progress for many years following treatment,[104] muscles undergoing necrosis with oedema, atrophy and eventual fibrosis. Sigimura et al.[63] noted changes on MR from 3 weeks to longer than 12 months after irradiation for pelvic malignancy. The homogeneous increase in signal intensity on T2-weighted images in a unilateral or bilateral distribution was seen in the pelvic sidewall muscles (Fig. 55.29). Chronic atrophic changes are also evident on CT with asymmetry or loss of muscle bulk.

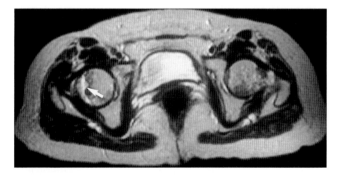

Figure 55.28. *Transaxial T2-weighted MR showing bilateral avascular necrosis of the femoral head following corticosteroid treatment and chemotherapy for Hodgkin's disease. Note double line sign in right femoral head (arrow) (see text).*

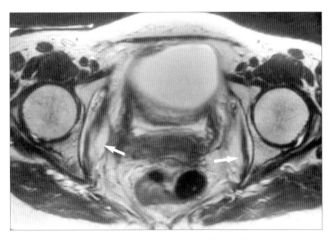

Figure 55.29. *Transaxial T2-weighted MR of the pelvis demonstrating bilateral homogeneous increase in signal intensity in the obturator internus muscles (arrows) following pelvic radiotherapy.*

Peripheral nerves

Radiation change to the lumbosacral plexus is uncommon, but has been reported in patients with gynaecological cancer who receive radiation doses in excess of 70 Gy to the whole pelvis.[104] The imaging features have not been clearly defined.

Blood vessels

Radiation damage to blood vessels occurs predominantly in the intimal layer with changes that are indistinguishable from atherosclerosis.[105] The irradiated artery shows focal or diffuse irregularity, stenosis or occlusion angiographically. Aneurysm formation and rupture may occur. Venous changes are infrequently reported but mesenteric venous occlusion has been noted following pelvic irradiation.[106]

Treatment effects on the growing skeleton

In children, skeletal abnormalities result not only from external beam radiation for solid tumours but also from total body irradiation in preparation for BMT.[107] The most striking effect is on growth and may result from damage to nerves, blood vessels, muscles and bones either alone or in combination.

Radiation-induced interruption of vertebral body growth gives typical radiographic features. The vertebral body height is reduced and there may be anterior beaking resembling the appearance of the mucopolysaccharidoses. Dense, sometimes multiple, growth arrest lines occur parallel to the vertebral end plates and occasionally there is a 'bone within a bone' appearance. The trabecular pattern is coarsened and the end plates are irregular. Asymmetrical vertebral development results in kyphosis and scoliosis, particularly when the spine and paravertebral muscles have been unevenly irradiated. The convexity of the scoliosis points away from the irradiated side (Fig. 55.30).

Changes evident in the pelvis are hypoplasia of the iliac blade and acetabulum predisposing to hip dislocation. The risk of slipped femoral capital epiphysis is increased and tends to occur at an earlier age than the idiopathic type.[90] Associated rib hypoplasia may also be observed.

Children treated with long-term methotrexate in low dose for acute lymphoblastic leukaemia and those treated with high-dose methotrexate for brain tumours[108] and osteosarcoma[109] are prone to methotrexate osteopathy, a syndrome of bone pain, osteopenia and pathological fracture. The radiographic features of osteopenia, dense provisional zones of calcification, pathological fractures (frequently metaphyseal) and sharply outlined epiphyses resemble those of scurvy,[110] but marked subperiosteal haemorrhage is absent.

The alkylating agent ifosfamide is nephrotoxic and can precipitate clinical and radiological hypophosphataemic rickets, particularly in patients with previous nephrectomy or pre-existing renal disease.[111]

Key points: musculoskeletal system

- Understanding the normal distribution of haemopoietic and fatty bone marrow is key to the interpretation of MR after chemo-radiotherapy

- Radiotherapy renders bone vulnerable to fracture, infection and impaired healing

- Insufficiency fractures of the sacrum, pubis, femoral neck and vertebral body can occur following chemoradiotherapy

- Avascular necrosis results from radiotherapy, chemotherapy, and corticosteroids used alone or in combination

- Radiotherapy affects skeletal muscle, peripheral nerves and blood vessels

- There are characteristic changes in the growing skeleton following radiotherapy

Second malignant neoplasms (see also Chapter 6)

Some long-term survivors of cancer are already genetically predisposed to further malignancy; for example, women who have suffered from ovarian cancer have a higher risk of breast, thyroid, endometrial and lung cancers. There is also a recognized risk of treatment-induced second malignancies.[112,113] This is highest after treatment for childhood cancer and the overall risk varies between 2 and 12% in survivors at 20 years.[114] Most tumours are musculoskeletal sarcomas, lymphomas, or leukaemia.[115,116] In the abdomen, hepatomas can occur in patients who have undergone

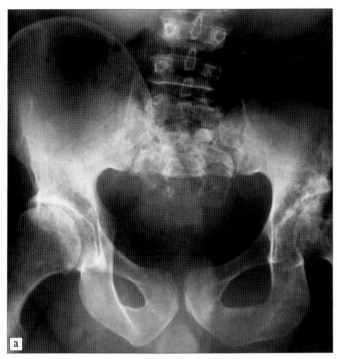
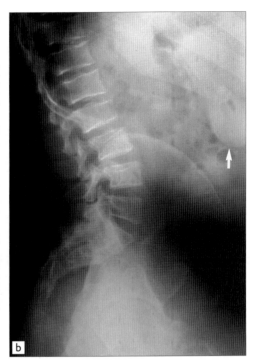

Figure 55.30. *Effects of radiotherapy on the growing skeleton. (a) Antero-posteror and (b) lateral radiographs of a 26-year-old man, treated with radiotherapy aged 2 years for Wilms' tumour. There is kyphoscoliosis and hypoplasia of the left ribs and left iliac blade. Characteristic vertebral body changes are seen (see text). The sacro-iliac joints are fused. Avascular necrosis of the left femoral head has occurred and there is secondary dysplasia of the acetabulum. Degenerative changes are present in the right hip joint. The left kidney is absent and there is compensatory hypertrophy of the right kidney (arrow).*

upper abdominal radiation therapy (Fig. 55.31) and, in the pelvis, at-risk organs are the bladder and rectum.[117] Patients who have had solid-organ transplantation are prone to post-transplantation lymphoproliferative disorder consisting of Epstein–Barr virus-induced B cell proliferation. The pattern of disease differs from other lymphomas, with extra-nodal and extrasplenic involvement (liver, small bowel, kidney and mesentery) being common.[118]

Radiation-induced sarcomas arise more frequently in soft tissues than in bone,[119] usually more than 10 years after radiotherapy, but with a wide time range of 3–55 years.[88] The most common cell types are: malignant fibrous histio-cytoma and osteosarcoma[119–121] (Fig. 55.32). The cardinal imaging feature is the presence of a new soft tissue mass within the radiation field. Therefore, it is necessary to obtain a histological diagnosis of any abnormal mass, particularly when there is a long time interval between the treatment of the primary lesion and the development of new symptoms. In bone, focal loss of the expected postradiation high signal intensity fatty marrow on T1-weighted images is an early finding. On plain radiographs or CT, a lytic destructive lesion is identified which may extend beyond the area of pre-existing postradiation atrophy.[88] Differentiation from postradiation osteomyelitis can be difficult and require biopsy. The presence of additional lesions outside the radiation field and a short latent period to the development of the lesion are indicative of metastatic disease.

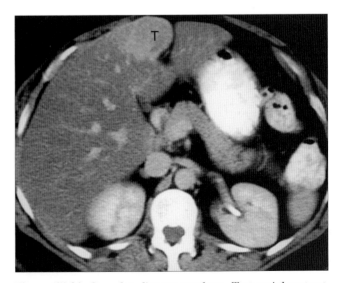

Figure 55.31. *Second malignant neoplasm. Transaxial contrast-enhanced CT of the liver in a patient with Hodgkin's disease who received chemotherapy and radiotherapy 10 years previously. There is a large mass (T) within the left lobe of the liver, which shows some enhancement on CT within an otherwise fatty liver. Biopsy of this lesion revealed hepatoma.*

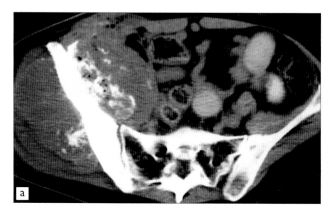

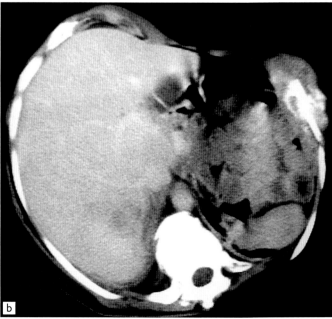

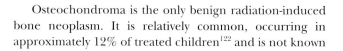

Figure 55.32. *Radiation-induced sarcoma. (a) Transaxial CT image of the pelvis showing a chondrosarcoma of the right iliac blade following radiotherapy for cervical carcinoma; (b) postcontrast transaxial CT image of the upper abdomen showing an osteosarcoma of the left 12th rib in an adult irradiated in childhood for Wilms' tumour. (Also note the absent left kidney, vertebral body changes and rib changes.)*

Osteochondroma is the only benign radiation-induced bone neoplasm. It is relatively common, occurring in approximately 12% of treated children[122] and is not known to undergo malignant degeneration. The imaging features are indistinguishable from the idiopathic type. This topic is discussed in detail in Chapter 53.

Summary

- Surgery, chemotherapy and radiation all induce changes in normal tissues

- Significant radiation damage occurs in 5–10% of patients and is divided into acute, subacute and chronic reactions

- Clinically, significant damage most frequently occurs in the gastro-intestinal and genito-urinary tracts

- Radiation damage to bowel includes mucosal lesions, fixation of bowel loops, motility disturbance, strictures and fistulae

- The bladder is the most radiation-sensitive organ in the urinary tract. Damage is seen in 20% of patients. Oedema, haemorrhage and necrosis lead to fibrosis

- Distinction of radiation damage from recurrent tumour relies on morphological appearances on CT, ultrasound and MR. Signal intensity changes and use of IV contrast on MR may be helpful but considerable overlap occurs

- [18]FDG PET and monoclonal antibody imaging have a role in the detection of recurrent tumour

- Radiation injury to the musculoskeletal system results in bone marrow atrophy, fractures, osteomyelitis, avascular necrosis, muscle atrophy and injury to fat, nerves and blood vessels

- Characteristic changes occur in the growing skeleton following radiotherapy

- The development of a second malignancy occurs in 2–12% of patients following treatment of childhood cancer and is usually musculoskeletal sarcoma, lymphoma or leukaemia

References

1. Fu K K. Biological basis for the interaction of chemotherapeutic agents and radiation therapy. Cancer 1985; 55(9 Suppl): 2123–2130

2. Rubin P. Law and order of radiation sensitivity. Absolute versus relative. In: Vaeth S M, Meyer J L (eds). Frontiers of Radiation Therapy and Oncology 1989; 23: 7–40

3. DeCosse J J, Rhodes R S, Wentz W B et al. The natural history and management of radiation-induced injury of the gastrointestinal tract. Ann Surg 1969; 170: 369–384

4. van Nagell R J, Maruyama Y, Parker J C et al. Small bowel injury following radiation therapy for cervical carcinoma. Am J Obstet Gynecol 1974; 118: 163–167

5. Graham J B, Abad R S. Ureteral obstruction due to radiation. Am J Obstet Gynecol 1967; 99: 409–415

6. Stockbrine M F, Hancock J E, Fletcher G H. Complications in 831 patients with squamous cell carcinoma of the intact uterine cervix treated with 3000 rads or more whole pelvis irradiation. Am J Roentgenol 1970; 108: 293–304

7. Mason G R, Dietrich P, Friedland G W et al. The radiological findings in radiation-induced enteritis and colitis. Clin Radiol 1970; 21: 232–247

8. Kimose H H, Fischer L, Spjeldnaes N et al. Late radiation injury of the colon and rectum. Surgical management and outcome. Dis Colon Rectum 1989; 32: 684–689

9. Pavy J J, Denekamp J, Letschert J et al. EORTC Late Effects Working Group. Late effects toxicity scoring: the SOMA scale. Radiother Oncol 1995; 35: 11–15

10. Krestin G P, Steinbrich W, Friedman G. Recurrent rectal cancer: diagnosis with MR imaging versus CT. Radiology 1988; 168: 307–311

11. Ebner F, Kresel H Y, Mintz M C et al. Tumour recurrence versus fibrosis in the female pelvis: differentiation with MR imaging at 1.5 T. Radiology 1988; 166: 333–340

12. Hawnaur J M, Johnson R J, Isherwood I, Jenkins J P. Gadolinium–DTPA in magnetic resonance imaging of bladder carcinoma. In: Bydder G, Felix R, Bücheler E et al (eds). Contrast Media in MRI. Medicom, 1990; 357–363

13. Dobson M J, Carrington B M, Collins C D et al. The assessment of the irradiated bladder using dynamic contrast-enhanced MR imaging. Clin Radiol 2001; 56: 44–48

14. Hircak H, Swift P S, Campos Z et al. Irradiation of the cervix uteri: value of unenhanced and contrast-enhanced MR imaging. Radiology 1993; 189: 381–388

15. Libutti S K, Alexander H R, Choyke P et al. A prospective study of 2-[18F] fluoro-2-deoxy-D-glucose/positron emission tomography scan, 99mTc-labelled arcitumomab (CEA-scan), and blind second-look laparotomy for detecting colon cancer recurrence in patients with increasing carcinoembryonic antigen levels. Ann Surg Oncol 2001; 8: 779–786

16. Seltzer M A, Barbaric Z, Belldegrun A et al. Comparison of helical computerised tomography, positron emission tomography and monoclonal antibody scans for evaluation of lymph node metastases in patients with prostate specific antigen relapse after treatment for localised prostate cancer. J Urol 1999; 162: 1322–1328

17. Makhija S, Howden N, Edwards R et al. Positron emission tomography/computed tomography imaging for the detection of recurrent ovarian and fallopian tube carcinoma: a retrospective review. Gynecol Oncol 2002; 85: 53–58

18. Sasson A R, Sigurdson E R. Surgical treatment of liver metastases. Semin Oncol 2002; 29: 107–118

19. Parikh A A, Curley S A, Fornage B D, Ellis L M. Radiofrequency ablation of liver metastases. Semin Oncol 2002; 29: 168–182

20. Sottsky T K, Ravikumar T S. Cryotherapy in the treatment of liver metastases from colorectal cancer. Semin Oncol 2002; 29: 183–191

21. Dromain C, de Baere T, Elias D et al. Hepatic tumors treated with percutaneous radio-frequency ablation: CT and MR imaging follow-up. Radiology 2002; 223: 255–262

22. Gervais D A, Fernandez-del Castillo C, O'Neill M J et al. Complications after pancreatoduodenectomy: imaging and imaging guided interventional procedures. Radiographics 2001; 21: 673–690

23. Petit P, Bret P M, Atri M et al. Splenic vein thrombosis after splenectomy: frequency and role of imaging. Radiology 1994; 190: 65–68

24. Yoshikawa J, Matsui O, Takashima T et al. Focal fatty change of the liver adjacent to the falciform ligament: CT and sonographic findings in five surgically confirmed cases. Am J Roentgenol 1987; 149: 491–494

25. Halvorsen R A, Korobkin M, Ram P C, Thompson W M. CT appearance of focal fatty infiltration of the liver. Am J Roentgenol 1982; 139: 277–281

26. White E M, Simeone J F, Mueller P R et al. Focal periportal sparing in hepatic fatty infiltration: a cause of hepatic pseudomass on US. Radiology 1987; 162: 57–59

27. Kissin C M, Bellamy E A, Cosgrove D O et al. Focal sparing in fatty infiltration of the liver. Br J Radiol 1986; 59: 25–28

28. Hirohashi S, Ueda K, Uchida H et al. Nondiffuse fatty change of the liver: discerning pseudotumour on MR images enhanced with ferumoxides – initial observations. Radiology 2000; 217: 415–420

29. Martín J, Puig J, Falcó J et al. Hyperechoic liver nodules: characterization with proton fat–water chemical shift MR imaging. Radiology 1998; 207: 325–330

30. Hale H L, Husband J E, Gossios K et al. CT of calcified liver metastases in colorectal carcinoma. Clin Radiol 1998; 53: 735–741

31. Young S T, Paulson E K, Washington K et al. CT of the liver in patients with metastatic breast carcinoma treated by chemotherapy: findings simulating cirrhosis. Am J Roentgenol 1994; 163: 1385–1388

32. King P D, Perry M C. Hepatotoxicity of chemotherapy. Oncologist 2001; 6: 162–176

33. Lassau N, Leclere J, Auperin A et al. Hepatic veno-occlusive disease after myeloablative treatment and bone marrow transplantation: value of gray-scale and Doppler US in 100 patients. Radiology 1997; 204: 545–552

34. Shirkhoda A. CT findings in hepatosplenic and renal candidiasis. J Comput Assist Tomogr 1987; 11: 795–798

35. Wharton J T, Delclos L, Gallager S et al. Radiation

hepatitis induced by abdominal radiation with the cobalt 60 moving strip technique Am J Roentgenol 1971; 117: 73–80

36. Cheng J C-H, Wu J-K, Huang C-M et al. Radiation-induced liver disease after three-dimensional conformal radiotherapy for patients with hepatocellular carcinoma: dosimetric analysis and implication. Int J Radiat Oncol Biol Phys 2002; 54: 156–162

37. Lawrence T S, Robertson, J M, Anscher M S et al. Hepatic toxicity resulting from cancer treatment. Int J Radiation Oncol Biol Phys 1995; 31: 1237–1248

38. Unger E C, Lee J K T, Weyman P J. CT and MR imaging of radiation hepatitis. J Comput Assist Tomogr 1987; 11: 264–268

39. Yamasaki S A, Marn C S, Francis I R et al. High-dose localized radiation therapy for treatment of hepatic malignant tumours: CT findings and their relation to radiation hepatitis. Am J Roentgenol 1995; 165: 79–84

40. Chiou S Y, Lee R C, Chi K H et al. The triple-phase CT image appearance of post-irradiated livers. Acta Radiol 2001; 42: 526–531

41. Capps G W, Fulcher A S, Szucs R A, Turner M A. Imaging features of radiation-induced changes in the abdomen. Radiographics 1997; 17: 1455–1473

42. Dailey M O, Coleman C N, Fajardo L F. Splenic injury caused by theraputic irradiation for Hodgkin's disease. Ann Int Med 1982; 96: 44–47

43. Weimann M, Becker G, Einsele H, Bamberg M. Clinical indications and biological mechanisms of splenic irradiation in chronic leukaemias and myeloproliferative disorders Radiother Oncol 2001; 58: 235–246

44. Friedman N B. Effects of radiation on the gastrointestinal tract, including the salivary glands, the liver, and the pancreas. Arch Pathol 1942; 34: 749–787

45. Levy P, Menzelxhiu A, Paillot B et al. Abdominal radiotherapy is a cause for chronic pancreatitis. Gastroenterology 1993; 105: 905–909

46. Taourel P G, Fabre J M, Pradel J A et al. Value of CT in the diagnosis and management of patients with suspected acute small-bowel obstruction Am J Roentgenol 1995; 165: 1187–1192

47. Kim K A, Park C M, Park S W et al. CT findings in the abdomen and pelvis after gastric resection Am J Roentgenol 2002; 179: 1037–1041

48. Muller-Scimpfle M, Brix G, Layer G et al. Recurrent rectal cancer: diagnosis with dynamic MR imaging. Radiology 1993; 189: 881–889

49. Kinkel K, Tardivon A A, Soyer P et al. Dynamic contrast-enhanced subtraction versus T2-weighted spin echo MR imaging in the follow-up of colorectal neoplasm: a prospective study of 41 patients. Radiology 1996; 200: 453–458

50. Dicle O, Obuz F, Cakmacki H et al. Differentiation of recurrent rectal cancer and scarring with dynamic MR imaging. Br J Radiol 1999; 72: 1155–1159

51. Stomper P C, D'Souza D J, Bakshi S P et al. Detection of pelvic recurrence of colorectal carcinoma: prospective, blinded comparison of Tc99m IMMU-4 monoclonal antibody scanning and CT. Radiology 1995; 197: 688–692

52. Ito K, Kato K, Tadokoro M et al. Recurrent rectal cancer and scar: differentiation with PET and MR imaging. Radiology 1992; 182: 549–552

53. Johnson K, Baksh A, Young D et al. Correlating computed tomography and positron emission tomography scans with operative findings in metastatic colorectal cancer. Dis Colon Rectum 2001; 44: 334–337

54. Ogunbiyi O A, Flanagan F L, Dehdashti F et al. Detection of recurrent and metastatic colorectal cancer: comparison of positron emission tomography and computed tomography. Ann Surg Oncol 1997; 4: 613–620

55. Whiteford M H, Whiteford H M, Ogunbiyi O A et al. Usefulness of FDG-PET scan in the assessment of suspected metastatic or recurrent adenocarcinoma of the colon and rectum. Dis Colon Rectum 2000; 43: 759–767

56. Saunders T H, Mendes Ribeiro H K, Gleeson F V. New techniques for imaging colorectal cancer: the use of MRI, PET and radioimmunoscintigraphy for primary staging and follow-up. Br Med Bull 2002; 64: 81–99

57. DuBrow R A. Radiation changes in the hollow viscera. Semin Roentgenol 1994; 24: 38–52

58. Rogers L F, Goldstein H M. Roentgen manifestations of radiation injury to the gastrointestinal tract. Gastrointest Radiol 1977; 2: 281–291

59. Mendeleson R M, Nolan D J. The radiological features of chronic radiation enteritis. Clin Radiol 1985; 36: 141–148

60. Taylor P M, Johnson R J, Eddleston B E et al. Radiological changes in the gastrointestinal and genitourinary tract following radiotherapy for carcinoma of the cervix. Clin Radiol 1990; 41: 165–169

61. Doubleday L C, Bernardino M E. CT findings in the perirectal area following radiation therapy. J Comput Assist Tomogr 1980; 4: 634–638

62. Ohtomo K, Shuman W P, Griffin B R et al. CT manifestation in the pararectal area following fast neutron radiotherapy. Radiol Medica 1987; 5: 198–201

63. Sugimura K, Carrington B M, Quivey J M, Hricak H. Postirradiation changes in the pelvis: assessment with MR imaging. Radiology 1990; 175: 805–813

64. Outwater E, Schieber M L. Pelvic fistulas: findings on MR images. Am J Roentgenol 1993; 160: 327–330

65. Barker P G, Lunniss P J, Armstrong P et al. Magnetic resonance imaging of fistula in ano: technique, interpretation and accuracy. Clin Radiol 1994; 49: 7–13

66. Spencer J A, Ward J, Beckingham I J et al. Contrast-enhanced MR imaging of perianal fistulas. Am J Roentgenol 1996; 167: 735–741

67. Ilancheran A, Monaghan J M. Pelvic lymphocyst: a 10-year experience. Gynecol Oncol 1988; 29: 333–336

68. van Sonnenberg E, Wittich G R, Casola G et al. Lymphoceles: imaging characteristics and percutaneous management. Radiology 1986; 161: 593–596

69. Razzaq R, Carrington B M, Hulse P A, Kitchener H C. Abdominopelvic CT scan findings after surgery for ovarian cancer. Clin Radiol 1998; 53: 820–824

70. Reed D H, Dixon A K, Williams M V. Ovarian conservation at hysterectomy: a potential diagnostic pitfall. Clin Radiol 1989; 40: 274–276

71. Marks L B, Carroll P R, Dugan T C, Anscher M S. The response of the urinary bladder, urethra and ureter to radiation and chemotherapy. Int J Radiat Oncol Biol Phys 1995; 31: 1257–1280

72. Johnson R J, Carrington B M. Pelvic radiation disease. Clin Radiol 1992; 45: 4–12

73. Cassady J R. Clinical radiation nephropathy. Int J Radiat Oncol Biol Phys 1995; 31: 1249–1256

74. Parkin D E. Lower urinary tract complications of the treatment of cervical carcinoma. Obstet Gynecol Surg 1989; 44: 523–529

75. Seymore C H, El-Mahdi A M, Schellhammer P F. The effect of prior transurethral resection of the prostate on postradiation urethral strictures and bladder neck contractures. Int J Radiat Oncol Biol Phys 1986; 12: 1597–1600

76. Rowley M J, Leach D R, Warner G A, Heller C G. Effect of graded doses of ionising irradiation on the human testis. Radiat Res 1974; 59: 665–678

77. Arrivé L, Change Y C F, Hricak H et al. Radiation-induced uterine changes: MR imaging. Radiology 1989; 170: 55–58

78. Grigsby P W, Russell A, Bruner D et al. Late injury of cancer therapy on the female reproductive tract. Int J Radiat Oncol Biol Phys 1995; 31: 1281–1299

79. Wallace W H, Shalet S M, Crowne E C et al. Ovarian failure following abdominal irradiation in childhood: natural history and prognosis. Clin Oncol 1989; 1: 75–79

80. Andrews C L. Evaluation of the marrow space in the adult hip. Radiographics 2000; 20: 527–542

81. Levine C D, Schweitzer M E, Ehrlich M S. Pelvic marrow in adults. Skeletal Radiol 1994; 23: 343–347

82. Ricci C, Cova M, Kang Y S et al. Normal age-related patterns of cellular and fatty bone marrow distribution in the axial skeleton: MR imaging study. Radiology 1990; 177: 83–88

83. Dawson K L, Moore S G, Rowland J M. Age related marrow changes in the pelvis: MR and anatomical findings. Radiology 1992; 183: 47–51

84. Stevens S K, Moore S G, Kaplan I D. Early and late bone marrow changes after irradiation: MR evaluation. Am J Roentgenol 1989; 154: 745–750

85. Otake S, Mayr N A, Veda T et al. Radiation induced changes in MR signal intensity and contrast enhancement of lumbosacral vertebrae: do changes occur only inside the radiation therapy field? Radiology 2002; 222: 179–183

86. Casamassima F, Ruggiero C, Caramella D et al. Hematopoietic bone marrow recovery after radiation therapy: MRI evaluation. Blood 1989; 73: 1677–1681

87. Yankelevitz D F, Henschke C I, Knapp P H et al. Effect of radiation therapy on thoracic and lumbar bone marrow. Evaluation with MR imaging. Am J Roentgenol 1991; 157: 87–92

88. Remeios P A, Colletti P M, Raval J K et al. Magnetic resonance imaging of bone after radiation. Magn Res Imag 1988; 6: 301–304

89. Disler D G, McCauley T R, Ratner L M et al. In-phase and out-of-phase MR imaging of bone marrow; prediction of neoplasia based on the detection of coexistent fat and water. Am J Roentgenol 1997; 169: 1439–1447

90. Libshitz H I. Radiation changes in bone. Semin Roentgenol 1994; 29: 15–37

91. Blumemke D A, Fishman E K, Kuhlman J E et al. Complications of radiation therapy: CT evaluation. Radiographics 1991; 11: 581–600

92. Rafii M, Firooznia H, Golimbu C et al. Radiation-induced fractures of the sacrum: CT diagnosis. J Comput Assist Tomogr 1988; 12: 231–235

93. Blomlie V, Lien H H, Iversen T et al. Radiation-induced insufficiency fractures of the sacrum: evaluation with MR imaging. Radiology 1993; 188: 241–244

94. Bonfiglio M. The pathology of fracture of the femoral neck following irradiation. Am J Roentgenol 1953; 70: 449–459

95. Moulopoulos L A, Dimopoulos M A. Magnetic resonance imaging of the bone marrow in hematologic malignancies. Blood 1997; 90: 2127–2147

96. Moulopoulos L A, Yoshimitsu K, Libshitz H I. MR prediction of benign and malignant vertebral compression fractures. J Magn Res Imaging 1996; 6: 667–674

97. Cuenod C A, Laredo J D, Chevret S et al. Acute vertebral collapse due to osteoporosis or malignancy: appearance on unenhanced and gadolinium-enhanced MR images. Radiology 1996; 199: 541–549

98. Wignall T A, Carrington B M, Logue J P. Post-radiotherapy osteomyelitis of the symphysis pubis: computed tomographic features. Clin Radiol 1998; 53: 126–130

99. Harper P G, Trask C, Souhami R L. Avascular necrosis of bone caused by combination chemotherapy without corticosteroids. Br Med J 1984; 288: 267–268

100. Mould J J, Adam N M. The problem of avascular necrosis of bone in patients treated for Hodgkin's disease. Clin Radiol 1983; 34: 231–236

101. Chan Lam D, Prentice A G, Copplestone J A et al. Avascular necrosis of bone following intensified steroid therapy for acute leukaemia and high-grade malignant lymphoma. Br J Haematol 1994; 86: 227–230

102. Gabriel H, Fitzgerald S W, Myers M T et al. MR imaging of hip disorders. Radiographics 1994; 14: 763–781

103. Rubin P, Probhasawat D. Characteristic bone lesions in post irradiated carcinoma of the cervix: metastases versus osteonecrosis. Radiology 1961; 76: 703

104. Gillete E L, Mahler P A, Powers B E et al. Late radiation injury to muscle and peripheral nerves. Int J Radiat Oncol Biol Phys 1995; 5: 1309–1318

105. Granmayeh M, Libshitz H I. Vascular system. In: Libshitz HI (ed). Diagnostic Roentgenology of Radiotherapy Change. Baltimore: Williams and Wilkins, 1979; 195–201

106. Dencker H, Holmdahl H, Lunderquist A et al. Mesenteric angiography in patients with radiation injury of the bowel after pelvis irradiation. Am J Roentgenol 1972; 114: 476–481

107. Fletcher B D, Crom D B, Krance R A et al. Radiation-induced bone abnormalities after bone marrow transplantation for childhood leukemia. Radiology 1994; 191: 231–235

108. Meister B, Gassner I, Streif W et al. Methotrexate osteopathy in infants with tumours of the central nervous system. Med Pediatr Oncol 1994; 24: 493–496

109. Ecklind K, Laor T, Goorin A M et al. Methotrexate osteopathy in patients with osteosarcoma. Radiology 1997; 2002: 543–547

110. Roebuck D J. Skeletal complications in pediatric oncology patients. Radiographics 1999; 19: 873–885

111. Raney B, Ensign L G, Foreman J et al. Renal toxicity of ifosfamide in pilot regimens of the Intergroup Rhabdomyarcoma Study for patients with gross residual tumour. Am J Pediatr Hematol Oncol 1994; 16: 286–295

112. Hutchison G B. Late neoplastic changes following medical irradiaton. Cancer 1976; 37: 1102–1107

113. Parker R G. Radiation-induced cancer as a factor in clinical decision-making (The 1989 Astro Gold Medal Address). Int J Radiat Oncol Biol Phys 1989; 18: 993–1000

114. Tucker M A, d'Angio G J, Boice J D et al. Bone sarcoma linked to radiotherapy and chemotherapy in children. N Engl J Med 1987; 317: 588–593

115. Messerschmidt G L, Hoover R, Young R C. Gynecologic cancer treatment: risk factors for therapeutically induced neoplasia. Cancer 1981; 48: 442–450

116. Quilty P M, Kerr G R. Bladder cancer following low- or high-dose pelvic irradiation. Clin Radiol 1987; 38: 583–585

117. Tucker M A, Frumeni J F. Treatment-related cancers after gynecologic malignancy. Cancer 1987; 60: 2117–2122

118. Pickhardt P J, Seigel M J. Post-transplantation lymphoproliferative disorder of the abdomen: CT evaluation in 51 patients. Radiology 1999; 213: 73–78

119. Wiklund T A, Blomquist C P, Räty I et al. Post-irradiation sarcoma: analysis of Nationwide Cancer Registry material. Cancer 1991; 68: 524–531

120. Huvos A G, Woodward H Q, Cahan W G et al. Post-irradiation osteogenic sarcoma of bone and soft tissues: a clinicopathological study of 66 patients. Cancer 1985; 55: 1244–1255

121. Sheppard D G, Libshitz H I. Post-radiation sarcomas: a review of the clinical and imaging features in 63 cases. Clin Radiol 2001; 56: 22–29

122. Libshitz H I, Cohen M A. Radiation-induced osteochondromas. Radiology 1982; 142: 643–647

Part VIII

THE IMMUNOCOMPROMISED HOST

Chapter 56

The immunocompromised host: clinical considerations

Jacqueline M Parkin

Introduction

Immunocompromised individuals comprise an increasing proportion of the patient population. There are several factors contributing to this change. Firstly, those with long-term immunosuppression are living longer. Improved management of organ transplant and rejection episodes has led to over 90% of renal transplant recipients surviving beyond 10 years. The advent of effective combination anti-retroviral therapy for human immunodeficiency virus (HIV) infection has extended survival of patients into decades. Management of malignancy with improved chemotherapeutic regimens and use of stem cell transplants or modified bone marrow transplants (BMTs) has led to prolonged survival of patients, but at the cost of long-term immune defects as a result of their therapies. A small but increasing population are those with congenital immunodeficiencies in whom gene therapy or BMT is now possible, and who are surviving long enough to develop malignancies, as well as those with common variable immunodeficiency whose management has been revolutionized by the availability of immunoglobulin replacement therapy. Secondly, an increasing number of patients are receiving immunosuppressive regimens, due to the extension of organ transplantation, especially heart–lung and liver, to a wider range of conditions and the broadening of use of immunomodulating therapies for autoimmune diseases, including those with a relatively high prevalence, such as rheumatoid arthritis, inflammatory bowel disease and connective tissue diseases. Thirdly, the development of new and more targeted immunosuppressive drugs [such as tacrolimus, micophenolate, monoclonal antibodies (mAb) to T-cell receptors CD3 and CD4 and cytokine antagonists] to interleukin-2 (IL-2) and tumour necrosis factor (TNF) or their receptors has led to the use of combination regimens. It is not infrequent for up to three agents to be used in the transplant setting, being clinically effective but intensely immunosuppressive.

The evolution in range and extent of immunosuppression in patients has significant implications for clinical care and diagnosis. Both the level of immunocompromise and time for which it is maintained are important factors predicting the development of tumours. The majority of patients receiving solid-organ transplant require lifelong immunosuppression. Malignancy is now the most significant factor in long-term morbidity and mortality, with a cumulative incidence of 60–70% at 25 years post-transplant. Patients with HIV infection on active antiretroviral therapy have persistent immunological abnormalities, meaning they may remain susceptible to cancers in the long term. The immunological effects of the newer immunosuppressives, such as anti-TNF therapies, have been shown not only in the response of Behçet's vasculitis and inflammatory bowel disease control, but also in the unwanted effects of increased incidence of opportunist infections with mycobacteria and fungi. The effects of such drugs, when used intermittently in young individuals over long periods of time, will not become clear for some years.

The understanding of the pathogenesis of some tumours in the immunocompromised is increasing and is improving diagnosis and management. Predisposing factors for the development of certain tumours, such as acquisition of Epstein–Barr virus (EBV) and the development of post-transplant lymphoproliferative disorders (PTLD), or pretransplant seropositivity for human herpesvirus Type 8 (HHV-8) and development of Kaposi's sarcoma (KS), are being identified. This leads to the potential for targeted screening of high-risk individuals for early diagnosis and treatment of tumours. Novel approaches to therapy have been developed, for example, clones of EBV-specific T-cells can be raised from bone marrow donors and stored in readiness to transfuse into the recipient should EBV-related lymphoproliferation develop. The role of imaging in immunocompromised patients is crucial in this respect to enable the earliest diagnosis of neoplasms. A better understanding of the time-course of the development of tumours in relation to transplant enables appropriate monitoring to be put into place at the right time. The major tumours associated with immunodeficiency often commence as a non-malignant proliferation; detecting and treating at this stage will stand a greater chance of success than when malignant transformation has taken place. Imaging also plays a central role in monitoring of response to therapy and early detection of relapse, which is unfortunately a frequent occurrence in these diseases.

Immune dysregulation and malignancy

In the beginning of the 20th century, even when understanding of the immune system was in its infancy, a potential function of the immune system in controlling carcinomas was recognized.[1] Half a century later, Burnet and Thomas developed their hypothesis that the immune system was continually searching out and destroying premalignant and malignant cells to prevent the development of cancer – the immune surveillance theory.[2–4]

Tumour immunosurveillance – immunoediting and tumour sculpture

Since its first description, there has been controversy over the clinical significance of the immunosurveillance concept in the elimination of malignant cells. There is no doubt that individuals with tumours mount specific antitumour responses to malignant cells, recognizing, for example, altered cell-surface molecules or re-expression of fetal antigens. This immune 'pressure' leads to selection of tumour variants with reduced immunogenicity as these are not destroyed by the cytotoxic T cell response. For example, loss of HLA expression by malignant cells diminishes the ability of T cells to recognize the abnormal cells. This process, by which the immune system drives changes in the immunophenotype of tumour cells, has been termed 'sculpting'. The immunoediting hypothesis combines the immunosurveillance and tumour-sculpting into one dynamic process of cancer–immune system interaction.[5]

The evidence cited for a proactive role of the immune system in tumour control is as follows:

- It is not uncommon for postmortem examinations to show the presence of small foci of cancers that were not clinically apparent in life
- Cancers may resolve 'spontaneously'
- Specific cytotoxic T cells are present in the blood and infiltrating tumour lesions in patients with established malignancy and the extent of this T cell response correlates with prognosis for some tumours
- There is an association of HLA-DR homozygosity
- Development of tumours is markedly enhanced in the immunosuppressed transplant population, this being documented very soon after the introduction of this technique,[6,7] and also in patients with primary immunodeficiency[8]

However, although antitumour responses are often demonstrated in patients, the level of clinically relevant surveillance and protection is unclear. Understanding of the relationship of cancer to immunodeficiency (type, level and duration) enables the hypothesis to be tested further. Cancer statistics within organ transplant registries and HIV studies enable this to be investigated with a relatively large number of individuals. Although it is certainly the case that malignancies are much more common, this rate varies from three- to 500-fold as only some cancers are significantly affected.

The immunodeficiency states that are particularly susceptible to cancer development are those in which cell-mediated immunity (T cell and macrophage function) is affected. Macrophages function to present antigens to T cells, which then initiate the immune response; CD4 (helper) T cells are the orchestrating cell and CD8 (cytotoxic) cells destroying virally-infected and tumour cells. The tumours observed in those with cell-mediated defects are mainly those with underlying viral pathogenesis, where there is up to many-fold increase in rate over the healthy population (Table 56.1). It is suggested that these represent the effects of opportunist infections and lack of control of viral replication leading to oncogenesis, rather than proof of the immunosurveillance theory. However, there is an increase, albeit much smaller, in other types of cancer. This suggests that the immune system may be playing a role, but that other factors are more prominent in the predisposition to these multifactorial diseases.

Association of specific tumours and immunodeficiency

Particularly high incidence ratios have been observed for non-Hodgkin's lymphoma (NHL), KS and carcinomas of the skin, genito-urinary and ano-genital regions in immunocompromised individuals with T cell defects, the major causes of which are listed in Table 56.2. These are prominent regardless of the underlying cause of the immunodeficiency. The Cincinatti Tumour Transplant Registry (CTTR) shows skin and lip cancers making up 40–50%; PTLDs 17%; KS 4%; and renal, cervical and ano-genital, hepato-biliary and various sarcomas.[9,10] There are similar findings in Scandinavian[11] and Australian and New Zealand registries.[12] As discussed, many of these cancers have a viral aetiology and are linked to infection with EBV, HHV-8 and human papilloma virus (HPV), respectively.[13,14] The risks for other cancers, which are less closely linked to an infectious origin, are also increased in the immunocom-

Table 56.1. *Major tumours in immunocompromised patients*

Skin cancer: non-melanomous	Squamous cell carcinoma, including ano-genital disease
	Basal cell carcinoma
Skin cancer	Melanoma
Lymphoma (mainly B cell)	Non-Hodgkin's lymphoma
	Body cavity-based lymphoma/ primary effusion lymphoma
	Castleman's disease
	Post-transplant lymphoproliferative disorder
	MALToma
Kaposi's sarcoma	

Table 56.2. *Immunodeficiencies associated with tumour development*

Congenital	**T cell/T and B cell combined defects**
	Duncan's syndrome and EBV-associated lymphoproliferative disease
	DiGeorge syndrome and skin cancer
	DNA repair defects
	Ataxia telangiectasia
Acquired	**B cell**
	Common variable hypogamma-globulinaemia and gut lymphoma
	T cell
	Human T cell lymphoma Type I (HTLV-I) and T cell lymphoma/leukaemia
	HIV infection
Immunodysregulation	**Autoimmune disease**
	Sjögren's syndrome
Iatrogenic immunosuppression	**Solid-organ transplant**
	Bone marrow transplant
	Treatment of inflammatory conditions
	Rheumatoid arthritis
	Connective tissue disease
	Inflammatory bowel disease

promised, but to a much lower extent. Follow-up of 925 patients in Australia and New Zealand who received cadaveric renal transplants from 1965 to 1998 showed increased risk ratios for colon, pancreatic, lung and endocrine neoplasms, in addition to malignant melanomas.[12] Studies in Northern Europe have shown similar findings,[11] with the addition of increased risk for cancers of the urinary tract.

It is expected that the development of tumours in the immunocompromised, as in other situations, is multifactorial and failure to control oncogenic organisms is important but not the only aspect. The immune system in immunocompromised individuals usually shows signs of chronic activation as the available cells combat the barrage of infectious agents to which the host is continually exposed. Continual activation makes lymphoid cells more prone to uncontrolled and/or malignant transformation, as shown in mucosa-associated lymphoid tissue lymphoproliferative disorders (MALTomas) thought to be caused by B cell activation in response to chronic *Helicobacter pylori* infection. Other important factors are decreased immunosurveillance against carcinogens; the failure of the immune system to eliminate malignant clones; environmental exposure, such as the rapid and profound effects of UV light exposure on the development of cutaneous squamous cell carcinoma in transplant recipients; genetic susceptibility; and potential carcinogenic effects of other drug therapies.

Key points: types of tumour in immunosuppressed individuals

- Mainly tumours with viral aetiology, especially:

- Lymphoproliferative disorders, PTLD, NHL

- Kaposi's sarcoma

- Squamous cell carcinoma (SCC) of skin and anogenital region

Drugs used for immunosuppression

An increasing range of immunosuppressive drugs is now available with effects on different elements of the immune system (Table 56.3). Regimens used in the control of transplant rejection target cell-mediated (T cell) responses, but most will often have additional immunological effects. For example, corticosteroids reduce T cell proliferation and function, but also reduce adhesion molecule expression causing functional neutrophil defects; anti-T lymphocyte drugs such as anti-thymocyte globulin, mAbs to CD3 or CD4, or those that affect IL-2 production (cyclosporin A and tacrolimus) will also affect antibody production to some extent as T cell help is needed for B cell functioning.

Effects of immunocompromise on the clinical presentation of tumours

Not only is the spectrum of tumour types different in immunocompromised host, but the clinical presentation is also affected by the limited immune response. This makes the diagnosis more challenging, yet the aggressive nature of the tumours, and the potential to control them by reducing immunosuppression, means that early diagnosis is crucial.

Many immunocompromised patients will be paediatric

Table 56.3. *Specific immunosuppressive agents*

Inhibitors of lymphocyte proliferation	Corticosteroids
	Purine synthesis inhibitors:
	Azathioprine
	Mycophenolate mofetil
IL-2 inhibitors	Calcineurin inhibitors:
	Cylosporin, tacrolimus
	CD25 (receptor antibody)
	Sirolimus (Rapamycin)
Anti-T lymphocyte antibodies	Antithymocyte globulin (ATG)
	Campath-1 H (humanized)
	Anti-CD3, anti-CD4
Anti-B lymphocyte antibodies	CD20
Anti-tumour necrosis factor/receptor	Infliximab, etanercept

or young adults who will present with tumours normally associated with the elderly, such as SCCs of the skin or NHL. The presentation is 'atypical' compared with the immunocompetent population:

- Tumours are commonly multifocal or disseminated at presentation, e.g. many tens of skin cancers or KS lesions are not unusual
- The site of disease may be unexpected, e.g. lymphoma is frequently extranodal
- Disease can be extremely aggressive, e.g. cutaneous SCC, which is very common in young transplant patients, carries a mortality of 5–15%; skin cancers recur in 5–8% cases and metastasize often within 2 years of excision

Key points: presentation of tumours in the immunosuppressed

- Tumours are often disseminated at presentation
- Tumours develop at unusual sites
- Types of tumours usually observed mainly in the elderly occur in young immunosuppressed patients
- Progression and recurrence may be more aggressive than in immunocompetent patient
- Tumours can respond to reduction in immunosuppression

Factors confounding diagnosis

There needs to be a high index of suspicion of tumours as there may be a lack of the normal clinical symptoms of disease due to lack of immune response to the tumour; for example, systemic 'B' symptoms of fever and sweats may not be observed in patients with HIV infection and lymphoma.

Concurrent opportunist infection is common and may confuse the diagnosis as this may be assumed to be the cause of the symptoms and signs, which are in reality due to the underlying tumour. This is further confounded as some of the therapies used for infections, which are common in the immunocompromised, such as rifampicin for tuberculosis, may also cause temporary shrinkage of lymphoma leading the clinician to assume that the enlarged lymph node was mycobacterial. Steroids used in high dose for control of rejection may also cause shrinkage of lymphoma, confusing the picture. Previously unrecognized tumours are emerging, such as body cavity lymphomas, particularly in HIV-infected individuals. This underlines the importance of aggressive investigation and re-investigation, often requiring tissue diagnosis.

Key points: factors confounding diagnosis

- Tumours may occur with acute onset within weeks of immunosuppression mimicking infection
- Multiple tumours of different type can occur concurrently in same site
- Co-existing opportunist infection may hinder diagnosis
- Drugs used for concurrent infection, e.g. rifampicin for tuberculosis or for suppression of graft rejection, and corticosteroids may cause temporary reduction in lymphoma lesions

Factors affecting development of tumours in immunocompromised individuals

Degree of immunosuppression

The development of malignancy appears to be dependent on both the level of immunosuppression and length of therapy. Cardiac transplant recipients tend to receive greater immunosuppression than other transplant patients and also show a greater incidence of tumour development, in particular NHL. There is a direct dose-dependent relationship between cyclosporin A therapy and development of skin cancers. The instigation of combination immunosuppressive therapies in transplant recipients was associated with an increased incidence of tumour development, which has been curtailed by better tailoring of the regimens. In addition, reduction of immunosuppressive therapy in transplant recipients or improvement in immune function with antiretroviral therapy in HIV infection can directly lead to improvement/resolution of KS, lymphoproliferative disorders and MALTomas.

Length of immunosuppression

The time over which immunosuppression is maintained is also a significant risk factor for tumour development.[15] Tumours that are clearly virally-driven (PTLDs and KS) develop rapidly post transplant (median development within 12 months) or, for KS in HIV infection, when the CD4 count declines. Other cancers show a median time to development of 46 months post transplant, with a continuing increase in incidence over following years. For example, the cumulative risk of skin cancer in renal transplants is determined to be 13–18% at 10 years, 34–50% at 20 years and 60–70% at 25 years.[16]

Geographical variation in incidence of tumours

The incidence of tumour types shows some difference geographically. This may reflect the use of different immunosuppressive regimens (the question has been raised as to whether some drugs are intrinsically more liable to increase susceptibility to tumours outside of the level of immunosuppression they induce), and it is possible that organ transplant type, immunosuppressive regimens and/or the prophylactic antiviral therapies that are used as standard of care may affect the range and incidence of tumours that develop. Environmental factors also are involved, the level of UV exposure being reflected in the higher rate of sun and skin cancer in Australia (45% at 10 years and 70% at 20 years)[17] compared to 30–40% at 20 years in Europe.

Key points: factors affecting development of tumours

- The development of malignancy is dependent on the level of immunosuppression: cardiac transplant patients, who receive the greatest immunosuppression, show the greatest incidence of tumours

- The length of immunosuppression is a risk factor for tumour development

- The incidence of tumour types varies geographically

Tumours commonly observed in solid-organ transplant recipients

Post-transplant lymphoproliferative disorder/disease

This is the commonest cancer in the first year post transplant, being overtaken by skin cancers at later stages. The incidence is 0.2–1% in renal, 2.5% in liver and 1.2–3% in cardiac transplantation.[18] The proliferation develops relatively rapidly, 70% occurring in the first 12 months, then a levelling of incidence at 0.03–0.4% in subsequent years. The allograft site is the most common focus of disease, but multiple organ involvement is also observed. The tumours are mainly B cell lymphoma, but vary from benign lymphoid hyperplasia to malignant lymphoma. However, the disease is patchy and may evolve rapidly requiring repeated sampling. The overall mortality is 35%,[19] but varies from 9 to 50%[20] depending on whether disease is non-neoplastic or malignant. There are differences in reported incidence of PTLD and these are likely to be due to variety of definitions used in the past. These have been clarified by consensus definitions[21] of the American Society of Transplant Surgeons (ASTS) and American Society of Transplant Physicians (ASTP).

The tumours are EBV-related in 70% of cases, tumour cells being positive for viral proteins. In addition to immunosuppression, particular risk factors are being EBV-sero-negative pretransplant and receiving an organ from a sero-positive donor.[22] An additional risk is young age (less than 14 years) at transplant, with 6.3–20% in paediatric cases.[20] However, young age may not be an independent risk factor, merely a surrogate for EBV sero-negativity. To combat this disease there is development of EBV transfer regimens to protect recipients post BMT, using EBV-specific T cell clones for adoptive transfer of immunity should PTLD emerge. Human herpesvirus Type 8 may be responsible for some of the lymphomas that are not related to EBV.[23]

There has been an increased incidence of PTLD since the introduction of heavily-immunosuppressive combination regimens and there is rapid development when OKT3 (a mAb to T cells) is used in regimens with median time to PTLD of 53 days post-therapy. Tacrolimus, as primary immunosuppressive therapy, may also be an additional risk in children.[20] Post-transplant lymphoproliferative disorder is clearly related to the level of immunosuppression and may resolve in up to 40% cases when drugs are stopped or reduced, depending on the level of malignant change.

MALTomas

MALTomas have been observed in heart, liver and kidney transplant patients. Although one of the more rare tumours in the transplant population, the incidence appears to be 10- to 100-fold higher than in the general population.[24] The tumour may be most common in liver transplant recipients. Unlike the lymphoproliferative disorders, these tumours are usually EBV-negative, low-grade and confined to the stomach or gastro-intestinal tract-associated tissue of pancreas or parotids. They occasionally metastasize. These tumours develop late in the course of transplantation, with a median of 5.2 years. Clinical response has been documented using various regimens of anti-Helicobacter treatment, reducing immunosuppressive regimen or local excision.

Skin cancers

Overall, these are the most common cancers in transplant recipients due to the year-on-year increase in incidence. Squamous cell and basal cell carcinomas account for >90% of all skin cancers.[25–28] Of these, SCC is most common, with a 65- to 250-fold increased incidence over general population. The rate is higher for men than women, but rare in people of Japanese origin. Basal cell cancer is increased by a factor of 10.[29]

Ultraviolet (UV) light exposure is critically important, the incidence being markedly higher in environments with high sunlight, lesions mainly confined to sun-exposed areas and a greater incidence in patients with pretransplant high UV exposure. There appears to be no specific drug risk (a link between azathioprine and skin cancers has not been conclusively proven in extensive studies), although there may be very rapid development when OKT3 is used in the regimen. Most squamous cell cancers are associated with histological features of HPV infection in the lesions and are often associated with concurrent cutaneous warts. Lesions may contain multiple strains of wart virus, and both oncogenic strains (16 and 18) and non-oncogenic strains are detected.

Genital or anal dysplasia and SCCs also show increased incidence in patients, with immunodeficiency of up to 100-fold.[30] The risk is higher in men than woman, and in those with multiple sexual partners and a history of sexually-transmitted infection, including herpes simplex virus and HPV, suggesting that a sexually-transmitted agent, presumably HPV, is involved in the pathogenesis. Smoking, which is known to produce local immunosuppressive effect on genital mucosal immunity, is an additional risk factor in transplant as in immunocompetent individuals.

Kaposi's sarcoma

The incidence of this tumour post transplant is 84- to 500-fold that in the general population. This tumour is due to proliferation of vascular or lymphatic endothelial cells. The vascular cells give rise to slit-like spaces that trap red cells, causing the typical purplish colour of the lesions. Cutaneous disease is the most common initial presentation. The lower limbs are commonly affected by lympho-oedema due to local lymph node involvement. The tumour is usually multifocal, polyclonal in origin and does not show characteristic features of malignancy in that metastasis does not occur. However, visceral involvement can cause life-threatening disease due to mechanical effects. Endo-

bronchial lesions can cause bronchial obstruction and recurrent infection in the lung beyond the lesion; parenchymal involvement causes shortness of breath and chronic cough; pleural lesions may lead to significant pleural effusions. Disease in the gastro-intestinal tract may be a cause of protein-losing enteropathy. The brain is characteristically spared. Human herpesvirus Type 8 is thought to be the causative virus[31] and there is a very close association with pretransplant infection with HHV-8.[32] The incidence of KS parallels the carriage of HHV-8, highest in those from the Mediterranean, Middle East and Central/Sub-Saharan Africa.

Melanoma

The incidence is three to four times higher in transplant recipients than the age-matched population. It is observed mainly in those with fair skin and more frequently in children. The median time to diagnosis is 5 years post transplant.

Key points: tumours common following solid-organ transplant

- PTLD is the commonest cancer in the first year post transplant; tumours are EBV-related in 70% of cases and young patients are particularly at risk

- Skin cancers (squamous and basal cell) are the commonest cancers in transplant recipients

- MALTomas are 10- to 100-fold more common following transplantation than in the general population

- KS is up to 500 times more common post transplant than in the general population

- Melanomas are three to four times more common in transplant recipients than in non-transplant recipients

Cancers in the non-transplant patient

Cancers in HIV infection[13]

The types of cancer observed in HIV-related immunodeficiency are very similar to those in transplant patients. However, KS is particularly frequent in homosexual men and patients from Sub-Saharan Africa, reflecting the higher rate of seropositivity to HHV-8 in these populations. A decrease in the incidence of new cases of KS in homosexual men was noted at the end of the 1980s/early 1990s. This was hypothesized to be due to reduced infection rate with HHV-8 due to changes in sexual practice. The success of combination antiretroviral therapy in reversing or preventing severe immunodeficiency in HIV-infected individuals has led to a marked decrease in the incidence of both KS and NHL, previously the two major cancers in this population. However, there are now cases being documented where lymphoproliferative disorders have emerged acutely during initiation of antiretroviral therapy. This may be an 'immunoreconstitution' phenomenon due to intense stimulation of lymphocytes by infectious antigen within the host, as the immune system regenerates. The rapidity of onset can mimic an acute tuberculous or bacterial infection within lymph nodes.

Ano-genital SCCs, however, may be an increasing problem in patients with HIV infection, who like the transplant patients have long-term immunodeficiency. The natural history of intraepithelial neoplasia within the cervix or anus is not yet clear in this situation, and regular monitoring of patients and treatment of premalignant lesions is required.

Other conditions

The impact on tumour development of more widespread and long-term use of immunosuppressive regimens in rheumatoid arthritis, inflammatory bowel disease, connective tissue disease, refractory asthma and psoriasis is as yet uncertain. Some of these patients may commence therapy at a young age and, therefore, have a high life-time exposure to immunosuppression. Older patients in the transplant setting appear to be particularly susceptible to rapid development of skin cancers and the use of immunosuppressive regimens in conditions common in older patients, such as rheumatoid arthritis, may be associated with an increase in such tumours.

Summary

■ Immunocompromised patients, especially those with T cell deficiencies, are highly susceptible to tumour development

■ Immunocompromised patients are increasing in numbers due to improved management of primary and acquired immunodeficiency disorders, increasing numbers of solid-organ transplantations and the application of an increasing number of highly immunosuppressive agents to a broadening population of patients with inflammatory diseases

■ Although the level and length of time of immunosuppression are the main predictors for the development of malignancies, environmental and host factors also play a role

■ The majority of tumours are related to failure to control oncogenic viruses such as EBV, HHV-8 and HPV

■ The clinical presentation of cancer in these populations is atypical and usually aggressive

■ Differentiation from opportunistic infections is challenging as tumours may mimic infection and multiple pathologies often occur concurrently

■ Early diagnosis significantly improves outcome; some cancers may be detected when the proliferation is still polyclonal and when reduction in immunosuppression alone can lead to regression of the tumour

References

1. Ehrlich P. Ueber den jetzigen Stand der Karzinomforschung. Ned Tijdschr Geneeskd 1909; 5: 273–290

2. Burnet F M. Cancer: a biological approach. Br Med J 1957; 1: 841–847

3. Thomas L. In: Lawrence H S (eds). Cellular and Humoral Aspects of the Hypersensitive States. New York: Hoeber-Harper, 1959; 529–532

4. Burnet F M. The concept of immunological surveillance. Prog Exp Tumor Res 1970; 13: 1–27

5. Dunn G P, Bruce A T, Ikeda H et al. Cancer immunoediting: from immunosurveillance to tumor escape. Nat Immunol 2002; 3: 991–998

6. Penn I. Malignant Tumors in Organ Transplant Recipients. New York: Springer-Verlag, 1970

7. Bouwes Bavinck J N, Claas F H, Hardie D R et al. Relation between HLA antigens and skin cancer in renal transplant recipients in Queensland Australia. J Invest Dermatol 1997; 108: 708–711

8. Gatti R A, Good R A. Occurrence of malignancy in immunodeficiency diseases. A literature review. Cancer 1971; 28: 89–98

9. Penn I. Post-transplant malignancies. Transplant Proc 1999; 31: 1260–1262

10. Penn L. Post-transplant malignancy. The role of immunosuppression. Drug Safety 2000; 23: 101–113

11. Birkeland S A, Storm H H, Lamm L U et al. Cancer risk after renal transplantation in the Nordic countries, 1964–1986. Int J Cancer 1995; 60: 183–189

12. Sheil A G R. In: Morris P J (ed). Kidney Transplantation. Philadelphia: WB Saunders, 2001; 558–570

13. Boshoff C, Weiss R. AIDS-related malignancies. Nat Rev Cancer 2002; 2: 373–382

14. Harward C A, Surentheran T, McGregor J M et al. Human papillomavirus infection and non-melanomous skin cancer in immunosuppressed and immunocompetent individuals. J Med Virol 2000; 62: 289–297

15. London N, Farmery S, Will E et al. Risk of neoplasia in renal transplant patients. Lancet 1995; 346: 403–406

16. Vial T, Descotes J. Immunosuppressive drugs and cancer. Toxicology 2003; 185: 229–240

17. Bouwes Bavinck J N, Hardie D R, Green A et al 1996. The risk of skin cancer in renal transplant recipients in Queensland, Australia. A follow-up study. Transplantation 1996; 61: 715–721

18. Opelz G, Henderson R. Incidence of non-Hodgkin's lymphoma in kidney and heart recipients. Lancet 1993; 342: 1514–1516

19. Niaudet P. Post-transplant lymphoproliferative disease following renal transplantation: a multicentre retrospective study of 41 cases observed between 1991 and 1996. French Speaking Transplantation Workshop. Transplant Proc 1998; 30: 2816–2817

20. Guthery S L, Heubi J E, Bucuvalas J C et al. Determination for Epstein–Barr virus-associated post-transplant lymphoproliferative disorder in pediatric liver transplant recipients using objective case ascertainment. Transplantation 2003; 73: 989–993

21. Paya C V, Fung J J, Nalesnik M A et al. Epstein–Barr virus-induced post-transplant lymphoproliferative disorders ASTS/ASTP EBV-PTLD Task Force and the Mayo Clinic organised International Consensus Development Meeting. Transplantation 1999; 68: 1517

22. Newell K A, Alonso E M, Whitington P F et al. Post-transplant lymphoproliferative disease in pediatric liver transplantation. Transplantation 1996; 62: 370–375

23. Kapelushnik J, Ariad S, Benharroch D et al. Post-renal transplantation human herpesvirus 8-associated lymphoproliferative disorder and Kaposi's sarcoma. Br J Haematol 2001; 113: 425–428

24. Shehab T M, Hsi E D, Poterucha J J et al. *Helicobacter pylori*-associated gastric MALT lymphoma in liver transplant patients. Transplantation 2001; 71: 1172–1175

25. Webb M C, Compton F, Andrews P A, Koffman G C. Skin tumours post-transplantation: a retrospective analysis of 28 years' experience at a single centre. Transplantation Proc 1997; 29: 828–830

26. Hiesse C, Rieu P, Kriaa F et al. Malignancy after renal transplantation: analysis of incidence and risk factors in 1700 patients followed during a 25-year period. Transplant Proc 1997; 29: 831–833

27. Winkelhorset J T, Brokelman W J, Tiggeler R G, Wobbes T. Incidence and clinical course of de novo malignancies in renal allograft recipients. Eur J Surg Oncol 2001; 27: 409–413

28. Sanchez E Q, Marubashi S, Jung G et al. De novo tumours after liver transplantation: a single-institution experience. Liver Transplant 2002; 8: 285–291

29. Euvrard S, Kanitakis J, Claudy A. Skin cancers after organ transplantation. N Engl J Med 2003; 348: 1681–1691

30. Penn I. Cancers of the anogenital region in renal transplant recipients: analysis of 65 cases. Cancer 1986; 58: 611–616

31. Jenkins F J, Hoffmann L J, Liegey-Dougall A. Reactivation of and primary infection with human herpesvirus 9 among solid-organ transplant recipients. J Infect Dis 2002; 185: 1238–1243

32. Catani P, Nanni G, Graffeo R et al. Pretransplantion human herpesvirus 8 seropositivity as a risk factor for Kaposi's sarcoma in kidney transplant recipients. Transplant Proc 2000; 32: 526–527

Chapter 57

The immunocompromised host: central nervous system

Jane Evanson

Introduction

Immunocompromised patients are susceptible to the development of lymphoid neoplasms within the central nervous system (CNS). The patients at risk of these malignancies include those with congenital immunodeficiencies (e.g. Wiskott–Aldrich syndrome) as well as those with acquired immunodeficiency. Acquired immunodeficiency may be the result of illness, e.g. lupus, or infection, e.g. acquired immunodeficiency syndrome (AIDS), or iatrogenic immunosuppression, e.g. after transplantation. Two specific groups of patients are susceptible to these lymphoid malignancies: patients with AIDS and those who have received solid-organ transplants. In both these groups of patients the lymphoid proliferations are thought to be due to an Epstein–Barr virus (EBV)-induced B-cell proliferation, which is unopposed by the suppressed T cells [suppressed either as a result of immunosuppressive drugs or human immunodeficiency virus (HIV) infection]. Transplant patients most commonly develop post-transplant lymphoproliferative disorders within the first 2 years after transplantation. The lymphoid proliferations in these patients have some similarities in imaging appearances, which is not unexpected given their identical pathogenesis. These appearances are often distinct from those of primary central nervous system lymphoma (PCNSL) in the immunocompetent patient. There does not seem to be any documented increased risk of primary glial neoplasms of the CNS in these patients.

Key points: general features

- Immunosuppressed patients are susceptible to lymphoid neoplasms in the CNS
- The neoplasms are typically EBV-related B-cell lymphomas
- AIDS patients and solid-organ transplant patients are at particular risk
- Symptoms are variable and non-specific

Primary CNS lymphoma in AIDS

It was recognized in the 1980s that patients with AIDS had an increased incidence of PCNSL. Overall, there has been an approximately threefold increase in the incidence of PCNSL in the last 20 years, most particularly in AIDS patients.[1] It had been previously estimated that up to 3% of all patients with AIDS would develop PCNSL;[1] however, since the introduction of highly active antiretroviral therapy (HAART), the risk of these patients developing PCNSL, or indeed any focal brain lesion, has reduced.[2] Nonetheless, PCNSL remains the second most common cause of focal brain lesions in AIDS patients with neurological symptoms, after cerebral toxoplasmosis.[2] Histologically, these PCNSLs are typically large cell B-cell non-Hodgkin's lymphomas; a minority are small cell Burkitt's type. Presenting symptoms are variable and non-specific but seizures, focal neurological deficit, or headache are most common. The initial identification of focal brain abnormalities on imaging (computed tomography (CT) or magnetic resonance (MR) imaging) will not distinguish PCNSL from toxoplasmosis or other entities such as tuberculosis (TB) granulomas or even progressive multifocal leucoencephalopathy (PML). Commonly, a trial of treatment for toxoplasmosis is the initial management, whilst awaiting serological tests and cerebrospinal fluid (CSF) analysis (if safe). Detection of EBV DNA in the CSF has high sensitivity and specificity for PCNSL,[3] whereas cytological examination of the CSF has a low sensitivity.[4]

The prognosis remains poor, with only 10% of those treated surviving beyond a year.[5] This is in comparison to the recent improvement in survival for AIDS patients treated for systemic (non-CNS) lymphoma.[5] PCNSL is rare in children with AIDS although a few cases are reported[6] and they also seem to be related to EBV; the intracranial lesions are similar to those seen in adults.

Imaging appearances of primary CNS lymphoma

Primary cerebral lymphomas in AIDS are commonly multifocal, 71% in a recent series.[7] Therefore, the number of lesions will not reliably differentiate PCNSL from toxoplasmosis. The most common appearance is that of a ring-enhancing mass(es)[7] (Fig. 57.1), the peripheral enhancement after gadolinium reflecting central necrosis of the lesion, presumably related to the relatively rapid growth of these lesions. They can occur both in the deep grey matter of the basal ganglia or the periventricular region as well as more peripherally in the cerebral hemispheres, and the location of the lesion(s) is not a useful distinguishing feature in differentiating PCNSL from other pathologies. Posterior fossa involvement is uncommon but recognized.[7] In the immunocompetent patient, PCNSL is typically solidly enhancing[8] (Fig. 57.2) but this is a less common, though recognized, appearance in the immunocompromised patient.[9] The mass effect and oedema with PCNSL is mild to modest and extensive oedema is not common.[7,9] It does seem there is an increased frequency of non-enhancing lymphoma in AIDS patients. Just over a quarter of lymphomatous lesions in a recent series did not show enhancement, and in some cases there were both enhancing and non-enhancing lesions present. It is well recognized that a small proportion of lymphomas will be non-enhancing[8] and it is important to remember that steroid administration can abolish enhancement in any CNS lymphoma. Small foci of haemorrhage, identified as high T1-weighted signal intensity prior to enhancement with contrast medium have been reported, as has a primary presentation with cerebral haemorrhage.[10] T2-weighted signal characteristics are variable;[7,9] the low T2-weighted signal intensity expected in very cellular neoplasms is not always striking.

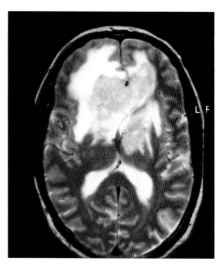

Figure 57.2. *Primary CNS lymphoma in an immunocompetent patient. Axial T2-weighted image shows a solid mass extending across the genu of the corpus callosum and extending around the margins of the lateral ventricles with modest oedema. There was homogeneous enhancement after contrast.*

Magnetic resonance is more sensitive than CT to the presence of PCNSL, but CT is often the first-line investigation in the acute setting (Fig. 57.3).

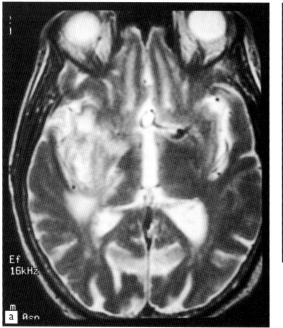
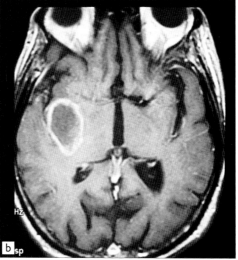

Figure 57.1. *(a) Primary CNS lymphoma in an AIDS patient. Axial T2-weighted image shows a mass in the right posterior temporal region. There is central high signal intensity compatible with necrosis and modest adjacent oedema for the size of the mass. The periphery of the lesion is of relatively low T2 signal intensity – a variable feature of primary CNS lymphoma. This was a solitary lesion. (b) Axial T1-weighted image post-gadolinium. The mass shows ring enhancement with central necrosis.*

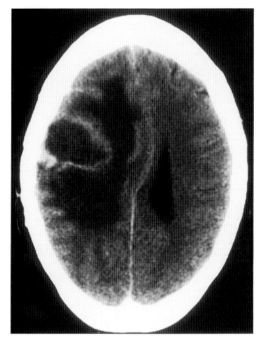

Figure 57.3. *Enhanced axial CT of biopsy-proven primary CNS lymphoma in an AIDS patient. There is a large ring-enhancing mass in the right frontal region with prominent vasogenic oedema.*

Differential diagnosis

Distinguishing between toxoplasmosis and PCNSL remains difficult (Fig. 57.4); whether the lesions are solitary or multiple will not allow accurate differentiation. Imaging findings should be correlated with results of other clinical investigations; examination of CSF for EBV DNA is a usefully sensitive and specific test for PCNSL.[3] Thallium-201

brain single-photon emission computed tomography (SPECT) might be useful, if available. Increased thallium uptake is seen in lymphomas, with reported sensitivities of 100% and specificities of 93%,[11] although other groups have since reported this technique as non-reliable[12] and it may be best to be guided by local experience. Combining thallium SPECT and EBV DNA analysis shows a high diagnostic accuracy for AIDS-related primary cerebral lymphoma.[13] The improved accuracy of CSF analysis has already reduced the requirement for cranial biopsy in these patients.[5] Positron emission tomography scanning using 2-[F-18]fluoro-2-deoxy-D-glucose ([18]FDG PET) is a promising technique, showing increased uptake in lymphoma compared to infective lesions.[14,15] Despite all these advances in non-invasive diagnostic techniques, there are still a significant proportion of these patients that will require a cranial biopsy to make the definitive diagnosis.

Other diagnoses to be considered include TB and PML. Multiple enhancing lesions of TB granulomata cannot be distinguished solely on imaging grounds from toxoplasmosis or multifocal enhancing lymphoma; CSF analysis may be contributory. Meningeal involvement suggests TB, cryptococcal meningitis or other infective processes. The incidence of PML in AIDS patients has not declined despite the introduction of HAART therapy, unlike both toxoplasmosis and PCNSL.[2] PML is a condition of demyelination due to JC polyoma virus and therefore manifests as areas of signal change within the white matter. Mutifocal areas of low T1 and high T2 weighting are seen in the white matter without mass effect and without enhancement (Fig. 57.5).[16] The lack of local mass effect should be a helpful identifying feature. The parietal lobe is the most commonly involved; however, frontal, periventricular, brain stem and posterior fossa involvement are all recognized.[17] In a few cases, faint periph-

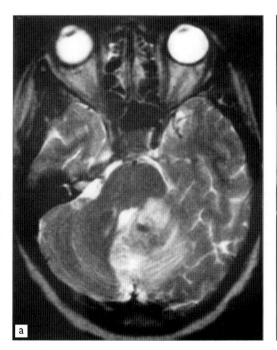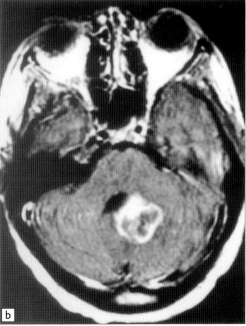

Figure 57.4.
Toxoplasmosis in an AIDS patient. (a) Axial T2-weighted image shows a relatively low signal intensity mass in the left cerebellar hemisphere with moderate oedema. (b) Axial T1-weighted image post gadolinium. Peripheral enhancement is evident; no other lesions were present. It is not possible to distinguish this from primary CNS lymphoma.

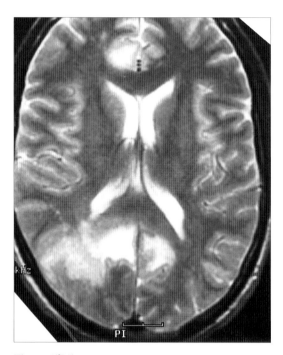

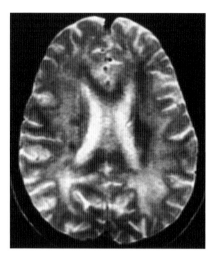

Figure 57.6. *HIV encephalopathy. Axial T2-weighted image shows diffuse symmetrical high signal intensity in the hemispheric white matter.*

Figure 57.5. *Progressive multifocal leuco-encephalopathy. Axial T2-weighted image shows focal areas of high signal intensity change within the white matter of both occipital lobes and the right frontal lobe. The adjacent cortex is spared and there is minimal mass effect. There was no enhancement after contrast. Multifocal non-enhancing primary CNS lymphoma could have this appearance, but more mass effect would be expected.*

eral enhancement has been noted[16] and enhancement may develop after commencing treatment with HAART.[18] Cerebrospinal fluid examination for the JC virus DNA has high specificity, in the order of 95%,[19] but in negative or doubtful cases a brain biopsy may still be needed. The lesions of PML are typically asymmetrical, which should help to distinguish it from HIV encephalopathy, which produces extensive symmetrical high signal intensity throughout the supratentorial white matter (Fig. 57.6).

Key points: central nervous system lymphoma

- Ring-enhancing mass lesions are typical imaging findings of CNS lymphoma

- Differential diagnosis includes infections, toxoplasmosis or TB

- AIDS patients are less at risk of CNS lymphoma since HAART treatment

- Lymphoma is the second most common intracranial mass lesion in AIDS patients

- Lymphoma lesions are often multiple and show ring enhancement

- CSF analysis, SPECT or [18]FDG PET all aid diagnosis

Post-transplantation lymphoproliferative disorder

Post-transplant lymphoproliferative disorder (PTLD) is a syndrome of uncontrolled lymphoid growth in the transplant patient. It occurs in approximately 2–3% of patients with solid-organ transplants.[20] Transplanted children are particularly susceptible, with frequencies as high as 10% reported.[21] Chronic immunosuppression in these patients allows an EBV-induced B-cell proliferation, and seronegativity for EBV at the time of transplantation is a risk factor.[22] It has a propensity to involve extranodal sites, particularly the allografted organ, gastro-intestinal tract, the thorax and the CNS. Central nervous system involvement is reported in between 10 and 25% of cases.[23,24] The prevalence of PTLD is highest in patients after lung transplant, followed in decreasing order of frequency by kidney, pancreas, heart and liver transplants.[25] PTLD has been reported at any time between 1 month and 10 years after transplantation,[26] although the majority occur within the first two transplant years. Definitive diagnosis of PTLD requires biopsy as it is vital to distinguish between the various histological types.[27] There is a pathological classification subdividing PTLDs into polymorphic and monomorphic forms, most of the monomorphic forms being B-cell non-Hodgkin's lymphomas. Subsequent to biopsy, full clinical staging and imaging as for lymphomas is required. The treatment strategy is dependent upon the histology. A reduction in immunosuppression is the initial approach and, in a subgroup of patients, this may be successful. However, chemotherapy, irradiation or monoclonal antibodies may be used subsequent to reduction of immunosuppression.[27,28] Survival is best in paediatric patients and those with localized disease; 5-year adult survival rates vary between 86[21] and 50%.[27]

The clinical presentation of PTLD has been grouped into three syndromes:[29]

- Infectious mononucleosis-like
- Isolated or multiple tumours
- Widespread fulminant disease

PTLD in the CNS usually presents as part of the isolated/multiple tumour syndrome and may present with seizures, focal neurological deficit or impaired mental state. It most commonly presents with isolated CNS involvement, rather than as part of diffuse systemic involvement with PTLD.

Imaging appearances of CNS involvement

Ring-enhancing mass lesions are the typical imaging findings of CNS involvement with PTLD. The features are similar to those described above of AIDS-related PCNSL, namely, ring-enhancement, central necrosis and location within both the deep or superficial structures of the cerebral hemispheres (Fig. 57.7). Posterior fossa involvement is uncommon but reported.[30] Lesions may be solitary or, less commonly, multifocal (Fig. 57.8). High T1 signal intensity before contrast (representing haemorrhage) is recognized.[30] The extent of associated vasogenic oedema is variable. The dense cellularity of lymphoproliferative abnormalities is often associated with relatively low T2 signal intensity in the peripheral cellular part of the tumour. However, these signal characteristics are not a reliable discriminator between PTLD and other infectious lesions. Meningeal abnormalities or durally based spinal lesions, which are typical of secondary lymphoma in immunocompetent patients, are unusual in PTLD but have been recognized (Fig. 57.9).

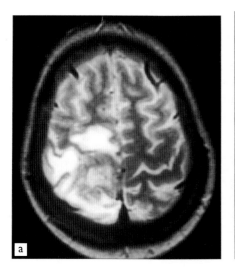
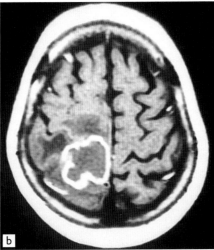

Figure 57.7. *(a) PTLD in a transplant patient. Axial T2-weighted image shows a right parietal mass lesion with central necrosis and adjacent oedema. The periphery of the lesion is of relatively low T2 signal intensity. (b) Axial T1-weighted image after gadolinium demonstrating ring enhancement.*

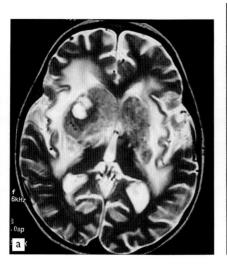
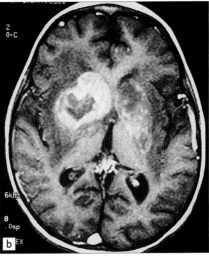

Figure 57.8. *(a) PTLD in a child post transplant. Axial T2-weighted image shows mass lesions in the periventricular region bilaterally; other lesions were present in the peripheral white matter (not shown). (b) Axial T1-weighted image shows ring enhancement on the right and patchy enhancement on the left.*

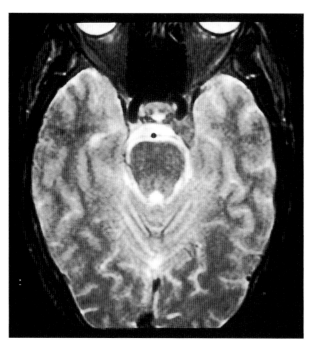

Figure 57.9. *Durally based PTLD in a patient with systemic PTLD. Axial T2-weighted image shows a subtle low signal intensity mass in the left cavernous sinus, which showed a little enhancement (not shown). These appearances are similar to those of secondary lymphoma seen in immunocompetent patients.*

The differential diagnosis of a ring-enhancing mass lesion in the CNS in a transplant patient must include infection. Fungal infections, particularly Aspergillosis, should be considered, along with Candida and histoplasmosis. Toxoplasmosis is less common in the transplant population than in the AIDS population. Ultimately, biopsy is necessary for diagnosis and to determine the appropriate treatment.

Differential diagnosis

A well-recognized complication of immunosuppressive therapies such as Cyclosporin A and Tacrolimus (FK506) is the posterior reversible encephalopathy syndrome (PRES).[31–33] PRES also usually presents with headaches, seizures or altered mental state. CT and MR imaging demonstrate symmetrical areas of vasogenic oedema, predominantly in the white matter of the parietal and occipital regions. PRES is also seen in patients with hypertensive encephalopathy, eclampsia,[34] thrombotic thrombocytopenic purpura[35] and in association with chemotherapy, specifically cisplatin,[36] interferon α,[31] intrathecal methotrexate[37] and in the treatment of acute lymphoblastic leukaemia in children.[38,39] It seems that a failure in cerebral autoregulation allows leakage of intravascular fluid producing vasogenic oedema. Diffusion imaging has confirmed that the signal intensity changes in this condition are due to vasogenic oedema, which can be completely reversed with treatment. In a few severe cases, however, infarction and permanent damage can result.[40]

Magnetic resonance appearances are those of high signal intensity on T2-weighted images within the white matter of the parieto-occipital regions bilaterally (Fig. 57.10). Despite the name, frontal lobe involvement is common[40] but the parieto-occipital involvement is typically more severe. Brain stem involvement indicates severe PRES.[40] Mass effect is minimal and enhancement is usually absent, although patchy enhancement has been reported.[32] The lack of enhancement should help in distinguishing between this syndrome and PTLD where enhancement is typical. White matter involvement is dominant but cortical involvement is also recognized.[41] Use of fluid attenuation inversion recovery (FLAIR) sequences increases the conspicuity of the cortical and subcortical involvement and should be used routinely in assessment of such cases.[41]

The MR changes and the symptoms of PRES are typically reversible, resolving fully after the adjustment of the immunosuppressant drugs, the treatment of hypertension or adjustment of chemotherapy.[41–43] If severe or unrecognized, the prognosis can be poor.

Head and neck involvement with PTLD

Patients with PTLD affecting the extracranial head and neck may present with cervical lymphadenopathy or with focal masses in Waldeyer's ring. The lymphadenopathy may present as a large nodal mass or an excess number of relatively normal-sized nodes. Necrosis within the nodes appears more common than in immunocompetent patients

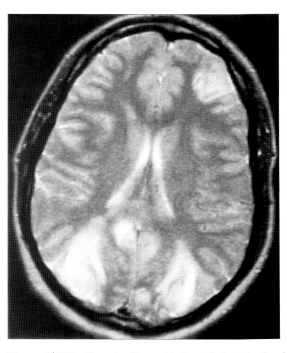

Figure 57.10. *Posterior Reversible Encephalopathy Syndrome (PRES) in a patient with eclampsia. Axial T2-weighted image shows the high signal intensity in the white matter of the parieto-occipital regions bilaterally. The cortex is relatively spared. There is a little involvement of the left frontal white matter.*

with lymphoma.[44] Sino-nasal and orbital masses may also be manifestations of PTLD.[45] Head and neck PTLD is usually associated with disease in the thorax and abdomen.[30]

Key points: post-transplantation lymphoproliferative disorder

- PTLD occurs in 2–3% of organ transplant patients
- CNS involvement is seen in 10–25% of cases
- Imaging with CT and MR typically shows ring enhancement
- Differential diagnosis typically includes aspergillus and candidiasis
- Immunosuppressant drugs can cause imaging abnormalities in the white matter

Summary

- Immunocompromised patients are susceptible to the development of lymphoid neoplasms
- Patients with acquired immunodeficiency in AIDS and postorgan transplantation are susceptible to lymphoid malignancies
- There has been a threefold increase in PCNSL in the last 20 years
- HAART has reduced the risk of PCNSL
- The prognosis of PCNSL is poor – 10% 1-year survival
- PCNSL is commonly multifocal
- Imaging with CT and MR usually shows a rim-enhancing mass(es)

- A small percentage of PCNSL masses are non-enhancing
- Differential diagnosis of PCNSL includes toxoplasmosis, TB and PML
- PTLD is a syndrome of uncontrolled lymphoid growth
- PTLD has the highest incidence in lung-transplanted patients
- 5-year survival ranges from 50 to 86%
- PTLD in the CNS usually presents as isolated involvement
- CT and MR show ring-enhancing lesions in PTLD
- The differential diagnosis includes PRES

References

1. Velasquez W S. Primary central nervous system lymphoma. J Neurooncol 1994; 20: 177–185
2. Ammassari A, Cingolani A, Pezzotti P et al. AIDS-related focal brain lesions in the era of highly active antiretroviral therapy. Neurology 2000; 55: 1194–1200
3. Bossolasco S, Cinque P, Ponzoni M et al. Epstein–Barr virus DNA load in cerebrospinal fluid and plasma of patients with AIDS-related lymphoma. J Neurovirol 2002; 8: 432–438
4. DeAngelis L M, Yahalom J, Heinemann M H et al. Primary CNS lymphoma: combined treatment with chemotherapy and radiotherapy. Neurology 1990; 40: 80–86
5. Sparano J A. Clinical aspects and management of AIDS related lymphoma. Eur J Cancer 2001; 37: 1296–1305
6. Del Mistro A, Laverda A, Calabrese F et al. Primary lymphoma of the central nervous system in two children with acquired immune deficiency syndrome. Am J Clin Pathol 1990; 94: 722–728
7. Thurnher M M, Rieger A, Kleibl-Popov C et al. Primary central nervous system lymphoma in AIDS: a wider spectrum of CT and MRI findings. Neuroradiology 2001; 43: 29–35
8. Johnson B, Fram E, Johnson P, Jacobowitz R. The variable MR appearance of primary lymphoma of the central nervous system: comparison with histopathologic features. Am J Neuroradiol 1997; 18: 563–572
9. Cordoliani Y S, Derosier C, Pharaboz C et al. Primary brain lymphoma in AIDS: 17 cases studies by MRI before stereotaxic biopsies. J Radiol 1992; 73: 367–376
10. Fukui M B, Livstone B J, Meltzer C C, Hamilton R L. Hemorrhagic presentation of untreated primary CNS lymphoma in a patient with AIDS. Am J Roentgenol 1998; 170: 1114–1115
11. Kessler L, Ruiz A, Donovan Post M J et al. Thallium-201 brain SPECT of lymphoma in AIDS patients: pitfalls and technique optimization. Am J Neuroradiol 1998: 19; 1105–1109
12. Licho R, Litofsky NS, Senitko M, George M. Inaccuracy of Tl-201 brain SPECT in distinguishing cerebral infections from lymphoma in patients with AIDS. Clin Nucl Med 2002; 27: 81–86

13. Antinori A, De Rossi G, Ammassari A et al. Value of combined approach with thallium-201 single-photon emission computed tomography and Epstein–Barr virus DNA polymerase chain reaction in CSF for the diagnosis of AIDS-related primary CNS lymphoma. J Clin Oncol 1999; 17: 554–560

14. Heald A E, Hoffman J M, Bartlett J A, Waskin H A. Differentiation of central nervous system lesions in AIDS patients using positron emission tomography (PET). Int J STD AIDS 1996; 7: 337–346

15. Villringer K, Jager H, Dichgans M et al. Differential diagnosis of CNS lesions in AIDS patients by FDG PET. J Comput Assist Tomogr 1995; 19: 532–536

16. Whiteman M L, Post M J, Berger J R et al. Progressive multifocal leukoencephalopathy in 47 HIV-seropositive patients: neuroimaging with clinical and pathologic correlation. Radiology 1993; 187: 233–240

17. Post M J, Yiannoutsos C, Simpson D et al. Progressive multifocal leukoencephalopathy in AIDS: are there any MR findings useful to patient management and predictive of patient survival? AIDS Clinical Trials Group, 243 Team. Am J Neuroradiol 1999; 20: 1896–1906

18. Thurnher M M, Post M J, Rieger A et al. Initial and follow-up MR imaging findings in AIDS-related progressive multifocal leukoencephalopathy treated with highly active antiretroviral therapy. Am J Neuroradiol 2001; 22: 977–984

19. Fong I W, Britton C B, Luinstra K E et al. Diagnostic value of detecting JC virus DNA in cerebrospinal fluid of patients with progressive multifocal leukoencephalopathy. J Clin Microbiol 1995; 33: 484–486

20. Nalesnik M A. Post-transplantation lymphoproliferative disorders (PTLD): current perspectives. Semin Thorac Cardiovasc Surg 1996; 8: 139–148

21. Shapiro R, Nalesnik M, McCauley J et al. Post-transplant lymphoproliferative disorders in adult and pediatric renal transplant patients receiving tacrolimus-based immunosuppression. Transplantation 1999; 68: 1851–1854

22. Ho M, Jaffe R, Miller G et al. The frequency of Epstein–Barr virus infection and associated lymphoproliferative syndrome after transplantation and its manifestations in children. Transplantation 1988; 45: 719–727

23. Lim G Y, Newman B, Kurland G, Webber S A. Post-transplantation lymphoproliferative disorder: manifestations in pediatric thoracic organ recipients. Radiology 2002; 222: 699–708

24. Chen J M, Michler R E. Heart xenotransplantation: lessons learned and future prospects. J Heart Lung Transplant 1993; 12: 869–875

25. Walker R C, Paya C V, Marshall W F et al. Pretransplantation seronegative Epstein–Barr virus status is the primary risk factor for post-transplantation lymphoproliferative disorder in adult heart, lung, and other solid organ transplantations. J Heart Lung Transplant 1995; 14: 214–221

26. Basgoz N, Preiksaitis J K. Post-transplant lymphoproliferative disorder. Infect Dis Clin North Am 1995; 9: 901–923

27. Nalesnik M A. Clinicopathologic characteristics of post-transplant lymphoproliferative disorders. Recent Results Cancer Res 2002; 159: 9–18

28. Benkerrou M, Durandy A, Fischer A. Therapy for transplant-related lymphoproliferative diseases. Hematol Oncol Clin North Am 1993; 7: 467–475

29. Malatack J F, Gartner J C Jr, Urbach A H, Zitelli B J. Orthotopic liver transplantation, Epstein–Barr virus, cyclosporine, and lymphoproliferative disease: a growing concern. J Pediatr 1991; 118: 667–675

30. Pickhardt P J, Wippold F J II. Neuroimaging in post-transplantation lymphoproliferative disorder. Am J Roentgenol 1999; 172: 1117–1121

31. Hinchey J, Chaves C, Appignani B et al. A reversible posterior leukoencephalopathy syndrome. N Engl J Med 1996; 334: 494–500

32. Schwartz R, Bravo S, Klufas R et al. Cyclosporine neurotoxicity and its relationship to hypertensive encephalopathy: CT and MR findings in 16 cases. Am J Roentgenol 1995; 165: 627–631

33. Truwit C, Denaro C, Lake J, DeMarco T. MR imaging of reversible cyclosporin A-induced neurotoxicity. Am J Neuroradiol 1991; 12: 651–659

34. Schwartz R B, Feske S K, Polak J F et al. Pre-eclampsia–eclampsia: clinical and neuroradiographic correlates and insights into the pathogenesis of hypertensive encephalopathy. Radiology 2000; 217: 371–376

35. Bakshi R, Shaikh Z A, Bates V E, Kinkel P R. Thrombotic thrombocytopenic purpura: brain CT and MRI findings in 12 patients. Neurology 1999; 52: 1285–1288

36. Ito Y, Arahata Y, Goto Y et al. Cisplatin neurotoxicity presenting as reversible posterior leukoencephalopathy syndrome. Am J Neuroradiol 1998; 19: 415–417

37. Yaffe K, Ferriero D, Barkovich A, Rowley H. Reversible MRI abnormalities following seizures. Neurology 1995; 45: 104–108

38. Cooney M J, Bradley W G, Symko S C et al. Hypertensive encephalopathy: complication in children treated for myeloproliferative disorders: report of three cases. Radiology 2000; 214: 711–716

39. Shin R K, Stern J W, Janss A J et al. Reversible posterior leukoencephalopathy during the treatment of acute lymphoblastic leukemia. Neurology 2001; 56: 388–391

40. Covarrubias D J, Luetmer P H, Campeau N G. Posterior reversible encephalopathy syndrome: Prognostic utility of quantitative diffusion-weighted MR images. Am J Neuroradiol 2002; 23: 1038–1048

41. Casey S O, Sampaio R C, Michel E, Truwit C L. Posterior reversible encephalopathy syndrome: utility of fluid-attenuated inversion recovery MR imaging in the detection of cortical and subcortical lesions. Am J Neuroradiol 2000; 21: 1199–1206

42. Schwartz R B, Mulkern R V, Gudbjartsson H, Jolesz F. Diffusion-weighted MR imaging in hypertensive encephalopathy: clues to pathogenesis. Am J Neuroradiol 1998; 19: 859–862

43. Dillon W P, Rowley H. The reversible posterior cerebral edema syndrome. Am J Neuroradiol 1998; 19: 591

44. Loevner L A, Karpati R L, Kumar P et al. Post-transplantation lymphoproliferative disorder of the head and neck: imaging features in seven adults. Radiology 2000; 216: 363–369

45. Gordon A R, Loevner L A, Sonners A I et al. Post-transplantation lymphoproliferative disorder of the paranasal sinuses mimicking invasive fungal sinusitis: case report. Am J Neuroradiol 2002; 23: 855–857

Chapter 58

The immunocompromised host: chest

Janet E Kuhlman

Introduction

Evaluation of the immunocompromised host is one of the most difficult tasks in all of oncologic imaging. Confronted with an acutely ill, oncologic patient with respiratory symptoms or fever, the clinician must consider a vast array of possible thoracic aetiologies, including onset of opportunistic lung infection, recurrence of the primary tumour in the chest, development of a secondary malignancy or complication of cancer therapy. Early detection of thoracic disease is critical in any number of clinical settings. First is the oncologic patient who becomes immunocompromised as the result of therapy. The patient will be susceptible to a variety of opportunistic infections as well as complications of treatment. Second is the non-oncologic, but severely immunosuppressed, patient who secondarily develops a neoplasm as the result of their immunosuppressed state. This category of patient includes solid-organ transplant recipients who are aggressively immunosuppressed to ward off transplant rejection, but then become susceptible to secondary malignancies and opportunistic infections. Also in this category are those individuals infected with the human immunodeficiency virus (HIV) who develop acquired immunodeficiency syndrome (AIDS)-related tumours and opportunistic infections as their immuno-suppression worsens. Prompt detection of occult thoracic disease whether due to malignancy, infection, or therapy complications in these immunocompromised patients lessens morbidity and lengthens an individual's survival.[1]

The oncologic patient with therapy-induced immunosuppression

Oncologic patients undergoing aggressive therapies, especially aplasia-producing chemotherapy, are at great risk for development of opportunistic infections. Such patients include those with leukaemia and lymphoma, and others with bone marrow and solid-organ tumours who undergo periods of profound neutropenia due to marrow-suppressing chemotherapy. Lesser, though still significant, degrees of immunosuppression are also induced by corticosteroids and other medications received as part of treatment as well as the debilitation that occurs with cancer; all of which conspire to lower the body's immune defence mechanisms.

When such patients present with unexplained fever or respiratory symptoms, the clinical situation is often grave, and rapid, accurate diagnosis is imperative. Although the first line of investigation is still the conventional chest film, additional imaging with thoracic computed tomography (CT) is indicated early because of the poor sensitivity and low specificity of chest X-rays. Numerous articles have reported on the usefulness of thoracic CT in detecting and characterizing opportunistic infections in the immuno-compromised host, including those with leukaemia, lymphoma, solid-organ tumours, and disorders treated with bone marrow transplantation (BMT), as well as those with AIDS.[1-14]

Thoracic CT, including thin-section or high-resolution CT (HRCT), aids in the early detection of lung infection in these patients, as well as in differentiating between the onset of infection versus recurrence of the primary tumour or development of a secondary malignancy or thoracic complication such as pulmonary drug toxicity. Computed tomography patterns and signs help to characterize the nature of the thoracic process and guide more invasive biopsy procedures to areas of the lung most affected for definitive diagnosis. Computed tomography is also helpful in monitoring the response of lung infection, primary tumour or secondary malignancy to appropriate therapy and in detecting relapse.

Searching for a source of infection, sepsis or fever in the immunocompromised host

How does CT help in the evaluation of the febrile immuno-compromised host (ICH)? Often, when the plain film is non-diagnostic, equivocal or complex, the CT shows more definitive findings, such as those seen on CT in cases of fungal infection, *Pneumocystis carinii* pneumonia (PCP), lung abscess, empyema, or septic emboli. In particular, in the immunocompromised oncologic patient, the transplant recipient or the debilitated patient with AIDS who is at risk for opportunistic infection, CT can play an important role in early detection of lung infections. As experience with thoracic CT has accumulated, recognizable patterns and signs of specific lung infections have emerged that narrow the differential diagnosis. Although many of these CT patterns are non-specific, in the right clinical setting they often suggest one type of infection over another, thus redirecting further diagnostic evaluation and appropriate therapy.

Opportunistic infection in the neutropenic patient

Invasive fungal disease and computed tomography signs of invasive pulmonary aspergillosis

Oncologic patients receiving aplasia-producing chemotherapy undergo varying lengths of bone marrow suppression and absolute neutropenia. The most profoundly neutropenic patients are those with leukaemia during induction chemotherapy. Such patients are susceptible to a variety of infections, including bacterial, viral, mycobacterial and fungal ones. While prophylactic use of broad-spectrum antibiotics often thwarts the onset of bacterial pneumonias in these patients, paradoxically the risk for fungal infections such as invasive pulmonary aspergillosis (IPA) increases as the period of absolute neutropenia lengthens.[1,3–5,7]

The CT findings of IPA in the patient with acute leukaemia who is undergoing aplasia-producing chemotherapy are recognizable and follow a typical pattern of progression and resolution[1,3–5,7] (Fig. 58.1). During the period of absolute neutropenia when fungal infection takes hold, the CT will show one or more inflammatory nodules or mass-like round or wedge-shaped opacities. Often a 'CT halo sign' surrounds one or more of the round lung opacities. This halo consists of a zone of intermediate CT attenuation that surrounds a mass or nodule. Pathologically, the halo zone is due to pulmonary haemorrhage from lung infarction caused by the Aspergillus organism. Aspergillus is an angioinvasive pathogen that has a propensity to invade and thrombose pulmonary blood vessels in areas of lung infection.[15,16] There are, of course, other types of angioinvasive infections, including those caused by mucormycosis, *Candida torulopsis* and angioinvasive Pseudomonas, and these too can produce similar CT findings, but IPA is by far the most frequent fungal pathogen to produce such CT findings in the aplastic, leukaemic patient. Prompt use of antifungal agents such as amphotericin B is usually indicated at the first sign of IPA infection and can stabilize the infection until bone marrow recovery occurs. Liposomal forms of amphotericin have now been developed that are better tolerated and cause less renal toxicity.[12] In addition, newer antifungal agents including azoles and caspofungin are now available as well.[12] With bone marrow recovery, the neutrophil count returns to normal, and the lung nodules due to IPA often cavitate and form air crescent signs, an indication that healing has begun. As the infection contin-

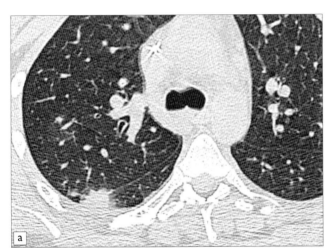
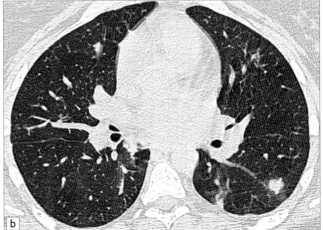
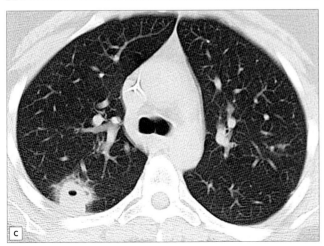

Figure 58.1. *CT features of invasive pulmonary aspergillosis in the immunocompromised oncologic patient. (a and b) A 30-year-old patient with AML and neutropenic fever. CT shows several inflammatory nodules with a surrounding CT 'halo sign' due to haemorrhagic infarction. As the bone marrow recovers and the neutrophil count returns to normal, lung nodules due to IPA often cavitate (c) or form air crescent signs, an indication of the onset of healing.*

ues to resolve, IPA nodules gradually diminish in size like resolving pulmonary infarcts, leaving behind thin-wall cysts or linear scars to the pleura.

A similar appearance of IPA can be seen in other susceptible hosts such as bone marrow and other organ transplant recipients who are receiving immunosuppressant agents.[10–12,14,17–19] In addition, several other forms of aggressive Aspergillus infection can be seen in these patients, including invasive tracheobronchitis and empyema.[10,11] Airway-invasive aspergillosis may present with 'tree-in-bud' opacities mimicking bronchiolitis or tuberculosis (TB) in its CT appearance.[12] Allogenic BMT recipients also develop acute graft versus host disease (GVHD), which can affect the lung and increases the risk for infections due to bacteria, cytomegalovirus (CMV) and Aspergillus.[12] Chronic GVHD is also associated with bronchiolitis obliterans, cryptogenic organizing pneumonia (COP) and infections in the lung.[12]

It is always important to remember that, depending upon the patient's immune status, the type of immune defect and the nature of the patient's underlying disease process, any number of other bacterial, viral, mycobacterial, protozoal and fungal species may cause pulmonary infection in the ICH patient. Geographic locality and history of recent travel may also provide clues to the most likely type of infection. In addition to IPA, other fungal infections due to *Candida albicans*, *Coccidioides immitis*, *Histoplasma capsulatum*, blastomycosis, coccidiomycosis and *Cryptococcus neoformans* may need to be considered.

In the ICH, thoracic CT may also detect other important non-pulmonary manifestations of fungal infection such as CT findings of oesophagitis or focal lesions in the liver or spleen, indicating a disseminated infection. Aspergillus and other fungal infections can disseminate to other organs including the liver, spleen, kidneys, adrenal glands, skin and to the brain causing brain abscesses.[17–19]

Key points: invasive pulmonary aspergillosis (IPA)

- IPA often results in a typical 'halo' sign on HRCT with lung opacities surrounded by a zone of intermediate signal intensity due to invasion and thrombosis in pulmonary vessels

- Other types of angioinvasive organisms can produce this appearance but IPA is by far the most common

- Several other forms of aggressive aspergillosis, including invasive tracheobronchitis and empyema, can occur in ICH

Septic emboli

Many oncologic patients are at risk for developing septic emboli because they are immunocompromised, have received a bone marrow or organ transplant, or simply have an indwelling catheter in place. Early detection, along with prompt administration of broad-spectrum antibiotics, is critical for good outcome. Unfortunately, the initial clinical diagnosis of septic emboli is not always straightforward. A detectable heart murmur may or may not be present, and blood cultures may remain negative or be suppressed by previously administered antibiotics. Early chest radiographic findings of septic emboli are often subtle, nonspecific, or obscured by poor quality portable chest films obtainable in ill patients. Computed tomography findings of septic emboli are often characteristic: multiple lung nodules or wedge-shaped opacities abutting the pleura with a peripheral distribution. Typically, the nodules show differing stages of cavitation and individual nodules may demonstrate a feeding vessel[20,21] (Fig. 58.2). Because CT overall is

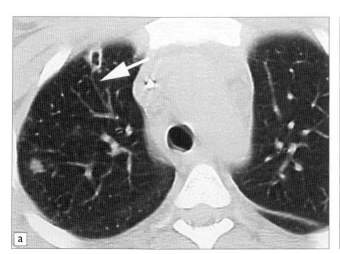
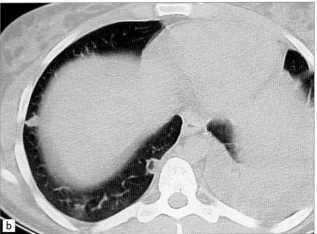

Figure 58.2. *CT features of septic emboli. (a and b) CT shows multiple peripheral lung nodules and pleural-based opacities. Typically, the nodules demonstrate varying stages of cavitation and individual nodules may demonstrate a feeding vessel sign (arrow). Blood cultures in this case grew Fusobacterium.*

more sensitive than plain films in detecting pulmonary nodules, septic emboli are more readily demonstrable with CT.[20,21]

Key point: septic emboli

■ Many oncological patients are at risk of septic emboli, which on CT typically are peripherally based nodules showing differing stages of cavitation

Pneumocystis carinii pneumonia

The prevalence of PCP infection in the susceptible oncologic and ICH has been dramatically reduced by the prophylactic use of trimethoprim/sulfamethoxazole (bactrim) in high-risk groups such as transplant recipients and individuals with AIDS. Still, PCP infection causes significant pulmonary disease and occurs in the setting of patient noncompliance with prophylaxis.[10]

Computed tomography is not used routinely to diagnose PCP, although its appearance on CT is often highly suggestive (Fig. 58.3). Rather the diagnosis is usually first suspected by clinical and chest radiographic findings and subsequently established through bronchoscopic sampling with lavage. In unsuspected or problematic cases, however, the patient may be referred to CT for evaluation of unexplained fevers or pulmonary symptoms. Computed tomography evaluation may also be requested in cases of known or suspected PCP when the patient fails to respond to appropriate therapy, in search of a compounding complication or evidence of a mixed infection. For these reasons, awareness of the spectrum of CT findings in PCP is still relevant.

The CT appearance of PCP is variable. By far the most common presentation is bilateral ground glass infiltrates that do not obscure bronchovascular bundles.[6,8] The resultant CT pattern is often patchy or mosaic in its distribution. Prominent interstitial markings develop in patients who have had multiple episodes of pneumocystis infection likely to be the result of fibrosis. There is also a cystic form of the PCP in which CT demonstrates one or more thin-walled cysts or cavities.[22–26] This cystic form may also be associated with disseminated PCP infection in which case calcifications in the liver, spleen, kidneys and enlarged lymph nodes may be seen on CT.[22–26]

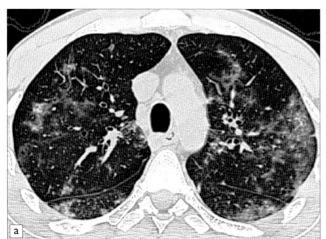
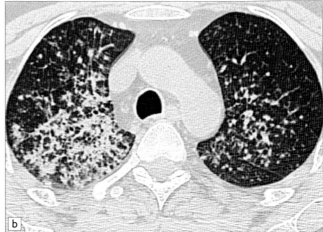
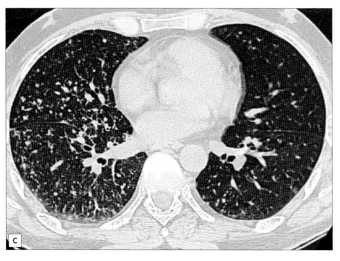

Figure 58.3. *CT features of PCP in two immunocompromised patients with AIDS. (a) A 41-year-old man with CD4 count of 15, fever and shortness of breath. CT shows a typical pattern of patchy bilateral ground glass opacities due to PCP that grew out of the patient's sputum. (b, c) A 38-year-old man with AIDS, an allergy to bactrim and a history of recurrent episodes of PCP. CT shows a more unusual pattern of PCP that is reticulonodular and miliary in appearance, one that can be seen with chronic, recurrent PCP.*

Spontaneous pneumothorax is a well-known complication of PCP infection and can be problematic to manage, particularly in the ICH patient, requiring mechanical ventilation.[27–29] Such pneumothoraces may be refractory to simple chest tube evacuation, and persistent air leaks may require invasive procedures such as pleurodesis, lung stapling or pleurectomy.

Key point: *Pneumocystis carinii* pneumonia

- The most common CT pattern of PCP is bilateral ground glass infiltration, but there is also a cystic form associated with intra-abdominal visceral calcification

---

Mycobacterium infection

The prevalence of mycobacterial infection is on the rise worldwide. The ICH patient is at risk for both *Mycobacterium tuberculosis* and atypical mycobacterial infections. The development of multidrug-resistant strains is a growing problem.[13]

Plain film findings and CT manifestations of TB in the ICH depend on the nature and severity of the patient's immunodeficiency. In the immunocompetent host, TB classically produces cavities and bronchogenic spread demonstrable as 'tree-in-bud' opacities on CT. These small opacities are inflamed bronchials that contain the inspissated caseous debris expelled from TB cavities in the lung.

In the ICH, however, mycobacterial infection may have a more varied and atypical appearance. Chest films and CT may demonstrate disease more reminiscent of primary TB, primary progressive TB, or miliary TB.[13,30–38] Cavities may still be seen, but often multiple pulmonary nodules or masses are seen instead. Mediastinal and hilar adenopathy as well as dissemination beyond the lungs to extrapulmonary sites are more likely to be encountered in the ICH.

Cytomegalovirus

Bone marrow, organ transplant recipients and patients with AIDS are particularly vulnerable to infection by CMV.[10–12,14,39,40] In the chest, CMV causes pneumonia, myocarditis and severe oesophagitis. Elsewhere, it may be the cause of hepatitis and gastro-intestinal ulcerations, in addition to viraemia.[39] Both reactivation of latent virus in the seropositive organ recipient and primary infection due to donor transmission of the virus represent significant problems.[39] Treatment of active, symptomatic CMV infection is with intravenous (IV) ganciclovir. Resistant strains of CMV have emerged. The radiographic and CT findings of CMV pneumonia are non-specific and mimic those of PCP. Both infections may be present simultaneously in the ICH. The most common manifestation of CMV lung infection is diffuse air-space disease, although ground glass infiltrates, nodular interstitial infiltrates, focal pneumonia and nodules have all been reported in this infection.[10,12,14,19]

Key points: tuberculosis and CMV

- In the ICH patient, mycobacterial infections have a variable appearance similar to that of primary TB, primary progressive TB, or miliary TB

- The radiographic appearances of CMV pneumonia are non-specific and mimic those of PCP

Thoracic complications in the ICH

Not all respiratory symptoms in the immunocompromised oncologic patient are due to infection or neoplasm. Other considerations not to be overlooked include thromboembolic disease and pulmonary drug toxicity as a cause of dyspnoea.

Pulmonary embolism

Especially in the oncologic and immunocompromised patient, the approach to diagnosing suspected pulmonary emboli has changed with the development and widespread dissemination of multidetector CT (MDCT) scanners. Spiral CT has a reported sensitivity for detecting central pulmonary emboli of 85–90% and specificity of greater than 90%.[41–46] Results from MDCT scans that are faster and use thinner slice thickness are likely to be even higher.[41–46] Although the accuracy of CT for detecting isolated, subsegmental emboli is not as good, the rapid diagnosis of clinically relevant large pulmonary emboli is expedited with CT.[41–46]

Multidetector CT findings of acute pulmonary emboli include: filling defects within contrast-enhanced pulmonary arteries and wedge-shaped lung opacities abutting the pleura due to pulmonary infarcts[47,48] (Fig. 58.4). 'Mosaic attenuation', a pattern of patchy lung CT attenuation, can indicate the presence of chronic thromboembolic disease. Chronic pulmonary emboli often appear as crescentic filling defects adherent to the walls of pulmonary arteries or as recanalized filling defects.[41,47]

Evaluation of suspected pulmonary emboli also involves looking for an embolic source; most often it is a deep venous thrombosis (DVT) in the lower extremities. Doppler ultrasound is an effective non-invasive method for diagnosing DVT that does not involve additional radiation exposure. However, this modality does not evaluate the deep pelvic veins or inferior vena cava (IVC), a common source of emboli in oncology patients. Computed tomography venography is an alternative method that involves scanning the lower extremities and the pelvis and up to the IVC if necessary. The study can be performed immediately following an MDCT study of the chest to rule out pulmonary embolism and uses only one dose of IV contrast. Computed tomography venography, however, does increase the gonadal radiation dose. Therefore, in younger patients, examination of the lower extremities with Doppler ultrasound is preferred.[49]

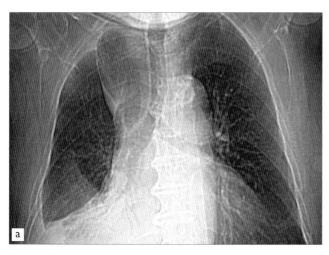
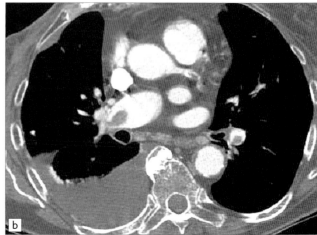

Figure 58.4. *Pulmonary thromboembolic disease in the immunocompromised oncologic patient. This female patient with breast cancer status post-mastectomy and chemotherapy presented with cough and shortness of breath. Considerations included infection due to pneumonia, recurrence of tumour in the lungs and pulmonary drug toxicity from chemotherapy. (a) The chest film was non-specific showing effusions and right lower lobe atelectasis. (b) Multidetector CT demonstrates multiple central pulmonary emboli as the cause of the patient's symptoms.*

Pulmonary drug toxicity

Pulmonary drug toxicity is a potential cause of respiratory symptoms in the oncologic patient who is receiving bleomycin, methotrexate, amiodarone, or other toxic agents to the lung. Early detection of drug-induced lung toxicity is critical before pulmonary damage becomes irreversible. Thoracic CT with HRCT may aid in the early detection of lung toxicity.

In cases of bleomycin lung, HRCT is more sensitive than chest radiographs in detecting early pulmonary toxicity. High-resolution CT accurately quantifies the extent of pulmonary damage and CT findings correlate well with measurements of impaired gas transfer and pulmonary function.[50–55]

Computed tomography features of bleomycin lung toxicity include reticulation, fibrotic bands and nodular opacities (Fig. 58.5). Initially, these nodular opacities are often mistaken for pulmonary metastases, opportunistic infection, or recurrent tumour.[50–55] Pulmonary toxicity often first affects the subpleural zone of the lung, those regions in the periphery of the lung and at the lung bases that parallel the pleural surfaces.[40–55] As the pulmonary toxicity progresses, the reticular and nodular opacities coalesce to form larger confluent opacities; diffuse, bilateral air-space disease can also be seen with acute bleomycin toxicity.[50,55]

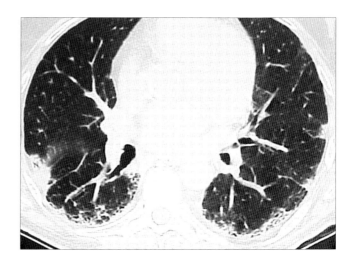

Figure 58.5. *CT features of bleomycin lung toxicity in the immunocompromised oncologic patient. A 71-year-old man with Stage IIB nodular sclerosing Hodgkin's disease developed bleomycin lung toxicity after receiving six cycles of ABV chemotherapy. CT shows peripheral reticulation and several irregular air-space opacities abutting the pleura due to bleomycin lung toxicity.*

Key points: pulmonary drug toxicity

- Chemotherapeutic agents are an important cause of respiratory symptoms in oncologic patients

- On HRCT, the features include nodules, reticulation, air-space disease and fibrotic bands

Organ transplantation: complications of infection and second malignancy

Thoracic imaging plays an important role in the ongoing surveillance of organ transplant recipients for oncologic complications.

Increasingly, the best hope for long-term survival for thousands of patients with end-stage organ failure is organ transplantation. Successful renal, lung, liver, heart, pancreas and intestinal organ transplantations have become routine at many major medical institutions. Advances in the treatment of organ rejection have improved the long-term survival of organ transplant recipients. Rejection is now detected earlier and treated aggressively with improved immunosuppression therapies.[10–12,14,56]

The major threats to survival for transplant recipients are often opportunistic infection and second malignancy.[10–12,14,17,18] Although these complications can occur at any time after transplantation, the relative frequency of specific complications varies depending on the degree of immunosuppression and the time elapsed from transplantation. Three major time periods of risk are recognized: the early postoperative period 0–30 days; the intermediate period during the first year post-transplantation; and the late period after 1 year following transplantation.[10–12,14,17,18,56]

During the early postoperative period, the primary concerns are infection, acute rejection and complications of the transplant surgery.[10–12,14,17–19] During the first year after transplantation, acute rejection and infection are the major complications.[10–12,14,17,19,56] After 1 year, chronic rejection and secondary malignancy become more important causes of morbidity and mortality.[10–12,14,17,18]

Although these time periods are somewhat arbitrary, organ transplant recipients usually require life-long immunosuppression and are therefore susceptible to infection, secondary malignancy and rejection at any time. The specifics of immunosuppression regimens vary from one transplant centre to another, and depend on the type of organ transplanted. Most use a combination of powerful immunosuppressive agents that may include corticosteroids, antisynthetic drugs (cyclosporine, tacrolimus) and antiproliferative agents (azathioprine, mycophenolate mofetil).[10–12,14,57]

Infection

Because life-long immunosuppression is usually required, the organ transplant recipient is always at risk for developing serious infection.[10–12,14] Immunosuppression is usually most profound during the first 3 months after transplantation when rejection risk is highest.[10–12,14,18,58] Infections may be due to viral, fungal, mycobacterial, bacterial and Mycoplasma pathogens.[10–12,14] Reactivation of latent CMV infection in the donor organ or reactivation of latent TB in the host can also occur.[57]

Infection that occurs within the first month post-transplantation is often bacterial or fungal in aetiology and the lungs are the most common site of infection.[10–12,14,18,57,59,60] Nosocomially acquired bacterial pneumonias are the most common and may be due to single or multiple pathogens including Staphylococcus aureus, Enterobacter and Gram-negative organisms such as Pseudomonas aeruginosa or Klebsiella pneumoniae.[10–12,14,17,58,61] More unusual bacterial infections due to anaerobes, Legionella, Listeria and Nocardia may also occur.[11]

Opportunistic infections due to Aspergillus, Candida, CMV, Legionella and other fungal species can occur at any time, but peak in incidence between 2 and 6 months post-transplantation.[10–12,14,18,60,62] Transplant recipients are also at risk for developing Pneumocystis carinii and Nocardia infections, although this risk has been substantially lowered by the prophylactic use of trimethoprim/sulfamethoxazole.[10–12,14,18,62] Ganciclovir is also given prophylactically to help prevent CMV infection.[10–12,14] Many other viruses have also been implicated as causes of pneumonia in transplant recipients.[10]

After the first 6 months, the risk of infection correlates directly with the degree of immunosuppression required to prevent organ rejection.[10–12,14] Those requiring only minimal immunosuppression are at lower risk, while those requiring high doses of corticosteroids and other agents are at high risk. Community-acquired pneumonias become more common especially those due to Pneumococcus and Haemophilus influenzae, but patients are still susceptible to opportunistic fungal and viral infections.[10–12,14]

As a result of immunosuppression, infections in organ transplant recipients are prone to dissemination from their primary site in the lung to form abscesses at other locations, including the soft tissues, muscles, liver, spleen, kidneys and brain.[10–12,14,17] Organ transplant recipients are also susceptible to infections of the sinuses and mastoid air cells and they may develop meningitis.[10–12,14,17]

Malignancy

The incidence of second malignancies in organ transplant recipients, including skin cancer and lymphoproliferative disease, is increased over the general population.[10–12,14,57,63] Cancer is second only to rejection as the most common cause of death in those recipients who survive longer than 1 year from transplantation.[17]

The most common secondary malignancies are skin cancers, lymphoproliferative disorders and visceral carcinomas.[17] Kaposi's sarcoma (KS) also occurs in these patients.[19]

Secondary neoplasms result from the body's depressed lymphocyte surveillance for cancer cells induced by immunosuppressant therapy and by infection with oncoviruses such as EBV.[10–12,14]

Skin tumours are primarily squamous cell carcinomas, and organ transplant recipients are encouraged to avoid direct sun exposure.

Secondary lymphoproliferative disorders include:

- Lymphoid hyperplasia
- Post-transplant lymphoproliferative disease (PTLD)
- Malignant lymphoma (mostly non-Hodgkin's in type) (Fig. 58.6)[10–12,14,19]

They are B cell in nature and associated with EBV infection.[64–66] The EBV infects B cells and causes them to proliferate. This proliferation goes unchecked because normal T cell control of B cells is markedly reduced by the immuno-

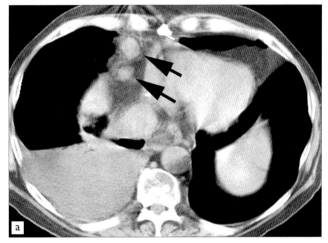

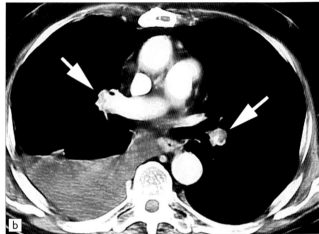

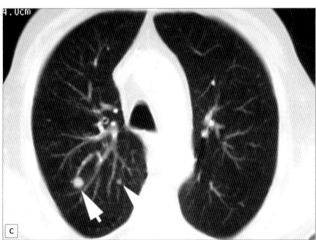

Figure 58.6. *Secondary neoplasms in two immunocompromised patients following heart transplantation – post-transplant lymphoproliferative disorder (PTLD) and lymphoma. (a and b) Thirteen months after cardiac transplantation, this 64-year-old man developed shortness of breath. CT shows a large right pleural effusion, bilateral pulmonary emboli (white arrows) and adenopathy in the right paracardiac region (black arrows). Cytology of the pleural effusion revealed monoclonal large cell lymphoma. (Image 58.6a reprinted with permission from Kuhlman J E. Thoracic imaging in heart transplantation. J Thorac Imaging 2003; 17:113-121.) (c) Eight months after cardiac transplantation, this 61-year-old man's CT shows new lung nodules (arrows). Open lung biopsy revealed PTLD.*

suppressant agents used to prevent organ rejection.[66] PTLD occurs in 1–20% of organ transplant recipients.[10,66] The frequency of PTLD varies with the type of organ transplant and is higher in lung and lung–heart transplant recipients than other organ recipients.[66] It is also higher in children who receive organ transplants and correlates with the severity of the immunosuppression regimen.[66]

PTLD and lymphoma in organ transplant recipients are often 'atypical' in presentation, and extranodal in location, either localized or disseminated.[17] Any organ may be involved, including the lung, liver, kidneys, spleen, gastrointestinal track, lymph nodes and cervical and tonsillar neck masses.[17,66] The site of the organ transplant will affect the likely sites of PTLD. For example, in patients receiving a single lung transplant, PTLD is more likely to occur in the chest and in the grafted organ.[66] Heart transplants appear to be an exception to this rule.[66] In the lung, PTLD or lymphoma usually present as one or more pulmonary nodules or masses, with or without adenopathy.[10–12,14,19,67] However, many patterns are seen including multiple or solitary nodules, air-space consolidation, hilar and mediastinal adenopathy, pleural and pericardial effusions.[10–12,14,66] Because infection in these patients produces similar find-

ings, biopsy to confirm the diagnosis is usually required.[66] PTLD may respond to reduction of immunosuppression and treatment with acyclovir.[10–12,14,66]

Lung cancer may also arise and grow rapidly in the immunosuppressed organ transplant recipient, and this patient population appears to be at increased risk for its development.[10,11,14,18,19,68–71] Most patients have been heavy smokers and advanced stages of tumour are the norm (Fig. 58.7).[10,11,14,18,19,68–71]

Key points: malignancy following organ transplantation

■ The most common malignancies following organ transplantation include skin cancers, lymphoproliferative disorders and visceral carcinomas

■ Lymphoproliferative disorders include PTLD, lymphoid hyperplasia and lymphoma

■ The frequency of PTLD is highest in lung and lung–heart recipients and is usually extranodal

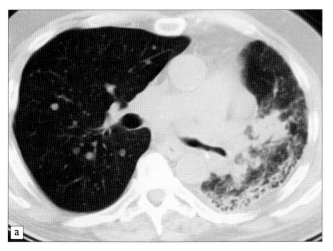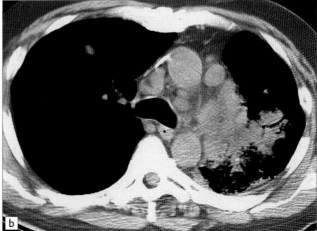

Figure 58.7. *Secondary neoplasm in the immunocompromised patient with previous lung transplant – lung cancer. This 62-year-old former smoker underwent orthotopic lung transplantation for bronchiectasis and pulmonary fibrosis in 1998. (a and b) A chest CT in 2001 showed that the patient had developed an aggressive left hilar mass, mediastinal adenopathy and multiple pulmonary metastases due to metastatic adenocarcinoma of the lung.*

Recurrence of primary disease

In addition to opportunistic infection and secondary malignancies, the primary disease may recur in the allografted organ. Documented recurrences of sarcoid, lymphangioleiomyomatosis, alveolar proteinosis, Langerhans' cell histiocytosis, desquamative interstitial pneumonitis and diffuse panbronchiolitis have been reported in lung transplant patients.[10]

AIDS-related tumours of the chest

Worldwide, more than 10 million people are infected with HIV and the numbers are growing.[72] As the pandemic continues to spread, no vaccine or cure for AIDS has been developed. Nevertheless, significant strides have been made in the treatment of AIDS-related diseases. Human immunodeficiency virus-infected individuals who have access to medications are living longer, primarily due to prophylactic treatments for opportunistic infections such as PCP and because of new antiretroviral agents.[13,73,74] Combination therapies using antiretroviral agents dramatically lower HIV virus burden and can reverse T-cell immunosuppression, thus radically changing the length of survival and quality of life of patients living with AIDS.[13,75]

The association between HIV infection and malignancies has been known since the early days of the epidemic.[76] Kaposi's sarcoma and non-Hodgkin's lymphoma are two AIDS-defining cancers that have a definite increased incidence in HIV-infected individuals. Invasive cervical carcinoma in the HIV-infected woman has recently been added to the list of AIDS-defining neoplasms as well.[76] Other tumours have been reported in association with HIV infec-

tion, including Hodgkin's lymphoma, testicular cancer, squamous cell cancer of the mouth and anus, lung cancer and hepatoma, among others.[77]

Neoplasms involving the chest in AIDS

AIDS-defining neoplasms that involve the chest include KS and AIDS-related lymphomas. Other lymphoproliferative disorders, such as AIDS-related lymphadenopathy syndromes (ARLS) and lymphocytic interstitial pneumonitis (LIP), are included in this discussion. Lung cancer and other non-AIDS defining malignancies of the chest are also addressed with respect to their differing manifestations in the HIV-infected individual.

Diagnostic approach to pulmonary/thoracic neoplasms in AIDS

Pulmonary disease in AIDS remains extremely common. Radiological diagnosis of thoracic diseases in AIDS is best done as an integrated approach that combines clinical information, radiographic and CT manifestations with a clear understanding of the natural history of AIDS.[78–84]

Diagnosis of pulmonary disease in AIDS is often challenging. Any number of opportunistic infections or neoplastic processes can present as pulmonary infiltrates, nodules, masses, lymphadenopathy or pleural effusions.[84] Atypical presentations and uncommon features confuse presentations and can delay diagnosis. Multiple pathogens and multifactorial disease often coexist in the lung (i.e. KS with PCP, lymphoma and a bacterial or disseminated fungal infection). Few radiographic features are specific.

Despite these discouraging facts, recognizable patterns of disease are seen in AIDS patients. Combining radiographic and CT pattern recognition with knowledge of the clinical presentation, CD4 count, underlying risk group, sex, race, geographic area and previous drug treatments narrows the diagnostic possibilities in many cases and expedites management decisions.[80,84,85]

It is perhaps most important to recognize that AIDS encompasses disease states that vary greatly in their degree of immunosuppression, from the asymptomatic HIV carrier to the end-stage terminal patient with AIDS. The degree of immune suppression often dictates the most likely pulmonary disease or neoplasm present in the patient.

HIV causes many defects in the immune system, the most devastating of which is the progressive destruction of CD4 helper T lymphocytes.[86] The CD4 count correlates well with the type of AIDS-related disease that is seen in the chest. Early in the course of HIV disease, when the CD4 count is still normal, virulent pathogens such as *M. tuberculosis* and encapsulated pyogenic bacteria successfully infect the lung. At this relatively early stage of AIDS, when immunosuppression is still not severe, KS may also develop.[85] Not until the CD4 count falls below 200–250 cells/mm^3 do opportunistic infections like PCP or disseminated fungal infections occur. When severe immunosuppression develops and CD4 counts drop below 50–100 cells/mm,^{3} less virulent pathogens such as CMV and *M. avium* complex (MAC) flourish.[86–88]

AIDS-related lymphomas tend to be seen at these later stages of immunosuppression. When a definitive diagnosis for pulmonary disease is required, diffuse opportunistic lung infections can often be diagnosed with induced sputums or bronchoscopy with broncho-alveolar lavage. More invasive procedures, such as transbronchial and open lung biopsies, are often avoided due to the increased complication rates in AIDS patients.[89] Focal lesions of the lung in the HIV-infected patient, whether due to neoplasm or infection, can be safely diagnosed with transthoracic needle-biopsy aspiration. These techniques have a high diagnostic yield for focal lung lesions in AIDS patients (85%) and carry an acceptable complication rate (28%).[90–92]

> ### Key point: pulmonary/thoracic neoplasms in AIDS
>
> ■ The degree of immune suppression in AIDS often dictates the most likely pulmonary disease or neoplasm. While immunosuppression is still not severe, KS may develop, whereas AIDS-related lymphomas tend to develop at later stages of immunosuppression

HAART and immune restoration syndrome

Patients who are treated with a combination regimen called highly active antiretroviral therapy (HAART) show dramatic decreases in their HIV viral load and increases in their CD4 counts, significantly reducing their HIV-related mortality.[13] However, with HAART's partial reconstitution of the immune system, the patient's cellular inflammatory response is also restored and this can lead to worsening of imaging findings due to certain infections such as mycobacterial disease. Patients with HIV and TB who receive HAART may demonstrate dramatic lymph node enlargement, worsening of lung disease and pleural effusions, which occur as the result of the restored inflammatory response.[13] Reports of newly diagnosed pulmonary sarcoid in HIV-infected patients receiving HAART have also appeared in the literature.[93]

Kaposi's sarcoma

Kaposi's sarcoma is a vascular neoplasm believed to arise from a mesenchymal cell of origin.[94,95] Its cause is not known,[96] but the histology of KS is characterized by scattered aggregates of spindle cells surrounding slit-like vascular spaces and extravasated red cells. In pulmonary KS, these aggregates proliferate within the interstitium of the lung, demonstrating a predilection for the peribronchial and perivascular lymphatics.[97–99] Several clinical varieties of KS exist:

- The classic form
- The endemic African version
- An acquired form associated with organ transplantation
- The AIDS-related variant

The classic form of the tumour was first described by M. Kaposi, a Hungarian dermatologist, in 1872. He noted most cases to be indolent tumours occurring in older men of Mediterranean or Eastern European heritage or Jewish background.[100,101] Disease was often localized to skin lesions of the lower extremities, but could spread to visceral involvement.[102] A more aggressive, 'endemic' form of the tumour was later recognized in children and young men in central Africa; and an acquired form was found in association with immunosuppression after organ transplantation.[100,102] 'Epidemic' or AIDS-related KS resembles the more deadly form of the tumour and is generally multifocal in its involvement; it affects to various extent:[96]

- The skin
- Mucous membranes
- Lymph nodes
- Gastro-intestinal tract
- Lung
- Visceral organs

In the USA and other industrialized countries, AIDS-related KS occurs almost exclusively in HIV-infected homosexual or bisexual men and their sexual partners (~95%). Only an estimated 3–4% of patients with HIV secondary to intravenous drug use or blood transfusion manifest KS and even fewer heterosexual HIV-infected women develop KS.[103–107] Over the last decade, the proportion of AIDS patients presenting with KS has declined from an estimated high of 30–40%[100] of the HIV-infected population to less than 15% of patients.[85,94,107–109] Although the incidence of KS as a presenting diagnosis of AIDS has declined, the prevalence of KS cases continues to increase as the pandemic spreads and AIDS patients live longer with KS from the time of diagnosis.[87,96] Changes in behaviour patterns among homosexual men may explain the decline in the number of new cases of KS;[81,107,109–111] it has long been hypothesized that an environmental or sexually transmitted cofactor is responsible along with HIV for the development of the disease.[85,103,112] In fact, recent discovery of human herpesvirus[8] in all forms of KS, including AIDS- and non-AIDS-related KS, suggests this may be the causal transmitted agent.[86]

Pulmonary involvement is estimated to occur in anywhere from 3.4 to 40% of patients with KS.[94,98,99,110–123] Pulmonary KS is found to be the cause of lung disease in 8–18% of AIDS patients with lung disorders, and KS is the cause of 10–45% of pleural effusions in AIDS patients.[94] In patients with skin KS and respiratory symptoms, 18–40% are found to have lung KS ante mortem, while an estimated 38–75% will have evidence of lung KS at autopsy.[94]

When pulmonary KS is present, there is usually widespread multisystem disease with disseminated KS involving the skin, mucous membranes, lymph nodes, visceral organs, bone marrow and gastro-intestinal tract.[99,111,119–122,124–126] Skin lesions are apparent on physical examination in 95% of AIDS patients with KS.[97,127,128] Exceptions do occur, however, with cases of isolated lung involvement due to KS reported in the literature.[99,112,119,122,129,130] More common, however, is the patient with relatively extensive pulmonary KS, who has limited disease elsewhere, with only a few isolated skin or mucous

membrane lesions on physical examination making the diagnosis more difficult to make. An estimated 5–23% of AIDS patients with pulmonary KS do not exhibit skin lesions and patients may have lymph node enlargement from KS without skin involvement.[94]

Definitive diagnosis of pulmonary KS can be problematic.[95] On bronchoscopy, characteristic blue-purple, violaceous, or cherry-red endobronchial papules are seen in only 30–45% of patients with lung KS.[95,103,114,124,128,131–133] Their absence does not exclude deeper involvement of the lung, as pulmonary KS can be entirely intraparenchymal.[103]

More invasive transbronchial biopsies are not commonly performed to confirm suspected KS, however. Unfortunately, transbronchial biopsies are positive in only 10–20% of cases, due to the patchy distribution of the disease.[95,97,103,114–116] Biopsies, even of superficial endobronchial lesions, may prove hazardous with significant bleeding occurring in 30% of attempts.[95,103,112]

Radiological appearances

Fortunately, chest film and CT findings of pulmonary KS often demonstrate a characteristic pattern of involvement that is distinct from opportunistic infections or lymphoma (Figs. 58.8–58.11).[98,110,123] These findings, taken in conjunction with physical examination and evidence of skin or mucous membrane KS, can often substantiate a diagnosis of pulmonary KS without the need for more invasive biopsy procedures.

Kaposi's sarcoma demonstrates a typical bronchovascular distribution of disease on plain films and even more strikingly on CT (Figs. 58.8, 58.9 and 58.11).[98,110,123,134,135] Chest film findings of KS include:

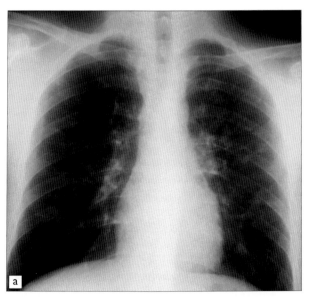
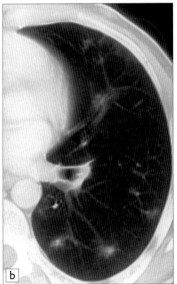
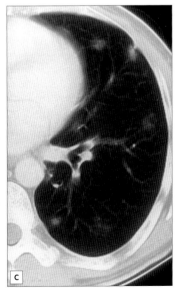

Figure 58.8. *A 32-year-old male homosexual with skin KS and early lung involvement. (a) Chest film shows subtle reticulonodular infiltrates radiating out from both hila, more prominent on the left than the right. (b and c) CT scan shows irregular, nodular opacities along the bronchovascular bundles due to pulmonary KS.*

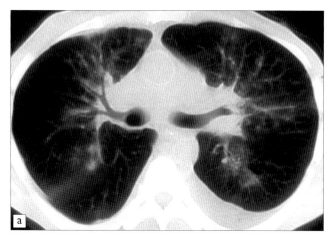

Figure 58.9. *CT features of pulmonary KS. (a and b) CT shows typical distribution of disease along the bronchovascular interstitium, radiating out from both hila. Note also the bilateral pleural effusions that are quite common in KS. In this patient the disease is more linear and less nodular in appearance. (c and d) More extensive pulmonary KS is present on this CT. The distribution of disease, however, is still strikingly along the bronchovascular bundles. There are also surrounding ground-glass infiltrates due to pulmonary haemorrhage.*

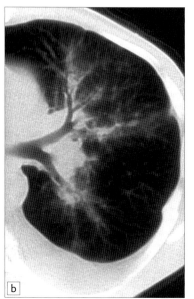
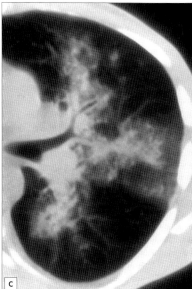
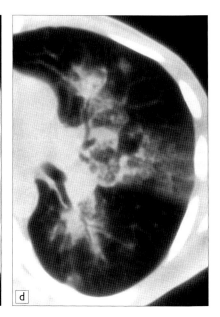

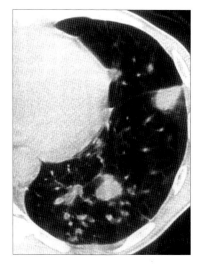

Figure 58.10. *A 44-year-old male with AIDS and pulmonary KS. This patient's CT scan demonstrates larger focal masses.*

- Reticulonodular infiltrates that are bilateral and more prominent in the perihilar and lower lung zones (Figs. 58.8 and 58.11)

- Thickening of the interstitial markings and septal lines (Fig. 58.12)
- Larger tumoural masses (Fig. 58.10)
- Focal areas of air-space consolidation or collapse as well as rapidly enlarging pleural effusions[95]

The chest film may be normal in 5–20% of patients with pulmonary KS.

Computed tomography findings of pulmonary KS include 'fluffy' or poorly marginated and irregular nodular opacities that are distributed along the bronchovascular bundles (Figs. 58.8, 58.9 and 58.12). Subpleural nodules and nodular thickening of the interlobular septa are also seen, all due to the tumour's propensity to involve the lymphatics in these locations (Fig. 58.12).[98,110,123,134,136] The pulmonary disease appears to radiate out from the pulmonary hilum and encase the bronchi and vessels (Figs. 58.9 and 58.12).[52] Parenchymal masses may also be seen, and both nodules and masses may be surrounded by a zone of ground glass attenuation which is probably due to haemorrhage (Figs. 58.9 and 58.10).[136] In one of the larger series of

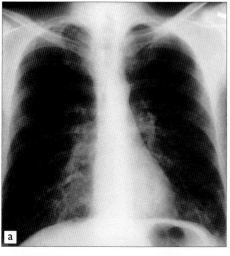
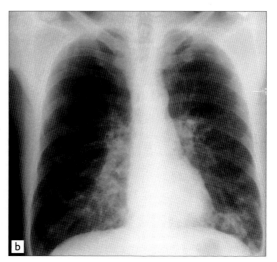
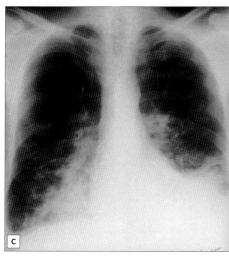

Figure 58.11. *A 49-year-old male with AIDS and progressive shortness of breath over a 6-month period. Chest films in April (a), May (b) and August (c) show the typical pattern of progression of pulmonary KS. Increasing reticulonodular, bibasilar and perihilar disease, more prominent in the lung bases, gradually worsens over the 6-month period. Bilateral pleural effusions appear and increase by August.*

patients with pulmonary KS, reported in the literature, including 53 patients with CT scans, the following findings were made:

- Multiple nodules in 79%
- Larger masses >2 cm in 53%
- A bronchovascular distribution of disease in 66%
- Pleural effusions in 55% (76% bilateral, 24% unilateral)
- Thickening of interlobular septa in 28% [136]

Associated features of thoracic KS include pleural effusions found in 30–67% of patients (Figs. 58.9, 58.11 and 58.12).[98,111,123,136] These effusions are frequently bloody on thoracocentesis or occasionally chylous due to lymphatic obstruction.

The reported frequency of lymph nodes in thoracic KS varies. Lymphadenopathy, in general, is seen in 30–35% of patients with KS.[102,112,136] On chest CT, lymphadenopathy may be identified in the axilla or mediastinum. Mediastinal lymph nodes were observed in 43% of cases in one series, but most nodes in the mediastinum were normal-sized nodes, with only 15% of cases demonstrating enlarged mediastinal nodes.[135] In another series, 53% of patients demonstrated axillary lymph nodes: 33% showed mediastinal nodes, 13% hilar nodes and 6% internal mammary nodes.[123] In general, the intrathoracic lymph nodes are not enlarged to the same extent as seen in cases of lymphoma, mycobacterial or fungal infections in AIDS. Lymphadenopathy due to KS has also been reported to demonstrate enhancement after bolus injection of IV contrast that exceeds that of skeletal muscle.[122,137] Other causes of enhancing lymph nodes include Castleman's disease, carcinoid tumour and angioimmunoblastic lymphadenopathy, but these entities are much less common than KS in AIDS.[137]

Computed tomography scans of the chest may also demonstrate evidence of extrapulmonary disease including: skin and subcutaneous nodules, bone metastases to the ribs, sternum, and thoracic vertebral bodies, and chest wall involvement by larger KS masses. Bone scans may fail to demonstrate osseous lesions due to KS, so radiographs, CT or MR imaging may be needed to diagnose early bone involvement.[96]

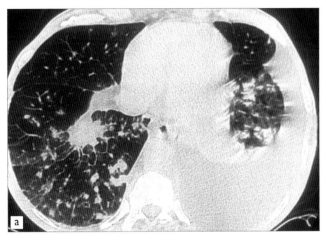
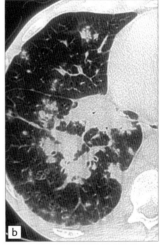
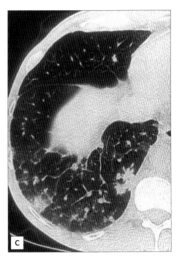

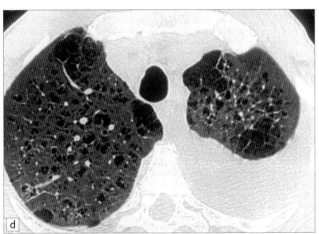
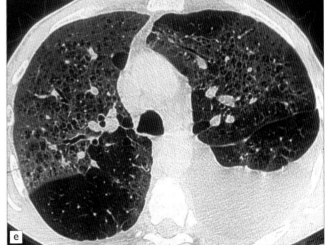

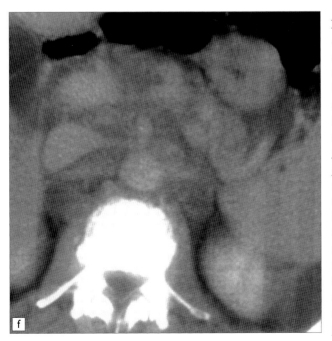

Figure 58.12. *A 49-year-old man with advanced AIDS, CD4 count less than 100 and multifactorial disease due to KS, PCP and disseminated M. avium-intracellulare (MAI). (a–c) CT shows characteristic findings of lung KS with nodular disease encasing the hilum and bronchi, thickening of the interlobular septa and pleural effusions. On bronchoscopy, the patient had bluish-red papules lining the mucosa of the airways compatible with the diagnosis of endobronchial and pulmonary KS. (d and e) Upper lung zones show ground glass attenuation bilaterally and cystic changes in the lung parenchyma. These changes are not seen in pulmonary KS, but are typical of PCP in AIDS. (f) CT scans through the upper abdomen revealed retroperitoneal adenopathy. The enlarged lymph nodes are low density on this contrast-enhanced CT scan and proved to be due to disseminated MAI infection. Kaposi's sarcoma does cause adenopathy, but the lymph nodes are not usually of low density after intravenous contrast, and may even demonstrate increased enhancement when compared to muscle. Low-density nodes in an AIDS patient should raise the question of mycobacterial infection either due to TB or atypical Mycobacterium, fungal infection, or possibly an AIDS-related lymphoma.*

The major differential diagnosis for pulmonary infiltrates in an AIDS patient with KS is opportunistic infection. Differentiating opportunistic infection from KS involving the lung can usually be done by careful examination of the chest radiograph, the CT scan and correlation with clinical signs and symptoms. In most cases where there is extensive skin KS and typical CT and chest film findings of lung KS, the diagnosis is confirmed with endoscopic visualization of endobronchial lesions and broncho-alveolar lavage (BAL) to exclude superimposed infection.[94] A superimposed infection in patients with pulmonary KS will be present in 17–27% of patients (Fig. 58.12).[94]

Presentation and course of KS in AIDS is highly variable. Patients who develop KS early at higher CD4 counts tend to have more indolent disease with slow progression. As the degree of immunosuppression advances, the virulence of KS increases as well, with disease becoming more explosive in some cases.[73]

Patients with pulmonary KS usually present with increasing dyspnoea and/or persistent non-productive cough that progresses over weeks to months; this is a clinical course more gradual in onset than most cases of opportunistic infection. Recurrent hemoptysis, stridor, or bronchospasm may indicate upper airway or endobronchial disease due to KS.[102] Pleuritic chest pain may indicate pleural or chest wall involvement by KS. Other non-specific symptoms include fever and weight loss which overlap with opportunistic infection.[102,138] Sputum production is not typical of pulmonary KS and is more likely to be due to opportunistic infection.

Most opportunistic infections in AIDS including PCP, mycobacterial and fungal infections do not demonstrate a striking bronchovascular distribution of disease like KS on plain films or CT. Pleural effusions are rarely seen in PCP infections, but may be seen with mycobacterial or fungal infections, lymphoma and lung cancer in AIDS patients. Adenopathy is also rare in PCP, unless the infection is disseminated, in which case the lymph nodes often show calcification. However, mycobacterial infection, fungal infection, AIDS-related lymphoma, lung cancer, or KS can all cause adenopathy in the chest. Necrotic or low-density lymph nodes, demonstrating rim enhancement with IV contrast, should suggest infection, particularly TB, other mycobacterial infection, or fungal infection (Fig. 58.12).

A number of features of KS can also be mimicked by one unusual infection that occurs in AIDS patients: bacillary angiomatosis. Skin nodules, visceral involvement, lytic bone lesions and hypervascularity with contrast enhancement can be seen in bacillary angiomatosis, a disseminated infection due to Rochalimaea henselae and R. quintana, bacilli in the same family of organisms causing cat-scratch fever.[96,139] Diagnosis of bacillary angiomatosis is made by skin biopsy or positive blood cultures in the presence of bacteraemia; the infection is effectively treated with antibiotics such as erythromycin or doxycycline.[139]

It is also important to remember that in the more advanced stages of AIDS, multiple diseases coexist simultaneously in the lung, making it almost impossible to exclude superimposed infection with one or more organisms in addition to involvement of the lung with KS (Fig. 58.12). Thus, bronchoscopy with BAL is often employed in patients with suspected pulmonary KS to exclude other treatable diseases such as superimposed opportunistic infection.

In problem cases, nuclear scintigraphy may provide some additional help. Pulmonary KS is thallium-avid, but does not accumulate gallium tracer. Opportunistic infections in AIDS do not accumulate thallium, but do accumulate gallium; and lymphoma accumulates both thallium and gallium.[113] Sequential thallium and gallium nuclear scintigraphy has been used to document the presence of extracutaneous KS and non-invasively to follow the response of visceral KS to treatment.[113,118]

The role of MR in the evaluation of patients with KS is limited, but one recent report has stated that pulmonary KS demonstrates enhancement with gadolinium on T1-weighted images, but low signal intensity on the long TE, T2-weighted images.[94,140]

Because the rate of progression of KS and its extent is quite variable, a staging system for KS which incorporates the extent of the tumour, the presence of symptoms, and the CD4 count has been advocated by the AIDS Clinical Trials Group.[141] Prognosis correlates with visceral involvement, including the extent of lung disease.[93] The median survival for patients with lung involvement is 6 months.[95] Patients with better prognosis are those with tumour limited to the skin, lymph nodes, or minimal oral lesions; a CD4 count greater than 200; no 'B' symptoms or opportunistic infections; and a Karnofsky performance status greater than or equal to 70%.[141]

Treatment of KS is palliative and aimed at slowing the progression of disease.[73,138] Therapy includes local measures and systemic methods.[73] Indications for treatment include: progressive dyspnoea, increasing effusions, impending obstruction of the airway.[95] In the chest, local treatments include pleurodesis of symptomatic pleural effusions and laser or radiotherapy for bleeding or obstructing airway or laryngeal lesions. Systemic methods of treatment include single or multi-agent chemotherapy, whole lung radiation, and alpha-interferon (IFN-α).[73] Widespread pulmonary KS has been treated with whole-lung radiation therapy or combination chemotherapy. Kaposi's sarcoma is radiosensitive and larger symptomatic masses can be treated with radiation therapy with response rates of 50–80%.[102] Alpha-interferon is often combined with zidovudine to treat KS early in AIDS because of the suppressive effects on both the tumour and viral cofactors. Unfortunately, IFN-α works less well as the CD4 count drops below 400 and the response time is relatively slow.[73,94,95,102,138] A number of chemotherapy protocols for treating KS have been used with moderate success in causing temporary regression of disease. Unfortunately, relapse occurs and remissions usually are of short duration.[95] Single agents are employed for early, limited disease and combinations of drugs including doxorubicin, vinblastine, vincristine, bleomycin and etoposide (VP-16) are used for more extensive disease.[31] Because pulmonary KS can cause death due to progressive respiratory failure, it is often treated with combination chemotherapy. Adriamycin, bleomycin, vincristine (ABV) treatment in this setting has a reported response rate in the lung of 80%.[102,137,142,143] New approaches to treatment, including targeting of lesions with liposomal doxorubicin and liposomal daunorubicin, are also being tested.[73,95]

No treatment for KS, however, has been shown to prolong survival, and all treatments cause myelosuppression increasing the risk of opportunistic infection as a complication.[94,95,102,144] Prophylactic treatment for PCP is mandatory and use of granulocyte–macrophage colony stimulating factor (GM–CSF) with chemotherapy may provide additional haematological support.[88,95] Overall prognosis of patients with pulmonary KS is poor with most patients succumbing to HIV-related infections or progressive respiratory failure.[102,117,145] Serial CT examinations are more accurate than plain films for determining response of the pulmonary KS to treatment on follow-up examinations.

Key points: Kaposi's sarcoma

- AIDS-related KS is of the 'epidemic' variety and resembles the more deadly form of the tumour

- AIDS-related KS occurs almost exclusively in homosexual or bisexual men and their sexual partners

- Skin lesions are present in the majority of AIDS patients with pulmonary KS

- Pulmonary KS can be entirely intraparenchymal, endobronchial papules are seen in only 30–45% of patients with lung KS, and transbronchial biopsies are positive in only 10–20% of cases due to the patchy distribution of the disease

- The rate of progression of KS is variable and the prognosis correlates with visceral involvement including the extent of lung disease – if there is lung involvement the median survival is 6 months

AIDS-related lymphomas (see also chapter 32)

AIDS-related lymphomas are usually seen as a late manifestation of AIDS,[146] often after the CD4 count has fallen below 50–100 cells/mm³ when the patient is in a state of severe immunosuppression.[87] An estimated 2–5% of AIDS patients are affected by an AIDS-related lymphoma, and the incidence of these tumours is increasing.[112,143,147–151] As prophylactic and antiretroviral therapies for AIDS patients have prolonged survival, the number of patients developing AIDS-related lymphomas is expected to continue to increase.[73,87,146] AIDS-related lymphomas are mostly non-Hodgkin's B-cell lymphomas – poorly differentiated large or anaplastic lymphomas, Burkitt's lymphoma and immunoblastic sarcomas.[146]

Various cofactors including oncoviruses such as Epstein–Barr that result in proliferation of B cells have been implicated as the cause of AIDS-related lymphomas.[148,152]

AIDS-related lymphomas are aggressive, rapidly growing tumours that present with widespread visceral involvement including extranodal sites (85%) such as bone marrow, bowel, liver/spleen, kidneys, CNS and skin.[100,143,148,153,154] The reported incidence of thoracic lymphoma in AIDS ranges from 6 to 40%.[152] The lung parenchyma is involved in approximately 10% of patients.[100] Lymphoma is the initial AIDS-defining illness in almost 80% of cases.[154]

Characteristics of AIDS-related lymphomas include high-grade, late-stage lymphoma at presentation and severe B symptoms.[146,152]

Thoracic manifestations of AIDS-related lymphomas are varied[100] and differ from the typical findings of lymphoma in the general population. Only 22–25% will demonstrate hilar or mediastinal lymph node involvement, the more typical findings of lymphoma in the general population (Fig. 58.13).[100,112,152] AIDS-related lymphomas also present in atypical patterns with chest wall masses, lytic bone lesions, pulmonary nodules and masses with or without lymphadenopathy (Fig. 58.14).[82,100] Pleural effusions are more common in AIDS-related lymphomas occurring in 30–50% of patients.[152] Lung involvement may take the form of nodules, masses, reticulonodular infiltrates or air-space consolidation.[152] Pulmonary nodules or masses are more common in AIDS-related lymphomas occurring in 10–30% of cases at the time of presentation (Fig. 58.14).[112,152] Lung nodules from lymphoma may be small or large, but they rarely cavitate so enabling differentiation from nodules due to infections; additionally, they are usually better marginated compared to the nodules in KS.[152] Lung masses due to lymphoma may also demonstrate very aggressive growth patterns.[100,152]

Staging of AIDS-related lymphomas includes CT examinations of the head, chest, abdomen and pelvis. Gallium scanning may also be used; however, increasingly ¹⁸FDG PET scanning is used to stage AIDS-related lymphomas (Fig. 58.15). Newer hybrid ¹⁸FDG PET–CT devices that combine both MDCT and dedicated ¹⁸FDG PET scanner are especially useful in staging these tumours. Initial staging also involves bone marrow aspiration and lumbar puncture for cytology.[148]

The prognosis for AIDS-related lymphomas is poor, although some (33–60%) will temporarily respond to chemotherapy.[148] Relapse rates are high and remission usually short-lived, with median survival of 5–7 months.[112,148,152] Combination chemotherapy with cyclophosphamide, doxorubicin, vincristine and prednisone (CHOP) is often used in conjunction with GM–CSF in an attempt to lessen myelosuppression while treating the lymphoma.[73]

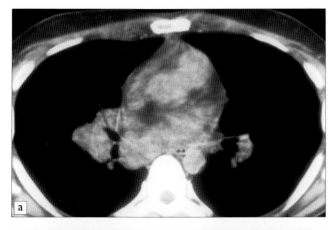

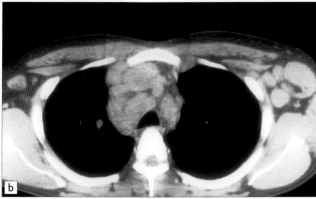

Figure 58.13. *A 35-year-old man with AIDS-related lymphoma. Bulky adenopathy is present in both axilla, the right hilum, and the mediastinum including the internal mammary nodes, the anterior mediastinum, the right paratracheal zone and the subcarinal area. Only 25% of AIDS-related lymphomas will demonstrate this pattern of nodal disease in the chest.*

Whether AIDS patients also have an increased risk for Hodgkin's lymphoma remains uncertain.[146] Some reports have shown an increased incidence in homosexual HIV-infected males, but overall incidence of Hodgkin's disease in AIDS has not been documented.[90] Hodgkin's disease in the setting of HIV infection, however, is atypical in its manifestations: patients present with tumours at more advanced stages of disease and with more aggressive histologies, usually of mixed cellularity types; and they present with more extranodal disease; additionally their Hodgkin's disease responds less well to treatment. Prognosis is significantly poorer in the HIV-infected patient with Hodgkin's disease than in the general population.[148,152]

Rare primary pulmonary T-cell lymphomas have been reported in HIV-infected patients. These tumours present as slow-growing pulmonary masses.[155]

Key points: AIDS-related lymphomas

- AIDS-related lymphomas (ARL) is usually seen when the patient is in a severe state of immunosuppression

- ARLs are most commonly non-Hodgkin's B-cell lymphomas, poorly differentiated, Burkitt's or immunoblastic

- ARL presents with atypical patterns with chest wall masses, lytic bone lesions, pulmonary nodules and masses. Only 22–25% have mediastinal or hilar lymph node involvement

- The prognosis for ARL is poor, relapse rates are high, remission short-lived and the median survival is 5–7 months

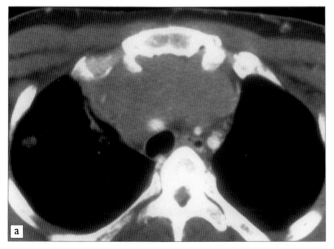

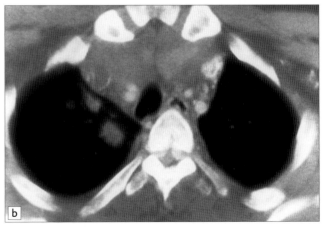

Figure 58.14. *A 45-year-old man whose AIDS-defining illness was this aggressive, non-Hodgkin's lymphoma. (a and b) CT scan shows a large infiltrative tumour in the anterior mediastinum encasing the vessels and obliterating the fat planes. Note also the multiple right pulmonary nodules found at presentation. Lymphoma in the general population rarely presents with pulmonary nodules, rather pulmonary spread is usually a late manifestation after treatment failure and recurrence. Not so in the AIDS patient who may present with pulmonary disease due to an AIDS-related lymphoma.*

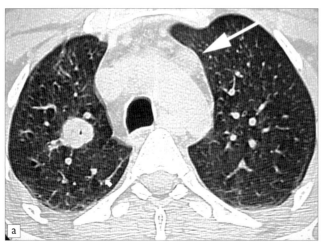
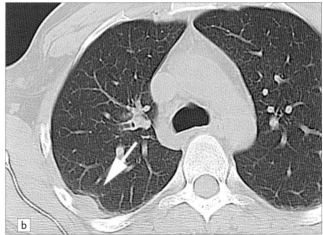
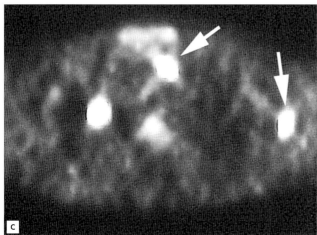
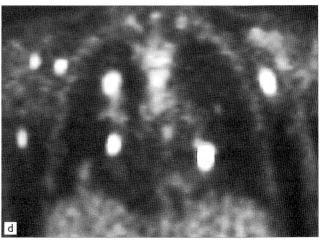
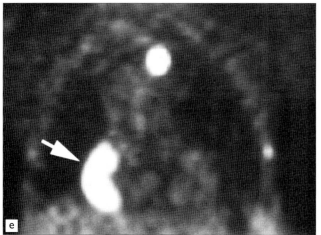

Figure 58.15. *A 36-year-old man with AIDS, CD4 count of 45 and viral load of 431,200. (a and b) CT showed multiple new pulmonary nodules including one in the right upper lobe (a) and one abutting the right pleura (b, arrow). Also present were some mildly enlarged lymph nodes in the anterior mediastinum. (a, arrow). (c–e) An ¹⁸FDG PET scan was performed. (c) Axial ¹⁸FDG PET image shows intense abnormal uptake in the right upper lobe nodule and in lymph nodes (arrows) in the mediastinum and left axilla. (d) Coronal ¹⁸FDG PET image shows abnormal uptake in multiple other lesions in the lungs and lymph nodes. (e) Coronal ¹⁸FDG PET shows abnormal uptake in a pericardial effusion (arrow) as well as in the lymph node in the upper mediastinum. Bronchoscopy with transbronchial biopsy of the right upper lobe nodule revealed large cell lymphoma. The entire ¹⁸FDG PET scan showed multiple lesions in the head, chest, abdomen and pelvis compatible with widely disseminated lymphoma. (Courtesy of Jannette Collins, MD, Med.)*

AIDS-related lymphadenopathy syndromes

Other HIV-associated lymphoproliferative disorders include AIDS-related adenopathy. Lymphadenopathy is a common finding in patients with AIDS and may be due to a variety of causes including:

- Infection (secondary to TB, *M. avium* complex, fungal infections, disseminated PCP)

- AIDS-related lymphomas
- The lymphadenopathic form of KS[156]
- Benign lymphoid hyperplasia[157]

Adenopathy due to lymphoid hyperplasia that occurs in the HIV-infected patients without an AIDS-defining illness is part of the AIDS-related complex (ARC) and the persistent generalized lymphadenopathy syndrome (PGL). Persistent generalized lymphadenopathy syndrome is lymphadenopathy present at two or more extra-inguinal, non-contiguous sites that persists for more than 3 months. No other AIDS-defining illnesses, infection, or drug reaction may be present to fit the criteria.[87]

These patients frequently demonstrate moderately enlarged lymph nodes on chest CT scans in the axilla, the supraclavicular region and the cervical neck region.

Extensive mediastinal adenopathy is not usually a manifestation of lymphoid hyperplasia or the PGL syndrome. When extensive mediastinal adenopathy is detected on CT or plain films, the differential diagnosis should include opportunistic infection particularly due to mycobacterial or fungal pathogens, an AIDS-related lymphoma, or rarely the lymphadenopathic form of KS.[82,156–159] Persistent generalized lymphadenopathy syndrome indicates chronic over-stimulation of B-cell production and a proportion of these patients will go on to develop an AIDS-related B lymphoma.[146]

Other features of mediastinal and hilar nodes may be helpful in narrowing the differential diagnosis. For example, enlarged lymph nodes due to mycobacterial infection, particularly TB, often demonstrate necrotic low-density centres and rim enhancement (Fig. 58.12). Such features, however, may also be seen in disseminated fungal infections and lymphoma.[158,159] Lymph nodes involved with KS may show enhancement greater than surrounding muscle or soft tissues when IV contrast is administered. Disseminated pneumocystis infection can cause large bulky mediastinal and hilar lymph nodes that demonstrate significant dystrophic calcification on CT.[26,160]

Lymphoid interstitial pneumonitis

Lymphoid interstitial pneumonitis is characterized pathologically by infiltration of the lung interstitium by lymphocytes and plasma cells.[112,161] This is an AIDS-defining pulmonary illness when it occurs in children and adolescents less than 13 years of age (Fig. 58.16). It has also been reported in adult patients with AIDS, primarily in blacks and Haitians.[112,161] On chest radiographs, LIP presents as bilateral reticular or reticulonodular pulmonary infiltrates (Fig. 58.16). Hilar and mediastinal lymphadenopathy may also be seen.[162] Lymphoid interstitial pneumonitis must be distinguished from PCP in the infant with AIDS. Pneumocystis pneumonia usually occurs within the first year of life, between the ages of 3 and 6 months. Lymphoid interstitial pneumonitis, on the other hand, is more likely to occur in the HIV-positive infant who is older than 1 year of age.[163,164] A closely related disorder is pulmonary lymphoid hyperplasia (PLH), which is in the spectrum of polyclonal B-cell lymphoproliferative disorders (PBLD) seen in HIV-infected children. In cases of PLH, hyperplastic lymphoid follicles proliferate around distal small airways. PLH may be seen with LIP. Epstein–Barr virus has been implicated as the infectious cofactor in both PLH and LIP.[87]

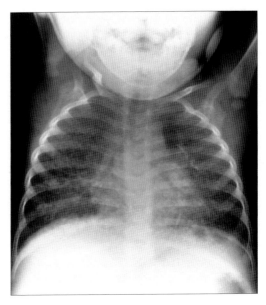

Figure 58.16. *Lymphocytic interstitial pneumonitis (LIP) in a child less than 13 years of age is an AIDS-defining illness. Chest film in this 1-year-old girl with AIDS shows typical LIP reticulonodular infiltrates bilaterally. (Reprinted with permission from Kuhlman J E. Pneumocystic infections: the radiologist's perspective. Radiology 1996; 198: 623–635.)*

Lung cancer in AIDS

Whether other malignancies such as lung cancer have an increased incidence in AIDS is uncertain.[4,5,96] A few small series of young male patients with AIDS and lung cancer have appeared in the literature.

Most, if not all, patients with lung cancer and AIDS are long-term smokers (90%) and male (97%) (Figs. 58.17 and 58.18).[76,79,165–170] The degree of immunosuppression and the CD4 count do not correlate well with the presence of lung cancer in HIV-infected patients, so if there is an increased association of lung cancer in AIDS it may be due to a direct oncogenic effect of HIV rather than through immunosuppression.[76,171] Lung cancer appears to occur at an earlier age in HIV-infected patients, and present at more advanced stages of disease.[76,79,167–170,172] The most common histology is adenocarcinoma (Fig. 58.17).[75,76,173] Prognosis is very poor with less than 1 year's survival after diagnosis.[76,168–171,174–179]

Radiographic manifestations of bronchogenic carcinoma in 30 HIV-infected patients were recently reviewed by Fishman et al.[167] Findings included a peripheral mass (60%) versus a central hilar or mediastinal mass (37%). One patient presented with a pleural mass. Peripheral tumours had a predilection for the upper lobes. Lymphadenopathy was identified in 63%, and pleural effusions in 33%. Peripheral tumours in three patients were mistaken for or hidden by inflammatory disease, so delaying diagnosis.[167] Distribution of cell types was as follows:

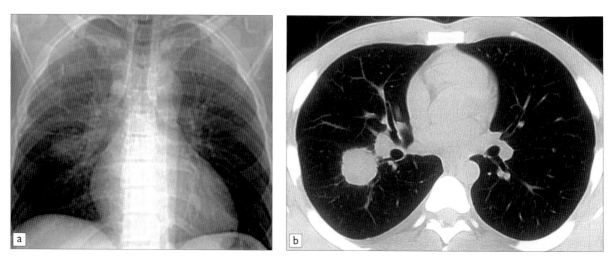

Figure 58.17. *A 27-year-old HIV-infected man who smokes. (a and b) A 3 cm mass is present in the perihilar region of the superior segment of the right lower lobe. Bronchoscopic biopsy revealed adenocarcinoma of the lung. In HIV-infected patients, lung cancer occurs at an earlier age, presents at more advanced stage and has a poorer prognosis. The most common cell type is adenocarcinoma.*

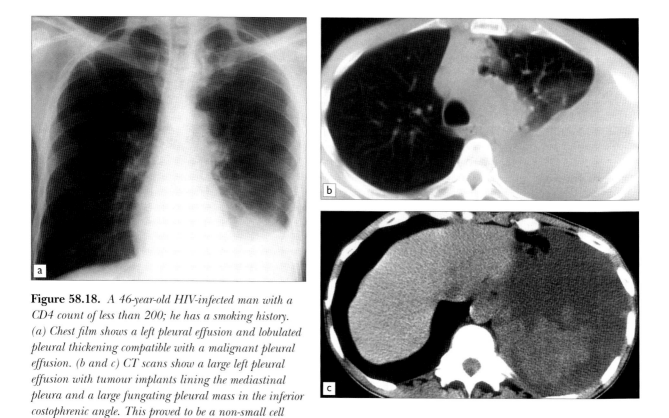

Figure 58.18. *A 46-year-old HIV-infected man with a CD4 count of less than 200; he has a smoking history. (a) Chest film shows a left pleural effusion and lobulated pleural thickening compatible with a malignant pleural effusion. (b and c) CT scans show a large left pleural effusion with tumour implants lining the mediastinal pleura and a large fungating pleural mass in the inferior costophrenic angle. This proved to be a non-small cell lung carcinoma. One of the more 'atypical' presentations of lung cancer in AIDS is one characterized predominantly by pleural disease.*

adenocarcinoma (43%), squamous cell (30%), adenosquamous (7%), small cell (7%), large cell (7%), mixed small and large cell (3%), poorly differentiated non-small cell (3%).[168] Only 20% of tumours were Stage I at presentation, while 20% were Stage III and 53% were Stage IV tumours.[168]

Similar findings have been noted in other series, including cases in which pleural disease and effusions were the predominant presenting manifestations of lung cancer (Fig. 58.18).[76,168]

Because delays in diagnosis of lung cancer have

occurred when focal lung lesions are assumed to be due to infection in an AIDS patient, any focal lesion which fails to respond to antibiotic treatment should be further evaluated.[170] Peripheral focal lung lesions are amenable to percutaneous transthoracic biopsy which has a high diagnostic yield of 85% for focal lung lesions.[92] Complication rate in this setting is acceptable and not higher than in non-HIV infected patients.[92]

Summary

- In the immunocompromised host or the immune-suppressed oncologic patient with respiratory symptoms of fever, diagnostic considerations include opportunistic lung infection, recurrence of the primary tumour, development of a secondary malignancy or complication of therapy. The degree of immune suppression often indicates the most likely pulmonary infection, neoplasm or disease

- In the patient with AIDS, KS can develop when immunosuppression is still not severe

- The major differential diagnosis for pulmonary infiltrates in an AIDS patient with KS is opportunistic infection – sputum production is not typical of pulmonary KS and is more likely due to opportunistic infection

- In the more advanced stages of AIDS, multiple diseases coexist simultaneously in the lung, making it almost impossible to exclude superimposed infection with one or more organisms in addition to involvement of the lung with KS

- ARL is usually a late manifestation of AIDS, often after CD4 counts have fallen below 50–100 cells/mm³

- Thoracic manifestations of ARL differ from the typical findings of lymphoma in the general population

- Causes of lymphadenopathy in AIDS include ARL, KS, lymphoid hyperplasia and opportunistic infection

- LIP is an AIDS-defining pulmonary illness where it occurs in children less than 13 years of age

References

1. Burch P A, Karp J E, Merz W G et al. Favorable outcome of invasive aspergillosis in patients with adult acute leukemia. J Clin Oncol 1987; 5: 1985–1993

2. Kuhlman J E. AIDS-related diseases of the chest. In: Kuhlman J E (ed). CT of the Immunocompromised Host. Contemporary Issues in Computed Tomography, vol 14. New York: Churchill Livingstone, 1991: 27–69

3. Kuhlman J E. Opportunistic fungal infection: the neutropenic patient with leukemia, lymphoma, or bone marrow transplantation. In: Kuhlman J E (ed). CT of the Immunocompromised Host. Contemporary Issues in Computed Tomography. New York: Churchill Livingstone, 1991; 5–25

4. Kuhlman J E, Fishman E K, Burch P A et al. Invasive pulmonary aspergillosis in acute leukemia: the contribution of CT to early diagnosis and aggressive management. Chest 1987; 92: 95–99

5. Kuhlman J E, Fishman E K, Burch P A et al. CT of invasive pulmonary aspergillosis. Am J Roentgenol 1988; 150: 1015–1020

6. Kuhlman J E, Fishman E K, Hruban R H et al. Diseases of the chest in AIDS: CT diagnosis. Radiographics 1989; 9: 827–857

7. Kuhlman J E, Fishman E K, Siegelman S S. Invasive pulmonary aspergillosis in acute leukemia: characteristic findings on CT, the CT halo sign, and the role of CT in early diagnosis. Radiology 1985; 157: 611–614

8. Kuhlman J E, Kavuru M, Fishman E K, Siegelman S S. *Pneumocystis carinii* pneumonia: spectrum of parenchymal CT findings. Radiology 1990; 175: 711–714

9. Naidich D P, Garay S M, Goodman P C. Pulmonary manifestations of AIDS. In: Federle M D, Megibow A J, Naidich D P (eds). Radiology of AIDS. New York: Raven Press, 1988; 47–76

10. Collins J. Imaging of the chest after lung transplantation. J Thorac Imag 2002; 17: 102–112

11. Fishman J E, Rabkin J M. Thoracic radiology in kidney and liver transplantation. J Thorac Imag 2002; 17: 122–131

12. Gosselin M V, Adams R H. Pulmonary complications in bone marrow transplantation. J Thorac Imag 2002; 17: 132–144

13. Saurborn D P, Fishman J E, Boiselle P M. The imaging spectrum of pulmonary tuberculosis in AIDS. J Thorac Imag 2002; 17: 28–33

14. Kuhlman J E. Thoracic imaging in heart transplantation. J Thorac Imag 2002; 17: 113–121

15. Hruban R H, Ren H, Kuhlman J E et al. Inflation-fixed lungs: pathologic–radiologic (CT) correlation of lung transplantation. J Comput Assist Tomogr 1990; 14: 329–335

16. Orr D P, Myerowitz R L, Dubois P J. Pathoradiologic correlation of invasive pulmonary aspergillosis in the compromised host. Cancer 1978; 41: 2028–2039

17. Knollmann F D, Hummel M, Hetzer R, Felix R. CT of heart transplant recipients: spectrum of disease. RadioGraphics 2000; 20: 1637–1648

18. Leung A N. Invited Commentary: Scientific Exhibit. RadioGraphics 1999; 19: 340–341

19. Knisely B L, Mastey L A, Collins J, Kuhlman J E. Imaging of cardiac transplantation complications. RadioGraphics 1999; 19: 321–339.

20. Huang R M, Naidich D P, Lubat E et al. Septic pulmonary emboli: CT–radiologic correlation. Am J Roentgenol 1989; 153: 41–45

21. Kuhlman J E, Fishman E K, Teigen C. Pulmonary septic emboli: diagnosis with CT. Radiology 1990; 174: 211–213

22. Kuhlman J E, Knowles M C, Fishman E K, Siegelman S S. Premature bullous damage in AIDS: CT diagnosis. Radiology 1989; 173: 23–26

23. Panicek D M. Cystic pulmonary lesions in patients with AIDS. Radiology 1989; 173: 12–14

24. Gurney J W, Bates F T. Pulmonary cystic disease: comparison of *Pneumocystis carinii* pneumatoceles and bullous emphysema due to intravenous drug abuse. Radiology 1989; 73: 27–31

25. Sandhu J, Goodman P C. Pulmonary cysts associated with *Pneumocystis carinii* pneumonia in patients with AIDS. Radiology 1989; 173: 33–35

26. Radin D R, Baker E L, Klatt E C et al. Visceral and nodal calcification in patients with AIDS-related *Pneumocystis carinii* infection. Am J Roentgenol 1990; 154: 27–31

27. Joe L, Gordin F, Parker R H. Spontaneous pneumothorax in *Pneumocystis carinii* infection. Arch Intern Med 1986; 146: 1816–1817

28. Goodman P C, Daley C, Minagi H. Spontaneous pneumothorax in AIDS patients with *Pneumocystis carinii* pneumonia. Am J Roentgenol 1986; 147: 29–31

29. Fleisher A G, McElvaney G, Lawson L et al. Surgical management of spontaneous pneumothorax in patients with acquired immunodeficiency syndrome. Ann Thorac Surg 1988; 45: 21–23

30. Amos A, Denning D, Katz D, Smith H. Computed tomography of chest in diagnosis of miliary tuberculosis. Lancet 1987; 1: 1269–1270

31. Auerbach O, Dail D H. Mycobacterial infections. In: Dail D H, Hammar S P (eds). Pulmonary Pathology. New York: Springer-Verlag, 1988: 173–188

32. Barnett S M. CT findings in tuberculous mediastinitis. J Comput Assist Tomogr 1986; 10: 165–166

33. Contreras M A, Cheung O T, Sanders D E, Goldstein R S. Pulmonary infection with nontuberculous mycobacteria. Am Rev Respir Dis 1988; 137: 149–152

34. Hauser H, Gurret J P. Miliary tuberculosis associated with adrenal enlargement: CT appearance. J Comput Assist Tomogr 1986; 10: 254–256

35. Im J G, Song K S, Kang H S et al. Mediastinal tuberculous lymphadenitis: CT manifestations. Radiology 1987; 164: 115–119

36. Kuhlman J E, Deutsch J H, Fishman E K, Siegelman S. CT features of thoracic mycobacterial disease. Radiographics 1990; 10: 413– 431

37. Marinelli D L, Albelda S M, Williams T M et al. Nontuberculous mycobacterial infection in AIDS; clinical, pathologic, and radiographic features. Radiology 1986;160: 77–82

38. Naidich D P, McCauley D I, Leitman B S et al. CT of pulmonary tuberculosis. In: Siegelman S S (ed). Computed Tomography of the Chest. New York: Churchill Livingstone, 1984; 175–217

39. Rubin R H. Prevention and treatment of cytomegalovirus disease in heart transplant patients. J Heart Lung Transplant 2000; 19: 731–735

40. Dee, P. AIDS and other forms of immunocompromise. In: Armstrong P, Wilson A G, Dee P, Hansell D M (eds). Imaging of Diseases of the Chest, 2nd edn. St Louis: Mosby, 1995; 253

41. Remy-Jardin M, Remy J, Wattinne L, Giraud F. Central pulmonary thromboembolism: diagnosis with spiral volumetric CT with the single breath hold technique – comparison with pulmonary angiography. Radiology 1992; 185: 381–387

42. Zeman R K, Silverman P M, Vieco P T, Costello P. CT angiography. Am J Roentgenol 1995; 165: 1079–1088

43. Remy-Jardin M, Remy J, Cauvain O et al. Diagnosis of central pulmonary embolism with helical CT: role of two-dimensional multiplanar reformations. Am J Roentgenol 1995; 165: 1131–1138

44. Goodman L R, Lipchik R J, Kuzo R S et al. Subsequent pulmonary embolism: risk after a negative helical CT pulmonary angiogram: prospective comparison with scintigraphy. Radiology 2000; 215: 535–542

45. Goodman L R, Curtin J J, Mewissen M W et al. Detection of pulmonary embolism in patients with unresolved clinical and scintigraphic diagnosis: helical CT versus angiography. Am J Roentgenol 1995; 164: 1369–1374

46. Gefter W B, Davis S D, Gurney J W et al. Thoracic radiology. Radiology 1996; 198: 926–931

47. Godwin J D, Webb W R, Gamsu G, Ovenfors C. Computed tomography of pulmonary embolism. Am J Roentgenol 1980; 135: 691–695

48. Balakrishnan J, Meziane M A, Siegelman S S, Fishman E K. Pulmonary infarction: CT appearance with pathologic correlation. J Comput Assist Tomogr 1989; 13: 941–945

49. Rademaker J, Griesshaber V, Hidajat N et al. Combined CT pulmonary angiography and venography for diagnosis of pulmonary embolism and deep vein thrombosis: radiation dose. J Thorac imaging 2001;16: 297–299

50. Bellamy E A, Husband J E, Blaquiere R M, Law M R. Bleomycin-related lung damage: CT evidence. Radiology 1985; 156: 155–158

51. Bellamy E A, Nicholas D, Husband J E. Quantitative assessment of lung damage due to bleomycin using computed tomography. Br J Radiol 1987; 60: 1205–1209

52. Fleischman R W, Baker J R, Thompson G R et al. Bleomycin-induced interstitial pneumonia in dogs. Thorax 1971; 26: 675–681

53. Nachman J B, Baum E S, White H, Cruissi F G. Bleomycin-induced pulmonary fibrosis mimicking recurrent metastatic disease in a patient with testicular carcinoma: case report of the CT scan appearance. Cancer 1981; 47: 236–239

54. Kuhlman J E. The role of chest computed tomography in the diagnosis of drug-related reactions. J Thorac Imaging 1991; 6: 52–61

55. Rimmer M J, Dixon A K, Flower C D R, Sikora K. Bleomycin lung: computed tomographic observations. Br J Radiol 1985; 58: 1041–1045

56. Hosenpud J D, Bennett L E, Keck B M et al. The Registry of the International Society for Heart and Lung Transplantation: sixteenth official report. J Heart Lung Transplant 1999; 18: 611–626

57. Winkel E, DiSesa V J, Costanzo M R. Advances in heart transplantation. Dis Mon 1999; 45: 62–87

58. Petri W A Jr. Infections in heart transplant recipients. Clin Infect Dis 1994; 18: 141–148

59. Fishman J A, Rubin R H. Infection in organ-transplant recipients. N Engl J Med 1998; 338: 1741–1751

60. Miller L W, Schlant R C, Kobashigawa R et al. 24th Bethesda conference: Cardiac transplantation. Task Force 5: Complications. J Am Coll Cardiol 1993; 22: 41–54

61. Austin J H, Schulman L L, Mastrobattista J D. Pulmonary infection after cardiac transplantation: clinical and radiologic correlations. Radiology 1989; 172: 259–265

62. Thaler SJ, Rubin R H. Opportunistic infections in the cardiac transplant recipient. Curr Opin Cardiol 1996; 11: 191–203

63. Penn I. Tumor incidence in human allograft recipients. Transplant Proc 1979; 11: 1047–1051

64. Armitage J M, Kormos R L, Stuart R S et al. Post-transplant lymphoproliferative disease in thoracic organ transplant patients: 10 years of cyclosporine-based immunosuppression. J Heart Lung Transplant 1991; 10: 877–886

65. Young L, Alfieri C, Hennessy K et al. Expression of Epstein–Barr virus transformation-associated genes in tissues of patients with EBV lymphoproliferative disease. N Engl J Med 1989; 321: 1080–1085

66. Lim G Y, Newman B, Kurlan G, Webber S A. Post-transplantation lymphoproliferative disorder: manifestations in pediatric thoracic organ recipients. Radiology 2002; 222: 699–708

67. Haramati L B, Schulman L L, Austin J H M. Lung nodules and masses after cardiac transplantation. Radiology 1993; 188: 491–497

68. Goldstein D J, Austin J H M, Zuech N et al. Carcinoma of the lung after heart transplantation. Transplantation 1996; 62: 772–775

69. Pham S M, Kormos R L, Landreneau R J et al. Solid tumors after heart transplantation: lethality of lung cancer. Ann Thorac Surg 1995; 60: 1623–1626

70. Johnson W M, Baldursson O, Gross T J. Double jeopardy: lung cancer after transplantation. Chest 1998; 113: 1720–1723

71. Delcambre F, Pruvot F R, Ramon P et al. Primary bronchogenic carcinoma in transplant recipients. Transplant Proc 1996; 28: 2884–2885

72. Mann J M, Welles S L. Global aspects of the HIV epidemic. In: De Vita V T, Hellman S, Rosenberg S A (eds). AIDS: Etiology, Diagnosis, Treatment and Prevention. Philadephia: Lippincott, 1988; 89–98

73. Conant M A. Management of human immunodeficiency virus-associated malignancies. Recent Results Cancer Res 1995; 139: 423–432

74. Osmond D, Charlebois E, Lang W et al. Changes in AIDS survival time in two San Francisco cohorts of homosexual men, 1983 to 1993. JAMA 1994; 271: 1083–1087

75. Mitchell D M, Miller R F. New developments in the pulmonary diseases affecting HIV-infected individuals. Thorax 1995; 50: 294–302

76. White C S, Haramati L B, Elder K H, Karp J, Belani C P. Carcinoma of the lung in HIV-positive patients: findings on chest radiographs and CT scans. Am J Roentgenol 1995; 164: 593–597

77. Safui B, Diaz B, Schwartz J. Malignant neoplasms associated with human immunodeficiency virus infection. Cancer J Clin 1992; 42: 74–95

78. Munoz A, Schrager L K, Bacellar H et al. Trends in the incidence of outcomes defining acquired immunodeficiency syndrome (AIDS) in the multicenter AIDS cohort study: 1985–1991. Am J Epidemiol 1993; 137: 423–438

79. Padhani A R, Kuhlman J E. Pulmonary manifestations of AIDS. Appl Radiol 1993; 22: 13–19

80. Kuhlman J E. Invited commentary. CT pattern recognition in AIDS. Radiographics 1993; 13: 785–786

81. Naidich D P. Pulmonary manifestations of HIV infection. In: Greene R (ed). Syllabus: A Categorical Course in Diagnostic Chest Radiology. Oak Brook, Illinois: Radiologic Society of North America, Inc, 1992; 135–155

82. Kuhlman J E. CT evaluation of the chest in AIDS. In: Thrall J H, Decker BC (eds). Current Practice of Radiology. Philadelphia: Mosby-Year Book Inc, 1993; 9–18

83. Gradon J D, Timpone J G, Schnittman S M. Emergence of unusual opportunistic pathogens in AIDS: A review. Clin Infect Dis 1992; 15: 134–157

84. Sider L, Gabriel H, Curry D R et al. Pattern recognition of the pulmonary manifestations of AIDS on CT Scans. Radiographics 1993; 13: 771–784

85. Katz M J, Hessol N A, Buchbinder S P et al. Temporal trends of opportunistic infections and malignancies in homosexual men with AIDS. J Infect Dis 1994; 170: 198–202

86. Weiss R A. Human herpesvirus 8 in lymphoma and Kaposi's sarcoma: now the virus can be propagated. Nat Med 1996; 2: 277–278

87. Nash G, Said J W, Nash S V, DeGirolami U. Short course: The pathology of AIDS. Mod Pathol 1995; 8: 199–217

88. Wang C Y E, Schroeter A L, Su W P D. Acquired immunodeficiency syndrome-related Kaposi's sarcoma. Mayo Clin Proc 1995; 70: 869–879

89. Trachiotis G D, Hafner G H, Hix W R, Aaron B L. Role of open lung biopsy in diagnosing pulmonary complications of AIDS. Ann Thorac Surg 1992; 54: 898–902

90. Hessol N A, Katz M H, Liu J Y et al. Increased incidence of Hodgkin's disease in homosexual men with HIV infection. Ann Int Med 1992; 117: 309–311

91. Gruden J F, Klein J S, Webb W R. Percutaneous transthoracic needle biopsy in AIDS: analysis in 32 patients. Radiology 1993; 189: 567–571

92. Scott W W Jr, Kuhlman J E. Focal pulmonary lesions in patients with AIDS: percutaneous transthoracic needle biopsy. Radiology 1991; 180: 419–421

93. Haramati L B, Lee G, Singh A et al. Newly diagnosed pulmonary sarcoidosis in HIV-infected patients. Radiology 2001; 218: 242–246

94. Cadranel J, Mayaud C. Intrathoracic Kaposi's sarcoma in patients with AIDS. Thorax 1995; 50: 407–414

95. Denton A S, Miller R F, Spittle M F. Management of pulmonary Kaposi's sarcoma: new perspectives. Br J Hosp Med 1995; 53: 344–350

96. Steinbach L S, Tehranzadeh J, Fleckenstein J L et al. Human immunodeficiency virus infection: musculoskeletal manifestations. Radiology 1993; 186: 833–838

97. White D A, Zaman M K. Pulmonary disease. Medical management of AIDS patients. Med Clin North Am 1992; 76: 19–44

98. Davis S D, Henschke C I, Chamides B K et al. Intrathoracic Kaposi's sarcoma in AIDS patients: radiographic–pathologic correlation. Radiology 1987; 163: 495–500

99. Sivit C J, Schwartz A M, Rockoff S D. Kaposi's sarcoma of the lung in AIDS: radiologic–pathologic analysis. Am J Roentgenol 1987; 148: 25–28

100. Goodman P C. Pulmonary manifestations of AIDS. Curr Probl Diagn Radiol 1988; 17: 81–89

101. Albini A, Mitchell C D, Thompson E W et al. Invasive activity and chemotactic response to growth factors by Kaposi's sarcoma cells. J Cell Biochem 1988; 36: 369–376

102. Cooley T P. Kaposi's sarcoma. In: Libman H, Witzburg R A (eds). HIV Infection: A Clinical Manual, 2nd edn. Boston: Little, Brown & Co, 1993; 354–367

103. Mitchell D M, Miller R F. Recent developments in the management of the pulmonary complications of HIV disease. Thorax 1992; 47: 381–390

104. Ognibene F P, Steis R G, Macher A M et al. Kaposi's sarcoma causing pulmonary infiltrates and respiratory failure in the acquired immunodeficiency syndrome. Ann Intern Med 1985; 102: 471–475

105. Zibrak J D, Silvestri R C, Costello P et al. Bronchoscopic and radiologic features of Kaposi's sarcoma involving the respiratory system. Chest 1986; 90: 476–479

106. Wahman A, Melnick S L, Rhame F S, Potter J D. The epidemiology of classic, African, and immunosuppressed Kaposi's sarcoma. Epidemiol Rev 1991; 13: 178–199

107. Beral V, Peterman T A, Berkelman R L, Jaffe H W. Kaposi's sarcoma among patients with AIDS: a sexually transmitted infection? Lancet 1990; 335: 123–128

108. Friedman-Kien A E, Saltzman B R. Clinical manifestations of classical, endemic African and endemic AIDS–associated Kaposi's sarcoma. J Am Acad Dermatol 1990; 22: 1237–1250

109. Montaner J S G, Le T, Hogg R et al. The changing spectrum of AIDS index disease in Canada. AIDS 1994; 8: 693–696

110. Naidich D P, McGuinness G. Pulmonary manifestations of AIDS: CT and radiographic correlations. Radiol Clin North Am 1991; 29: 999–1017

111. Naidich D P, Garay S M, Leitman B A et al. Radiographic manifestations of pulmonary disease in acquired immunodeficiency syndrome (AIDS). Semin Radiol 1987; 22: 14–30

112. Heitzman E R. Pulmonary neoplastic and lymphoproliferative disease in AIDS: a review. Radiology 1990; 177: 347–351

113. Lee V W, Fuller J D, O'Brien M J et al. Pulmonary Kaposi sarcoma in patients with AIDS: scintigraphic diagnosis with sequential thallium and gallium scanning. Radiology 1991; 180: 409–412

114. Hanson P J V, Hancourt-Webster J N, Grazzard B G et al. Fibroscopic bronchoscopy in the diagnosis of pulmonary Kaposi's sarcoma. Thorax 1987; 42: 269–271

115. Lau K Y, Rubin A, Littner M et al. Kaposi's sarcoma of the tracheobronchial tree: clinical bronchoscopic and pathologic features. Chest 1986; 89: 158–159

116. Pitchenick A E, Fischl M A, Saldoma M. Kaposi's sarcoma of the tracheobronchial tree: Clinical bronchoscopic and pathologic features. Chest 1985; 87: 122–124

117. Gill P J, Akil B, Colletti P et al. Pulmonary Kaposi's sarcoma: clinical findings and resulting therapy. Am J Med 1989; 87: 57–61

118. Lee V W, Rosen M P, Baum A et al. AIDS-related Kaposi sarcoma: findings on thallium-201 scintigraphy. Am J Radiol 1988; 151: 1233–1235

119. Garay S M, Belenko M, Fazzini E et al. Pulmonary manifestations of Kaposi's sarcoma. Chest 1987; 91: 39–43

120. Antman K, Nadler L, Mark E J et al. Primary Kaposi's sarcoma of the lung in an immunocompetent 32-year-old heterosexual white man. Cancer 1987; 54: 1696–1698

121. Kornfeld H, Axelrod J L. Pulmonary presentation of Kaposi's sarcoma in a homosexual patient. Ann Rev Respir Dis 1983; 127: 248–249

122. Herts B R, Megibow A J, Birnbaum B A et al. High-attenuation lymphadenopathy in AIDS patients:

significance of findings at CT. Radiology 1992; 185: 777–781

123. Wolff S D, Kuhlman J E, Fishman E K. Thoracic Kaposi's sarcoma in AIDS: CT findings. J Comput Assist Tomogr 1993; 17: 60–62

124. Meduri G U, Stover D E, Lee M et al. Pulmonary Kaposi's sarcoma in the acquired immune deficiency syndrome. Clinical, radiographic, and pathologic manifestations. Am J Med 1986; 81: 11–18

125. Zibrak J D, Silvestri R C, Costello P et al. Bronchoscopic and radiologic features of Kaposi's sarcoma involving the respiratory system. Chest 1986; 90: 476–479

126. White D A, Stover D E. Pulmonary effects of AIDS. Clin Chest Med 1988; 9: 363–535

127. Franquet T, Gimenez A, Caceres J et al. Imaging of pulmonary–cutaneous disorders: matching the radiologic and dermatologic findings. Radiographics 1996; 16: 855–869

128. Longo D L. Kaposi's sarcoma and other neoplasms. Ann Intern Med 1984; 100: 92–106

129. Caray S, Belenko M, Fazzini E, Schinella R. Pulmonary manifestations of Kaposi's sarcoma. Chest 1987; 91: 39–43

130. Nash G, Fligiel S. Kaposi's sarcoma presenting as pulmonary disease in the acquired immunodeficiency syndrome: diagnosis by lung biopsy. Hum Pathol 1984; 15: 999–1001

131. Pitchenik A F, Fischl M A, Saldana M J. Kaposi's sarcoma of the tracheobronchial tree: clinical, bronchoscopic and pathologic features. Chest 1985; 87: 122–124

132. Hanson P J V, Hancourt-Webster J N, Grazzard B G, Collins J V. Fibroscopic bronchoscopy in the diagnosis of pulmonary Kaposi's sarcoma. Thorax 1987; 42: 269–271

133. Lau K Y, Rubin A, Littner M, Krauthammer M. Kaposi's sarcoma of the tracheobronchial tree: clinical, bronchoscopic and pathologic features. Chest 1986; 89: 158–159

134. Naidich D P, Tarras M, Garay S M et al. Kaposi's sarcoma: CT–radiographic correlation. Chest 1989; 96: 723–728

135. Khalil A M, Carette M F, Cadranel J L et al. Intrathoracic Kaposi's sarcoma: CT findings. Chest 1995; 108: 1622–1626

136. Hartman T E, Primack S L, Muller N L, Staples C A. Diagnosis of thoracic complications in AIDS: accuracy of CT. Am J Roentgenol 1994; 162: 547–553

137. Herts B R, Megibow A J, Birnbaum B A et al. High-attenuation lymphadenopathy in AIDS patients: significance of findings at CT. Radiology 1992; 185: 777–781

138. Wagner R P, Farber H W. Pulmonary manifestations. In: Libman H, Witzburg RA (eds). HIV Infection: A Clinical Manual, 2nd edn. Boston: Little, Brown & Co, 1993; 124–145

139. Tappero J W, Koehler J E, Berger T G et al. Bacillary angiomatosis and bacillary splenitis in immunocompetent adults. Ann Int Med 1993; 118: 363–365

140. Khalil A M, Carette M F, Cadranel J L et al. Magnetic resonance imaging (MRI) findings in pulmonary Kaposi's sarcoma: a series of 10 cases. Eur Respir J 1994; 7: 1285–1289

141. Krown S E, Metroka C, Werntz J C. AIDS Clinical Trials Group Oncology Committee. Kaposi's sarcoma in the acquired immune deficiency syndrome: a proposal for uniform evaluation, response and staging criteria. J Clin Oncol 1989; 7: 1201–1207

142. Gill P S, Alcil B, Colletti P et al. Pulmonary Kaposi's sarcoma: clinical findings and results of therapy. Am J Med 1989; 87: 57–61

143. Nyberg D A, J Effrey R B Jr, Federle M P et al. AIDS-related lymphomas: evaluation by abdominal CT. Radiology 1986; 159: 59–63

144. Krigel R L, Friedman-Kien A E. Kaposi's sarcoma. In: De Vita V T, Hellman S, Rosenberg S A (eds). AIDS: Etiology, Diagnosis, Treatment and Prevention. Philadelphia: Lippincott, 1988; 245–261

145. White D A, Matthay R A. Noninfectious pulmonary complications of infection with the human immunodeficiency virus. Am Rev Resp Dis 1989; 140: 1763–1787

146. Gaidano G, Dalla-Favera R. Molecular pathogenesis of AIDS-related lymphomas. Adv Cancer Res 1995; 67: 113–120

147. Hessol N A, Katz M H, Liu J Y et al. Increased incidence of Hodgkin's disease in homosexual men with HIV infection. Ann Intern Med 1992; 117: 309–311

148. Cooley T P. Aids-related lymphoma. In: Libman H, Witzburg R A (eds). HIV Infection: A Clinical Manual, 2nd edn. Boston: Little, Brown & Co, 1993; 368–375

149. Kaplan L D, Abrams D I, Feigal E et al. AIDS associated non-Hodgkin's lymphoma in San Francisco. JAMA 1989; 261: 719–724

150. Pluda J M et al. Development of non-Hodgkin's lymphoma in a cohort of patients with severe human immunodeficiency (HIV) infection on long-term antiretroviral therapy. Ann Intern Med 1990; 113: 276–282

151. Moore R D, Kessler H, Richman D D et al. Non-Hodgkin's lymphoma in patients with advanced HIV infection treated with zidovudine (Abstract). 7th International Conference on AIDS, Florence, June, 1991

152. Dodd G D, Greenler D P, Confer S R. Thoracic and abdominal manifestations of lymphoma occurring in the immunocompromised patient. Radiol Clin N Am 1992; 30: 597–610

153. Meduri G U, Stein D S. Pulmonary manifestations of acquired immunodeficiency syndrome. Clin Infect Dis 1992; 14: 98–113

154. Radin D R, Esplin J A, Levine A M, Ralls P W. AIDS-related non-Hodgkin's lymphoma: abdominal CT findings in 112 patients. Am J Roentgenol 1993; 160: 1133–1139

155. Kohler C A, Gonzales-Ayala E, Rowley P et al. Primary pulmonary T-cell lymphoma associated with AIDS: the syndrome of the indolent pulmonary mass lesion. Am J Med 1995; 99: 324–326

156. Kuhlman J E, Fishman E K, Knowles M G et al. Disease of the chest in AIDS: CT diagnosis. Radiographics 1989; 9: 827–857

157. Bottles K, McPhaul L W, Volberding P. Fine-needle aspiration biopsy of patients with the acquired immunodeficiency syndrome (AIDS): experience in an outpatient clinic. Ann Int Med 1988; 108: 42–45

158. Radin D R. Intraabdominal Mycobacterium tuberculosis vs Mycobacterium avium-intracellulare infections in patients with AIDS: distinction based on CT findings. Am J Roentgenol 1991; 156: 487–491

159. Radin D R. Disseminated histoplasmosis: abdominal CT findings in 16 patients. Am J Roentgenol 1991; 157: 955–958

160. Groskin S A, Massi A F, Randall P A. Calcified hilar and mediastinal lymph nodes in an AIDS patient with *Pneumocystis carinii* infection. Radiology 1990; 175: 345–346

161. Travis W D, Fox C H, Devaney K O et al. Lymphoid pneumonitis in 50 adult patients infected with the human immodeficiency virus: lymphocytic interstitial pneumonitis versus nonspecific interstitial pneumonitis. Hum Pathol 1992; 23: 529–541

162. Rubinstein A. Pediatric AIDS. Curr Probl Pediatr 1986; 16: 361–409

163. Marquis J R, Bardeguez A D. Imaging of HIV infection in the prenatal and postnatal period. Clin Perinatal 1994; 21: 125–147

164. Simonds R J, Lindegren M L, Thomas P et al. Prophylaxis against *Pneumocystis carinii* pneumonia among children with perinatally acquired human immunodeficiency virus infection in the United States. N Engl J Med 1995; 332: 786–790

165. Braun M A, Killam D A, Remick S C et al. Lung cancer in patients seropositive for human immunodeficiency virus. Radiology 1990; 175: 341–343

166. Moser R J III, Tenholder M F, Ridenour R. Oat-cell carcinoma in transfusion-associated acquired immunodeficiency syndrome. Ann Intern Med 1985; 103: 478

167. Fishman J E, Schwartz D S, Sais G J et al. Bronchogenic carcinoma in HIV-positive patients: findings on chest radiographs and CT scans. Am J Roentgenol 1995; 164: 57–61

168. Braun M A, Killam D A, Remick S C, Ruckdeschel J C. Lung cancer in patients seropositive for human immunodeficiency virus. Radiology 1990; 175: 341–343

169. Sridhar K S, Flores M R, Raub W A Jr, Saldana M. Lung cancer in patients with human immunodeficiency virus infection compared with historic control subjects. Chest 1992; 102: 1704–1708

170. Tenholder M F, Jackson H D. Bronchogenic carcinoma in patients seropositive for human immunodeficiency virus. Chest 1993; 104: 1049–1053

171. Shiramizu B, Hendier B G, McGrath M S. Identification of a common clonal human immunodeficiency virus integration site in human immunodeficiency virus associated lymphomas. Cancer Res 1994; 34: 2069–2072

172. Monfardini S, Vaccher E, Pizzocaro G et al. Unusual malignant tumours in 49 patients with HIV infection. AIDS 1989; 3: 449–452

173. Fraire A E, Awe R J. Lung cancer in association with human immunodeficiency virus infection. Cancer 1992; 70: 432–436

174. Chan T K, Aranda C P, Rom W N. Bronchogenic carcinoma in young patients at risk for acquired immunodeficiency syndrome. Chest 1993; 103: 862–864

175. Nguyen V Q, Ossorio M A, Roy T M. Bronchogenic carcinoma and the acquired immunodeficiency syndrome. J Ky Med Assoc 1991; 89: 322–324

176. Karp J, Profeta G, Marantz P R, Karpel J P. Lung cancer in patients with immunodeficiency syndrome. Chest 1993; 103: 410–413

177. Fraire A E, Awe R J. Lung cancer in association with human immunodeficiency virus infection. Cancer 1992; 70: 432–436

178. Vaccher E, Tirelli U, Spina M et al. Lung cancer in 19 patients with HIV infection (letter). Ann Oncol 1993; 4: 85–86

179. Biggar R J, Burnett W, Miki J, Nasca P. Cancer among New York men at risk of the acquired immunodeficiency syndrome. Int J Cancer 1989; 43: 979–985

Chapter 59

The immunocompromised host: abdomen and pelvis

Alec J Megibow

Introduction

Acquired immunodeficiency syndrome (AIDS) occurs in every part of the world; the epidemic has spared no socio-economic segment of the population. As of the year 2000, there were an estimated 800,000–900,000 human immunodeficiency virus (HIV)-infected individuals living in the USA, with approximately 40,000 new infections occurring each year. In the UK, approximately 31,000 cases and 15,000 cumulative deaths have been reported to the World Health Organization (WHO) as of December 1999 (Epidemiological Factsheet for UK, 2000 edition, WHO). Approximately three quarters of the cases occur in men; 1% are reported in children. Since the beginning of the epidemic, the United States Centers for Disease Control estimate that 448,000 had died by the year 2000.

As the disease entity was recognized 'early' in the USA, a large volume of case experience has accrued. Imaging has maintained a peripheral, but important, role in the evaluation of these patients. Because of the overlap of radiological findings in neoplastic and non-neoplastic diseases encountered in the patient with AIDS, the major role of imaging has been first to localize sites of disease and second to attempt to guide therapy to the site of disease which is most treatable and has the most significant morbidity.[1,2] In these patients, neoplastic diseases are not the source of immediate life-threatening clinical situations. Radiologists should be familiar with the predictable appearances of neoplasms and their distribution so that they will not be confused with other clinical entities.

Kaposi's sarcoma (KS) and non-Hodgkin's lymphoma (NHL) account for virtually all of the neoplasms seen by oncologists who treat AIDS patients. No statistically significant association between AIDS and other cancers has been established. However, several cancers occur in the abdomen and pelvis with approximately twice the frequency compared to the general population:

- Squamous cell cancer of the anal canal (but not cervical)
- Leiomyosarcoma
- Hodgkin's disease
- Testicular cancer[3,4]

Kaposi's sarcoma preferentially affects homosexual men. The risk varies by geographic area, suggesting that there is an environ-mental co-factor for KS in addition to HIV. Despite intensive investigation, the responsible co-factor has not been identified conclusively. Human immune deficiency virus-associated NHL affects all HIV transmission groups, and the risk of NHL increases with duration of HIV infection and age.

The radiological features of each will be described for the abdomen. Differential diagnostic considerations will be catalogued at the end of the chapter.

Pathology and clinical background

The appearance of KS in a young homosexual male was the first reported case which led to the recognition of the AIDS epidemic.[5] One of the earliest descriptive radiological series was derived from this clinical material.[6]

The clinical course of AIDS-related KS is highly variable, ranging from minimal, non-progressive disease to a course characterized by explosive growth. Ninety-five percent of patients with KS will display cutaneous lesions.[7] After the skin, the most frequently involved organs by KS are lymph nodes and the gastro-intestinal tract, including oral cavity, and the lungs.[8–10] The tumour is derived from lymphatic endothelia and is associated with gastro-intestinal luminal lesions in at least 40% of patients. Its presence generally does not alter overall survival in AIDS.[11] The most frequently involved sites in decreasing frequency are the small intestine, stomach and colon. Early stages of KS in the gastro-intestinal tract are not as easily recognized as they are in the skin or lymph nodes.[8]

The overall incidence of NHL continues to increase in the UK and in the USA (see Chapter 32). The incidence of NHL is greatly increased in HIV-infected individuals; the vast majority being clinically aggressive B cell-derived neoplasms (similar to Burkitt's lymphoma). Approximately 80% arise systemically (nodal and/or extranodal), and the remaining 20% arise as primary central nervous system (CNS) lymphomas. Extranodal sites of involvement include:[12]

- Gastro-intestinal tract (54%)
- Liver (29%)
- Kidney (11%)
- Adrenal gland (11%)
- Lower genito-urinary tract (11%)
- Spleen (7%)
- Peritoneum and omentum (7%)
- Pancreas (5%)
- Epidural space (4%)
- Bone (3%)
- Muscle (10%)

The gastro-intestinal tract is a common site of involvement in AIDS-related lymphoma (ARL). The most common presentations of gastro-intestinal NHL are:

- Abdominal pain (77%)
- Abdominal tenderness (77%)
- Weight loss (77%)
- Gastro-intestinal bleeding (38%)

The most common sites of gastro-intestinal involvement are:[13]

- The large bowel (46%)
- Ileum (39%)
- Stomach (23%)

Gastro-intestinal lymphomas are usually symptomatic and require treatment, unless the patient's overall state of debilitation precludes therapeutic intervention. Clinical symptoms include change in bowel habits, rectal bleeding, unremitting weight loss, abdominal pain, abdominal tenderness, peripheral lymphadenopathy, cachexia and hepatosplenomegaly. Obstruction, perforation and bleeding may occur in patients with luminal involvement, whereas hepatic or biliary disease may lead to jaundice. There is a strong correlation with the presence of significant symptomatology and the presence of definable lesions in patients with gastro-intestinal ARL.[11,14]

Radiological imaging of the abdomen – an overview

The AIDS patient is most frequently referred for imaging to evaluate an acute change in symptomatology. Because the case definition of AIDS is partially dependent on the clinical diseases afflicting the patient, the underlying disease(s) will be known at the time of imaging.[1,15] Therefore, the role of the imaging study is more accurately characterized as localization (for biopsy) and pattern (suggestive of diagnosis).

In Western countries, computed tomography (CT) is the most widely used imaging technique for a global overview of the entire abdomen and pelvis, facilitating the recognition of the distribution and patterns and segregating the multiple diseases often present in these individuals.[16–18] Radin analysed the computed tomography scans with abnormal findings in 259 patients with HIV infection which revealed the following findings: mycobacterial infection ($n=87$), lymphoproliferative disease ($n=63$), KS ($n=17$), fungal infection ($n=17$), hepatocellular disease ($n=13$), *Pneumocystis carinii* infection ($n=8$), other disorders ($n=39$), or unknown ($n=30$). Abnormal findings included lymph node enlargement ($n=159$), hepatomegaly ($n=100$), splenomegaly ($n=62$), luminal mass or wall thickening ($n=61$) and low attenuation lesions in the liver ($n=50$) or spleen ($n=55$). Diagnoses thought to account for CT findings were made in 247 (95%) of the 259 patients. In another more recent study comprised of 339 HIV-positive patients, 278 (82%) showed abnormal abdominal findings on CT. Median survival was 29 months. Splenomegaly ($n=147$), hepatomegaly ($n=144$) and lymphadenopathy ($n=111$) were the most common abdominal findings on CT but lacked prognostic relevance. Main determinants of survival were a low CD4(+)-T lymphocyte count, the presence of the hepatic masses, pathologic lymphadenopathy and ascites.[19]

Ultrasound is most commonly used when CT is not available. Ultrasound, in countries such as Sub-Saharan Africa, may represent the extent of imaging resources. In a series of 414 patients undergoing 684 ultrasound studies, abnormalities were detected in 264 of the 399 studies available for review. Abnormalities include splenomegaly ($n=124$), lymphadenopathy >3 cm ($n=83$), gallbladder/bile duct abnormalities ($n=80$), hepatomegaly ($n=77$), and ascites ($n=54$). Clinical indications with the highest frequency of abnormal findings included hepatosplenomegaly ($n=337$) and abnormal liver function tests ($n=270$).[20] Abdominal pain, fever of unknown origin, hepatosplenomegaly, lymphadenopathy and abnormal liver function tests were the most frequent clinical indications for imaging in an audit of ultrasound utilization in 900 HIV-positive patients in Central Africa. The AIDS group of patients had a significantly higher proportion of splenomegaly, hepatomegaly, lymphadenopathy, biliary tract abnormalities, gut wall thickening and ascites than those who were HIV-positive. There were no differences in renal or pancreatic abnormalities.[21]

Barium radiography is reserved for patients with symptoms directly related to the gastro-intestinal tract and oesophagus.[22] Double-contrast barium oesophagography is sensitive and specific for Candida infections and identification of patterns of ulceration suggesting viral oesophagitis.

Magnetic resonance is useful for patients with potential allergy to intravenous (IV) contrast. For neoplastic abdominal diseases in AIDS patients, MR offers little value over

CT. There is no significant large-scale reported experience with 2-[F-18]fluoro-2-deoxy-D-glucose positron emission tomography ([18]FDG PET) scanning in these individuals.

Careful examination technique is critical to successful detection and characterization of abdominal AIDS pathology. All CT scans should be performed with sufficient oral contrast to uniformly distend and outline the entire small bowel. Intravenous contrast, administered with a power injector, is critical for the detection of solid-organ pathology and characterization of lymph nodes. Barium studies will be requested for the evaluation of intestinal mucosa. In this regard, double-contrast techniques are mandatory. While there may be some increase in the detection of small bowel pathology with enteroclysis techniques, these patients are generally too debilitated to justify naso-duodenal intubation.

Kaposi's sarcoma

Alimentary tract

In AIDS patients, KS rarely presents in the gastro-intestinal tract without cutaneous manifestations. Kaposi's sarcoma is associated with luminal lesions in at least 40% of patients. Gastro-intestinal EKS is usually asymptomatic but may bleed, obstruct or become the lead point of an intussusception.[11,23] Intestinal perforation may rarely occur.[24]

Kaposi's sarcoma is recognized by the presence of nodules of varying size. Careful fluoroscopic evaluation will show these lesions to arise within the submucosa of the alimentary canal. As opposed to classic KS, few of the nodules display the so-called 'bull's eye' appearance. In advanced disease, the nodules coalesce and present as infiltrating lesions, which can cause contour abnormalities simulating varices. The lesions are best visualized with double-contrast radiography.

The differential diagnosis is generally not problematic. Multiple submucosal lesions may be seen in a variety of metastatic tumours to the gut wall, but these are not likely in the AIDS patient. Infiltration commonly occurs in the stomach and the appearance can simulate advanced gastric lymphoma. The endoscopic appearance is characteristic.

Liver and spleen

Kaposi's sarcoma affects the liver in approximately one third of patients with cutaneous disease.[7] The lesions are rarely visualized at CT. Sporadic reports have appeared characterizing the lesions as low attenuation masses against a background of enhanced hepatic parenchyma. They have been reported to present in close association with portal vein branches. Imaging rarely demonstrates EKS in the spleen. Because of the relatively minor importance of EKS splenic involvement, establishing its presence is rarely pursued.

Several types of lesions can produce small lucencies within the liver in the AIDS patient. Most common differ-

ential considerations include microabscesses,[25] mycobacterial disease[26] and bacillary angiomatosis.[27]

Lymph nodes

Lymphadenopathy is the most frequent abnormality encountered in KS. Differential diagnosis of the cause of adenopathy is critical because it may be caused by treatable disease. Kaposi's sarcoma has a distinctive appearance on CT scans on which the lymph nodes show bright enhancement after IV contrast medium (Fig. 59.1). This can be ascribed to vascular hyperplasia within the lymph nodes displaying interweaving fascicles of spindle cells, extravasated red blood cells, vascular slits and deposition of haemosiderin.[8] The positive predictive value of hyperattenuating adenopathy for EKS was shown recently to be 79%; findings statistically significant at the 95% confidence interval.[28] The distribution of adenopathy is not specific. Most cases we have seen involve retroperitoneal and pelvic lymph nodes. There is a high frequency of inguinal and femoral node involvement, relating to lymphatic drainage from the lower extremities. In many patients, CT will show characteristic 'streaky' soft tissue attenuation and infiltration in the inguinal fat. This results in obscuration of the borders of the femoral vessels and nodes (Fig. 59.2). It should be noted that there is an association of Castleman's disease and EKS. Because the lymphadenopathy seen in Castleman's disease brightly enhances following contrast administration, it can be confused with KS.[29]

Other sites

Pancreatic involvement in AIDS occurs in 90% of patients. However, it is usually asymptomatic.[30] Most pancreatic disease is non-neoplastic in origin. Kaposi's sarcoma can produce a tumorous infiltration of the pancreatic head, which can be confused with pancreatic ductal adenocarcinoma. Diagnosis may be made by identification of human herpesvirus Type 8 (HHV-8) in pancreatic juice or bile, and

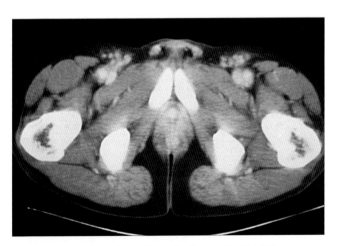

Figure 59.1. *KS: enhanced lymphadenopathy. Brightly enhanced inguinal adenopathy, isodense with pelvic vessels.*

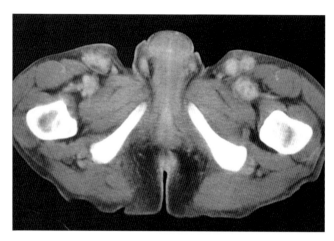

Figure 59.2. *KS: infiltrative changes in inguinal fat. Inguinal and femoral adenopathy, isodense with pelvic vessels. Note the streaky increased density in the inguinal fat. This finding is typical of KS and may persist in the absence of adenopathy.*

successful clinical outcome is possible by intensive antiviral and cytostatic treatment.[31]

Key points: Kaposi's sarcoma (KS)

■ Gastro-intestinal KS is seldom present without skin KS

■ KS of the gastro-intestinal tract usually manifests as nodules

■ Liver and spleen involvement is rarely demonstrated on imaging

■ Lymph nodes infiltrated with KS typically show intense enhancement following IV contrast medium injection

■ There is an association between Castleman's disease and EKS

■ Although most pancreatic disease in patients with AIDS is non-neoplastic, EKS can infiltrate the pancreatic head

AIDS-related lymphoma

Alimentary tract

There is a wide spectrum of radiological abnormalities seen in the gastro-intestinal tract in patients with ARL. In a large review of CT findings in patients with ARL, the gastro-intestinal tract was shown to be the most common site of the disease.[12] Of interest are the almost mirror-like sites of involvement compared to non-AIDS gastro-intestinal lymphoma (see Chapter 32). In ARL, distal involvement is common, with the stomach being least frequently affected.

In large urban practice settings, over half of patients

with intestinal lymphoma will actually prove to have AIDS.[32] One will usually see an obvious thickening of the wall of the affected segment of bowel (Fig. 59.3). Ulceration may occur. Correlation with barium radiological patterns suggests that mural infiltration and irregular fold thickening are the most common manifestations. AIDS-related lymphoma rarely results in mucosal infiltration (as seen in 'Mediterranean lymphomas'), the endo-exoenteric forms, or in so-called aneurysmal dilatation typically seen in non-AIDS patients.[33] AIDS-related lymphoma is more frequently associated with concurrent solid-organ involvement as opposed to non-ARL.[32] Conversely, the presence of lymphadenopathy is unusual.

Even though there are no 'typical' appearances to gastro-intestinal lymphomas, the lesions are often large or extensive at presentation. Computed tomography alone can detect the disease and it is rarely necessary to use barium radiography or endoscopy (Fig. 59.4). Barium is used to validate equivocal findings. Barium studies are cost-

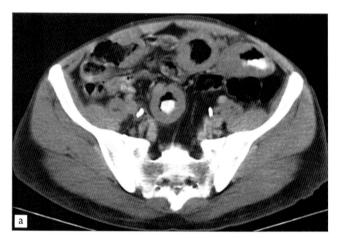

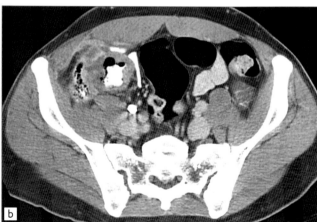

Figure 59.3. *ARL: small bowel. (a and b) Images from CT studies in two different patients reveal focal, variable, segmental, soft tissue attenuating wall thickening indicative of enteric ARL. No barium correlation is necessary to establish the aetiology. Note the lack of peritumoural adenopathy frequently accompanying similar lesions in non-ARL cases.*

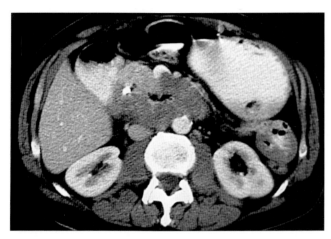

Figure 59.4. *ARL: duodenum. The patient had presented with obstructive jaundice. On the contrast-enhanced CT scan a bulky low attenuation mass surrounds the irregular, ulcerated duodenal lumen. The mass invades the superior mesenteric vein. Notice the discretely defined borders of the enhanced pancreatic parenchyma.*

effective because, when present, the disease is usually obvious. If CT reveals a finding which is subtle or equivocal, it is usually due to unfilled or undistended bowel loops.

Bulky perirectal lymphomas are virtually unique in ARL. Huge central pelvic masses massively thicken the rectal wall, and displace the lower pelvic viscera (Fig. 59.5).[34]

In our experience, these patients are often seen by their physician complaining of tenesmus or other related symptomatology, suggesting a perianal or perirectal abscess. An apparent fluctuant mass may be palpated. When aspiration fails to reveal pus, the patient is referred for imaging localization and the entire extent of the lesion becomes immediately apparent.

Liver and spleen

The liver is the second most frequent abdominal site of radiologically detectable ARL. Focal splenic and hepatic involvement is more common in both AIDS-related Hodgkin's disease (10%) and ARL (26%) than reported in the non-AIDS population.[35] Moderate or marked hepatomegaly (cephalocaudal span >20 cm) and splenomegaly (cephalocaudal span >15 cm) is unusual without demonstrable focal masses. Most hepatic involvement is seen in association with multicentric, extranodal disseminated disease. However, primary hepatic lymphoma has been reported.[36]

Focal liver lesions in ARL present as well-defined round masses which in our experience range from 1 to 3 cm in size. We have not seen conglomerate solitary masses. The periphery of the lesion is not sharply circumscribed as in 'typical' metastatic disease. The lesions almost always display a uniform attenuation value slightly less than that of enhanced hepatic parenchyma. Their detection requires contrast-enhanced CT performed during peak hepatic enhancement (Fig. 59.6). In approximately 10% of cases, the lesions will have varying amounts of central low attenuation, presumably necrosis. On unenhanced and contrast-enhanced CT, the lesions were hypodense in all cases; a thin enhancing rim can be identified in scattered cases. The presence of this feature does not correlate with the size of the lesions. On sonography, the masses are deceptively hypoechoic (typical of lymphomatous lesions elsewhere), but display poor through-transmission. AIDS-related lymphoma is most frequently multiple within the liver. On MR, the lesions appear hypointense on T1-weighted images and hyperintense on T2-weighted images.[37]

Splenic lesions are large (>1.5 cm) masses with a homogeneous attenuation similar to the liver lesions. This is the only radiologically detectable form of the disease. Unlike

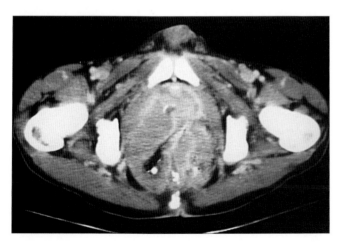

Figure 59.5. *ARL: rectum. This is a typical appearance of ARL involving rectum on CT with lateral spread throughout the pelvis.*

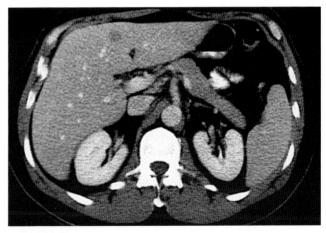

Figure 59.6. *ARL: liver. The lesion seen in the medial segment of the left lobe is typical of hepatic ARL on CT. Note the lack of a discrete border and the minimal contrast against enhanced hepatic parenchyma. Meticulous scanning technique in terms of hepatic enhancement is necessary to detect these findings.*

non-AIDS lymphoma, splenic infiltration and enlargement is uncommon. Splenomegaly as an isolated finding may be indicative of other abnormalities. Diffuse enlargement probably reflects haematopoietic or reticulo-endothelial hyperplastic states as opposed to neoplastic infiltration.

Genito-urinary disease

Renal lymphoma is usually a manifestation of disseminated disease and is often asymptomatic. Occasionally, the kidney(s) may be the major or only demonstrable site of disease, which may then present with a variety of urological symptoms. The imaging studies should be tailored according to the presenting symptoms and prior history. Currently, CT with IV contrast material enhancement is the study of choice for both the evaluation of renal involvement as well as staging of the disease. When necessary, CT or sonography may be used to guide percutaneous needle biopsy of suspicious masses.[38] Most renal disease is seen in the context of multicentric non-nodal involvement. However, primary renal lymphoma has been reported.[39] Multiple bilateral homogeneously attenuating soft tissue masses, similar to lymphomatous renal involvement seen in non-ARL, are visualized (Fig. 59.7). We have not seen renal ARL present as diffuse nephromegaly, a well-documented manifestation in non-ARL (see Chapter 32).

Adrenal enlargement may signal lymphomatous involvement of these structures. The patients do not have clinical or chemical evidence of adrenal malfunction. Function is not compromised during or following systemic treatment.

Although lymphomas may affect any portion of the genito-urinary tract, focal masses along transitional epithelium are rare. Lower genito-urinary involvement, when seen, manifests as sheet-like infiltration of the lower pelvic viscera. The fat planes between the bladder, seminal vesicles and prostate are blurred by the dense soft tissue sheets of infiltrating neoplasm. As the disease is treated, follow-up imaging will show the normal visceral contours emerging from the pelvic infiltration.

Lymph nodes

Although extranodal involvement is the hallmark of ARL, nodal disease does occur. Radin et al. found lymphadenopathy in 41 of 72 patients with ARL and with focal abdominal abnormalities on CT scanning.[12] However, these authors did not establish that *all* of the adenopathy was due to lymphoma. In our experience, one must be wary of assuming that adenopathy in patients with extranodal abdominal ARL is due to lymphoma. When confronted with this finding, we recommend biopsy of an accessible node to confirm that the patient is not harbouring a second disease (most frequently mycobacterial). Gallium scanning is also useful in identifying the nodes as lymphomatous. Conversely, if clinical symptomatology and laboratory data do not support infection, one could treat the lymphoma and monitor nodal response. A more complete discussion of lymphadenopathy is presented in the previous section on KS.

Other sites

AIDS-related lymphoma may present within the peritoneal cavity (Fig. 59.8). The features are identical to any metastatic lesion within the peritoneal cavity including omental caking.[40] Peritoneal lymphomatosis may be seen in non-AIDS lymphomas as well. Peritoneal lymphomas are a rare subtype of AIDS-associated NHL, occurring with less severe immune deficiency than for other NHLs. The increased frequency among persons with prior KS suggests a common aetiology, presumably infection with KS-associated herpes virus, as found in primary effusion lymphoma.[41]

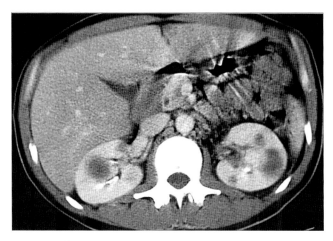

Figure 59.7. *ARL: kidneys. There are bilateral homogeneous soft tissue masses in the kidneys. This is virtually pathognomonic of lymphoma. The appearances of ARL are identical to non-ARL.*

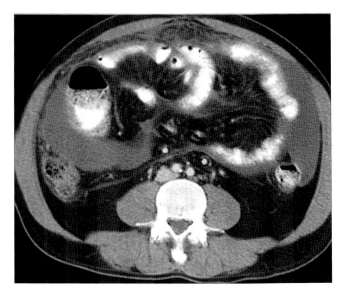

Figure 59.8. *ARL: peritoneal cavity. CT scan showing changes typical of peritoneal carcinomatosis with loculated ascites and omental caking are seen. Bowel appears normal. There is no adenopathy.*

Non-Hodgkin's lymphoma may involve the pancreas presenting as a focal mass which may obstruct the common bile duct.[30]

Key points: AIDS-related lymphoma

- The gastro-intestinal tract is the most common site of involvement; the sites of involvement are unlike those in non-AIDS gastro-intestinal lymphoma

- The appearances are non-specific; distal gastro-intestinal tract involvement is common and the disease is usually bulky

- Bulky perirectal lymphoma is almost unique to AIDS

- Focal liver and spleen abnormalities are common in ARL and usually range in size from 1 to 3 cm

- Renal ARL is most commonly manifest as multiple masses

- Even in visceral involvement by ARL, lymphadenopathy may be due to other causes

- Peritoneal lymphomas are a rare subtype of ARL and occur with increased frequency in patients with a history of EKS

Complications of therapy

Patient survival has been significantly improved in recent years with advent of new classes of antiretroviral agents and protease inhibitors. While these therapies can have a multitude of side-effects common to all patients receiving chemotherapy, two specific effects deserve special mention: development of renal calculi and AIDS-related lipodystrophy.

Renal calculi

Patients treated with protease inhibitors such as indinavir sulphate form radiolucent calculi. Crystallization and stone formation are demonstrated in as many as 20% of patients taking the medication. This can result in renal colic requiring hospitalization. Patients present with nausea or vomiting and haematuria. Imaging studies confirmed obstruction in all patients with radiolucent (indinavir) and/or radio-opaque stones due to the presence of calcium oxalate. Indinavir calculi are radiolucent on CT scanning. The diagnosis is suspected when there is evidence of hydronephrosis and perinephric stranding.[42,43]

Changes in fat distribution

Marked abnormalities of fat distribution have been reported in HIV patients undergoing antiviral therapies. Reported changes include: abdominal fat accumulation, breast enlargement, thick necks, buffalo humps, multiple lipomatous growths, cushingoid features, centralized fat redistribution and mesenteric, omental, and retroperitoneal fat accumulation. Some subjects switched or stopped their antiretroviral therapy, others underwent surgery to remove the fat and many considered their symptoms disabling.[44]

One of the more disconcerting side-effects of effective viral control therapy relates to a significant redistribution of body fat. The general term, 'lipoatrophy syndrome; is applied to these disorders. Extreme depletion of facial fat and accumulation of abdominal fat occurs. The morphologic changes add to the patient's self-consciousness. CT scanning is employed to evaluate fat redistribution so that appropriate dietary measures can be instituted.[45] The distribution of these changes is particularly offensive to patients in that the thinning of the extremities and increase in girth may break treasured anonymity. These patients are, furthermore, at risk for complications of obesity including diabetes, premature heart disease and pancreatitis. While several aetiologic factors have implicated, an increased association with the use of highly active retroviral therapy (HAART) with agents such as stavudine and indinavir is recognized.[46]

Computed tomography scanning in these patients reveals extensive accumulation of intra-abdominal fat with little subcutaneous fat.[47] Because increased loss of bone density occurs, follow-up studies using bone densitometry are also employed.

Liver fat content may be a more sensitive and specific predictor of insulin resistance than subcutaneous or intra-abdominal fat. Liver fat content can be measured with proton spectroscopic MR.[48]

Key points: complications of therapy

- New antiretroviral drugs are associated with renal calculi and AIDS-related lipodystrophy

- 20% of patients on some drugs develop renal calculi which may be radiolucent

- Marked changes in fat distribution can occur with the use of HAART, including abdominal fat accumulation and subcutaneous atrophy

Summary and differential diagnosis

The major differential diagnoses confronting the clinician caring for the patient with AIDS is between infectious or neoplastic disease. Based on imaging findings alone, differentiation is frequently impossible, and often imaging serves as a guide for needle aspirations or tissue biopsies. There are several 'rules' which may direct the investigation:

■ Most visceral masses greater than 1 cm are due to ARL

■ Liver lesions such as tuberculosis, micro-abscesses, bacillary angiomatosis, etc. produce lesions in the 0.3–10 mm range

■ Involvement of solid organs with these entities will produce a myriad of lesions, whereas lymphomas produce only few

■ Organ enlargement is not typical of ARL

■ Lymphadenopathy is rare in ARL in marked contradistinction to non-ARL. Lymphadenopathy is common in mycobacterial diseases and in KS. In the latter entity, one may see high attenuation in the nodes in approximately 80% of cases

■ Kaposi's sarcoma rarely produces significant masses in the gastro-intestinal tract

■ Liver and spleen involvement are well established at autopsy, but rarely produce disease recognizable by current imaging methods

■ Virtually all patients suspected of KS lesions by imaging will have cutaneous manifestations of the disease

■ Although the hallmark of gastro-intestinal pathology on CT scanning is mural thickening, non-neoplastic disease can be separated from neoplastic abnormalities by visualization of oedema in the bowel wall; its visibility is enhanced by IV contrast administration

■ The radiologist must be aware that, more often than not, multiple diseases will be present in the same individual

■ New antiviral drugs are associated with renal calculus and lipodystrophy

References

1. Gore R M, Miller F H, Yaghmai V. Acquired immunodeficiency syndrome (AIDS) of the abdominal organs: imaging features. Semin Ultrasound CT MR. 1998; 19: 175–189

2. Chui D W, Owen R L. AIDS and the gut. J Gastroenterol Hepatol 1994; 9: 291–303

3. Biggar R J, Rabkin C S. The epidemiology of AIDS-related neoplasms. Hematol Oncol Clin North Am 1996; 10: 997–1010

4. Rabkin C S. Epidemiology of AIDS-related malignancies. Curr Opin Oncol 1994; 6: 492–496

5. Friedman-Kien A E. Disseminated Kaposi's sarcoma syndrome in young homosexual men. J Am Acad Dermatol 1981; 5: 468–471

6. Rose H S, Balthazar E J, Megibow A J et al. Alimentary tract involvement in Kaposi sarcoma: radiographic and endoscopic findings in 25 homosexual men. Am J Roentgenol. 1982; 139: 661–666

7. Federle M P, Nyberg D A, Hulnick D H, Jeffrey R Jr (eds). Malignant Neoplasms: Kaposi's Sarcoma, Lymphoma, and Other Diseases with Similar Radiographic Features. New York: Raven, 1988

8. Amazon K, Rywlin A M (eds). Systemic Manifestations of Kaposi's Sarcoma. Philadelphia: Lea & Febiger, 1988

9. Dezube B J. Acquired immunodeficiency syndrome-related Kaposi's sarcoma: clinical features, staging, and treatment. Semin Oncol 2000; 27: 424–430

10. Dezube B J. Clinical presentation and natural history of AIDS-related Kaposi's sarcoma. Hematol Oncol Clin North Am 1996; 10: 1023–1029

11. Friedman S L. Kaposi's sarcoma and lymphoma of the gut in AIDS. Baillieres Clin Gastroenterol 1990; 4: 455–475

12. Radin D R, Esplin J A, Levine A M, Ralls P W. AIDS-related non-Hodgkin's lymphoma: abdominal CT findings in 112 patients. Am J Roentgenol 1993; 160: 1133–1139

13. Knowles D M. Etiology and pathogenesis of AIDS-related non-Hodgkin's lymphoma. Hematol Oncol Clin North Am 1996; 10: 1081–1091

14. Cappell M S, Botros N. Predominantly gastrointestinal symptoms and signs in 11 consecutive AIDS patients with gastrointestinal lymphoma: a multicenter, multiyear study including 763 HIV-seropositive patients. Am J Gastroenterol 1994; 89: 545–549

15. Pantongrag-Brown L, Nelson A M, Brown A E et al. Gastrointestinal manifestations of acquired immunodeficiency syndrome: radiologic–pathologic correlation. Radiographics 1995; 15: 1155–1178

16. Jeffrey R Jr. Abdominal imaging in the immunocompromised patient. Radiol Clin North Am 1992; 30: 579–596

17. Megibow A J, Wall S D, Balthazar E J, Rybak B J (eds). Gastrointestinal Radiology in AIDS Patients. New York: Raven, 1988

18. Radin R. HIV infection: analysis in 259 consecutive patients with abnormal abdominal CT findings. Radiology 1995; 197: 712–722

19. Knollmann F D, Maurer J, Grunewald T et al. Abdominal CT features and survival in acquired immunodeficiency. Acta Radiol 1997; 38: 970–977

20. Smith F J, Mathieson J R, Cooperberg P L. Abdominal abnormalities in AIDS: detection at US in a large population. Radiology 1994; 192: 691–695

21. Tshibwabwa E T, Mwaba P, Bogle-Taylor J, Zumla A. Four-year study of abdominal ultrasound in 900 Central African adults with AIDS referred for diagnostic imaging. Abdom Imaging 2000; 25: 290–296

22. Wall S D. Gastrointestinal imaging in AIDS: luminal gastrointestinal tract. Gastroenterol Clin North Am 1988; 17: 523–533

23. Chalasani N, Wilcox C M. Gastrointestinal hemorrhage in patients with AIDS. AIDS Patient Care STDS 1999; 13: 343–346

24. Yoshida E M, Chan N, Chanyan C, Baird R M. Perforation of the jejunum secondary to AIDS-related gastrointestinal Kaposi's sarcoma. Can J Gastroenterol 1997; 11: 38–40

25. Murray J G, Patel M D, Lee S et al. Microabscesses of the liver and spleen in AIDS: detection with 5-MHz sonography. Radiology 1995; 197: 723–727

26. Schneiderman D J. Hepatobiliary abnormalities of AIDS. Gastroenterol Clin North Am 1988; 17: 615–630

27. Mohle-Boetani J C, Koehler J E, Berger T G et al. Bacillary angiomatosis and bacillary peliosis in patients infected with human immunodeficiency virus: clinical characteristics in a case–control study. Clin Infect Dis 1996; 22: 794–800

28. Herts B R, Megibow A J, Birnbaum B A et al. High-attenuation lymphadenopathy in AIDS patients: significance of findings at CT. Radiology 1992; 185: 777–781

29. Saif M W. Castleman disease in an HIV-infected patient with Kaposi's sarcoma. AIDS Read 2001; 11: 572–576

30. Chehter E Z, Longo M A, Laudanna A A, Duarte M I. Involvement of the pancreas in AIDS: a prospective study of 109 post-mortems. AIDS 2000; 14: 1879–1886

31. Menges M, Pees H W. Kaposi's sarcoma of the pancreas mimicking pancreatic cancer in an HIV-infected patient. Clinical diagnosis by detection of HHV 8 in bile and complete remission following antiviral and cytostatic therapy with paclitaxel. Int J Pancreatol 1999; 26: 193–199

32. Balthazar E J, Noordhoorn M, Megibow A J, Gordon R B. CT of small-bowel lymphoma in immunocompetent patients and patients with AIDS: comparison of findings. Am J Roentgenol 1997; 168: 675–680

33. Levine M S, Rubesin S E, Pantongrag-Brown L et al. Non-Hodgkin's lymphoma of the gastrointestinal tract: radiographic findings. Am J Roentgenol 1997; 168: 165–172

34. Ioachim H L, Weinstein M A, Robbins R D et al. Primary anorectal lymphoma. A new manifestation of the acquired immune deficiency syndrome (AIDS). Cancer 1987; 60: 1449–1453

35. Nyberg D A, Jeffrey R Jr, Federle M P et al. AIDS-related lymphomas: evaluation by abdominal CT. Radiology 1986; 159: 59–63

36. Scerpella E G, Villareal A A, Casanova P F, Moreno J N. Primary lymphoma of the liver in AIDS. Report of one new case and review of the literature. J Clin Gastroenterol 1996; 22: 51–53

37. Rizzi E B, Schinina V, Cristofaro M et al. Non-Hodgkin's lymphoma of the liver in patients with AIDS: sonographic, CT, and MRI findings. J Clin Ultrasound 2001; 29: 125–129

38. Eisenberg P J, Papanicolaou N, Lee M J, Yoder I C. Diagnostic imaging in the evaluation of renal lymphoma. Leuk Lymphoma 1994; 16: 37–50

39. Tsang K, Kneafsey P, Gill M J. Primary lymphoma of the kidney in the acquired immunodeficiency syndrome [see comments]. Arch Pathol Lab Med 1993; 117: 541–543

40. Maya M M, Fried K, Gendal E S. AIDS-related lymphoma: an unusual cause of omental caking [letter]. Am J Roentgenol 1993; 160: 661

41. Mbulaiteye S M, Biggar R J, Goedert J J, Engels E A. Pleural and peritoneal lymphoma among people with AIDS in the United States. J Acquir Immune Defic Syndr 2002; 29: 418–421

42. Kohan A D, Armenakas N A, Fracchia J A. Indinavir urolithiasis: an emerging cause of renal colic in patients with human immunodeficiency virus. J Urol 1999; 161: 1765–1768

43. Schwartz B F, Schenkman N, Armenakas N A, Stoller M L. Imaging characteristics of indinavir calculi. J Urol 1999; 161: 1085–1087

44. Mann M, Piazza-Hepp T, Koller E et al. Unusual distributions of body fat in AIDS patients: a review of adverse events reported to the Food and Drug Administration. AIDS Patient Care STDS 1999; 13: 287–295

45. Saint-Marc T, Partisani M, Poizot-Martin I et al. Fat distribution evaluated by computed tomography and metabolic abnormalities in patients undergoing antiretroviral therapy: preliminary results of the LIPOCO study. AIDS 2000; 14: 37–49

46. Lichtenstein K A, Ward D J, Moorman A C et al. Clinical assessment of HIV-associated lipodystrophy in an ambulatory population. AIDS 2001; 15: 1389–1398

47. Gellett L R, Haddon L, Maskell G F. CT appearances of HIV-related lipodystrophy syndrome. Br J Radiol 2001; 74: 382–383

48. Sutinen J, Hakkinen A M, Westerbacka J et al. Increased fat accumulation in the liver in HIV-infected patients with antiretroviral therapy-associated lipodystrophy. AIDS 2002; 16: 2183–2193

Part IX

NEW HORIZONS IN IMAGING

Chapter 60

Magnetic resonance lymphography

Willem Deserno, Mukesh Harisinghani and Jelle Barentsz

Introduction

Lymph node metastases have a significant impact on the prognosis of patients with pelvic malignancies. In prostate cancer, for example, even micro-metastases in a single node may exclude surgical cure by the available treatment protocols and in bladder cancer, more than five lymph node metastases or extracapsular growth preclude curative surgical treatment.[1] Thus, the status of the lymph nodes largely dictates the management of the primary tumour.

Cross-sectional imaging modalities lack the desired sensitivity for identifying metastases as they largely rely on size criteria, and small metastases in normal-sized nodes can be missed. Surgical open pelvic lymph node dissection (PLND), considered to be the only reliable method of assessing lymph node status, is an invasive procedure associated with potential complications and side-effects. In addition, in prostate cancer it may have no therapeutic value. Laparoscopic PLND, although less invasive, is time-consuming, expensive, involves, hospitalization and also requires a long prolonged learning curve for the surgeon.[2] For prostate cancer, therefore, there is great pressure to identify those patients with a low risk of pelvic node metastases in whom a PLND would be of little value and hence could be avoided. Recently, it has been shown, that in patients with prostate-specific antigen (PSA) <10 ng/ml, Gleason score <7 and Stage II disease on digital examination, the risk of lymph node metastases is less than 1%. Therefore, node dissections and non-invasive imaging can be avoided in this group.[3] Nevertheless, in the remaining patients, approximately 56% of the population with prostate cancer, lymph node dissection still has to be performed, as both computed tomography (CT) and magnetic resonance (MR) imaging have limited sensitivity.[4] In bladder cancer, radiological cross-sectional staging techniques, combined with cystoscopic histologic biopsy to assess local stage and grade, can make a moderately accurate prediction of the presence of lymph node metastasis. However, information obtained in this way does not provide any information regarding the number and extent of nodal metastases.

Imaging methods

A non-invasive, reliable method for detecting and staging nodal metastasis would reduce unnecessary surgery. Currently, there are four imaging techniques for nodal staging: CT, MR, 2-[F-18]fluoro-2-deoxy-D-glucose positron emission tomography ([18]FDG PET) and MR imaging after injection of ultrasmall superparamagnetic iron oxide particles (USPIO-MR).

Computed tomography and magnetic resonance imaging

CT and MR imaging do not have adequate sensitivity or specificity for the reliable detection of lymph node metastases in pelvic cancer; for example, in prostate cancer reports in the literature indicate that the sensitivity for both techniques is in the region of 36%.[4] The reason for this low sensitivity is the use of size as the only criterion to distinguish benign from malignant lymph nodes on both CT and MR. A threshold for the upper limit of normal for a pelvic node is generally regarded as 10 mm for an oval node and 8 mm for a round node.[5] Contrast enhancement with CT and MR is not helpful for characterizing enlarged nodes as both benign and malignant nodes may enhance.[6] Magnetic resonance signal intensity differences between benign and malignant nodes are also unreliable.

Thus, in routine clinical practice, staging PLND remains the only reliable method of assessing lymph node status in prostate and bladder cancer and the technique continues to have an important place in the management protocol.

[18]FDG PET

Although very promising in detecting nodal metastases in lung cancer, the role of [18]FDG PET scanning is limited in the detection of nodal involvement in urological cancers. This is partly because [18]FDG is excreted through the urinary tract[7] and partly because [18]FDG uptake is relatively low in metastatic nodes in bladder and prostate cancer. Although the sensitivity of [18]FDG PET is slightly better (67%) than CT and unenhanced MR imaging,[8,9] this improvement in sensitivity is not sufficient for the technique to replace PLND.

Key points: standard imaging techniques

■ Cross-sectional imaging techniques are unreliable for detecting nodal metastases in pelvic cancers

■ Intravenous (IV) contrast medium cannot be used to distinguish benign from malignant nodes on MR and CT

■ [18]FDG PET is more sensitive than CT or MR for detecting involved nodes in prostate and bladder cancer but cannot replace PLND

■ PLND remains the preferred technique for diagnosis of nodal involvement in pelvic cancers

USPIO-MR imaging

USPIO particles with a long plasma circulation time have been shown to be suitable as a MR contrast agent for IV MR lymphangiography.[10,11] After IV injection, the USPIO particles are taken up by macrophages and transported to the interstitial space and from there through the lymph vessels to the lymph nodes (Fig. 60.1). Once within normally functioning nodes, these particles reduce the signal intensity of normal nodal tissue as a result of the T1 and T2* susceptibility effect of iron oxide, thus producing a signal intensity drop or *negative* enhancement. In areas of lymph nodes containing malignant cells, macrophages are replaced by cancer cells and therefore in these areas there is no uptake of the USPIO particles. In addition, due to increased vascular permeability in cancer tissue, there is leakage of USPIO particles into the malignant metastatic areas, which produces a low local concentration and non-clustering of USPIO particles at these sites.[12] Through their T1-relaxivity this can induce an increase in signal intensity on T1-weighted images, producing *positive* enhancement.[13–15] Thus the ability of post-USPIO-MR imaging to identify metastatic areas in lymph nodes depends primarily on the degree of uptake of USPIO by the macrophages in normal lymph node tissue and the leakage of USPIO particles into the metastatic environment. Twenty-four hours after IV injection of USPIO, normal lymph nodes and malignant tissue have different signal intensity on MR imaging and therefore this non-invasive technique may permit the detection of metastatic deposits in normal-sized nodes (Figs. 60.1 and 60.2).[13]

Magnetic resonance lymphography-USPIO

Imaging technique

Essential imaging sequences required for USPIO-enhanced MR include two- or three-dimensional gradient-echo (GRE) T1-weighted, two-dimensional axial T2-weighted fast or turbo spin-echo (f/tSE) and two-dimensional axial GRE T2*-weighted sequences which should be performed before and 24 hours after the administration of USPIO. Although the default plane for imaging is generally considered to be the axial plane, a plane parallel to the psoas mus-

cle – the 'obturator' plane – provides essential information (Fig. 60.3). This plane allows visualization of lymph nodes along the vessels, which results in better distinction between nodes and vessels and is optimal for separating different lymph node chains and regions (Fig. 60.4). In addition, the first area in which the nodes are removed at PLND, the so-called 'obturator' region, can be well depicted in this 'obturator' plane.

A three-dimensional T1-weighted GRE sequence may also be added for presurgical mapping of nodes. Such a three-dimensional sequence allows determination of nodal locations, nodal shape and size.

T1- and T2-weighted sequences are useful for anatomic localization and node detection. In addition, T1-weighted sequences help to identify hilar fat within the node, which may mimic nodal metastases on T2- and T2*-weighted sequences (Fig. 60.5). High-resolution gradient-echo T2*-weighted sequences are essential for the final evaluation of USPIO uptake, and thus the detection of small metastases.

Key points: USPIO characteristics and imaging technique

■ After IV injection, USPIO particles are taken up by macrophages and transported to the lymph nodes

■ USPIO particles with macrophages reduce the signal intensity of normal nodal tissue due to the T1- and T2* susceptibility effect of iron oxide

■ Malignant cells within a lymph node replace macrophages and therefore malignant foci do not show a signal intensity reduction following injection of USPIO

■ Minimal leakage of USPIO into the malignant area also accounts for lack of signal intensity drop in metastatic foci

■ MR sequences should include GRE T1-weighted, T2-weighted fast or turbo spin-echo and GRE T2*-weighted sequences

■ An imaging plane parallel to the psoas muscle – the 'obturator' plane – provides essential information for detecting and characterizing nodal metastases

Imaging strategies

Timing of postcontrast examination

The optimal time for the post-USPIO-MR examination is 24–36 hours after the injection. This time lag is essential to allow sufficient accumulation of USPIO within the nodes. If imaging is performed prematurely, lack of sufficient nodal uptake in normal nodes may lead to erroneous interpretation as malignant nodes.

It may be considered unnecessary to perform a pre-USPIO-MR examination but if this initial phase of the examination is excluded then it is mandatory to apply addi-

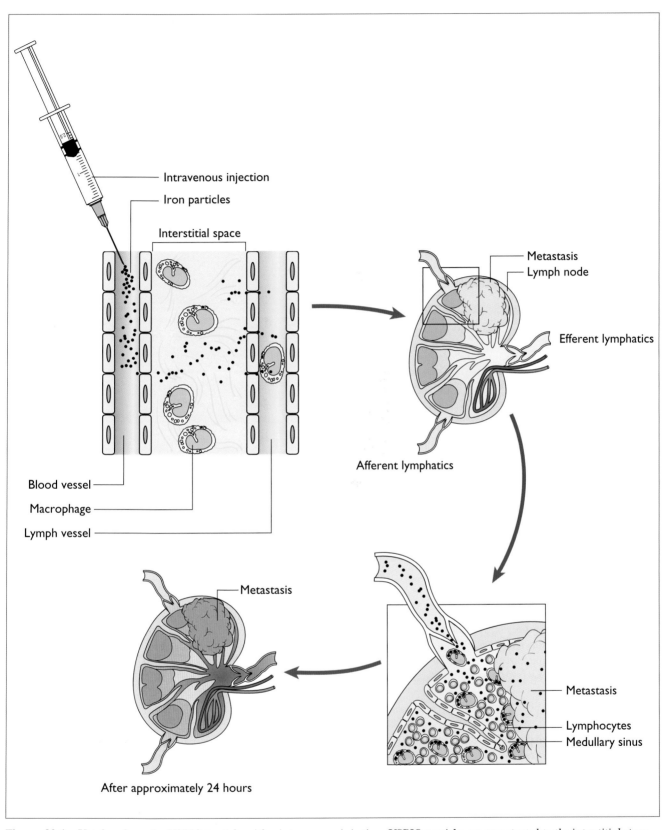

Figure 60.1. *Uptake scheme for USPIO particles. After intravenous injection, USPIO particles are transported to the interstitial space (1) and through lymph vessels into the node (2). There is accumulation of USPIO particles in normal nodal tissue within macrophages (3). Therefore a normal node will have a low signal intensity 24–36 hours after contrast injection, whereas metastases will have unchanged or slightly higher signal intensity (4). Thus normal and metastatic nodes can be differentiated (see also Fig. 60.2).*

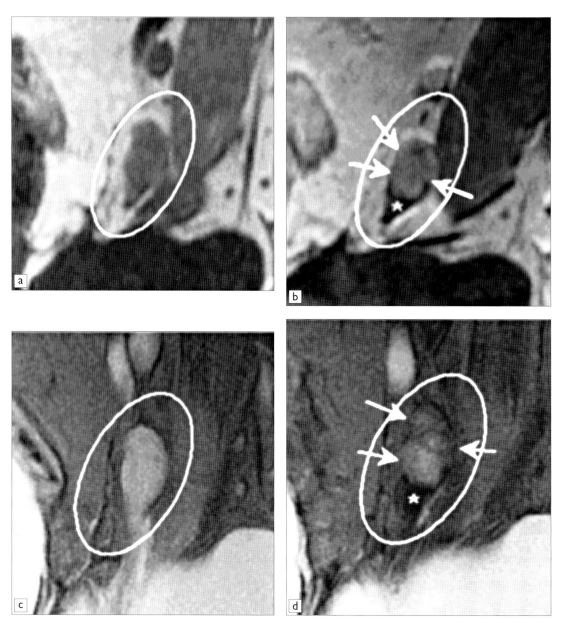

Figure 60.2. *Signal intensities of a partially involved metastatic node (11 × 18 mm). (a) Pre-USPIO T1-weighted image. Both normal and metastatic nodal tissue have homogeneous intermediate signal intensity (SI). (b) Identical post-USPIO image. The metastatic area has higher SI (arrows) and normal nodal tissue lower SI (*). (c) T2*-weighted image. The entire node has homogeneous high signal intensity. (d) Identical post-USPIO image. Metastatic area (arrows) has a persisiting high SI and normal nodal tissue has a lower SI (*).*

tional sequences insensitive to USPIO, to evaluate nodal size. This cannot be done with sequences which are too sensitive to iron (e.g. T1- or T2*-weighted GRE images) because this will result in overestimation of the nodal size due to 'blurring' (Fig. 60.6). For this reason a T1-weighted f/tSE sequence is preferred as it is insensitive to USPIO.

Slice thickness
Accurate characterization of nodes with USPIO needs high spatial resolution scanning. One of the important factors affecting the resolution is slice thickness. Scanning with thinner slices reduces partial volume artefacts and allows detection of small metastatic foci within the nodes. The use of ultra thin slices is, however, limited by the limitations of signal-to-noise. In addition, also the in-plane resolution plays an important role. Recommended minimal voxel size is 0.5 × 0.5 × 3.0 mm.

Optimizing imaging parameters on T2* sequences
USPIO shortens T1- and T2* values. The shortening of the T1-value increases signal intensity whereas shortening of the T2*-value decreases signal intensity. Thus imaging

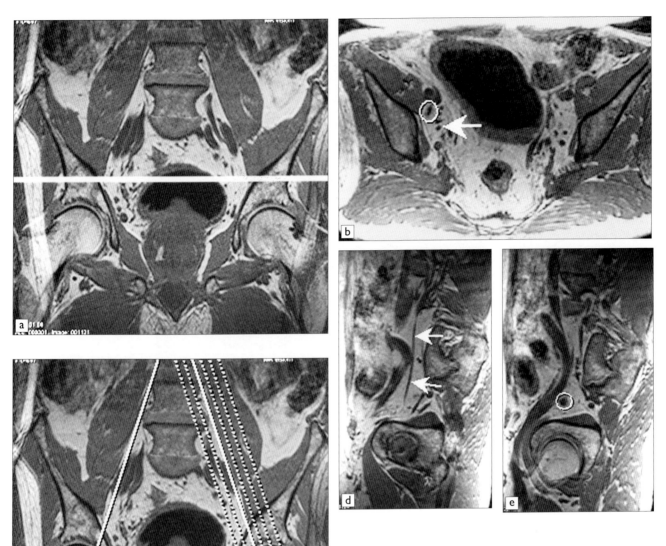

Figure 60.3. *Planes for nodal imaging. Pre-USPIO T1-weighted three-dimensional images, (a and c) coronal, (b) axial, (d) 'obturator' left plane, (e) 'obturator' right plane. Plane of (b) is presented in (a), and plane (d) and (e) are shown in (c). Stippled lines show images of left 'obturator' sequence. On (b), axial plane node (2×5 mm) (circle) is difficult to separate from vessels and the obturator nerve (arrow). Node (circle), vessels and nerve (arrows) are more easily recognized on 'obturator' images (d and e).*

detection of USPIO can be based upon pulse sequences sensitive to either its T1- or its T2* effect, but not to both. Indeed, a balanced sequence can obscure the presence of USPIO in a lymph node. As the primary concern is lymph node characterization and estimating nodal tumour burden, the goal is to enhance T2* weighting while limiting T1 influence. A long TR or small flip angle keeps the T1 effects from masking the T2* effect for imaging of lymph nodes.

Optimizing time-to-echo for T2 sequence*
As imaging of normal lymph nodes with USPIO relies on signal intensity drop from susceptibility, choosing an optimal time-to-echo (TE) value is important for making the correct diagnosis. Just as imaging earlier than 24 hours may result in erroneous interpretation, imaging with a suboptimal short TE may provide inadequate signal intensity drop, resulting in erroneous interpretation. Time-to-echo values should be long enough to enhance the susceptibility from normal accumulation of USPIO within nodes. Time-to-echo values ranging between 18 and 24 msec are reliable for detecting minimal USPIO accumulation within the nodes.

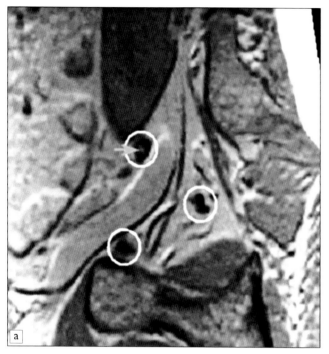

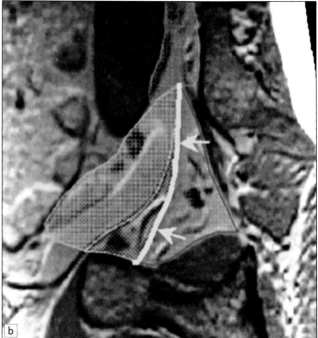

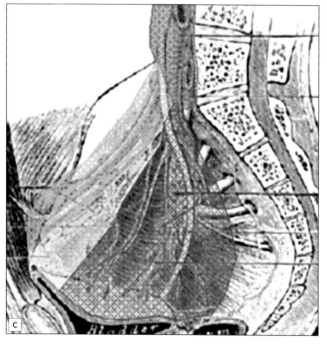

Figure 60.4. *Lymph node regions. On (a) and (b), 'obturator' T1-weighted post-USPIO images, vessels are bright and normal nodes are black (circles). Some nodes have a bright centre, which is caused by a fatty hilum (yellow arrow). In (b), regions are displayed. (c) Schematic drawing. The obturator region (yellow) is medial and dorsal to the external iliac vessels, ventral to the obturator nerve, cranial to the pelvic bone and caudal to the internal–external iliac bifurcation. The obturator region is part of the external iliac region. The rest of the external iliac region (green) is located in between, ventral and lateral to the external iliac vessels. The internal iliac region (blue) is dorsal to the obturator nerve, up to the internal iliac vessels. The common iliac region is cranial to the internal–external iliac bifurcation.*

Key points: imaging strategies

- The optimal time for the post-USPIO-MR examination is 24–36 hours after the injection

- If a precontrast examination is not performed it is essential to obtain T1-weighted f/tSE images to measure nodal size

- Recommended minimal voxel size for high resolution images is $0.5 \times 0.5 \times 3.0$ mm

- USPIO shortens T1- and T2* values. Optimal sequences should enhance T2* weighting while limiting T1 influence

- TE values ranging between 18 and 24 msec are reliable for detecting minimal USPIO accumulation within the nodes

Image interpretation

In Figures 60.7 and 60.8, an overview is presented of normal and metastatic nodes on pre- and post-USPIO-MR

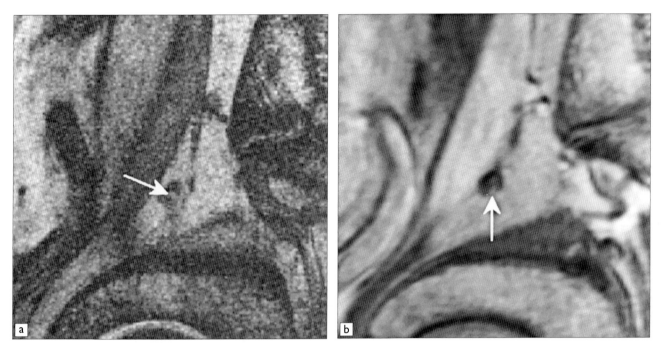

Figure 60.5. *Hilar fat mimicking small metastases. (a) T2*-weighted post-USPIO GRE image shows low signal intensity node with a central area of high signal intensity (arrow), which could represent a metastasis. (b) Three-dimensional T1-weighted GRE image also shows a high signal intensity area which looks like the continuation of perinodal fat on the caudal side (arrow). Histopathology confirmed that this node was a benign node with a fatty hilum.*

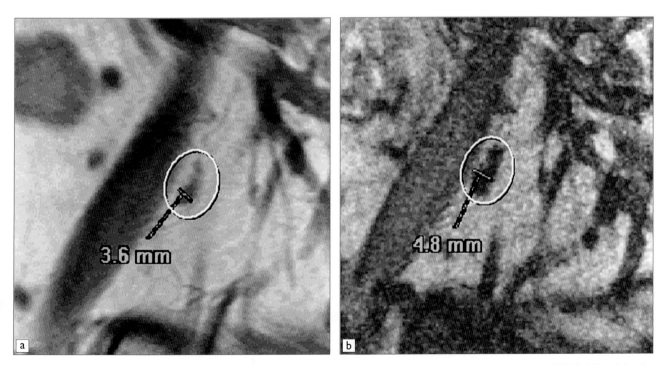

Figure 60.6. *'Blurring' on a T2*-weighted GRE sequence. This 'blurring' makes nodes appear larger. (a) Post-USPIO T1-weighted t/fSE sequence. Due to lack of sensitivity for USPIO the node does not appear black and its size can be reliably measured. (b) Post-USPIO T2*-weighted sequence. This sequence is sensitive to USPIO, the node is black and it looks bigger than on (a) (4.8 vs 3.6 mm). Therefore the t/fSE sequence may be used to provide a 'pre'-USPIO image for nodal measurement.*

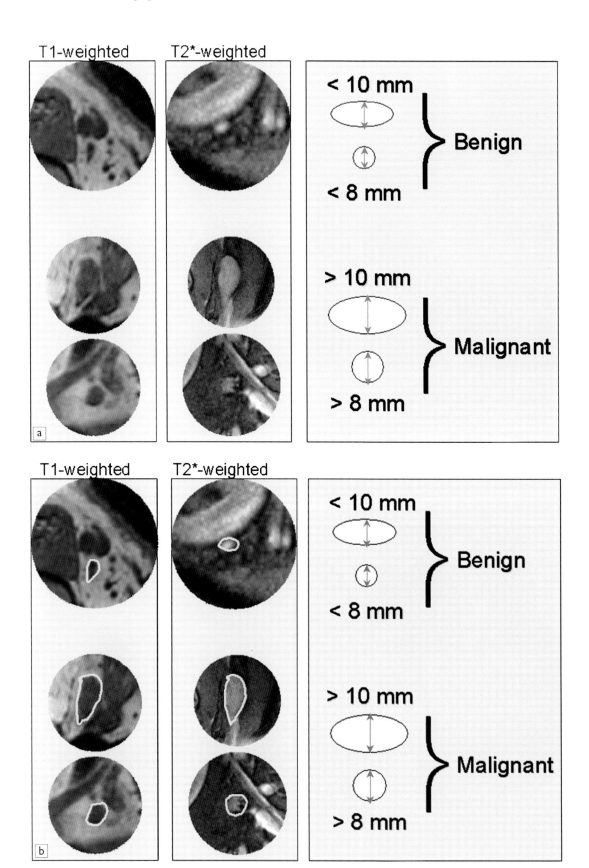

Figure 60.7. *(a) Nodes on pre-USPIO-MR imaging. On T1-weighted images both normal and metastatic nodes have intermediate signal intensity. On T2*-weighted images, both normal and metastatic nodes have high signal intensity. A node is metastatic if the axial diameter is more than 10 mm in a spherical node and more than 8 mm if the node is round. (b) Nodes on pre-USPIO-MR imaging. Nodes are highlighted.*

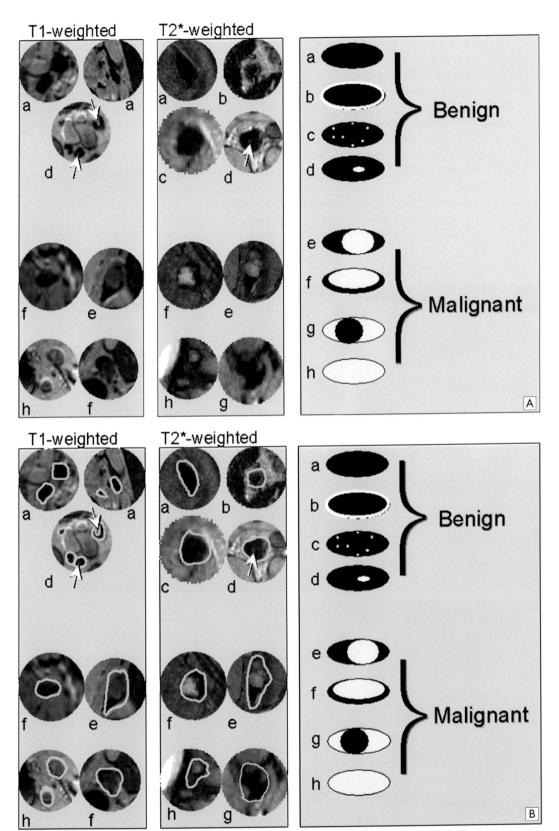

Figure 60.8. (A) Nodes on post-USPIO-MR imaging. On T1-weighted images, normal nodes have low and metastases have intermediate to high signal intensity. On T2*-weighted images normal nodes have low and metastases have high signal intensity. Normal nodes are entirely black (a), may show a slightly bright rim (b), minimal 'speckles' (c), or a high signal intensity area in the centre on T1-weighted images (d) (arrows), which is typical for hilar fat. Metastases show an area of lack of low signal intensity. This can be small (e), large (f and g), or be the entire node (h). (B) Nodes on post-USPIO-MR imaging. Nodes are highlighted in yellow.

imaging. Nodal shape and size should be evaluated on pre-USPIO images or post-USPIO images with low susceptibility for USPIO (e.g. T1-weighted t/fSE sequence). According to size criteria, a node should be considered to be metastatic if its maximum short axis axial diameter is more than 10 mm in a spherical-shaped node and more than 8 mm in a round node. However, if an enlarged node shows uniform low signal intensity on post-USPIO-MR, it should be also regarded as benign (Fig. 60.9). Indeed, all nodes visualized with uniform low signal intensity on post-USPIO images should be diagnosed as non-metastatic.

On T1-weighted sequences a focal area of high signal intensity may be observed in the centre of benign nodes due to normal hilar fat (Figs. 60.5 and 60.8). Furthermore,

tiny intermediate/high signal intensity speckles may be present in normal nodes usually caused by noise (Fig. 60.8). Finally, a higher signal intensity rim may also be found in normal nodes (Fig. 60.8).[16] However, if a node shows one or more focal areas of lack of low signal intensity, especially on high-resolution T2*-weighted sequences, the node should be regarded as containing malignant foci.

Pitfalls

The threshold using current 1.5T MR systems with a phased-array body coil for detecting metastases is 2–3 mm in 5-mm diameter nodes (Fig. 60.10). For recognizing smaller metastases (1–2 mm), the resolution is too low and noise may mimic small metastases. This means that very small metas-

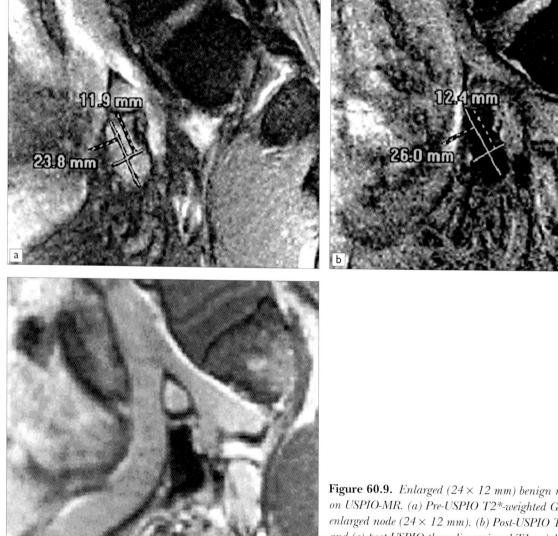

Figure 60.9. *Enlarged (24 × 12 mm) benign node, true negative on USPIO-MR. (a) Pre-USPIO T2*-weighted GRE image shows an enlarged node (24 × 12 mm). (b) Post-USPIO T2*-weighted GRE and (c) post-USPIO three-dimensional T1-weighted GRE images. The node has a low signal intensity which suggests that the node is benign. Histopathology confirmed a hyperplastic benign node. On (b), the nodal length is larger due to USPIO susceptibility.*

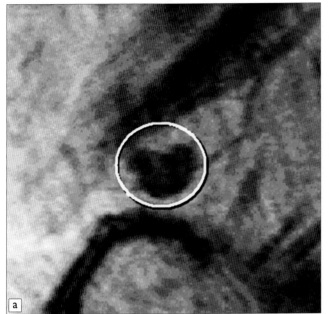
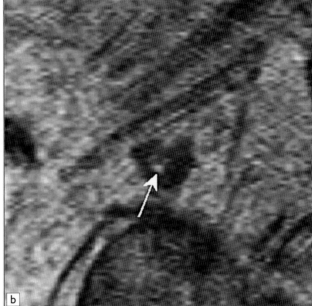

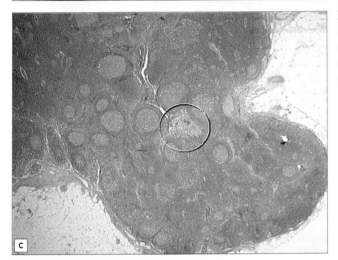

Figure 60.10. *Very small (2 mm) metastasis recognized on post-USPIO-MR. (a) T1-weighted tSE image. This sequence shows the node (circle) without central hilar fat. (b) Post-USPIO T2*-GRE image. This shows a central high signal intensity area (arrow). (c) Histopathology confirmed a 2 mm central metastasis (circle).*

tases are difficult to recognize. Reported sensitivity in >5 mm nodes is 41%.[17] False positive diagnoses may be seen in areas within a node which lack normal nodal tissue, such as foci of fibrosis following irradiation (Fig. 60.11). A fatty hilum may also be misinterpreted as a metastatic deposit (Fig. 60.5). False positive examinations may also occur if sequences which are less sensitive for USPIO are used (e.g. using a T2-w t/fSE sequence) (Fig. 60.12).

Key points: interpretation

- All lymph nodes with uniform low signal intensity on post-USPIO images should be diagnosed as non-metastatic

- A focal area of high signal intensity in the centre of a node on T1 weighting represents normal hilar fat

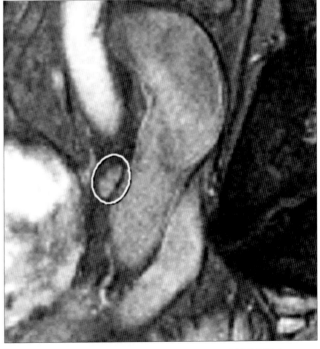

Figure 60.11. *False positive node on a post-USPIO-MR image following radiotherapy. Post-USPIO T2*-weighted image showing a high signal intensity node (circle). Histopathology revealed a benign fibrotic node.*

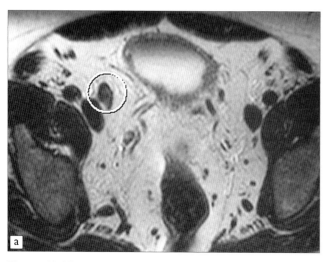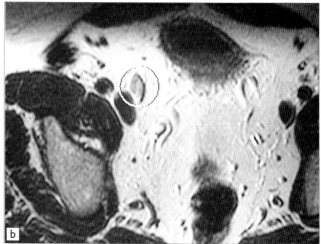

Figure 60.12. *False positive node due to technique. (a) Post-USPIO T2-weighted t/fSE sequence. This shows an 8 × 12 mm node (circle) with a relatively high signal intensity. (b) Post-USPIO T2*-weighted sequence. On this sequence the TE is too short and the high signal intensity of the node (circle) is suggestive of a metastasis. However, histology showed a benign node. Neither sequence was sensitive enough for the detection of iron.*

- A high signal intensity rim may be found in normal nodes

- Focal areas of lack of low signal intensity within a node, especially on high-resolution T2*-weighted sequences, should be regarded as malignant foci

- The threshold for detecting metastases is 2–3 mm in 5-mm diameter nodes

- False positive examinations may occur due to fibrosis, fatty replacement and the use of sequences insensitive to USPIO

Clinical value

When using a high-resolution MR technique, small metastases (3–7 mm) can be prospectively recognized in small (5–10 mm) lymph nodes.[17] These small lymph nodes would be considered to be normal on plain MR or CT examinations. In addition, enlarged benign nodes can be correctly recognized. Furthermore, USPIO can identify large malignant nodes and extracapsular extension and, if the node is not too small (i.e. >8 mm in diameter), the presence of malignancy can be confirmed by image-guided biopsy in approximately 70% of the cases.

Novel three-dimensional reconstruction techniques would be of particular value in displaying and analysing the massive amount of high-resolution data. In this context it should be feasible to display both normal and abnormal lymph nodes and their location with respect to important surgical landmarks such as vessels, obturator nerves and ureters in three-dimensions (Fig. 60.13).

In the future, when MR lymphography becomes more widely available, the technique may allow reliable selection of patients for prostatectomy, cystectomy, or radiotherapy without the need for invasive and costly procedures such as open and laparoscopic PLND.

For example, Fowler and Whitmore showed that 12% of all node-positive patients and 5% of all patients subjected to PLND have positive nodes missed at PLND because they are located solely in the internal iliac or common iliac region and therefore are not included in the modern modified PLND for prostate cancer.[18] An important advantage of imaging with USPIO is that all nodal sites are visualized and thus involvement of nodes in the internal iliac or common iliac chains can be predicted preoperatively. Harisinghani and Barentsz showed that, in nine out of a total of 80 patients with prostate cancer in which post-USPIO-MR imaging suggested metastases outside the classical field of lymph node resection and who underwent more extensive exploration, true metastases were confirmed at these sites in all patients.[15] In bladder cancer, USPIO-MR imaging may improve visualization of all the sites of metastatic involvement. This is important information for the urologist because removal of all these metastatic nodes contributes to the curative potential of surgery.[19]

The accuracy of USPIO-MR imaging of pelvic nodes in prostate cancer has recently been reported in a series of 80 patients.[15] Of the 63 nodes involved, 45 did not fulfil the conventional criteria for diagnosing nodal involvement. The sensitivity of USPIO-MR was 90.5% and the specificity was 97.8%. These excellent results show the enormous potential of MR lymphography as a new non-invasive diagnostic tool, not only for the detection of nodal involvement in pelvic cancers but also for the detection of lymph node metastases in other anatomical sites.

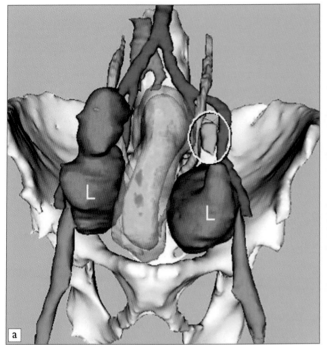

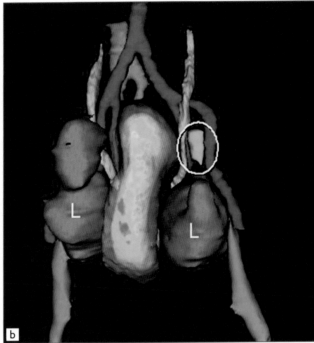

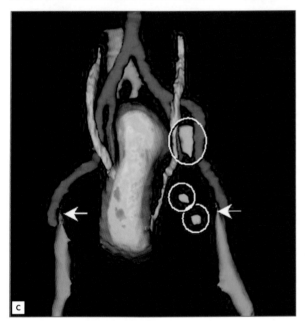

Figure 60.13. *Three-dimensional segmentation of pelvis, vessels, ureters, nodes and lymphocoeles. Segmentation of three-dimensional T1-weighted GRE sequence in patient after laparoscopic nodal dissection. (a) Showing pelvis, vessels, ureters, lymphocoeles compressing the bladder and enlarged node in obturator region (green), this is same node as in Figure 60.2. (b) Pelvic bones are removed. (c) Lymphocoeles are removed. Now two more nodes (circles) in internal iliac region, and compression sites of both external iliac veins are visible (arrows). All nodes were metastatic.*

Key points: clinical value

- The sensitivity of USPIO-MR imaging is 90.5% and the specificity is 97.8% for the detection of nodal metastases in prostate cancer
- MR lymphography may allow reliable selection of patients for prostatectomy, cystectomy or radiotherapy

Conclusion

High-resolution MR imaging after IV injection of USPIO allows the detection of small and otherwise undetectable lymph node metastases in patients with pelvic cancer. However, thorough knowledge of sequence parameters and imaging planes, lymph node anatomy, appearance of normal and abnormal nodes and pitfalls is essential for accurate diagnosis of nodal involvement.

Summary

- Cross-sectional imaging techniques are unreliable for detecting nodal metastases in pelvic cancers

- [18]FDG PET is more sensitive than CT or MR imaging for detecting involved nodes in prostate and bladder cancer but cannot replace PLND

- PLND remains the preferred technique for diagnosis of nodal involvement in pelvic cancers

- The optimal time for the post-USPIO-MR examination is 24–36 hours after the injection

- USPIO shortens T1- and T2* values. Optimal sequences should enhance T2* weighting while limiting T1 influence

- All lymph nodes with uniform low signal intensity on post-USPIO images should be diagnosed as non-metastatic

- A focal area of high signal intensity in the centre of a node on T1 weighting represents normal hilar fat

- A high signal intensity rim may be found in normal nodes

- Focal areas of lack of low signal intensity within a node should be regarded as malignant

- The threshold for detecting metastases is 2–3 mm in 5–10 mm diameter nodes

- False positive examinations may occur due to fibrosis, fatty replacement and the use of sequences insensitive to USPIO

- The sensitivity of USPIO is 90.5% and the specificity is 97.8% for the detection of nodal metastases in prostate cancer

- The clinical value of MR lymphography as a non-invasive technique is currently being evaluated

- MR lymphography may allow more accurate selection of patients for surgery

References

1. Mills R D. Pelvic lymph node metastases from bladder cancer: outcome in 83 patients after radical cystectomy and pelvic lymphadenectomy. J Urol 2001; 166: 9–23

2. Narayan P, Fournier G, Galendran V et al. Utility of preoperative serum prostate-specific antigen concentration and biopsy Gleason score in predicting risk of pelvic lymph node metastases in prostate cancer. Urology 1994; 4: 519–524

3. Crawford E D, Batuello J T, Snow P et al. The use of artificial intelligence technology to predict lymph node spread in men with clinically localized prostate carcinoma. Cancer 2000; 88: 2105–2109

4. Wolf J S, Cher M, dalla 'Era M et al. The use and accuracy of cross-sectional imaging and fine-needle aspiration cytology for detection of pelvic lymph node metastases before radical prostatectomy. J Urol 1995; 153: 993–999

5. Jager G J, Barentsz J O, Oosterhof G O et al. Pelvic adenopathy in prostatic and urinary bladder carcinoma: MR imaging with a three-dimensional T1-weighted magnetization-prepared-rapid gradient-echo sequence. Am J Roentgenol 1996; 167: 1503–1507

6. Barentsz, J O, Jager G J, van Vierzen P B et al. Staging urinary bladder cancer after transurethral biopsy: value of fast dynamic contrast-enhanced MR imaging. Radiology 1996; 201: 185–193

7. Pieterman R M, Van Putten J W G, Meuzelaar J J et al. Preoperative staging of non-small-cell lung cancer with positron-emission tomography. N Engl J Med 2000; 343: 254–261

8. Bachor R, Kotzerke J, Reske S N, Hautmann R. Lymph node staging of bladder neck carcinoma with positron emission tomography. Urologe 1999; 38: 46–50

9. Heicappell R, Muller Mattheis V, Reinhardt M et al. Staging of pelvic lymph nodes in neoplasms of the bladder and prostate by positron emission tomography with 2-[(18)F]-2-deoxy-D-glucose. Eur Urol 1999; 36: 582–587

10. Vassallo P, Matei C, Heston W D W et al. AMI-227-enhanced MR lymphography: usefulness for differentiating reactive from tumor-bearing lymph nodes. Radiology 1994; 193: 501–506

11. Weissleder R, Elizondo G, Wittenberg J et al. Ultrasmall paramagnetic iron oxide: an intravenous contrast agent for assessing lymph nodes with MR imaging. Radiology 1990; 175: 494–498

12. Gerlowski L E, Jain R K. Microvascular permeability of normal and neoplastic tissues. Microvasc Res 1986; 31: 288–305

13. Bellin M F, Roy C, Kinkel K et al. Lymph node metastases: safety and effectiveness of MRI with ultrasmall superparamagnetic iron oxide particles. Initial clinical experience. Radiology 1998; 207: 799–808

14. Chambon C, Clement O, Le Blanche A et al. Superparamagnetic iron oxides as positive MR contrast agents: in vitro and in vivo evidence. Magn Reson Imaging 1993; 11: 509–519

15. Harisinghani M, Barentsz J, Hahn P et al. Noninvasive detection of clinically occult lymph-node metastases in prostate cancer. N Engl J Med 2003; 348: 2491–2499

16. Koh D M, Brown G, Temple L et al. USPIO-MR imaging

of mesorectal lymph nodes in rectal carcinoma: initial observations. Radiology 2003, in press

17. Guimares R, Clement O, Bittoun J et al. MR lymphography with super paramagnetic nanoparticles in rats: pathologic basis for contrast enhancement. Am J Roentgenol 1994; 162: 201–207

18. Fowler J E, Whitmore W F. The incidence and extent of

pelvic lymph node metastases in apparently localized prostatic cancer. Cancer 1981; 47: 2941–2945

19. Leissner J, Hohenfellner R, Thuroff J W, Wolf H K. Lymphadenectomy in patients with transitional cell carcinoma of the urinary bladder; significance for staging and prognosis. Br J Urol 2000; 85: 817–823

Chapter 61

Imaging angiogenesis: clinical implications

Anwar R Padhani

Introduction

Angiogenesis, the sprouting of new capillaries from existing blood vessels, and vasculogenesis, the de novo generation of blood vessels, are the two primary methods of vascular expansion by which nutrient supply to tissues is adjusted to match physiological needs. Angiogenesis is an essential component of several normal physiological processes that include menstrual cycle changes in the ovaries and uterus, organ regeneration, wound healing and the spontaneous growth of collateral vessels in response to ischaemia.[1] Pathological angiogenesis is an integral part of a number of disease states (e.g. rheumatoid arthritis, age-related macular degeneration, proliferative retinopathy, psoriasis) and is critical for growth of primary malignant tumours and for the development of metastases.[2] The importance of tumour angiogenesis has been well recognized by clinical oncologists for many years but it is only recently that radiologists have become interested in the topic. This is because the potential of imaging to characterize neovasculature non-invasively has become realized. This chapter describes the process of tumour angiogenesis and features unique to tumour microvasculature. Emphasis will be placed on the technique of dynamic contrast medium-enhanced MR imaging (DCE-MRI).[3–5] Comparison of DCE-MRI with other imaging techniques that are able to depict the angiogenic status of tumours in situ, including macromolecular contrast media (MMCM)-enhanced MR,[6] blood oxygen level-dependent (BOLD)-MR[7] and functional computed tomography (CT),[8] is addressed. In addition, the potential of positron emission tomography (PET) to image angiogenesis is briefly discussed. The clinical potential of angiogenesis imaging will be highlighted and ongoing challenges of functional imaging techniques as clinical and research tools will be explored.

Tumour angiogenesis

Angiogenesis involves a cascade of events in which mature, resting host endothelial cells are stimulated to proliferate to form new blood vessels. The angiogenic phenomenon is a complex multistep process involving many growth factors (cytokines) and interactions between varieties of cell types (Fig. 61.1). A detailed review of the processes initiating and

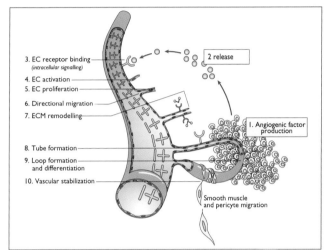

Figure 61.1. *Angiogenesis, the cascade of events. Activation of host endothelium cells by angiogenic stimuli results in a series of events leading to the formation of a vascular plexus that supplies oxygen and nutrients to tumours. Adapted from The Angiogenesis Foundation (www.angio.org). EC, endothelial cell; ECM, extracellular matrix.*

controlling both regulated and unregulated neoangiogenesis is beyond the scope of this chapter and interested readers are directed to other comprehensive texts where further information can be found.[9,10] However, a few pertinent observations are in order.

It is well established that diffusion distances for oxygen and other nutrients in tissues are of the order of 150 microns.[11] As tumours grow, an initial avascular phase is followed by neovascularization which permits further tumour growth. Although some tumours co-opt native vessels from the start and are apparently well vascularized,[12] it is clear that tumour growth beyond 1–2 cubic millimetres requires vascular in-growth. The primary stimulus for new vessel formation is presumed to be hypoxia. In tumours, there are often areas of high angiogenic activity with regions of hypoxia occurring because of the disparity between blood flow, nutrient delivery and oxygen consumption.[13,14] Tissue angiogenesis is invoked by expression of proangiogenic growth factors (cytokines) and by suppression of antiangiogenic factors; this is known as the balance hypothesis for the 'angiogenic switch' (Fig. 61.2). Expression of angiogenic cytokines can be induced as a response to hypoxic

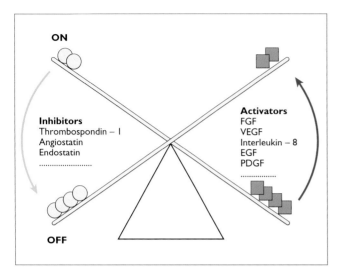

Figure 61.2. *The balance hypothesis for the angiogenic switch. It is the balance of proliferative (antiapoptotic) and proapoptotic factors that determines the state of angiogenesis at this level. FGF, fibroblast growth factor; VEGF, vascular endothelial growth factor; EGF, epidermal growth factor; PDGF, platelet-derived growth factor. (Reproduced with permission from Hanahan D, Folkman J. Cell 1996; 86: 353–364.)*

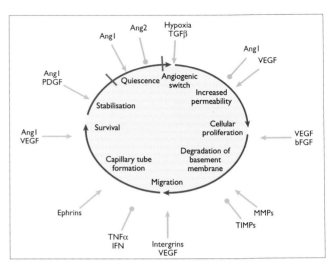

Figure 61.3. *The angiogenic cascade and major mediators of angiogenesis. Stimulators ↓; inhibitors !. Ang, angiopoietin; bFGF, beta fibroblast growth factor; IFN, interferon; TIMP, tissue inhibitor of matrix metalloproteinases (MMP); TNF, tumour necrosis factor; VEFG, vascular endothelial growth factor; PDGF, platelet-derived growth factor. (Adapted from Kaban K. Hematol Oncol Clin N Am; 2002; 16: 1125–1171.)*

stress, by hormonal stimulation, but can also result from activation of oncogenes.

The process of angiogenesis in normal tissues is well organized[15,16] and therefore differs from that in tumours in which the process is disorganized and chaotic. This is probably due to imbalances in the mix of pro- and antiangiogenic cytokines. The precise nature of this imbalance is not completely understood and is probably multifactorial with significant variation between different tumours. The factors involved in angiogenesis can be classified according to the role they play in the process.[17] Many tumours secrete high levels of proangiogenic cytokines, including vascular endothelial growth factor (VEGF) and fibroblast growth factor (FGF). At least 15 proangiogenic cytokines are known about and most are secreted by tumour cells. Importantly, proangiogenic factors serve as survival factors for proliferating endothelial cells. Tumours also produce antiangiogenic factors (e.g. angiostatin, endostatin and thrombospondins), many of which suppress angiogenesis at metastatic sites but not of the primary tumour.[18,19] Apoptosis (programmed cell death) is important in angiogenesis. Antiangiogenic factors are proapoptotic for proliferating endothelial cells. It is the net balance of positive (proliferative and antiapoptotic) and negative regulators of angiogenesis (proapoptotic) that determine the state of angiogenesis at the local level.

The angiogenic process in tumours (Fig. 61.3) begins when normal vessels become activated by VEGF; within minutes vasodilatation and increased permeability to macromolecular serum proteins occurs. Extravasation of plasma proteins leads to deposition of a provisional extra-cellular matrix (ECM), which will facilitate endothelial cell migration. In response to angiogenic stimuli such as VEGF and FGF, endothelial cells at first proliferate and degrade their basement membrane. Prior to endothelial proliferation and migration, activated vessels show local shedding of pericytes and smooth muscle cells. These perivascular cells are essential for maintaining vascular integrity but also further suppress endothelial cell proliferation. Proliferation, migration and elongation of endothelial capillaries require degradation of the ECM, and endothelial cells thus activated release a number of proteolytic enzymes, including metalloproteinases (MMPs). The sprouting and migration of endothelial cells is mediated by vascular cell adhesion molecules such as integrins. Tube formation follows, leading to the generation of a functional but immature endothelial plexus. The final stages of angiogenesis include stabilization, remodelling and maturation of the new vessels by recruitment of pericytes and smooth muscle cells.[20] Angiopoietin-1 (Ang1) plays an important role in the recruitment of smooth muscle cells and pericytes. Ephrins play an important role in the fusion of smooth muscle cells and pericytes to endothelial tubes.

Key points: tumour angiogenesis

- Angiogenesis is critical for tumour growth
- The primary stimulus for angiogenesis in tumours is hypoxia

- Tumours cannot grow beyond the size of 1–2 mm³ without a blood supply

- Angiogenesis is invoked by proangiogenic (e.g. VEGF and FGF) and suppressed by antiangiogenic factors (e.g. angiostatin and endostatin)

- New vessels develop as a result of proliferation and elongation of endothelial cells to form tube-like structures. These become remodelled, mature and stabilize by recruitment of pericytes and smooth muscle cells

Tumour vascular characteristics

There are many different features of tumour vascularity which are characteristic of malignancy. These characteristics permit distinction of malignant vascularity from benign vascularity using functional imaging techniques. The structural and functional characteristics of malignant tumours are illustrated in Fig. 61.4a and b and include:

- Spatial heterogeneity and chaotic structure – no hierarchy of vascular structures is observed, with abrupt changes in diameter and blind-ending vessels, particularly within the centres of tumours. Few structurally complete arteries or veins are found with sinusoidal capillary plexuses prevailing. The remodelling of the vasculature seen in inflammation or wound healing is largely missing
- Poorly formed, fragile vessels with high permeability to macromolecules, due to the presence of large endothelial cell gaps or fenestrae,[21] incomplete basement membrane and relative lack of pericytes or smooth muscle associations with endothelial cells[16]
- Arteriovenous shunting, high vascular tortuosity and vasodilatation[22]
- Intermittent or unstable blood flow (with acutely collapsing vessels)[23] and areas of spontaneous haemorrhage
- Extreme heterogeneity of vascular density with areas of low vascular density mixed with regions of high angiogenic activity[22]
- Structural abnormalities of new tumour vessels lead to pathophysiological changes within the confines of the tumour. These alterations in pathophysiological parameters are the underlying factors leading to the visualization of tumours on contrast-enhanced imaging. These pathophysiological changes include an increase in:
Capillary permeability
Volume of extravascular extracellular space
Interstitial pressure
Tumour perfusion

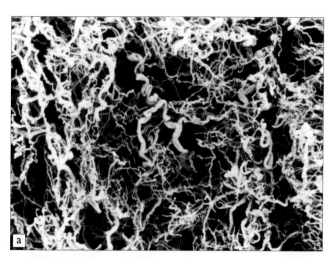

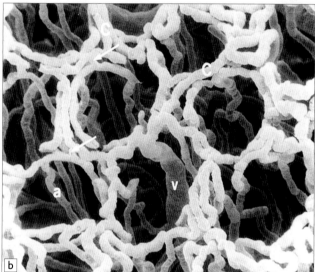

Figure 61.4. (a) Electron micrograph showing tumour microvasculature. Note chaotic structure of vessels with areas of dense microvasculature and areas where vessels are sparse. (b) Normal mucosal vessels: arterioles (a); capillaries (c); venules (v). Note symmetrical hierarchical structure of normal colonic mucosal vasculature. (Reproduced with kind permission of Professor Moritz Konerding, Anatomisches Institut, Mainz University, Germany.)

Biological and clinical importance of tumour angiogenesis

Sustained tumour growth in solid tissues cannot occur without vascular support.[19] Transgenic animal tumour model experiments have shown that progression from an *in situ* to invasive cancer is accompanied by the onset of angiogenesis.[24] There are a number of clinical examples where vascularization has been related to tumour progression (e.g. in the change from breast ductal carcinoma *in situ* to invasive cancer).[25] Immunohistochemical techniques show changes consistent with this observation; for example, expression of the endothelial cell-specific tyrosine kinase receptor, Tie-2 (TEK), is increased during the transition from benign to invasive cancer.[26] Patient prognosis is related to angiogenesis; elevated tumour levels of VEGF are associated with poorer overall prognosis in breast cancer.[27–29] Immunohistochemical staining measurement of angiogenic activity by microvessel density (see below) has been shown to be an important prognostic factor for overall survival that is independent of other known prognostic variables, including stage, grade and lymph node status in a number of cancer types.[30] Additionally, vascular access is essential for a tumour to be able to metastasize to distant sites.[24]

Key points: tumour vascular characteristics

- Tumour vessels show spatial heterogeneity and a chaotic non-hierarchical structure

- Tumour vessels are fragile, highly permeable and show intermittent and heterogeneous blood flow

- Structural abnormalities of new vessels result in pathophysiological changes. These changes form the basis of contrast enhancement patterns observed in malignant tumours

- Progression from in situ cancer to invasive cancer is dependent on angiogenesis

- In human tumours, prognosis is related to angiogenesis

Methods of assessing angiogenesis

Current methods of assessing angiogenesis can be considered as either direct or indirect. The most frequently used direct method is microvessel density (MVD) counting after the immunostaining of endothelial cells using a variety of antibodies that include Factor VIII-related antigen, CD34 and CD31.[31] This technique requires tumour tissue, usually obtained from operative specimens, and is limited by the inability to provide information on the functional state of the vasculature.

Recently, indirect or surrogate methods of assessing angiogenesis such as blood levels of angiogenic factors (VEGF, FGF)[32] and imaging methods have been developed. Advantages of indirect methods are that they are non-invasive, can be performed with the tumour in situ and may be used to monitor response to treatment. Indirect techniques may be semiquantitative or quantitative and, in the case of imaging, the functional status of the vasculature can be assessed. It is important to note that implanted tumour xenograft data show that there is a discrepancy between perfused and visible microvessels; a variable 20–85% of microvessels are perfused at any given time. This results in

a difference between histological MVD and what is described as the 'true or functional vascular density'.[33]

Imaging angiogenesis: comparisons of methods

Several imaging techniques are able to assess human tumours with respect to their angiogenic status (Table 61.1). Both CT and MR have the advantage of good spatial resolution (frequently equal to that of corresponding morphological images), they are minimally invasive and involve little patient risk. The signal intensity and contrast-to-noise ratios of MR images are high and both CT and MR are more readily available than PET or xenon inhalation CT. In general, MR data acquisition is quick and thus can be incorporated into routine patient studies. Importantly, MR is sensitive to small vessel function, depending on the technique used, whereas PET is dominated by information from larger vessels. Magnetic resonance techniques are also sensitive to a variety of pathophysiological parameters, including blood flow, microvessel permeability and diameter, tissue oxygenation (BOLD) and metabolism which when taken together can inform on the tumour microenvironment. The tumour microenvironment describes the oxygenation, pH, metabolic and energetic status of the tumour and is defined by the oxygen and nutrient supply and drainage of metabolites, which depend themselves on tumour vascularization, tumour blood flow and the transport of substances across the interstitial space.

Computed tomography can be performed with contrast medium to measure vascular characteristics including blood flow, blood volume, mean fluid transit time and capillary permeability in a variety of organs and tumours.[34–36] Functional CT can show alterations in tissue perfusion that may reflect underlying malignancy, even when there is no gross anatomical abnormality present.[8] However, there has so far been little validation of functional CT with accepted surrogates of angiogenesis; poor anatomical coverage, increased sensitivity to physiological motion and radiation remain potential drawbacks. There are a few key differences between functional perfusion imaging with CT and DCE-MRI. In principle, both techniques sequentially observe the passage of a bolus of contrast medium through a region of interest and allow quantification of the profile of tissue enhancement. Depending on the technique used, dynamic CT techniques yield high-quality information based predominantly on the first pass of contrast (absolute perfusion, blood volume), whereas the most commonly used MR technique (T1-weighted DCE-MRI) samples a volume of interest less frequently but over a longer period of time and yields parameters that reflect microvessel perfusion, permeability and extracellular leakage space.

Ultrasound imaging can identify vascular features in tumours at different levels of resolution (40–200 μm diameter vessels) depending upon the technique employed.[37,38]

Table 61.1. *Commonly available functional imaging techniques for angiogenesis evaluation*

Technique	Measured parameters	Pathophysiological correlates	Advantages	Disadvantages
Contrast-enhanced MRI (DCE-MRI)	Contrast medium uptake rate Transfer rates Extracellular volume Relative perfusion	Vessel density Permeability Perfusion Extravascular space	Availability High spatial resolution Registered anatomy	Image quality can be affected by respiration Surrogate measures requiring validation
Doppler ultrasound techniques	Pulsatile index (PI) Resistive index (RI) Acceleration index (AI) Peak systolic flow velocity (V_{max}) Patterns of flow	Global 'flow' Vascular resistance Vascularity	Availability Non-invasive Easily repeatable Low cost	Unable to image microvasculature Operator dependence No signal at low flow Restricted anatomical access
Computed tomography	Peak gradient in tissue and arteries Perfusion Blood volume Permeability	Perfusion Blood volume Permeability	Availability Quantitative	Limited in number of slices Some methodology problems
Positron emission tomography (PET)	Perfusion Blood volume Specific vascular markers	Perfusion Blood volume	Quantitative Repeatable	Expensive Limited availability

Contrast-enhanced ultrasound using an intravascular agent can generate indices of blood flow, blood volume, or vascularity within malignant tissue that correlate well with intravascular red blood cell velocities.[39,40] Targeted imaging using ultrasound-mediated destruction of microbubbles can visualize vessels at high resolution within the tumour vascular tree.[41] To date, however, there has been little validation of ultrasound with accepted histological surrogates of angiogenesis;[38] poor accessibility to certain anatomic regions (e.g. lungs and brain) and operator dependence are other outstanding issues. Positron Emission Tomography can also be used to evaluate tumour metabolism, hypoxia as well as blood flow and volume.[42] A number of radiotracers are available to characterize neoplastic tissues including ^{15}O-labelled water and carbon monoxide to quantify tissue perfusion and blood volume, respectively.[43,44] PET is considered by many to be the gold standard for non-invasive measurement of tissue perfusion but there are few tumour data outside the brain. PET methods are limited by high cost, limited availability of equipment and poor anatomic resolution. Furthermore, the short lives of radio-isotopes require that a cyclotron and onsite radio-chemistry be present.

Key points: methods of assessing angiogenesis

- Direct measurement of angiogenesis is performed by MVD counting using immunostaining techniques

- The true vascular density differs from the histological MVD because a variable 25–85% of tumour vessels are perfused at any one time

- Indirect measurement of angiogenesis can be performed non-invasively using MR, CT, ultrasound and PET

Magnetic resonance methods of assessing angiogenesis

Magnetic resonance can be used experimentally to characterize microvasculature, providing information about tumour microvessel structure and function.[6,45–47] Magnetic resonance techniques can be divided into non-enhanced and contrast media-enhanced methods.[48] The latter can be further divided by the type of contrast medium utilized:

- Low molecular weight agents (<1,000 Daltons) that rapidly diffuse in the extracellular fluid space (ECF agents)
- Large-molecular agents (>30,000 Daltons) designed for prolonged intravascular retention (macromolecular contrast media, MMCM, or blood pool agents)
- Agents intended to accumulate at sites of concentrated angiogenesis mediating molecules[49]

Tumour angiogenesis can also be analysed using intrinsic BOLD contrast MR.[7] DCE-MRI utilizing low molecular weight contrast agents, MMCM- and BOLD-MR techniques are reviewed in more detail below.

Key points: magnetic resonance imaging methods of assessing angiogenesis

- MR contrast techniques can assess microvasculature by contrast- and non-contrast-enhanced methods

- Contrast-enhanced methods most commonly utilize low molecular weight agents

- Large molecular weight agents are not yet widely available and are designed for prolonged vascular retention

Low molecular weight extracellular space contrast agents kinetics

DCE-MRI is able to distinguish malignant from benign and normal tissues by exploiting differences in contrast agent behaviour. When a bolus of paramagnetic, low molecular weight contrast agent passes through a capillary bed, it is transiently confined within the vascular space (Fig. 61.5). This 'first pass' includes the arrival of contrast medium and can last many cardiac cycles. Within the vascular space, paramagnetic contrast media produces magnetic field (Bo) inhomogeneities that result in a decrease in the signal intensity of surrounding tissues. In most tissues except the brain, testes and retina, the contrast agent rapidly passes into the extravascular–extracellular space (EES; also called leakage space – v_e) at a rate determined by the permeability of the microvessels, their surface area and by blood flow. In tumours, a variable 12–45% of the contrast media can leak into the EES during the first pass.[50] The transfer constant (K^{trans}) describes the transendothelial transport of low molecular weight contrast medium by diffusion (Fig. 61.6).

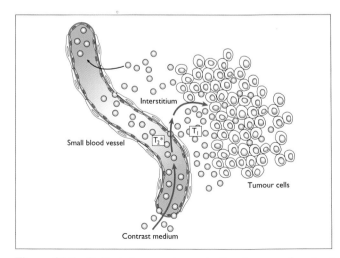

Figure 61.5. *Stylized diagram demonstrating passage of contrast agent through tissue and MR actions.*

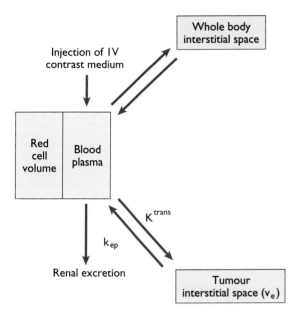

Figure 61.6. *Body compartments accessed by low molecular weight contrast media.*

Three major factors determine the behaviour of low molecular weight contrast media in tissues during the first few minutes after injection:

- Blood perfusion
- Transport of contrast agent across vessel wall
- Diffusion of contrast medium in the interstitial space

If the delivery of the contrast medium to a tissue is insufficient (flow-limited situations or where vascular permeability is greater than inflow) then blood perfusion will be the dominant factor determining contrast agent kinetics and K^{trans} approximates to tissue blood flow per unit volume.[51] The latter situation is commonly found in extracranial tumours. If tissue perfusion is sufficient and transport out of the vasculature does not deplete intravascular contrast medium concentration (non-flow limited situations, e.g. in areas of fibrosis or normal brain tissues) then transport across the vessel wall is the major factor that determines contrast medium kinetics (K^{trans} then approximates to permeability surface area product).

As low molecular weight contrast media do not cross cell membranes, the volume of distribution is effectively the EES (v_e). Contrast medium also begins to diffuse into tissue compartments further removed from the vasculature including areas of necrosis and fibrosis. Over a period typically lasting several minutes to hours, the contrast agent diffuses back into the vasculature (described by the rate constant or k_{ep}) from where it is excreted (usually by the kidneys although some ECF contrast media have significant hepatic excretion). When capillary permeability or surface area is very high, the return of contrast medium is typically quick resulting in fast washout. Contrast medium elimina-

tion from very slow-exchange tissues such as fibrosis and areas of necrosis occurs slowly, explaining the persistent delayed enhancement characteristic of some tumours, e.g. cholangiocarcinoma and in breast cancer.[52]

Magnetic resonance sequences can be designed to be sensitive to the vascular phase of contrast medium delivery (so-called T2* methods which reflect on tissue perfusion and blood volume).[53,54] Similarly, sequences sensitive to the presence of contrast medium in the EES reflect on microvessel perfusion, permeability and extracellular leakage space (so-called T1 methods). These two methods are compared in Table 61.2.

Key points: general features of low molecular weight contrast agents

- Contrast medium is transiently confined to the vascular bed during the 'first pass' following intravenous injection of a bolus

- In most tissues, contrast medium rapidly passes into the extravascular space (leakage space v_e) through gaps between vessel endothelium cells

- The transfer constant (K^{trans}) describes the transendothelial transport of low molecular weight contrast medium by diffusion

T2*-weighted dynamic magnetic resonance

Data acquisition

Perfusion-weighted images can be obtained with 'bolus-tracking techniques' that monitor the passage of contrast material through a capillary bed.[53,54] The decrease in signal intensity of tissues can be observed with susceptibility-weighted T1- or T2*-weighted sequences, the latter providing greater sensitivity and contrast to perfusion effects (Fig. 61.7). In this context, spin-echo sequences are more sensitive to capillary blood flow compared with gradient-echo sequences, which incorporate signals from larger vessels.[55] The degree of signal loss observed is dependent on the vascular concentration of the contrast agent and microvessel size[56] and density. The signal-to-noise ratio (SNR) of such images can be improved by using high doses of contrast medium (i.e. ≥0.2-mmol/kg body weight).[57] High specification, echo-planar-enabled MR systems capable of rapid image acquisition are required to adequately characterize these effects. However, such studies are possible on conventional MR systems using standard gradient-echo sequences but are limited to fewer slices.

Quantification

Tracer kinetic principles can be used to provide estimates of relative blood volume (rBV), relative blood flow (rBF) and mean transit time (MTT) derived from the first-pass of contrast agent through the microcirculation (Fig. 61.8).[53,54,58]

Table 61.2. *Comparison of T2*- and T1-weighted dynamic contrast-enhanced MR techniques*

	T2*-weighted imaging	**T1-weighted imaging**
Tissue signal intensity change	Darkening	Enhancement
Duration of effect and optimal data acquisition	Seconds/subsecond	Minutes/2–25 seconds
Magnitude of effect	Small	Larger
Optimal contrast medium dose	≥0.2 mmol/kg	0.1–0.2 mmol/kg
Quantification method used	Relative more than absolute	Relative and absolute
Physiological property measured	Perfusion/blood volume	Transendothelial permeability, capillary surface area, lesion leakage space, blood flow
Kinetic parameters derived	Blood volume and flow, transit time	Transfer and rate constants, leakage space
Pathological correlates	Tumour grade and microvessel vessel density	Microvessel density
		Vascular endothelial growth factor (VEGF)
Clinical MR applications	Lesion characterization – breast, liver and brain	Lesion detection and characterization
	Non-invasive brain tumour grading	Improving accuracy of tumour staging
	Directing brain tumour biopsy	Predicting response to treatment
	Determining brain tumour prognosis	Monitoring response to treatment
	Monitoring treatment, e.g. radiotherapy	Novel therapies including antiangiogenic drugs
		Detecting tumour relapse

These variables are related by the central volume theorem equation (BF = BV/MTT). A number of conditions of the central volume theorem cannot be met in biological tissues. For example, injection time is not instantaneous and as the arterial input function is not typically measured, these parameter estimates are qualitative or 'relative'. Recently, quantification of these parameters has been undertaken in normal brain and low-grade gliomas by simultaneous monitoring of the concentration of contrast agent in a large neck or brain vessel and quantification of perfusion parameters.[59,60]

Limitations

Recirculation of contrast medium can impair the calculation of T2*-weighted parameters (Fig. 61.7). Other physiological effects that hinder accurate measurements include non-laminar flow, which arises from the presence of irregular calibre vessels, non-dichotomous branching and high vascular permeability, which leads to increased blood viscosity (from haemoconcentration). In addition, factors such as machine stability, patient motion and intrinsic patient variables, particularly cardiac output and upstream stenoses, can affect the computations. The quantification techniques described above also cannot readily be applied to areas of marked blood–brain barrier breakdown or to extracranial tumours with very leaky blood vessels. This is because the T1-enhancing effects of gadolinium (Gd) chelates can counteract T2* signal intensity-lowering effects, resulting in falsely low blood volume values in very

leaky vessels. Quantitative imaging is thus most reliable when used for normal brain and non-enhancing brain lesions (e.g. low-grade gliomas) because the contrast medium is retained within the intravascular space. One solution to overcoming these problems is to use non-gadolinium susceptibility contrast agents based on the element dysprosium or USPIOs, which have strong T2* effect but a weak T1 effect.[61,62] Other solutions to counter T1-enhancing effects of gadolinium chelates include idealized model fitting (Fig. 61.8) and pre-dosing with contrast medium to saturate the leakage space. The latter two techniques are favoured by the author and illustrative images of computed rBV, rBF and rMTT for breast cancer are shown in Figure 61.8.

Clinical experience

T2*-weighted perfusion mapping techniques are best suited to investigation of the brain and over recent years have progressively entered into neurological clinical practice.[63–66] In the World Health Organization (WHO) grading system for classifying cerebral gliomas, neovascularization, cellular and nuclear pleomorphism cell density and necrosis are key histological features. Areas of high tumour relative cerebral blood volume (rCBV) are readily visible in patients with brain gliomas (Fig. 61.9)[65,67] and appear to correlate with mitotic activity (information on tumour grade) and vascularity but not with cellular atypia, endothelial proliferation, necrosis or cellularity.[65] rCBV maps have been shown to have a high negative predictive value in

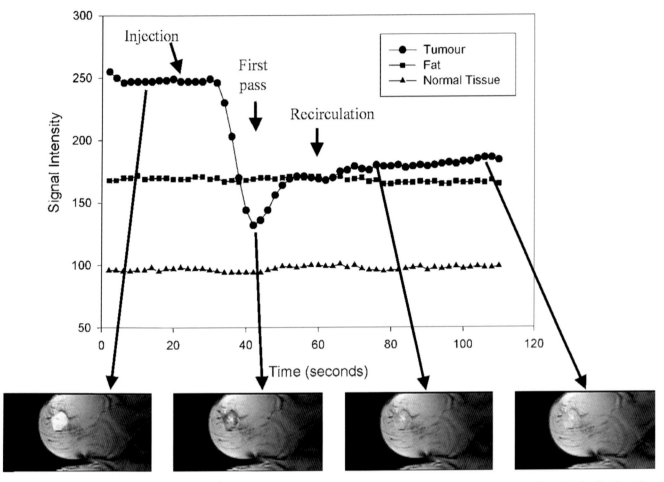

Figure 61.7. *Typical T2*-weighted DCE-MRI study. A patient with breast cancer (same patient illustrated in Figs. 61.8, 61.10 and 61.12). First pass T2* susceptibility effects cause marked darkening of the tumour with no alteration in signal intensity of fibroglandular breast parenchyma or fat. The first pass and recirculation phases can clearly be seen.*

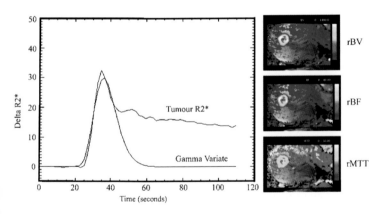

Figure 61.8. *Model fitting of T2*-weighted data and parametric map formation (same patient as illustrated in Figs. 61.7, 61.10 and 61.12). T2* signal intensity data from Fig. 61.7 is converted into R2* (1/T2*) and then fitted with a gamma variate function. Parametric maps representing blood flow kinetics [relative blood volume (top), relative blood flow (middle) and mean transit time (bottom)] are derived on a pixel-by-pixel basis.*

excluding the presence of high-grade tumour in untreated patients regardless of their enhancement characteristics on T1-weighted MR. In low-grade gliomas, homogeneous low rCBV is found, whereas higher-grade tumours display both low and high rCBV components.[68] rCBV images can also be used to direct stereotactic biopsy, to distinguish radiation necrosis from recurrent disease, to determine prognosis and for monitoring response to radiotherapy.

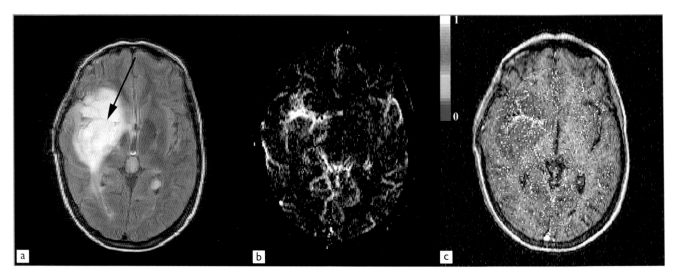

Figure 61.9. *Combined blood volume and permeability MR of low-grade glioma with high blood volume. Data obtained by the Clinical Magnetic Resonance Research Group at the Royal Marsden Hospital, London. (a) Axial FLAIR MR of an untreated Grade II low-grade astrocytoma. There is a large mass in the right cerebral hemisphere with moderate mass effect. A large blood vessel can be seen traversing the mass (arrow). (b) The high signal intensity, rounded areas in the trigone of the left lateral ventricle and in the midline posteriorly are due to cerebrospinal fluid pulsations. Relative cerebral blood volume map at the same slice location derived from a T2* measurement following contrast medium administration. The tumour is noted to be markedly hypervascular particularly around the central blood vessel. The blood volume is increased in a heterogeneous pattern with a blood volume equal to or greater than cortical grey matter. (c) Transfer constant map (colour scale 0–1/min) in the same patient shows that the blood–brain barrier is intact. This glioma subsequently transformed into a high-grade tumour (Grade III).*

Key points: T2*-weighted dynamic magnetic resonance

- T2*-weighted dynamic MR can provide perfusion-weighted images

- rBV, rBF and MTT can be derived from T2*-weighted sequences

- T2*-weighted perfusion imaging is most suited to investigation of brain tumours because the contrast medium is largely retained within the cerebral vascular circulation

T1-weighted dynamic magnetic resonance imaging

Data acquisition

Extracellular contrast media readily diffuse from the blood into the EES of tissues at a rate determined by the permeability of the capillaries and their surface area. Shortening of T1 relaxation rate caused by contrast medium is the mechanism of tissue enhancement. Most DCE-MRI studies employ gradient-echo sequences to monitor the tissue-enhancing effects of contrast media (Fig. 61.10). This is because gradient-echo sequences have good contrast medium sensitivity, high SNR and data acquisition can be performed rapidly. The degree of signal enhancement seen on T1-weighted images is dependent on a number of patho-

physiological and physical factors. These include tissue perfusion, capillary permeability to contrast agent, volume of the extracellular leakage space, native T1-relaxation rate of the tissue, contrast agent dose, imaging sequence used and parameters utilized and on machine scaling factors.

Quantification

Signal enhancement seen on a dynamic acquisition of T1-weighted images can be assessed in two ways: by the analysis of signal intensity changes (semiquantitative) and/or by quantifying contrast agent concentration change using pharmacokinetic modelling techniques. Semiquantitative parameters describe tissue signal intensity enhancement using a number of descriptors. These parameters include onset time (time from injection or appearance in the arterial tree to the arrival of contrast medium in the tissue), gradient of the upslope of enhancement curves, maximum signal intensity and washout gradient. As the rate of enhancement is important for improving the specificity of examinations, parameters that include an additional time element are also used [e.g. maximum intensity time ratio (MITR)[69] and maximum focal enhancement at one minute[70,71]]. The uptake integral or initial area under the time signal curve (initial AUC) has also been studied.[72] For example, Kuhl et al.[73] have successfully correlated the shape of time signal intensity curves with breast lesion histology. Semiquantitative parameters have the advantage of being relatively straightforward to calculate but have a number of

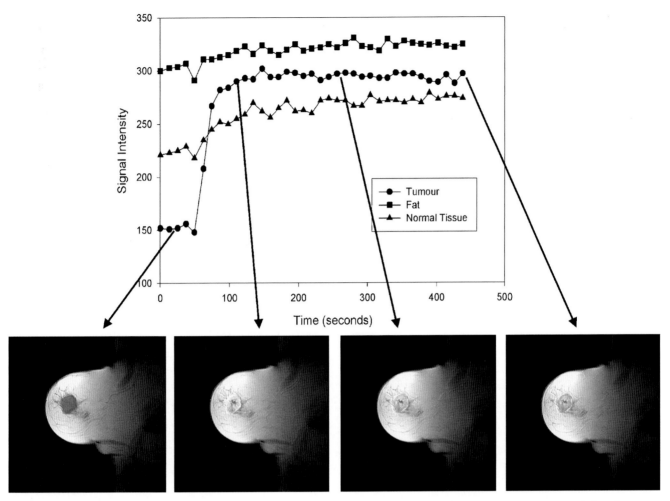

Figure 61.10. *Typical T1-weighted DCE-MRI study (same patient as illustrated in Figs. 61.7, 61.8 and 61.12). Marked and sustained, early ring-like enhancement of the central breast tumour is seen compared to the gradual increase in signal intensity of fibroglandular breast parenchyma and fat. The shape of the curve is markedly different to that seen on T2*-weighted imaging in Fig. 61.7.*

limitations. These limitations include the fact that they do not accurately reflect contrast medium concentration in the tissue of interest and can be influenced by scanner settings (including gain and scaling factors). Semiquantitative parameters have a close but complex and undefined link to underlying tissue physiology and contrast agent kinetics. These factors limit the usefulness of semiquantitative parameters and render comparisons between patients and systems difficult (*vide infra*).

Quantitative techniques use pharmacokinetic modelling techniques that are usually applied to tissue contrast agent concentration changes. Signal intensity changes observed during dynamic acquisition are used to estimate contrast agent concentration *in vivo*.[74,75] Concentration–time curves are then mathematically fitted using one of a number of recognized pharmacokinetic models and quantitative kinetic parameters are derived (Fig. 61.11). For a detailed discussion on pharmacokinetic modelling techniques, the reader is directed to a recent review by Tofts.[76] Examples of modelling parameters include the volume

transfer constant of the contrast agent (K^{tran}) – formally called permeability-surface area product per unit volume of tissue), leakage space as a percentage of unit volume of tissue (v_e) and the rate constant (k_{ep} also called K_{21}). These standard parameters are related mathematically ($k_{ep} = K^{trans}/v_e$) (Fig. 61.6).[51]

Quantitative parameters are more complicated to derive than semiquantitative parameters. The model chosen may not exactly fit the data obtained (Fig. 61.11), and each model makes a number of assumptions that may not be valid for every tissue or tumour type.[51,76] Nonetheless, if contrast agent concentration can be measured accurately and the type, volume and method of administration are consistent, then it is possible to compare pharmacokinetic parameters acquired serially in a given patient and in different patients imaged at the same or different scanning sites.[77,78]

Clinical validation
Many studies have attempted to correlate tissue MR enhancement with immunohistochemical MVD measurements.

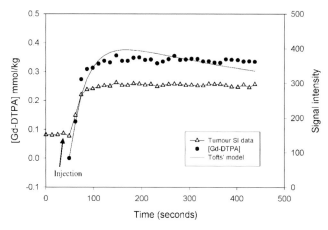

Figure 61.11. *Converting signal intensity into contrast concentration and model fitting. Data obtained from the patient as illustrated in Figs. 61.7, 61.8, 61.10 and 61.12. Contrast medium injection took place after the third data point. Quantification of time signal intensity data (Δ) into contrast agent concentration (●) is performed first according to the method described by Parker et al.[75] The model fitting procedure (continuous line) is done using the Tofts model.[77] Note that model fitting to contrast agent concentration data is not perfect. Calculated quantified parameters are transfer constant = 0.82/min, leakage space 47%, rate constant = 1.74/min.*

Some MR studies have shown broad correlations between T1 kinetic parameters estimates and MVD,[79–82] whereas others have found no correlation.[83,84] Recently, VEGF, a potent vascular permeability and angiogenic factor (see above), has been implicated as an additional explanatory factor which determines MR signal intensity enhancement. Knopp et al.[85] reported that MR vascular permeability to contrast media closely correlated with tissue VEGF expression in breast tumours. The importance of the role of VEGF in determining MR enhancement is supported by the spatial association of hyperpermeable capillaries detected by MMCM-MR and VEGF expression on histological specimens.[86] A correlation between serum VEGF levels and rectal tumour K^trans values has also been reported.[87] Furthermore, the observation that MR kinetic measurements can detect suppression of vascular permeability after antiVEGF antibody[88] and after the administration of inhibitors of VEGF signalling,[89] lends weight to the important role played by VEGF in determining MR enhancement. Other characteristics that have been correlated with enhancement patterns include the degree of stromal cellularity and fibrosis[52,90] and tissue oxygenation.[84,91]

Clinical experience
Analysis of enhancement seen on T1-weighted DCE-MRI is a valuable diagnostic tool in a number of clinical situations. The most established role is in lesion characterization where it has found a role in distinguishing benign from malignant breast and musculoskeletal lesions.[70,92] Dynamic T1-

weighted MR studies have also been found to be of value in staging gynaecological malignancies, bladder and prostate cancers.[93–96] Recently, enhancement parameters have been shown to predict prognosis in patients with cervical cancers; that is, tumours with fast initial rate of enhancement or high vascular flow permeability were more likely to have a poorer prognosis[97] despite having a higher radiotherapy response rate.[98] DCE-MRI studies have also been found to be of value in detecting tumour relapse in the presence of fibrosis within treated tissues of the breast and pelvis.[99–106]

DCE-MRI is also able to predict response or monitor the effects of a variety of treatments. These include neo-adjuvant chemotherapy in bladder and breast cancers and bone sarcomas.[107–111] In breast cancer, for example, it has been shown repeatedly that a progressive decrease in transendothelial permeability accompanies tumour response to chemotherapy and that an increase or no change in permeability can predict non-responsiveness (Figs. 61.12 and 61.13).[111,112] Other treatments that can be monitored include radiotherapy in rectal and cervix cancers,[87,113–115] androgen deprivation in prostate cancer[110] and vascular embolization of uterine fibroids.[116–118] A number of studies have recently reported on the use of T1-weighted DCE-MRI for monitoring the effects of antiangiogenic/antivascular treatments (Fig. 61.14).[89,119] All these response assessment studies show that successful treatment results in a decrease in the rate of enhancement and that poor response results in persistent abnormal enhancement, however judged (semiquantitatively or quantitatively). The lack of specificity of DCE-MRI as a tumour response variable (i.e. it can be affected by most treatments) may reflect the fact that tumour cell kill, no matter how achieved, ultimately results in vascular shut down due to the loss of proangiogenic cytokine secretion, which in turn leads to apoptosis of proliferating endothelial cells.

Key points: T1-weighted dynamic magnetic resonance

- ■ T1-weighted techniques provide both semiquantitative and quantitative data

- ■ Semiquantitative parameters are not accurate for comparing data between patients and between different scanners

- ■ Quantitative data more accurately reflect pathophysiological processes and can be used to compare data serially in a given patient and between different patient groups

- ■ DCE-MRI is useful for distinguishing malignant from benign breast lesions and for monitoring response to treatment of primary breast tumours

- ■ DCE-MRI may be used to distinguish benign from malignant musculoskeletal masses

- ■ DCE-MRI may be helpful for staging, monitoring response and detecting relapse in pelvic malignancies

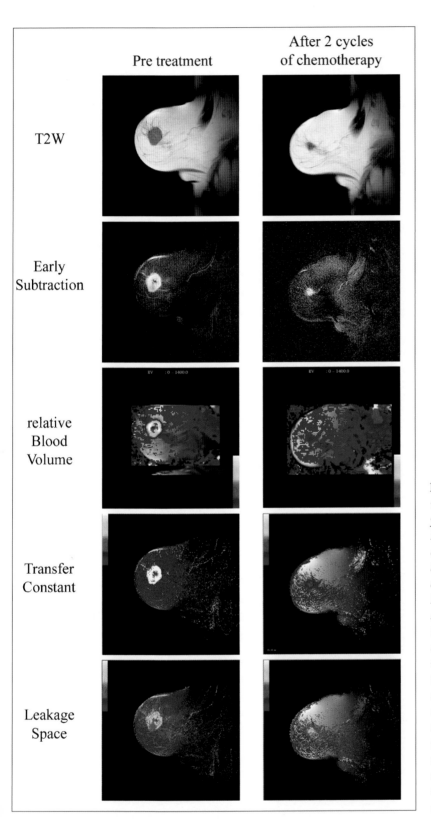

Pre treatment

After 2 cycles
of chemotherapy

T2W

Early
Subtraction

relative
Blood
Volume

Transfer
Constant

Leakage
Space

Figure 61.12. *Monitoring chemotherapy response of breast cancer with DCE-MRI. A 52-year old postmenopausal woman with a Grade III invasive ductal cancer of the breast. Columns depict sample images at identical slice positions before and after two cycles of FEC (5-fluorouracil, epirubicin, cyclophosphamide) chemotherapy. Rows depict T2-weighted anatomical images, subtraction images (obtained by subtracting MRI image acquired at 100 seconds after contrast agent administration from baseline image), relative blood volume map (see Fig. 61.8), transfer constant map (colour range 0–1/min) and leakage space (maximum v_e 100%). With treatment, the number of enhancing pixels is seen to decrease on the subtraction images, with a reduction in relative blood volume and transfer constant. Leakage space changes are least marked. This patient had a complete clinical and radiological response to treatment after six cycles of chemotherapy.*

Magnetic resonance with macromolecular weight contrast media

Extracellular space contrast agents have a high first pass extraction fraction in both normal and abnormal tissues.[50] Macromolecular weight contrast media have molecular sizes that approximate to some serum proteins and have minimal first pass extraction fraction in normal vessels and therefore appear well suited to the measurement of tumour macromolecular hyperpermeability.[50,120,121] Macromolecular weight contrast media are probably delivered to the

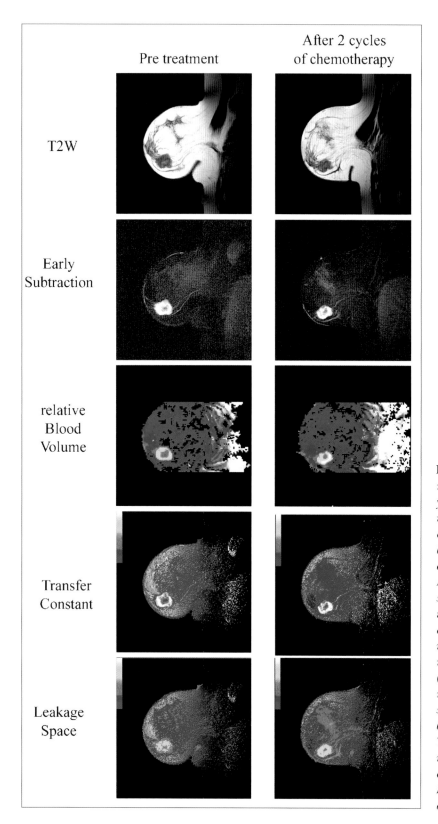

Figure 61.13. *Monitoring chemotherapy non-response of breast cancer with DCE-MRI. A 39-year old premenopausal woman with a Grade III invasive ductal cancer of the breast. Columns depict sample images at identical slice positions before and after two cycles of FEC (5-fluorouracil, epirubicin, cyclophosphamide) chemotherapy. Rows depict T2-weighted anatomical images, subtraction images (obtained by subtracting MR image acquired at 100 seconds after contrast agent administration from baseline image), relative blood volume map, transfer constant map (colour range 0–1/min) and leakage space (maximum v_e 100%). With treatment, the number of enhancing pixels is unchanged on the subtraction images, with no change in relative blood volume, transfer constant or leakage space. This patient had a stable clinical and radiological response to treatment after 6 cycles of chemotherapy and macroscopic, invasive Grade III ductal cancer was noted at pathological evaluation.*

interstitial space by non-specific vesicular transport (vesiculo-vacuolar organelles) or through transendothelial channels.[122] Only preclinical validation of MMCM techniques appears in the literature but approval of agents for human use is expected soon. Albumin-(Gd-DTPA)$_{30}$ is the prototype MMCM (70–90 kDa) but this agent has been found to be immunogenic and has significant retention in the liver and bone.[123] Polylysine-(Gd-DTPA) is not readily biodegradable, which also makes it unsuitable for human use. Other Gd-based MMCM (e.g. Gadomer 17 and the

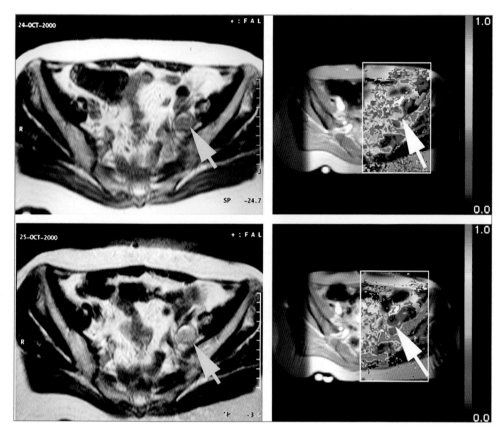

Figure 61.14. *Significant changes in tumour transfer constant following antivascular targeting treatment. Left column: axial T2-weighted MR through the mid-pelvis shows a large, left inferior hypogastric lymph node (arrow) in a patient with malignant peritoneal carcinoma unchanged over a period of a day. Right column: transfer constant map (maximum transfer constant displayed 1.0/min) before (top) and 4 hours after (bottom) administration of Combretastatin (52 mg/m²). A marked reduction in transfer constant is seen in the lymph node particularly in its centre.*

macromolecular Gd-DOTA derivate P792) are currently in advanced clinical trials and licensing for human use for these agents is expected in the near future. Ultrasmall superparamagnetic iron oxide particles (diameter 20–30 nm) have been investigated as MMCM for the evaluation of angiogenesis.[124,125]

Key points: macromolecular contrast agents

- MMCM have molecular sizes that approximate to some serum proteins

- MMCM are well suited to the measurement of tumour macromolecular hyperpermeability

- Currently, MMCM-MR remains in the animal research arena

Imaging vascular function using haemoglobin as a contrast agent

Analysis of vascular function can be accomplished by using deoxyhaemoglobin as an intrinsic, paramagnetic contrast agent (BOLD contrast).[7] Gradient-echo T2*-weighted sequences that are sensitive to changes in blood volume, blood flow and blood oxygenation are used. Blood oxygen level-dependent contrast can be used for mapping changes in blood volume fraction, and vascular functionality associated with angiogenesis.[126,127] Vascular function can be evaluated by analysis of BOLD contrast changes in response to hyperoxia and hypercapnia.[7] Clinical application of this technique by Taylor and colleagues[128] has revealed high signal enhancements in response to carbogen (5% CO_2, 95% O_2) inhalation in human tumours. The primary advantage of BOLD techniques is that there is no need to administer contrast material. Measurements can be repeated as needed with almost no limitation. Blood oxygen level-dependent contrast is not sensitive to fluctuation in permeability. A major reservation for intrinsic contrast imaging is the low contrast-to-noise ratio in the images obtained.

Key points: haemoglobin as a contrast agent

- Deoxyhaemoglobin can be used as an intrinsic contrast agent (BOLD)

- Gradient-echo T2*-weighted sequences sensitive to functional abnormalities associated with angiogenesis are utilized

- BOLD imaging techniques are not currently in routine clinical practice

Future impact of imaging angiogenesis on clinical practice

The data presented in this review show the potential utility of angiogenesis imaging techniques in a variety of clinical situations which include lesion detection, characterization, staging, treatment response and evaluation of residual disease. To date, most studies have been undertaken in breast, musculoskeletal and pelvic cancers.[70,92,99–106] The majority of clinical studies to date have been performed in selected (usually small) patient groups and more studies with sufficient power to define the exact clinical role of these new techniques are required. Examples of such large-scale studies currently underway include screening women at high genetic risk of breast cancer and comprehensive staging of breast cancer.[129]

DCE-MRI techniques will play an important role in the functional assessment of patients treated by antiangiogenic/antivascular therapies.[130] Antiangiogenic drugs prevent the formation of neovasculature and thus require continuous treatment inducing long-term changes in the vasculature. Early drug trials have reported very low toxicity compared with chemotherapy. In contradiction, vascular targeting drugs cause rapid vascular damage that can result in haemorrhagic necrosis of tumours. Their effect on vasculature is reversible, often within hours of a single treatment, and thus requires intermittent administration. Early drug trials have shown that vascular targeting drugs have significant toxicity. The number of antiangiogenic/antivascular compounds entering clinical trials is rapidly increasing, each aimed at different points in the angiogenesis and metastatic cascade.[17] The efficacy of treatment could vary between tumours, and thus the choice of optimal treatment will require information on the biology and functional status of the tumour vasculature. Non-invasive characterization of the angiogenic status of specific tumours may allow rational selection of such treatments. Because antiangiogenic treatments have lower toxicity compared with antivascular treatments and chemotherapy, toxicity-based selection of dose may not be appropriate. The biologically active dose can be defined with DCE-MRI by showing quantitative biological effects specified by a mechanism-based knowledge of drug action. The intrinsic redundancy of signalling mechanisms associated with angiogenesis will lead to partial or complete resistance of the tumour vessels to therapy. Interest in imaging techniques that can provide early indicators of effectiveness at a functional or molecular level has therefore increased. Tumour response to treatment can be detected by imaging techniques that are capable of monitoring changes in perfusion, blood volume or microvessel permeability (Fig. 61.14). Finally, monitoring the therapeutic effects of antiangiogenic therapy is expected to be harder to detect and quantify. This is because antiangiogenic treatments may not result in substantial reductions in tumour volume and conventional size measurements of response may be insensitive or markedly delayed even when there is a significant biological effect. Imaging-based approaches are therefore likely to be valuable for monitoring long-term treatment as well.

Key points: future impact on clinical practice

- Antiangiogenic drugs prevent the development of new tumour blood vessels
- Vascular targeting agents destroy tumour vessels
- DCE-MRI will have an important role in assessing the efficacy of antiangiogenic and antivascular agents

Challenges for angiogenesis imaging techniques

A variety of imaging techniques can evaluate microvascular structure and function but the different parameters measured and different methodologies used for interpreting the data make meaningful comparison between different techniques, different tissue types and different imaging centres very difficult. In order to progress the use of functional imaging in clinical practice, the clinical imaging community must agree on a limited number of examination types and analysis protocols for each modality. This will then permit techniques to be validated and used in clinical trials appropriately. Standardized methods for quantified T1-weighted MR data collection have recently been published.[48,131]

Another issue which needs to be addressed is that of data collection in body parts where there is a large degree of *physiological movement*, such as the lungs and liver. Some techniques, for example PET, are unable to demonstrate heterogeneity within tumours at high spatial resolution and physiological motion appears less of a problem. However, for CT and MR, the presence of motion can invalidate functional vascular parameter estimates.

A practical question posed by many is whether it is necessary to quantify imaging data to answer clinical questions. Simple morphologic contrast enhancement patterns and semiquantitative analyses already work well in a number of clinical situations.[73] However, semiquantitative diagnostic criteria cannot be utilized between centres, particularly when different equipment and sequences are used. *Quantification techniques* aim to minimize errors that can result from the use of different equipment and imaging protocols. Quantification techniques also enable the derivation of kinetic parameters that are based on some understanding of physiological and pathophysiological processes and therefore can provide insight into tumour biology. For example, quantification techniques are preferred when evaluating novel angiogenic interventions.

Measurement error is the variation between measurements of the same quantity on the same individual. An estimate of measurement error determines whether a change in observation represents a real change. Data addressing the precision and measurement variability of angiogenesis imaging techniques is urgently needed and should be an integral part of any new prospective study that evaluates functional response to therapy. Factors that determine measurement error for a given technique also need to be defined. Any imaging assay of tumour microvascular characteristics must be rigorously *validated* against accepted surrogates of angiogenesis. Unfortunately, no single imaging assay or surrogate is able to adequately reflect the whole spectrum of events involved in angiogenesis. Commonly used and appropriate surrogates include histological MVD[31] and vascular maturation index (VMI).[132] Similarly, the imaging assays need to be tested against each other in order to determine their relative utility.

Analysis and presentation of imaging data needs to take into account the heterogeneity of tumour vascular characteristics. Some imaging studies utilize user-defined regions of interest (ROI). Region of interest methods yield graphical outputs with good SNR, but lack spatial resolution and are prone to partial volume averaging errors. In its simplest form, an ROI encompassing the whole tumour is drawn from which an average enhancement curve is extracted. This method ignores heterogeneity of tumour enhancement and many authors have commented that whole-tumour ROI assessment may be inappropriate, particularly for the evaluation of malignant lesions where heterogeneous areas of enhancement are diagnostically important.[65,71,75] Pixel mapping has a number of advantages, including the appreciation of heterogeneity of enhancement and removal for the need to selectively place user-defined ROIs. The risk of missing important diagnostic information and of creating ROIs that contain more than one tissue type is reduced. An important advantage of pixel mapping is the ability to match tumour vascular characteristics spatially such as blood volume, blood flow, permeability and leakage space (Figs. 61.12 and 61.13). Such displays provide unique insights into tumour structure, function and response. Pixel mapping techniques have the disadvantages of having poor SNRs and require specialist software for their generation.

Conclusion

There are well-defined clinical needs to develop non-invasive imaging assays of tumour angiogenesis. Computed tomography scanners are widely available and software for processing data reflecting angiogenesis is freely available or can be readily purchased. Magnetic resonance techniques potentially have greater sensitivity and flexibility. DCE-MRI is the only one of a number of MR techniques that can evaluate tumours with respect to the state of the functional microcirculation. DCE-MRI techniques using ECF agents are far from ideal in this regard and MMCM may well prove superior in the long term. There are a number of challenges that must be met before these techniques can become mainstream diagnostic and research tools. Angiogenesis imaging techniques potentially have widespread clinical applications and their development has been driven by advances in novel anticancer discovery programmes, many of which target the functioning tumour microvasculature. Given the lead-time between the development of a new therapeutic approach or drug in the laboratory and its evaluation in the clinic, radiologists need now to evaluate fully the current and evolving imaging methods for assessing tumour microvascular function.

Summary

- Tumours cannot grow beyond the size of 1–2 mm^3 without a blood supply

- The primary stimulus for angiogenesis is hypoxia

- Angiogenesis is invoked by proangiogenic (e.g. VEGF and FGF) and depressed by antiangiogenic factors (e.g. angiostatin and endostatin). New vessels develop as a result of proliferation and elongation of endothelial cells to form tube-like structures

- Progression from *in situ* cancer to invasive cancer is dependent on angiogenesis

- Tumour vessels show spatial heterogeneity and a chaotic non-hierarchical structure. They are fragile, highly permeable and show intermittent and heterogeneous blood flow

- Structural abnormalities of new vessels result in pathophysiological changes. These changes form the basis of contrast enhancement patterns observed in malignant tumours

- In human tumours, prognosis is related to angiogenesis

- Direct measurement of angiogenesis is performed by MVD counting using immunostaining techniques

- The true vascular density differs from the histological MVD because only 25–85% of a tumour is perfused at any one time

- Indirect measurement of angiogenesis can be performed non-invasively using MR, CT, ultrasound and PET

- MR contrast techniques can assess microvasculature by contrast- and non-contrast-enhanced methods

- Contrast-enhanced MR methods most commonly utilize low molecular weight agents; large (macro)molecular weight agents (MMCM) are designed for prolonged vascular retention

- MMCM are well suited to the measurement of tumour macromolecular hyperpermeability and, currently, MMCM remain in the animal research arena

- In most tissues, low molecular contrast medium rapidly passes into the extravascular space (leakage space v_e) through gaps in the tumour vessel endothelium

- The transfer constant (K^{trans}) describes the transendothelial transport of low molecular weight contrast medium by diffusion

- Relative blood volume (rBV), relative blood flow (rBF) and mean transit time (MTT) can be derived from T2*-weighted sequences

- T2*-weighted perfusion imaging is most suited to investigation of brain tumours because the contrast medium is largely retained within the cerebral vascular circulation

- T1-weighted techniques provide both semiquantitative and quantitative data

- Semiquantitative parameters are not accurate for comparing data between patients examined on different scanners

- Quantitative data more accurately reflect pathophysiological processes and can be used to compare data serially in a given patient and between different patient groups

- DCE-MRI is useful for distinguishing malignant from benign lesions, for staging, for monitoring response to treatment and for detecting relapse in selected cancers

- DCE-MRI has a useful clinical role in the evaluation of breast, musculoskeletal, pelvic and brain tumours

- Deoxyhaemoglobin can be used as an intrinsic contrast agent (BOLD). Gradient-echo T2*-weighted sequences are utilized which are sensitive to functional vascular abnormalities associated with angiogenesis including hypoxia and blood flow

- Antiangiogenic drugs prevent the development of new tumour blood vessels

- DCE-MRI will have an important role in assessing the efficacy of antiangiogenic and antivascular agents

Acknowledgements
The support of Cancer Research UK and the Childwick Trust who support the work of the Clinical Magnetic Resonance Research Group at the Royal Marsden Hospital (where some of the illustrated work originates) and at the Paul Strickland Scanner Centre, respectively, is gratefully acknowledged. I am grateful to Dr Jane Taylor for assistance in the preparation of the illustrative material for this chapter.

References

1. Conway E M, Collen D, Carmeliet P. Molecular mechanisms of blood vessel growth. Cardiovasc Res 2001; 49: 507–521

2. Folkman J. Angiogenesis in cancer, vascular, rheumatoid and other disease. Nat Med 1995; 1: 27–31

3. Parker G J, Tofts P S. Pharmacokinetic analysis of neoplasms using contrast-enhanced dynamic magnetic resonance imaging. Top Magn Reson Imaging 1999; 10: 130–142

4. Padhani A R. Dynamic contrast-enhanced MRI in clinical oncology: current status and future directions. J Magn Reson Imaging 2002; 16: 407–422

5. Knopp M V, Giesel F L, von Marcos H et al. Dynamic contrast-enhanced magnetic resonance imaging in oncology. Top Magn Reson Imag 2001; 12: 301–308

6. Brasch R, Turetschek K. MRI characterization of tumors and grading angiogenesis using macromolecular contrast media: status report. Eur J Radiol 2000; 34: 148–155

7. Howe F A, Robinson S P, McIntyre D J et al. Issues in flow and oxygenation dependent contrast (FLOOD) imaging of tumours. NMR Biomed 2001; 14: 497–506

8. Miles K A. Functional computed tomography in oncology. Eur J Cancer 2002; 38: 2079–2084

9. Haroon Z A, Peters K, Greenberg C et al. Angiogenesis and oxygen transport in solid tumors. In: Teicher B (ed). Antiangiogenic Agents in Cancer Therapy. 1998; 3–21

10. Voest E E, D'Amore P A. Tumor angiogenesis and microcirculation. New York: Marcel Dekker, 2001

11. Gray L H, Conger A D, Ebert M. The concentration of oxygen dissolved in tissues at the time of irradiation as a factor in radiotherapy. Br J Radiol 1953; 26: 638–648

12. Holash J, Wiegand S J, Yancopoulos G D. New model of tumor angiogenesis: dynamic balance between vessel regression and growth mediated by angiopoietins and VEGF. Oncogene 1999; 18: 5356–5362

13. Secomb T W, Hsu R, Braun R D et al. Theoretical simulation of oxygen transport to tumors by three-dimensional networks of microvessels. Adv Exp Med Biol 1998; 454: 629–634

14. Raleigh J A, Calkins-Adams D P, Rinker L H et al. Hypoxia and vascular endothelial growth factor expression in human squamous cell carcinomas using pimonidazole as a hypoxia marker. Cancer Res 1998; 58: 3765–3768

15. Lawrence W T. Physiology of the acute wound. Clin Plast Surg 1998; 25: 321–340

16. Benjamin L E, Golijanin D, Itin A et al. Selective ablation of immature blood vessels in established human tumors follows vascular endothelial growth factor withdrawal. J Clin Invest 1999; 103: 159–165

17. Kaban K, Herbst R S. Angiogenesis as a target for cancer therapy. Hematol Oncol Clin North Am 2002; 16: 1125–1171

18. Hahnfeldt P, Panigrahy D, Folkman J, Hlatky L. Tumor development under angiogenic signaling: a dynamical theory of tumor growth, treatment response, and postvascular dormancy. Cancer Res 1999; 59: 4770–4775

19. Folkman J. New perspectives in clinical oncology from angiogenesis research. Eur J Cancer 1996; 32A: 2534–2539

20. Darland D C, D'Amore P A. Blood vessel maturation: vascular development comes of age. J Clin Invest 1999; 103: 157–158

21. Dvorak H F, Nagy J A, Feng D et al. Vascular permeability factor/vascular endothelial growth factor and the significance of microvascular hyperpermeability in angiogenesis. Curr Top Microbiol Immunol 1999; 237: 97–132

22. Dewhirst M W. Angiogenesis and blood flow in solid tumors. In: Teicher B (ed). Drug Resistance in Oncology. New York: Marcel Dekker, 1993; 3–24

23. Braun R D, Lanzen J L, Dewhirst M W. Fourier analysis of fluctuations of oxygen tension and blood flow in R3230Ac tumors and muscle in rats. Am J Physiol 1999; 277 (2 Pt 2): H551–568

24. Rak J W, St Croix B D, Kerbel R S. Consequences of angiogenesis for tumor progression, metastasis and cancer therapy. Anticancer Drugs 1995; 6: 3–18

25. Gilles R, Zafrani B, Guinebretiere J M et al. Ductal carcinoma in situ: MR imaging–histopathologic correlation. Radiology 1995; 196: 415–419

26. Peters K G, Coogan A, Berry D et al. Expression of Tie2/Tek in breast tumour vasculature provides a new marker for evaluation of tumour angiogenesis. Br J Cancer 1998; 77: 51–56

27. Gasparini G, Toi M, Miceli R et al. Clinical relevance of vascular endothelial growth factor and thymidine phosphorylase in patients with node-positive breast cancer treated with either adjuvant chemotherapy or hormone therapy. Cancer J Sci Am 1999; 5: 101–111

28. Obermair A, Kucera E, Mayerhofer K et al. Vascular endothelial growth factor (VEGF) in human breast cancer: correlation with disease-free survival. Int J Cancer 1997; 74: 455–458

29. Linderholm B, Tavelin B, Grankvist K, Henriksson R. Vascular endothelial growth factor is of high prognostic value in node-negative breast carcinoma. J Clin Oncol 1998; 16: 3121–3128

30. Weidner N. Tumoural vascularity as a prognostic factor in cancer patients: the evidence continues to grow. J Pathol 1998; 184: 119–22

31. Vermeulen P B, Gasparini G, Fox S B et al. Quantification of angiogenesis in solid human tumours: an international consensus on the methodology and criteria of evaluation. Eur J Cancer 1996; 32A: 2474–2484

32. Kerckhaert O A, Voest E E. The prognostic and diagnostic value of circulating angiogenic factors in cancer patients. In: Voest E E, D'Amore P A (eds).

Tumor Angiogenesis and Microcirculation. New York: Marcel Dekker, 2001; 487–500

33. Endrich B, Vaupel P. The role of microcirculation in the treatment of malignant tumors: facts and fiction. In: Vaupel P (ed). Blood Perfusion and Microenvironment of Human Tumors. Berlin: Springer-Verlag, 1998; 19–39

34. Blomley M J, Coulden R, Bufkin C, Lipton M J, Dawson P. Contrast bolus dynamic computed tomography for the measurement of solid organ perfusion. Invest Radiol 1993; 28 (Suppl 5): S72–77; discussion S78

35. Miles K A, Leggett D A, Kelley B B et al. In vivo assessment of neovascularization of liver metastases using perfusion CT. Br J Radiol 1998; 71: 276–281

36. Harvey C, Dooher A, Morgan J, Blomley M, Dawson P. Imaging of tumour therapy responses by dynamic CT. Eur J Radiol 1999; 30: 221–226

37. Ferrara K W, Merritt C R, Burns PN et al. Evaluation of tumor angiogenesis with US: imaging, Doppler, and contrast agents. Acad Radiol 2000; 7: 824–839

38. Cheng W F, Lee C N, Chu J S et al. Vascularity index as a novel parameter for the in vivo assessment of angiogenesis in patients with cervical carcinoma. Cancer 1999; 85: 651–657

39. Correas J M, Bridal L, Lesavre A et al. Ultrasound contrast agents: properties, principles of action, tolerance, and artifacts. Eur Radiol 2001; 11: 1316–1328

40. Jakobsen J A. Ultrasound contrast agents: clinical applications. Eur Radiol 2001; 11: 1329–1337

41. Cosgrove D, Eckersley R, Blomley M, Harvey C. Quantification of blood flow. Eur Radiol 2001; 11: 1338–1344

42. Blankenberg F G, Eckelman W C, Strauss H W et al. Role of radionuclide imaging in trials of antiangiogenic therapy. Acad Radiol 2000; 7: 851–867

43. Wilson C B, Lammertsma A A, McKenzie C G et al. Measurements of blood flow and exchanging water space in breast tumors using positron emission tomography: a rapid and noninvasive dynamic method. Cancer Res 1992; 52: 1592–1597

44. Leenders K L. PET: blood flow and oxygen consumption in brain tumors. J Neuro-oncol 1994; 22: 269–273

45. Bhujwalla Z M, Artemov D, Glockner J. Tumor angiogenesis, vascularization, and contrast-enhanced magnetic resonance imaging. Top Magn Reson Imaging 1999; 10: 92–103

46. Gillies R J, Bhujwalla Z M, Evelhoch J et al. Applications of magnetic resonance in model systems: tumor biology and physiology. Neoplasia 2000; 2: 139–151

47. Neeman M, Provenzale J M, Dewhirst M W. Magnetic resonance imaging applications in the evaluation of tumor angiogenesis. Semin Radiat Oncol 2001; 11: 70–82

48. Brasch R C, Li K C, Husband J E et al. In vivo monitoring of tumor angiogenesis with MR imaging. Acad Radiol 2000; 7: 812–823

49. Weissleder R, Mahmood U. Molecular imaging. Radiology 2001; 219: 316–333

50. Daldrup HE, Shames DM, Husseini W et al. Quantification of the extraction fraction for gadopentetate across breast cancer capillaries. Magn Reson Med 1998; 40: 537–543

51. Tofts P S, Brix G, Buckley D L et al. Estimating kinetic parameters from dynamic contrast-enhanced T(1)-weighted MRI of a diffusable tracer: standardized quantities and symbols. J Magn Reson Imaging 1999; 10: 223–232

52. Matsubayashi R, Matsuo Y, Edakuni G et al. Breast masses with peripheral rim enhancement on dynamic contrast-enhanced MR images: correlation of MR findings with histologic features and expression of growth factors. Radiology 2000; 217: 841–848

53. Barbier E L, Lamalle L, Decorps M. Methodology of brain perfusion imaging. J Magn Reson Imaging 2001; 13: 496–520

54. Sorensen A G, Tievsky A L, Ostergaard L et al. Contrast agents in functional MR imaging. J Magn Reson Imaging 1997; 7: 47–55

55. Simonsen C Z, Ostergaard L, Smith D F et al. Comparison of gradient- and spin-echo imaging: CBF, CBV, and MTT measurements by bolus tracking. J Magn Reson Imaging 2000; 12: 411–416

56. Dennie J, Mandeville J B, Boxerman J L, Packard et al. NMR imaging of changes in vascular morphology due to tumor angiogenesis. Magn Reson Med 1998; 40: 793–799

57. Bruening R, Berchtenbreiter C, Holzknecht N et al. Effects of three different doses of a bolus injection of gadodiamide: assessment of regional cerebral blood volume maps in a blinded reader study. Am J Neuroradiol 2000; 21: 1603–1610

58. Rosen B R, Belliveau J W, Buchbinder B R et al. Contrast agents and cerebral hemodynamics. Magn Reson Med 1991; 19: 285–292

59. Wenz F, Rempp K, Brix G et al. Age dependency of the regional cerebral blood volume (rCBV) measured with dynamic susceptibility contrast MR imaging (DSC). Magn Reson Imaging 1996; 14: 157–162

60. Wenz F, Rempp K, Hess T et al. Effect of radiation on blood volume in low-grade astrocytomas and normal brain tissue: quantification with dynamic susceptibility contrast MR imaging. Am J Roentgenol 1996; 166: 187–193

61. Moseley M E, Vexler Z, Asgari H S et al. Comparison of Gd- and Dy-chelates for T2 contrast-enhanced imaging. Magn Reson Med 1991; 22: 259–264

62. Reimer P, Schuierer G, Balzer T, Peters P E. Application of a superparamagnetic iron oxide (Resovist) for MR imaging of human cerebral blood volume. Magn Reson Med 1995; 34: 694–697

63. Cha S, Lu S, Johnson G, Knopp E A. Dynamic susceptibility contrast MR imaging: correlation of signal intensity changes with cerebral blood volume measurements. J Magn Reson Imaging 2000; 11: 114–119

64. Maeda M, Itoh S, Kimura H et al. Tumor vascularity in

the brain: evaluation with dynamic susceptibility-contrast MR imaging. Radiology 1993; 189: 233–238

65. Aronen H J, Gazit I E, Louis D N et al. Cerebral blood volume maps of gliomas: comparison with tumor grade and histologic findings. Radiology 1994; 191: 41–51

66. Siegal T, Rubinstein R, Tzuk-Shina T, Gomori J M. Utility of relative cerebral blood volume mapping derived from perfusion magnetic resonance imaging in the routine follow up of brain tumors. J Neurosurg 1997; 86: 22–27

67. Sugahara T, Korogi Y, Kochi M et al. Correlation of MR imaging-determined cerebral blood volume maps with histologic and angiographic determination of vascularity of gliomas. Am J Roentgenol 1998; 171: 1479–1486

68. Aronen H J, Glass J, Pardo F S et al. Echo-planar MR cerebral blood volume mapping of gliomas. Clinical utility. Acta Radiol 1995; 36: 520–528

69. Flickinger F W, Allison J D, Sherry R M, Wright J C. Differentiation of benign from malignant breast masses by time-intensity evaluation of contrast enhanced MRI. Magn Reson Imaging 1993; 11: 617–620

70. Kaiser W A, Zeitler E. MR imaging of the breast: fast imaging sequences with and without Gd-DTPA. Preliminary observations. Radiology 1989; 170: 681–686

71. Gribbestad I S, Nilsen G, Fjosne H E et al. Comparative signal intensity measurements in dynamic gadolinium-enhanced MR mammography. J Magn Reson Imaging 1994; 4: 477–480

72. Evelhoch J L. Key factors in the acquisition of contrast kinetic data for oncology. J Magn Reson Imaging 1999; 10: 254–259

73. Kuhl C K, Mielcareck P, Klaschik S et al. Dynamic breast MR imaging: are signal intensity time course data useful for differential diagnosis of enhancing lesions? Radiology 1999; 211: 101–110

74. Parker G J, Baustert I, Tanner S F, Leach M O. Improving image quality and T(1) measurements using saturation recovery turboFLASH with an approximate K-space normalisation filter. Magn Reson Imaging 2000; 18: 157–167

75. Parker G J, Suckling J, Tanner S F et al. Probing tumor microvascularity by measurement, analysis and display of contrast agent uptake kinetics. J Magn Reson Imaging 1997; 7: 564–574

76. Tofts P S. Modeling tracer kinetics in dynamic Gd-DTPA MR imaging. J Magn Reson Imaging 1997; 7: 91–101

77. Tofts P S, Berkowitz B, Schnall M D. Quantitative analysis of dynamic Gd-DTPA enhancement in breast tumors using a permeability model. Magn Reson Med 1995; 33: 564–568

78. den Boer J A, Hoenderop R K, Smink J et al. Pharmacokinetic analysis of Gd-DTPA enhancement in dynamic three-dimensional MRI of breast lesions. J Magn Reson Imaging 1997; 7: 702–715

79. Stomper P C, Winston J S, Herman S et al. Angiogenesis and dynamic MR imaging gadolinium enhancement of malignant and benign breast lesions. Breast Cancer Res Treat 1997; 45: 39–46

80. Hawighorst H, Knapstein P G, Weikel W et al. Angiogenesis of uterine cervical carcinoma: characterization by pharmacokinetic magnetic resonance parameters and histological microvessel density with correlation to lymphatic involvement. Cancer Res 1997; 57: 4777–4786

81. Tynninen O, Aronen H J, Ruhala M et al. MRI enhancement and microvascular density in gliomas. Correlation with tumor cell proliferation. Invest Radiol 1999; 34: 427–434

82. Buckley D L, Drew P J, Mussurakis S et al. Microvessel density of invasive breast cancer assessed by dynamic Gd-DTPA enhanced MRI. J Magn Reson Imaging 1997; 7: 461–464

83. Hulka C A, Edmister W B, Smith B L et al. Dynamic echo-planar imaging of the breast: experience in diagnosing breast carcinoma and correlation with tumor angiogenesis. Radiology 1997; 205: 837–842

84. Cooper R A, Carrington B M, Loncaster J A et al. Tumour oxygenation levels correlate with dynamic contrast-enhanced magnetic resonance imaging parameters in carcinoma of the cervix. Radiother Oncol 2000; 57: 53–59

85. Knopp M V, Weiss E, Sinn H P et al. Pathophysiologic basis of contrast enhancement in breast tumors. J Magn Reson Imaging 1999; 10: 260–266

86. Bhujwalla Z M, Artemov D, Natarajan K et al Vascular differences detected by MRI for metastatic versus nonmetastatic breast and prostate cancer xenografts. Neoplasia 2001; 3: 143–153

87. George M L, Dzik-Jurasz A S, Padhani A R et al. Non-invasive methods of assessing angiogenesis and their value in predicting response to treatment in colorectal cancer. Br J Surg 2001; 88: 1628–1636

88. Pham C D, Roberts T P, van Bruggen N et al. Magnetic resonance imaging detects suppression of tumor vascular permeability after administration of antibody to vascular endothelial growth factor. Cancer Invest 1998; 16: 225–230

89. Thomas A, Morgan B, Drevs J et al. Pharmacodynamic results using dynamic contrast-enhanced magnetic resonance imaging, of two phase I studies of the VEGF inhibitor PTK787/ZK 222584 in patients with liver metastases from colorectal cancer. Proc Am Soc Clin Oncol 2001; A279

90. Yamashita Y, Baba T, Baba Y et al. Dynamic contrast-enhanced MR imaging of uterine cervical cancer: pharmacokinetic analysis with histopathologic correlation and its importance in predicting the outcome of radiation therapy. Radiology 2000; 216: 803–809

91. Lyng H, Vorren A O, Sundfor K et al. Assessment of tumor oxygenation in human cervical carcinoma by use of dynamic Gd-DTPA-enhanced MR imaging. J Magn Reson Imaging 2001; 14: 750–756

92. van der Woude H J, Verstraete K L, Hogendoorn P C et

al. Musculoskeletal tumors: does fast dynamic contrast-enhanced subtraction MR imaging contribute to the characterization? Radiology 1998; 208: 821–828

93. Liu P F, Krestin G P, Huch R A et al. MRI of the uterus, uterine cervix, and vagina: diagnostic performance of dynamic contrast-enhanced fast multiplanar gradient-echo imaging in comparison with fast spin-echo T2-weighted pulse imaging. Eur Radiol 1998; 8: 1433–1440

94. Barentsz J O, Jager G J, van Vierzen P B et al. Staging urinary bladder cancer after transurethral biopsy: value of fast dynamic contrast-enhanced MR imaging. Radiology 1996; 201: 185–193

95. Jager G J, Ruijter E T, van de Kaa C A et al. Dynamic TurboFLASH subtraction technique for contrast-enhanced MR imaging of the prostate: correlation with histopathologic results. Radiology 1997; 203: 645–652

96. Huch Boni R A, Boner J A, Lutolf U M et al. Contrast-enhanced endorectal coil MRI in local staging of prostate carcinoma. J Comput Assist Tomogr 1995; 19: 232–237

97. Hawighorst H, Weikel W, Knapstein P G et al. Angiogenic activity of cervical carcinoma: assessment by functional magnetic resonance imaging-based parameters and a histomorphological approach in correlation with disease outcome. Clin Cancer Res 1998; 4: 2305–2312

98. Mayr N A, Yuh W T, Magnotta V A et al. Tumor perfusion studies using fast magnetic resonance imaging technique in advanced cervical cancer: a new noninvasive predictive assay. Int J Radiat Oncol Biol Phys 1996; 36: 623–633

99. Gilles R, Guinebretiere J M, Shapeero L G et al. Assessment of breast cancer recurrence with contrast-enhanced subtraction MR imaging: preliminary results in 26 patients. Radiology 1993; 188: 473–478

100. Kerslake R W, Fox J N, Carleton P J et al. Dynamic contrast-enhanced and fat suppressed magnetic resonance imaging in suspected recurrent carcinoma of the breast: preliminary experience. Br J Radiol 1994; 67: 1158–1168

101. Mussurakis S, Buckley D L, Bowsley S J et al. Dynamic contrast-enhanced magnetic resonance imaging of the breast combined with pharmacokinetic analysis of gadolinium-DTPA uptake in the diagnosis of local recurrence of early stage breast carcinoma. Invest Radiol 1995; 30: 650–662

102. Kinkel K, Tardivon A A, Soyer P et al. Dynamic contrast-enhanced subtraction versus T2-weighted spin-echo MR imaging in the follow-up of colorectal neoplasm: a prospective study of 41 patients. Radiology 1996; 200: 453–458

103. Hawnaur J M, Zhu X P, Hutchinson C E. Quantitative dynamic contrast enhanced MRI of recurrent pelvic masses in patients treated for cancer. Br J Radiol 1998; 71: 1136–1142

104. Dao T H, Rahmouni A, Campana F et al. Tumor recurrence versus fibrosis in the irradiated breast:

differentiation with dynamic gadolinium-enhanced MR imaging. Radiology 1993; 187: 751–755

105. Heywang-Kobrunner S H, Schlegel A, Beck R et al. Contrast-enhanced MRI of the breast after limited surgery and radiation therapy. J Comput Assist Tomogr 1993; 17: 891–900

106. Blomqvist L, Fransson P, Hindmarsh T. The pelvis after surgery and radio-chemotherapy for rectal cancer studied with Gd-DTPA-enhanced fast dynamic MR imaging. Eur Radiol 1998; 8: 781–787

107. Barentsz J O, Berger-Hartog O, Witjes J A et al. Evaluation of chemotherapy in advanced urinary bladder cancer with fast dynamic contrast-enhanced MR imaging. Radiology 1998; 207: 791–797

108. Reddick W E, Taylor J S, Fletcher B D. Dynamic MR imaging (DEMRI) of microcirculation in bone sarcoma. J Magn Reson Imaging 1999; 10: 277–285

109. van der Woude H J, Bloem J L, Verstraete K L et al. Osteosarcoma and Ewing's sarcoma after neoadjuvant chemotherapy: value of dynamic MR imaging in detecting viable tumor before surgery. Am J Roentgenol 1995; 165: 593–598

110. Padhani A R, MacVicar A D, Gapinski C J et al. Effects of androgen deprivation on prostatic morphology and vascular permeability evaluated with MR imaging. Radiology 2001; 218: 365–374

111. Knopp M V, Brix G, Junkermann H J, Sinn H P. MR mammography with pharmacokinetic mapping for monitoring of breast cancer treatment during neoadjuvant therapy. Magn Reson Imaging Clin N Am 1994; 2: 633–658

112. Padhani A R, Hayes C, Assersohn L et al. Response of breast carcinoma to chemotherapy – MR permeability changes using histogram analysis. In: International Society for Magnetic Resonance in Medicine, 8th Scientific meeting, Denver, Colorado, 2000; 2160

113. Devries A F, Griebel J, Kremser C et al. Tumor microcirculation evaluated by dynamic magnetic resonance imaging predicts therapy outcome for primary rectal carcinoma. Cancer Res 2001; 61: 2513–2516

114. de Vries A, Griebel J, Kremser C et al. Monitoring of tumor microcirculation during fractionated radiation therapy in patients with rectal carcinoma: preliminary results and implications for therapy. Radiology 2000; 217: 385–391

115. Mayr N A, Yuh W T, Arnholt J C et al. Pixel analysis of MR perfusion imaging in predicting radiation therapy outcome in cervical cancer. J Magn Reson Imaging 2000; 12: 1027–1033

116. Burn P R, McCall J M, Chinn R J et al. Uterine fibroleiomyoma: MR imaging appearances before and after embolization of uterine arteries. Radiology 2000; 214: 729–734

117. Jha R C, Ascher S M, Imaoka I, Spies J B. Symptomatic fibroleiomyomata: MR imaging of the uterus before and after uterine arterial embolization. Radiology 2000; 217: 228–235

118. Li W, Brophy D P, Chen Q et al. Semiquantitative assessment of uterine perfusion using first pass dynamic contrast-enhanced MR imaging for patients treated with uterine fibroid embolization. J Magn Reson Imaging 2000; 12: 1004–1008

119. Galbraith S M, Taylor N J, Maxwell R et al. Combretastatin A4 phosphate reduces tumour blood flow in animal and man, demonstrated by MRI. Proc Am Soc Clin Oncol 2001; A279

120. Su M Y, Muhler A, Lao X, Nalcioglu O. Tumor characterization with dynamic contrast-enhanced MRI using MR contrast agents of various molecular weights. Magn Reson Med 1998; 39: 259–269

121. Roberts T P, Roberts H C, Brasch R C. Optimizing imaging techniques to reduce errors in microvascular quantitation with macromolecular MR contrast agents. Acad Radiol 1998; 5 (Suppl 1): S133–136

122. Dvorak A M, MacGlashan D W Jr, Morgan E S, Lichtenstein L M. Vesicular transport of histamine in stimulated human basophils. Blood 1996; 88: 4090–4101

123. Schmiedl U, Ogan M, Paajanen H et al. Albumin labeled with Gd-DTPA as an intravascular, blood pool-enhancing agent for MR imaging: biodistribution and imaging studies. Radiology 1987; 162: 205–210

124. Turetschek K, Roberts T P, Floyd E et al. Tumor microvascular characterization using ultrasmall superparamagnetic iron oxide particles (USPIO) in an experimental breast cancer model. J Magn Reson Imaging 2001; 13: 882–888

125. Turetschek K, Huber S, Floyd E et al. MR imaging characterization of microvessels in experimental breast tumors by using a particulate contrast agent with histopathologic correlation. Radiology 2001; 218: 562–569

126. Abramovitch R, Dafni H, Smouha E et al. In vivo prediction of vascular susceptibility to vascular endothelial growth factor withdrawal: magnetic resonance imaging of C6 rat glioma in nude mice. Cancer Res 1999; 59: 5012–5016

127. Neeman M, Dafni H, Bukhari O et al. In vivo BOLD contrast MRI mapping of subcutaneous vascular function and maturation: validation by intravital microscopy. Magn Reson Med 2001; 45: 887–898

128. Taylor N J, Baddeley H, Goodchild K A et al. BOLD MRI of human tumor oxygenation during carbogen breathing. J Magn Reson Imaging 2001; 14: 156–163

129. Brown J, Buckley D, Coulthard A et al. Magnetic resonance imaging screening in women at genetic risk of breast cancer: imaging and analysis protocol for the UK multicentre study. UK MRI Breast Screening Study Advisory Group. Magn Reson Imaging 2000; 18: 765–776

130. Padhani A R, Neeman M. Challenges for imaging angiogenesis. Br J Radiol 2001; 74: 886–890

131. Evelhoch J, Brown T, Chenevert T et al. Consensus recommendation for acquisition of dynamic contrast-enhanced MRI data in oncology. In: Proceedings of the International Society of Magnetic Resonance in Medicine, Denver, Colarado, 2000; 1439

132. Eberhard A, Kahlert S, Goede V et al. Heterogeneity of angiogenesis and blood vessel maturation in human tumors: implications for antiangiogenic tumor therapies. Cancer Res 2000; 60: 1388–1393

Chapter 62

Molecular imaging in cancer treatment: positron emission tomography

Nishi Gupta and Patricia Price

Introduction

The term molecular imaging can be broadly defined as the 'in vivo characterization and measurement of biological processes at the cellular and molecular level'.[1] The explosion in molecular imaging in oncology has emerged from the joining of two powerful forces. Great strides have been made in molecular science to increase our knowledge of tumour biology, particularly with regard to the molecular basis of cell cycle control and proliferation, with cancer viewed as a series of biological processes rather than a single disease entity. This has coincided with extensive advances in nuclear imaging technology, based on improved electronics, greater computing power, better sensitivity, resolution and new tracers for key molecules that facilitate cancer growth and development.[2] New insights into the genetic and molecular biological basis of cancer have resulted in a fundamental reordering of drug discovery and therapeutic approaches from empirical observations, towards rational drug discovery based on molecular sites of action. Treatment strategies have therefore altered to assimilate the evolving identification of abnormal pathways in cancer biology. This has required a paradigm shift in the demands on imaging, from solely providing rigid structural and anatomical details with conventional X-rays, to providing *in vivo* methods to detect and characterize cellular and biochemical changes in the cancer cell itself. Such imaging techniques will not only assist in the diagnosis of malignancy, but assess the efficacy of novel treatments such as gene therapy, enable earlier response detection to therapy, particularly to cytostatic drugs, contribute to logical drug development, visualization of specific molecular pathways such as apoptosis and angiogenesis, as well as answering important questions in clinical translational research.

Over the last 10 years, the potential role of positron emission tomography (PET) in molecular imaging has become increasingly recognized in the clinical and preclinical settings. The advantages of PET in this context manifests from its unrivalled sensitivity, providing quantitative kinetic information down to the subpicomolar level, with high specificity and temporal resolution,[3,4] although spatial resolution is less compared to magnetic resonance (MR) imaging and computed tomography (CT).[5]

The process of PET imaging involves replacement of a molecule in a compound of interest with a positron emitting isotope without modifying pharmaceutical, biological or biochemical properties (PET probe or radiotracer). Radiotracers are usually produced in a cyclotron and most have short half-lives (see Table 62.1), which is ideal for clinical studies by producing a high initial signal intensity, minimizing radiation exposure to the patient and allowing multiple scans in the same subject. The radiotracer is injected into the patient after the patient has been positioned in the PET scanner for image acquisition (Fig. 62.1). The positrons that are emitted from decay of the isotope interact with a positively charged electron locally, resulting in the simultaneous release of two 511 KeV gamma rays at 180° to one another (Fig. 62.2), which are recorded by a ring of external detectors, with the inference that the decay event occurred between the two opposing detectors.

Positron emission tomography images are reconstructed tomographically after correction for attenuation and detector efficiency. Advanced, complex mathematical modelling has been developed to derive quantitative data[6-8] of, for example, delivery and retention components, combining information from time radioactivity curves in regions of interest from dynamic PET images and continuous and discrete sampling of arterial blood. One limitation of PET analysis is that it is not possible to distinguish between radiolabelled metabolites and radiolabelled parent as they both produce an identical signal on the image.

Table 62.1. *Cyclotron-generated positron emitters*

Radioisotope	Half-life	Positron decay (%)
Carbon-11	20.4 min	99.8
Copper-62	9.7 min	97.8
Copper-64	12.7 h	19.3
Fluorine-18	109.8 min	96.9
Gallium-68	68.1 min	90
Iodine-124	4.2 days	25
Nitrogen-13	10 min	100
Oxygen-15	2.03 min	99.9

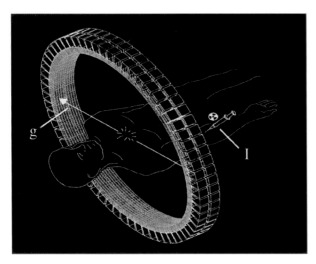

Figure 62.1. *Patient in PET scanner. Intravenous injection (I) of radiolabelled tracer. Two 511 KeV gamma rays (g) are emitted simultaneously and at 180° to one another, are recorded by a ring of detectors. (Courtesy of Imaging Research Solutions Ltd.)*

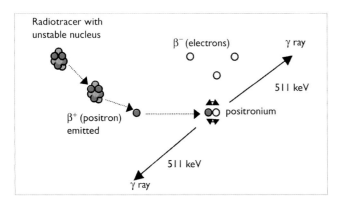

Figure 62.2. *The basic principles of PET. The unstable nucleus decays naturally by emitting a positron (blue) to leave a stable nucleus. The positron travels a short distance in tissue before colliding with a surrounding electron (yellow) and forms a positronium. Almost instantaneously, the positronium disintegrates, forming two gamma rays (γ).*

Approaches to extract the parent contribution from total measured radioactivity include performing a separate radiolabelled metabolite scan[9] or employing mathematical modelling of metabolites.[10]

Positron emission tomography imaging with 2-[F-18]fluoro-2-deoxy-D-glucose ([18]FDG PET) has dominated the field of oncology for the last two decades. An observation by Warburg in the 1930s that malignant tumours have increased glycolytic rate compared to normal tissue was followed in the 1980s with studies by Di Chiro, who showed that the degree of malignancy of cerebral tumours was correlated with their [18]FDG uptake.[11–13] After systemic delivery, [18]FDG initially follows the same metabolic pathway as glucose, and is transferred into cells by specific glucose transporters (GLUT-1) and is then phosphorylated into

[18]FDG-6-phosphate by hexokinase. Unlike glucose, [18]FDG-6-phosphate is trapped and accumulates within the cell as it lacks a hydroxyl group and cannot act as a substrate for further glycolysis.[14,15] Although [18]FDG uptake is not specific to neoplastic cells, the role of [18]FDG in current clinical applications in oncology is diverse and includes:

- Preoperative detection and staging of disease
- Detection of recurrence
- Differentiation between recurrence and scarring post treatment
- Evaluating response to treatment[16]
- Determination of biopsy site

Despite the fact that 95% of all clinical PET scans use [18]FDG,[17] the future challenge for PET imaging lies in the development of novel PET radiotracers (or molecular PET probes) to fulfil its expectation in the arena of molecular imaging and cancer treatment. The complexities of PET require a multidisciplinary approach with involvement of experts from molecular biology, chemistry, pharmacology, genetics, physics, imaging sciences, computer sciences and clinical oncology to achieve this goal. This chapter will give an overview of the new advances and potential opportunities that PET imaging can offer in a wide range of molecular processes and treatment strategies in oncology.

Key points: molecular imaging in positron emission tomography

- ■ Inherent sensitivity and specificity of PET constitute its most important strengths

- ■ PET is a complex technology requiring an expert, multidisciplinary, interactive team

- ■ The current emphasis on [18]FDG PET scanning may compromise the emergence of new PET molecular imaging methodology

- ■ Molecular imaging with PET can offer a huge resource to the current evolving concepts of cancer treatment

Drug development

Positron emission tomography is evolving as a unique tool for drug development in oncology for improving both the efficacy of established treatments and new cancer drugs. Drug discovery has undergone a revolution in cancer medicine with better knowledge of possible therapeutic approaches led primarily by identification of specific processes responsible for malignant cellular transformation. Combinatorial chemistry, another new technology, has grown at a tremendous rate to produce a plethora of novel treatments.[18] However, drug development is still a protracted and expensive business. It is estimated that, of 5,000 potential drugs screened, only one drug is successfully approved and introduced into the market.[19] In addition, the candidate drug finally selected takes an average of 10 years of development before proceeding to clinical trial, necessitating an investment of several million pounds.[20] Consequently, there is a need for an additional method of evaluating promising new drugs and optimizing existing treatment strategies. There is greater awareness that PET has a major role to play in expediting drug development in the preclinical and clinical settings, which may substantially reduce the costs that are currently incurred. Furthermore, with the introduction of small animal PET scanners, initial pharmacokinetic studies may be performed in suitable animal models, with more rapid translation to human testing.

The objectives of drug development are clearly defined. The principal aim involves the optimum delivery of drug to the tumour with minimal exposure to normal tissue, thereby achieving maximum therapeutic benefit. This requires accurate monitoring of drug pharmacology, including pharmacokinetics (absorption, distribution, metabolism and elimination) and pharmacodynamics (tumour response, enzyme induction or inhibition etc). At present, these parameters are measured by analysis of blood and urine samples and occasionally using biopsy specimens of relevant tissue.

There are a number of generic issues in drug development that can be addressed by PET:

- Does the drug sufficiently distribute to target (tumour) and how much goes to normal tissue?
- How is the drug eliminated from tumour and normal tissue?
- Does the drug modulate its target in a predictable way?
- Is the drug efficacious?

Despite extensive application in psychiatry and neurology in drug evaluation, PET has not yet reached its full potential in cancer therapeutics. This section will review some previous and ongoing applications of PET imaging in drug pharmacology.

5-Fluorouracil

5-Fluorouracil (5-FU) has been in use in oncology for over 40 years, most frequently in colorectal cancer for which it is the single most important drug. 5-Fluorouracil is a fluorinated pyrimidine that needs to be metabolized to nucleotides to exert its antineoplastic effect. The two pathways of greatest importance for this are:[21]

- Reduction of DNA synthesis by inhibition of the enzyme thymidylate synthase (TS) by the 5-FU anabolite, 5-fluoro-2′deoxyuridine-5′monophosphate (FdUMP)

- Impaired function of RNA after incorporation of another 5-FU anabolite, fluorouridine 5′-triphosphate (FUTP), into RNA

Up to 80% of systemically administered 5-FU is degraded through catabolism by dihydropyrimidine dehydrogenase (DPD) to α-fluoro-β-alanine (FBAL).[22] Despite the many years of experience in treating metastatic colorectal cancer with 5-FU either alone in differing schedules, or in combination therapy, response rates remain below 30%.[23]

[18]fluorine radiolabelled 5-FU (5-[18F]FU) has been the most successfully studied anticancer drug by PET in animals and man. A relationship between tumour uptake of 5-FU and response first seen in mice has been reproduced in man using PET methodology.[24] A group in Heidelberg found that colorectal liver metastasis with a high uptake of 5-[18F]FU at 2 hours, as indicated by a standardized uptake value (SUV) of more than 3, had a negative growth rate, whereas those with an SUV of less than 2 had tumour progression.[25] This association has been confirmed in MR spectroscopy (MRS) studies where an increase in intratumoural half-life of 5-FU was tightly correlated with clinical response in man.[26,27]

Saleem et al. investigated the strategy of combining 5-[18F]FU with eniluracil,[28] a known inhibitor of DPD.[29] There was a marked reduction in radiotracer uptake in the liver and kidney after eniluracil administration, suggesting a decrease in production of FBAL as expected with eniluracil. Following metabolite correction, the levels of 5-[18F]FU and anabolites were found to be higher in liver metastasis after eniluracil treatment. This study illustrates how PET can provide *in vivo* imaging of the postulated action of a novel enzyme inactivator (Fig. 62.3).

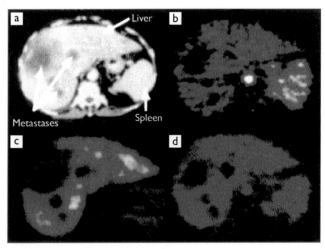

Figure 62.3. *Typical transabdominal CT (a) and corresponding PET blood flow (b) and PET ^{18}F-fluorouracil images without eniluracil (c) and after eniluracil (d), showing liver, spleen and multiple hepatic metastases. (Reproduced with permission from* The Lancet, *Elsevier Ltd.)*

One reason for poor tumour response rates of 5-FU is because tumour masses typically exhibit abnormal blood vessel networks.[30] This can substantially reduce perfusion in tumours compared to normal tissue, which consequently can restrict and impair drug delivery. Previous work by our group has underlined the importance of blood flow in determining initial 5-[^{18}F]FU uptake and retention at 1 hour.[31]

A combination of carbogen (95% O_2 and 5% CO_2) and nicotinamide, an amide of vitamin B3, showed an increase in blood flow in superficial tumour masses in man measured with laser Doppler probes.[32] Carbogen has been administered to mice bearing subcutaneous RIF-1 tumours whilst receiving 5-FU chemotherapy, and an increase in 5-FU uptake secondary to changes in tumour blood flow and pH detected by MRS was found in larger tumours.[33] To answer the important question whether the same relationship exists in man, our group studied 5-[^{18}F]FU uptake in patients with metastatic colorectal cancer undergoing chemotherapy with 5-FU who also received carbogen and nicotinamide. A 50% increase in tumour perfusion and a 30% increase in 5-[^{18}F]FU delivery was observed in liver metastasis after administration of carbogen and nicotinamide.[34] This demonstrates that PET can provide valuable information on physiological biomodulation of an existing drug.

Thymitaq™ (nolatrexed, AG337)

Thymitaq™ is a non-classical TS inhibitor, an enzyme crucial for the replication of thymidine and DNA synthesis as mentioned. Cells can overcome this cytotoxicity by incorporating extracellular thymidine into DNA, the salvage pathway,[35] which can give an indication of response to TS inhibition. A PET kinetic strategy was devised to quantitate this salvage pathway using radiolabelled thymidine (2-[^{11}C]thymidine) in vivo using PET scanning. Patients with advanced gastro-intestinal malignancies imaged 1 hour after Thymitaq™ treatment had an increased intratumoural uptake of 2-[^{11}C]thymidine compared to controls.[36] This coincided with an increase in peak plasma concentrations of the drug in treated patients, which is a more conventional method of assessing TS inhibition. This suggests that PET imaging can provide pharmacodynamic data for new drugs.

Key points: drug development

- PET is evolving as a unique tool for drug development

- It is estimated that, of 5,000 potential drugs screened, only one drug is successful and introduced into clinical practice

- The principal aim of drug development is the optimum delivery of drug to the tumour with minimal exposure to normal tissue to achieve maximum benefit

- Accurate monitoring of drug pharmacology (pharmacokinetics and pharmacodynamics) with PET is now being explored

- Pharmacokinetics refers to drug absorption, distribution, metabolism and elimination

- Pharmacodynamics refers to tumour response, enzyme induction or inhibition, etc.

- 5-Fluorouracil and Thymitaq™ have been studied extensively with PET in advanced gastro-intestinal malignancy

Tumour proliferation

The standard technique to assess tumour response to anticancer treatment is with conventional imaging modalities such as X-ray, ultrasound or CT. These methods rely principally on changes in anatomical criteria such as tumour dimensions (unilateral or bilateral) or volume to determine whether therapy has been a success or failure. In addition, any residual tumour mass may be partially or completely composed of necrotic, apoptotic or inflammatory tissue or viable tumour cells, which can confound interpretation of results. After the instigation of chemotherapy or radiotherapy regimens, there may often be a delay of 2–3 months before any obvious signs of tumour response are apparent, which impedes decisions on rapid treatment modification when there has been no response. The new opportunities being offered in cancer medicine such as antiangiogenic agents or gene therapy may be cytostatic and treatment will not invariably lead to a reduction in tumour size. There is a clinical need for an alternative strategy of response assessment and, with an emphasis on earlier prediction and detection of pharmacodynamics end-points, for faster screening of novel drugs.

Change in tumour size is preceded by important biochemical changes, including a decrease in cellular proliferation and/or an increase in cellular death rate and subsequent decline in the number of viable tumour cells.[37] One of the most accurate measures of response remains serial biopsy,[38,39] but this is obviously impractical and has limitations in itself, including potential sampling errors, particularly in tumours which are intrinsically heterogeneous.

Many of these drawbacks can be overcome with functional PET imaging. ^{18}FDG has been the most used radiotracer in this field so far. The increased demands of glycolysis in neoplastic cells compared to benign cells and consequent higher uptake of ^{18}FDG has been used to infer information on tumour growth and proliferation. Numerous in vitro and in vivo studies in humans have demonstrated that the uptake of ^{18}FDG is related to tumour grade in a range of malignancies. In general, low-grade, slowly proliferating tumours have less [18]FDG uptake than is seen in poorly differentiated, rapidly growing tumours.[40–42] However, non-cell division-related tumour cell activities require a supply of energy, as do inflammatory cells such as macrophages and neutrophils,[43] making glucose metabolism an ambiguous measure of tumour proliferation.[44]

These issues have led to the introduction of two thymidine-based radiotracers which are emerging as leading candidates to measure tumour proliferation with PET:

- Radiolabelled thymidine
- 3'-Deoxy-3'-^{18}F]fluorothymidine

Radiolabelled thymidine

Thymidine is a pyrimidine nucleotide that is unique as it is a precursor only for DNA and not for RNA, as with other nucleotides, and is a logical choice to act as a molecular PET probe to image DNA proliferation (Fig. 62.4). Thymidine incorporated into DNA is either derived from the exogenous pathway and is transported into the cell or is produced locally by the cell itself via the *de novo* pathway. Unless there is a shortage of thymidine precursor, the rate of DNA synthesis depends on the rate of proliferation of the tissue, and not on the concentration of thymidine.[45] Since the 1950s, tritiated thymidine (^{3}H]thymidine) has been used in this capacity to measure cell growth and elucidate the cell cycle using autoradiography.

Initially, thymidine was radiolabelled in the methyl-5-position as methyl-^{11}C]thymidine. In murine models, a significant correlation was demonstrated between methyl-^{11}C]thymidine uptake and tumour grade.[46] An association was also observed clinically in patients with non-Hodgkin's lymphoma.[47] However, PET imaging with ^{11}C]thymidine

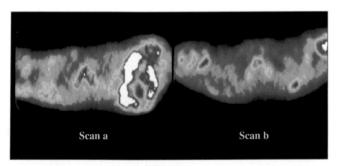

Figure 62.4. *Patient with Ewing's sarcoma in the upper thorax and shoulder. A 2-[11C]thymidine PET image (a) before and (b) after chemotherapy. The white area indicates the region of highest uptake. Resection revealed almost complete histological response corresponding with the post treatment 2-[11C]thymidine PET image. (Reproduced with permission from PET for Drug Development and Evaluation, Kluwer Academic Publishers.)*

has yielded poor results because of the production of a large number of labelled metabolites making it difficult to attribute the acquired tissue signal to thymidine alone.[48]

A more promising approach has been the use of thymidine labelled in the 2-C position (2-^{11}C]thymidine). This leads to fewer labelled metabolites than in corresponding methyl thymidine scans making interpretation of the scan easier.[49] Vander Borght et al. has shown that 2-^{11}C]thymidine uptake had a significant relationship with normal tissue proliferation in a partially hepatectomized rat model of regenerating liver.[50,51]

The principal metabolite of 2-^{11}C]thymidine in blood and tissue is ^{11}C]O_2,[51] which is rapidly eliminated by the lungs and can be assayed in exhaled air with high temporal resolution.[52] Our group has developed a technique to correct the tissue signal for ^{11}C]O_2 metabolite by performing a radiolabelled bicarbonate ([H11]CO_3^-) scan.[9] This allows for the final data to be analysed quantitatively.

A preliminary study to investigate the use of 2-^{11}C]thymidine PET scans to measure early response after initiation of chemotherapy was undertaken in six patients. This demonstrated a decline in cellular 2-^{11}C]thymidine uptake at 1 week in patients who had successful therapy. Patients with progressive disease had little alteration in thymidine uptake.[53]

Another study has directly correlated a histopathological measure of DNA proliferation with 2-^{11}C]thymidine uptake in 17 chemotherapy naïve patients with advanced intra-abdominal malignancy.[54] The results showed a significant relationship between fractional retention of 2-^{11}C]thymidine at 60 minutes with Molecular Immunology Borstel 1 (MIB-1), an *ex vivo* measure of tumour proliferation. MIB-1 detects the presence of Ki_{67}, an antibody raised against a nuclear antigen found in proliferating cells.

3'-Deoxy-3'-^{18}F]fluorothymidine

Unlabelled 3'-Deoxy-3'-fluorothymidine (FLT), a thymidine analogue, was initially evaluated as a chemotherapeutic agent for leukaemia,[55] before its exceptional anti-HIV activity was discovered.[56] Toxicity deterred further progression as a clinical treatment in both diseases.[57]

However, certain features of FLT suggested that it could be a suitable tracer for imaging cell proliferation with PET after radiolabelling with ^{18}F]fluorine. The most important aspect is that after FLT has permeated the cell membrane it undergoes monophosphorylation, catalysed by the enzyme thymidine kinase 1 (TK1).[58] This represents the penultimate step in DNA synthesis. To ascertain the ability of ^{18}F]FLT to measure TK1 activity, Rasey et al. performed *in vitro* experiments with A549 human lung cancer cells and found a strong correlation between ^{18}F]FLT uptake and TK1 activity.[59] As TK1 activity also has a positive relationship with cellular proliferation,[60] [18]F]FLT uptake is being assessed as a marker of tumour proliferation.

The first PET imaging with ^{18}F]FLT was performed in 1998 in animals and a patient with non-small cell lung cancer (NSCLC). [^{18}F]FLT was specifically taken up in proliferating tissues, including tumours and the bone marrow (Fig. 62.5).[61] A further [^{18}F]FLT PET study in 30 patients with solitary pulmonary nodules found a significant correlation between [^{18}F]FLT uptake and proliferative activity as determined by Ki_{67} immunostaining.[62] A similar relationship between [^{18}F]FLT uptake and Ki_{67} has been established *in vivo* in 10 patients with NSCLC.[63]

The main advantage of [^{18}F]FLT compared to 2-[^{11}C]thymidine is that there are fewer metabolites produced, allowing easier analysis of data. Quantitative data have not yet been obtained with [^{18}F]FLT, and it remains to be seen how applicable this would be.

Key points: tumour proliferation

■ Change in tumour size is preceded by important biochemical changes, including a decrease in cellular proliferation and/or an increase in cellular death rate

■ Antiangiogenic agents or gene therapy may be cytostatic and treatment may not lead to a reduction in tumour size

■ Leading candidates to measure tumour proliferation with PET are radiolabelled thymidine and FLT

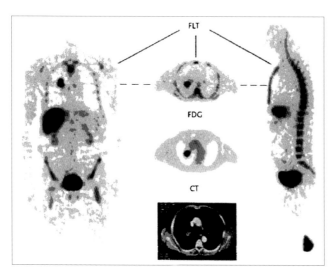

Figure 62.5. *Images of a patient with non-small cell lung cancer obtained after the injection of 50 MBq of [^{18}F]FLT using a GE Advance tomograph (Milwaukee, WI, USA). Coronal (left), sagittal (right) and transverse images of FLT are shown in comparison to transverse FDG and CT images. FLT images were obtained as successive 6-min bins, each covering 15 cm of the body, between 60 and 110 min post injection. All PET images are attenuation corrected. Uptake is noted in the tumour, normal marrow, bladder and liver. ^{18}F activity is also seen in a urinal in the lower portion of the sagittal image. The patient was imaged after the injection of 400 MBq of ^{18}FDG on another day, where tumour, but not marrow, uptake is noted. (Reproduced with permission from Nature Medicine, Nature Publishing Group.)*

Gene expression

Remarkable progress in genetic engineering has been made to develop and clarify knowledge about cascades of gene expression and interaction between gene and gene products. This has been accompanied by the exciting prospect of gene manipulation in cancer treatment by either transferring appropriate genes into abnormal cells or by detection of endogenous gene expression for clinical translation and diagnosis.[64] However, without improving the ability to monitor and quantitate the degree of gene expression, which can currently only be achieved with biopsy specimens, the field of gene therapy would continue to face significant obstacles for routine use. Imaging gene expression is important for monitoring the location(s), magnitude and time variation of gene expression from gene-therapy vectors, and can be important to measure efficacy of treatment and to answer questions pertaining to optimization of treatment:[65]

• Has gene transfer been successful?
• Is gene expression localized to the target tissue or organ, and is this optimal?
• Is there sufficient transgene expression to obtain a therapeutic effect?
• Is there unwanted toxicity resulting from gene expression?
• When pro-drug treatment is to be initiated, when is the most effective time to commence it?
• How long does the gene expression persist in the target or any other tissues?

Two major approaches have been developed for monitoring the gene expression using PET methodology:

• Direct imaging of endogenous genes or molecules
• Indirect imaging, where there is 'linking' of the expressed therapeutic gene to a 'PET reporter gene' which 'reports' back on the status of expression of the gene of interest when properly linked

Direct imaging
Direct imaging of gene expression can be accomplished by developing radiolabelled probes that bind selectively to highly specific regions of the product of the expressed gene (e.g. protein, mRNA, or DNA).[66,67] However, the advancement of this method of gene expression imaging is limited by the lack of specific and suitably labelled PET probes currently available.[68]

Indirect imaging
More progress has been made with indirect imaging of gene expression utilizing reporter genes despite its greater complexity.[69] Indirect imaging falls into two distinct categories: enzyme-based or receptor-based. In both cases, indi-

rect imaging involves simultaneous expression between both the reporter gene and therapeutic gene product after construction of a cassette linking these genes that can be transfected into specific cells using a vector. This can be achieved in several ways:

- A single vector encoding for both transcribed genes in one mRNA, which is then translated into two proteins
- An inducible bi-directional vector can be used which initiates the transcription of both the therapeutic and the reporter gene
- The reporter and therapeutic gene can be delivered using two separate vectors
- A fusion protein containing both the therapeutic and reporter protein can be used

All of these approaches are dependent on having a useful PET reporter gene and radiolabelled probe.[17] The paradigm for enzyme-based gene expression is the herpes simplex virus type 1 thymidine kinase gene (HSV1-tk), and is illustrated in Fig. 62.6. The HSV1-tk gene encodes for the enzyme, HSV1-TK, that can phosphorylate radiolabelled derivatives of thymidine [e.g. iodinated 2′-fluoro-2′-deoxy-1-β-D-arabinofuranosyl-5-iodo-uracil or ([*I]-FIAU)] which acts as the PET probe after transportation into cells. In cells where HSV1-TK has been expressed, the radiolabelled phosphorylated probe (i.e. [*I]-FIAU(PO$_4$)) is effectively 'trapped' (as it does not readily cross the cell membrane), and so accumulates within the cell, emitting a radioactive signal that reflects level of HSV1-TK enzyme activity and HSV1-tk gene expression.[69] The HSV1-tk gene vector with [*I]-FIAU as the tracer has imaged gene expression in the liver and in transfected tumour cells.[70,71]

Where gene expression uses the model of receptor imaging, the reporter gene is a receptor that 'irreversibly' traps the complementary radiolabelled PET probe in the transduced cell. An example of a receptor PET reporter gene is the dopamine type 2 receptor (DR2),[72] which has

been validated in animals. Other reporter genes, including those that encode stomatostatin receptor[73] and Na/I symporter (NIS gene),[74] have been examined in preliminary studies. All of these PET reporter genes work on the premise of binding to a suitable radiotracer producing sufficient, proportional accumulation of PET signal within the region for further analysis.

Studies in imaging reporter-gene expression in human subjects have only recently started. The HSV1-TK gene vector can also be used as a therapeutic 'suicide' gene in combination with the pro-drug, ganciclovir. In this scenario, a cell expressing HSV1-TK enzyme will commit suicide on exposure to ganciclovir under appropriate conditions.[75] To assess the extent of gene expression and predict therapeutic potency, intratumoural liposomal HSV1-tk gene vector was infused into recurrent glioblastomas of five patients.[76] Dynamic PET scanning with [^{124}I]FIAU was performed at baseline and after gene vector application and ganciclovir treatment commenced 4 days after vector infusion. Results showed that in one in five patients there was accumulation of [^{124}I]-FIAU activity within the observed tumour after HSV1-tk infusion, and this corresponded to an area of intratumoural necrosis on an ^{18}FDG PET scan performed after ganciclovir treatment (Fig. 62.7). These preliminary findings show that non-invasive FIAU PET imaging of HSV1-tk expression is feasible in patients and that vector-mediated gene expression may predict therapeutic effect.

Key points: gene expression

- Imaging gene expression is important for monitoring the location(s), magnitude and time variation of gene expression from gene-therapy vectors

- Imaging may be important to measure efficacy of gene therapy and to answer questions pertaining to optimization of treatment

- Direct imaging of gene expression can be accomplished by developing radiolabelled probes that bind selectively to highly specific regions of the product of the expressed gene

- Indirect imaging of gene expression utilizing reporter genes is more useful than direct gene imaging despite its greater complexity

- Indirect imaging falls into two distinct categories: enzyme-based or receptor-based

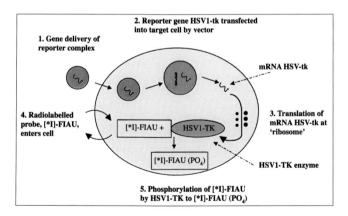

Figure 62.6. *Diagram illustrating the paradigm of imaging gene expression with the PET reporter gene, HSV1-tk.*

Markers of hypoxia

Tumour hypoxia, resulting from inadequate and chaotic blood supply to neoplastic tissue, is an important prognostic indicator and a crucial factor in cancer therapy outcome to radiotherapy and some chemotherapy treatments.

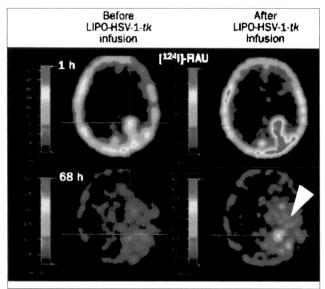

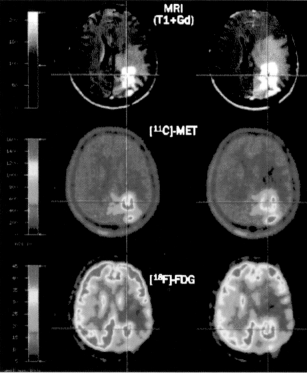

Figure 62.7. *Co-registration of FIAU PET, MET PET, [18]FDG PET and MR before (left column) and after (right column) vector application. The region of specific [[124]I]FIAU retention (68 h) within the tumour after liposome-HSV1-tk-complex transduction (white arrow) showed the signs of necrosis (cross-hairs, right column; reduced methionine uptake [MET] and glucose metabolism [[18]FDG]) after ganciclovir treatment. (Reproduced with permission from* The Lancet, Elsevier Ltd.)

Oxygen mediates the biological effects of ionizing radiation and the response of cells to radiation depends strongly on the availability of oxygen. This 'oxygen effect' was first recognized by Mottram in 1936.[77] Gray[78] studied the influence of oxygen in mammalian tissue in detail and discovered

that, typically, hypoxic cells were 2.5–3 times more radioresistant than well-oxygenated cells. Assessment of tumour hypoxia prior to radiation therapy would provide a rational means to identify the outcome of radiation therapy in patients and to offer alternative radiotherapy strategies that may be more effective.

Preliminary clinical studies with Eppendorf pO_2 histographs have shown significant correlation between median pO_2 of tumours and their response to therapy.[79–81] However, limitations of microelectrode probes to measure tumour hypoxia are that it is invasive, has poor reproducibility, can only access superficial tumours and may overestimate degree of hypoxia in necrotic tissue.[82]

Non-invasive markers of hypoxia for PET imaging fall into two categories: 2-nitroimidazole analogues and non-nitroimidazole agents. 2-Nitroimidazole analogues contain the moiety azomycin and can covalently bind to cellular molecules upon reduction in hypoxic cells, e.g. [18]fluorine-labelled misonidazole ([^{18}F]MISO). Non-nitroimidazole markers, such as Cu(II)-diacetyl-bis(N^4-methylthio-semicarabaone) (Cu-ATSM), are a complex of copper bis(thiosemicarbazones) that rely on the reduction of chelated metal for their selective deposition in hypoxic tissue.[83]

In PET, the most experimental and clinical experience of hypoxic imaging has been gained by studying [^{18}F]MISO (Fig. 62.8a).

[^{18}F]MISO has been shown to accumulate in hypoxic tissue in inverse portion to tissue oxygenation.[84] Under hypoxic conditions, the rate of [^{18}F]MISO binding can be up to 28 times more than in normoxic cells.[85] Subsequent biodistribution studies defined hypoxia as tissue-to-blood [^{18}F]MISO ratio of 1 : 4, 2 hours after radiotracer administration.[86] In a study of 37 patients with lung, head and neck and prostate cancer, hypoxia was present in 97% of the tumours studied and the extent of hypoxia varied

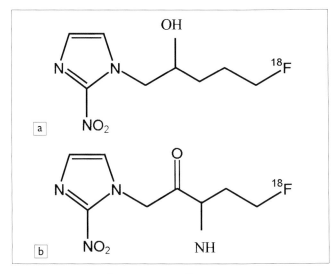

Figure 62.8. *(a) [^{18}F]MISO; (b) [^{18}F]FETA.*

markedly between tumours in the same site or of the same histology. Hypoxia was also distributed heterogeneously between regions within a single tumour. The intra- and intertumour variability indicate the importance of making oxygenation measures in individual tumours and the necessity to sample as much of the tumour volume as possible.[87]

However, there are three main problems with imaging with [^{18}F]MISO:

- There is lack of contrast between tumour and normal tissue uptake of [^{18}F]MISO due to poor cellular uptake of [^{18}F]MISO in vivo[88]
- [^{18}F]MISO is cleared from normal tissue over a 2-hour period. These slow kinetics delay imaging and result in low count rate studies with images of reduced quality[88]
- High rates of metabolism of [^{18}F]MISO limit its use to permit quantitative analysis[89]

Recent research has reported on the synthesis of a new 2-nitroimidazole derivative, [^{18}F]fluoroetanidazole ([^{18}F]FETA) (Fig. 62.8b), a monofluorinated congener of etanidazole. [^{18}F]FETA demonstrates oxygen-dependent binding and retention in tumours that is very similar to that for [^{18}F]MISO in vitro, and may offer the advantage in imaging hypoxic tumours because it is less rapidly metabolized in vivo. In addition, brain-to-blood ratios indicate that [^{18}F]FETA readily crosses the blood–brain barrier and may have a role in assessment of gliomas.[90–92]

The latest development in nitroimidazoles for PET imaging of hypoxia is fluorine-labelled 2-(2-nitro-1[H]-imidazol-1-yl)-N-(2,2,3,3,3-pentafluoropropyl)-acetamide ([^{18}F]EF5). In rat tumour models, [^{18}F]EF5 distributed evenly in normal tissues with higher uptake in tumours visualized. Again, activity was located in the brain, and plans are underway to initiate a research project to determine the safety and preliminary evidence for the efficacy of this preparation in patients with brain tumours.[93]

Several recent studies have concentrated on the use of Cu-ATSM as a hypoxic marker. Cu-ATSM is retained in ischaemic tissue but rapidly diffuses out of normoxic tissue and uptake has been correlated with tumour pO$_2$ in small animal models.[94] Compared with [^{18}F]MISO, Cu-ATSM exhibits more efficient uptake and superior washout kinetics in hypoxic and normoxic cells, with higher contrast levels obtained 10–15 minutes post injection. The positron-emitting isotope ^{60}CU-ATSM has been used to predict response in patients with NSCLC with encouraging results.[95] Systems are being developed to integrate Cu-ATSM delineated hypoxic regions in tumours and to deliver higher doses of radiotherapy to these smaller subvolumes using intensity-modulated radiotherapy (IMRT).[96]

Key points: tumour hypoxia

- Tumour hypoxia is an important prognostic indicator
- Tumour hypoxia is a crucial factor in cancer therapy outcome
- Hypoxic cells are 2.5–3 times more radio-resistant than well-oxygenated cells
- Non-invasive markers of hypoxia for PET imaging fall into two categories: 2-nitroimidazole analogues and non-nitroimidazole agents
- Most experimental and clinical experience of hypoxic PET imaging has been gained by studying the 2-nitroimidazole analogue [^{18}F]MISO

Angiogenesis

Tumours do not grow beyond 1–2 mm^3 in size without the development of new blood vessels.[97] Angiogenesis, which is the growth of blood vessels either from existing vasculature or from de novo generation of blood vessels, is imperative to allow tumour cells to increase their nutrient supply, proliferate and survive, even though the new vessels often have structural and functional abnormalities compared to normal tissue. Numerous experimental animal models have demonstrated that angiogenesis is one of the most critical steps for progression of the primary tumour, as well as metastatic dissemination.[98] Although angiogenesis remains a complex, multistep process, great strides have been made in the last few years to elucidate its molecular mechanism in much greater detail. Many cytokines implicated in this pathway have been discovered, including vascular endothelial growth factor (VEGF), whose levels are upregulated in several cancers such as breast, colon, ovarian and lung, and which may have prognostic significance.[99,100] There are two evolving categories of treatment that interfere with tumour vasculature for therapeutic benefit:

- Antiangiogenic agents, which inhibit new endothelial cell development and subsequent formation of capillary networks
- Antivascular drugs, which disrupt existing endothelial cells, leading to destruction of the tumour blood vessel architecture

Both treatment strategies have proved attractive, with the development of numerous therapeutic agents with antiangiogenic or antivascular activity.

Antiangiogenesis

The main restriction in the increasing number of new antiangiogenic drugs is the limited availability of surrogate markers of therapeutic efficacy. The outcome of antiangiogenic drugs is difficult to determine as there is a wide range of mechanisms by which they can prevent neo-genesis or neo-vascularization. Effective therapy may not lead to any substantial reduction in tumour size, rendering conventional imaging modalities unable to determine response. Positron emission tomography methods are being developed to measure parameters related to the angiogenic phenotype. Vascular endothelial growth factor is one of the most potent cytokines mediating angiogenesis,[101] and is secreted in response to hypoxia by tumour cells.[102] One study has demonstrated the feasibility of imaging VEGF using an anti-VEGF antibody labelled with iodine 124 ([124I]-VG76e) in mice bearing human xenografts. *Ex vivo* biodistribution confirmed antibody localization within tumour (Fig. 62.9).[103] Such PET imaging may help identify patients with high tumoural expression of VEGF, allowing appropriate selection for treatment with antiangiogenic drugs and provide an accurate marker of treatment response. Recent effort has concentrated on developing radiolabelled antagonists to the integrin, $\alpha_v\beta_3$. $\alpha_v\beta_3$ is highly expressed on acti-

vated endothelial cells and plays a crucial part in new vessel formation.[104] It binds to the tripeptide sequence arginine–glycine–aspartic acid (RGD) of various extracellular matrix proteins and, by blocking these interactions, can result in inhibition of tumour-induced angiogenesis.[105,106] A radiolabelled glycopeptide of RGD, [18F]Galacto-RGD, showed accumulation in $\alpha_v\beta_3$ receptor-positive tumours in mice using small animal PET scanning (Fig. 62.10).[107] Further studies need to be undertaken to determine the clinical potential of [18F]Galacto-RGD PET in patients undergoing antiangiogenic treatment.

Antivascular

The end-point of antivascular activity is easier to define as the direct consequence of destruction of tumour vasculature is a reduction in tumour perfusion. Therefore the effect of newer antivascular agents may be monitored by changes in blood flow.[108] [15O]-labelled water ([15O]H$_2$) has been utilized extensively and with good reproducibility in dynamic PET studies to quantify normal tissue and tumour blood flow *in vivo* using an input function derived from continuous arterial sampling over the period of imaging.[109–112] Positron emission tomography blood flow scans have contributed to the clinical evaluation of a novel antivascular agent, Combretastatin A4 Phosphate (CA4P), a tubulin-binding agent, which induces rapid and selective blood flow reductions in experimental tumour systems by possible cytotoxic effects on proliferating endothelial

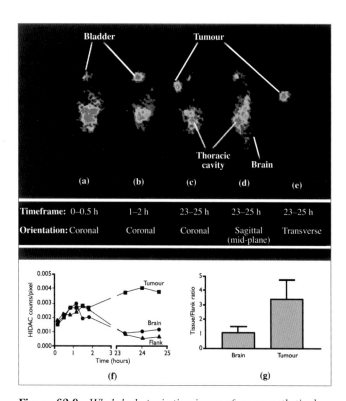

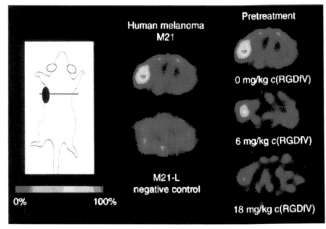

Figure 62.9. *Whole-body projection image of an anaesthetized HT1080-26.6 tumour-bearing mouse at selected time-points after an intravenous injection of [124I]SHPP-VG76e (16 µCi). The tumour was implanted subcutaneously on the rear dorsum of the mouse. PET images were acquired with the mouse positioned prone using a HIDAC PET scanner. The panels show selected 0.5-mm-thick slices through the image volume. Images were visualized using Analyze software. Image intensities have been scaled to the maximum signal intensity for each panel. (Reproduced with permission from Cancer Research, American Association of Cancer Research.)*

Figure 62.10. *Transaxial small animal PET images of nude mice bearing human melanoma xenografts. Images were acquired 90 min after injection of approximately 5.5 MBq of [18F]Galacto-RGD. The top left image shows selective accumulation of the tracer in the $\alpha_v\beta_3$-positve (M21) tumour on the left flank. In contrast, no focal tracer accumulation is visible in the $\alpha_v\beta_3$-negative (M21-L) control tumour (bottom left image). The three images on the right were obtained from serial [18F]Galacto-RGD PET studies in one mouse. These illustrate the dose-dependent blockade of tracer uptake by the α_v-selective cyclic pentapeptide cyclo(-Arg-Gly-Asp-D-Phe-Val-). (Reproduced with permission from Cancer Research, American Association of Cancer Research.)*

cells.[113–116] Eight patients treated with CA4P in a Phase I trial had [^{15}O]H$_2$ PET scanning before, 30 minutes after and 24 hours after the first infusion of CA4P. Results showed a 30–60% temporary reduction in tumour blood flow at the higher dose level of CA4P, corroborating data obtained in animal studies[117,118] (see also Chapter 61).

Key points: angiogenesis

- Tumours do not grow beyond 1–2 mm^3 in size without the development of new blood vessels

- Many cytokines implicated in angiogenesis have been discovered including VEGF

- VEGF is secreted in response to hypoxia by tumour cells

- Antiangiogenic agents inhibit new endothelial cell development

- Antivascular drugs disrupt existing endothelial cells

- Effective therapy may not lead to any substantial reduction in tumour size, rendering conventional imaging modalities unable to determine response

- PET imaging may identify patients with high tumoural expression of VEGF, allowing appropriate selection for treatment with antiangiogenic drugs

- PET imaging may provide an accurate marker of treatment response

- Antivascular activity can be measured as a reduction in tumour perfusion

Receptor detection and drug interactions

Advances in tumour biology characteristics have revealed that many cell-surface and intracellular receptors are upregulated in cancer cells. The detection of these receptors can provide important additive information on diagnosis and prognosis. As they are often the targets of inhibitory effects of hormones and growth factors that exert their therapeutic effect by interacting with these receptors, identification might help in selection of patients suitable for hormonal therapy and in assessing response. Positron emission tomography can be used to image relevant receptors and study drug-receptor interactions *in vivo* with either appropriately radiolabelled receptor binding hormones or antibodies, avoiding the necessity of recurrent invasive tumour biopsies which may also be prone to errors of tumour sampling. Receptor studies can either be direct (labelling the molecule of interest) or indirect (displacement of radioligand by the molecule of interest). The regional kinetics of radioligands can be used to derive val-

ues for receptor number (B_{max}), affinity (K_d) and binding potential (B_{max}/K_d).[119] With the production and availability of radioligands of different receptors in various types of cancers (e.g. breast, prostate and neuro-endocrine), receptor studies are now being performed in oncology.

Oestrogen

The most extensively studied receptor is the intracellular steroid oestrogen receptor (ER). 16α-[^{18}F]fluoro-17β-oestradiol (FES), an oestrogen analogue, has been widely used to assess ER status in breast tumours *in vivo* (Fig. 62.11a and b).

Good overall agreement between *ex vivo* ER assays and FES uptake has led to the conclusion that FES PET provides direct information on ER status.[120] A decrease in the uptake of FES in metastatic breast cancers after the administration of tamoxifen has been visualized, demonstrating the presence of functional ERs in the tumour.[121] The reduction in FES uptake after tamoxifen was significantly greater in patients who responded to hormonal therapy.[122] A further study correlating ER status with treatment response observed a group of patients with ER-positive biopsies but FES-negative PET scans who had poor response to hormone therapy, suggesting identification of a subset of patients with hormone refractory disease despite ER-positive biopsies.[123] FES PET imaging has therefore opened up an intriguing

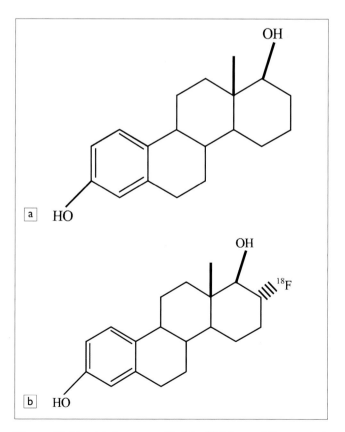

Figure 62.11. *(a) Oestrogen; (b) 16α-[^{18}F]fluoro-17β-oestradiol (FES).*

new way to monitor receptor function and response to hormonal therapy in patients with breast cancer at a cellular level.[124] In addition, FES has also been utilized in meningiomas where FES uptake correlated with immunohistochemical measurement of ER status from biopsies.[125]

Androgen

The androgen receptor (AR) is a key biomolecule in the biology of prostate cancer and has been targeted by PET for radiolabelling and subsequent imaging to aid diagnosis and therapeutic planning. [18]F has been used to label several hormone analogues, including 16β-[18F]fluoro-5a-dihydrotestosterone (FDHT), 16β-[18F]-substituted testosterone, 16α- and 16β-[18F]7α-methyl-nortestosterone, 20-[18F]fluoro-R1881 (metribolone) and 20-[18F]fluoromiboloerone.[126–128] In man, AR expression has been studied with PET using FDHT. In a group of patients with progressive androgen-independent prostate cancer, the majority of active lesions have been visualized with FDHT using PET. The impact of the expression of the AR on response of individual lesions to AR targeted anticancer drug therapies is being explored.[129]

Neuroendocrine

Neuroendocrine tumours expressing somatostatin receptors have been imaged using PET with radiolabelled ocreotide, a somatostatin analogue. [64]Copper-labelled ocreotide PET scanning has shown promising results in patients with carcinoid and islet cell tumours.[130] [68]Gallium- and [66]Gallium-labelled ocreotide analogues are currently undergoing imaging trials in patients and animals, respectively.[131,132] [18F]fluoro-ethyl-siperone, a PET tracer with a high affinity for D_2 dopamine receptors, has been used to image non-functioning pituitary adenomas to distinguish them from craniopharyngiomas and meningiomas, in vivo, which do not possess these receptors.[133]

Epidermal growth factor

Epidermal growth factor receptor (EGFR) is frequently overexpressed in malignancies. Strategies to target EGFR include monoclonal antibodies to prevent ligand binding and small molecule inhibitors of the tyrosine kinase activity to stop autophosphorylation and downstream intracellular signalling, e.g. Iressa.[44] A preliminary in vitro study has successfully prepared [11C]-6-acrylomido-4-(3,4-dichloro-6-fluoroa-nilino)quinazoline (MLO3) as a potential PET biomarker for EGFR.[134] In vivo visualization of EGFR-expressing tumours could allow for non-invasive patient selection and response assessment for those undergoing such treatment.

Antibodies

Antibodies are also a potential tracer for targeting cell-surface receptors. Although primarily explored for imaging with gamma cameras and single-photon emission CT (SPECT), newer small animal studies and clinical trials are starting to use positron-labelled antibody fragments. Monoclonal antibodies developed against specific antigen targets are problematic because their relatively slow clearance from blood leads to images with very high background signals, even up to 1 week after injection. Systematic construction of engineered antibody fragments for, e.g., carcinoembryonic antigen (CEA), has developed. Although they have less affinity to CEA, they are more rapidly cleared in blood because of their smaller size. Humanized versions of these engineered antibodies have been labelled with [76]bromine and [64]copper, and mouse tumour xenografts imaging has been performed with micro PET.[135–137]

Radiolabelled antibody fragments have also been developed to identify the cell surface antigen receptor to C-erb2, a proto-oncogene product that has prognostic and therapeutic implications in breast cancer, with [124]iodine for PET imaging.[138] Again, this may assist in targeting appropriate patient therapy.

Key points: receptor detection and drug interactions

- Advances in tumour biology characteristics have revealed that many cell-surface and intracellular receptors are upregulated in cancer cells

- Hormones and growth factors exert their therapeutic effect by interacting with these receptors

- PET can be used to image relevant receptors and study drug–receptor interactions in vivo with appropriately radiolabelled receptor binding hormones or antibodies

- Appropriately radiolabelled receptor binding hormones and antibodies being studied include oestrogen, androgen, neuro-endocrine somatostatin receptors and EGF

Apoptosis

Deregulation of cellular proliferation and suppression of mechanisms controlling programmed cell death (apoptosis) are believed to be important preliminary molecular events in the development of cancer.[139] Therapeutic strategies in cancer treatment are commonly mediated by initiation of apoptotic pathways, and apoptosis is thought to be the likely mechanism behind the cytoreductive effects of standard chemotherapy and radiotherapy regimens. A measure of apoptosis is desirable to predict and monitor tumour response to therapy. An early occurrence in the apoptotic cascade is the selective exposure of phosphatidylserine (PS) on the external surface of the cell; PS is a membrane-associated intracellular phospholipid normally expressed internally on the plasma bilayer membrane.[140,141] Recombinant human Annexin V (rh-AnnexinV), an endogenous protein, has been shown to bind avidly to membrane-bound PS[142] and was labelled initially with fluorescein for *in vitro, ex vivo* apoptotic assays, but now, with 99m-Technetium (Tc-99m-AnnexinV) to permit imaging of apoptosis *in vivo* using SPECT.[143,144] A recent study in 15 patients (with lung, lymphoma and breast cancer), evaluating early response following one cycle of chemotherapy by Tc-99m-AnnexinV imaging found no uptake of Tc-99m-AnnexinV in tumour prechemotherapy. However, 1–3 days post-treatment, seven patients showed uptake of Tc-99m-AnnexinV at tumour sites, in whom four had complete response and three had partial response as correlated with [18]FDG PET and CT images. Conversely, six out of eight patients with no significant postchemotherapy uptake of Tc-99m-AnnexinV had progressive disease. The two breast cancer patients demonstrated poor tracer uptake but actually had partial response, suggesting selective use of Tc-99m-AnnexinV apoptotic imaging in lymphoma and lung follow-up.[145] However, Tc-99m-AnnexinV SPECT analysis relies on visual interpretation of static and planar images, resulting in qualitative or semiquantitative data. Current developments are emerging to radiolabel AnnexinV with iodine-124[146] and fluorine-18[147] for use as potential apoptotic probes in PET studies. This will have the added advantage of not only allowing quantitative analysis but also producing dynamic, three-dimensional images. These radiotracers are being validated in preclinical studies, and will be of greater benefit in assessing the efficacy of treatment options at an early time point.

Key points: apoptosis

- Apoptosis is defined as programmed cell death

- Apoptosis is probably the mechanism behind the cytoreductive effects of standard chemotherapy and radiotherapy regimes

- An early occurrence in the apoptotic cascade is the selective exposure of phosphatidylserine (PS) on the external surface of the cell

- Tc-99m-AnnexinV SPECT imaging has been explored to measure apoptosis

- Iodine-124 and fluorine-18 AnnexinV are potential PET apoptotic probes

Other applications of imaging

Choline

Alteration of choline metabolism, a constituent of the phospholipid bilayer cell membrane, has recently been evaluated as a marker of malignant transformation.[148] Extracellular choline is phosphorylated to phosphocholine by choline kinase after it is transported into cells. This commits choline to phosphatidylcholine biosynthesis, which is an essential signalling molecule for cell growth and essentially 'traps' the extracellular choline within the cell, hence its attraction for PET imaging. Whilst little is known of the mechanisms that regulate choline kinase activity or phosphocholine production, choline kinase dysregualtion is frequently found in a variety of human tumours such as lung, colorectal and prostate tumours, and increased activity of choline kinase is found in panels of human cancer-derived cell lines compared to non-malignant cells.[149] This has supported the role of PET with radiolabelled choline as a tumour marker.

Clinical studies have been conducted with methyl-[^{11}C]-labelled choline. It appears to be of particular interest in urological tumours where methyl-[^{11}C]choline has higher uptake in bladder and prostate cancer than [18]FDG.[150–153] In addition, better visualization is obtained of urinary tract malignancies as there is minimal renal excretion of the tracer.[150]

Another study has compared methyl-[^{11}C]choline uptake with histopathological specimens and gadolinium-enhanced MR, in 22 patients with brain tumours. The methyl-[^{11}C]choline PET scans differentiated between high- and low-grade gliomas, and areas of methyl-[^{11}C]choline accumulation were larger than areas enhanced with MR in some patients. However, methyl-[^{11}C]choline was unable to distinguish low-grade gliomas from benign lesions.[154] This suggests that a combination of methyl-[^{11}C]choline PET scanning and MR will allow more accurate diagnosis of high-grade gliomas.

Multidrug resistance

Acquired multidrug resistance (MDR) represents a major cause of chemotherapy failure in cancer treatment with certain classes of drugs, in particular compounds such as anthracyclines, vinca alkaloids and taxanes.[155,156] The molecular mechanism for this resistance has been identified as overexpression of the P-glycoprotein (Pgp), a plasma membrane transporter, encoded for by the MDR gene.[157,158] These proteins reduce intracellular accumulation of cytotoxic agents and diminish the efficacy of chemotherapy. Attempts have been made to examine this process further using radiolabelled pharmaceuticals, in conjunction with strategies to decrease the activity of Pgp. Technetium-99m Sestamibi (Tc-99m-Sestamibi), a substrate for Pgp, has been utilized in SPECT studies to image the blockade of the Pgp-mediated transport after suppression of the Pgp pump.[159] *In vivo* PET studies involved in evaluation of MDR have been confined to experimentation in animals. [^{11}C]-labelled drugs such as [^{11}C]-verapamil and [^{11}C]-daunorubicin[160] and [^{11}C]-colchicine[161] have been investigated and are additional tools for the quantification of Pgp-mediated transport with PET. A potential use of such agents would be to select patients who could benefit from the addition of Pgp modulators which are being designed.[162]

Summary

- Huge advances have been made in molecular science to determine the complex processes underlying tumour biology

- Abnormal cellular and molecular pathways are being targeted to provide a novel and rational basis for cancer treatment

- A fundamental change in the requirements of imaging is necessary to meet the current challenges posed by these new treatment strategies in cancer medicine

- Molecular imaging with PET is a valuable technique that can address many questions related to this emerging field *in vivo*, such as:

  - Characterization of pharmacodynamic end-points

  - Pharmacokinetic imaging of drugs

  - Determination of mechanism of action of drugs

  - Early assessment of tumour response

  - Direct evaluation of tumour proliferation, particularly beneficial with cytostatic therapy

  - Receptor, antibody or choline detection can assist in diagnosis, prognosis and treatment decisions

  - Patient selection for specific treatments such as antiangiogenesis and hypoxic modulation

- Small animal PET scanners can give essential information on radiolabelled molecular probes prior to testing in humans

References

1. Weissleder R, Mahmood U. Molecular imaging. Radiology 2001; 219: 316–333
2. Larson S M. Molecular imaging in oncology: the diagnostic imaging 'revolution'. Clin Cancer Res 2000; 6: 2125
3. Jones T. The imaging science of positron emission tomography. Eur J Nucl Med 1996; 23: 807–813
4. Jones T. The spectrum of medical imaging. Eur J Cancer 2002; 38: 2067–2069
5. Price P. PET as a potential tool for imaging molecular mechanisms of oncology in man. Trends Mol Med 2001; 7: 442–446
6. Patlak C S, Blasberg R G, Fenstermacher J D. Graphical evaluation of blood-to-brain transfer constants from multiple-time uptake data. J Cereb Blood Flow Metab 1983; 3: 1–7
7. Peters A M. Graphical analysis of dynamic data: the Patlak–Rutland plot. Nucl Med Commun 1994; 15: 669–672
8. Cunningham V J, Jones T. Spectral analysis of dynamic PET studies. J Cereb Blood Flow Metab 1993; 13: 15–23
9. Gunn R N, Yap J T, Wells P et al. A general method to correct PET data for tissue metabolites using a dual-scan approach. J Nucl Med 2000; 41: 706–711
10. Mankoff D A, Shields A F, Graham M M et al. A graphical analysis method to estimate blood-to-tissue transfer constants for tracers with labeled metabolites. J Nucl Med 1996; 37: 2049–2057
11. Warburg O. The metabolism of tumours. New York, NY: Richard Smith, 1931; 129–169
12. Di Chiro G, DeLaPaz R L, Brooks R A et al. Glucose utilization of cerebral gliomas measured by [18F] fluorodeoxyglucose and positron emission tomography. Neurology 1982; 32: 1323–1329
13. Di Chiro G. Brain imaging of glucose utilization in cerebral tumours. Res Publ Assoc Res Nerv Ment Dis 1985; 63: 185–197
14. Nelson C A, Wang J Q, Leav I et al. The interaction among glucose transport, hexokinase, and glucose-6-phosphatase with respect to 3H-2-deoxyglucose retention in murine tumour models. Nucl Med Biol 1996; 23: 533–541
15. Smith T A. Mammalian hexokinases and their abnormal expression in cancer. Br J Biomed Sci 2000; 57: 170–178
16. Young H, Braum R, Cremerius E et al. Measurement of clinical and subclinical tumour response using [18F]-fluorodeoxyglucose and positron emission tomography: review and 1999 EORTC recommendations. European Organization for Research and Treatment of Cancer (EORTC) PET Study Group. Eur J Cancer 1999; 35: 1773–1782
17. Gambhir S S. Molecular imaging of cancer with positron emission tomography. Nat Rev 2002; 2: 683–693
18. Leonard K A, Deisseroth A B, Austin D J. Combinatorial chemistry in cancer drug development. Cancer J 2001; 7: 79–83
19. Tatum J L, Hoffman J M. Congressional update: report from the Biomedical Imaging Program of the National Cancer Institute. Imaging drug development. Acad Radiol 2000; 7: 1007–1008
20. Cambell B. Drug development and positron emission tomography. In Comar D (ed). PET for Drug Development and Evaluation. Dordrecht: Kluwer Academic Publishers, 1995; 1–24
21. Myers C E. The pharmacology of the fluoropyrimidines. Pharmacol Rev 1981; 33: 1–15

22. Pinedo H M, Peters G F. Fluorouracil: biochemistry and pharmacology. J Clin Oncol 1988; 6: 1653–1664

23. Meta-analysis Group in Cancer. Efficacy of intravenous continuous infusion of fluorouracil compared with bolus administration in advanced colorectal cancer. J Clin Oncol 1998; 16: 301–308

24. Shani J, Wolf W. A model for prediction of chemotherapy response to 5-fluorouracil based on the differential distribution of 5-[18F]fluorouracil in sensitive versus resistant lymphocytic leukemia in mice. Cancer Res 1977; 37: 2306–2308

25. Dimitrakopoulou-Strauss A, Strauss L G, Schlag P et al. Fluorine-18-fluorouracil to predict therapy response in liver metastases from colorectal carcinoma. J Nucl Med 1998; 39: 1197–1202

26. Presant C A, Wolf W, Albright M J et al. Human tumour fluorouracil trapping: clinical correlations of in vivo 19F nuclear magnetic resonance spectroscopy pharmacokinetics. J Clin Oncol 1990; 8: 1868–1873

27. Presant C A, Wolf W, Waluch V et al. Association of intratumoural pharmacokinetics of fluorouracil with clinical response. Lancet 1994; 343: 1184–1187

28. Saleem A, Yap J, Osman S et al. Modulation of fluorouracil tissue pharmacokinetics by eniluracil: in vivo imaging of drug action. Lancet 2000; 355: 2125–2131

29. Schlisky R L, Hohneker J, Ratain M. Phase 1 clinical and pharmacological study of eniluracil plus fluorouracil in patients with advanced colorectal cancer. J Clin Oncol 1998; 16: 1450–1457

30. Vaupel P, Kallinowski F, Okunieff P. Blood flow, oxygen and nutrient supply, and metabolic microenvironment of human tumours: a review. Cancer Res 1989; 49: 6449–6465

31. Harte R J, Matthews J C, O'Reilly S M et al. Tumour, normal tissue, and plasma pharmacokinetic studies of fluorouracil biomodulation with N-phosphonacetyl-L-aspartate, folinic acid, and interferon alfa. J Clin Oncol 1999; 17: 1580–1588

32. Powell M E, Hill S A, Saunders M I et al. Effect of carbogen breathing on tumour microregional blood flow in humans. Radiother Oncol 1996; 41: 225–231

33. McSheehy P M, Robinson S P, Ojugo A S et al. Carbogen breathing increases 5-fluorouracil uptake and cytotoxicity in hypoxic murine RIF-1 tumours: a magnetic resonance study in vivo. Cancer Res 1998; 58: 1185–1194

34. Gupta N, Saleem A, Osman S et al. Carbogen and nicotinamide selectively increase blood flow index (BFI) and 5-fluorouracil (5-FU) delivery in human tumors. Proc Am Soc Clin Oncol 2002; 21: 124, 493a

35. Jackman A L, Taylor G A, Calvert A H et al. Modulation of anti-metabolite effects. Effects of thymidine on the efficacy of the quinazoline-based thymidylate synthetase inhibitor, CB3717. Biochem Pharmacol 1984; 33: 3269–3275

36. Wells P, Gunn R, Hughes A et al. The in vivo quantitation of thymidine salvage by positron emission tomography (PET) as a pharmacodynamic endpoint for thymidylate synthase (TS) inhibition. Proc Am Soc Clin Oncol 2001; 20: 88, 349a

37. Krohn K A, Mankoff D A, Eary J F. Imaging cellular proliferation as a measure of response to therapy. J Clin Pharmacol 2001; 41: 96S–103S

38. Feldman L D, Hortobagyi G N, Buzdar A U et al. Pathological assessment of response to induction chemotherapy in breast cancer. Cancer Res 1986; 46: 2578–2581

39. Chang J, Powles T J, Allred D C et al. Biologic markers as predictors of clinical outcome from systemic therapy for primary operable breast cancer. J Clin Oncol 1999; 17: 3058–3063

40. Buck A C, Schirrmeister H H, Guhlmann C A et al. Ki-67 immunostaining in pancreatic cancer and chronic active pancreatitis: does in vivo FDG uptake correlate with proliferative activity? J Nucl Med 2001; 42: 721–725

41. Avril N, Menzel M, Dose J et al. Glucose metabolism of breast cancer assessed by 18F-FDG PET: histologic and immunohistochemical tissue analysis. J Nucl Med 2001; 42: 9–16

42. Vesselle H, Schmidt R A, Pugsley J M et al. Lung cancer proliferation correlates with [F-18]fluorodeoxyglucose uptake by positron emission tomography. Clin Cancer Res 2000; 6: 3837–3844

43. Kubota R, Yamada S, Kubota K et al. Intratumoural distribution of fluorine-18-fluorodeoxyglucose in vivo: high accumulation in macrophages and granulation tissues studied by microautoradiography. J Nucl Med 1992; 33: 1972–1980

44. Van de Wiele C, Lahorte C, Oyen W et al. Nuclear medicine imaging to predict response to radiotherapy: a review. Int J Radiat Oncol Biol Phys 2003; 55: 5–15

45. Cleaver J E. Thymidine metabolism and cell kinetics. Front Biol 1967: 43–100

46. Larson S M, Weiden P L, Grunbaum Z et al. Positron imaging feasibility studies. I: Characteristics of [3H]thymidine uptake in rodent and canine neoplasms: concise communication. J Nucl Med 1981; 22: 869–874

47. Martiat P, Ferrant A, Labar D et al. In vivo measurement of carbon-11 thymidine uptake in non-Hodgkin's lymphoma using positron emission tomography. J Nucl Med 1988; 29: 1633–1637

48. Goethals P, van Eijkeren M, Lemahieu I. In vivo distribution and identification of 11C-activity after injection of [methyl-11C]thymidine in Wistar rats. J Nucl Med 1999; 40: 491–496

49. Shields A F, Mankoff D, Graham MM et al. Analysis of 2-carbon-11-thymidine blood metabolites in PET imaging. J Nucl Med 1996; 37: 290–296

50. Vander Borght T M, Lambotte L E, Pauwels S A, Dive C C. Uptake of thymidine labeled on carbon 2: a potential index of liver regeneration by positron emission tomography. Hepatology 1990; 12: 113–118

51. Vander Borght T, Lambotte LE, Pauwels S A et al. Noninvasive measurement of liver regeneration with

positron emission tomography and [2-11C]thymidine. Gastroenterology 1991; 101: 794–799

52. Gunn R N, Ranicar A, Yap J T et al. On-line measurement of exhaled [11C]CO$_2$ during PET. J Nucl Med 2000; 41: 605–611

53. Shields A F, Mankoff D A, Link J M et al. Carbon-11-thymidine and FDG to measure therapy response. J Nucl Med 1998; 39: 1757–1762

54. Wells P, Gunn R N, Alison M et al. Assessment of proliferation in vivo using 2-[(11)C]thymidine positron emission tomography in advanced intra-abdominal malignancies. Cancer Res 2002; 62: 5698–5702

55. Blau I W, Elstner E, Waechter M et al. Sensitivity of CFU-GM from normal human bone marrow and leukaemic clonogenic cells (CFU-L) from blood of patients with myelogenous leukaemia to 3′-deoxy-3′-fluorothymidine in comparison to 3′-azido-3′-deoxythymidine. Blut 1989; 59: 455–457

56. Kong X B, Zhu Q Y, Vidal P M et al. Comparisons of anti-human immunodeficiency virus activities, cellular transport, and plasma and intracellular pharmacokinetics of 3′-fluoro-3′-deoxythymidine and 3′-azido-3′-deoxythymidine. Antimicrob Agents Chemother 1992; 36: 808–818

57. Flexner C. Relationship between plasma concentrations of 3′-deoxy-3′-fluorothymidine (alovudine) and antiretroviral activity in two concentration-controlled trials. J Infect Dis 1994; 170: 1394–1403

58. Eriksson S, Kierdaszuk B, Munch-Peterson B et al. Comparison of the substrate specificities of human thymidine kinase 1 and 2 and deoxycytidine kinase toward antiviral and cytostatic nucleoside analogs. Biochem Biophys Res Commun 1991; 176: 586–592

59. Rasey J S, Geierson J R, Wiens L W et al. Validation of FLT uptake as a measure of thymidine kinase-1 activity in A549 carcinoma cells. J Nucl Med 2002; 43: 1210–1217

60. Ellims P H, Van der Weyden M B, Melley G et al. Thymidine kinase isoenzymes in human malignant lymphoma. Cancer Res 1981; 41: 691–695

61. Shields A F, Grierson J R, Dohmen B M et al. Imaging proliferation in vivo with [F-18]FLT and positron emission tomography. Nat Med 1998; 4: 1334–1336

62. Buck A K, Schirrmeister H, Hetzel M et al. 3-deoxy-3-[(18)F]fluorothymidine-positron emission tomography for noninvasive assessment of proliferation in pulmonary nodules. Cancer Res 2002; 62: 3331–3334

63. Vesselle H, Grierson J, Muzi M et al. In vivo validation of 3′deoxy-3′-[(18)F]fluorothymidine ([(18)F]FLT) as a proliferation imaging tracer in humans: correlation of [(18)F]FLT uptake by positron emission tomography with Ki-67 immunohistochemistry and flow cytometry in human lung tumours. Clin Cancer Res 2002; 8: 3315–3323

64. Gillies R J. In vivo molecular imaging. J Cell Biochem Suppl 2002; 39: 231–238

65. Blasberg R. PET imaging of gene expression. Eur J Cancer 2002; 38: 2137–2146

66. Tavitian B, Terrazzino S, Kuhnast B et al. In vivo imaging of oligonucleotides with positron emission tomography. Nat Med 1998; 4: 467–471

67. Tavitian B. In vivo antisense imaging. Q J Nucl Med 2000; 44: 236–255

68. Younes C K, Boisgard R, Tavitian B. Labelled oligonucleotides as radiopharmaceuticals: pitfalls, problems and perspectives. Curr Pharm Des 2002; 8: 1451–1466

69. Tjuvajev J G, Avril N, Oku T et al. Imaging herpes virus thymidine kinase gene transfer and expression by positron emission tomography. Cancer Res 1998; 58: 4333–4341

70. Tjuvajev J G, Stockhammer G, Desai R et al. Imaging the expression of transfected genes in vivo. Cancer Res 1995; 55: 6126–6132

71. Gambhir S S, Herschman H R, Cherry S R et al. Imaging transgene expression with radionuclide imaging technologies. Neoplasia 2000; 2: 118–138

72. MacLaren D C, Gambhir S S, Satyamurthy N et al. Repetitive, non-invasive imaging of the dopamine D2 receptor as a reporter gene in living animals. Gene Ther 1999; 6: 785–791

73. Rogers B E, McLean S F, Kirkman R L et al. In vivo localization of [(111)In]-DTPA-D-Phe1-octreotide to human ovarian tumour xenografts induced to express the somatostatin receptor subtype 2 using an adenoviral vector. Clin Cancer Res 1999; 5: 383–393

74. Groot-Wassink T, Aboagye E O, Glaser M et al. Adenovirus biodistribution and noninvasive imaging of gene expression in vivo by positron emission tomography using human sodium/iodide symporter as reporter gene. Hum Gene Ther 2002; 13: 1723–1735

75. Moolten F L. Suicide genes for cancer therapy. Sci. Med 1997; 4: 16–25

76. Jacobs A, Voges J, Reszka R et al. Positron-emission tomography of vector-mediated gene expression in gene therapy for gliomas. Lancet 2001; 358: 727–729

77. Mottram J C. A factor of importance in the radiotherapy of tumours. Br J Radiol 1936; 9: 606–614

78. Gray L H, Conger A D, Ebert M et al. Concentration of oxygen dissolved in tissues at the time of irradiation as a factor in radiotherapy. Br J Radiol 1953; 26: 638–638

79. Brizel D M, Dodge R K, Clough R W et al. Oxygenation of head and neck cancer: changes during radiotherapy and impact on treatment outcome. Radiother Oncol 1999; 53: 113–117

80. Brizel D M, Sibley G S, Prosnitz L R et al. Tumour hypoxia adversely affects the prognosis of carcinoma of the head and neck. Int J Radiat Oncol Biol Phys 1997; 38: 285–289

81. Hockel M, Schlenger K, Aral E et al. Association between tumour hypoxia and malignant progression in advanced cancer of the uterine cervix. Cancer Res 1996; 56: 4509–4515

82. Khalil A A, Horsman M R, Overgaard J. The importance of determining necrotic fraction when studying the effect of tumour volume on tissue oxygenation. Acta Oncol 1995; 34: 297–300

83. Lewis J S, McCarthy D W, McCarthy T J et al. Evaluation of 64Cu-ATSM in vitro and in vivo in a hypoxic tumour model. J Nucl Med 1999; 40: 177–183

84. Yeh S H, Liu R S, Wu L C et al. Fluorine-18 fluoromisonidazole tumour to muscle retention ratio for the detection of hypoxia in nasopharyngeal carcinoma. Eur J Nucl Med 1996; 23: 1378–1383

85. Rasey J S, Koh W J, Grierson J R et al. Radiolabelled fluoromisonidazole as an imaging agent for tumour hypoxia. Int J Radiat Oncol Biol Phys 1989; 17: 985–991

86. Koh W J, Rasey J S, Evans M L et al. Imaging of hypoxia in human tumours with [F-18]fluoromisonidazole. Int J Radiat Oncol Biol Phys 1992; 22: 199–212

87. Rasey J S, Koh W J, Evans M L et al. Quantifying regional hypoxia in human tumours with positron emission tomography of [18F]fluoromisonidazole: a pretherapy study of 37 patients. Int J Radiat Oncol Biol Phys 1996; 36: 417–428

88. Lewis J S, Welch M J. PET imaging of hypoxia. Q J Nucl Med 2001; 45: 183–188

89. Varagnolo L, Stokkel M P, Mazzi U et al. 18F-labeled radiopharmaceuticals for PET in oncology, excluding FDG. Nucl Med Biol 2000; 27: 103–112

90. Barthel H, Brown G, Wilson H et al. In vivo evaluation of [18F]Fluoroetanidazole for imaging tumour hypoxia with positron emission tomography (PET). Br J Cancer 2002; 86: S13 (Abstract 1.2)

91. Barthel H, Brown G, Wilson H et al. {18F}Fluoroetanidazole for imaging modulated tumour hypoxia with positron emission tomography (PET). World J of Nucl Med 2002; 1: S103 (Abstract 220)

92. Rasey J S, Hofstrand P D, Chin L K et al. Characterization of [18F]fluoroetanidazole, a new radiopharmaceutical for detecting tumour hypoxia. J Nucl Med 1999; 40: 1072–1079

93. Ziemer S, Evans S M, Kachur A V et al. Noninvasive imaging of tumour hypoxia in rats using the 2-nitroimidazole (18)F-EF5. Eur J Nucl Med Mol Imaging 2003; 30: 259–266

94. Lewis J S, Sharp T L, Laforest R et al. Tumour uptake of copper-diacetyl-bis(N(4)-methylthiosemicarbazone): effect of changes in tissue oxygenation. J Nucl Med 2001; 42: 655–661

95. Dehdashti F, Mintun J S, Lewis R et al. Evaluation of tumour hypoxia with Cu-60-ATSM and PET. J Nucl Med 2000; 41: 34P

96. Chao K S, Bosch W R, Mutic S et al. A novel approach to overcome hypoxic tumour resistance: Cu-ATSM-guided intensity-modulated radiation therapy. Int J Radiat Oncol Biol Phys 2001; 49: 1171–1182

97. Folkman J. Tumour angiogenesis: therapeutic implications. N Engl J Med 1971; 285: 1182–1186

98. Folkman J. What is the evidence that tumours are angiogenesis-dependent? J Natl Cancer Inst 1990; 82: 4–6

99. Miller K D, Sweeney C J, Sledge G W Jr. Redefining the target: chemotherapeutics as antiangiogenics. J Clin Oncol 2001; 19: 1195–1206

100. Poon R T, Fan S T, Wong J. Clinical implications of circulating angiogenic factors in cancer patients. J Clin Oncol 2001; 19: 1207–225

101. Ferrara N. VEGF and the quest for tumour angiogenesis factors. Nat Rev Cancer 2002; 2: 795–803

102. Shweiki D, Itin A, Soffer D et al. Vascular endothelial growth factor induced by hypoxia may mediate hypoxia-initiated angiogenesis. Nature 1992; 359: 843–845

103. Collingridge D R, Carroll V A, Glaser M et al. The development of [(124)I]iodinated-VG76e: a novel tracer for imaging vascular endothelial growth factor in vivo using positron emission tomography. Cancer Res 2002; 62: 5912–5919

104. Stromblad S, Cheresh D A. Integrins, angiogenesis and vascular cell survival. Chem Biol 1996; 3: 881–885

105. Westlin W F. Integrins as targets of angiogenesis inhibition. Cancer J 2001; 7: S139–143

106. Brooks P C, Stromblad S, Klemke R et al. Antiintegrin alpha v beta 3 blocks human breast cancer growth and angiogenesis in human skin. J Clin Invest 1995; 96: 1815–1822

107. Haubner R, Wester H J, Weber W A et al. Noninvasive imaging of alpha(v)beta3 integrin expression using 18F-labeled RGD-containing glycopeptide and positron emission tomography. Cancer Res 2001; 61: 1781–1785

108. Anderson H, Price P, Blomley M et al. Measuring changes in human tumour vasculature in response to therapy using functional imaging techniques. Br J Cancer 2001; 85: 1085–1093

109. Beaney R P, Lammertsma A A, Jones T et al. Positron emission tomography for in vivo measurement of regional blood flow, oxygen utilisation, and blood volume in patients with breast carcinoma. Lancet 1984; 1: 131–134

110. Lammertsma A A. Positron emission tomography and in vivo measurements of tumour perfusion and oxygen utilisation. Cancer Metastasis Rev 1987; 6: 521–539

111. Wilson C B, Lammertsma A A, McKenzie C G et al. Measurements of blood flow and exchanging water space in breast tumours using positron emission tomography: a rapid and noninvasive dynamic method. Cancer Res 1992; 52: 1592–1597

112. Anderson H, Price P. Clinical measurement of blood flow in tumours using positron emission tomography: a review. Nucl Med Commun 2002; 23: 131–138

113. Dark G G, Hill S A, Prise V E et al. Combretastatin A-4, an agent that displays potent and selective toxicity toward tumour vasculature. Cancer Res 1997; 57: 1829–1834

114. Tozer G M, Prise V E, Wilson J et al. Combretastatin A-4 phosphate as a tumour vascular-targeting agent: early effects in tumours and normal tissues. Cancer Res 1999; 59: 1626–1634

115. Prise V E, Honess D J, Stratford M R et al. The vascular response of tumour and normal tissues in the rat to the vascular targeting agent, combretastatin A-4-phosphate, at clinically relevant doses. Int J Oncol 2002; 21: 717–726

116. Chaplin D J, Hill S A. The development of combretastatin A4 phosphate as a vascular targeting agent. Int J Radiat Oncol Biol Phys 2002; 54: 1491–1496

117. Anderson H, Yap J T, Price P. Measurement of tumour and normal tissue (NT) perfusion by positron emission tomography (PET) in the evaluation of antivascular therapy: results in the phase I study of combretastatin A4 phosphate (CA4P). Proc Am Soc Clin Onco 2000; 19: 179a

118. Griggs J, Metcalfe J C, Hesketh R. Targeting tumour vasculature: the development of combretastatin A4. Lancet Oncol 2001; 2: 82–87

119. Cunningham V J, Lammertsma A A. Radioligand studies in brain: kinetic analysis of PET data. Med Chem Res 1994; 5: 79–96

120. Dehdashti F, Mortimer J E, Siegal B A et al. Positron tomographic assessment of estrogen receptors in breast cancer: comparison with FDG-PET and in vitro receptor assays. J Nucl Med 1995; 36: 1766–1774

121. McGuire A H, Dehdashti F, Siegal B A et al. Positron tomographic assessment of 16alpha-[18F] fluoro-17beta-estradiol uptake in metastatic breast carcinoma. J Nucl Med 1991; 32: 1526–1531

122. Dehdashti F, Flanagan F L, Mortimer J E et al. Positron emission tomographic assessment of 'metabolic flare' to predict response of metastatic breast cancer to antiestrogen therapy. Eur J Nucl Med 1999; 26: 51–56

123. Mortimer J E, Dehdashti F, Siegal B A et al. Positron emission tomography with 2-[18F]Fluoro-2-deoxy-D-glucose and 16alpha-[18F]fluoro-17beta-estradiol in breast cancer: correlation with estrogen receptor status and response to systemic therapy. Clin Cancer Res 1996; 2: 933–939

124. Flanagan F L, Dehdashti F, Siegel B A. PET in breast cancer. Semin Nucl Med 1998; 28: 290–302

125. Moresco R M, Scheithauer B W, Lucignani G et al. Oestrogen receptors in meningiomas: a correlative PET and immunohistochemical study. Nucl Med Commun 1997; 18: 606–615

126. Liu A J, Katzenellenbogen J A, Van Brocklin H F et al. 20-[18F]fluoromibolerone, a positron-emitting radiotracer for androgen receptors: synthesis and tissue distribution studies. J Nucl Med 1991; 32: 81–88

127. Liu A, Carlson K E, Katzenellenbogen J A. Synthesis of high-affinity fluorine-substituted ligands for the androgen receptor. Potential agents for imaging prostatic cancer by positron emission tomography. J Med Chem 1992; 35: 2113–2129

128. Bonasera T A, O'Neil J P, Xu M et al. Preclinical evaluation of fluorine-18-labeled androgen receptor ligands in baboons. J Nucl Med 1996; 37: 1009–1015

129. Larson S M. Measuring response to therapy with molecular imaging. Eur J Cancer 2002; 7 (Suppl): S12

130. Anderson C J, Dehdashti F, Cutler P D et al. 64Cu-TETA-octreotide as a PET imaging agent for patients with neuroendocrine tumours. J Nucl Med 2001; 42: 213–21

131. Henze M, Schuhmacher J, Hipp P et al. PET imaging of somatostatin receptors using. J Nucl Med 2001; 42: 1053–1056

132. Ugur O, Kothari P J, Finn R D et al. Ga-66 labeled somatostatin analogue DOTA-DPhe1-Tyr3-octreotide as a potential agent for positron emission tomography imaging and receptor mediated internal radiotherapy of somatostatin receptor positive tumours. Nucl Med Biol 2002; 29: 147–157

133. Lucignani G, Losa M, Moresco R M et al. Differentiation of clinically non-functioning pituitary adenomas from meningiomas and craniopharyngiomas by positron emission tomography with [18F]fluoro-ethyl-spiperone. Eur J Nucl Med 1997; 24: 1149–1155

134. Ben-David I, Rozen Y, Ortu G et al. Radiosynthesis of ML03, a novel positron emission tomography biomarker for targeting epidermal growth factor receptor via the labeling synthon: [11C]acryloyl chloride. Appl Radiat Isot 2003; 58: 209–217

135. Lovqvist A, Sundin A, Ahlstrom H et al. 76Br-labeled monoclonal anti-CEA antibodies for radioimmuno positron emission tomography. Nucl Med Biol 1995; 22: 125–131

136. Lovqvist A, Sundin A, Ahlstrom H et al. Pharmacokinetics and experimental PET imaging of a bromine-76-labeled monoclonal anti-CEA antibody. J Nucl Med 1997; 38: 395–401

137. Wu A M, Yazaki P J, Tsai S et al. High-resolution microPET imaging of carcinoembryonic antigen-positive xenografts by using a copper-64-labeled engineered antibody fragment. Proc Natl Acad Sci USA 2000; 97: 8495–8500

138. Bakir M A, Eccles S, Babich J W et al. c-erbB2 protein overexpression in breast cancer as a target for PET using iodine-124-labeled monoclonal antibodies. J Nucl Med 1992; 33: 2154–2160

139. Evan G I, Vousden K H. Proliferation, cell cycle and apoptosis in cancer. Nature 2001; 411: 342–348

140. Verhoven B, Krahling S, Schlegel R A et al. Regulation of phosphatidylserine exposure and phagocytosis of apoptotic T lymphocytes. Cell Death Differ 1999; 6: 262–270

141. Blankenberg F G, Tait J, Ohtsuki K et al. Apoptosis: the importance of nuclear medicine. Nucl Med Commun 2000; 21: 241–250

142. van Heerde W L, de Groot P G, Reutelingsperger C P. The complexity of the phospholipid binding protein Annexin V. Thromb Haemost 1995; 73: 172–179

143. Blankenberg F G, Katsikis P D, Tait J F et al. In vivo detection and imaging of phosphatidylserine expression during programmed cell death. Proc Natl Acad Sci U S A 1998; 95: 6349–6354

144. Blankenberg F G, Katsikis P D, Tait J F et al. Imaging of apoptosis (programmed cell death) with 99mTc annexin V. J Nucl Med 1999; 40: 184–191

145. Belhocine T, Steinmetz N, Hustinx R et al. Increased uptake of the apoptosis-imaging agent (99m)Tc recombinant human Annexin V in human tumours after one course of chemotherapy as a predictor of

tumour response and patient prognosis. Clin Cancer Res 2002; 8: 2766–2774

146. Glaser M, Collingridge D, Aboagye E et al. Iodine-124 labelled Annexin-V as a potential radiotracer to study apoptosis using positron emission tomography. Appl Radiat Isot 2003; 58: 55–62

147. Zijlstra S, Gunawan J, Burchert W. Synthesis and evaluation of a 18F-labelled recombinant Annexin V derivative, for identification and quantification of apoptotic cells with PET. Appl Radiat Isot 2003; 58: 201–207

148. Aboagye E O, Bhujwalla Z M. Malignant transformation alters membrane choline phospholipid metabolism of human mammary epithelial cells. Cancer Res 1999; 59: 80–84

149. Ramirez de Molina A, Rodriguez-Gonzalez A, Gutierrez R et al. Overexpression of choline kinase is a frequent feature in human tumour-derived cell lines and in lung, prostate, and colorectal human cancers. Biochem Biophys Res Commun 2002; 296: 580–583

150. de Jong I J, Pruim J, Elsinga P H et al. Visualisation of bladder cancer using (11)C-choline PET: first clinical experience. Eur J Nucl Med Mol Imaging 2002; 29: 1283–1288

151. de Jong I J, Pruim J, Elsinga P H et al. Visualization of prostate cancer with 11C-choline positron emission tomography. Eur Urol 2002; 42: 18–23

152. Picchio M, Landori C, Messa C et al. Positive [11C]choline and negative [18F]FDG with positron emission tomography in recurrence of prostate cancer. Am J Roentgenol 2002; 179: 482–484

153. Hara T, Kosaka N, Kishi H. PET imaging of prostate cancer using carbon-11-choline. J Nucl Med 1998; 39: 990–995

154. Ohtani T, Kurihara H, Ishiuchi S et al. Brain tumour imaging with carbon-11 choline: comparison with FDG PET and gadolinium-enhanced MR imaging. Eur J Nucl Med 2001; 28: 1664–1670

155. Zijlstra J G, de Vries E G, Mulder N H. Drug resistance in medical oncology. Neth J Med 1987; 30: 85–93

156. Bellamy W T, Dalton W S, Dorr R T. The clinical relevance of multidrug resistance. Cancer Invest 1990; 8: 547–562

157. Germann U A, Pastan I, Gottesman M M. P-glycoproteins: mediators of multidrug resistance. Semin Cell Biol 1993; 4: 63–76

158. Gottesman M M, Pastan I. Biochemistry of multidrug resistance mediated by the multidrug transporter. Annu Rev Biochem 1993; 62: 385–427

159. Hendrikse N H, Franssen E J, van de Graaf W T et al. Visualization of multidrug resistance in vivo. Eur J Nucl Med 1999; 26: 283–293

160. Elsinga P H, Franssen E J, Hendrikse N H et al. Carbon-11-labeled daunorubicin and verapamil for probing P-glycoprotein in tumours with PET. J Nucl Med 1996; 37: 1571–1575

161. Levchenko A, Mehta B M, Lee J B et al. Evaluation of 11C-colchicine for PET imaging of multiple drug resistance. J Nucl Med 2000; 41: 493–501

162. Brady F, Luthra S, Brown G et al. Radiolabelled tracers and anticancer drugs for assessment of therapeutic efficacy using PET. Curr Pharm Des 2001; 7: 1863–1892

Chapter 63

Molecular imaging in cancer treatment: magnetic resonance imaging

Andrzej Dzik-Jurasz

Introduction

All living organisms from unicellular bacteria to the most complex must perform several critical functions including growth, respiration, reproduction, locomotion, digestion, excretion and possess a mechanism(s) through which they sense their environment. These processes occur at the cellular level and are mediated via molecular events. It is these very mechanisms that molecular imaging aims to visualize. The fundamental building block of all organisms is the cell. Each cell has the capability to carry out the functions listed above but as organisms became more complex so cells began to take on dedicated roles (i.e. red blood cells and neurones).

Cells typically consist of a nucleus that contains the full complement of genetic material in the form of chromosomes. These chromosomes are contained within a *nuclear envelope* segregating nuclear from extra-nuclear material. Outside the nucleus are specialized organelles whose proportion will vary depending on the specific role of that cell. A cell interacts with its environment via a *semi-permeable membrane*. Although highly lipophilic substances, such as general anaesthetics, cross this barrier with ease the majority of interactions occur via membrane receptors that have components extending out of and into the cell. Groups of cells will be contained within an extracellular matrix whose composition again will depend on the tissue in question.

Ultimately, the function and fate of any cell depends on the interaction between the proteins coded for by its genes and its surrounding environment. These genes carry the chemical instructions that code for the proteins that determine the structure and function of that cell and the organism as a whole. It is generally accepted that, in the majority of instances, the flow of instructions runs from genes and is expressed in the proteins coded for by those genes. Any alteration in the mechanism of this global process can result in advantage or disadvantage to the organism. Advantage, for example, could be gained through an enhanced ability to reproduce, whilst we usually classify disadvantage as disease. Clearly, cancer confers no advantage to an organism.

With the advent of molecular medicine and the sequencing of the human genome,[1,2] a real need has arisen to image molecular events *in vivo*.[3] Strategically, the importance of developing molecular imaging as part of radiological research and practice has been highlighted in statements from the National Cancer Institute,[4,5] National Institute of Health and several bodies representing the radiological community.[6–8]

Currently, the imaging of molecular events *in vivo* by MR imaging remains firmly within the experimental field in which a sizeable literature is beginning to accumulate. It is only a matter of time though before those experimental techniques begin translation into the clinic, making it necessary for radiologists to become acquainted with subjects outside their usual curriculum. Molecular imaging, by necessity, requires a multidisciplinary approach incorporating elements of molecular and cell biology, genetics, chemistry and biophysics. The subject matter is considerable and therefore this chapter does not seek to be comprehensive but representative. A brief overview is given of molecular, cell and tumour biology and the physical properties characterizing the tumour microenvironment, followed by a discussion of the current state and future directions of molecular imaging.

Molecular and cell biology: targets for molecular imaging

In this section the key concepts of molecular and cell biology are reviewed. As an aid to the nomenclature, the reader is referred to an excellent glossary on the subject.[9]

Chemical and structural background

The sum total of the genomic information characterizing an organism resides in DNA (deoxyribonucleic acid), although eukaryotes (organisms whose cellular DNA is contained within a nuclear envelope) also possess a small 16,569 base pair circular mitochondrial DNA. Structurally, DNA is composed of a double helix (Fig. 63.1), most commonly in the B-DNA form describing a right-handed helix just over 10 base pairs per turn. Alternating sugars (deoxyribose in the case of DNA) and phosphates make up the backbone of each strand of DNA. A base and a sugar are termed a *nucleoside*, whilst a base, sugar and phosphate com-

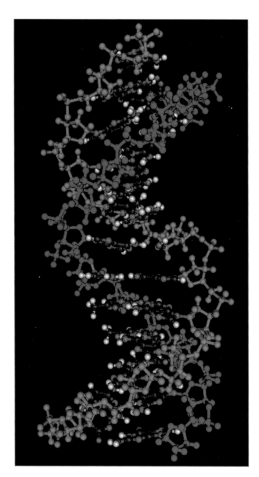

Figure 63.1. *A short section of DNA demonstrating the typical helical and central rung structure. The two strands of DNA are depicted in blue and purple and the atoms of the central rung are in grey, red and white. The bases in the central rung are complementary, with adenine binding to thymine and guanine to cytosine via hydrogen bonding. The structure is based on crystallographic work[10] and has protein data bank identification 1GSE.*

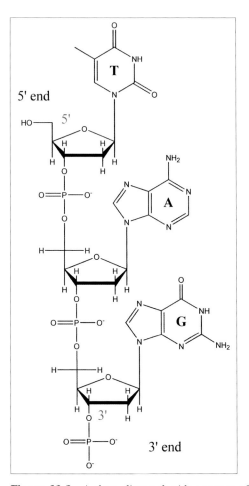

Figure 63.2. *A short oligonucleotide sequence of thymine, adenine and guanine with the 3′ and 5′ ends of the sequence indicated on the diagram. The 5′ and 3′ terms refer to the position of the nucleotide bases relative to the sugar molecule. The convention is that the 5′ end indicates the start of a DNA strand and the 3′ the end. The 3′ and 5′ carbons are indicated in red.*

plex is termed a *nucleotide*. Nucleotides are linked to each other via a phosphodiester link. The bases are attached to the sugars and include the pyrimidines, cytosine and thymine, and the purines, adenine and guanine. In RNA (ribonucleic acid), uracil replaces thymine. Strands of DNA are antiparallel and complementary. In order to create an energetically stable structure, adenine pairs via hydrogen (non-covalent electrostatic) bonding to thymine and cytosine binds to guanine, giving DNA its characteristic central rung structure. The exclusive complementarity binding of adenine to thymine and cytosine to guanine is also referred to as Watson–Crick base pairing. A nucleotide sequence therefore has one end where the 5′ carbon is not linked to another sugar, whilst the other end of the molecule has a 3′ carbon lacking a phosphodiester link (Fig. 63.2). The 5′–3′ concept is essential for understanding DNA replication and translation. A set of three bases termed a *codon* defines one of the 20 amino acids that make up the polypeptide and

protein structures of the body whilst the region of DNA coding a specific polypeptide is termed a *gene*. Many base sequences in chromosomes do not code for genes and are termed 'nonsense' sequences, whilst other non-coding regions possess specific functions, such as UAA, UAG and UGA, which terminate transcription.

The transcription of a segment of gene DNA into its protein product involves the intermediary of RNA. In the majority, RNA is single stranded and exists in three forms:

- Messenger RNA (mRNA) carries the complementary DNA base pair sequence of a gene
- Transfer RNA (tRNA) carries amino acids to ribosomes
- Ribosomal RNA (rRNA) is involved in the interaction between mRNA and tRNA during protein synthesis

In the nucleus, DNA is packaged into a *nucleosome* consisting of eight histone proteins with 146 DNA base pairs wound one and three quarter times around a nucleosome. This nucleoprotein complex creates the *chromatin* structure that becomes condensed during metaphase into a *chromosome* recognizable at light microscopy. During the metaphase stage of mitosis, each chromosome consists of two symmetrical *chromatids* attached at the *centromere*. Giemsa staining of chromatids results in dark and light G-bands that can be identified on the short (p) and long (q) arm of a chromosome. The *karyotype* therefore defines the specific number and form of chromosomes unique to a species. Human cells, for example, contain 46 chromosomes, 44 of which are autosomes (22 matching pairs numbered 1–22) and two of which are the sex chromosomes

(XX for female and XY for male). Finally, the *genome* refers to the complete genetic make-up of an individual or organism and consists of approximately 3×10^9 base pairs in humans coding in the region of 30,000 genes.

DNA replication (Fig. 63.3)

The general mechanisms behind DNA replication are now well understood and follow an ordered pattern. DNA *helicase* stimulates separation of the two DNA strands in conjunction with DNA *gyrase*, which aids in unwinding the double helix. Once created, the single-stranded DNA is stabilized by binding proteins. RNA is the primer for DNA synthesis and occurs when short strands of RNA, termed *primers*, base pair with DNA. DNA *polymerases* (Pols) then catalyse the addition of nucleotides to a pre-existing strand

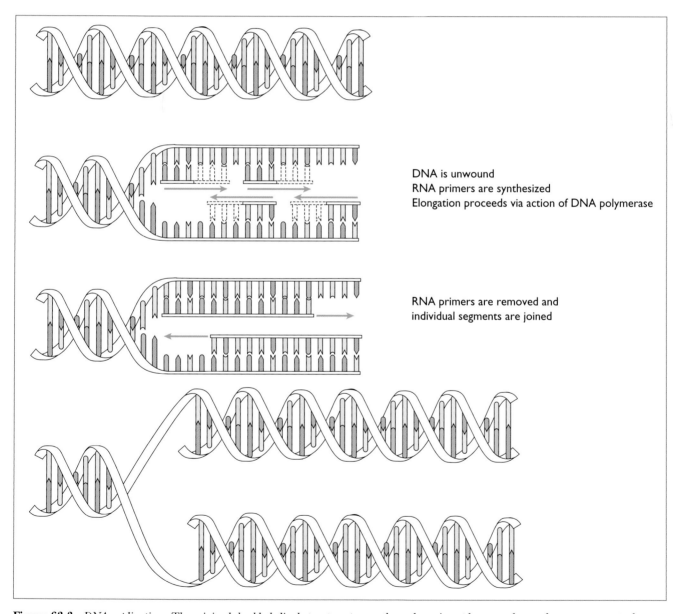

DNA is unwound
RNA primers are synthesized
Elongation proceeds via action of DNA polymerase

RNA primers are removed and
individual segments are joined

Figure 63.3. *DNA replication. The original double helical structure passes through various phases under nuclear enzyme control, resulting in the creation of a copy of the original.*

of DNA or primer RNA. Mismatched base pairs can be removed now and the *3′-5′ exonuclease* characterizes the efficient editing of DNA available to the cell. A *5-3′ exonuclease* removes the RNA primer and repairs double-stranded DNA if necessary.

Cell cycle (Fig. 63.4)

In eukaryotes, the cell cycle has two periods, *mitosis* and *interphase*, with cell division occurring during mitosis whilst cell growth and DNA replication occur during interphase. Interphase is further divided into the *G1* phase where the cell prepares for DNA synthesis, *S* phase when DNA synthesis occurs and the *G2* phase. Although cells in the *G0* phase will often remain metabolically active, they do not proceed through the cell cycle (i.e. neurones).

Gene transcription and protein synthesis (Fig. 63.5)

The transcription of the *antisense* strand of DNA to mRNA consists of initiation in which RNA polymerases bind to promoter sites, subsequently elongate and, finally, terminate. Numerous proteins control transcription that occurs mostly at the level of initiation in eukaryotes. Characteristically, up to 95% of the human genome is non-coding for protein products. A gene consists of coding regions termed *exons* and non-coding areas termed *introns*. Introns begin with GT and end with AG, whilst UTRs (untranslated regions) flank the upstream part (the 5′ end) of the first exon and the downstream (3′ end) of the last exon. The rate of gene transcription is usually regulated by DNA sequences outside of the transcription unit which are termed *cis-acting control elements*. These areas do not encode proteins but act as binding sites for DNA-binding proteins that control replication. These *cis*-regions tend to be clustered in the promoter and enhancer regions of most genes, with certain DNA sequences occurring with greater regularity than others such as the TATA and CAAT box. These sequences together with other binding sites and proteins define the rate of transcription.

Transcription begins at the 5′ end of the mRNA that becomes capped by 7-methylguanosine and is termed the *CAP* end. Immediately beyond the CAP at the 5′ end is a *leader* sequence sited next to an *initiation* codon (often ATG). The whole gene (exons and introns) is then transcribed until a stop sequence is encountered, indicating the end of the translated region. This is followed by a UTR, usually in the form of a polyadenylated sequence signalling cleavage. The introns are then excised and the exons sliced whilst still in the nucleus.

The *translation* into proteins occurs via the ribosomal machinery in the cytoplasm. Mechanistically, the ribosome moves relative to the mRNA and has three binding sites for tRNA termed the *acceptor, peptidyl* and *exit* sites. Translation begins with binding of the ribosome to the AUG initiation codon on mRNA, with synthesis subsequently driven by elongation factors. Each codon on mRNA is recognized by a specific anticodon on tRNA carrying the appropriate amino acid. The amino acids are joined together to form the protein product by peptidyl transferase with the catalysis being driven by the RNA molecules in the ribosome. On reaching a termination codon, the polypeptide is completed and the ribosome falls off. The protein product is still not fully functional at this point and, in most circumstances, undergoes post-translational processing (e.g. proteolytic cleavage, glycosylation, phosphorylation and transportation to the intracellular compartment appropriate for its function). The three-dimensional structure of a protein, for example, is essential to its biological role and considerable research is currently directed towards understanding its mechanisms. This is partly encompassed in the work of *proteomics* to which the computing power of *bioinformatics* is being applied.[11]

Biomolecular techniques

The power and speed of molecular *in vitro* techniques has greatly increased recently and is providing unprecedented insight into gene expression. The resulting information is now being channelled to the rational design of molecular imaging targeting agents.[12] Two key methodologies include:

- Polymerase chain reaction (PCR)
- Microarray analysis

Polymerase chain reaction (Fig. 63.6)

This is a method by which a sequence of DNA is amplified to provide sufficient quantities of product for further analysis. Three steps are involved in the process. DNA is first denatured at 95°C causing its double-stranded structure to separate. Second, oligonucleotide (short single-stranded nucleotides) *primers* (usually 15–25 base pairs in length) are added at 55°C that anneal with the single strands of DNA.

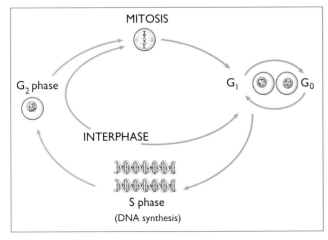

Figure 63.4. *A schematic of the cell cycle.*

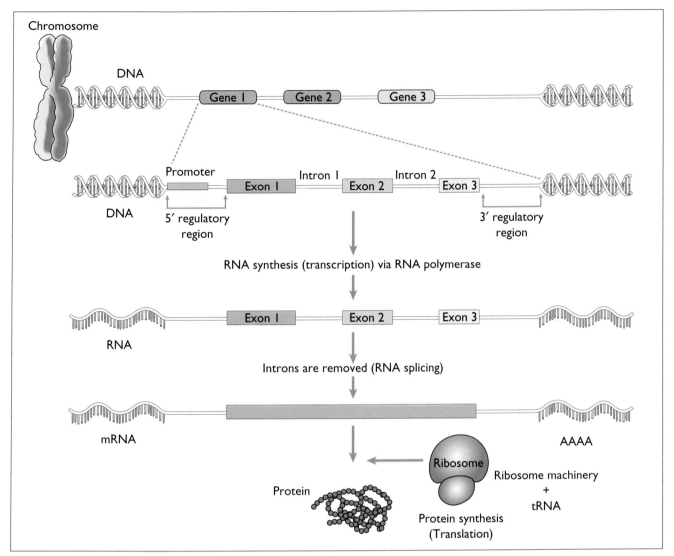

Figure 63.5. *Gene structure and expression. Each chromosome carries a variety of genes that together constitute the organism's genotype. Each gene consists of exons and introns and specialized regulatory regions at its 5′ and 3′ ends. RNA is synthesized from DNA via the process of transcription that is catalysed principally by RNA polymerase. Transcription begins at the 5′ end and continues towards completion at the 3′ end. The new mRNA molecule is processed by splicing, capping (at the 5′ end) and polyadenylation at the 3′ end. A protein is finally constructed when the mRNA is translated using the ribosomal machinery and tRNA to assimilate the requisite amino acid structure of the protein.*

Third, in a step controlled at 72°C, DNA polymerases extend the primers creating an identical complementary strand. This three-stage cycle has an amplification factor of 2^n where n is the number of times the three-stage process is repeated. A 2^{30}-fold amplification is therefore gained after 30 cycles. It is therefore due to this extraordinary specificity and sensitivity – essentially only one copy of a DNA sequence is required as a template – as to why the technique has revolutionized not only cancer but diagnostic and forensic research.

Microarray analysis (Fig. 63.7)

This technique has revolutionized gene analysis and is likely to impact on clinical management in the future.[13] In comparison to other methodologies used to study gene expression, the novel features of microarray analysis are:

- Assessment of global gene expression patterns in cells
- Miniaturization and automation of the method
- Development of bioinformatics and software for handling and analysing the very complex data sets that are generated

Microarrays are manufactured either as DNA spotted onto a glass slide or as oligonucleotides synthesized on to a silica glass slide (photolithography). The methodology is based on the *hybridization* of oligonucleotides representing indi-

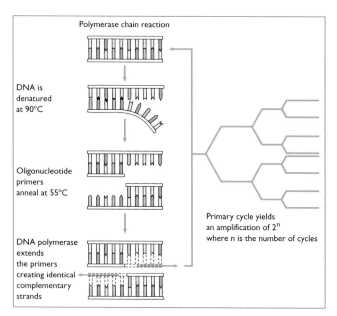

Figure 63.6. *The polymerase chain reaction cycle and amplification. The amplification process can yield enough material for further analysis from as little as a drop (0.4 ml) of blood.*

vidual genes with fluorescently labelled *cDNA* (complementary DNA, that is DNA synthesized from an RNA template). The revolutionary aspect of the technique is in the miniaturization of the process. Up to half a million oligonucleotides are synthesized on a microarray chip measuring less than 2 cm². The expression of up to 15,000 genes can therefore be analysed on a single slide. The use of microar-

rays has already begun to have an impact on oncological practice. It was therefore possible, for example, to distinguish between acute lymphoid and myeloid leukaemia[14] by analysing the expression profiles of 6,817 genes from either blood or bone marrow samples. Although diagnostically useful, there was no prognostic information to be gained from the data. Microarray studies have since been able to prognostically subclassify diffuse large B-cell lymphoma[15] and similar studies have now been reported for melanoma,[16] breast[17] and colorectal cancer.[18]

Tumour biology – the cellular perspective

An extensive literature exists on cancer biology and the reader is referred to several excellent texts[19–22] on the subject. Several essential principles of cancer biology are, however, worth summarizing. The majority of human cancers are generated by mutations in cellular genes and cancer is therefore a genetic disease. A mutation may be sporadic or inherited but ultimately results in the over- or underexpression of a particular gene that has either a direct or downstream effect on cellular and, ultimately, tissue function. Mutations occur as a result of uncorrected errors in DNA replication, often following damage from chemical or physical carcinogens. Carcinogenesis is characterized by multiple steps that often take several decades to be manifested clinically as a tumour. The basis for the process is the concept of clonal escape and dominance. In other words, once a mutation develops in a cell line, that and subsequent generations are more likely to progress towards a clinically manifest tumour. The process is

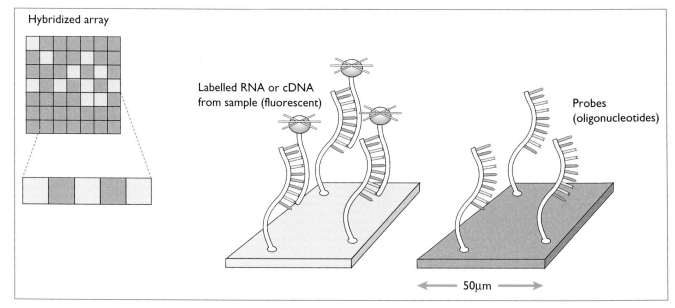

Figure 63.7. *Schematic of a DNA microarray chip. DNA microarrays consist of thousands of DNA probes arranged as an array. Each probe is complementary to a different mRNA (or cDNA). The mRNA that is isolated from a tissue is converted to fluorescently labelled cDNA and used to hybridize the array. The advantage of the technique is its ability to probe the expression of thousands of genes from a sample in one experiment.*

therefore analogous to Darwinian selection such that a stochastically determined mutation results in an inheritable trait conferring a survival and replicative advantage.[23,24] It is estimated that four to seven rate-limiting stochastic events ('hits') characterize the development of most adult-onset solid tumours. Environmental agents such as retroviruses are a rare cause of cancer in humans, but not so DNA viruses, which are now recognized as important carcinogenic agents and include human papilloma virus (cervical cancer), hepatitis B virus (hepatocellular carcinoma) and Epstein–Barr virus (Burkitt's lymphoma).

Oncogenes are genes whose cellular functions are activated by the carcinogenic process and are dominant at the cellular level. The protein product of the oncogene, the *oncoprotein*, may either be structurally abnormal such as mutant Ras exhibiting a single amino acid substitution or be overexpressed like c-MYC in malignant B cells.

Tumour suppressor genes are genes whose functions are inactivated by mutation and act in a recessive fashion at the cellular level. Two common suppressor genes are retinoblastoma (Rb) and p53. The Rb protein (Fig. 63.8) is a nuclear phosphoprotein with DNA-binding activity and influences cell proliferation via the action of transcription factors. p53 (Fig. 63.9), often termed the 'guardian of the genome', acts as a cell cycle checkpoint protein. It does this primarily by activating genes with growth suppression activity. Interestingly, neither p53 nor Rb is necessary for normal cell growth.

A cancer cell is therefore endowed with certain characteristic traits or hallmarks. Hanahan and Weinberg enumerate six neoplastic traits:[27]

- Self-sufficiency in growth signals
- Insensitivity to antigrowth signals

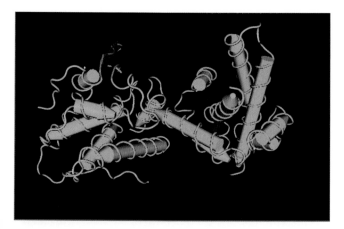

Figure 63.8. *Schematic cartoon of the crystal structure of the retinoblastoma tumour-suppressor pocket domain bound to a nine-residue peptide determined by X-ray crystallography.[25] The product of the retinoblastoma gene is a nuclear phosphoprotein with DNA binding activity that influences cell proliferation. The structure has the protein data bank identification 1GUX.*

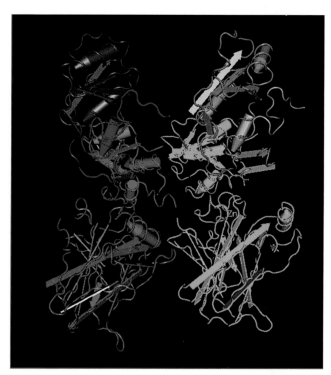

Figure 63.9. *Schematic cartoon of the structure of a human 53BP1–p53 complex determined by X-ray crystallography.[26] 53BP1 is a DNA damage response protein that binds to the DNA binding domain of p53. p53 is important in health and disease. In health it acts as a cell cycle checkpoint protein whilst over 50% of cancers demonstrate mutation in p53. Protein function is determined by amongst others its polypeptide sequence but its three-dimensional disposition is equally crucial to function.*

- Apoptosis
- Limitless replicative potential
- Sustained angiogenesis
- Tissue invasion and metastasis

Self-sufficiency in growth signals

Normal cells require an exogenous signal mediated via diffusible chemical signals and cell receptors to undergo active proliferation. Neoplastic cells are characterized by a loss of this dependence and will often generate their own growth signals through the activation of appropriate oncogenes. Alterations can therefore occur in the extracellular signal, the cellular receptors and the downstream mechanisms initiated by those signals.

Insensitivity to antigrowth signals

Just as normal cells respond positively to a growth stimulus, so antigrowth signals limit replication by control of entry into the cell cycle. Signals received by cells from the environment are sensed by cellular receptors and processed mostly via the retinoblastoma protein, a commonly mutated suppressor gene in cancer.

Apoptosis

Apoptosis is the process of programmed cell death and is characterized histologically by cytoplasmic condensation, DNA and chromatin fragmentation and cellular disintegration, resulting in apoptotic bodies that ultimately become phagocytosed. It is also the process by which several conventional anticancer agents mediate their cell kill effects. The most common strategy for cancer cells to evade apoptosis is via mutation of the p53 suppressor gene. The result is that the normal activation of the enzymatic intracellular cascade system resulting in apoptosis is absent in transformed cells.

Limitless replicative potential

This refers to a loss of a cell-autonomous programme carried by most mammalian cells that limits the number of divisions available to the cell. The mechanism is normally mediated through gradual loss of telomeric DNA at each cell cycle. It is unsurprising therefore that telomeres are maintained in almost all cancers.

Sustained angiogenesis

Angiogenesis determines the growth of new blood vessels. Tumour cells activate the angiogenic switch by favouring the induction of angiogenesis over its inhibition. This is mediated principally via the overexpression of vascular endothelial growth factor (VEGF) and acidic and basic fibroblastic growth factor (a/bFGF). These polypeptides mediate their action by binding to endothelial transmembrane tyrosine kinase that cascades and amplifies the intracellular signal downstream. The inhibition of the angiogenic pathways, including that of tyrosine kinase, is currently a focus of considerable therapeutic interest.

Tissue invasion and metastasis

Metastatic disease accounts for 90% of cancer deaths.[28] The mechanisms are highly complex and remain incompletely understood. In principal, several proteins anchoring cells to their surrounds are altered in malignancy. For example, the function of E-cadherin, a cell-to-cell interaction molecule, is commonly lost in the majority of epithelial cancers. In addition, upregulation of several extracellular proteases with concomitant downregulation of their inhibitors has been described. Clearly, the neoplastic process is highly complex at the cellular and molecular level but potentially provides numerous therapeutic and imaging targets.

Tumour microenvironment – imaging surrogate markers of molecular events

The structural and molecular complexity so evident at the cellular level exists at the level of the tumour microenvironment. The tumour microenvironment is a dynamic system in which there is biophysical and metabolic heterogeneity both spatially and temporally. There is therefore a continuous interaction between tumour cells, the cellular and humoral host response, the vascularity of the tumour and the extracellular matrix (Fig. 63.10). In addition, the phenotype of the tumour will vary with alterations in gene expression. The ability of MR to probe the physical and metabolic characteristics makes this compartment an important target for the application of molecular imaging strategies.[29] It is partially this complexity in the tumour microenvironment that limits morphological imaging in the prediction and prognosis of cancer to treatment.[30] Solid tumours, for example, display several physical barriers that limit the delivery of therapeutics.[31,32] The vascularity of a tumour is known to exhibit considerable heterogeneity and can display a flow greater, equal to or less than that in normal tissue.[33] Hypoxia[34] and acidosis are two further characteristics of the tumour microenvironment that can significantly influence the outcome of anticancer therapies[35] and lead to a more aggressive phenotype.[29] The majority of MR studies examining the tumour microenvironment have been conducted in animal systems where the limitations of intervention and field strength are not as restrictive as in humans. Other than tumour vascularity, tumour hypoxia has been studied using gradient-echo imaging, often in an attempt to elicit a blood oxygen level-dependent (BOLD) effect in response to inhaled carbogen ($95\%\ O_2 + 5\%\ CO_2$) in animals[36] and humans.[37] Oxygen tension maps have been acquired using ^{19}F-MR in animals,[38] whilst in humans, hypoxic imaging markers based on fluorinated nitroimidazoles[39] are currently being evaluated. The *in vivo* assessment of tumour pH by MR is based mostly on spectroscopic work. ^{31}P-MRS (MR spectroscopy), for example, demonstrated that tumours tend to be acidic extracellularly, and neutral or alkaline intracellularly.[40] Interestingly, pH-sensitive MR contrast agents have been described[41] and there is work currently in progress examining the use of magnetization transfer together with paramagnetic agents[42] in the measurement of pH. The current limitation in the sensitivity of MR to direct molecular events has led for the search for surrogate markers of these events. The recent interest in therapeutic targeting of molecular events expressed at the level of the microenvironment has added further impetus to the development of functional MR techniques. None more so than in imaging antiangiogenic therapy and it is in this field that MR of a surrogate molecular event has found greatest success.[43,44] A correlation was demonstrated, for example, by our group between an MR measure of capillary leakiness and response to conventional chemotherapy[45] in patients with locally advanced rectal tumour. In addition, that same study demonstrated a linear correlation between serum VEGF and the capillary leakiness, suggesting that the vascular parameters measured by MR are reflective of the underlying angiogenic process. The validation of the vascular MR parameters is an important task that is currently under intensive investigation.[44] In addition, further work is required to confirm the association between capillary leakiness and response as conflicting results have been published.[46] Finally, it is worth mentioning the role of quantitative diffusion-weighted imaging

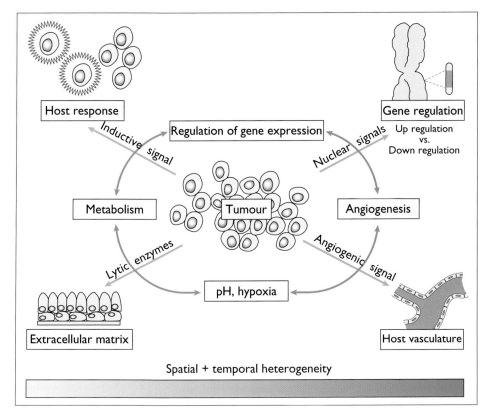

Figure 63.10. *The tumour microenvironment is a complex entity that varies spatially and temporally. The various interacting and competing elements are illustrated in this schematic.*

(DWI). Diffusion-weighted imaging records the translational freedom of motion of a water molecule. At the field strengths typically used in humans, a low apparent diffusion coefficient (ADC) suggests a more cellular environment than a high ADC. From animal studies,[47] it is known that the ADC is a surrogate marker of necrosis. A limited number of human studies in patients with glioma[48,49] have described that an initial rise in the ADC of the tumour in response to therapy is an earlier measure of response than morphological size change. With improved methodology it is likely that extracranial tumours will be studied quantitatively such as rectal cancers in which the mean pretreatment ADC of the tumour was strongly associated with response to chemotherapy and chemoradiotherapy.[50]

Key points: general points

■ Molecular imaging records events occurring on the molecular and cellular scale

■ Molecular imaging is broadly categorized into imaging surrogate markers and/or direct molecular events

■ Cancer is characterized by an autonomous clonal proliferation of cells with loss of normal cellular control mechanisms

■ Molecular events characterizing neoplasia are complex and occur at the level of the cell, microenvironment and organism. Molecular imaging targets reside at all levels

Visualizing molecular events: the challenge to magnetic resonance imaging

At 1.5T, barely one in a million nuclei reside in an energy configuration that contributes to a nuclear MR (NMR) signal. Methods that amplify the NMR signal have therefore been a focus of research for some time and are likely to remain so for molecular imaging. At 1.5T, drugs and metabolites can on average be detected down to 0.1–0.2 mM. The concentration of substances at the molecular/receptor level are often in the nano- to picomolar range and therefore, even with an increased field strength, there will be a disparity of several orders of magnitude in signal sensitivity. Despite this restriction, *in vivo* imaging of molecular events by MR has been described in animal systems. These can broadly be categorized into four fields:[51]

- Gene expression
- Angiogenesis and apoptosis
- Cell tracking
- Phenotyping of transgenic mice

Gene expression (Fig. 63.11)

Gene expression has been imaged by enzymes used as imaging markers or via a receptor-mediated approach. In the enzymatic approach, the *transfection* of several cell lines with *wild-type* and *mutant* tyrosinase gene was detected as a result

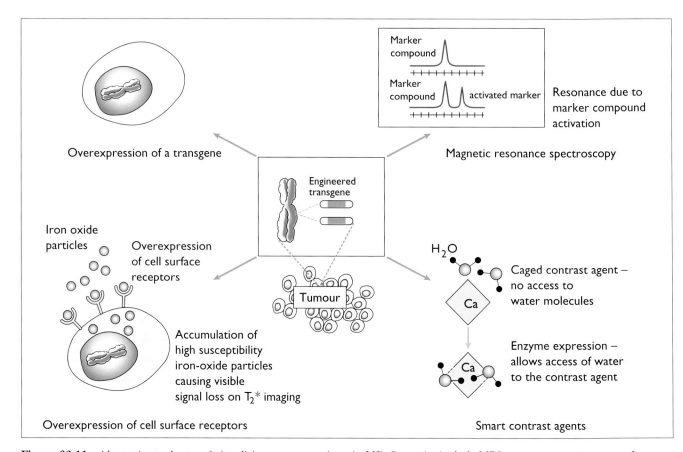

Figure 63.11. *Alternative pathways of visualizing gene expression via MR. Strategies include MRS, smart contrast agents and overexpression of cell surface receptors. The methods are all characterized by a significant alteration in local relaxivity as a result of gene expression.*

of the high metal binding capacity of melanins resulting from the initial catalysis of tyrosine to dioxyphenyl alanine (DOPA).[52,53] In other words, the successful insertion of the human tyrosinase gene into an experimental cell genome was detected as a result of the accumulation of iron leading to a shortening of the cellular T1. The result was an increase in the signal intensity from cells on T1 imaging. A conceptually alternative approach was used to image the expression of an exogenous β-galactosidase gene transferred to a *Xenopus laevis* (African claw-toed frog) embryo. In this instance, a gadolinium construct was synthesized (Fig. 63.12) such that the access of water was restricted to the gadolinium ion by a galactopyranosyl ring that was cleaved only in the presence of the expressed enzyme.[54] The enzymatic cleavage permitted closer access of water molecules to the gadolinium ion, resulting in a 51% shortening in the T1.

An alternative strategy for imaging gene expression has been to stimulate the production of cell surface receptors that internalize particulates or compounds that alter the local magnetic field. This has been successfully demonstrated at 1.5T in an animal model using monocrystalline iron oxide nanoparticles (MIONS).[55] Tumours overexpressing a mutated cell surface transferrin receptor implanted into a murine model showed a fivefold increase

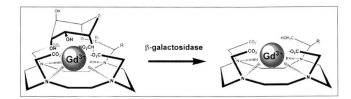

Figure 63.12. *Schematic depicting the transition of a 'smart' contrast agent[54] from a state of low to high relaxivity. The agent works on the principle that the gadolinium(III) ion of the construct remains shielded from bulk water protons until the galactopyranosyl ring is cleaved by the action of β-galactosidase. (Structure courtesy of Prof. T. Meade, Northwestern University, USA.)*

in the uptake of MIONS. The result was that the mutated transferrin-positive receptor tumours demonstrated significant signal loss on T2*-weighted gradient-echo imaging, whilst the wild-type tumour showed none.

In addition to imaging, MRS has successfully monitored gene expression. Magnetic resonance spectroscopy is a powerful *in vivo* research technique[56] that has been applied in oncology to the study of endogenous[57] and anticancer drug metabolism.[58] The strength of MRS lies in the sensitivity of an NMR visible nucleus to its local magnetic field. Because this will vary with the make-up of the chemical environment, MRS is sensitive to changes in chemical structure. By this approach, cytosine deaminase (CD) gene expression was demonstrated in a mouse bearing a human tumour xenograft.[59] Cytosine deaminase is not a normal constituent of mammalian cells and therefore a yeast CD was engineered into a human colon carcinoma cell line and then inoculated subcutaneously into the animal model. *In vivo* CD expression was inferred because the ^{19}F signature of 5-fluorocytosine (a substrate of CD) resonates at a slightly different chemical shift (approximately 1.1 ppm upfield) to its product 5-fluorouracil (5-FU). The study was important because it demonstrated the feasibility of monitoring the therapeutic approach termed *gene-directed enzyme prodrug therapy*.[60] In this case, the 5-fluorocytosine was the pro-drug and 5-FU the activated drug. Imaging marker genes is not confined to ^{19}F-MRS and the *transduction* of arginine kinase via a recombinant viral vector has been demonstrated using ^{31}P-MRS.[61] Arginine kinase is the invertebrate correlate of creatine kinase and catalyses the formation of phospho-arginine from ATP and arginine. Therefore, two weeks following injection of an adenoviral vector containing the arginine kinase gene, a detectable ^{31}P-MR resonance attributable to phosphoarginine was detected in the treated hind limb of the animal model. This example simply reinforces the use of a characteristic resonance to monitor gene expression. Technically, these studies are feasible at 1.5T and current gene therapy trials are a good opportunity to translate laboratory work into the clinic.

Tracking cell motion and distribution

The tracking of cell motion and distribution currently depends on labelling a marker cell with a paramagnetic or superparamagnetic agent. Applications include fate-mapping in embryology[62] but clinical applications are likely to impact in fields such as stem cell therapy.[63,64] The labelling of cells with macromolecular complexes of gadolinium are relatively inefficient and invasive. However, a recently described technique is likely to result in a high-efficiency internal labelling of cells.[65] The cellular internalization of a superparamagnetic nanoparticle iron oxide contrast agent was facilitated by a TAT sequence added to the construct. The TAT protein is an HIV (human immunodeficiency virus) polypeptide that internalizes complexes into cells at a significantly increased rate. The nanoparticle was a construct of dextran cross-linked iron oxide (CLIO) to which the TAT sequence had been conjugated. The particles internalized into several cell lines including CD34+ progenitor cells and mouse neural progenitor cells. The resulting contrast was intense enough that cells were imaged in phantoms at 14 T.

Imaging angiogenesis and apoptosis

The importance of these two mechanisms to the progression, outcome and targeting of molecular therapies has

already been mentioned (see above). The targets for putative imaging agents include markers expressed on the altered neo-endothelial surface of tumour vessels and specific molecular markers of apoptosis. For example, in addition to increased tortuosity and permeability, angiogenic vessels express characteristic proteins such as the *integrin* $\alpha_v\beta_3$. Targeted contrast agents exhibiting paramagnetic[66] or superparamagnetic[67] properties have been conjugated to an $\alpha_v\beta_3$ antibody and have been shown to characterize malignant endothelium *in vivo*. Alternatively, cells induced into apoptosis via anticancer treatment were imaged at 9.4 T[68] using iron oxide nanoparticles conjugated with the C_2 domain of synaptotagmin I (Fig. 63.13). The C_2 domain was used because of its known binding to the plasma membrane of apoptotic cells. Because many chemotherapeutic agents mediate their anticancer action via induction of apoptosis, such a targeted imaging agent could, for example, be investigated as a novel marker of response.

Targeting molecular events: gadolinium-based designer agents for the amplification of the magnetic resonance signal

The imaging of molecular events requires not only the specific binding of a targeted agent but an adequate amplification of the NMR signal. Several approaches were described

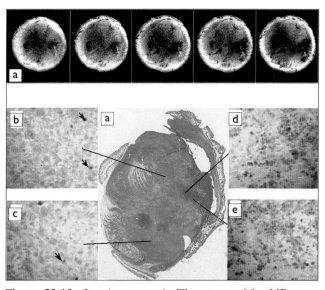

Figure 63.13. *Imaging apoptosis. The top row of five MR images demonstrates the progressive signal loss in a treated mouse tumour following administration of the synaptotagmin I C_2 domain-superparamagnetic iron oxide construct. The micrograph below demonstrates histology in the same tumour. Apoptotic nuclei are highlighted with black arrows together with representative high field images from different regions in the tumour (b–e). (Reproduced with permission from the author and Nature Publishing Group.)*

in the previous section and this section will summarize the strategies currently being explored by researchers developing gadolinium-based agents for this purpose. These strategies are often generic and can be applied individually or increasingly in combination with several imaging modalities including positron emission tomography (PET), optical imaging and ultrasound.[65]

The paramagnetic enhancement of an NMR signal arises from the unpaired electrons in the outer shell of the gadolinium(III) ion, the strength of the effect being based on the considerably greater magnetic moment of an electron compared to that of a nucleus. The electronic magnetic moment is transferred via a dipole ('through space') interaction to a nucleus (i.e. a water proton) within the gadolinium's inner and/or outer sphere of influence. The effect occurs across very short distances and falls off with the inverse of the sixth power of the distance (r^{-6}). The nucleus so influenced then exchanges with the bulk solvent, resulting in a propagation of the effect throughout a given compartment (i.e. the extracellular space). The principal issues involved in the rational design of targeted contrast agents[69] include optimizing the T1 relaxivity, delivering the compound to its site of action and estimating the minimum concentration of gadolinium required to elicit a detectable change in signal intensity.

A gadolinium(III) complex optimized for maximum relaxivity will ideally have a short exchange lifetime but long rotational correlation time, a long electronic relaxation time and a maximum number of complexed water molecules.[70,71] In animal systems, simply binding gadolinium to albumin increases water proton T1 relaxivity by one order of magnitude. A particularly interesting application in the prolongation of the rotational correlation time was the entrapment of gadolinium units inside the inner spherical cavity of apoferritin.[72] In this construct (Fig. 63.14), water diffuses freely through the 4 Å pores of the apoferritin propagating the considerably increased T1 relaxivity of the construct over that of individual gadolinium units.

There have been several reports in which gadolinium was targeted in such a way as to provide the highest density of contrast agent at the desired site of action. For example, a biotinylated monoclonal antibody was constructed (Fig. 63.15) specific to the $\alpha_v\beta_3$ epitope expressed on endothelium.[66] The purpose of the biotin conjugate was to bind a liposome–gadolinium complex via an avidin moiety (avidin binds very strongly to biotin). The specificity to $\alpha_v\beta_3$ therefore resides in the antibody and the gadolinium is targeted and concentrated by the binding of the gadolinium-loaded liposome to the antibody via the avidin–biotin complex. An additional increase in T1 relaxivity results partly from the gadolinium acquiring the rotational correlation time of the liposome. A related approach exploited the overexpression of sialic acid on the cell surface of many tumours to create a contrast agent binding directly to the overexpressed sialic acid.[75]

Irrespective of binding specificity, there will be a thresh-

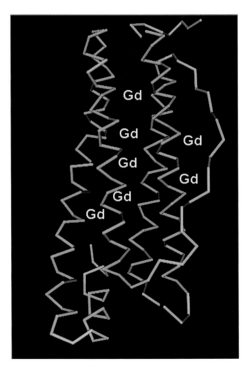

Figure 63.14. *An apoferritin complex[72] has the advantage of conferring high relaxivity and targeting capabilities on the entrapped gadolinium. The structure of the apoferritin was determined by X-ray crystallography.[73,74]*

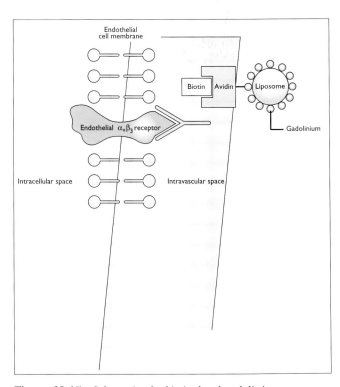

Figure 63.15. *Schematic of a biotinylated gadolinium nanoparticle attached to an $\alpha_v\beta_3$ endothelial receptor.[66,67,69] The antibody recognizes and binds to the $\alpha_v\beta_3$ epitope on the endothelial cell surface.*

old concentration below which a signal will be undetectable. It has been estimated that on commercial systems cell surface receptor visualization requires 10^2–10^3 paramagnetic chelates per receptor.[76] In addition, it has been demonstrated that a concentration of 10–100 μM can be visualized intracellularly.[77] In recent work, Aime et al.[69] reported that in the order of 2×10^9 gadolinium molecules per cell with relaxivities in the order of 4–5/s/mM are necessary to detect contrast variation at 7 T. On the other hand, internalization of 4–5×10^7 gadolinium complexes expressing a relaxivity of 80/s/mM will visualize cells. Encouragingly, it is estimated that using the apoferritin approach described above only a few tens of millions of gadolinium units would be required, that is four to five times fewer atoms than for a MION.[69]

Finally, it is briefly worth examining probes activated by a specific molecular event. In most instances these are compounds activated by specific receptors and substrate–ligand interactions. The cleavage of the galactopyranosyl ring protecting a central gadolinium moiety[54] is one example already mentioned. Recently, a construct has been described in which the water proton relaxivity was altered by a molecular conformational change (Fig. 63.16) induced by a calcium ion.[78,79] The significant role of calcium in several physiological signalling mechanisms suggests this contrast agent could be of particular value in vivo. The final example involves a contrast agent designed to be solubilized on enzymatic cleavage.[69] In this system, the insoluble element is Gd-DTPA (gadolinium diethylenetriamine pentaacetic acid) functionalized with a long aliphatic chain, the aliphatic chain conferring the insolubility of the compound in water. The complex becomes soluble and acquires increased T1 relaxivity following enzymatic (esterase) cleavage of the aliphatic (hydrophobic) chain. Potential clinical application includes nodal assessment as such particles are anticipated to undergo phagocytosis and be cleaved by macrophage esterases.

Although this chapter has focused on molecular imaging via MR, it is essential to appreciate that other physical imaging modalities (including PET, optical imaging,

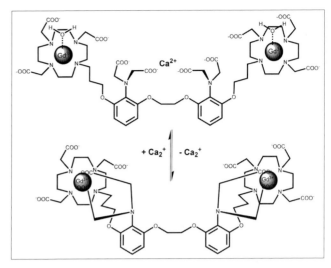

Figure 63.16. *Schematic of the proposed conformational change in a gadolinium-based agent whose relaxivity is altered in the presence of calcium ions.*[78] *(Structure courtesy of Prof. T. Meade, North Western University, USA.)*

ultrasound and computed tomography) will contribute individually and in combination to the study of molecular events in vivo. The reader should also bear in mind that other technologies only recently applied to biological NMR hold the promise of visualizing molecular events in vivo.[80]

Key points: targeting molecular events

- Gene expression, cell motion and elements of angiogenesis and apoptosis can be imaged in vivo by MR

- Tackling limitations of signal sensitivity will be a principal feature of molecular MR imaging research

- A considerable increase in targeted molecular contrast agents based on paramagnetic and superparamagnetic agents is expected

Summary

- Molecular imaging aims to visualize events on the molecular scale. In vivo this is done using surrogate markers or by direct visualization

- Neoplasia is a complex process occurring across several orders of scale. Molecular imaging can be applied to each level

- Many structural, physical and biochemical processes are altered in cancer. Inevitably, one process influences

another, resulting in a cooperative network spanning several properties/features/processes. The robust characterization of a tumour in vivo will inevitably require multifunctional information. MR in combination with other imaging modalities can begin to address these issues

- Molecular imaging incorporates several disciplines. A successful outcome will depend on the cooperation of members from the life, physical and medical sciences

Acknowledgements

I would like to thank Mr David Collins and Professor Mel Greaves for their critical review of the manuscript and Professor Tom Meade and Professor Kevin Brindle for contributing illustrations to this chapter.

References

1. Venter J C, Adams M D, Myers E W et al. The sequence of the human genome. Science 2001; 291: 1304–1351

2. Lander E S, Linton L M, Birren B et al. Initial sequencing and analysis of the human genome. Nature 2001; 409: 860–921

3. Weissleder R, Mahmood U. Molecular imaging. Radiology 2001; 219: 316–333

4. Hoffman J M, Menkens A E. Molecular imaging in cancer: future directions and goals of the National Cancer Institute. Acad Radiol 2000; 7: 905–907

5. Clarke L P, Croft B Y, Menkens A et al. National Cancer Institute initiative for development of novel imaging technologies. Acad Radiol 2000; 7: 481–483

6. Sullivan D C. Biomedical imaging symposium: visualizing the future of biology and medicine. Radiology 2000; 215: 634–638

7. Hillman B J, Neiman H L. Translating molecular imaging research into radiologic practice: summary of the proceedings of the American College of Radiology Colloquium, April 22–24, 2001. Radiology 2002; 222: 19–24

8. Li K C. Biomedical imaging in the postgenomic era: opportunities and challenges. Acad Radiol 2002; 9: 999–1003

9. Wagenaar D J, Weissleder R, Hengerer A. Glossary of molecular imaging terminology. Acad Radiol 2001; 8: 409–420

10. Hoehn S T, Turner C J, Stubbe J. Solution structure of an oligonucleotide containing an abasic site: evidence for an unusual deoxyribose conformation. Nucleic Acids Res 2001; 29: 3413–3423

11. Bayat A. Bioinformatics. Br Med J 2002; 324: 1018–1022

12. Hogemann D, Ntziachristos V, Josephson L, Weissleder R. High throughput magnetic resonance imaging for evaluating targeted nanoparticle probes. Bioconjug Chem 2002; 13: 116–121

13. Aitman T J. DNA microarrays in medical practice. Br Med J 2001; 323: 611–615

14. Golub T R, Slonim D K, Tamayo P et al. Molecular classification of cancer: class discovery and class prediction by gene expression monitoring. Science 1999; 286: 531–537

15. Alizadeh A A, Eisen M B, Davis R E et al. Distinct types of diffuse large B-cell lymphoma identified by gene expression profiling. Nature 2000; 403: 503–511

16. Clark E A, Golub T R, Lander E S, Hynes R O. Genomic analysis of metastasis reveals an essential role for RhoC. Nature 2000; 406: 532–535

17. Perou C M, Sorlie T, Eisen M B et al. Molecular portraits of human breast tumours. Nature 2000; 406: 747–752

18. St Croix B, Rago C, Velculescu V et al. Genes expressed in human tumor endothelium. Science 2000; 289: 1197–1202

19. Yarnold J R, Stratton M R, McMillan T J (eds). Molecular Biology for Oncologists. London: Chapman and Hall, 1996

20. King R J B. Cancer Biology. Harlow: Prentice Hall, 2000

21. Greaves M. Cancer: the Evolutionary Legacy. Oxford: Oxford University Press, 2001

22. Bradley J, Johnson D, Rubinstein D. Molecular Medicine. Oxford: Blackwell Science Ltd, 2001

23. Gould S J. The Structure of Evolutionary Theory. Cambridge, Massachusetts: Harvard University Press, 2002

24. Greaves M. Cancer causation: the Darwinian downside of past success? Lancet Oncol 2002; 3: 244–251

25. Lee J O, Russo A A, Pavletich N P. Structure of the retinoblastoma tumour-suppressor pocket domain bound to a peptide from HPV E7. Nature 1998; 391: 859–865

26. Joo W S, Jeffrey P D, Cantor S B et al. Structure of the 53BP1 BRCT region bound to p53 and its comparison to the Brca1 BRCT structure. Genes Dev 2002; 16: 583–593

27. Hanahan D, Weinberg R A. The hallmarks of cancer. Cell 2000; 100: 57–70

28. Sporn M B. The war on cancer. Lancet 1996; 347: 1377–1381

29. Gillies R J, Raghunand N, Karczmar G S, Bhujwalla Z M. MRI of the tumor microenvironment. J Magn Reson Imaging 2002; 16: 430–450

30. Husband J E, Gwyther S J, Rankin S. Monitoring tumor response. Abdom Imaging 1999; 24: 618–621

31. Jain R K. Transport of molecules in the tumor interstitium: a review. Cancer Res 1987; 47: 3039–3051

32. Jain R K. Delivery of molecular and cellular medicine to solid tumors. J Controlled Release 1998; 53: 49–67

33. Vaupel P, Kallinowski F, Okunieff P. Blood flow, oxygen and nutrient supply, and metabolic microenvironment of human tumors: a review. Cancer Res 1989; 49: 6449–6465

34. Hockel M, Vaupel P. Tumor hypoxia: definitions and current clinical, biologic, and molecular aspects. J Natl Cancer Inst 2001; 93: 266–276

35. Molls M, Vaupel P (eds). Blood Perfusion and Microenvironment of Human Tumors. Implications for Clinical Radio-oncology. Berlin: Springer, 2000

36. Neeman M, Dafni H, Bukhari O et al. In vivo BOLD contrast MRI mapping of subcutaneous vascular function and maturation: validation by intravital microscopy. Magn Reson Med 2001; 45: 887–898

37. Taylor N J, Baddeley H, Goodchild K A et al. BOLD MRI of human tumor oxygenation during carbogen breathing. J Magn Reson Imaging 2001; 14: 156–163

38. Zhao D, Constantinescu A, Jiang L et al. Prognostic radiology: quantitative assessment of tumor oxygen dynamics by MRI. Am J Clin Oncol 2001; 24: 462–466

39. Aboagye E O, Kelson A B, Tracy M, Workman P. Preclinical development and current status of the fluorinated 2-nitroimidazole hypoxia probe N-(2-hydroxy-3,3,3-trifluoropropyl)-2-(2-nitro-1-imidazolyl) acetamide (SR 4554, CRC 94/17): a non-invasive diagnostic probe for the measurement of tumor hypoxia by magnetic resonance spectroscopy and imaging, and by positron emission tomography. Anticancer Drug Des 1998; 13: 703–730

40. Gillies R J, Liu Z, Bhujwalla Z. 31P-MRS measurements of extracellular pH of tumors using 3-aminopropylphosphonate. Am J Physiol 1994; 267: C195–203

41. Zhang S, Wu K, Sherry A D. A novel pH-sensitive MRI contrast agent. Angew Chem Int Ed Engl 1999; 38: 3192–3194

42. Aime S, Barge A, Delli Castelli D et al. Paramagnetic lanthanide(III) complexes as pH-sensitive chemical exchange saturation transfer (CEST) contrast agents for MRI applications. Magn Reson Med 2002; 47: 639–648

43. Padhani A R. Functional MRI for anticancer therapy assessment. Eur J Cancer 2002; 38: 2116–2127

44. Padhani A R, Neeman M. Challenges for imaging angiogenesis. Br J Radiol 2001; 74: 886–890

45. George M L, Dzik-Jurasz A S, Padhani A R et al. Non-invasive methods of assessing angiogenesis and their value in predicting response to treatment in colorectal cancer. Br J Surg 2001; 88: 1628–1636

46. de Vries A, Griebel J, Kremser C et al. Monitoring of tumor microcirculation during fractionated radiation therapy in patients with rectal carcinoma: preliminary results and implications for therapy. Radiology 2000; 217: 385–391

47. Lemaire L, Howe F A, Rodrigues L M, Griffiths J R. Assessment of induced rat mammary tumour response to chemotherapy using the apparent diffusion coefficient of tissue water as determined by diffusion-weighted 1H-NMR spectroscopy in vivo. MAGMA 1999; 8: 20–26

48. Chenevert T L, Stegman L D, Taylor J M et al. Diffusion magnetic resonance imaging: an early surrogate marker of therapeutic efficacy in brain tumors. J Natl Cancer Inst 2000; 92: 2029–2036

49. Mardor Y, Roth Y, Lidar Z et al. Monitoring response to convection-enhanced taxol delivery in brain tumor patients using diffusion-weighted magnetic resonance imaging. Cancer Res 2001; 61: 4971–4973

50. Dzik-Jurasz A, Domenig C, George M et al. Diffusion MRI for prediction of response of rectal cancer to chemoradiation. Lancet 2002; 360: 307–308

51. Allport J R, Weissleder R. In vivo imaging of gene and cell therapies. Exp Hematol 2001; 29: 1237–1246

52. Weissleder R, Simonova M, Bogdanova A et al. MR imaging and scintigraphy of gene expression through melanin induction. Radiology 1997; 204: 425–429

53. Simonova M, Wall A, Weissleder R, Bogdanov A Jr. Tyrosinase mutants are capable of prodrug activation in transfected nonmelanotic cells. Cancer Res 2000; 60: 6656–6662

54. Louie A Y, Huber M M, Ahrens E T et al. In vivo visualization of gene expression using magnetic resonance imaging. Nat Biotechnol 2000; 18: 321–325

55. Weissleder R, Moore A, Mahmood U et al. In vivo magnetic resonance imaging of transgene expression. Nat Med 2000; 6: 351–355

56. Smith I C P, Stewart L C. Magnetic resonance spectroscopy in medicine: clinical impact. Prog Nucl Mag Res Sp 2002; 40: 1–34

57. Leach M O. Introduction to in vivo MRS of cancer: new perspectives and open problems. Anticancer Res 1996; 16: 1503–1514

58. Findlay M P, Leach M O. In vivo monitoring of fluoropyrimidine metabolites: magnetic resonance spectroscopy in the evaluation of 5-fluorouracil. Anticancer Drugs 1994; 5: 260–280

59. Stegman L D, Rehemtulla A, Beattie B et al. Noninvasive quantitation of cytosine deaminase transgene expression in human tumor xenografts with in vivo magnetic resonance spectroscopy. Proc Natl Acad Sci USA 1999; 96: 9821–9826

60. Niculescu-Duvaz I, Cooper R G, Stribbling S M et al. Recent developments in gene-directed enzyme prodrug therapy (GDEPT) for cancer. Curr Opin Mol Ther 1999; 1: 480–486

61. Walter G, Barton E R, Sweeney H L. Noninvasive measurement of gene expression in skeletal muscle. Proc Natl Acad Sci USA 2000; 97: 5151–5155

62. Jacobs R E, Fraser S E. Magnetic resonance microscopy of embryonic cell lineages and movements. Science 1994; 263: 681–684

63. Rafii S, Lyden D, Benezra R et al. Vascular and haematopoietic stem cells: novel targets for anti-angiogenesis therapy? Nat Rev Cancer 2002; 2: 826–835

64. Park K I, Ourednik J, Ourednik V et al. Global gene and cell replacement strategies via stem cells. Gene Ther 2002; 9: 613–624

65. Lewin M, Carlesso N, Tung C H et al. Tat peptide-derivatized magnetic nanoparticles allow in vivo tracking and recovery of progenitor cells. Nat Biotechnol 2000; 18: 410–414

66. Sipkins D A, Cheresh D A, Kazemi M R et al. Detection of tumor angiogenesis in vivo by alphaVbeta3-targeted magnetic resonance imaging. Nat Med 1998; 4: 623–626

67. Anderson S A, Rader R K, Westlin W F et al. Magnetic resonance contrast enhancement of neovasculature with alpha(v)beta(3)-targeted nanoparticles. Magn Reson Med 2000; 44: 433–439

68. Zhao M, Beauregard D A, Loizou L et al. Non-invasive detection of apoptosis using magnetic resonance

imaging and a targeted contrast agent. Nat Med 2001; 7: 1241–1244

69. Aime S, Cabella C, Colombatto S et al. Insights into the use of paramagnetic Gd(III) complexes in MR-molecular imaging investigations. J Magn Reson Imaging 2002; 16: 394–406

70. Aime S, Botta M, Fasano M, Terreno E. Lanthanide(III) chelates for NMR biomedical applications. Chem Soc Rev 1998; 27: 19–29

71. Lauffer R B. Paramagnetic metal-complexes as water proton relaxation agents for NMR imaging: theory and design. Chem Rev 1987; 87: 901–927

72. Aime S, Frullano L, Geninatti Crich S. Compartmentalization of a gadolinium complex in the apoferritin cavity: a route to obtain high relaxivity contrast agents for magnetic resonance imaging. Angew Chem Int Ed Engl 2002; 41: 1017–1019

73. Gallois B, Granier T, Langlois D'Estaintot B et al. X-ray structure of recombinant horse L-chain apoferritin at 2.0 angstrom resolution: Implications for stability and function. J Biol Inorg Chem 1996; 2: 360

74. Michaux M A, Dautant A, Gallois B et al. Structural

investigation of the complexation properties between horse spleen apoferritin and metalloporphyrins. Proteins 1996; 24: 314–321

75. Lemieux G A, Yarema K J, Jacobs C L, Bertozzi C R. Exploiting differences in sialoside expression for selective targeting of MRI contrast reagents. J Am Chem Soc 1999; 121: 4278–4279

76. Nunn A D, Linder K E, Tweedle M F. Can receptors be imaged with MRI agents? Q J Nucl Med 1997; 41: 155–162

77. Ahrens E T, Rothbacher U, Jacobs R E, Fraser S E. A model for MRI contrast enhancement using T1 agents. Proc Natl Acad Sci USA 1998; 95: 8443–8448

78. Li W H, Parigi G, Fragai M et al. Mechanistic studies of a calcium-dependent MRI contrast agent. Inorg Chem 2002; 41: 4018–4024

79. Li W H, Fraser S E, Meade T J. A calcium sensitive magnetic resonance imaging contrast agent. J Am Chem Soc 1999; 121: 1413–1414

80. Cherubini A, Bifone A. Hyperpolarised xenon in biology. Prog Nucl Mag Res Sp 2003; 42: 1–30

Index